TREATMENT
IN GENERAL PRACTICE

BY

HARRY BECKMAN, M.D.

Professor of Pharmacology at Marquette University
School of Medicine, Milwaukee, Wis

SECOND EDITION
REVISED AND ENTIRELY RESET

PHILADELPHIA AND LONDON
W. B. SAUNDERS COMPANY
1935

Copyright, 1930, by W. B. Saunders Company

Copyright, 1934, by W. B. Saunders Company

All Rights Reserved

This book is protected by copyright. No part of it
may be duplicated or reproduced in any manner
without written permission from the publisher

Reprinted July, 1934

Reprinted May, 1935

MADE IN U. S. A.

PRESS OF
W. B. SAUNDERS COMPANY
PHILADELPHIA

DEDICATED TO

ANNA SERENIUS BECKMAN

PREFACE TO THE SECOND EDITION

In the revision I have had always two leading-strings to my pen: one that tugged it to include with meticulous care all that has proved, or fairly promises to prove, its worth in treatment since the appearance of the first edition of the book; and another that pulled it ruthlessly across the pages in slashing marks of deletion. Space has been found without increasing the size of the volume, for a presentation of the following entities not included previously: Acetylsalicylic acid (aspirin) poisoning; agranulocytosis; blackwater fever; bronchomycosis; cyanide poisoning; erysipeloid; food allergy; gasoline and kerosene poisoning; hiccup; hyperinsulinism (hypoglycemia) and dysinsulinism; hypothyroidism without myxedema; lead poisoning; lymphogranuloma inguinale (climatic bubo); malnutrition; methyl chloride poisoning; onchocerciasis; oriental sore, dermal and mucocutaneous leishmaniasis; prophylaxis of gonorrhea in the female; serum sensitization and desensitization; simple achlorhydric anemia; strongyloides infection; tear gas burns; tetany; varicose ulcer; and a section on vehicles and incompatibilities.

It has been obligatory to deal with the bibliography in a most high-handed manner, for in order to include the host of new references all those names no longer specifically mentioned in the text have had to be omitted from the final list; a necessary step which has been taken somewhat grudgingly. Yet I find that with the passing years an increasing incisiveness has come upon me—whether for good or ill is not quite clear—so that I am ever more closely gripped by the old council

> Whate'er the preconceptions are—Be brief;
> So lively words apprise the willing brain
> And there hold fast in confident belief;
> All surfeits from the sated bosom drain.
> —Horati, De Arte Poetica.

HARRY BECKMAN

MILWAUKEE, WIS.

7

PREFACE

The neglect of thorough and painstaking teaching of therapeutics in this country is not so often the subject of serious consideration in our medical councils as it well might be. With only a few notable exceptions, the medical schools seem content if there is presented within their halls, usually to Junior students who have had as yet practically no contact with the sick, a ridiculously inadequate course of lectures, the rest being left to the teachers in the departments of medicine, pediatrics, obstetrics, etc. And these latter seem to shift the responsibility largely onto the gods, not through any culpability upon their part, but simply because in their immersion in the task of acquainting the student with the prodigious methodology of modern diagnosis, no time is left for an exhaustive consideration with him of the treatment of disease. Hence it is that the therapeutic credo of the average young practitioner today contains but two articles: one, that there are certain therapeutic principles that invariably hold and that they need to be varied only in detail in the handling of particular diseases; and, the other, that the art of treatment is one that "comes" if only one has mastered the art of diagnosis.

It is in an attempt to shake, however feebly, the false foundations of these beliefs that the present book has been written. In it each of the principal diseases of man, exclusive of those that by prescriptive right belong within the domain of the legitimate specialties, has had its own peculiar therapy described, as that therapy has been evolved out of the experience of physicians all over the world. The true authors of the book, then, are those men and women whose names appear in the Bibliography. Whenever possible I have presented their work in their own words, but often it has been necessary to abstract and to condense, and not infrequently to present a subject in a manner and perhaps even from a point of view that has apparently little in common with that held by those who reported the original trials and observations. Always, however, I have looked upon myself merely as an editor, and I hope that no more than editorial liberties have been taken in any portion of the book. Of course it has not been possible to keep my own opinion invariably in the background; hence I elected in the beginning to write in the first person so that there might be at no time any confusion as to whose work or views were being presented.

Very humbly I recognize that the rather lengthy presentations of controversies that are to be found here and there in the book will give much offense to all save those who, like myself, have been even more disturbed by the indolent type of pedagogy that seeks sanctuary in the shameful words: "Upon this point we can say very little as the authorities are at present in disagreement." Only as I have thought and taught through the years have I been able to write, a limitation which I suppose every author recognizes. As for the many other shortcomings of the book, I can only assure the reader that, no matter how grievous he finds them, they can in no wise affect him so deeply as they do me, for only I can know with what bright hopes the work was planned and begun several years ago.

To my wife I am deeply indebted for that intelligent and indefatigable assistance which is so invaluable in bringing a task of this sort to completion.

HARRY BECKMAN.

MILWAUKEE, WIS.

9

CONTENTS

INFECTIOUS DISEASES

DISEASES CAUSED BY FLUKES

DISEASES CAUSED BY WORMS

DISEASES OF ALLERGY

DEFICIENCY DISEASES

DISEASES OF METABOLISM

DISEASES OF THE GASTRO-INTESTINAL TRACT

DISEASES OF THE RESPIRATORY TRACT

DISEASES OF THE KIDNEY

DISEASES OF THE BLOOD-FORMING ORGANS

DISEASES OF THE CIRCULATORY SYSTEM

DISTURBANCES OF THE THYROID GLAND

GENITO-URINARY INFECTIONS AND STONE

DISEASES OF THE NERVOUS SYSTEM

DISEASES OF THE SKIN

OPIUM AND COCAINE ADDICTION

ACUTE POISONING

BURNS

OBSTETRICS

CONTENTS

MISCELLANY

TREATMENT IN GENERAL PRACTICE

INFECTIOUS DISEASES

ANTHRAX

(Woolsorters' Disease, Malignant Pustule)

Anthrax is an acute infectious disease of animals, especially herbivora, caused by *Bacillus anthracis*. It is transmissible to man, in whom it appears either in the cutaneous, pulmonary or gastro-intestinal form. Workers in hide, hair, bristles, wool, horn, and bone are particularly susceptible, but it may be contracted by butchers, veterinarians, farm laborers and others in contact with animals. It is also not infrequently contracted from contact with an infected shaving brush. The symptoms of the pulmonary and gastro-intestinal forms are not characteristic, but the pustule and edema occurring in the cutaneous form are of a type which hardly admits of mistaking it for anything else.

Anthrax was described by Hippocrates (460–370 b. c.) in one of the books of Epidemic Diseases thought to have been the authentic work of the Coan master, and it appears to have been well known during the period (732–1096 a. d.) of Arabian and Jewish ascendency in medicine; but it is of interest to note that Galen (131–201 a. d.) had mistaken Hippocrates' description for that of erysipelas. The strange periodic malady of the middle ages, *Malum Malannum*, may have been anthrax, which is known with certainty to have been epidemic in the early seventeenth century. I believe the first complete treatise on the disease was that of Chabert, in 1780. Koch demonstrated his cultures of the bacillus in 1876, the organism having been discovered by Davaine in 1850.

THERAPY

The criteria for ideal anthrax therapy, as laid down by Regan, are: that it should (1) be applicable to the various forms and locations of the disease, (2) have the lowest mortality rate, (3) be as specific as possible, (4) possess no danger of generalizing the local infection, (5) offer the least amount of scarring and deformity, (6) cause a minimum of pain, (7) entail the shortest absence from employment.

Surgical Treatment.—Excision has been the most commonly used method of treatment, but it has been so often combined with serum or cautery or the use of chemical caustics, that it is difficult to tell to which the results are mostly attributable. Some such treatment as the following, described by Dudley, is recommended by most text-books of surgery:

As soon as the diagnosis is made, the skin is scrubbed gently with soap and rinsed thoroughly with sterile water. The skin is painted with aqueous 8 per cent, or stronger, phenol (carbolic acid) solution, and rinsed with alcohol. Next the lesion is painted with collodion to avoid contamination of the incision. Eight per cent phenol is injected into the tissues all around the lesion to wall off the infective process. From 3 to 5 syringefuls of solution (about 60 cc.) will be sufficient. One-fourth inch outside of this phenolized zone, 5 or 6 syringefuls of 25 per cent alcohol are injected. These injections are usually made within 1½ inches of the center of the lesion. The line of incision is painted with 8 per cent phenol, and an area from $2\frac{1}{2}$ to $3\frac{1}{2}$ inches in diameter is excised. After the excision, the base and edges of the wound are painted with pure phenol (95 per cent), which is immediately neutralized with absolute alcohol. The surface is cleansed with alcohol, and a wet dressing of boric acid, alcohol or hypertonic saline solution, is applied. If this excision fails to stop the process, free incisions are made into the tissues along the course of the edema, and gauze drains are put in.

Though surgical excision and incision continues to be the treatment most frequently employed, its limitations and disadvantages have been repeatedly shown. The most frequent source of danger is the difficulty of accurately defining the area to be excised, especially when the edema and induration are marked, for microscopical sections have at times shown bacilli far beyond the limits of the pustule in the edematous zone. To excise less than the entire area is to subject the patient to the pain and discomfort of the operation without a compensatory certainty of cure; again, Nature's barrier zone may be broken down and the blood and lymph channels opened, increasing the danger of a general dissemination of the malady. From an esthetic point of view it is also objectionable, for if the lesion is large an extensive surface is left devoid of skin, requiring subsequent skin grafting to prevent scar formation. Symmers, of Bellevue Hospital, is so impressed by the likelihood of precipitating fatal sepsis by surgical interference, that he has recently stated: "If no serum is available the lesion should be covered with a bit of sterile gauze to collect the secretions, but otherwise left absolutely alone." The statistics of Schwartz upon this point of absolute noninterference, however, are not reassuring, for of 10 patients given symptomatic treatment and rest, 9 died.

Antianthrax Serum.—As a result of the use of antianthrax serum in the treatment of the disease, several authorities have reported a decided lowering of the mortality rate, especially in France, Italy and Russia. Thus Sclavo reports a striking fall in the death rate in Italy, from 24 to 6 per cent following the use of the serum; in Russia (Rosener) it has been reduced from 14 to 8 per cent. It has been little used in the United States compared with England, South America and the Continent. The serum, which is made by immunizing horses against virulent anthrax organisms, has been shown experimentally to contain protective antibodies. It is administered subcutaneously, intramuscularly or intravenously, and has recently been shown to be additionally effective if injected locally into the lesion simultaneously with the systemic injection.

Regan has reported 16 cases in which he has used the serum in the United States, 14 of whom were saved. He ascribes all failures to the following factors: (1) Use too late in the course of the disease (*i. e.*, in the practically moribund), (2) too small doses, (3) failure to repeat injections frequently, (4) use in persons with such chronic diseases as alcoholism, nephritis, syphilis, myocarditis, etc. The treatment which he has devised with the aim of preventing or combating sepsis, counteracting the toxemia, and causing the subsidence of the local lesion, is outlined in Table 1.

By local therapy is meant the injection of 2 to 3 cc. at three or four equidistant points so as to circumscribe the lesion, the needle being inserted into the red indurated border just beyond the blanched zone.

Unfortunately the cost of this treatment is very high, as the production and marketing of the serum seem to entail considerable expense.

Normal Beef Serum.—In the Argentine, Krause and his collaborators, Penna and Cuenca, have reported on the treatment employed by them, which has astoundingly reduced the mortality. Ordinary beef serum, which has been sterilized by heating it twice for half an hour at 56 C., is employed, without other measures; the pustule and sepsis are said to subside under it

TABLE 1.—USE OF ANTHRAX SERUM

In absence of anthrax septicemia (as revealed by blood culture)

	Intravenous dose.	Number.	Intervals.
Mild cases with little constitutional symptoms, small lesion, no edema.	50 cc.	3 or 4	8 to 12 hours
	Subsequent injections at 12- to 24-hour intervals, usually not more than a total of 6. Local therapy (see below) every 12 to 24 hours.		
Moderate cases with definite constitutional symptoms, medium lesion, moderate edema.	50 to 80 cc.	3 or 4	8 hours
	Subsequently every 12 hours, usually a total of 6 or 8. Local every 12 hours.		
Severe cases with marked constitutional symptoms, large lesion, extensive edema.	80 to 100 cc.	3 or 4	6 to 8 hours
	Subsequently 50 cc. every 12 hours. Local every 6 to 8 hours.		

In presence of anthrax septicemia.			
	100 to 150 cc.		3 or 4 hours
	Continued to improvement or death. Local every 4 to 6 hours.		

even more promptly and surely than when antianthrax serum is used. The serum is injected subcutaneously in doses of 30 to 50 cc., and this is repeated in twelve, twenty-four or thirty-six hours as the case may require. Anaphylaxis is even more rare with beef serum than with horse serum. In 1917–18 these workers reported a series of 200 cases of anthrax thus treated, with a mortality of only 0.5 per cent, while during the previous ten-year period the mortality in 250 cases otherwise treated had been 10 per cent. Despite the fact the Ligniéres, in the Argentine, and Kolmer, Wanner and Koehler, in the United States, have questioned the efficacy of this treatment on theoretical and experimental grounds, the actual clinical results of Krause deserve a far greater recognition than they have had.

Other Measures.—Chief among the many other measures employed against this dread disease are: the use of live steam, the application to the lesion of powdered ipecac, cauterization with potassium hydroxide, and the injection of an extract made from a culture of *Bacillus pyocyaneus*, thought to be antagonistic to *Bacillus anthracis*. All of these have had their day and are more or less discarded. Warringsholz (1932) has recently advocated the giving of creolin by mouth, claiming that the danger of such use has been greatly exaggerated: for the adult 2 teaspoonfuls are given in soup every two hours; every three hours as the fever begins to decrease.

ASIATIC CHOLERA

Asiatic cholera is an acute specific infectious disease, caused by the *Vibrio cholerae,* and involving primarily the lower portion of the ilium. It is characterized by vomiting, profuse, effortless diarrhea, muscular cramps, collapse, and suppression of urine. The whole course of the disease from its onset to death may be only a few hours to a few days, though a certain number of those who survive the first period of collapse go into a typhoid-like state which may prove fatal. Convalescence is slow, especially in Europeans.

The "rice-water" stools, so characteristic of this disease, were first shown to contain epithelium from the walls of the small intestine about one hundred years ago (Horner, 1834). Despite the still unsatisfactory state of our therapy in this disease, it has been much studied in the past; so long ago as 1848 the great Russian military surgeon, Pirogoff, performed 800 autopsies upon victims of the malady in one year in St. Petersburg. In 1854, John Snow, who had stated that the disease was water-borne and that the causative agent entered the body through the mouth, was able to prove his point by having the handle of a certain pump removed during a severe epidemic in London, with the result that the incidence of new cases at once began to decline.

This disease has always been epidemic, and sometimes pandemic, in many parts of Asia, where its incidence is still very high. The first invasion of Europe and America was in 1826–37; Heinrich Heine has most realistically described the scenes which ensued when Paris was suddenly struck. There were many subsequent epidemics in that century; in 1892, the epidemic in Hamburg was one of the first outbreaks of disease of any sort to be fought upon the new principles laid down by the bacteriological discoveries of Koch. During the World War and the subsequent starvation period, cholera constituted a major medical problem for Russia and the Central Powers. The recent investigations of Gill and Lal tentatively incriminate the housefly as an important transmitting agent of the disease.

THERAPY

The mortality in cholera varies distinctly in different epidemics and also rises to a peak during a given epidemic, but under ordinary conditions, with patients coming under treatment when already collapsed, a mortality of 50 to 75 per cent may be expected; when they report earlier, proper treatment may restrict the mortality to from 25 to 30 per cent. As stated by Sellards, the three objects of treatment are, (1) relief of toxemia, (2) restoration of fluid, (3) prevention of acidosis and uremia.

Relief of Toxemia.—(*a*) *Antiserums.*—"For many years no significant results were obtained with antiserums to cholera. The recognition by both French and German bacteriologists that the cholera vibrio produces a soluble toxin, and the utilization of this toxin as well as the bacteria themselves in immunization, has given an antiserum which in recent epidemics, particularly in Russia (Salimbeni), has seemed very efficacious."—Gay (1923).

(*b*) *Kaolin.*—I quote from an editorial which appeared in the Journal of the American Medical Association during the World War (64, 1991, 1915):

"Aluminum silicate, kaolinum, fullers' earth and bolus alba are various names under which the essentially same substance is familiar to physicians. In 1906, Stumpf of Wurzburg published a detailed report of his experience with it in cholera under the title 'A Reliable Method of Treating Asiatic Cholera and Severe Infectious Cholera Morbus, and the Importance of Bolus Alba (kaolin) in the Treatment of Certain Bacterial Infections.' His attention was early attracted to the possible disinfecting virtues of clay by his observation that cadavers exhumed after being buried in clay soil were always in a remarkable state of preservation in comparison with those in other soil. At that time his experience with the kaolin covered eight years. He believed that it owed its efficiency in bacterial infections to its action in depriving the bacteria of a suitable culture medium while mechanically burying them alive, separating them from the mucosa and other tissues by a protecting, comparatively impermeable coating. He applied it as a remedy to extensive septic wounds, putrid leg ulcers and the like. Stumpf experimented on himself to determine the harmlessness of the finely pulverized kaolin taken internally in large amounts, and found that it was well tolerated. He administered it in cases of cholera, and found that colics and tendency to vomit were at once arrested. The dose given was 125 Gm. of the most finely pulverized kaolin poured on top of half a tumbler of water. After the powder sank to the bottom of the glass, it was thoroughly stirred in with a spoon, and the whole amount taken at once or within a few minutes. After an interval of three hours, the same dose was repeated. Infants were given proportionately smaller doses. . . .

"In the present European war, the physicians in the German and Austrian armies are using large amounts of kaolin to combat dysentery and cholera, and according to Stumpf, the microscopic findings in the feces of the patients treated fully warrant its use. Wolff-Eisner, from his experience in the war, believes that kaolin has been triumphant in the treatment of cholera. He tabulates 25 cases, showing almost immediate stopping of diarrhea in dysentery and typhoid after a dose of a double spoonful each of kaolin and charcoal had been taken from one to three times a day. In severer cases, the proportion of kaolin was doubled. He regards the kaolin-charcoal treatment as a kind of immunotherapy, basing his belief on Hofmeister's dictum that all the phenomena of immunity are colloid chemical reactions. He believes that the kaolin binds toxins which are beyond the reach of serotherapy. . . . "

Restoration of Fluid.—This is of extreme importance, since the profound fall in blood pressure, cyanosis and loss of elasticity in the skin, restlessness of the patient and loss of the voice, are doubtless largely due to dehydration. Restoration of this fluid accomplishes the most gratifying results in cases not already moribund. Sellards says that the average patient requires the intravenous injection (vomiting precludes the oral route) of 2 liters of salt solution every six to eight hours for one or two days.

Prevention of Acidosis and Uremia.—In cholera the urine is extremely acid and the individual's tolerance to alkalis is enormously increased. This acidosis is closely associated with the acute nephritis and uremia. During the stage of collapse, 0.5 per cent sodium bicarbonate and 0.5 per cent sodium chloride should be used intravenously. As the stage of reaction sets in the quantity of bicarbonate should be increased to 1.5 or 2 per cent and the chloride omitted; these bicarbonate injections should be continued until the urine becomes alkaline or is very liberally secreted. It is stated that the early and persistent use of alkalis has practically eliminated death from uremia in cholera.

PROPHYLAXIS

Vaccine.—Vaccines prepared from killed cholera vibrios have been used for many years, but it is difficult to determine the exact degree of their efficacy. The vaccine made at the government laboratory at Bombay contains 8000 million killed organisms per cubic centimeter, 0.5 cc. is administered subcutaneously at the first dose, and 1 cc. at the second. It is being issued in increasing amounts in India year by year, and the few reports that are published are distinctly favorable. The local and general reactions are very mild. The immunity is evanescent, apparently lasting only about six months; it begins on the ninth or tenth day after the first inoculation.

During the World War the Central Powers had considerable experience with the vaccine on the Eastern front. Hoffman (quoted by Wayson) reported that among the German troops when advancing in the regions of the Bug and Rokitano marshes, the mortality among the uninoculated was from 35 to 50 per cent, while among those inoculated it was from 0 to 20 per cent. Kaup (also quoted by Wayson) stated that after the Austrian soldiers had been inoculated, the morbidity was from 1 to 5 per cent, though the exposure was great, and that the course was quite mild when the disease had been contracted. It is significant that a Polish newspaper, in commenting on a winter epidemic of cholera in Poland at that time, remarked, "Cholera seems to be a disease which attacks the civil population and spares soldiers."

Bacteriophage.—D'Herelle, who was appointed by the British government to head a special mission to study cholera in India, has reported the results of his work there; the following is from the Paris letter to the Journal of the American Medical Association (90, 783, 1928):

"The bacteriophage of the vibrio of cholera, when it is found associated with the latter, engages in a struggle with the vibrio and often comes off victorious. The cholera patients who recover spontaneously are those who have in advance an abundance of bacteriophages in the intestine. One finds in India, in the Punjab, entire villages completely free from cholera, though an epidemic rages around them, owing to the fact that the drinking water in these villages contains the bacteriophage in abundance. D'Herelle succeeded in eradicating the disease and immunizing the population of large areas by transferring to the wells of the country merely from 30 to 40 cc. of the cultures of the bacteriophage, which he easily obtained. The mode of treatment is simple. A culture is prepared of the bacteriophage that is found in the stools of convalescents. These cultures are somewhat peculiar in that the bacteriophage can feed only on living matter, and, furthermore, only on that to which it is habituated. In this manner, its activity can be increased so that it will completely destroy in a few hours the bacterial cultures. Later, all that need be done is to administer a few cubic centimeters by mouth in repeated doses. As it finds an abundant food supply in the infected intestine, it develops easily, and a cure is effected with surprising rapidity, corresponding to the speed with which it destroys the vibrios. In Rajiana, which has some 3000 inhabitants, there were 56 cases of cholera, from July 3 to July 22. The treatment was begun, July 21; there were 4 new cases, July 23, but not a single case after that. In Lalpura, with 1500 inhabitants, there were 39 cases from July 23 to July 26; July 28, there was just 1 new case and the epidemic was ended. The most curious thing is that the persons thus treated disseminate the bacteriophage by their stools deposited on top of the ground and thus aid in stamping out the epidemic. D'Herelle was the hardest put to it in treating the grave cases, the patients being for the most part moribund, and these were just the cases in which his aid was sought. There was a mortality of 8 per cent in the patients treated and of 62 per cent in those not treated. It appears, therefore, that the prophylaxis of cholera will consist henceforth in combating an epidemic of the vibrion septique with an epidemic of its parasite, the bacteriophage, which, when enhanced by cultivation, rapidly destroys the vibrio. If these statements are confirmed, this will certainly be one of the greatest conquests of bacteriology."

Unfortunately, these early bright promises have not been fulfilled in all instances, and the profession in India and elsewhere is divided in its opinion of the efficacy of this new method. The outstanding contribution recently has been the laying down of the dictum that there are three types of bacteriophage and that, as no one gives a permanent lysis of a cholera culture and a mixture of two does so only rarely, a mixture of the three types is absolutely necessary for effective prophylaxis and treatment. So far no artificial mixture of this sort, of sufficient stability to be satisfactory, has been prepared; natural mixtures from patients have unquestionably both greater stability and potency.

In India the difficulty of judging the effectiveness of the new methods is very great because the village headmen do not report the presence of the disease until several persons have died; the effect of giving bacteriophage upon a large scale in the early cases is therefore still not clearly known, while the conclusions drawn from the results obtained in later cases must always be subject to a reasonable doubt, for cholera mortality always drops toward the end of an epidemic. However, two areas of large population have recently come under quasi-experimental conditions, and Col. Morison, a close student of the subject, has been willing to say: "On the final outcome of this experiment [*i. e.*, after a period of years] it may be possible to say whether in areas not amenable to sanitation, to control of the water supplies, or to preventive vaccination, we may depend on an attack on the disease through an agent active against the vibrio itself, which the first cases of an epidemic can be made to distribute as they ordinarily distribute the cholera vibrio." Col. Mackie states that, in 1933, feeling at Calcutta is still sharply divided for and against the efficacy of phage.

Bacteriophage in Treatment.—The method of administration, as described typically by Asheshov, Khan and Lahiri, is very simple. The bacteriophage is stocked in 50-cc. bottles and 5-cc. ampules; the undiluted substance which is an almost tasteless and odorless clear fluid, is taken by sipping in amounts of 4 cc. at a time at thirty-minute intervals in the beginning. Two bottles are taken in the first sixteen hours, and after the first twenty-four hours one bottle in the next forty-eight hours is considered sufficient. If one of the 5-cc. ampules is given intravenously for quicker action it must be well diluted with a saline solution containing 120 grains of sodium chloride to the pint of water.

BLACKWATER FEVER

I hesitate to commit myself on the delicate question of blackwater fever; indeed, I shall only state that there is a certain type of pernicious malaria (known as "hemoglobinuric fever") characterized by hemoglobinemia and the passing of large quantities of blood into the urine—which some observers hold not to be malaria at all. The interesting researches of Thompson (1922–24) in Rhodesia produced strong evidence in favor of *Plasmodium falciparum* as the causative organism in all cases, but some observers hold that the syndrome may appear occasionally in benign tertian and exceptionally in quartan cases. Perhaps malaria with a tendency to blackwater has a different etiology from the ordinary form of the disease, and may be caused by a specific plasmodium—*P. tenue* Stephens, as suggested by Sinton. Strickland and his collaborators believe that several varieties of mosquitoes may be grouped into the single species *A. funestus,* which is capable of modifying the malarial parasites so as to make them more apt to provoke blackwater. Or the disease may be a plasmodium infection complicated with some other parasite, such as Bartonella, or by an unknown virus. However, everything revealed in most of the careful studies of the occurrence of blackwater fever— such as the painstaking work of Whitmore, for instance, in the West Indies and Central America, and of many others in Africa, India and elsewhere— supports the belief, held by many physicians, that the disease is caused by neglected chronic malaria; nevertheless, Schüffner (1931) has placed the Malaria Commission of the League of Nations on record as opposed to the view that, in India at least, blackwater is merely a complication of malaria. Schilling and Jossmann have observed a case in a patient with general paralysis who had been inoculated in Berlin with benign tertian; James, Nicol and Shute (1932) have added two more cases inoculated with subtertian in England.

THERAPY

Most writers do not favor the use of quinine, believing that the drug is either the provocative factor or increases the severity of the symptoms by increasing hemolysis. As a result of his exhaustive review of the 832 cases notified in Nigeria between 1899 and 1929, Connal (1930) concludes that quinine may be acquitted of specific complicity in the production of the disease, and that it is more fitting to stress the fact that by its proper employment in prophylaxis and in the treatment of malaria, no case would proceed to the chronic condition of infection which is the precursor of blackwater fever. Yorke's trenchant comment upon this should be quoted: "It would really be interesting, if not advantageous, if the author would be good enough to state precisely what he regards to be adequate quinine treatment and adequate quinine prophylactic treatment." A large experience has caused Brem, and Deeks and James, all of the Isthmian Canal Commission, to advise against its use during an attack. In Deaderick's series of 2007 cases treated with quinine there was a mortality of 25.5 per cent, while in the 1183 cases treated without quinine there was a mortality of but 10.4 per cent. One must ever be on guard, however, against *post hoc ergo propter hoc* reasoning from statistical studies. Deaderick does not hold that quinine should never be used, but states that the only conditions in which it is indicated are: First, where the parasites show no tendency to disappear after forty-eight hours from onset; and second, in the infrequent cases of intermittent hemoglobinuria where the outbreak corresponds with parasitic sporulation.

Cort (1929) has had excellent results with neoarsphenamine in a small series of cases: 0.15 Gm. every day for three days, then 0.3 Gm. after an interval of three days, then weekly doses of 0.3 Gm. for three or four weeks, then the same dose two weeks apart for three to six months. In a few instances the treatment seemed to aggravate the hemoglobinuria temporarily, but usually convalescence was rapid. Cort feels that the increased use of alkalis in these cases was especially helpful, which is in accord with the observation of many physicians. Cooke and Willoughby (1929) write: "Judging from the results of these two cases it appears that immediate transfusion with sodium bicarbonate solution is indicated in all cases of blackwater fever to curtail the duration of the attack, to prevent blockage of the kidney tubules, and to avoid suppression of urine." Additional transfusions—from 10 to 20 ounces of a sodium bicarbonate solution of 150 grains to the pint is perhaps the average dosage employed, sometimes followed by half the fluid quantity of 5 per cent glucose solution—are considered indicated if there is no improvement within twenty-four hours. Low, Cooke and Martin (1928) feel that in desperate cases the fear of causing more hemolysis should not prevent the employment of blood transfusion. They apparently saved a moribund case in this way, but Manson-Bahr and Sayers (1927) failed in their case, though the first of the transfusions remarkedly revived the patient.

For a consideration of the use of plasmoquine in blackwater fever, see page 110.

Munoz, quoted by Cardamitis, reported, in 1920, the cure of 5 grave cases under intravenous injection of mercuric cyanide. Others have reported similar experiences since, and Cardamitis (1926) added another grave case to the list, with prompt recovery after three intravenous injections of 0.01 Gm. of mercuric cyanide in five days.

CATARRHAL FEVER
(Common Cold, Grippe, Influenza)

I am in entire agreement with Fantus, who says that to draw a sharp distinction between common colds, grippe and influenza is futile; hence to embrace the whole group I have adopted the term "catarrhal fever," as advocated by him. That the ordinary cold, grippe (or nonepidemic influenza) and epidemic influenza are different manifestations of one and the same thing may be debated profitably by bacteriologists and immunologists, but from the standpoint of practical handling of the cases the point is not a controversial one. The successful treatment of all three is the successful prophylaxis of their complications.

Catarrhal fever is an acute infectious disease the exact primary causative organism of which is not as yet known, though in view of recent investigations it would seem that the virus is filtrable. It exists endemically as the common cold and grippe, and periodically and pandemically as virulent influenza. Both the cold and grippe occur with greatest frequency during winter and spring. The virulent type of influenza shows no predilection for season when first it appears, but always in the second and third waves which invariably characterize a pandemic there is a definite increase in incidence during the inclement months. The symptoms are almost too well known to warrant description here: typical "cold in the head," headache, chilliness, pains all over the body, especially in the back and legs, impairment of taste and smell, a nonproductive cough with considerable soreness behind the sternum, fever, malaise, etc. The variability of these symptoms largely determines our diagnosis: if the attack is mild, it is a "cold," if severe, grippe; if the latter, and occurring during an epidemic, it is influenza.

Influenza derives its name from the fact that during medieval times, when it was widely spread by the crusades, it was looked upon as a cosmic or celestial "influence" (*influentia coeli*). The correlative occurrence of lethargic states was definitely noted by Fernel in the sixteenth century. Influenza was common in both the new and old world throughout the seventeenth and eighteenth centuries, in the latter century being dubbed *influenza* by the English and *grippe* by the French. The malady was more or less epidemic throughout the nineteenth century and pandemic in 1830–33, 1836–37, 1847–48, 1889–90. The visitation of 1918–19 is well known to most readers of this book.

PROPHYLAXIS

Chilling of any portion of the body and excessive fatigue both no doubt lower the resistance to the infection and should therefore be avoided, especially during the inclement months. The crowding together of large numbers of people in closed spaces doubtless facilitates the spread of the disease, but whether prohibition of such meetings during an epidemic really affects the total morbidity is doubtful, since it would seem that a given epidemic of influenza persists until all who are not immune have become so or have died. Such prohibitions are justified, however, in that they doubtless delay the incidence in many cases until the virulence of the virus has been somewhat attenuated by a lessening of the rapidity of its passage through the human host. I am not at all convinced that any of the vaccines, whether of the mixed type or composed of the so-called "influenza" bacilli, have been shown to be of positive value in preventing the disease. Gay's discussion of the subject, as it contains an excellent bibliography, should be consulted by the interested reader. The use of the gauze mask and the antiseptic nasal spray have yet to prove their cases in *carefully controlled* clinical experiments; and, despite all the pother about it in the advertisements, there is not as yet any scientific evidence that excess of any of the vitamins—be it A or D or what have you—will prevent a cold, or grippe or "flu," or have any effect in curing it.

THERAPY

Symptomatic Treatment.—There are two chief indications, to keep the patient warm and to make him comfortable. The first of these can only be met by putting him to bed, and this applies as well for the common cold as for grippe or epidemic influenza. I think that all those who had extensive experience in the pandemic of 1918–19, and were not seeking to show that some particular drug as used by them was marvellously efficacious, will agree with the statement that the occurrence of serious complications (which is the only thing to be feared in this disease, since influenza itself is practically never fatal) was confined almost exclusively to those who either would not or could not go to bed at once on the appearance of symptoms. Though loath to overburden an already slogan-weary world, my intense conviction on this point tempts me to advocate a facetious placard for display in all offices and factories: "Go home when you feel it!" I believe the industrial world would suffer far less economically when next the disease is rife among us if the individual who insists upon tottering about as long as he can were subjected to open scorn for his action. And the beam in our own eye? Who among us has not "stuck" at his post on the ward or in the clinic, or in the immensely more arduous pursuit of private practice, when he should really have been in bed with the "flu"? Surely to err here on the side of too much early care is to err not at all.

The patient, then, should be kept warm in bed, but whether it is necessary to carry this to the point of causing him to sweat is a moot point. The question was certainly answered in the affirmative in the beginning at least of the recent pandemic, for salicylates and other diaphoretics were so generally employed by physicians that the laity looked upon drenching sweats as one of the characteristic symptoms of the disease. One wonders how many patients were submitted to fatal chillings by this means. Many very competent clinicians deserted the excessive use of these drugs in treating the later waves of the disease. In the beginning, however, some such capsule as the following, to be repeated every three hours for only a few doses, will greatly relieve the patient's discomfort:

℞. Acetylsalicylic acid	gr. v	0.3
Phenacetin	gr. iiss	0.15
Caffeine citrate	gr. ss	0.03

A "hot toddy" of whisky, sugar and hot water is of value to many patients in the beginning, causing a mild diaphoresis, a considerable amelioration of the general bodily weariness, and a grateful lessening of apprehension; there is no contraindication, despite all that emasculated reformers among us have said to the contrary. The old-fashioned Dover's powder (powder of ipecac and opium, U. S. P.) used very much to be employed for this purpose; the dose is 5 to 8 grains (0.3 to 0.5 Gm.).

For the relief of the substernal tightness and pain, a mustard poultice is frequently employed. This is conveniently made by spreading between two layers of thin muslin a paste made by mixing equal parts of ordinary household mustard and wheat flour stirred together with warm water; it will not be nearly so effective if made with hot water. Prepared plasters which are very convenient to use may be purchased at drug-stores. Whether the prepared or home-made article is used, it should be left in place over the upper part of the sternum until the skin becomes quite red, which usually requires from fifteen to thirty minutes.

Relief of the cough will also lessen the chest discomfort, but it should be remembered that therapy here should be in the direction of loosening and not drying the cough, for experience would seem to show that to dry up a cough, or to lessen the patient's sensitiveness to it by repeated doses of an opiate, is to invite the most feared complication, namely, pneumonia. This is not to be taken to mean that opiates are never to be used; on the contrary they are frequently of value but, instead of using them in small doses routinely in conjunction with a cough mixture, they should be withheld when possible until the patient shows signs of fatigue from the cough and restlessness, and then a full dose may be given sufficient to ensure several hours of satisfying, strength-renewing rest. Among the expectorants ammonium chloride is probably the most certain in its action. Some such preparation as the following, which contains approximately 8 grains of the drug to each teaspoonful, is usually effective if given every *two* hours:

℞. Ammonium chloride................................ ʒiv   15.0
    Syrup of citric acid................................ ʒj   30.0
    Water to make...................................... ʒiv   120.0

Frequently the drug is used as in the following prescription, in which the "brown mixture"—containing too little of its active ingredients (paregoric, tartar emetic and spirits of nitrous ether) to be usually effective alone—very satisfactorily supplements the action when used as a vehicle:

℞. Ammonium chloride................................ ʒiv   15.0
    Compound mixture of glycyrrhiza to make............ ʒiv   120.0
    Label: 1 teaspoonful every two to three hours.

It must not be forgotten, however, that this patient *is* being given an opiate here.

If the ammonium chloride nauseates, sodium citrate may be substituted in 10- to 15-grain doses; this drug has the added advantages that it is a diuretic and indirectly an alkali. Or 2 or 3 drops of a saturated solution of sodium or potassium iodide may be given in water every two hours, but bearing in mind the frequent occurrence of iodism, the interval between doses should be lengthened as soon as possible. The syrup of hydriodic acid is well taken by children in doses scaled down from 1 drachm according to size and age. Fantus has found the iodide effect to be most pleasantly obtained in children by giving Sajodin in doses of 1 grain (0.06) mixed with sugar, 5 grains (0.3), and 10 per cent of cacao, preferably in the form of sweet tablets, though powders will do if tablets are not available. Syrup of ipecac is frequently used also. The U.S.P. expectorant dose is 12 minims, but this is too large if the drug is to be repeated often, which is the only way to get results with it. Therefore the best dosage is 5 to 8 minims every two hours and nausea is unlikely to occur.

℞. Syrup of ipecac................................... ʒiv   15.0
    Aqueous elixir of glycyrrhiza to make.............. ʒiv   120.0
    Label: 1 teaspoonful every two hours.

For a child, with its preference for sweets, the syrup of glycyrrhiza had best be substituted, or any of the other vehicles liked by children may be used: syrup of raspberry, syrup of tolu (vanilla-like flavor), syrup of cacao (chocolate flavor), syrup of cinnamon.

When it is felt that a full effective amount of an opiate should be incorporated in the cough mixture, some such prescriptions as the following may be written (the doses are for adults, of course):

℞. Pantopon... gr. iss   0.10
    Syrup of thiocol to make........................... ʒiv   120.00
    Label: 1 teaspoonful every three hours.

The pantopon is present here in $\frac{1}{20}$-grain doses; for a note on the syrup of thiocol, see page 243.

℞. Codeine sulphate................................. gr. viiss   0.45
    Ammonium chloride................................ ʒiv   15.00
    Syrup of citric acid................................ ʒj   30.00
    Water to make...................................... ʒiv   120.00
    Label: 1 teaspoonful every three to four hours.

There is approximately ¼ grain of codeine sulphate and 8 grains of ammonium chloride per dose here; a larger amount of codeine may be needed.

Terpin hydrate is best reserved for the type of cough in which there is excessive secretion. It may be given in 4-grain doses in powders or capsules or in the form of the Elixir of Terpin Hydrate (N. F.), which latter contains 1 grain of the drug to the teaspoonful; it is well to bear in mind that this elixir contains 42 per cent of alcohol.

As in all other fevers, water should be liberally given. The patient should take at least ½ tumblerful every hour while awake. It is often easier to induce the taking of this much fluid if it is given in the form of lemon- or orangeade. This fruit juice, since it is potentially alkaline, also helps to meet what is generally looked upon as a definite indication, namely, the necessity to overcome acidosis. Whether this acidosis actually exists, or whether the effectiveness of "alkalinizing the patient" is only an unfounded clinical tradition, is not definitely answered so far as I am aware. Ten or 15 grains of sodium bicarbonate added to the glass of lemonade will help in accomplishing this desired result. In those cases in which there is nausea and vomiting, fluids should be given by rectum. From 2 to 8 ounces, according to the patient's size, of a 2 per cent sodium bicarbonate solution may be given as a retention enema every two to four hours until the stomach will retain water.

And now the question of the initial cathartic. I well remember my late professor of medicine as, with serious mien, he said to us many a time in class, "Gentlemen, I *always* prescribe calomel on the first visit," and then, with a sly twinkle in his eyes, "or on the second." And doubtless he did just that. But why? Certainly if a cathartic is to be used at all it had best be calomel, or at least not a saline, for Macht and Finesilver have conclusively shown in both laboratory and clinic that the taking of a saline cathartic prevents the absorption, and therefore the effect, of other drugs taken simultaneously or quite some time later. But why give a cathartic at all when we know the debilitating effect of a purge even in a well individual? Some time ago the following facetious letter, which has caused me much amusement, appeared in the Journal of the American Medical Association; I quote almost *in toto:*

"*To the Editor:*—I appeal to the fountainhead of medical knowledge for information on a subject of greatest personal and community importance. Shall I take a physic? And shall I give a physic to practically all my patients? I have not taken a physic for nearly fifteen years and am in perfect health. My intestinal exit operates as faithfully as the inlet, with an almost unvarying ratio of three to one. Traffic occasionally slows up a bit and as a consequence terminal unloading facilities may be put to some test, but this is never extreme and there have been no failures nor needed repairs. Once in a long time I have a cold but in no instance has a cold ever slowed up deliveries. Years ago I always took a physic for my colds, which always did two ugly things to me: They always gave me a bellyache and disturbed my regular evacuating habits. My colds without physics are just as brief as those subjected to the foregoing complications.

"Now as to my patients. They all want a 'thorough cleaning out' and 'a change in diet.'" Regarding diet, "I am frequently distressed with my inability to supply new formulas and combinations; but I am not now asking for any relief in this particular. However, I do want enlightenment on the contention that if the patient suddenly shows a little fever or a subnormal temperature, or restlessness, or tympanites, or a collapsed abdomen, or frequency of bowel movements or a total stoppage, or numbness of the first three fingers on the right side, or anorexia, or a gluttonous appetite, or nausea, with or without vomiting, or a sudden dislike for the male parent, that such a patient should at once have a physic. And if so, what? and when? and how long?

"A new treatise on skin disease just came to my notice, and in going through it in a quick review, my memory may not serve me perfectly but I can now recall just one condition that did not require a 'purge,' a 'physic' or a complete overhauling of the eliminating machinery, and that was freckles. I was pleased, as I have freckles and it may be safe to go right on neglecting my bowels as heretofore with safety. I have no more trouble keeping my bowels regular than my nose Roman, and I have about come to the conclusion that, colds or no colds, I need plastics for my nose just as frequently as physics for my bowels, and that's that.

"Such limited reading of last editions as I do gives me scant support for my aversion) purges and 'thorough cleaning out of the intestinal tract.' My frequent contact with physicians convinces me that I do far less cleaning out than they do, and when it comes to toning up a liver with laxatives I am almost a total failure. I try. In this community one simply must be able to do considerable in the way of toning up livers. It seems that we live in the toneless liver belt; and since Marshall Field established that the customer is always right, we must tone 'em up as per general request, or they will get another toner. I do not know whether the people or the physicians established this belt, but it's here alright and we live in the center of it. . . . At a recent meeting of our society I informed my confrères . . . that I was making no effort to transform my 'cold' cases into dysentery cases, and now I wish I had not for I fear I lost caste or something . . ."

E. O. HARROLD, M. D.

Well, well! But this matter should be put to the test. Macdonald has recently made the attempt and, though his series was small and not subject to very rigid control, he has shown that during an epidemic of mild catarrhal fever occurring in an industrial plant, the loss of time among those who had taken an initial cathartic was 14.3 per cent greater than among those not so dosing themselves. Can the matter not be definitely settled during our next pandemic or during the next great war when considerable epidemics are certain to occur among troops under ideal conditions for carefully controlled clinical experiments?

Other Measures.—These are legion, and so diverse have been the offerings of drugs having specific value, both in the United States and other countries, that I believe none of them merit description. Considerable hope was felt for a time following the report, in 1924, of the American Army surgeons, Vedder and Sawyer, that they had found inhalations of chlorine to have a distinctly curative value in common colds, influenza, whooping cough and other respiratory diseases in which the infecting organisms are located on the surface of the mucous membranes of the respiratory passages. Unfortunately, other investigators have been unable entirely or even in the main to confirm this finding. For instance, in the two clinics established by the Health Commissioner of New York City for the purpose of studying the use of chlorine, Harris has stated that only 6.5 per cent of 506 persons with various respiratory diseases reported themselves as cured by the gas, in contrast to 71.4 per cent of 931 patients reported cured in the original paper of Vedder and Sawyer. Diehl's findings are likewise not impressive. He studied the results of the chlorine treatment of 425 students with "colds" compared with the "medical" treatment of a group of 392 similarly afflicted. Of the entire series, 51.4 per cent of those treated with chlorine and 47.9 per cent of those given medical treatment recovered in three days; while 73.3 per cent of those treated with chlorine and 72.6 per cent of those with medical treatment recovered within a week.

A new, purely symptomatic type of therapy, which has been considerably used in Germany in recent years, is the intramuscular injection of ether. An ampule containing $\frac{1}{2}$ cc. of ether and $\frac{1}{2}$ cc. of olive oil, to which has been added a small amount of a local anesthetic, is injected on the evening of the first and second days and repeated if necessary on the fourth and fifth evenings. In Strehl's (1932) enthusiastic report of 150 cases, the following seem to be the outstanding results: a feeling of bodily comfort replaces the chilliness, the cough becomes much less wracking and more productive and the breathing easier; the fever falls and the initial slight feeling of euphoria soon gives way to sleep in most cases. All of this sounds very well and the treatment is probably at least harmless in properly selected cases but there is some indication in the reports that the sense of dryness and burning in the mouth, nose and throat can sometimes be very objectionable. The champions of this therapy consider it to be contraindicated if there are signs of bronchial congestion.

Many patients in the mild attacks of catarrhal fever are principally made uncomfortable by the excessive nasal secretions and the feeling of fulness in the head. Both these symptoms can be greatly relieved by the use of an oil spray, such as the following:

℞.	Thymol	gr. ss	0.03
	Menthol	gr. iv	0.24
	Eucalyptol	♏x	0.60
	Liquid petrolatum	℥ij	64.00

This will require the use of the oil nozzle on the atomizer, or, if preferred, 5 drops or so of the mixture may be placed well back in each nostril with the patient recumbent. Or a few drops of 10 per cent of menthol in alcohol may be inhaled from a handkerchief. A teaspoonful of the following inhalant may be vaporized by pouring scalding water upon it in a previously heated cup; with his head low over the cup, and a large towel enclosing both, the patient breathes with mouth open. Sometimes the feeling of stuffiness is only increased by such a steamy inhalant; exposure should be avoided for an hour after its use. The housewife will be grateful if forewarned that both the cup and spoon are very difficult to clean after their employment for this purpose.

℞.	Oil of pine needles	℥iv	16.0
	Tincture of benzoin to make	℥iv	128.0

If desired, creosote (℥ ss) may be added to the above, but as it is a mixture of phenols there is some reason to believe that if used too freely it may cause some damage to the kidneys. For bed-ridden patients, Means and Lerman have found it convenient to place the above ingredients in an ordinary teakettleful of boiling water on a chair beside the bed; a length of large rubber tubing is stuck onto the spout and the patient takes the free end into his mouth, thus getting the full effect of the medicated steam without having to put his neck into an uncomfortable position.

Complications.—The most frequent complications are acute sinusitis, otitis media, mastoiditis, purulent bronchitis, bronchiectasis, and pneumonia. Bearing in mind that catarrhal fever patients die from the complications and not from the disease *per se*, the employment of the treatment as outlined in the last few pages ("coddling" treatment as Fantus has styled it) offers our best hope of holding down the mortality, designed as it is to prevent the occurrence of complications. Of course so far as is possible the patient should be isolated from sources of secondary infection.

CEREBROSPINAL FEVER

(Epidemic Cerebrospinal Meningitis, Meningococcus Meningitis, Spotted Fever)

Cerebrospinal fever is an infectious disease which occurs sporadically or in epidemics and is caused by the *Meningococcus* (*Diplococcus intracellularis*); infection probably takes place by droplet transfer from an active case or from a healthy carrier. Symptomatically, and indeed perhaps pathologically, it can be divided into three stages, the first two of which are unfortunately not often recognized. The first stage may simply be a carrier stage without symptoms, or there may be a tonsillitis, pharyngitis, or sinusitis, or a conjunctivitis with discharge containing the causative organism. In the second stage the patient goes to bed, where he lies curled on his side, knees up and head bent toward them; he is extremely apathetic, loses both play of feature and modulation of voice, and when urged will complain in monosyllables of being "sore" all over his body. It is during this stage that the rash appears. In the third stage the diagnosis is most frequently made. Here there is the bursting headache, chilliness and erratic fever, possibly delirium or coma (in children, of course, often convulsions), cloudiness of the spinal fluid, with increase in pressure unless block has occurred, and the well-known Kernig's and other signs. The disease is characterized by what an irate friend of mine once called an "unnecessary tendency" toward complications, such as panophthalmitis, endocarditis and pericarditis, pneumonia, otitis media, internal hydrocephalus, etc. Relapses occur in perhaps one fourth of all cases; cases which run an entirely atypical course for several weeks are also not uncommon.

So far as I am aware the first published accounts of cerebrospinal fever were those of Gaspard Vieusseaux (1805) at Geneva, and L. Danielson and E. Mann (1806) in Massachusetts. In 1811, the American, Elisha North, published a large monograph on the subject. Weichselbaum discovered the causative organism in 1887, and Flexner introduced the antiserum in 1909. The periods when the disease has been most rife are the following: 1805–30, 1837–50, 1854–74, 1904 to the present.

THERAPY

The frequent drainage of the spinal canal, without other treatment, was the sheet anchor of therapy in the days prior to the world-wide epidemic of 1904, when we had no specific treatment for this disease. And indeed there are still those who maintain its superiority to the use of serum. I cannot but feel that the dangers of the serum treatment are grossly exaggerated, though it must be admitted that some danger there surely is. Here are the figures, however: During the preserum period the recorded mortality in the United States was about 80 per cent, in France 75 per cent, in England 70 per cent, and in Germany 60 per cent. Since the use of serum became widespread, the gross mortality everywhere has been reduced to about 30 per cent, and in some epidemics it has been brought much lower even than this.

The Use of Serum.—Antimeningococcus serum is prepared by immunizing horses with different strains of meningococci. Polyvalent serum should always be used as the superiority of the monovalent serum over the polyvalent serum made in the United States has not been demonstrated. It is important to bear in mind, however, that serums from different sources oftentimes vary in their potency against a given case of the disease. This difference was well shown in the recent World War. At the beginning of the outbreak of epidemic meningitis in the British armies, the antiserum used failed to reduce the mortality below 40 per cent, except in the London district, where it was reduced to 18.5 per cent. Trial of this London serum elsewhere quickly showed its superior effectiveness wherever used. The experience in the Salt Lake City, Utah, epidemic of 1929, as reported by Anderson, was of a similar nature. If a patient does not respond to an injection of serum as it is felt he should, a new supply from a different source should be obtained at once.

The importance of the early administration of the serum is well shown in Table 2.

Intraspinal Injection.—Intraspinal injection of serum should be made about once in every twenty-four hours in the average case; in very severe cases it may be repeated every twelve hours for three or four doses and there-

TABLE 2.—EFFECT OF SERUM ON MORTALITY IN CEREBROSPINAL MENINGITIS

Treatment began.	Flexner, per cent.	Netter, per cent.	Dopter, per cent.	Christo-manos, per cent.	Levy, per cent.	Flack, per cent.
Before third day...............	18.1	7.1	8.2	13.0	13.2	9.09
From fourth to seventh day....	27.2	11.1	14.4	25.9	20.4	
After seventh day.............	36.5	23.5	24.1	47.0	28.6	50.0

after every twenty-four hours until the symptoms markedly decline. The average case probably requires four to eight doses, but it may sometimes be necessary to administer as many as twenty before the fluid becomes sterile; two successive sterile fluids at twenty-four-hour intervals is a satisfactory indication for stopping treatment. "If, however, the symptoms do not improve after the fluid becomes sterile, and the serum has been temporarily discontinued, it is well to resume the injections, as they may be due to a localized meningitis with adhesions which may be favorably influenced by the continued use of the serum" (J. B. Neal, Meningitis Div., N. Y. C. Dept. of Health). Bunim and Wies (1933) feel that in resistant cases the addition of 5 cc. of fresh normal human serum might advantageously be made, for its complement content, to each 15 cc. of the antimeningococcus serum. When the serum is discontinued a daily or every other day spinal drainage is of value in lessening the tendency toward a hydrocephalic block, and is also of value in enabling one to detect early signs of recrudescence. In making the spinal injection enough fluid should be withdrawn by lumbar puncture to reduce the pressure to normal, i. e., until the flow is about 1 drop per minute; this amount is usually from 20 to 60 cc. Then introduce the serum, warmed to body temperature, the amount to be from 5 to 10 cc. less than the amount of spinal fluid withdrawn; the usual amount is between 20 and 40 cc. Let it run in by gravity, never by forcible injection. Also the needle should be left in place for a few minutes to see whether grave symptoms are going to occur, such as rapid and irregular pulse, cyanosis and respiratory embarrassment. These symptoms can usually be overcome by the prompt withdrawal of fluid; artificial respiration may have to be resorted to for a time. It is well to give a hypodermic of morphine and atropine before the injection.

If, correctly performed, spinal puncture fails to produce fluid, it is fair to assume, what will be true in most cases, that hydrocephalic block has taken place. This complication demands immediate drainage by puncture of the cisterna magna and introduction of serum there. This is usually easy to accomplish in children, but in adults the skull will oftentimes have to be trephined in order to draw off fluid and replace it with serum. We thus actually place antibodies where they are greatly needed, but it should be remembered that in replacing the fluid with serum in this way we are in a measure stultifying ourselves, for the relief of pressure itself is of tremendous importance. Bearing in mind the work of Weed and McKibben, who have shown that the intravenous injection of hypertonic solutions of certain electrolytes and crystalloids causes a transient rise and then a very pronounced fall in the spinal fluid pressure, would it not be well to make injections of this sort a matter of routine in the cases, as suggested by Haden? He has reported 2 cases in which the slow injection of several hundred cubic centimeters of 25 per cent glucose solution over a long period of time seemed to be an important factor in the favorable outcome. Fay has found that magnesium sulphate solution, 1½ ounces of crystals in water by mouth or 3 ounces of crystals in 6 ounces of water by rectum, has given marked relief from symptoms of intracranial pressure in other conditions. Could not this simple procedure be utilized also? Recently, Stookey, Elliott and Teachenor have introduced the conception that extreme edema of the cord is the cause of spinal block in many instances, having encountered the condition *post mortem* in 4 out of 17 cases in infants. They feel that since beginning the use of concentrated glucose solution (50 per cent) intravenously where block of this nature has been diagnosed they have seen a reestablishment of the circulation of the cerebrospinal fluid take place.

Intravenous Injection.—The combination of intravenous injections of serum with the intraspinal injections has been much advocated of late. It would seem rational and advisable to give serum intravenously in all cases were it not for the fact that the intravenous injection is often associated with a more severe systemic reaction than attends the intraspinal injection. In adults this reaction is rarely followed by serious consequences, but Blackfan believes the danger to be so great in children that he prefers in them to give it intravenously only in cases in which the organism persists or reappears in the blood stream. Herrick's experience with this combined therapy in adults at one of the large army cantonments was most gratifying. In 137 cases treated by intraspinal methods alone, the mortality was 34.3 per cent; in 128 cases treated by a combination of intraspinal and intravenous therapy, the mortality was 14.8 per cent. He says: "The intravenous treatment must be employed with boldness, yet with care. One must be prepared to give from four to eight massive injections by vein of from 80 to 150 cc. during the acute stages of the disease or a period of from two to four days. There is much more danger in insufficient than in excessive intravenous serum administration. We have, in fact, in 128 cases so treated, had no serious serum effects. Our regrets have been that serum was not more freely used in many of the early cases.

"The desensitization by subcutaneous injection of 1 cc. of serum one hour before the introduction of serum into the vein and the cautious injection of the first 15 cc. at the rate of 1 cc. per minute are the secrets of safe intravenous serum therapy. Immediate stopping of the injection with the appearance of dyspnea, pallor, cyanosis, vomiting, weak, rapid or irregular pulse or other immediate serum effects is essential. Renewal of the attempt after two or three hours is rarely unsuccessful. Even those patients thoroughly sensitized to serum by earlier courses of treatment can be treated safely with these precautions. It is desirable to give morphine and atropine before the injection, but they are not absolutely necessary."

One cubic centimeter of epinephrine hydrochloride, 1: 1000 solution, is useful in combating the alarming symptoms.

Serum-fluid Substitution.—In an attempt to accomplish the substitution of serum for infected cerebrospinal fluid, Lyon (1932) has introduced serum into the ventricles above while simultaneously withdrawing the purulent fluid from the spinal subarachnoid space below. The method, which has succeeded very well in his hands and will most likely be given an extensive trial, is as follows:

"A new 19- or 20-gauge Luer lumbar puncture needle 7 cm. long was introduced into the right ventricle. The stylet was left in place, the patient turned on his left side and a lumbar puncture performed with a new 20-gauge Luer needle. A 100-cc. Luer syringe, connected by a rubber tube 20 cm. long, was attached then to the lumbar puncture needle and the baby placed in a position of normal extension. Then with the patient still on the left side a 100-cc. Luer syringe barrel was connected to the needle in the ventricle by a rubber tube 20 cm. long. This syringe barrel contained 90 cc. of antimeningococcus serum to which had been added 1 cc. of neutral phenolphthalein. The weight of the dependent plunger at the lumbar puncture

3

needle combined with that of a column of serum at the ventricle from 10 to 30 cm. high provided the only pressure employed. After from 65 to 70 cc. of purulent fluid had been withdrawn and about 55 cc. of serum introduced, the dye appeared in the fluid from the lumbar puncture needle. Both syringes were then disconnected from their respective needles and the fluid from each allowed to flow until it dropped at the rate of approximately 30 drops per minute. This rate was considered an indication of essentially normal pressure. Approximately 0.5 cc. of fluid escaped from the ventricular needle before pressure there was normal. Then the needle was withdrawn. In a short time the fluid from the lumbar region indicated a return to normal pressure, approximately 2 cc. having escaped before this occurred. The lumbar needle was then withdrawn. The usual febrile reaction occurred. Small amounts of fluid were withdrawn from time to time for study and for the relief of pressure. Cultures and smears were made to determine when sterilization of the fluid occurred. Forty-eight hours following the first substitution, the procedure was repeated except that the patient was placed on his right side and the left ventricle tapped. Approximately 15 cc. more of fluid was removed than was introduced. Following the second administration spinal drainage was done with decreasing frequency and the progress in the spinal fluid characteristics noted. . . .

"In spite of the age of the five infants treated, and the severity of their infections, an early and complete recovery occurred in each case. The cerebrospinal fluid was sterilized within twenty-four to forty-eight hours following the first substitution of antimeningococcus serum. The duration of the illness was shortened. There were no sequelae. A large initial dosage of serum combined with an extensive withdrawal of contaminated cerebrospinal fluid was obtained. The resulting concentration of serum was high and an intimate contact of serum with meningococci was provided. Early sterilization of the fluid occurred. In each case, two serum substitutions affected a clinical cure. Fewer injections of serum were required. In this manner it was possible to avoid the complications resulting from the repeated administration of serum intrathecally.

"The substitution of serum by this method did not produce any untoward effects in the patients so treated. Vomiting, convulsions, cardiac or respiratory embarrassment, etc., did not occur. There was no increased depression or aggravation of the clinical condition at any time. The output of cerebrospinal fluid in response to serum injected was greater than obtained by other methods of administration. This was a favorable adjunct to therapy as it provided excellent lavage of the cerebrospinal fluid spaces. Spinal drainage, when indicated, prevented difficulties from increased fluid pressure. In the forty-eight-hour period following the introduction of serum, as little fluid as possible was withdrawn, in an attempt to maintain throughout that period a high concentration of serum."

Intracarotid Injection of Pregl's Iodine Plus Serum.—Stimulated by the preliminary studies of Kolmer, Crawford (1932) has reported the administration of Pregl's colloidal iodine solution in 6 cases that had shown unfavorable response to specific serum; there were 4 recoveries.

"*Case 3.*—E. W., a woman, aged twenty-nine, admitted to the Henry Ford Hospital, June 19, 1929, had typical signs and symptoms of meningococcus meningitis. The medical treatment was active, consisting of 353 cc. of specific serum given intraspinally, intravenously and by cistern. The course became unfavorable, the patient becoming semicomatose and delirious. The cell counts and cultures indicated poor response to the treatment. Surgical aid was requested and we injected 10 cc. of Pregl's solution of iodine and 15 cc. of specific serum into each carotid artery, followed by cistern puncture on the ninth, eleventh, and thirteenth days of the disease. The condition improved noticeably after each injection and the cultures became negative the day after the third injection. The patient made a complete recovery and left the hospital on the twentieth day."

Crawford believes that Pregl's solution may be given safely in doses of 20 to 30 cc. daily for three or four days, but no longer nor in any higher dosage. "With that dosage and duration there should be some improvement if it is going to help." He mentions the case of a young girl in whom an acute hemorrhagic nephritis was found at autopsy after a dose of 50 cc. on three successive days.

Other Measures.—Morphine should be given without stint to disturbed patients to control violent symptoms during the first twenty-four to forty-eight hours. Large amounts are well tolerated. Chloral hydrate and the bromides are also useful.

Relapse.—In the relapses and recrudescences which so frequently occur in epidemic meningitis the entire cycle of treatment must be repeated with the same meticulous care used in the initial course.

CHICKENPOX

(Varicella)

Chickenpox is an acute infectious, and very highly contagious, disease of unknown etiology, which attacks nearly all children at some time during their early years. A great many serious students are at the present time attempting to show a causal relationship between it and herpes zoster (shingles), but they have not met with success as yet. The malady is characterized by the sudden appearance of a vesicular rash usually without any prodromal or accompanying constitutional symptoms; when the latter do appear they are extremely mild. The rash may be differentiated from that of smallpox (a feat not always so easy of accomplishment as this glib statement would indicate!) by the fact that it begins on the back or some part of the trunk whence it spreads to the whole of the body, including the scalp, but is seen on the face and palms and soles only occasionally, and then to the extent of only a few lesions; that several stages of the eruption may be seen at one time, to wit, erythematous maculopapules, clear vesicles, turbulent vesicles, somewhat pustular vesicles, and crusted vesicles; and by the fact that these vesicles are unilocular (collapse completely after a single needle puncture) and are not umbilicated.

The incubation period varies from four to more than twenty days but the vast majority of cases develop within twelve to fourteen days after exposure. One attack practically always protects for life. So far as is known to me there is no racial immunity to chickenpox.

The disease was first described by Ingrassias (1553), but the most famous of the early treatises is that of Heberden (1767), which contains his original illustrations. Attention was first attracted to the possible relationship of chickenpox to herpes by Bokay in 1892.

THERAPY

Chickenpox is constitutionally a mild affair and usually requires no treatment. For control of the itching recourse may be had to the measures employed in smallpox (see p. 166). After-scarring is very infrequent.

PROPHYLAXIS

Chickenpox in adults, if not actually a serious malady, is certainly more incapacitating than it is in children, from which it would seem advisable to permit all youngsters to contract it in order to become immune before they reach maturity. Recently, however, studies have been made in the prophylaxis of the disease which find their justification in the fact that its extreme contagiousness sometimes makes it an "unpleasant complication among groups of children in hospitals" (Schamberg). The measures employed are vaccination and injection with convalescent serum.

Vaccination.—The vaccination of exposed individuals with the contents of chickenpox vesicles was introduced in Germany by Kling in 1913, but from the subsequent reports of Cooke, Handrik, Rabinoff, Michael, Greenthal, Meyer-Stromfeldt, Waddell and Eley, Hess and Unger, Mitchell and Ravenel, and others, it is very unlikely that the method can be counted upon to control institutional outbreaks where immediate protection of children already exposed, rather than permanent immunization, is desired. Indeed, Soldin, in Germany, and Hoffmann, in Switzerland, both feel that this type of vaccination actually only induces a mild attack of the disease and that vaccinated children can be infectious for nonvaccinated ones. However, the method is still being studied; the technic follows:

"To secure the best results, vaccination should be performed on the first or second day of exposure. The contents of a fresh vesicle is drawn into a capillary tube (after cleansing the vesicle with alcohol and saline solution and wiping dry with cotton). The contents of the tube is expressed onto the forearm of the patient to be vaccinated, and forty or fifty punctures through this fluid are made with a sterile needle; the needle merely punctures the epidermis and no blood is obtained. The procedure is practically painless and can be done in a minute or two. The fluid is allowed to dry on the arm and seals the punctures. If a 'take' occurs, it will be noticed that between the eighth and thirteenth day a papule appears at the site of vaccination. This rapidly changes to a vesicle and then to a crust which later drops off, leaving in some instances a scar which resembles the scar remaining after smallpox vaccination. There is usually no fever or discomfort from the vaccination. Precautions are taken to avoid the use of vesicle fluid from syphilitic patients."

Convalescent Serum.—In 1923, Blackfan, Petersen and Conroy introduced the use of convalescent serum in the prophylaxis of chickenpox, and reported that among 42 susceptible children to whom 5 cc. of this serum had been given within five days of exposure, 7 contracted a mild form of the disease and 35 escaped without symptoms. Weech (1924) treated 9 infants, of whom 8 did not contract the disease and the ninth had only an extremely mild attack which did not develop until after the unusually long incubation period of twenty-two days. Mitchell and Ravenel treated 68 children, of whom only 4 developed the disease, and in these also the incubation period was abnormally long. It would seem that the best dose is 4 to 10 cc., given intramuscularly into the lateral aspect of the thigh. Reactions of any moment apparently do not occur. The careful studies of Gordon and Meader (1929) have demonstrated that the serum furnishes a high degree of protection if obtained within one month of the appearance of the donor's eruption; obtained thereafter it is less efficient, and after five months confers protection in only a third of the immunized susceptible patients. The blood is centrifuged, the serum from several donors pooled, passed through a Berkfeld filter and, after sterility tests over seven days, bottled in 15 cc. vials. When stored in the ice-box the serum thus prepared is said not to lose its potency up to four months. Such serum confers a brief passive immunity upon approximately 90 per cent of susceptible exposed individuals.

COMMON COLD

(See Catarrhal Fever)

DENGUE

(Breakbone Fever)

Dengue is an acute fever of unknown origin which occurs endemically and sometimes epidemically in warm countries. Boylon, of Java, first described it in 1779, and the American, Benjamin Rush, in 1780. Graham, in Beyrouth, Syria, in 1903, first suggested that it is mosquito borne, and Cleland and Bradley, working in Sydney, Australia, in 1928, clearly showed it to be transmitted by the yellow fever mosquito, *Stegomyia fasciata*. In the Philippines, where the morbidity rate of dengue fever is and always has been high for American troops, much in regard to its transmission, incubation period and immunity has recently been brought to light (see Siler, Hall and Hitchens; Holt and Kintner; Simmons, St. John and Reynolds in the Bibliography). In the last few years it has several times been epidemic in the southern United States, the 1922 epidemic in Louisiana comprising, according to Scott, some 30,000 cases; Levy says that there were 500,000 cases in Texas between June and December. In the Greek epidemic of 1928, there developed 239,000 cases in Athens alone in one month. The disease is usually not very difficult to diagnose for it never develops in the absence of mosquitoes and consequently is never present after frost. However, yellow fever must always be borne in mind, and some quite competent observers maintain that it is an abortive form of this disease, though it seems to me that the evidence is insufficient. The characteristic onset is sudden, with severe headache and pain behind the eyeballs, muscle and joint ache and usually excruciating backache, extreme fatigue, a rapid rise of temperature and pulse rate, and a constant leukopenia, this latter of great diagnostic importance. On the third day the temperature falls rapidly, usually accompanied by sweats, diuresis and nosebleed, and the patient feels much improved. However, on the fifth day the process recurs and there is usually a third definite attack also. During the second effervescence a rash of varied character appears on the body in most cases. The second and third attacks are milder than the first; sometimes, however, the intermissions do not occur. A fourth attack is extremely rare. Convalescence is often quite protracted. Apparently one bout of dengue confers a high degree of immunity of about one year's duration.

THERAPY

Here, as in its kindred affection yellow fever, we have an endemic and epidemic mosquito-borne disease which, in its characteristic symptoms and capacity for debilitating at a stroke large numbers of people, cries aloud for specific therapy. But in vain. Indeed, because the disease itself is rarely fatal and seldom gives rise to serious complications (save in aged and debilitated individuals and in pregnant women), evidence of serious application to a study of its symptomatic treatment is all but lacking in the literature. One reads that salicylates give great relief from pain though sometimes morphine is necessary, that the bowels should be "freely opened" and "fever treatment" applied, that the heart should be guarded against severe strain during convalescence. Verily, verily, here is a plea for distinguished service.

All attempts at protective vaccination have so far met only with failure.

DIPHTHERIA

Diphtheria is an acute infectious disease, caused by *Bacillus diphtheriae*, which is endemic in larger centers and often becomes epidemic during the winter months. It occurs chiefly in children. In the beginning of the attack the patient is but moderately indisposed, having a little soreness of the throat and slight elevation of temperature. However, the typical membrane soon begins to form in the throat and by the third or fourth day is quite thick and may cover a considerable part of the fauces. Absorption of toxins from the local lesion gives rise to profound constitutional symptoms, and there may be definite degeneration of the heart muscle, kidneys and peripheral nerves. Bronchopneumonia is a complication in nearly all the fatal cases. Average cases, if properly treated with antitoxin, show a rapid subsidence of severe symptoms and are fully convalescent in seven to ten days. In especially virulent cases, or those not properly treated, the symptoms may gradually increase in intensity to about the sixth day, when there will be considerable obstruction to the nose and throat by the spreading membrane, a massive cervical adenitis and cellulitis, rapid and feeble pulse, and perhaps subnormal temperature. Then coma supervenes upon the profound sepsis and finally death. In that type of the disease in which the membrane first appears in the posterior part of the nasal cavity, and in the laryngeal type, where the symptoms are respiratory from the beginning, the prognosis is especially poor.

According to the Babylonian Talmud (352–427 A. D.), the ancient Hebrews so much feared diphtheria that upon the discovery of the first case in a community the *shofar* was blown; for all other contagious diseases it was sounded only after the third case was reported. The classical description was that of Aretaeus the Cappadocian (*circa* 100 A. D.). Aëtius, in the sixth century, mentions paralysis of the palate as a sequel. A number of epidemics of the Middle Ages were described by prelates of the period; during the Renaissance and well up into the eighteenth century the Spaniards and Italians particularly concerned themselves with its description. I believe that the first recorded cases in America occurred in Massachusetts in 1659. To me it seems a strange thing that the diminished liability to the disease after adolescence was apparently not recorded in the literature before the publication of Heberden's famous *Commentaries* in 1802. Bretonneau gave the disease its present name in 1826, but the laryngeal and pharyngeal types were not recognized as being the same malady until 1880. Von Behring introduced antitoxin in treatment in 1894 and toxin-antitoxin in immunization in 1913. The present pandemic developed in the middle of the last century and has reached all parts of the world, though it is unquestionably very much more prevalent in colder climates, especially the north temperate zone, than in the tropics. A little before the turn of the century a slight decline in incidence set in, but the rate has not fallen generally and in recent years has indeed risen in some countries; mortality, however, has considerably diminished, and it is but a question of time until the newer immunization methods will effect a similar reduction in the world morbidity figures.

THERAPY

Antitoxin Treatment.—Before the discovery of antitoxin the mortality from diphtheria was about 40 per cent; since its use this figure has been gradually reduced, and now varies between 5 and 10 per cent. Its efficiency depends upon the administration of a sufficient dose as soon as possible to prevent the action of the toxin upon the heart and nervous system. If treated with antitoxin within the first twenty-four hours nearly every patient can be saved. Delay of two, three, or four days may mean irreparable injury to vital organs by the absorbed toxin, which cannot be neutralized by subsequent administration of even enormous doses of antitoxin. The data, taken from Ker (quoted by Zingher), are well displayed in the following table (Table 3):

TABLE 3.—RELATION OF MORTALITY IN DIPHTHERIA TO TIME OF ADMINISTRATION OF ANTITOXIN

Day of illness.	Number of patients.	Deaths.	Percentage of mortality.
First.....................................	329	5	1.52
Second....................................	2269	77	3.39
Third.....................................	2407	165	6.85
Fourth....................................	1612	176	10.91
Fifth.....................................	911	136	14.92
Sixth.....................................	416	54	12.98
Seventh...................................	320	53	16.56
Later.....................................	327	50	15.29
Total....................................	8591	716	8.33

The first injection should be large enough to control the disease. One large dose given early is far more efficacious than the same amount in divided doses. The usual site for subcutaneous injection is the infrascapular region. Very sick patients, those who have only received antitoxin after delay, or patients in whom the disease is progressive because of an insufficient first dose, should be given a large intravenous injection whenever feasible. In this way the full value of the antitoxin is obtained at once; the absorption from the subcutaneous injection is so slow that many hours must elapse before any great amount of antitoxin finds its way into the general circulation.

The following table gives the doses recommended by the New York City Department of Health (Table 4):

TABLE 4.—AMOUNT OF ANTITOXIN REQUIRED IN THE TREATMENT OF DIPHTHERIA

	Mild cases.	Moderate.	Severe.*	Malignant.*
Infants 10 to 30 pounds in weight (under two years)	2000 units to 3000 units	3000 units to 5000 units	5000 units to 10,000 units	7500 units to 10,000 units
Children 30 to 90 pounds in weight (under fifteen years)	3000 units to 4000 units	4000 units to 10,000 units	10,000 units to 15,000 units	10,000 units to 20,000 units
Adults 90 pounds and over in weight	3000 units to 5000 units	5000 units to 10,000 units	10,000 units to 20,000 units	20,000 units to 40,000 units

* When given intravenously one half the amount stated.

Cases of laryngeal diphtheria, moderate cases seen late at the time of the first injection, and cases of diphtheria occurring as a complication of the exanthemata should be classified and treated as "severe" cases.

In all cases a single dose of the proper amount, as indicated in the schedule, is recommended.

It is recommended that the methods of administration be as follows:

Mild Cases: Subcutaneous or intramuscular.

Moderate Cases: Intramuscular or subcutaneous.

Severe Cases: Intravenous or intramuscular.

Malignant Cases: Intravenous.

When the antitoxin has been administered early enough and in sufficient dose to be fully effective, a striking improvement is soon seen, as manifested by a fall in temperature and a favorable change in the character of the cardiac and nervous symptoms. Within twenty-four hours of the injection of the antitoxin the membrane stops spreading, begins to soften and loosen, and the swelling of the mucous membrane subsides. Zingher says: "In some cases the membrane apparently spreads and the alarmed physician is tempted to give a second dose of antitoxin. What has really happened, however, is that the area of mucous membrane which corresponds to the extending portion of false membrane has been injured by the toxin previous to the injection of the antitoxin, and the appearance of the fibrinous exudate is simply the later manifestation of the damage that has already taken place."

Combined Antitoxin, Glucose and Insulin in Severe Cases.—It is extremely exceptional for a case of diphtheria not to respond to antitoxin given early and in adequate dosage, but it is common hospital experience to encounter such failures in cases that have come under treatment too late. Several years ago, Edmunds and Cooper found experimentally that the intravenous introduction of glucose solution was almost certain to save the life of a dog severely poisoned by diphtheria toxin, and Schwentker and Noel (1930) have confirmed the observations of others and added evidence of their own to show that profound changes in carbohydrate metabolism in the human are caused by this toxin in severe cases. There is an exhaustion of glycogen from the liver and from the specialized conducting tissue of the heart with a simultaneous rise in blood sugar; this is sometimes followed by a period of hypoglycemia, and then there occurs a final hyperglycemia due to toxic depression of the pancreas and other sources of insulin supply. Benn, Hughes and Alstead (1932) have now shown that following intravenous injection of dextrose solution in these cases, the delayed return of the blood-sugar curve to normal is comparable to what occurs in diabetes; they are able to report a carefully controlled series of hypertoxic cases in which the judicious use of dextrose and insulin to supplement the antitoxin has resulted in a notable reduction in mortality. In setting down their method here I wish to point out that it is available for use only where repeated estimations of the blood sugar can be made; to inject insulin in diphtheria without adequate laboratory control would be extremely dangerous as a hypoglycemic reaction might easily be mistaken for a cerebral complication of the disease.

Method.—"1. Immediately on admission: (*a*) Intramuscular injection of antitoxin (32,000 to 56,000 units[1]). (*b*) Preliminary blood-sugar estimation.

"2. One hour after admission: (*a*) Intravenous injection of antitoxin (32,000 to 100,000 units). (*b*) Intravenous injection of dextrose (20 Gm. of glucose in 50 per cent solution). Serum and dextrose are given together with several 20-cc. syringes *very slowly* at 37 C. The serum is in concentrated form and undiluted.

"3. Ten minutes after intravenous dextrose, second blood-sugar estimation.

"4. One hour after intravenous dextrose, third blood-sugar estimation.

"5. One and a half hours after intravenous dextrose, fourth blood-sugar estimation.

"6. Two hours after intravenous dextrose, fifth blood-sugar estimation.

"7. If the two-hour blood-sugar estimation shows a slow return to normal a suitable dose of insulin is given intramuscularly (10 to 30 units). Subsequent treatment consists in giving glucose by mouth in all cases where the cooperation of the patient can be obtained. Commonly, children receive, diluted in lemonade, from 4 to 8 ounces of glucose by mouth daily for at

---

[1] Much higher doses than are employed by most authorities.—H. B.

least the first ten days after admission, and in some cases for three or four weeks. If the patient refuses, or is unable to tolerate, glucose by mouth, 40 to 100 Gm., in 50 per cent solution, are given intravenously during each twenty-four hours.

"Transient glycosuria after the initial dose of dextrose appears to be rare in the severely toxic cases, but was almost invariably present in the moderately toxic cases. Albumin was found in the urine at some stage of the disease in all the moderately and severely toxic cases.

"Dosage with insulin depends on the degree of toxemia as estimated by the initial dextrose-tolerance test. In accordance with the practice of Schwentker and Noel, 1 unit of insulin is given for every 1 to 2 Gm. of dextrose, and it is then injected twice daily until the patient has passed the stage of acute toxemia."

Deleterious Effects of Antitoxin Injections.—In a rather large proportion of cases an urticarial rash with a slight rise in temperature occurs from two to seven days after the injection; rarely other types of rash with more severe constitutional symptoms. Entirely distinct from these slight effects, from which recovery always ensues, are occasional severe disturbances. Park says: "A few minutes after an injection about one in every thousand persons develops a rapid and feeble pulse, nausea and a feeling of suffocation. With stimulation and, if necessary, artificial respiration, recovery soon ensues. Those who frequently suffer from attacks of asthma are liable to an attack after an antitoxin injection. There have also been recorded a few deaths. These have occurred chiefly and perhaps wholly in cases of status lymphaticus. About one death has occurred for every 70,000 persons injected, and these deaths, with possibly two exceptions, have followed the first serum injection. The fear of repeating a serum injection because of having sensitized the patient is almost wholly groundless. There need be no fear in giving a second intramuscular or subcutaneous injection to any person who has not suffered severely from the first. The only difference in the effects of the two injections will be that the serum reaction will follow almost immediately the second injection."

An intravenous injection may be followed by a chill and an accompanying rise of temperature lasting about two hours. Osgood has shown that the liability to chill is slightly greater when the antitoxin has been diluted with saline solution before injecting. If a second injection is given intravenously after a considerable lapse of time, it should be given even more slowly than the first.

Patients who have a history of asthma and are suspected of being hypersensitive to horse serum, or who have had antitoxin some time previously, should be given a preliminary intradermal test: One fortieth of 1 cc. of the antitoxin diluted 1: 100 with sterile salt solution is injected intradermally on the flexor surface of the forearm. Individuals who are unusually susceptible to horse serum will show within five to ten minutes, at the site of the test, a large urticarial wheal surrounded by a distinct areola. In these cases intravenous or intramuscular injections should be avoided and the antitoxin be given subcutaneously in doses of 0.1 cc. every twenty minutes until the total amount has been administered.

All of these reactions are becoming less frequent because in the refined and concentrated antitoxins now obtainable the causative globulins have been largely removed by precipitation. One cc. of epinephrine hydrochloride, 1: 1000 solution, is useful in combating the alarming symptoms.

Cardiac Complications.—It is doubtless true that heart failure is today the most common cause of death in diphtheria, though I believe the question is not entirely settled whether the circulatory failure is primarily of cardiac or vascular origin. This fact, however, is incontrovertible: *practically all* *these cardiac deaths occur in cases where antitoxin has been withheld too long or given in too feeble dose.* The usual circulatory stimulants are of little avail here. Because of the degenerative changes in the heart muscle digitalis is looked upon as more or less contraindicated; in attempting to determine the position of the drug in animal experimentation, Edmunds and Cooper and Myers have found it to be protective in dogs poisoned by diphtheria toxin, but Gold *et al.* found it of no value in cats.

It is the part of wisdom to continue heart vigilance for several weeks following diphtheria and, even though the patient has to all appearances grown strong, to insist that he return gradually to full physical activity.

Local Treatment.—The nose and throat are nowadays left very much alone, though a gargle or spray of saline or Dobell's solution is sometimes employed. Wesselhoeft says that hot glucose irrigation of the throat every three hours greatly reduces the foul odor in a diphtheria ward; if done very gently it is apparently very soothing.

The Period of Quarantine.—The patient should be kept isolated until two successive nose and throat cultures prove negative. Attempts to lessen the length of this period are usually made by the employment of Dobell's solution and other mild antiseptics. If the cultures continue positive for several weeks, guinea-pig inoculations should be made to determine the virulence of the organisms. If they are nonvirulent, quarantine can be raised. A few years ago it was reported that the use of lactic acid organisms in the spray, or naturally soured milk as a gargle, would shorten the quarantine period. I believe it is now conceded that the lactic acid bacilli only hasten the disappearance of the diphtheritic membrane, but do not produce cultures negative to *Bacillus diphtheriae.*

Paralysis.—In general, the various types of paralyses so commonly associated with diphtheria are estimated to occur in from 10 to 25 per cent of all the cases. That of the swallowing muscles which sometimes occurs in the height of a severe case requires nasal or parenteral feeding. Diaphragmatic paralysis is rare and nearly always fatal. The more usual type of postdiphtheritic paralysis, that of the arms or legs, comes on in from one to six or seven weeks and is usually transient. Recovery may be hastened by massage and the use of strychnine sulphate in tonic doses. As this condition sometimes precedes late cardiac failure the patients should be kept perfectly quiet. Of course antitoxin "big and early" will prevent these paralyses; in those appearing after convalescence is established it is not indicated.

Emergency Relief in Laryngeal Cases.—The dyspnea is caused by one or more of the following: A partially detached membrane which has been drawn down into the lumen of the glottis; obstruction by tenacious mucopurulent secretion; edema of the inflamed subglottic tissues; spasm of the glottis. The measures available for the relief of this very serious condition— removal of membrane with forceps or with an applicator introduced through the laryngoscope; intubation, tracheotomy, aspiration—will not be described here as they are all highly specialized procedures which can only be learned upon the cadaver and in the ward and not from the pages of a book.

PROPHYLAXIS

It is probable that diphtheria will never be conquered by antitoxin alone for two reasons: the frequent delay in making the diagnosis, and the menace of the ever-present carrier. Therefore any successful measures directed toward the prevention of the disease must be recognized as of the highest value. Only the intervention of the World War prevented us from completely realizing a number of years ago that such preventive measures were at hand. In 1913 von Behring announced that he had succeeded in developing antitoxin in a small number of persons by injecting them with neutralized toxin. Though announced as an original discovery by him, this was really only a repetition in the human of the results which had been obtained in laboratory animals by a number of workers during the preceding fifteen years or more. Then came the dark years, and it was only in 1920 that Bieber published his analysis of the inoculated cases showing the method to be practicable. More recently toxoid has been developed, and we now know quite definitely the degree of effectiveness and the best means of employing these measures. Before the age of six months many babies are protected against diphtheria if their mothers are immune, but fully 95 per cent of children are susceptible when they reach the age of one year, as shown by the Schick test. From that time on susceptibility slowly declines, as "natural" immunity is slowly acquired, until at the age of seventeen only about 18 per cent are susceptible. Beyond this age susceptibility does not seem to decrease, for from 10 to 20 per cent of adults show a positive Schick reaction. These figures are true only for individuals living in the more crowded cities; in rural sections the percentage of susceptibility is much higher for both children and adults. Zingher has stated that among nurses coming into training schools from small towns and rural sections, the Schick test is positive in 40 to 80 per cent.

Now for a statement *seriatim* of a few pregnant facts amply attested by observations on several hundred thousand children and adults:

Over 80 per cent of all cases of diphtheria occur in children under the age of ten.

Over 64 per cent of all cases and over 80 per cent of all deaths from diphtheria occur in children under the age of five.

An overwhelming majority of all persons, of whatever age, receiving proper prophylactic treatment become immune.

The implied professional duty is obvious:

Immunize all children from six months to six years of age.

In the very laudable efforts to immunize all susceptible school children, which are being made in many large cities, this most susceptible age-group is being omitted because it has not yet reached the schools. In the hands of the private practitioner largely rests the responsibility of immunizing these preschool youngsters. The task is simplified in that the Schick test may be omitted for the reason that they are practically all susceptible; however, all children should be Schick-tested from three to six months after being immunized, for Blum has recently shown that a variable proportion of infants retain the passive immunity inherited from their mothers as long as nine months—this group will not have been protected by the injections because of the inability to graft an active immunity upon a preexisting passive one.

Tonsillectomy and Immunity.—It is a rather general impression which does not entirely lack statistical confirmation, that diphtheria is relatively rare in children whose tonsils have been removed, but evidence that an increase in immunity, as evidenced by an alteration in the Schick reaction, follows upon the tonsillectomy is not yet convincing: Schick and Topper concluded that the operation increases the production of immunity in residents of a densely overpopulated area, but Wheeler, Doull and Frost failed to confirm the findings under comparable conditions, and Burton and Balmain found no supporting evidence in children living in a residential, nonrural, noncongested area.

Comparison of Toxin-antitoxin and Toxoid ("Anatoxin").[1]—The toxin-antitoxin mixture of von Behring consists in a standardized preparation of

---

[1] Beckman, H.: Review of Toxin-Antitoxin and Toxoid in Diphtheria Immunization, Arch. Pediat., 50, 211, 1933. Brought up to date, the article is included here with the kind permission of the Editor of the journal in which it appeared.

diphtheria toxin neutralized by antitoxin so that the toxic properties are lost but the antigenic properties remain. The toxoid preparation, introduced by Ramon in 1923, is a diphtheria toxin modified by the addition of 3 to 4 per cent of commercial solution of formaldehyde and incubated at from 38 to 40 C. for four to six weeks; like the toxin-antitoxin mixture, this toxoid has lost its toxicity but retains its antigenic properties.

Results.—Toxoid is rapidly replacing toxin-antitoxin in immunization because of its greater efficiency, as indicated in the following table. It will be noted that the results of Park and his co-workers in New York City do not appear among the toxin-antitoxin statistics though they are admittedly somewhat better than those which do find a place in the table; this omission is deliberately made because of the belief that the New York City officials enjoy the use of a mixture which is more potent in its immunizing properties than that available to physicians throughout the country as a whole.

TABLE 5.—COMPARISON OF TOXIN-ANTITOXIN AND TOXOID IN DIPHTHERIA IMMUNIZATION
Toxin-antitoxin.

Observer.	Date.	Number of patients.	Percentage immunity obtained.
Schwartz and Janney............	1925	2,364	85
	1926	11,493	62
	1927	8,874	75
	1928	471	69
Dick and Dick.................	1929	100	82
Harrison.....................	1930	355	64
Schwartz and Janney...........	1930	361	78
Total......................		24,018	73.5 Average

Toxoid.

Zingher......................	1925	100	98
Lereboullet *et al*...............	1926	1,414	95
Bloomberg and Fleming.........	1927	32	94
Frankl *et al*..................	1928	163	100
Weinfeld and Cooperstock......	1929	83	92
Dick and Dick.................	1929	100	94
Harrison.....................	1930	475	95
Schwartz and Janney...........	1930	128	98
	1931	200	99
Greengard....................	1931	117	98
Ray.........................	1931	333	98
Park and Schroder.............	1932	243	94
Total......................		3,388	96.2 Average

Technic and Reactions.—*Toxin-antitoxin:* One cc. of toxin-antitoxin mixture is injected subcutaneously once each week for three weeks. Constitutional and local reactions following the injections are negligible in the infant; slight and infrequent in the young child; moderate or rather severe in perhaps 10 per cent of older children; and slight, moderate or quite severe in a large percentage of adults. In children of school age about 10 per cent develop fairly sore arms and a slight rise in temperature; about half of these feel miserable enough to stay at home from school for one day, a small number for two days. *Toxoid:* In the table above (Table 5), most of the observers had given two injections each of 1 cc. with an interval of three weeks between, but in some instances a third injection had been made with the same dosage and time interval. Most students of the matter believe that the routine administration of this third injection is unnecessary but that if given to those subjects who at the end of six months still show positive reactions to the Schick test it will probably immunize most of this small remaining number; however, it is certainly worthy of note that Ramon, who originated this method of immunization, is still thoroughly convinced that three doses should be given always. Some physicians, while using only a total dose of 2 cc., spread it out over three injections at three-week intervals instead of two at the same intervals; Ray (1931) has very successfully injected a large series of children from three months to fifteen years of age with two 1-cc. doses with only an interval of ten days between. Toxoid contains no horse or other serum but it nevertheless causes reactions similar to but occasionally, in adults, more severe than those caused by toxin-antitoxin; these reactions are probably due to the content of media and bacterial protein and it may also be that an allergic tendency in some individuals plays a part. Ramon's collected data on over 1,000,000 injections show that general reactions are extremely rare in children under eight years of age, and that local reactions of any moment occur very infrequently; that 20 to 40 per cent of persons over that age have slight reactions, 10 to 15 per cent moderate reactions, and 1 to 5 per cent strong reactions. An intracutaneous test dose of 0.1 cc. of the toxoid diluted with salt solution (1 in 20) is sometimes given and the toxoid then withheld from those who show a positive skin reaction; such skin-test solutions are distributed with some of the commercial preparations. Experience has shown that unduly severe reactions in adults may be avoided if the regular doses are preceded by two preliminary doses of 0.1 and 0.25 cc. of the undiluted toxoid at an interval of one week.

Serum Sensitization.—A possible objection to toxin-antitoxin administration is that the approximately 0.001 cc. of horse antitoxin in the immunizing dose might sensitize the child to a later administered dose of any antiserum made from the horse; the studies of Gordon and Creswell lend some support to this apprehension. But Spicer reviewed a series of patients who had received scarlet fever or diphtheria antitoxin and noted no greater incidence of serum reactions in those who had previously received toxin-antitoxin; Bauer and Wilmer reached essentially the same conclusion, and they furthermore noted no ill effects when toxin-antitoxin was administered to asthmatic individuals. However, immunizing mixtures made from goat and sheep serum are now available, and Park, though convinced that the fear of sensitization is largely unwarranted, considers it wise to use these newer preparations.

Toxin-antitoxin as Substitute for Schick Test.—"When toxin-antitoxin is accurately standardized, a full dose, injected just under the skin of the anterior surface of the arm, acts both as an immunizing injection and as a substitute for the Schick test. The result in the older children is not quite so accurate an index of immunity as that from the Schick test, but the error is on the safe side. This slight difference is due to the fact that a dose of suitable toxin-antitoxin is a little more toxic than the Schick test dose, and also to occasional nonspecific protein reactions. We have found that this use of toxin-antitoxin is a very valuable help among the school children of New York City, since without using the Schick test we are enabled to save fully 50 per cent of them from the second and third injections, as they are shown by their negative reactions to be immune. The readings are not made until the fifth or sixth day, to allow, in most cases, for the disappearance of the pseudoreactions, which are more pronounced than with the Schick test. The sixth day is also a suitable time for the second injection in those who require it" (Park and Schroder, 1932).

Deterioration.—Toxoid is quite stable, but toxin-antitoxin should unquestionably be used as fresh as possible; ageing causes the mixture to lose much of its effectiveness though it does not increase its toxicity. Freezing causes the separation and precipitation of some of the antitoxin, thus leaving an appreciable amount of the toxin unneutralized; however, it is doubtful if this ever occurs sufficiently to be in the least dangerous.

Reimmunization.—All individuals should be given a Schick test six months after being immunized, and all those found to be still positive can then be reimmunized by either one of the two methods with reasonable assurance that the second trial will be a success in most instances. Preliminary desensitization should precede the second series of injections.

Duration of Immunity.—It would seem that immunity is retained at least as long as six years in from 75 to 95 per cent of immunized individuals. Children seem to hold on to their immunity somewhat better than adults.

Toxin-sodium Ricinoleate.—Larson and his co-workers have been experimenting for a number of years with the detoxifying properties of sodium ricinoleate in the attempt to eliminate the danger of sensitization to foreign substances, since the sodium ricinoleate is not antigenic. This combination, however, has no advantages over toxoid and is being used scarcely at all at present.

Percutaneous Method (Löwenstein).—Löwenstein, in Vienna, believes that in order to secure absolute immunity against diphtheria, antibacillary as well as antitoxic action must be obtained; he has therefore advocated the use of an ointment which contains both toxoid and an unfiltered culture of dead diphtheria bacilli. On the Continent, a controversy of considerable proportions has arisen regarding the rationale of the new departure, but Besredka, in Paris, has stated his belief in the possibility of a genuine vaccination being accomplished in this manner. It will be very interesting to watch for a possible perfection of the method—whether or not the alleged antibacillary action is ultimately shown to occur—for if effective amounts of toxoid can be gotten into the blood stream in this manner, the use of the ointment will certainly become the method of choice. So far, the small number of reports indicate an immunizing efficiency of about 70 per cent. The ointment is rubbed into the larger absorbing surfaces of the body three to five times at intervals of a week. The preparation is not yet commercially available in this country; Abt and Feingold (1931) have reported results obtained with ointment sent to them by Löwenstein, and Park and Schroder's supply (1932) was made by them in their own laboratory.

Toxoid Plus Alum.—The studies of Park and his associates in this country and Saunders in Ireland indicate that the addition of 0.1 to 0.2 per cent of alum to toxoid greatly increases its effectiveness, 2 doses of 1 cc. being given with a one-week interval. Further large-scale studies will be awaited with interest. Graham, Murphree and Gill (1933) have also reported favorably upon the use of a toxoid completely precipitated by larger amounts of alum, the washed precipitate being then made up in such volume that one injection of 5 to 10 units seemed to confer satisfactory protection.

Prophylaxis with Antitoxin in Nonimmune Exposed Cases.—After the toxin-antitoxin injections immunity develops rather slowly; many of the children do not react negatively to the Schick test until six to twelve weeks have elapsed. In a few the interval is much longer. Formerly, it was the routine practice to give an immunizing dose of antitoxin to children who had been exposed to diphtheria and who had not been immunized. Nowadays, it is more customary to wait awhile, watching the child carefully for the early signs of the disease and then giving a suitable therapeutic dose of antitoxin should they appear. This change of policy has followed the repeated observation that even a small dose of the serum may cause an alarming reaction or render the patient sensitive to a therapeutic dose subsequently administered. Of course if the child cannot be watched, it should be given 1000 units of ordinary treatment antitoxin as soon as possible; this establishes an immediate passive immunity which lasts for about three weeks.

THE CARRIER

In a variable proportion of cases the organisms persist in the nose and throat through convalescence and even for a long time after the patient has become clinically well. Treatment of these carriers is very difficult, for the application of strong caustic antiseptics only seems to improve the culture medium for the bacilli and lengthen the period during which the patient remains positive. All of the milder antiseptics have their advocates, such as diluted Dobell's solution as spray or gargle and 10 to 25 per cent argyrol as a swab, or simply hot irrigations with normal saline. In 1921, Gray and Meyer reported on the systematic use of mercurochrome in 90 carriers. They used 1 per cent solution as a routine application by means of a medicine dropper, spray or swab, and 2 per cent in the more resistant cases. When patients complained of the application of the drug by the nasal swab, they used the medicine dropper and had them hold their head back for a minute or two after the application until the drug passed back into the nasopharynx. They relied on the medicine dropper in the nasal tract almost entirely and on the swab for the tonsils. In patients with nasal obstructions the nasal spray was utilized in endeavoring to place the germicide in contact with the organisms. The treatment was given twice daily. Eighty-eight of the 90 cases were rendered negative in an average of 12.7 days. The minimum standard set before a patient was considered carrier-free was three consecutive negative cultures taken at forty-eight-hour intervals, the third culture being secured at least twenty-four hours after the last local treatment. Gentian violet has also been employed very successfully by Saurman in a small number of cases. He directs that the patient, on awakening and immediately after the three meals and once during the evening, should have the nares and fauces well cleansed with saline solution, either by douche or spray, and that immediately thereafter the nares and fauces should be sprayed with a 2 per cent aqueous solution of gentian violet from an ordinary atomizer. Inspection should verify that the dye has reached every part that can be seen. The parents should be assured that the stain on skin, mucous membrane and teeth is not permanent. Godfrey, of the New York Department of Health, has recently pointed out that gentian violet makes it possible to obtain negative cultures for several days after its use, but that if cultures are taken a week or more after discontinuing treatment they are liable to be positive again. I think this is a very unfortunate criticism since it tends to discountenance a very promising method before it has had a fair trial. After obtaining three consecutive negatives by any other method, are we in the habit of reexamining routinely in a week or so? And if we did, how many who were permanently noncarriers should we ever find?

In 1916, the publications of Hektoen and of Rappaport drew attention to the use of kaolin for the removal of bacteria from the nose and throat by adsorption. One hundred patients thus treated were discharged an average of 7.84 days sooner than the control hundred who were not treated— a shortening of their time in hospital by 23.4 per cent. They describe their method as follows:

"As crude kaolin, which is moist and lumpy, has not the adsorptive power of the thoroughly dried and finely powdered product, the crude material is first thoroughly dried for several days in a bacteriological incubator. The lumps are then broken up and the powder passed through a fine flour sieve. This stock is kept in the incubator, and each morning the small amount necessary for the day's treatment is taken to the patient's room. On damp days it is necessary, for best results, to take kaolin from the incubator oftener—two or three times during the day. The point of this is that kaolin must be perfectly dry and finely powdered when applied, else the results will be disappointing.

"Whenever possible, the application of kaolin should be started as soon as the acute symptoms have subsided. The kaolin must be distributed thoroughly over the surface to be treated. When the mucous membranes are normal, this is attained more easily than when there is some pathologic condition present, such as enlarged tonsils, adenoids, or nasal disease and obstruction; here the thorough application of kaolin to the involved surface is difficult and often impossible. In small children—of less than three years of age—kaolin is best applied directly to the nasal mucous membrane, even when the bacilli are in the pharynx, as the powder works its way through the nasopharynx into the throat. The powder is blown into the nose by means of a rubber bulb attached to a glass tube with a tapering end that fits the nostril. Six treatments at two-hour intervals during the day is the practice, as a rule. To a large extent the powder remains in the nose, holding the organisms it has already taken up and preventing the kaolin of the next treatment from reaching the mucous surface; hence it is necessary at each treatment to remove the old kaolin before more is introduced. For this purpose a mild alkaline spray does very well, such as solution of sodium bicarbonate and sodium biborate, 2 per cent each.

"In the case of older persons, the powder is best applied to the pharynx by having the patient swallow it. Four half-teaspoonful doses at two-hour intervals, six times during the day, are given as a rule. The kaolin remains in the mouth and pharynx for some minutes, a sufficient time for it to take up the organisms with which it comes in contact. . . .

"Before dismissal of any patients as free from bacilli, the cultures from nose and throat must be negative for at least three consecutive days after the discontinuation of the kaolin treatment, which is continued for from two to five days after the first diphtheria-free culture. . . .

"In 20 per cent of the patients receiving nasal insufflations of kaolin, the nasal cultures became sterile, usually in from three to five days. Although in the pharynx, the tonsillar crypts, pillars, and other folds and irregularities afford excellent hiding places for the bacteria, rendering their removal more difficult, the larger number of this series became free of diphtheria bacilli, in from two to four weeks of treatment with kaolin. . . . "

In the throat carriers, tonsillectomy is said to be effective. Meader states that the condition was cured by the removal of the tonsils in about 80 per cent of his series; Dudley's recent findings are to the effect that the carrier rate is 20 per cent in "normals" and only 10 per cent in tonsillectomized individuals. In about the same proportion of cases x-ray would seem to be curative, according to Withers, Ranson and Humphrys.

The prevalent enlightened opinion is that carriers of virulent diphtheria bacilli are potential spreaders of the disease. That this belief is warranted is occasionally shown in outbreaks which can be definitely traced to such a carrier; as witness the epidemic in Austin, Texas, a few years ago, which Graham and Golaz found to be due to the milk distributed by a certain dairy and to one particular employee of that dairy. But actually how often are these carriers of the virulent organism responsible for outbreaks of the disease? Park writes, from his large experience in New York City, "By following up certain rather large groups of these carriers, I have come to the definite conclusion that although organisms from them are virulent in guinea-pigs, they are not what one might call 'catching'; they do not produce diphtheria, but they immunize the persons in whose throat they exist. For this reason I believe that carriers who have not recently received the bacilli from active cases are beneficial rather than harmful." Let us look at a few of the studies. An examination made by Doull and Fales of combined nose and throat cultures from 7790 children, selected at random from schools situated in the northeastern section of Baltimore during the period November, 1921, to June, 1922, resulted in the demonstration of 1.75 per cent carriers of virulent diphtheria organisms. There was no significant difference in the incidence of carriers among children with a previous history of diphtheria and those with no such history. The further work of Doull and Lara with this material fails to show any significant distinction between the risk of attack for those exposed respectively to carriers classified as "virulent," "avirulent," and "not tested." In Lewis' record for New Haven, Connecticut, there is evidence that virulent carriership does not depend upon having had in person, or having had contact with, an active case; it may be acquired from contact with an avirulent carrier. Meader's record for two years in Detroit shows 129 virulent carriers returning to 76 schools, in contact with about 1924 persons, with no case of diphtheria developing. He says: "Therefore we feel quite justified in assuming that diphtheria carriers who have not been exposed to a known case of diphtheria may be ignored from a public health point of view." McGuire and Hitchens report that cultures were made from the throats of 1080 students at one of the Citizens Military Training Camps, and that in 0.83 per cent of the cultures virulent diphtheria bacilli were found, indication that nearly 1 per cent of the young men coming to the camp were virulent carriers of this organism. The Schick test for susceptibility was made on 833 of the students, with the result that 55 per cent of them reacted positively, indicating the absence of immunity. In spite of this high rate of susceptibility and the number of persons in close association with them carrying diphtheria bacilli in their throats, no clinical diphtheria developed during the training period. And abroad? Haidvogl and Wiltschke have reported that in Graz, Steiermark, about 20 per cent of the healthy infants and young children and 10 per cent of the older children are carriers, and that 66 per cent of adults exposed to infection become carriers; while in Denmark, Christiansen is reiterating that negative findings as to diphtheria bacilli in the nose and pharynx are not dependable, for many convalescents leave the hospital still harboring the organisms notwithstanding several negative cultures, and that the number of virulent carriers is even greater among those who have not had the disease.

I take the liberty of reaffirming that toxin-antitoxin and toxoid *immunize* and antitoxin *cures*.

DYSENTERY

Nearly all of the notable writers since that able Byzantine compiler, Alexander of Tralles (525–605 A. D.), have left accounts of dysentery. During the Thirty Year War in the seventeenth century it ravaged the Continent and England, where the great Sydenham among others described it. The disease continued widely prevalent throughout the eighteenth century in Europe, and, following Clive's victorious campaigns in India, the varieties encountered by British medical officers there began to be described. Shiga discovered the bacillus which bears his name in 1897, Kruse in 1900, Flexner

4

in 1900; the bacilli of Strong and Musgrave, and the Y-bacillus of Hiss and Russell, in 1900–1903. Lambl probably saw the causative ameba of the protozoan type of the disease in 1860 when he discovered *Giardia intestinalis*, but the definite differentiation between epidemic bacillary dysentery and endemic amebic dysentery was made by Koch (1883) and Kartulis (1886–91) in Egypt.

AMEBIC TYPE

Amebic dysentery is an infectious disease caused by *Entameba histolytica*. The other allied parasites, *E. coli* and *E. nana*, are rarely if ever, pathogenic. *E. histolytica* causes more or less extensive areas of ulceration throughout the large bowel, and entering the blood stream is sometimes carried to the liver or brain, in either of which sites it may cause serious abscess. By extension, lung involvement sometimes occurs; indeed, pulmonary amebiasis apparently without a "primary" liver abscess is not unknown, but the contention that the amebae may spread all over the body and infect most organs still lacks parasitological proof. The disease is propagated in the human by ingestion of the encysted form of the organism which has been passed from the bowel of an actively infected individual. It usually begins gradually with intermittent attacks of· bloody, mucoid diarrhea, without nausea or loss of appetite, and with only moderate tenesmus and abdominal pain. In improperly treated cases, or in those which do not respond to treatment, the diarrhea finally becomes chronic, secondary bacterial invasion of the bowel occurs, the patient becomes anemic and emaciated, and in a few years is exhausted out of life. Granulomas of the lower bowel, resembling carcinoma in many respects, have been reported a number of times. A complement-deviation test, useful in diagnosis, is in the process of development.

Since amebic dysentery is well known to be endemic in India, Egypt, West Africa, the Philippines and other tropical and subtropical countries, it has commonly been supposed that it occurs only in these regions. However, Kaplan, Williamson and Geiger reported 38 cases from the Cook County Hospital in Chicago during the year 1926, and the reports of Brown and others show that many patients are treated at the Mayo Clinic who have never been far away from their homes in the northern states and Canadian provinces. In the autumn of 1933 the disease was admitted to be epidemic in Chicago; doubtless, because of the World's Fair, amebae have been widely disseminated throughout the land and henceforth amebic dysentery should be suspected in every case of severe or intermittent diarrhea wherever seen.

THERAPY

Among the many remedies which have been used in the treatment of this serious disease, ipecac and its derivatives, the arsenicals, yatren, and chaparro amargosa, have shown themselves to be the most effective. I shall describe below some of the more successful methods of using these and a few other drugs, but the reader should bear in mind that students of the disease look upon its treatment as being still far from perfect.

Ipecac.—The use of sufficient powdered ipecac for effective amebicidal action is precluded because of the violent vomiting which is caused. Salol-coated pills have not been uniformly satisfactory. The drug is at present used principally in two forms: emetine hydrochloride and emetine bismuth iodide, both prepared from its active principle, emetine. The routine formerly most frequently followed was to give an injection of emetine hydrochloride twice daily (at each dose, $\frac{1}{2}$ grain for the adult, $\frac{1}{6}$ grain for children of eight, and $\frac{1}{12}$ grain for younger children), and at the same time 1 grain of emetine bismuth iodide in gelatin capsule or salol-coated tablet after each meal. It was hoped that the hypodermically administered emetine would reach the deeply embedded amebae, while the orally administered salt destroyed those that were free in the lumen of the colon. The treatment was used for about ten days and after the lapse of a week cautiously repeated. Subcutaneous injection of the hydrochloride is sometimes followed by pain, discoloration of the skin and even slough; deep injection into the gluteal region is to be preferred. Emetine bismuth iodide often causes nausea and vomiting and has to be omitted. Nowadays, since the reporting of quite a number of cases of severe poisoning, the above dosage is no longer considered safe for routine use. Emetine bismuth iodide is omitted and the hydrochloride is employed about as follows: one injection daily (1 grain for the adult, ⅓ grain for children of eight, ⅙ grain for younger children) for six days, and then one injection of just one half these doses daily for the next six days. The adult will then have received 9 grains, which is close to what is considered to be the safe amount to be administered in one course—10 grains. During the rest period of ten days or more, other drugs may be given; then the injections may be repeated, or the emetine bismuth iodide (which contains 20 per cent emetine) may be given in 1-grain dose three times daily for ten days.

Willmore and Martindale give auremetine, a combination of emetine and auramine periodides devised by them in 1926, in 1-grain gelatin capsules four times daily after food on alternate days for seven days, and then one dose daily until a total of 40 to 60 grains (2.5 to 4 Gm.) has been given. This drug is said to be much less depressing than emetine.

There are few diseases which respond so quickly to any therapy as does amebic dysentery to emetine, both physician and patient being usually much cheered by the rapid subsidence of symptoms following the first few doses— then come the relapses. It is a fortunate patient indeed who gets an early and complete cure by the use of this drug alone, for its effectiveness is limited not only by the poisonous nature of its action if too long continued but also by the fact that the ameba undoubtedly becomes emetine-fast much as the Spirochaeta pallida becomes arsenic-fast.

The intravenous use of emetine hydrochloride is commonly referred to as too dangerous for routine practice. However, the work of Deuskar in India would seem to cast doubt upon the correctness of this position. He has given altogether over 1000 intravenous injections in 70 cases. Nine injections, each of 1 grain (0.06 Gm.), are given on nine consecutive days, followed by an interval usually of six days, after which another series of six injections is given. Thus at the end of the course each patient has received a total of 15 grains (1 Gm.). Deuskar describes the method as very effective, simple, painless, and safe.

The use of a retention enema of ipecac has been advocated off and on through the years. It was probably first described by Cecikas in Greece. The technic successfully used by Lawson in the United States is described as follows: "Our method of procedure is to put 60 or even 120 grains of powdered ipecac into about 24 ounces of water; this is kept hot for an hour, but not allowed to boil. After washing out the bowel with warm water, this whole preparation, without filtering, is given slowly by rectum to be retained as long as possible. If there is much pain and tenesmus, only part of this can be given. In a few of our cases there was some discomfort and the treatment had to be slowed down."

The partial failure of all emetine methods to satisfactorily cure amebic colitis is probably partially explained by the fact that the active harmful parasites are located at the base and undermined edges of ulcers which are plugged up with a thick, tenacious substance consisting of mucus, blood, degenerated mucosa, and dead and dying amebae and their secretions.

Ordinary enemas do not clean out these plugs, but active saline catharsis does remove much of the débris, as can be observed through the sigmoidoscope. The ideal treatment would seem to consist, therefore, in thoroughly cleaning out the ulcer craters by means of saline catharsis, and then the rapid diffusion of the destructive agent through the whole bowel so that every ulcer will be treated. Not long ago Andresen described the transduodenal method employed by him for the past seven years. I reprint his technic and comments here in the belief that the method, with proper controls, should be given a thorough trial on a large scale.

"(1) The patient is put on a nutritious lacto-farinaceous diet, with frequent feedings, such as would be used in a case of peptic ulcer, for two or three days preceding the treatment and throughout its course. (2) In the morning after a twelve-hour fast, a regulation duodenal tube is passed well in the patient's duodenum, its location being determined by the usual methods, preferably by x-ray. The tube may have to be passed the night before where much pylorospasm exists. (3) The pylorus is encouraged to close by giving the patient 4 or 5 ounces of cold milk to drink alongside the tube. (4) A Jutte transduodenal lavage is performed—500 cc. of a 10 per cent aqueous solution of sodium and magnesium sulphates, at a temperature of 105 F., is allowed to run slowly through the tube into the duodenum. This usually produces a copious, watery evacuation in from twenty to thirty minutes, and can be shown to clean out the ulcer bases very satisfactorily. (5) Twenty minutes after administration of the hypertonic salt solution, there is poured down the tube a suspension of 1 drachm of powdered ipecac in about 50 cc. of plain warm water, and this is followed by 50 cc. more of water to wash out the tube. The tube is best left in situ for an hour, as in its removal a little ipecac might be carried into the stomach and occasion very persistent vomiting. (6) One and one-half to two hours after the administering of the ipecac, the patient resumes his feedings, which are pushed even though no appetite is present. (7) These treatments are repeated daily for seven days, and are followed by an interval of seven days, and then another seven days' course of treatment.

"Our results have been most encouraging. Within forty-eight hours a weak, toxic patient, with twenty to thirty bloody, painful evacuations in twenty-four hours, begins to look brighter, puts on weight and may have no bowel movements except the large liquid stool following the transduodenal enema. During the second week, when no treatments are given, the patient is usually constipated, requiring soothing laxatives. The ulcers heal with remarkable rapidity, being hardly noticeable within a few days after treatment has been instituted. The stools have consistently failed to show either active or encysted amebae, even after the first week of treatment. Owing to the type of patients treated by us, mostly seamen of foreign ships, leaving our port as soon as they get well enough, we have not been able to follow our cases as they should be followed."

Emetine Poisoning.—The drug is undoubtedly a general protoplasmic poison, the chief depressing effect being upon the heart and vessels; the cause of death in most instances is heart failure, which is unaffected by digitalis or any of the other stimulants. Individuals seem to vary in their susceptibility—which unfortunately cannot be determined before treatment is begun—and death can apparently occur quite suddenly without warning symptoms. So far, studies of the minimum lethal dosage in animals have not been shown to be directly applicable to the human, but the dictum of Vedder (1914) that 10 grains (0.65 Gm.) should not be exceeded in one course in an adult has been amply confirmed by the experience of recent years.

Young and Tudhope have shown that emetine "neuritis" is in fact a myositis. Emetine diarrhea, which is not easily distinguishable from that which characterizes the disease in which the drug is being used, has been observed. Cumulative effects wear away after discontinuance of the drug, but patients should be returned to the ambulatory state only slowly to guard against cardiac disasters. Pregnancy, as well as cardiovascular disease, is considered to contraindicate the drug; in infants it is not usually used.

Arsenicals.—(a) *Stovarsol (Acetarsone, N.N.R., Spirocide).*—Of late years the arsenicals suitable for intravenous use have had an increasing vogue, being used in conjunction with some scheme of emetine therapy, or alone as in the treatment of syphilis. More promising than these intravenous drugs, however, is stovarsol, for it can be given by the mouth. Following the original publication of Marchoux of the Pasteur Institute, in 1923, a number of authors have reported enthusiastically on the use of the drug. Johns and Jamison describe the results in a series of 46 cases in New Orleans. These cases ranged from the acute fulminating down to the very chronic variety, and in all of them there was complete relief from dysenteric symptoms in three to six days following the introduction of the drug. Of these cases they selected a group who had received fairly uniform doses of stovarsol for an extended period of observation in order to arrive at some definite information regarding ultimate cures. Of this series of 27 patients, 4 were apparently cured by the administration of 0.75 Gm. (about 12 grains) of stovarsol daily for seven days; 16 with the administration of two such courses of treatment, with a seven-day rest interval between courses; 1 with three courses; 4 with four courses; and 1 with seven courses. One patient received eight courses, but relapsed within a few days following the completion of each course. Twenty-one of these patients had remained well and free of parasites for an average period of 3.8 months at the time of their writing; 5 had relapsed after remaining well for an average of 3.9 months. A little emetine was used in a few of the cases, but probably not enough to influence the findings. In his latest communication, Marchoux records the cure of 59 cases with only two failures, and recommends the continuous use of the drug over a period of four weeks. However, many physicians are now preferring to combine stovarsol with emetine hydrochloride, giving full doses of each drug on alternate days for two weeks.

(b) *Treparsol.*—This drug has been little used as yet. Brown and Osterberg (1931) recommend 4 grains (0.25 Gm.) two or three times daily, not to exceed a total of 48 grains (3 Gm.).

(c) *Carbasone.*—Reed and his associates (1932) in California have been carefully investigating this drug, which has not been very generally employed as yet. They describe satisfactory results with a dosage of 4 grains (0.25 Gm.) twice daily for ten days, given in gelatin capsules by mouth.

(d) *Reactions.*—There have been some reports of various dermatoses and even exfoliative dermatitis following the administration of stovarsol and treparsol, as would be expected when using such powerful organic arsenicals. Carbasone, as pointed out by Leake, contains a modified amino group in the para position to the arsenic and hence may be found on more extensive use to be injurious to the optic tract.

Chaparro Amargosa.—The merits of this substance as an amebicide were well established by J. W. Nixon in 1893, but it was neglected until P. I. Nixon again called attention to the drug in 1914. The latter Nixon reported 10 cases in which it had been most effectively used in the form of an infusion made by boiling the whole plant—roots, branches, foliage and fruit—in water for from thirty to sixty minutes. Six to 8 ounces of this infusion, which should have the color of weak tea, are given by mouth before meals and at bedtime; in addition 500 to 2000 cc. are introduced into the rectum twice daily, the patient being instructed to retain the solution as long as possible. The virtues of this "bitter bush" are known to the natives of many tropical regions; I am informed that the active principle has been isolated in a Mexican laboratory and is now available under the name of "Castamargina."

Oil of Chenopodium.—Two cc. of this drug are given together with 1½ ounces of castor oil at a single dose. Or the oil of chenopodium may be emulsified with acacia and administered by rectum. In such cases the anal mucosa must be protected with petrolatum, and it is well to terminate the injection with 2 ounces of inert oil. The buttocks should be elevated, the enema given slowly and with great care, the first dose not exceeding 8 ounces in the adult. This enema should be retained for an hour if possible. If the parts are well protected with petrolatum, the patient does not suffer from the intense burning sensations which would otherwise accompany the expulsion of the enema.

Barnes and Cort have reported a series of cases from Siam in which the results were equally as good as those obtained by the use of emetine. It would seem to be especially advantageous to use in ambulatory cases for the reason that it is not depressing to the circulation. Also the whole dose is taken at one time; indeed, in working among native populations, the two oils already combined can be sent to distant patients who could not otherwise be reached by treatment. A point to be remembered is that oil of chenopodium should not be repeated in full dose under two or three weeks because of the possibility of renal irritation.

Quinine.—This drug has been used for a long time for rectal irrigations with more or less success. One or 2 liters of 1: 1000 to 1: 2500 aqueous solution of the sulphate are employed. Quite severe cinchonism not infrequently follows its use by this route. *In vitro*, quinine kills amebae in dilution of 1: 20,000, whereas emetine kills in dilution of 1: 100,000. However, Brooke has well pointed out that this advantage of emetine is more apparent than real for the reason that quinine can be given in from five to ten times as large dose as emetine. He has employed quinine sulphate quite satisfactorily by mouth, giving 20 to 30 grains daily for six days and repeating after an interval of a week. Quinine is always available, and is certainly much cheaper than the emetine preparations.

Salicylic Acid.—This drug is used in the form of a 2 per cent solution of sodium salicylate by rectal enema. The dose for an adult is 3¼ drachms (13 Gm.) sodium salicylate in 650 cc. of water. Lutsch, in Africa, extols the method for the prompt relief of pain and tenesmus. He gives 5 grains (0.3) of calomel and allows nothing but barley water the first day and later a little boiled milk. Six hours or more afterward he gives the salicylate enema and repeats it the second and fourth or third and fifth days. The enema should be of body temperature and retained for half an hour. For a child a year old he uses only 90 cc. of the solution.

Yatren-105 and Anayodin (Chiniofon, N.N.R.).—These two drugs which are apparently identical, iodine compounds (sodium iodohydroxyquinolinesulphonate), have been quite extensively employed in the tropics in recent years, and apparently with considerable success. Thonnard-Neumann and Valera (1930) have reported a careful study of their use *per orum*, 30 patients receiving yatren and 25 anayodin. Both drugs were used in the form of coated pills of 4 grains (0.25 Gm.); they found that the anayodin pills deteriorated more rapidly in storage under tropical conditions than the yatren. I quote their method:

"After a presumptive clinical diagnosis of amebiasis or chronic amebic dysentery has been made, a saline cathartic is given at bedtime, which serves simultaneously as a provocative for the stool examination which follows the next morning. When the diagnosis is established, one or two pills three times daily, depending on the condition of the patient, are given. This dose is increased the following day to two or three pills three times daily; and this dosage is continued for five days. Then a second stool examination is performed and, if no amebae are found, a second treatment of two pills three times daily is carried out for a period of five more days preceded by an interval of three days' rest. If the second stool examination still shows amebae, three pills three times daily are given over the same period. With very few exceptions one need not exceed the daily dose of nine pills. If the general condition of the patient permits, he can follow this treatment without interruption of work. No severe restriction in diet, other than eggs, is necessary during the treatment of chronic cases. Both yatren and anayodin produced, in the majority of our cases, frequent soft or liquid evacuations of a greenish color; which, in some instances, were accompanied by colicky pains. Such complaints were more pronounced among the patients with acute symptoms. As a rule, small doses (1 to 2 drachms) of paregoric produced sufficient amelioration of symptoms to warrant continuance of the treatment without interruption. No toxic symptoms were seen even after prolonged use of the drugs."

Most workers are now giving the yatren by rectum and emetine bismuth iodide at the same time by mouth. Willoughby and Aslett (1931) report the very successful treatment of 150 cases, giving 10 ounces (300 cc.) of a 2½ per cent solution of the yatren preceded by one hour by a 1-pint (500 cc.) enema of 2 per cent solution of sodium bicarbonate; the yatren enema is retained for five to eight hours. Full doses (3 grains daily for the adult) of emetine bismuth iodide are given by mouth during the ten days which one such course of treatment lasts.

Vioform, N.N.R.—David *et al.* (1933) have been studying this drug, which differs only slightly from chiniofon, being iodochlorhydroxyquinoline. They give it in capsules of 4 grains (0.25 Gm.) each, a total dose of ½ ounce (15 Gm.) being given orally in two courses of 12 grains (0.75 Gm.) daily for ten days with a week's rest period between. In their 47 unselected cases, clinical "cure" resulted in 38; no evidences of toxicity from the drug were noted.

Kurchi.—Infusions made from the bark and seeds of the kurchi plant have long been popular antidysenteric remedies in India and Burma. Acton and Chopra have concluded that very superior results can be obtained with the drug; using 4 grains (0.25 Gm.) of kurchi bismuth iodide twice daily by mouth for ten days they cured 12 of 18 cases. However, I believe that most authorities have not so well succeeded with it; Reed (1932), for instance, has given 8 grains (0.5 Gm.) daily for ten days to 5 chronic amebiasis sufferers without relieving symptoms or clearing their stools, even temporarily, of the organisms.

Bismuth Subnitrate.—Deeks introduced this drug in 1914 following his experience in Panama. James (1925), who believes that it in some way indirectly affects the amebae, advocates the combined use of emetine and bismuth, and some of the physicians of the United Fruit Company, in which employ the combination has had its most extensive use, feel that it surpasses all other therapeutic measures. The bismuth subnitrate is given in quite heroic doses: in severe cases, 3 drachms (12 Gm.) in effervescent water every three hours, day and night. Some such prescription as the following might be used:

R. Bismuth subnitrate .... ℥vj   180.0
     Sodium bicarbonate .... ℥j   30.0
    Mix and divide into 30 powder papers (blue).
     Tartaric acid .... ℥j   30.0
    Divide into 30 powder papers (white).
    Label: Stir contents of 2 blue papers in half glass of water; dissolve contents of 2 white papers in separate half glass of water; mix the two and drink while effervescing.

The content of bismuth per powder is 1½ drachms. The amount of tartaric acid is purposely slightly in excess of that needed to cause effervescence with the bicarbonate, the object being to render the suspension pleasantly acid in taste. Citric acid could have been substituted in slightly smaller quantity, but it effloresces (*i. e.*, loses its water of crystallization) in warm atmosphere—not a very serious objection to its use.

In chronic cases, one or two doses of the bismuth are given daily for a month or more after convalescence has been established.

Rivanol.—This is a yellow acridine dye for which considerable claims have been made in recent years. But Biggam and Arafa, in Cairo (1930), have found the recommended concentration for rectal use of 1: 2000 to be very irritating, and lower concentrations were not lethal to the amebae. Given orally, even in doses as high as 1½ grains (0.075 Gm.) thrice daily, it was disturbing neither to the patient nor the parasite. However, they write:

"Marked relief from symptoms was experienced in most cases during the course of treatment, tenesmus, blood, mucus and diarrhea soon disappearing, usually to return shortly after stopping the rivanol. We consider that the antispasmodic and antiseptic action of the drug may with advantage be utilized for the relief of colic and tenesmus, and for assisting in cleansing the bowel of some of the super-added infection in various dysenteric conditions where lower bowel symptoms are a marked feature of the disease."

The Carrier of Endamoeba Histolytica.—The British suffered heavy casualties from amebic dysentery in the Gallipoli campaign. They therefore gave a number of their protozoologists intensive training, and placed in their hands large numbers of sufferers from chronic dysentery who were concentrated in special hospitals. Allan has tabulated some interesting statistics from the reports of Archibald, Hadfield, Logan and Campbell, of the Royal Army Medical Corps. Of 31,000 British troops returned from the Near East, 9.8 per cent were carriers of *E. histolytica*. Of 7000 troops and civilians without any history of bowel trouble, examined in the eastern Mediterranean area, 10.5 per cent were infected; and of 5000 troops examined on the western front, 8.9 per cent were carriers. Among the Americans, Kofoid, Kornhauser and Plato found by subjecting 2300 troops, just returned to New York from France, to one examination that 12.8 per cent were infected. The actual number of these troops who carried the organisms was probably from 24 to 36 per cent, since it is known that one examination will uncover only from one third to one half of the actual number infected, or the number that six examinations will uncover. Craig's (1932) "very conservative" estimate is that there are 1,200,000 people in the United States infected with *E. histolytica*.

The above statistics amply show forth the magnitude of the carrier problem in this disease. Many of these carriers are well individuals who do not know that they are harboring the organism, many more are chronic sufferers from dysentery of long standing, while a few show only vague, atypical symptoms and are only discovered on the sudden development of a liver abscess. In the treatment of these carriers we can only employ the remedies, singly or in combination, that have been described for use in the acute sufferer from the disease. Many observers of considerable experience emphasize the importance of repeated examinations of carriers who have been apparently cured. Dobell found that 90 per cent of relapses in treated carriers occur within three weeks; but they may occur later.

Complications.—Abscess of the lung and of the brain require the usual treatment for these conditions plus the systemic use of emetine. Peritonitis, perforation, or severe bowel hemorrhage requires complete rest or immediate surgery, largely depending on the patient's condition. In regard to abscess of the liver there is now some difference of opinion. It was formerly held that as soon as the diagnosis is made, radical surgical operation must be performed. Now many operators, after establishing surgical drainage, frequently irrigate the cavity with 1: 1000 emetine solution. The general tendency, however, seems to be to substitute aspiration for the larger operation. Recently several students of the disease have stated their belief that the systemic use of emetine alone is capable of curing abscess of the liver and bringing about absorption of the pus, even in the absence of surgical interference. In his third Lettsomian lecture, delivered in 1922, Sir Leonard Rogers stated that he had long thought that emetine alone was capable of curing these abscesses, but added that it is clearly advisable to hasten recovery by removing the sterile pus. "This," says Hodson, "only serves to show how strong is surgical tradition." The latter's studies have shown the literature to be quite rich in cases in which the diagnosis had been undoubted and in which the results of systemic emetine treatment alone have been even more remarkable for their rapidity and completeness than in those treated with aspiration and emetine. He says that the sound surgical maxim that abscesses require to be opened does not apply here for the reason that these so-called "abscesses" have sterile contents, in contradistinction to the ordinary pyogenic abscess. Therefore, since there is no delay in decision as to the success or failure of the emetine-alone treatment, he feels that in all cases surgery should be delayed until the systemic treatment has been given a fair chance. On the other hand, Manson-Bahr and Morris do not believe that the drug alone has ever cured liver abscess. In Chen, von Gorder and Yuan's (1931) careful study of 48 cases, aspiration with administration of emetine proved to be the method of choice; the total mortality of the series was 20.8 per cent, 32 per cent for cases operated upon and 9.9 per cent for the nonoperated. The question is of course still *sub judice*, but one cannot escape the feeling that the emetine therapists begin to crowd the surgeons here; the other drugs have not as yet seriously challenged emetine in the treatment of the complications.

BACILLARY TYPE

Bacillary dysentery is an infectious disease caused by *Bacillus dysenteriae*, of which there are two main species and very many related varieties. The cases range in severity from very mild to fulminating choleraic types. In the average case the onset is sudden with rise in temperature, severe abdominal pain and tenesmus, early appearance of bloody and mucous diarrhea, and the symptoms of toxemia and dehydration. There is diffuse inflammation of the colon and lower part of the ileum, with ultimately necrosis and extensive ulceration. Some of the cases become chronic. Adults between twenty and thirty and infants under two years of age are the most susceptible. The disease is endemic in the tropics, but may become epidemic anywhere during periods of crowding, bad sanitation, and privation. Flies, contaminated food and water, and human carriers are the agents of its dissemination. Bacillary dysentery prevailed on all fronts during the World War, being especially disastrous in Gallipoli in 1915. It would seem that both in the Philippines and in Haiti, where dysentery is a very serious problem, the bacillary type is predominant and often becomes epidemic; indeed, it is now believed by many observers that most tropical dysentery is of the bacillary and not the amebic type. The mortality varies widely with the locality and the particular outbreak, being from 2 to 80 per cent. Death is caused by toxemia, or later in the disease by peritonitis or inanition; heart failure or intercurrent pneumonia is frequently the cause during epidemics. The disease is notorious for the invalidism it causes.

THERAPY

The patient must be kept as quiet as possible since the very frequent stools are terribly wearing even though there were no toxemia. To keep him warm will sometimes tax the ingenuity of nurse and physician. Diet is of great importance. Proteins are especially poorly borne; also, it is advisable to use foods leaving very little coarse residue to pass over the inflamed mucosa of the bowel. Albumen water and thin gruels are usually employed in the beginning; milk is well borne in only exceptional cases. A return to full diet must be made very cautiously in the convalescent, for many relapses are chargeable to dietary indiscretions.

Perhaps it were well to repeat in this place that the mortality varies quite considerably, and that therefore the results obtained by any worker with a given remedy can be adjudged only by considering the success or failure of the remedy in the particular outbreak with which he is concerned. Mild cases, since they almost certainly recover whatever the treatment, cannot be fairly used in evaluating therapy in this disease.

Cathartics.—The attempt is made to lessen absorption of toxins by thoroughly washing out the bowel with cathartics and keeping it washed out. Sodium or magnesium sulphate is given in a dose of 60 grains (2 teaspoonfuls of saturated solution) every hour day and night until a watery stool containing fecal matter is obtained; thereafter it is administered every four hours. The treatment seems to considerably lessen toxemia, though it has its opponents. Graham advises the concomitant introduction of normal saline, since the tendency of the cathartic is to hasten dehydration of the patient. Certainly this seems to be rational therapy. He gives 300 cc. intravenously and 500 cc. subcutaneously for the first few days. Also he has used 5 per cent glucose solution intravenously; this supplies much needed nutriment in addition to the fluid. Perhaps this double use of salts, plus the occasional hypodermic injection of $\frac{1}{100}$ grain (0.6 mg.) atropine sulphate is the most satisfactory way of checking the pain and tenesmus which are often so severe. I believe it is nowadays conceded that calomel only serves to increase the tenesmus.

Castor oil to replace the saline cathartics has won a number of widely scattered advocates lately. Boase, in East Africa, considers it of great value when administered in repeated small doses. De Bellard reports a number of prompt recoveries under castor oil treatment in a region in Venezuela where the mortality was regularly from 40 to 80 per cent. He gives 60 cc. (2 ounces) at once and 4 cc. (1 drachm) every daytime hour the second and third day, repeating if necessary.

Adsorbents.—Kaolin and charcoal are used in the hope of adsorbing some of the toxins, in which capacity it would seem that they are oftentimes quite effective. Kaolin may be used in quantities up to 300 Gm., best given stirred up in a pint of hot tea to be drunk during the course of the day. The charcoal, up to 80 Gm. or more daily, may be added to this or given separately. Animal is preferred to vegetable charcoal as the large particles of the latter may be irritating.

Lactose.—Whitmore considers milk sugar useful in that it probably inhibits the activity of the dysentery bacilli by favoring the growth of acid-producing bacteria. An ounce (32 Gm.) or more may be given during the day if the patient will take it.

Serum.—The polyvalent serum usually employed is obtained by immunizing horses to the Shiga-Kruse bacilli and toxins, and also to the Flexner and other similar strains which do not produce exotoxins. Flexner states that "in cases of ordinary severity, a single subcutaneous dose may be followed by such marked alleviation of the symptoms as not to call for repetition. In other and severer cases the dose may need to be repeated in from twelve to twenty-four hours, and again in forty-eight hours.

"The effects of the injection of the serum tend to appear promptly. They consist first in the amelioration, often within a few hours, of the nervous symptoms and the general prostration. Usually within twenty-four hours the tenesmus and the colic disappear and the stools become markedly reduced in number. Along with this improvement there goes diminution in the blood and mucus content of the discharges, coincident with which there is a return of their feculent character. According to the severity of the attack, the stools return to normal in from two to five days.

"Acute cases of bacillary dysentery are especially subject to the serum treatment, but cases in their second or third week may still be favorably influenced, as may also relapses in the course of convalescence from acute attacks."

The use of large doses of 50 to 150 cc. is now being advocated. The dose should be diluted with an equal volume of normal saline and given intravenously, very slowly of course. The intravenous route is replacing the intramuscular because these large doses are very painful when placed in the buttocks. Smyly describes the technic of detecting and proceeding in the case of an individual highly sensitive to horse serum:

"The patient's sensitiveness to serum should be tested before the *first* dose by an intracutaneous injection of 0.02 cc. of 10 per cent serum. A positive reaction appears within an hour, and consists of a wheal surrounded by a red areola. If this is present, the patient must be desensitized by a series of gradually increasing doses given hypodermically at intervals of half an hour, commencing with 0.025 cc. The quantity is doubled each time until 1 cc. is given. If there is no reaction, 0.1 cc. may be given intravenously and followed at half-hour intervals by an injection of a dose just double that of each preceding injection."

About half of the patients given serum will develop serum sickness from seven to ten days later, usually accompanied by joint involvement. As arthritis is a common complication of this type of dysentery, it is difficult to determine whether serum actually increases its incidence as is maintained by some observers.

In the Shiga types of the disease which prevail in Eastern countries, and sometimes appear in Europe, I think there can be no doubt regarding the efficacy of the serum, for in many outbreaks the mortality is reported to have been reduced as much as 30 to 40 per cent. Lantin (1930) has also concluded, from his considerable experience in the Philippines, that the serum is in general effective there. In America and western Europe these fortunate results are not so often obtained. Indeed, this is to be expected since a large number of strains of the Flexner type of bacilli cause the disease in these countries, and it is hopeless to expect a stock serum to contain antibodies for all of them. For instance in the series of cases in children studied by Josephs and Davison in Baltimore, Birmingham and Boston in 1919 and 1920, serotherapy neither influenced the mortality nor the course of the disease. Also Nolf, in describing the several epidemics which occurred in the Belgian armies during 1917 and 1918, is most emphatic in declaring that the serum was of no use. However, favorable reports have appeared, such as those of Finlayson and of Waller in England, Klesk and Pribaum, respectively, in Germany, and Flexner in the United States. I think Smyly's position is a fair one: in mild cases which are likely to improve in any case, the cost of the serum plus the probability of serum sickness may be weighed in the balance before serum therapy is begun. In severe cases there should be no hesitancy in giving it in large doses, early, and in the vein.

Vaccine.—Nolf, above referred to, has become an enthusiastic advocate of the use of vaccines in treating the Flexner type. Where possible to isolate a dysenteric germ from the intestine, he made and employed an autogenous vaccine; otherwise he used a vaccine made from a bacillus of the Flexner type killed by heat. In the beginning he obtained good results by giving this vaccine subcutaneously, starting at 10,000 and increasing sometimes to as high as 5 to 10 billion organisms. The reaction was moderate usually but sometimes severe. He later used the intravenous route of introduction exclusively. He says of the intravenous dosage and results: "We applied the treatment . . . to all those in whom the course of the disease made one fear the development of the ulcerative form, that is to say, in every case in which, after one week, a dietetic and drug treatment had not brought about a cure, or at least promise of a speedy cure.

"The doses were given at four-day intervals, the initial dose being regularly 10,000 germs, then 30,000, then 50,000, then 100,000, etc. In general the betterment of the patient did not long delay. The fever dropped by lysis, with some recrudescences more or less marked on the day of the vaccine therapy and the next day; and the intestinal symptoms improved coincidently. In many cases of moderate intensity a complete cure was effected when the dose of 500,000 was reached. In the more refractory cases, it was necessary to push the vaccine up to about 10 million.

"In 52 cases treated in this way we had only two deaths. All the other patients left the hospital cured, except two whom military necessity forced us to send away too soon. We have no doubt that in these cases also the continuation of the treatment would have resulted in a cure in a relatively short time. By vaccinotherapy we were thus able to avoid the dangerous tendency toward chronicity which in 1917 [the year before—H. B.] was produced in a number of our patients. This last result we considered particularly gratifying."

Alivisatos attributes the rapid improvement in 111 out of 117 cases to the administration of a polyvalent vaccine by mouth. He used 20 to 30 drops on the first day, 50 drops on the second, and 60 to 70 drops on the third day—all fractioned in two or more doses. Glukhoff, Volkova, Erusalimchik, and Panina, in Russia, used vaccine by the oral route in a severe epidemic among 81 children and adults. Of those treated with vaccine, 7.7 per cent died; serum, 27 per cent; otherwise treated, 17 to 32 per cent. The vaccine, in the form of tablets, was prepared with both Shiga and Flexner bacilli, each tablet containing 100,000 millions of the organisms. The tablets were dissolved in water or sodium chloride solution and taken on an empty stomach. In grave cases five, even six tablets were given in a day. The treatment was continued from two to six days; in a few instances eleven days. Within the first day of the treatment they report that the stools became less frequent and the general condition improved. By the second day the blood in the stools decreased, disappearing entirely by the seventh day in over half of the patients. Experiments on the rabbit, conducted at the same time, indicated local immunity of the intestine following administration of the vaccine.

Bacteriophage.—It must be admitted that most of the evidence regarding the use of this agent in the treatment of bacillary dysentery shows it to be of no value. The study in Australia of Burnet, McKie and Wood (1931) to wit: an infection almost wholly of the Flexner type, treated with highly active, polyvalent, anti-Flexner strains of bacteriophage, including d'Herelle's own *Bact-dysenterie-phage*. Results, in 25 treated cases the mortality was 44 per cent, in 33 untreated controls it was 27 per cent. Taylor's observations in India (Shiga type) were of a similar nature.

Apple Diet.—In Germany there has recently developed, out of an "altes

Volksmittel," the so-called Moro-Heisler apple diet for the treatment of all sorts of diarrheal conditions in infants and young children. Its success has been so great that it will undoubtedly replace most of the other methods of handling these cases; I include a description of it here because it has begun to be used in adults also, among others in a few cases of severe bacillary dysentery. (See the following in the Bibliography: Moro, E.; Wolff, S.; Schreiber; Bogdanovic, P.; Hartwich, A.; Urbanitzky.) The method consists simply in feeding, during two days, ripe mellow apples which have been peeled, freed from seeds and core, and grated. Apparently this is fed *ad libitum* to adults; in children as much as 100 to 300 Gm. per meal, five meals or more per day. Nothing else may be eaten during this time, but water may be drunk and saline or glucose solutions injected if necessary in dehydrated patients. After the two apple days it is considered advisable to return to full diet gradually during two days in which a diet rich in protein and poor in milk and fats is ordered; tea, cocoa made with water instead of milk, zwieback, toast from stale bread with very little butter, bananas, cottage cheese, soups poor in fat but with eggs added, potatoes, lean meats of all sorts. If the diarrhea reappears on this diet, or after return to full feeding, a repetition of the apple diet usually completes the cure.

All observers stress the point that the apples must be mellow; in Germany there has already appeared a commercial preparation of grated apples, "Aplona," which is said to be made from certain sorts of apples which have proved to be the best.

Chronic Cases.—Rest and careful dietary measures are most important in these cases. Appendicostomy and washing out from above used to be much advocated, but since it has been amply shown that the entire colon can be filled from below I do not believe it is any longer a rational treatment. Smyly says that cecostomy, with the opening of an artificial anus to give the colon complete rest for three months, may prove a satisfactory treatment in exceptional cases. Most patients respond to less heroic measures in a shorter time. The silver salts are principally used locally: an enema of 500 cc. of a 1:100 argyrol (mild silver protein) solution, or 1:500 protargol (strong silver protein). Copper sulphate is frequently used in 0.5 per cent strength, or 2 per cent tannic acid solution. These solutions, the silver salts especially, stimulate an acute reaction and a reparative process, but the balance between inflammation and repair is not always easy to strike; they should therefore not be repeated too often. Ten per cent silver nitrate, rarely stronger, may be applied directly to the rectal ulcers.

Nolf also reports favorably upon the use of his intravenous vaccine method in chronic cases.

PROPHYLAXIS

Vaccines have been shown to be protective up to a few months, but are little used because of the dangerous reactions which often follow the parenteral use of vaccines made with Shiga bacilli. A number of attempts to modify them have not been entirely satisfactory. In 1924, however, Gauthier reported the results of his campaign against dysentery among refugees from Asia Minor arriving in Greece, to whom he gave polyvalent vaccines containing 3 billions of germs per cubic centimeter per mouth. As far as he was able to ascertain, *no infection occurred among the 29,800 persons thus vaccinated*. The doses used were 1 cc. for adults, 0.5 cc. for children over two years, and 0.25 cc. under two years, repeated on three successive days. It must be taken at least one hour before a meal. The serum of his patients agglutinated the bacilli from the third day; the maximum agglutination was on the eighth day, it then decreased progressively for two or three months. His findings have been substantiated. Antonovsky vaccinated by the mouth

1000 persons with a morbidity rate of 0.3 per cent, while it remained 3.11 per cent among 1768 not vaccinated. During the sojourn of the Dutch ship *Trump* in French waters, in 1925, there was an epidemic of dysentery aboard in which 50 cases had occurred within six weeks. Costa, Boyer and van Deinse report that after all the 348 men were vaccinated by the mouth only one mild case developed. A daily dose of 1 cc. of the vaccine was given for three days in succession.

In the United States, Wilkins and Wells, profiting by the preliminary report of Lucus and Amoss, have distinctly advanced the position of immunization in this disease by showing that it is perfectly feasible to use prophylactic vaccine subcutaneously provided it is made from the Flexner type of bacilli only. Among the 70 children vaccinated by them there were only mild local reactions, except in 2 cases. These 2 general reactions, which were not very severe, could be attributed to the improper preservation of the vaccine for a time. They prepared the vaccine by isolating bacilli from one of the cases and growing them on agar slants for eighteen hours, after which a suspension of 1 billion bacilli in 1 cc. was made with physiologic sodium chloride solution containing 0.25 per cent phenol. The organisms were killed by heating for one hour at 60 C. Three doses of 250, 500 and 1000 million, respectively, were given subcutaneously at intervals of three days. The dysentery outbreak was quite sharply checked.

The present status of bacteriophage in the prophylaxis of dysentery is about the same as in Asiatic cholera (see p. 22).

FLAGELLATE DYSENTERY

(Giardiasis (Lambliasis), Balantidiosis)

In dysenteries of the bacillary and amebic types in the tropics certain flagellate organisms are frequently also present in the intestinal discharges. It is recognized, however, that these organisms are themselves capable of causing symptoms. Chief among these flagellates are *Cercomonas hominis*, *Trichomonas intestinalis, Lamblia intestinalis* (*Giardia*), and *Balantidium coli*, this last alone being able to actually invade the intestinal wall. The disorder caused by this group of parasites is characterized by the frequent passage of liquid or semisolid stools, of good color though often foul odor, and only rarely containing a little mucus or a tinge of blood. The cases are nearly always chronic with frequent symptomless remissions. Constitutional evidences of infection are not always present, though the patients are often emaciated and weak. Many domestic animals and man are carriers and disseminators of the disease.

In late years it has been several times pointed out that flagellate diarrheas are encountered in other than tropical countries. At least some of the cases of "trench diarrhea" during the late war were caused by these organisms. In Germany, Lickint believes that the organisms are propagated principally in the coal mining sections under the same unhygienic conditions in which hookworm disease is found in northern countries. In Smithies' series of 71 uncomplicated cases, many of the patients have lived all their lives in the northwestern United States.

THERAPY

Emetine and the arsenicals, as used in the treatment of amebiasis (see p. 50), and the anthelmintic drugs, are only partially successful. Smithies claims that the flagellates are readily destroyed by the evening administration of 5 to 15 grains (0.3 to 1 Gm.) of calomel followed by 2 ounces (64 Gm.) of Epsom salt the next day, these doses of calomel to be repeated about every five days, according to the indications furnished by the stool examinations. Enemas of 1 per cent argyrol (mild silver protein), 0.2 per cent protargol (strong silver protein), 2 per cent tannic acid, and 0.1 per cent quinine sulphate are used with indifferent success. Cort, in Siam, has even given enemas of 15 cc. of oil of chenopodium in 150 cc. of olive oil; such medication should not, of course, be repeated under ten days to two weeks. Chase and Tasker report considerable success with the administration, both by mouth and by enema, of Merck's medicinal methylene blue (methylthionin chloride). It is essential that only the medicinally pure drug be used, as that ordinarily employed in the laboratory contains traces of zinc. They give 2 grains (0.12 Gm.) every three hours by mouth and once, or preferably twice, a day an enema of 500 cc. of 1: 500 up to 1: 200 aqueous solution of the drug, this to be retained for fifteen minutes. Chantriat (1932), who believes that lambliasis is in the majority of cases a cholecystitis or duodenitis secondarily complicated by enterocolitis, advocates the frequent administration of dilute hydrochloric acid to neutralize the alkalinity of the duodenal biliary fluid. Petrowych (1931) lavages the duodenum periodically with 25 per cent magnesium sulphate solution. Tsuchiya and Andrews (1930) have been successful with two 4-grain (0.25 Gm.) tablets of stovarsol daily for six days. Sorge (1931) has given 3 grains (0.2 Gm.) of naphthalene, purified by sublimation, three times daily after meals. Whittingham claims that fully 50 per cent of the cases can be cured by employing a judicious combination of purgation, anthelmintics, emetine and colonic lavage.

Certainly all observers are agreed that *Balantidium coli* is the most resistant organism of the lot. Greene and Scully report that they have apparently corrected a number of these cases by making a simple dietary adjustment. Two and one-half quarts (2.5 liters) of whole milk were given during the day, so divided that small portions were taken at regular intervals. After several days the milk was supplemented by the addition of one or two soft eggs. The only drug used was bismuth subnitrate in 15-grain (1 Gm.) doses during the first day or two to relieve the cramps and check the diarrhea. Later, when the bowels became sluggish, stewed fruits were given. There was rapid improvement in the general condition, the stools were cleared of *B. coli*, and the patients were returned to normal diet without any difficulty.

EPHEMERAL FEVER

(Febricula)

Certain fevers of one or at most three days' duration, unaccompanied by any demonstrable causative lesion, and disappearing as rapidly as they appear, have long been denoted "ephemeral" fevers for want of a better name. Sometimes there is nausea, vomiting, colic, and perhaps chills. It has been thought that exposure to sewage gas and foul odors from other sources is responsible for this type of fever, but it is extremely likely that as our diagnostic means and skill improve they will all eventually be recognized as abortive attacks of one of the clearly recognized infectious diseases.

The fevers of unknown origin frequently seen in youngsters following a sudden change of environment probably belong in this category.

THERAPY

Nothing, of course, has been evolved beyond the usual palliative measures designed to ease such slight symptoms as are met with here.

EPIDEMIC PLEURODYNIA
(Devil's Grip)

Epidemic pleurodynia is an acute infectious disease characterized by a sudden onset with excruciating pain at the site of the attachment of the diaphragm to the anterior thoracic wall on either side, or in the epigastrium; marked increase in rate and decrease in amplitude of respirations; several degrees of fever; and rather constant headache, but rarely pain elsewhere. The pain usually leaves within twenty-four hours as suddenly as it came; the fever also subsides, the patient breaks out into a sweat and, being greatly relieved, falls into a refreshing sleep. There is often an attack of lessened severity one or two days later, but a third seizure is rare. Children seem to be more susceptible to the disease than adults.

This entity first appeared in Virginia in 1888 and was described by Dabney. It then apparently disappeared until July, 1923, when Kelly (quoted by Payne and Armstrong) reported its reappearance in the same State. By the end of the summer there were officially reported nearly 1000 cases in Virginia, as well as a number in New York City in persons who had not been out of that city. In the summer of 1924 it was again reported to be epidemic, this time along the New York and New Jersey coasts and in Pennsylvania. At this time Small found in the blood of several patients an organism much resembling the malaria parasite. In the succeeding summer (1925) Churchill, Landis and Glusker reported an epidemic disease of a similar nature along the same seacoast, but this time further north, in Cape Cod, Massachusetts. The latter authors suggest that pleurodynia may be a temperate zone form of dengue, and offer evidence strongly implicating certain woods mosquitoes heretofore looked upon as innocent of disease bearing.

THERAPY

The patient wishes to lie undisturbed, as every movement of the trunk causes an agonizing twinge of pain. In a few cases, hot or cold applications are a sufficient analgesic measure, but usually some drug has to be used in addition. Acetanilid, 3 grains (0.18 Gm.), acetphenetidin (phenacetin), 5 grains (0.3 Gm.), antipyrine (phenazone, B.P.), 5 grains (0.3 Gm.), acetylsalicylic acid (aspirin), 10 grains (0.6 Gm.), have all been effectively used at three- to four-hour intervals. Amidopyrine (pyramidon), 5 grains, would be slower in asserting itself, but the single dose would perhaps suffice for the twenty-four hours. In the severer cases morphine must be resorted to.

Small states that the prompt exhibition of quinine sulphate in doses of 3 to 5 grains (0.18 to 0.3 Gm.) every two hours until 20 to 30 grains (1.2 to 1.8 Gm.) have been given, appears to terminate the disease specifically and to prevent the recurrence of paroxysms. He directs that half this daily dosage should be maintained for a period of one week after the temperature has become normal. I have found no other record of this felicitous use of the drug.

EPIDEMIC SORE THROAT
(Septic Sore Throat, "Glandular Fever")

This is the type of sore throat which appears in the winter and spring in explosive epidemic and is directly traceable to the ingestion of milk, or milk products, which are contaminated with *Streptococcus epidemicus*. The symptoms in the individual are sudden onset of chilliness, malaise, headache and vague body pains, high rise of temperature and swelling of the cervical lymphatic glands. The throat is extremely painful, swollen, congested, and usually shows a diffuse, thin grayish exudate. The most frequent complications (in from 2 to 6 per cent) are glandular suppuration, otitis media, peritonsillar abscess and arthritis. In some cases a scarlatiniform rash appears. The mortality in some epidemics has been as high as 3 per cent. In most cases the symptoms subside in a few days, but the patient remains prostrated for some time longer. A recurrence several days after resuming activity is not uncommon.

THERAPY

Attempts at a specific therapy, by the employment of antistreptococcic serum and vaccines, have only met with failure so far as I know. Dobell's solution (Compound Solution of Sodium Borate, N.F.) diluted one half with water, or Alkaline Aromatic Solution, N.F. (which much resembles the nostrum, "Glycothymoline," so beloved of the lay public—*and* the profession?) is usually very gratefully received by the patient when used as a spray. Cold packs about the throat often give much relief. Otherwise the symptomatic handling of these cases does not differ markedly from that of catarrhal fever, discussed elsewhere in this book.

ERYSIPELAS

Erysipelas is an acute disease characterized by a spreading erythematous skin lesion plus more or less profound constitutional symptoms. It is known to be caused by several definite strains of *Streptococcus hemolyticus*, which is believed to enter a preexisting skin abrasion. Mucous membrane cases are rare. Active adults in the middle decades, persons who have recently undergone a major operation, and women in the puerperium are the most frequent victims; however, individuals of any age and either sex are liable to the disease. Some persons manifest an especial susceptibility (perhaps because of some nasal or other focus of infection) and have many attacks during their lives. In the aged the constitutional symptoms are frequently very slight. The face is more often affected than any other portion of the body.

The onset is sudden with high rise of temperature, malaise, headache, sometimes vomiting, and not infrequently delirium. The skin lesion appears coincidently with the constitutional symptoms. The typical lesion is a red, swollen area with sharply demarcated and elevated border; small, flamelike extensions along the lymphatic channels are usually seen beyond this border. There is often a scattering of small vesicles throughout the affected area. The lesion spreads rapidly, and as it extends the earlier affected portions subside and desquamate. Sometimes localized abscesses form in the border, or the whole region may be undermined with pus. The pain, often quite severe, is of the burning order. The swelling in typical cases is very considerable. The fever usually persists for two or three days and then falls by lysis or crisis, usually several days before the complete subsidence of the skin symptoms. However, one cannot make any definite prediction in regard to the course of the fever, and indeed the whole clinical picture may persist, with relapse after relapse, for several weeks instead of the usual duration of four to eight days.

This disease, though contagious and serious enough, does not tend to become epidemic and has not been given great attention by medical writers through the ages. Hippocrates did not describe it, though Galen, through mistake, accepted his account of anthrax as applying to erysipelas. It is extremely likely that some of the cases of ergotism, which were so numerous

during the Middle Ages, were really this disease. Fehleisen showed the streptococcus to be causative in 1883; Tunnicliff definitely separated the streptococci of scarlet fever and erysipelas in 1920–27.

THERAPY

Local Measures.—The application of cold compresses is usually soothing.
Sometimes the making of the compress with saturated solution of magnesium
sulphate, instead of plain water, affords astounding relief from the burning
pain. The salt probably lessens swelling by reason of its hypertonicity
(it saturates at 50 per cent), and in addition it depresses the sensory nerve
endings. The compress should be covered with oiled silk and renewed
every two hours. Hallay powders his cases with sodium bicarbonate. From
10 to 20 per cent of ichthyol in an ointment in some cases exerts an analgesic
effect. Hydrous wool fat (lanolin) should be used as a base because its ad-
hesiveness permits of long application. Painting the skin beyond the border
of the lesion with tincture of iodine or a strong solution of silver nitrate, is
said sometimes to stop the advance of the process. Recently Eldridge has
reported upon the satisfactory use of mercurochrome. He applied a 5 per
cent aqueous solution to the whole affected area once daily until the eruption
was well on its way toward subsidence. Tendency to spread ceased almost
at once and the duration of the disease, as well as the occurrence of serious
complications, was considerably reduced. His cases were already hospitalized
and could therefore be treated early. Adams has had about the same success
with daily applications of brilliant green.

Collodion.—In 1918, Avata and Woodyatt described the very successful
use of collodion in treating erysipelas at one of the army camps in the United
States. Their technic follows:

"Collodion, U.S.P. (nonflexible), is painted with a cotton swab or brush
to form a stripe half an inch wide and from half an inch to an inch in
advance of the line of induration, in such a way that the diseased area is
completely circumscribed. The collodion stripe is painted over repeatedly
until, when dry, it makes a deeply constricted furrow not broken or imperfect
at any point. On the following days the collodion line is inspected for
breaks, cracks or inadequate constriction at any point; if found, these are
repaired by further coats of collodion. When enough collodion is used to
produce a continuous and sufficiently deep (from $\frac{1}{2}$ to $\frac{3}{4}$ inch) linear constriction of the skin, the erysipelatous induration advances to the collodion,
but not beyond it. The collodion is left in place until the temperature and
swelling have wholly subsided. If there is a break in the collodion line or
if the skin constriction is too shallow the disease may pass through or under
it. Presumably a successful result depends on a complete constriction of the
lymphatics of the skin through which the infection travels. . . . Within the
circumscribed area the inflamed skin swells intensely, at first appearances
more intensely than in noncircumscribed cases; but this is mainly an appearance due to the contrast between the swollen area and the line of depression
caused by the collodion. . . . Patients have not complained more of discomfort or the sensation of tightness, when so treated, than those not
circumscribed."

A total of 104 cases were treated by magnesium sulphate compresses,
and by "general measures, such as are rational in any febrile condition."
Twenty-three of these cases were in addition collodion treated. The comparative results are shown in the table (Table 6).

Ultraviolet Irradiation.—Ude and Platou (1930) report that ultraviolet
irradiation with the quartz mercury vapor lamp produced a clinical arrest of
the disease in 92 per cent of their 79 hospitalized cases. The exposure time
varies with the efficiency of the lamp, but is approximately twice the time

TABLE 6.—COLLODION TREATMENT OF ERYSIPELAS

	Collodion cases.	All others.
Average stay in hospital	15 days	30.4 days
Average febrile period	3.5 days	8.1 days
Average maximum temperature	103 F.	104.5 F.
Incidence of complications	0.0 per cent	15.3 per cent

required to produce a mild erythema on normal skin with the burner at 8 inches from the lesion. Their new burner required four minutes to accomplish this, but it was later necessary to increase the time to ten or twelve minutes. A 1-inch margin around the diseased area is included in the field; the eyeballs should be protected by black paper. One exposure usually sufficed, but the treatments may be repeated at two-day intervals. These results are so excellent that one may perhaps be excused for remaining a bit sceptical until they are confirmed in an equally large series of severe cases.

Local Use of Immune Serum.—Following the method of Rivers and Tillet, who showed that infiltration of the skin with normal or immune serum renders the area thus treated quite refractory to infection with hemolytic streptococci, Musser has reported 14 cases in which he infiltrated the skin around the borders of the erysipelatous process with antistreptococcal serum, much as in local anesthesia. In most of the cases he found that the process would extend to the infiltrated area and then stop. The method did not, however, seem to have much immediate effect on the general toxic symptoms. Bearing in mind Regan's success with the local and systemic employment of serum, coincidently, in anthrax (p. 18), one wonders whether somewhat the same method may not eventually prove to be the most effective way of using serum in the treatment of erysipelas.

Radiotherapy.—Good results have been obtained with both x-rays and ultraviolet rays, the latter especially; daily suberythema doses are used, covering considerable adjacent skin as well as the diseased area.

Systemic Measures.—*Antitoxin.*—In 1926, Birkhaug introduced the use of erysipelas streptococcus antitoxin, made by immunizing horses against the toxins of the organism. He reported astonishing results in 60 cases. Since that time antitoxin has been adopted for routine treatment to the exclusion of all other methods in Bellevue Hospital in New York City, where there is maintained perhaps the largest and most active erysipelas service in the world. Symmers and Lewis have described the results in 131 cases thus treated at the Bellevue, in comparison with 107 cases treated during the corresponding season of the year before the antitoxin method was adopted.

Of 111 cases of facial erysipelas, 85.6 per cent were cured in from three to seven days and 9.9 per cent in from eight to twenty-one days, with a mortality of 4.5 per cent; whereas, in the other series of 92 cases, 33.7 per cent were cured in from two to seven days, 47.8 per cent in from eight to eighteen days, and 12 per cent in from twenty-three to fifty-four days, the mortality being 6.5 per cent.

Of the 20 body cases treated with antitoxin, 60 per cent were cured in from three to seven days, 30 per cent in from eight to sixteen days, with a mortality of 10 per cent; whereas, in the other series of 15 cases, 46.6 per cent were cured in from seven to fifteen days and 13.3 per cent in from twenty-five to fifty-eight days, mortality being 40 per cent.

Thus it will be seen that not only the mortality has been reduced by the use of antitoxin; the length of the patient's stay in hospital has been likewise affected, which is very important. In the Bellevue series the sojourn was reduced in time more than 53 per cent. The incidence of abscesses seems to be about the same, whether antitoxin is used or not. Also the antitoxin confers no lasting immunity, recurrent attacks occurring with the same frequency as in cases treated by other methods.

Antitoxin Technic.—In the beginning they used the intravenous route for the introduction of the serum at Bellevue, but after several accidents they now prefer, and use exclusively, the intramuscular route. Twenty-five cc. is injected at the moment of the patient's admission, repeating usually at intervals of twenty-four hours until the erysipelatous blush disappears, the edema is dissipated and the temperature is normal. Sometimes one injection suffices, but oftener two or three are necessary, occasionally more.

It is of interest to note that when Symmers and Lewis began their study of the method it was planned to inject every other case as admitted, the alternate cases being treated by other methods, for control, by Dr. W. C. Lusk. However, "after a period of critical observation, Dr. Lusk requested that all of the cases be treated by antitoxin—this after an experience in the treatment of erysipelas as large as, perhaps larger than, that of any other physician on the American continent."

Eley has reported the successful use of the serum in a series of 33 infants. Dosage: 10 cc. intramuscularly, repeated daily so long as the lesion persists; in grave cases an initial dose of the unconcentrated form of the serum to be given intravenously (no intoward reactions were observed). Foote considers that, in addition, prompt transfusion of blood is important in cases in the newborn.

Convalescent Serum.—The use of convalescent serum was first made at the Providence (R. I.) City Hospital in 1919, but not reported by Jordan and Dustin until 1924. (Unknown to these authors, Kaiser had reported its use in a single case in 1915.) Of their methods and results they write as follows:

"Convalescent erysipelas serum is sterile serum from the blood of patients convalescing from uncomplicated erysipelas. The blood is collected in a wide mouth bottle by means of a simple suction apparatus made from a two-hole stopper, two L-shaped glass tubes, and two short sections of rubber tubing. A large intravenous needle is fitted to one of the rubber tubes by means of an adapter. The whole apparatus is autoclaved before using, and the blood and serum are handled, so far as practical, with sterile apparatus. One of the arm veins is used, and not more than 200 cc. of blood is taken even from large adults.

"Patients who have had a normal temperature for at least a week, and who show practically complete clinical recovery without complications, are chosen. Only patients with negative blood Wassermann reactions have been selected.

"The blood is allowed to stand in the ice-box for from thirty-six to forty-eight hours. At the end of this time the clot is firm and the clear serum can be poured or pipetted off without the admixture of many red cells. The serum is centrifuged in sterile tubes at high speed to separate the few suspended red cells. The serum is then transferred to sterile ampules of suitable size, and sealed. A further yield of serum can be obtained by squeezing the clot and centrifuging to separate the red cells. This serum is always more or less colored by hemolysis, but it is as effective as the clear serum. No preservative is added. The sealed ampules are heated to 56 C. for one hour on three consecutive days. Serum prepared in this way has been kept in the ice-box for months without losing its potency. Ampules have been opened and cultures found sterile. It is advisable, however, in case serum is to be left for any length of time, to add tricresol, 0.3 to 0.4 per cent, as a preservative.

"Because of the difficulty in keeping a sufficient supply of convalescent erysipelas serum on hand, it has been used only in selected cases. The patients have been those seen early in the disease, those showing an extension of the process after a period of improvement, or those who have been severely toxic. Practically all the serum has been given intramuscularly, as intravenous serum therapy is not in favor at this hospital. The maximum dose has been 40 cc., the minimum 10 cc., and the average, 14.5 cc. The dose has been varied according to the size of the patient and the clinical condition. From 15 to 20 cc. seems a fair dose for the average adult with no complications. [Their case histories reveal that a second dose has been given in but one instance; the patient recovered very quickly, though the prognosis had 'seemed extremely bad.'—H. B.]

"Eighteen patients have been treated. Of these, 3 died, 2 showed questionable improvement, and 13 showed very decided improvement. Only cases in which a marked improvement was shown in the temperature chart and in the clinical aspect have been counted as successful. The 3 patients who died were moribund on admission to the hospital."

Vaccines.—Benson's (1930) study of 235 carefully controlled acute cases has shown conclusively that vaccines of no sort whatever have any value in this disease.

Milk Injections.—On the Continent, the injection of milk for the production of a nonspecific protein reaction is often resorted to. Frehse (1931) describes the method and results:

"According to the condition of the patient, we inject into the gluteal region from 3 to 10 cc. of milk that has been sterilized in the water bath. There then generally occurs a rise in temperature, with or without a chill, then a critical fall in temperature—this within twelve to twenty-four hours. Redness, swelling, heat and the sense of tension usually subside quickly. When that is not the case—as occasionally happens—the temperature usually rises again quickly. In these cases we have repeated the injection with a larger dose."

Intravenous Mercurochrome.—Young has collected the reports of 32 cases of erysipelas that were treated by the intravenous use of mercurochrome. Of these, 28 were cured or improved, 1 was only temporarily improved, and in 3 cases the drug failed entirely. The almost immediate cessation of febrile and irritant symptoms and the great rapidity with which the skin lesion cleared up, was said to have been quite remarkable in most of the cases. For technic, see the article on Sepsis (p. 163).

Iron.—The tincture of ferric chloride has long been regarded as having specific value in the treatment of erysipelas. It is given in a dose of 15 to 25 minims (1 to 1.5 cc.) by the mouth every two hours. Oftentimes its use has to be abandoned because of gastric irritation. If it has been studied in an extensive series of cases I am not aware of the fact, though I have seen very satisfactory results follow its use in several cases in my own experience.

Prevention of Recurrent Attacks.—Birkhaug is at present studying the matter of active immunization against recurrent attacks of erysipelas by means of biweekly intramuscular injections of 500, 5000, and 50,000 skin test doses of the extracellular and intracellular toxin produced by the particular strain of *Streptococcus hemolyticus* which he holds responsible for the disease. These injections appear to produce in the patient's blood serum a rapidly increasing concentration of antitoxin. In his preliminary report he states that 24 patients with definite histories of frequent recurrent attacks of erysipelas have been actively immunized by means of this toxic filtrate, and that persons among these who previously suffered habitual attacks of the disease from every sixth to twelfth week have been free from subsequent recurrent attacks over a period approaching two years. Amoss (1931) undertook a similar immunization of 14 patients who had experienced 35 attacks in the two years preceding the experiment; in the 11 who survived the two years of observation and immunization there occurred only two attacks of erysipelas.

ERYSIPELOID

Erysipeloid is a disease which has been shown to be caused by a modified form of the organism, *Erysipelothrix suis*, which causes swine erysipelas, a bacillus that is apparently either pathogenic or saprophytic throughout the animal kingdom. In America most of the cases have been reported from the Atlantic seaboard, with a few from the Great Lakes region, and have nearly all been in fish-handlers and the handlers of the flesh of swine in packing houses—but the exceptions exhibit a wide gamut of possibilities, such as injury of the hand in the bed of a dried creek, skinning a rabbit, carrying an opossum by the tail! The disease is characterized by the appearance, after an incubation period of two days, of a sharply circumscribed, quadrangular, bluish-red lesion on the skin at the site of the infecting injury, and by constitutional symptoms which are usually very mild; however, cellulitis, lymphangitis and lymphadenopathy may occur, and the appearance of a diffuse erythema accompanied by the symptoms of sepsis have been reported. The majority of cases run a self-limited course of about three weeks, but in Germany there has been observed a chronic form of the disease which is characterized by polyarthritis and vegetative endocarditis and in America some of the cases have been observed to start up again in previously uninvolved areas after a short period of apparent cure.

THERAPY

The only distinctive treatment which has been developed consists in the preliminary trials of a specific antiserum. Callomon, in Germany, recommends the injection of 10 to 20 cc. of this serum subcutaneously in the affected arm, and describes good results, both when using it in treatment and as a prophylactic measure immediately after the accidental inoculation. In America, Klauder and Harkins (1931), and Ritchie and Becker (1931) have induced healing of the lesions in about five days following a single injection of 25 cc. into the gluteal region. However, the incidence of serum sickness has been particularly high after the systemic use of this serum, and its local use has recently been substituted with apparently equally good results. From 0.25 to 0.5 cc. is injected into numerous areas about the advancing border; sometimes the injections have to be repeated after a few days, or new areas must be freshly injected. A local reaction usually follows these injections: swelling, pain in the joints of the involved hand, urticaria near the site, and sometimes tenderness and enlargement of the lymph nodes draining the site.

FOOT AND MOUTH DISEASE

Foot and mouth disease is a highly contagious malady of domestic hoofed animals; a few cases have also been seen among wild rats, and cats, hedgehogs, and perhaps other rodents can be experimentally infected. It is caused by a filtrable virus which is sometimes transmitted to man through the medium of infected milk or milk products. The cases are rare. Among livestock the disease is widespread in Europe, South America and other parts of the earth; the United States has several times been threatened with serious epidemics, which have been stamped out by mass killing, immediate burial, and rigid quarantine. Recent studies in England have shown that dressed carcasses of infected animals may retain their infectivity even after ten weeks of refrigeration.

That great man, Girolamo Fracastoro (1484–1553)—who wrote the first complete description of syphilis, foresaw clearly the modern conception of the bacterial causation of disease, and performed many other feats of original genius—described the first recorded epidemic of foot and mouth disease. And, indeed, since his time there has not been a great deal written upon it in the strictly medical press. In 1898, Löffler and Frosch proved experimentally that the malady is caused by a filtrable virus. I give Clough's summary of the symptoms: "A mild febrile infectious disease, characterized by the appearance of an erythema and a superficial vesicular eruption over the mucous membrane of the mouth and on the skin of the hands and feet; by salivation, by swelling, burning and paresthesia of the affected parts, with subsequent desquamation; and by healing of the ulcers without scar formation."

THERAPY

Treatment consists in the use of antiseptic mouth washes such as 1: 2000 potassium permanganate. The silver nitrate stick may be applied to the ulcers just as in the treatment of canker sores. I fancy the lotion of calamine and zinc (see p. 166) would be soothing when applied to the lesions on the body surface. Very little has been written about the treatment of the disease; all attempts to influence its course by the intravenous introduction of dyes or other antiseptic substances have met only with failure.

GANGOSA
(See Yaws)

GERMAN MEASLES
(See Measles)

GLANDERS
(Farcy; Malleus)

Glanders is an infectious disease of horses and mules. It is caused by *Bacillus mallei,* and is communicable to man. The cases in man, which are fortunately rare for the disease is extremely fatal, are nearly all contracted directly from a diseased animal, though the danger of laboratory infection with the organism is very great, as was dolefully reemphasized in Prague, in 1924, when three well-known scientists succumbed to the disease within a brief period. The outbreak which they were investigating claimed in all seven deaths (in 7 cases), all deriving from one infected horse. Acute glanders in man may begin with symptoms indicative of almost any of the other infectious diseases, which makes early diagnosis very difficult; however, Symmers says: "The occurrence of symptoms of an acute infective disease in an individual who comes in contact with horses and who presents multiple abscesses in the skin or in the mucous membrane of the nose, with deep-seated pain or tenderness, indicative of abscesses in muscle tissues, tendon sheaths, fascia or periosteum, with or without joint symptoms, should suggest the diagnosis of glanders in spite of the extreme rarity of the disease, and confirmation should be sought in isolation of the causative bacillus and guinea-pig inoculation." There is also a chronic form of the disease.

It is thought that the strange affliction of animals and men during the ninth to twelfth century called *Malum Malannum* because of its recurrence in troublous years, was either anthrax or glanders. Solleysel described the transmission of the disease from horse to horse in 1664. The classical monograph on the disease in man is that of Rayer, in 1837. Löffler discovered the causative organism in 1882.

THERAPY

There is no specific treatment for glanders in man. The palliative measures directed to the relief of the general constitutional symptoms do not merit special description here; they are such as are applied in any other fulminating condition. It is said to be advisable to excise the local nodule where possible, though in a recent (1926) outbreak of 7 cases in eastern Austria, 5 terminated fatally though the original focus was eliminated in each case. A grave disease, then, for which we have no remedy.

GLANDULAR FEVER
(Acute Mononucleosis)

Glandular fever is an infectious and probably contagious disease characterized by intermittent fever which continues for two or three weeks, complaints of general malaise, sweats, sore throat, general enlargement of the superficial lymph nodes, perhaps a rash, and a mononuclear leukocytosis. The patients are chiefly children and young adults. The causative organism has not been isolated. The disease was first described by Filatow in 1886; first definitely envisaged as an acute mononucleosis by Sprunt and Evans, in 1920. Recently cases have been reported from the tropics (Philippines, China) which had hitherto been thought free from this affection.

THERAPY

There are. no drugs or biologicals which have any specific value. The treatment is symptomatic, with recovery occurring in practically all cases, though the swelling of the glands may last for a long time.

GRIPPE
(See Catarrhal Fever)

HYDROPHOBIA
(Rabies)

Hydrophobia is an acute infectious disease chiefly encountered in dogs, though many other animals are susceptible. The disease is caused by a filtrable virus which is associated with the so-called "Negri bodies" that develop in cells within the central nervous system of infected animals. A rabid animal, biting another, transmits the virus in the saliva. In the island of Trinidad, in 1931, it was proved that the vampire bat is capable of transmitting the virus between infected cattle and man, both of which this loathsome fellow feeds upon. Not all bitten individuals, whether animal or man, develop the disease, but once the symptoms appear a fatal termination, after terrible suffering, is certain.

There is little mention of hydrophobia between the classical description of Aëtius, a physician at the Byzantine Court in the sixth century, A. D., and the keener observers of the eighteenth century, such as Boerhaave and his famous pupil, van Swieten, the creator of the Vienna clinic. Pasteur's first preventive vaccination with the attenuated virus of the disease was performed upon the Alsatian shepherd-boy, Joseph Meister, in July, 1885. The specific cell inclusions were discovered in the central nervous system by Negri in 1903–04, and successfully cultured by Noguchi in 1913. Many years ago Sir Victor Horsley predicted that rabies could be stamped out by the muzzling of all dogs; this has often been put to the test in relatively small communities (occasionally throughout an entire national domain) and always with complete success, but a world-wide attack upon the disease in this way has yet to be organized.

Symptoms in the Dog.—The first sign is usually a change in disposition, the animal becoming increasingly restless and snappy. Then a great thirst develops, the attempts to swallow being embarrassed by a progressive paralysis of the pharyngeal muscles; salivation becomes marked and the mouth may "foam"; there is depravity of appetite and a tendency to emit low howls followed by a series of unnatural barks during which the jaws do not close; and the animal starts out on a long excursion without definite destination, usually traveling at a rapid pace and biting many inanimate and animate objects encountered en route. Finally there supervenes the paralytic stage, which ends in death; it begins in the hind legs. The disease runs its course in from two to eight days. In so-called "dumb" rabies, drowsiness and paralysis are more marked from the beginning, and death is mercifully quicker.

Rabies is particularly dangerous in cats for these animals, when infected, often slink into a dark retreat from which they fly out at the passer by, inflicting severe face wounds.

Symptoms in Man.—I quote Williams' description: "Furious rabies is the most frequent form in man. For about forty-eight hours there are usually indefinite nervous symptoms, such as a sensation of constriction in the throat, or difficulty in walking or breathing, or precordial anxiety, or neuralgic pains. The temperature is slightly increased, 100.4 to 102.2 F. (38 to 39 C.). The fear of water usually develops, due to painful spasm from attempts to swallow. Characteristic reflexes may be caused by a draft of air (aerophobia), or loud noises (hyperacusis). Remissions usually occur, except in the very severely infected cases. After about forty-eight hours the excitement increases, accompanied by hallucinations and even mania, though usually no attempt is made to injure others. The mind is clear between attacks. The voice becomes hoarse, but there is no real barking. The eyes may show photophobia, nystagmus, strabismus, and unequally dilated pupils. Vomiting usually occurs. The patient may die suddenly during this stage after one to four days, but he usually passes into the paralytic stage, with muscles relaxed, jaw dropped, ropy saliva flowing, and finally into a comatose condition. Death occurs in about two to eighteen hours. Just before death the temperature may reach 107.6 to 111.2 F. (42 to 44 C.).

"Dumb rabies is less frequent in man than in lower animals. Its recognition is particularly necessary, so that it may be differentiated from the paralysis which very rarely occurs during or just after the Pasteur treatment.

The onset may be convulsive, but the lower extremities feel very heavy and numb; then there quickly develops a condition of ataxia and progressive paralysis. Death occurs in from two to eight days from heart paralysis."

THERAPY

Treatment of the Dog.—A dog manifesting characteristic symptoms of hydrophobia should be at once killed and his head shipped, either packed in ice or in equal parts of glycerin and water, to the nearest laboratory equipped to make a confirmatory search for the Negri bodies. All animals definitely known to have been bitten by him should also be destroyed. If, however, the dog is only suspected of having the disease he should not be killed but quarantined for observation, for a negative laboratory examination at this time would only leave the diagnosis in doubt. There need be no fear that he will recover from a "light" case during the period of quarantine; all animals having rabies *die;* an animal showing no symptoms after three weeks in quarantine is an animal that has not had the disease.

Treatment of the Human.—*Local Treatment.*—The wound should be cauterized at once with phenol or fuming nitric acid. There is good reason to believe that this local treatment has been of benefit, especially in the more dangerous bites about the face and fingers, and in cases where the early institution of vaccine treatment is not possible.

Vaccine Treatment.—The incubation period of the disease in man is usually fourteen to one hundred days (though Hajare (1933) has recorded a case developing after fourteen months). It is during this period that the proper use of prophylactic vaccine will prevent the disease in the vast majority of cases; indeed, the failures constitute less than $\frac{1}{2}$ of 1 per cent. One may safely wait for the appearance or not of symptoms in a quarantined dog before starting the treatment, unless the bite has been received on the face or hands, in which case, owing to the short incubation period following wounds at either of these sites, the physician is usually well advised to begin treatment at once—unless, of course, he is firmly convinced of the dog's innocence. Pregnant and nursing women may be treated with safety.

Antirabic vaccine or antirabic virus is rabbit virus which has been rendered practically nonvirulent for man by passage through a long series of these animals and treated in various ways to decrease the infectivity still further. The methods commonly used in the United States are those of Pasteur (as modified by the Hygienic Laboratory, U. S. Public Health Service), Högyes, Semple, Fermi, Harris, and Cummings, and are described in "New and Nonofficial Remedies." It is no longer necessary to send a patient at great expense to a "Pasteur Institute" for treatment, as any physician can administer the vaccine in the improved form in which it now appears on the market. Most of the pharmaceutical houses send out the vaccine in syringes containing 2 to 3 cc. ready for injection when the accompanying sterile needle is attached. The contents of a syringe is administered daily over a period of fourteen to twenty-eight days according to the severity of the case (*i. e.*, the location and extent of the wound). The first package of seven syringes is sent by special delivery, the others following at proper intervals; it is well to keep the packages in the refrigerator.

The duration of immunity in man after vaccine treatment is probably no more than fourteen months, though to be sure there are very few available data on the subject. A person bitten a year or more after taking the Pasteur treatment should again go through a full course of injections. Remlinger and Bailly (1931) have reported an instance of four full antirabies treatments in four years; a second case of three treatments in four years; and a third of two treatments in seventeen years. There were no anaphylactic accidents in any of the cases.

I do not believe that the vaccine *per se* is actually responsible for any of the varied symptoms manifested by patients taking the Pasteur treatment. In my own case, despite the fact that treatment was begun early and that the vaccine was for the most part self-administered, I was the victim of a certain unwonted apprehension, and was thoroughly weary of the irksome routine long before the course was completed. In the layman these things might easily make for a quite variegated display of neuroses. I found the intramuscular injections into the buttocks distinctly less painful than those placed subcutaneously in the abdomen.

Postvaccinal Paralysis.—Two serious symptoms, however, do sometimes occur during or following the treatment; they are paralysis and polyneuritis. Recovery is the rule, though a few persons have died in the paralysis. The percentage incidence of these severe symptoms varies so widely in the numerous published reports that it is difficult to state a normal or average expectancy. However, it is never high enough to be considered a contraindication to the treatment.

Treatment of the Developed Case.—This can only be directed toward a relief of the suffering, as no cure of a proved case has ever been accomplished to my knowledge. Five per cent cocaine solution will give relief if sprayed well down into the pharynx. Large doses of chloral hydrate and sodium bromide, 30 to 50 grains (1.8 to 3 Gm.) of each, may be given in a few ounces of water by rectum. Opiates should be freely used, or light general anesthesia maintained to the end.

INFECTIOUS JAUNDICE
(Epidemic Jaundice, Weil's Disease)

This is an acute infectious disease caused by *Spirochaeta icterohemorrhagiae* (*Leptospira icterohemorrhagiae* of Noguchi). The symptoms are quite characteristic. There is abrupt onset with vomiting, headache, fever, muscular pains, especially in the calf, and great prostration; sometimes there is a transient stiffness of the neck; conjunctival injection is practically always present and labial herpes is frequent. The jaundice may appear very early and is usually present by the fourth day; with its appearance the liver becomes tender and swollen; the spleen may be palpable. The urine contains bile, albumin and casts, though there is believed to be no permanent kidney injury. The fever continues high for about ten days and then falls to normal in two or three days, accompanied by a subsidence of the other symptoms. In one fourth to one third of the cases there is a return of the fever, unaccompanied by other symptoms, this second fever running an intermittent course of three days to as many weeks. Convalescence is characterized by depression and is usually very protracted.

The causative organism is present in the blood up to the seventh day and in the urine throughout the febrile period and perhaps longer. The same organism is found in rats the world over and it is significant that most recorded epidemics have occurred in individuals who have passed some time in wet, rat-infested places, such as military trenches and civilian excavations, natural swimming pools, mines, etc. However, such insects as bedbugs, mosquitoes and horseflies have been shown not to be intermediary hosts. Buchanan has found a natural habitat of the causal agent outside the animal body. He demonstrated its presence in the slime taken from the roof of an infected mine, in a region which he believed to be inaccessible to rats. In a recent (1931) epidemic among laborers in the Andamans, the onset of the first case was six days after the beginning of work in a *Leptrospira* infected swamp and the last case appeared eight days after the work had stopped.

Weil first described this disease in 1886, and Ryukichi Inada and Yutaka Ido discovered the causative organism in 1914. The reports of sporadic and epidemic cases are quite numerous in the European and Asiatic medical literatures, but, despite the presence of infected rats, few cases have been recorded in the United States.

THERAPY

Specific therapy is sadly lacking in this disease, in which the mortality, though usually between 5 and 10 per cent, may reach as high as 32 per cent in some epidemics. One would be hopeful of the intravenous arsenicals here, but they have failed; indeed, some cases have been made worse by their use, probably because of the state of the liver. Vanni's work with animals, in Italy, indicated that tartar emetic might be found of value in the chemotherapy of the disease, but so far I have found no study of its worth in the human. Bismuth, too, has been experimented with in the guinea-pig, by Uhlenhuth and Seiffert, but not yet in man.

INFLUENZA
(See Catarrhal Fever)

KALA-AZAR
(Visceral Leishmaniasis, Dumdum Fever)

This disease, which is a very ancient one, is common in certain parts of India, in China, Indo-China, Arabia, all around the shores of the Mediterranean, southern Russia, and South Africa. It is extremely rare in the Western Hemisphere; the few reported cases were all imported. It is caused by *Leishmania donovani,* a protozoan organism, and everywhere that the disease is encountered in man it occurs in dogs also, except, according to Young, in India and China. The sandfly is not yet irrevocably incriminated as vector, but, as shown in Wenyon's (1932) excellent review, the evidence against the fellow is so overwhelming that one begins to wonder whether the missing evidence is not some factor or factors not directly concerned in the actual process of transmission. It has already been demonstrated that for each locality there must be the right sandfly and the right strain of the parasite: in India the local strain of *Leishmania donovani* and *Phlebotomus argentipes,* in North China the Chinese *L. donovani* and *P. major* var. *chinensis,* in Sicily and Malta *L. infantum* and *P. perniciosus,* in Palestine *L. tropica* and *P. papatasii,* and in Bagdad *L. tropica* and *P. sergenti.* The organisms, however they may enter the body, embed themselves in the endothelial cells lining blood and lymph vessels, whence they burst into the blood or lymph stream to be engulfed by other endothelial cells or by leukocytes.

The onset is usually insidious, though it may be acute. Usually the first complaint is of several bouts of fever with increasing weakness. In one fourth to one third of the cases the fever is of the double-remittent type, *i. e.,* with a rise and fall twice or thrice in the twenty-four hours; in the majority of cases it is of a very irregular sort. Emaciation and anemia (proportionate reduction in red cells and hemoglobin) are pronounced and there is a striking leukopenia. Sometimes the body assumes a dusky hue (kala-azar: "black sickness"). Great enlargement of the spleen, and later enlargement of the liver, cause the abdomen to be markedly protuberant.

Daily rigors are common, though other pronounced symptoms are rare. Diarrhea is usually, though not always, due to concomitant bacillary, amebic, or flagellate dysentery. The febrile periods are followed after two to six weeks by afebrile periods, and then further attacks of fever. Obtaining the organisms by splenic puncture is often necessary in order to rule out typhoid fever and malaria. Kala-azar has decimated whole populations in its time. It is said that Indian villagers have burned alive many of its victims, after first stuporizing them with alcohol, in the attempt to stamp out the disease. About 90 per cent of the untreated cases succumb in two months to two years.

THERAPY

Tartar Emetic.—Antimony, in the form of either antimony-sodium-tartrate or antimony-potassium-tartrate, is looked upon as a specific in this disease, but the treatments must be faithfully persisted in in order to obtain cure. This is sometimes difficult of accomplishment for the reason that the patient feels so well after awhile that he discontinues treatment before the desired course has been completed. Also the complications, chief among which are bronchopneumonia and cancrum oris, are often fatal even in patients under treatment. It is believed that a 30- to 60-grain (2 to 4 Gm.) course of tartar emetic, distributed over a period of three months, is sufficient to sterilize an adult of Leishmania parasites. The drug is given intravenously in 1 or 2 per cent concentration, in either water or physiologic saline solution, at intervals of two or three days. The solution is usually sterilized in the autoclave, though it has been pointed out that serious symptoms may arise from the formation of decomposition products of the drug when submitted to high temperatures. It may also be sterilized by passage through the Chamberland filter. The addition of 0.25 per cent of phenol after sterilization prevents the growth of molds which sometimes add to the toxicity of the preparation. Extreme care must be exercised in giving the injection, for even a very small amount placed outside the vein is very painful and causes a brawny induration which ruins the site for subsequent injections.

The occurrence of dizziness, coughing, vomiting, marked diarrhea, muscle and joint pains, pronounced slowing of the heart and frightening cessation of the respirations, severe headaches and rigors—are signs that the limit of tolerance has been reached, and that thereafter the dosage of the drug must either be reduced or its administration suspended altogether for a time. Some of the cases of intercurrent pneumonia seem to be directly due to the injection of the drug. A somewhat rare complication is acute arthritis, which usually beneficently influences the course of the primary affection.

Young (1927) gives the distribution of the total dosage for adults and for children, as employed in the Peking Union Medical College Hospital (Table 7).

Archibald, writing of the experiences of himself and others in the Sudan, states that it is the feeling there (1923) that a dose of 2 Gm. is correct for sterilization, but that it might well be distributed over a longer period than three months. Analyzing the fatal results which have occurred among several cases that from a clinical point of view should not have succumbed, he believes that in those cases characterized by progressive asthenia death is directly attributable to the drug, even though the patient has not shown the classical symptoms of intolerance listed above. Col. Biggar, Principal Medical Officer, Egyptian Army, has altered the treatment, as follows: The first dose of 0.5 grain (0.03 Gm.) is followed after *seven* days by 1 grain (0.06 Gm.) and subsequently 1 to 1.5 grains (0.06 to 0.09 Gm.) at *ten-* to *fourteen*-day intervals. This method is considered comparatively safe and would seem to be curative even in advanced stages of the disease, for at the time of Archibald's report it had to its credit a lower mortality than the more

TABLE 7.—TARTAR EMETIC DOSAGE IN KALA-AZAR

Time.	Adults.		Children 10 to 15 years.		Children under 10 years	
	Cc. of 2 per cent sol.	Gm. of drug.*	Cc. of 2 per cent sol.	Gm. of drug.*	Cc. of 2 per cent sol.	Gm. of drug.*
First week 1st injection........	1.5	0.03	1.0	0.02	0.5	0.01
2nd injection...............	2.0	0.04	1.0	0.02	0.5	0.01
3rd injection...............	2.5	0.05	1.5	0.03	1.0	0.02
Second week 1st injection......	3.0	0.06	1.5	0.03	1.0	0.02
2nd injection........	3.0	0.06	2.0	0.04	1.5	0.03
3rd injection	3.0	0.06	2.0	0.04	1.5	0.03
Third week 3 injections of......	3.5	0.07	2.5	0.05	2.0	0.04
Fourth week 3 injections of.....	4.0	0.08	3.0	0.06	2.5	0.05
Fifth week 3 injections of	4.5	0.09	3.0	0.06	2.5	0.05
Sixth week 3 injections of......	4.5	0.09	3.5	0.07	2.8	0.056
Seventh week 3 injections of....	5.0	0.10	3.5	0.07	2.8	0.056
Eighth week 3 injections of.....	5.0	0.10	3.8	0.076	3.0	0.06
Ninth week 3 injections of......	5.5	0.11	3.8	0.076	3.0	0.06
Tenth week 3 injections of.....	5.5	0.11	3.8	0.076	3.0	0.06
Eleventh week 3 injections of...	6.0	0.12	4.0	0.08	3.3	0.066
Twelfth week 3 injections of....	6.0	0.12	4.0	0.08	3.3	0.066
Total.....................	...	3.27	...	2.27	...	1.81

* This column is added by me—H. B.

intensive method. However, Napier, whose experience in the therapy of the disease is probably unrivaled, does not advocate this dosage, and Findlay (1930) sums up his excellent review of the subject thus: "The injections are given on alternate days throughout the course of treatment. Although it is permissible to extend the interval by one day in certain cases, the injections must never be given less frequently than twice a week."

In infants, in whom intravenous therapy is sometimes impossible, administration of the tartar emetic is often quite difficult. Saha (1931) has reported the successful treatment of five cases with rectal injections, introducing 2 cc. of a 0.25 per cent solution after cleansing the rectum with normal saline. The dose is increased 2 cc. in an injection given every second day until 8 cc. have been given; then increasing 1 cc. in an injection every fourth day to 12 cc. in children up to three years; in a girl of ten years he went up to 24 cc. Rectal irritation was not caused. Most authorities consider that both oral and rectal administration usually fail because antimony is absorbed in insufficient quantities, which may cause the infecting organisms to become antimony resistant or "fast." Intramuscular injection is very painful and almost invariably causes necrosis. Intraperitoneal injection in very dilute solution in physiologic saline has been used successfully by Smyly in the cure of a case of kala-azar in an infant, aged six months; however, Caronia (1930), whose experience in the disease is vast, has pointed out that he does not feel obliged to seriously consider the method because of the at least potential danger of setting up a severe peritoneal inflammation.

Pentavalent Antimony Compounds.—The high toxicity of tartar emetic, the fact that it can only be given intravenously, that the time required for the administration of a complete course is very long, and that many cases are completely resistant to it from the very start—these things have made it far from an ideal drug with which to attempt the eradication of a disease affecting many hundreds of thousands of people as does kala-azar. Therefore the search has been constantly going on for a better drug, which seems now to have been found in the form of certain pentavalent antimony compounds that are salts of *para*-aminophenylstabinic acid, or substitution products of the same. These compounds are certainly much less toxic than tartar emetic; they can be given in larger doses, thus reducing the average time required for treatment from two or three months to about three weeks (or to eight or ten days in the case of neostibosan, which can be administered daily); and they are suitable for intramuscular injection. Also, they are apparently much more effective than the earlier drug, there being fewer relapses among those treated with the pentavalent compounds and a considerably lower death rate: 4.2 per cent in Napier's series of 167 cases treated with six different pentavalent compounds as compared with 14.4 per cent in his series of 139 tartar-emetic-treated cases. Unfortunately, the new drugs are much more expensive than the tartrates, but it is very likely that the recently developed protein graph method of studying progress with them will greatly help in determining the best conditions of their use (see Findlay, G. M., in the Bibliography). I shall attempt here only a brief résumé of the present status of the chief of these new compounds in the treatment of this most grave of the tropical fevers.

Stibenyl.—This is the first of the pentavalent compounds to be employed clinically and it apparently remains the one most employed around the Mediterranean littoral and in the Near East; but it has been a failure in Asia, probably because of its unsuitability for export to the tropics. (See the following references in the Bibliography: Caronia; Foti and Javarone; Moragas y Garcia; Martinez; Giraud and Massot; Smorodintsev; Korchitz.) The dosage range for children, who are the principal victims of the disease in the regions in which this drug is employed, is from 0.03 to 0.1 Gm., sometimes going as high as 0.15 Gm. There are reports of cures following six to ten injections on alternate days, also reports of other cases in which the courses extended over several months.

Urea Stibamine.—This drug has been much used in Asia. The total amount of the salt given does not usually much exceed 2 Gm., though in exceptional cases it has been run up as high as 10 Gm. In Brahmachari's (1931) series of 125 cases, the intensive treatment of adults extended over six to nine days during which the daily dose given intravenously varied between 0.025 and 0.2 Gm. In Napier's series (1927–29) the average number of injections given was twelve.

Stibamine Glucoside (Neostam).—Not used as much as some of the other compounds. Average total dose usually does not much exceed 2 Gm., but in Napier's (1929) series, among 16 patients receiving an average total of more than 4 Gm., there was but one relapse. Struther's (1927) dosage is probably typical: beginning with 0.05 Gm., increasing at each injection by 0.05 Gm. until a maximum of 0.2 Gm. is reached; however, Napier gives an initial dose of 0.1 Gm., a second dose of 0.2 Gm., and 0.25 Gm. for each subsequent dose.

Urea Stibol.—Apparently very little used. Chopra *et al.* (1928) report the same dosage as with urea stibamine.

Amino Stiburea.—In Napier's series, the average total dose was 2.4 Gm., the average number of injections was twelve, and the average number of days under treatment was twenty-nine. The minimum total dose which produced cure for Hodgson, Sen and Das (1928) was 1.5 Gm., the average 2.99 Gm.

Stibosan (von Heyden 471).—In Napier's series (1926) of 104 cases, the average total dosage was 2.78 Gm., the average number of injections (three times weekly) was 13.3, and the maximum dose was 0.3 Gm.

Neostibosan (von Heyden 693 b).—This drug, which is the newest of the lot, is probably going to prove the best. Napier and Mullick (1929), in India, give a daily intramuscular injection of 0.3 Gm. for eight days, the total dose therefore being 2.4 Gm. Struthers (1931), in Tsinan, feels that the Chinese patient will not tolerate quite such high individual doses. In his series of 87 cases, the initial adult dose was 0.1 Gm. intravenously and subsequent doses of 0.2 to 0.3 Gm., sometimes daily and sometimes every other day; the average total dose was 2.63 Gm. and the average time under treatment was 23.3 days. In children, both intravenous and intramuscular injections were given, the initial dose of 0.05 Gm. being followed on alternate days by 0.2 Gm.; average total dose, 2.1 Gm., and the average time under treatment, thirty-two days.

Reactions.—The principal reactions are vomiting, diarrhea, hepatitis (necessitating immediate cessation of the treatment), and anaphylactic-like symptoms somewhat resembling those of the nitritoid reaction to the arsphenamines. None of these reactions are upon the whole as severe as those seen during the use of tartar emetic, nor do they occur with anything like as great frequency; neostibosan seems to be the least offender of the group, being particularly unlikely to cause vomiting.

Cancrum Oris.—In a few cases the slough may be removed and granulation successfully stimulated by the application of silver nitrate, in the beginning as the stick and later in solutions of decreasing strength.

ORIENTAL SORE, DERMAL AND MUCOCUTANEOUS LEISHMANIASIS

Dermal leishmaniasis, seen principally in India, responds favorably to the antimonial drugs, but the mucocutaneous type of the disease, which is prevalent in South America, is much more resistant; indeed, Findlay says, "A specific treatment for mucocutaneous leishmaniasis has yet to be found." All of the organic arsenicals have been tried with indifferent success; so also many other drugs: quinine, Bayer-205, etc. That is to say, the gamut of specifics is being run in the hope of finding one that will cure the disease. Some observers (de Rezende, 1925) have found curettage and the local application of 80 per cent lactic acid superior to any other treatment.

In Oriental sore, while it is certain that the antimony preparations are of considerable value, it is apparent that they do not exhibit the high degree of specificity seen in kala-azar. Since the disease is not fatal and usually pursues a self-limited course of from six to eighteen months, many students of the subject doubt the advisability of combating it with such potentially dangerous drugs. Emetine hydrochloride has been injected in solution subcutaneously and intracutaneously around and beneath the lesion; Sinderson (1925) obtained excellent results with a 2 per cent solution and one injection only in a series of 147 cases. Berberine sulphate is also successfully injected locally. Karamchandani (1927), using ¼ grain (0.015 Gm.) dissolved in 1.5 cc. of distilled water, obtained healing in fourteen days in 5 cases, as compared with eighteen days in a tartar-emetic-treated series—a significant difference when the nature of the two types of treatment is taken into account. Warma (1931) and de Castro (1931) have confirmed these results. Devi states that of eighteen sores on 12 patients, six healed completely after one injection, five after two injections, and five after three injections.

LEPROSY

(Lepra, Hansen's Disease)

Leprosy is a chronic infectious and very mildly contagious disease generally considered to be caused by *Bacillus leprae,* though Koch's postulates with regard to the organism have not as yet been acceptably fulfilled. Its origin is lost in antiquity but it is known to have been quite prevalent in southern Europe in the early centuries of the Christian era and in the Middle

Ages was pandemic in England as well as all over the Continent. The early Spanish and Portugese navigators, and later the thriving slave trade, brought it to the Western Hemisphere. The segregation of victims in hundreds of leprosariums, and perhaps other factors, slowly stamped it out in Europe, where it now exists endemically and sporadically in only a relatively few localities. At the present time it is very prevalent in the tropics all around the world, especially in regions of great moisture. In China and Japan it abounds, tropical South America has very many cases, it is endemic and has been epidemic in the East and West Indies and the mid-Pacific Islands; according to Rogers and Muir the incidence in equatorial Africa (130: 1000 of population) is higher than anywhere else in the world. In India, Muir, the leading authority upon the disease, has stated (1929) that a careful though limited survey has shown in that country between half a million and a million lepers; others place the number between one and three millions.

In the United States endemic foci are known to exist in certain of the southern, middle western and western states; and in Canada there are also foci. A conservative estimate of the prevalence of leprosy in continental United States made by the United States Public Health Service, in 1930, places the number at about 1200. At the National Leprosarium, at Carville, Louisiana, there are more than 300 patients always under treatment. During the thirty-four years' existence of this institution, 1894–1929, there were 718 admissions, of which number 215 were foreign-born and 503 native-born; in the period 1920–31, 84 individuals have been paroled as no longer a menace to public health. In New York City I had 7 cases under observation at one time and know that as many more were being treated in each of several other large clinics. The disease may occur at any age but it most frequently makes its appearance between the tenth and thirtieth years. It is more prevalent among males, but it is not hereditary nor does the susceptibility to the disease seem to be transmitted to the offspring. Contagion is very slight; indeed, little is known about the way in which leprosy is contracted, for though prolonged and close contact under unhygienic conditions seems to be necessary, conjugal cases are not significantly frequent. It is most interesting to note, however (Hasselmann-Kahlert, 1931), that in the Philippines, where the children of lepers are separated from their parents after six months, 10 to 15 per cent of them become infected from their mothers before that time.

The prodromal symptoms are not characteristic. In the "nodular" form of the disease progressive nodular infiltration of the skin takes place usually on the face and hands first. Later the other portions of the body are affected. It is the ulceration of some of these nodules, with ultimate necrosis of the deeper structures, which causes the mutilation that so terribly characterizes the disease. The mucous membrane of the pharynx, larynx, and often the conjunctiva and deeper eye structures are also affected. In the "nervous" form the skin lesions are macular and are definitely anesthetic. There is also nodular invasion of the nerve trunks with ultimate serious loss of sensibility. Contractures of the tendons, following trophic changes in various muscle groups, cause the typical "leper claw." A "mixed" form of the disease is frequent, in which the patient is seen using without pain horribly mutilated portions of his body. The name "lazarine" leprosy is given to a form characterized by pemphiginous lesions apparently independent of the other phenomena of the malady. The duration of untreated leprosy is very variable. It may last ten to twenty years, often longer in the pure nervous type. Intercurrent infections carry off many of the cases.

THERAPY

When leprosy was rampant during the Middle Ages and well up into the period of the Renaissance, as many as possible of its victims were accommodated, and wretched accommodations they must have been, in the leprosariums which were present in hundreds all over Europe. The objects of segregation at that period were two: to get the poor, loathsome creatures out of sight of the world until they died; and to stamp out the disease by preventing contact of the affected with the unaffected. But in the tropical countries where leprosy is so prevalent today among the natives of the lower strata, this idea of segregation never has been popular, and consequently we find but a very small proportion of the world's lepers gathered together in especially provided leprosariums in the twentieth century. And it is a sad commentary upon our present-day civilization, a fact very humbling to our scientific pride, indeed, that these modern victims of so ancient a disease have been offered no more relief from their suffering than were their ancestors who perished of their uncleanness so long, long ago. As of old, where possible we have herded them together and, "out of sight, out of mind," have sought to make merry as best we could. Till yesterday—when was born the hopeful phrase, "a possible cure for leprosy!" Still wabbly upon its legs, insecure of its hold upon life, one feels that the shine of victory upon its face should be quickly described, ere with a gasp it and hope again are gone.

Chaulmoogra Oil.—Chaulmoogra oil is obtained by expression from the seeds of a handsome East Indian tree, *Taraktogenos kurzii*, and a very similar substance, hydnocarpus oil, is obtained from *Hydnocarpus wightiana*. Both of these oils differ from other oils in being composed chiefly of the glycerol esters of two unsaturated fatty acids named chaulmoogric acid and hydnocarpic acid. The terms "chaulmoogra oil" and "hydnocarpus oil" are used interchangeably as the two oils are essentially the same, though in India, where the seeds of *H. wightiana* are likely to be more freshly gathered, "hydnocarpus oil" is probably the preferable term. In this article I shall use the name "chaulmoogra oil" as meaning either of these substances.

The chaulmoogra plant is among man's oldest known remedies. Regarding its first employment as a specific, Major-General Sir Patrick Hehir relates a pretty little legend sometimes current in India: "This legend is at the moment rather absorbing, connecting a fragment of the early history of medicine in India with the most up to date medical research. Rama, a king of Benares, was afflicted with leprosy, relinquished his throne in favor of his son, and disappeared into the jungle, in which he lived on roots and herbs, and especially on the leaves of the Kalaw tree [probably the Burmese name for *Taraktogenos kurzii*—H. B.]; he eventually recovered completely. One day he accidentally met the Princess Piya in the jungle; she had been banished from the kingdom of her father, also on account of suffering from leprosy. Rama effected her cure by feeding her on the fruit, root, and leaves of the Kalaw tree, married her, and erected a new city in the place where these trees grew. The lady by way of showing her gratitude presented the devoted Rama with twin sons on 16 occasions—so the story goes." The discovery of the virtue of these seeds, or of the oil expressed from them, is therefore in no sense a modern triumph, but up until almost the present time its usefulness has been very much limited by the fact that in curative quantities taken over a long period it gives rise to a gastrointestinal irritation intolerable to almost everyone. Modern science has placed the treatment on a much more hopeful basis by devising more acceptable methods of administration—which, it must be remarked, are all still more or less in the experimental stage. With the description of the current methods of treatment which follows, I beg to state that I am by no means satisfied, but it is the best summary of the subject that I have been able to prepare. According to plans made at a session of the Council of the League of Nations, in 1931, an international center for research in leprosy is to be established in Rio de Janeiro; it is my belief that persons appointed by this center will travel over the world and present us with an exhaustive report of the leprosy therapy as everywhere encountered.

Tourtelles of Cairo, as long ago as 1899, used chaulmoogra oil subcutaneously, but his work attracted very little attention. Heiser, while in Manila some fifteen years later, seems to have been the first one to use the oil intramuscularly, and the formula consisting of chaulmoogra oil, camphorated oil and resorcin, proposed by Mercado and Heiser, was much discussed during the period 1914–16. Independently, Rogers in India had used orally with some success a mixture of the fatty acids from the oil, which he called collectively "gynocardic acid," and later employed the sodium salts of these acids as soluble soaps, both subcutaneously and intravenously. Then, in 1919, Holman and Dean in Hawaii fractionated chaulmoogra oil by saponification and, instead of using the undesirable soaps, employed the liquid ethyl esters obtained from the fatty acids. In 1920 Walker and Sweeney demonstrated experimentally that chaulmoogra oil has a specific bactericidal activity for acid-fast bacilli *in vitro*.[1]

At the present time these esters, as well as the oil itself, are being tried on a very large scale and in various ways in leper colonies throughout the world; they are usually mixed with other substances to lessen the pain of injection and to increase the effectiveness of the chaulmoogric principles. I shall list the results obtained by some of these methods in the hands of workers scattered along a very "far-flung battle line."

Oil and Camphor (Wilson in Korea).—From his large experience in the treatment of leprosy, Wilson writes in 1923 as follows:

"Every Saturday afternoon each leper in the Kwanju Leper Home gets an injection of from 3 to 8 cc. of hot chaulmoogra oil with 1 per cent camphor. We start on 3 cc., and in three months reach to from 5 to 8 cc., according to the size and strength of the patient, or giving them about all they can well bear, the patient himself being the judge. The injection is made into the buttocks and not very deep. We found that occasionally a deep injection becomes infected, and a deep abscess is far worse than a shallow one. Since the lepers have learned to be more careful, we rarely ever get an abscess these days, though in their early days of doing this work they were not so careful and had some trouble. There is no excuse for an abscess.

"The oil is heated on a water-bath; then enough camphor is added to make 1 per cent camphor. The camphor should first be macerated, and then added. In cold weather this solidifies, and must be heated and melted before injecting. Just after the injection, the lepers must bathe, and then they are to rest until Monday morning. Usually Monday they are ready to take up their various duties again and suffer no inconvenience. No other treatment is given except as some other condition requires."

Writing again in 1926, he says:

"We have seen apparent cures in 30 per cent in spite of the fact that many of our cases have come in in the advanced stages. We find that more

---

[1] It is interesting to note that the ethyl and other esters of chaulmoogric acids were first prepared by Power and his collaborators, during their extended investigation of the chemistry of chaulmoogra oil at the Wellcome Chemical Research Laboratories in London from 1904 to 1907, but "notwithstanding the previous preparation of the esters by Power and the ancient use of chaulmoogra oil in leprosy [I am quoting Morrow, Walker and Miller], Ludwig Taub of Elberfeld, Germany, obtained patent rights in Germany in 1909 for the preparation of esters of chaulmoogra acids and their use in therapeutics. This patent right was assigned to a German chemical company, which put the ethyl esters on the market under the trade name of 'antileprol.' A little later, patent rights were obtained in Great Britain and the United States. Following the war, and the confiscation of German patent rights, the alien property custodian sold the rights of this patent in the United States to the Winthrop Chemical Company of New York, which is preparing and distributing the ethyl esters of chaulmoogra acids under the trade name of 'chaulmestrol.' "
"Chaulmestrol" is described in New and Nonofficial Remedies, 1933, page 135.

than 75 per cent of our patients have the disease arrested so that they can take an active part in some form of work. The lepers are all the better for it. They can take the oil with less interference and pain if working. Our lepers are required to produce all their garden vegetables. Most of the patients can scratch the earth and plant a few seeds, which acts like a tonic for them. Our lepers also erect all buildings, make brick and tile, and do carpentry, tinning, blacksmithing, and other jobs. I am firmly convinced that the old way of isolating lepers as hopeless incurables with nothing to do is a mistake. They should be given some active occupation and taught to help produce part of their care at least. The active life is the thing for the leper today."

The Esters and Iodine Intramuscularly Plus the Fatty Acids and Iodine by Mouth (McDonald and Dean in Hawaii; Wade, Lara and Nicolas in the Philippines).—The standard treatment employed at Kalihi Hospital was described by McDonald in 1920, as follows: "The weekly intramuscular injection of the ethyl esters of the entire fatty acids of the whole oil with 2 per cent of iodine by weight chemically combined, the dosage of which begins with 1 cc. and is increased by 1 cc. at every second or third injection until we reach from 2 to 6 cc., according to the age and weight of the patient. Internally, patients receive in capsule form the mixed fatty acids carrying 2.5 per cent iodine in chemical combination; the fatty acids, rather than their ethyl esters, because they better conform to the normal digestive process which precedes fat absorption; we are therefore using by mouth a predigested oil or fat which is semisolid at room temperature and, in capsule, very easy to take. Its dosage begins with $\frac{1}{6}$ Gm. per hundred pounds of the patients weight, three times a day, an hour or two after meals. This is gradually increased every two weeks until the maximum of 1 Gm. per hundred pounds of weight per dose is reached. Of these two forms of administration, we have gradually come to regard the injection as the vastly more important of the two. . . . It should be said for the fatty acids, however, that we consider them the most efficient form of the oil ever devised for internal use. We go for weeks at a time without a single complaint of digestive disturbance. We are sometimes asked why we add the iodine, but confess that we find ourselves unable to furnish an especially substantial defensive reason. It was used by our predecessors here, as also by others elsewhere, and was considered decidedly beneficial; it has an old and respectable reputation for effecting catabolic or retrograde metabolism, with a tendency to promote in the economy the absorption of inflammatory and hyperplastic products. Then, too, the fatty acids of chaulmoogra oil are unsaturated acids and therefore capable of taking up iodine to form chemical compounds having none of the irritating properties of free iodine."

Carefully controlled experiments later reported by McDonald and Dean show that patients taking injections progress just as well without taking the capsules in addition. They say: "It is very doubtful whether the inconvenience and expense attached to the oral administration is justified in view of the results obtained. The individual on standard treatment receives about six times as much material in capsules as he does by injection, and in spite of this fact it would appear that it is the injected material which is almost wholly responsible for arresting the disease. The preparation of the material which goes into the capsules, and the filling of them, entail considerable expense which does not appear to be justified."

According to the showing of McDonald and Dean, 50 per cent of the patients who had been in Kalihi Hospital during the period January 1, 1920, to March 15, 1921, had recovered and been paroled. Up to May, 1921, there had been no recurrence in any patient paroled since October 1, 1918. I am not aware of these statistics having been brought up to date.

Touching on the *raison d'être* of the iodine inclusion, Wade, Lara and Nicolas have shown in the Philippines, in 1924, that the plain ethyl esters are irritating, particularly to the tissues at the point of injection and to the respiratory tract, so much so as seriously to limit the intensiveness of the treatment. Iodized preparations are much less irritating locally and they also cause fewer complaints of general symptoms. The 2 per cent iodized ethyl ester preparation, heretofore generally used, has, according to their data, certain minor but not insignificant disadvantages over the plain drug. The 0.5 per cent iodized preparation is in several respects distinctly superior to the 2 per cent and, unlike this, in no important way compares disadvantageously with the plain drug.

Ester, Olive Oil and Creosote (Cochrane in India; Wade in the Philippines).—Cochrane states, after completing a tour of leprosariums in India in 1926, that the treatment which is meeting with the most success there is either the ester or oil mixed with creosote. The ester mixture has the following proportions: ester 50 parts, olive oil (free from fatty acids) 50 parts, double distilled creosote 4 parts. The injections are given twice a week by the method of subcutaneous infiltration as advocated by the School of Tropical Medicine of Calcutta. This method, as described by Rogers and Muir, is as follows: The needle is inserted beneath an area of diseased skin and pushed forward *in the subcutaneous tissue* to the hilt. A small fraction of the mixture is then injected, the needle is withdrawn for a short distance and reinserted at another angle to the hilt, and another fraction injected; and so on until all of the mixture is distributed. Similar distributions from a single puncture may then be made under other portions of the lesion. Pressure must be made to prevent escape of the fluid upon withdrawing the needle. While applying this pressure, gentle massage should be made over the infiltrated area so as to distribute the mixture and hasten absorption. Care must be taken that the mixture is placed in loose subcutaneous tissue and that the needle does not enter a vein or pierce a nerve. The dose should begin at 1 cc. and increase by increments of $\frac{1}{2}$ cc. at each dose. In individuals getting large doses of 10 to 15 cc., it is well to give but 4 cc. in this manner and the excess intramuscularly. The immediate result of infiltration is a certain amount of local swelling and induration of the infiltrated area, which begins to subside within three or four days. The advantages of the method are stated to be: "(1) There is local counterirritation applied to the lesions, as well as absorption of the drug and its generalized effect; (2) absorption takes place more quickly as it gets injected over a large surface; (3) a large selection of sites is available for injection, an important point if the treatment has to be carried on for a very long time."

Wade's experience with creosote in the Philippines has been that the addition of this substance (10 per cent) to the plain esters reduces the local irritation to almost, though not quite, the same degree as does 0.5 per cent iodine, and permits increased medication. The only noteworthy drawback for the creosoted preparations is an apparently greater tendency to cause respiratory tract irritation.

Ester and Iodine, Ester and Creosote, and Mercado Mixture (Rodriguez and Lara in the Philippines).—During the semester ending March, 1924, the following preparations were being used at the Culion Leper Colony: (1) Esters with 0.5 per cent iodine, (2) esters with 10 per cent creosote, (3) esters with 0.5 per cent iodine and 10 per cent creosote, and (4) Mercado mixture (chaulmoogra oil 60 cc., camphorated oil 60 cc., resorcin 4 Gm.). Rodriguez states that the iodized esters are giving the best results but that the value of creosote is in his opinion not yet definitely established. Wade has elsewhere stated that the combination of creosote and iodine, as used in preparation (3), has no distinct advantage and has certain disadvantages because of which its use is not justified except in those cases in which it can be shown to have an unexpected therapeutic superiority. In agreement with the experience of others, Rodriguez finds that improvement is rather slow under the Mercado mixture. However, this mixture, has a definite place in the treatment of leprosy, for, with the possible exception of the pure chaulmoogra oil, it is the only drug available that can be given with some degree of safety when nephritis is present as a complication. The mixture is used intramuscularly with a wide range of dosage, from ½ to 6 cc., depending upon the patient's condition.

At the Culion Leper Colony, Lara reports that 6300 patients have been treated from July, 1921, to June, 1927, and that about 20 per cent of these have not received systematic treatment on account of complications. Sixteen per cent of all cases that have received treatment from six months to six years have been paroled or discharged as cured. A recent personal communication from Dr. Lara, who is Chief Physician of the Colony, brings the figures up to January 1, 1928, and raises the cures to 18 per cent. This is still significantly lower than the figures reported from some other colonies, but it should be pointed out that most of these other reports were based on the treatment of a much smaller number of cases. Mercado reported 46 per cent cures in 52 cases, Rogers 41 per cent in 51 cases, Neill 31 per cent in 394 cases, Rabello 32 per cent in 57 cases. Wilson, to be sure, reports 30 per cent in about 1000 cases, but the duration of treatment and the criteria for cure are not described. Furthermore, the type of patient varies considerably in different institutions. The Culion cases were nearly all of long standing, an average duration of eight years; in children the showing has been much better, more than 50 per cent of 70 cases becoming negative, according to Nicolas and Roxas-Pineda (1928).

Leprosy Fever and Acute Eruptions.—In a certain proportion of cases, depending upon the stage of the disease in which treatment is inaugurated, there develops a bout of fever with an acute diffuse leprous eruption. The patients are usually decidedly ill in the beginning of this attack and oftentimes do not return to their former state for several weeks. Most observers have passed over these acute attacks as of no moment since the patients generally recover, but to Muir they have been of great interest. He has of late championed the view that few people die of leprosy, indeed that it is a self-healing disease, and that the only reason for treating it at all is to stimulate the earlier consummation of the process of resolution. In regard to the significance of these acute attacks under treatment, he says:

"In acute infectious diseases the multiplication of the causal organism is synchronous with acute toxic symptoms, toxins being set free by the bacilli as they multiply and in proportion to their numbers. In leprosy, however, the multiplication of bacilli may go on rapidly with but few toxic symptoms . . . and high numbers of bacilli may be present in the skin while the patient retains comparatively good health. On the other hand, acute febrile and other toxic symptoms may occur while the number of bacilli is still small.

"The apparent cause of this is that, as the bacilli multiply, they secrete a glutinous substance which fastens the newly formed bacilli to the bacillary mass or to the cells lining the lymph spaces, and this substance, which envelops the bacilli, prevents the setting free of toxins. Under certain circumstances, however, changes take place either locally or throughout the body which affect the bacilli and their glutinous matrix, toxins are set free, and febrile and other symptoms occur. Not only are toxins set free, but bacilli also are often set free and carried to other parts of the body where, under favorable circumstances, they form new foci and lead to a further extension of the disease.

"What the circumstances are which bring about the above-mentioned changes in the bacilli and their matrix I do not intend to discuss here, suffice it to say that the injection of certain drugs, the application of counter-irritation, and various febrile diseases are among the commonest causes."

Muir's Principles of Treatment.—Based upon his views of the immunity reaction in leprosy, Muir has laid down certain principles of treatment which I shall give here in his words:

"(*a*) *In the first stage* we have the disease in a limited form with few bacilli in the body, little or no acquired immunity, and either diminished general resistance (temporary or permanent) or the presence of some other condition which is favorable to the increase of the disease. Attention in this stage must therefore be directed to: (1) The diagnosis and removal of whatever diseased condition, environment, or unsuitable diet is lowering the general tissue resistance or making the tissues a suitable medium for the growth of the lepra bacillus. (2) The induction of immunity by the injection of antigens. Defatted acid-fast bacilli may prove useful. (3) The destruction of lepra bacilli by the injection of preparations of fatty acids. I have found the esters of the fatty acids of hydnocarpus and chaulmoogra oils specially useful for this purpose. Counterirritation by infiltrating esters into the subcutaneous tissue under skin and nerve lesions or by the external application of such substances as trichloracetic acid (a 1 in 3 solution in distilled water painted onto lesions every six or ten days)." He is at present, 1933, using for infiltration ethyl esters washed with steam and iodized to remove their irritating properties, as in the Philippines.

"(*b*) *In the second stage* the same remedies should be used but with more care. The bacilli are plentiful and there is grave danger that, in the absence of acquired immunity, further dissemination of the disease may take place, as is frequently the case if violent reactions are allowed to occur. Even greater stress must be laid upon the necessity of increasing the general resistance. Theoretically, antigens in the form of defatted acid-fast bacilli should be useful, but I have not yet had sufficient experience of their value to speak with confidence. Trichloracetic acid used as mentioned above is very valuable. The esters of the fatty acids are very useful, but they must be used with great care especially if the general health is not good.

"(*c*) *In the third stage,* where a fair degree of immunity has been acquired, all the above-mentioned forms of treatment should be pressed. Vaccines, however, are not of much use as compared with the other forms of treatment. Considerable reactions are generally followed by marked improvement and there is not the danger of an increase of the disease which there is in the second stage. Large injections of the esters of fatty acids may be given, and, when these do not have sufficient reaction-producing effect, the reaction level may be lowered by the oral administration of potassium iodide, beginning with a daily dose of $\frac{1}{2}$ grain and gradually working up the dose to the limit of the patient's tolerance. Many patients will react with small doses of the esters when under the influence of potassium iodide in whom large doses of the esters without iodide produce no reaction. This effect is dependent on the presence of large numbers of lepra bacilli in the body. Many leprous patients will complain of severe pains in the limbs and head after the administration of $\frac{1}{4}$ to 1 grain daily for a few days. It is then well to stop its administration for a few days and to renew it after the pains have subsided. In all the stages of leprosy regulation of diet, abundance of exercise, and careful regulation of the bowels are absolutely essential if good results are to be obtained. . . .

"It is highly important to be able to recognize what stage of the disease a patient has reached. This can only be done with any certainty by the clinical appearance of the lesions."

The Plancha, or Infiltration, Method of Treatment.—At Culion it is felt that the marked increase in the number of negatives released in very recent years is due to the general adoption of this form of treatment, which consists essentially in making multiple *intradermal* injections of antileprosy drugs directly into leprous skin lesions (see Lara; Lara and Nicolas; Velasco *et al.* in the Bibliography).

Choice of Preparations.—Only two drugs are recommended: (*a*) the purified chaulmoogra oil from which most of the free fatty acids and volatile impurities have been removed by treatment with alkali and steam; and (*b*) refined ethyl esters to which 0.5 per cent of iodine has been added and the mixture heated until it becomes brown.

Dosage.—It is considered that the total dose that can safely be given in any one treatment should not exceed twice the size of the standard intramuscular dose of 4 to 5 cc., though some patients can tolerate up to 15 to 20 cc. Leakage has been estimated to be from 15 to 20 per cent of the amount injected.

Technic.—"Since in the majority of cases a considerable number of injections is required, the patient should be spared as much pain as possible, its painfulness being the only important drawback to the method. A fine (No. 23 or 24), sharp, stiff needle and a 5 cc. syringe with a metal guard are used with the ethyl esters . . . which are thin and easy to inject; with the purified oil and the various oil mixtures, which are thicker preparations, a No. 22 needle and a 2 cc. syringe are preferable. Large needles, besides causing more pain, provide a ready outlet for the injected drug, to prevent the escape of which a more or less considerable number of collodion applications is required.

"The area to be infiltrated is first painted with tincture of iodine and alcohol. With the drug in the syringe and the needle in place, the latter is first held at an acute angle with the surface of the area to be infiltrated, with the point directed toward, and at a distance of about 1 cm. from, the lower border of the lesion, if the infiltration is to be made from below upward, or, similarly, at the upper border of the lesion if the infiltration is made from above downward. The object in directing the needle downward is to minimize subsequent leakage of the drug injected. The needle is then pushed through the epidermis into the corium, and a sufficient amount of the drug is injected to produce a sharply defined wheal of about 1 sq. cm., about 0.1 cc. Larger wheals are more painful and are followed by a more prolonged tissue reaction.

"The distance between the individual punctures should be about 2 cm. when a large area is to be infiltrated at one sitting, or when the injections are made on the face, close to the eyelids. One week later, after the tissue reaction has largely subsided, the intervening spaces are similarly treated. In this way a moderate degree of reaction, that does not incapacitate the patient for his ordinary duties, is maintained. When the lesions are few and small, the injections should be made 1 cm. apart, so that the lesions may become thoroughly infiltrated. The reaction thus produced is more intense, but is seldom severe enough to affect the normal routine of the patient. This form of infiltration is preferably made every other week, alternating with the intramuscular injections.

"In the case of hard nodules, which are difficult to infiltrate, the drug is also injected all around the lesions.

"During the process of infiltration an assistant carefully wipes off any blood and drug that may ooze from the punctures, with a moist, sterile, or iodine-treated, cotton ball. With the new method of infiltration it is seldom necessary to use collodion to prevent leakage of the drug—a definite economy when thousands of cases are treated."

The entire cutaneous surface is divided arbitrarily into three regions—

head and neck, trunk, and extremities—and these are treated in succession, so that sufficient time is allowed for the tissue reaction to subside before the treatment is repeated in one or other of the remaining regions. Only the eyelids and the external genitalia cannot be infiltrated.

Drugs Other Than Chaulmoogra.—Various of the metals, copper, mercury, antimony, tellurium, gold, have been tried in the treatment of leprosy—as crystalloids, colloids, inorganic and organic salts. Occasional successes have been obtained with all of them, but I doubt if these isolated instances warrant description here.

MALARIA
(Paludism, Chills and Fever, Ague)

This day relenting God
   Hath placed within my hand
A wondrous thing; and God
   Be praised. At His command

Seeking His secret deeds
   With tears and toiling breath
I find thy cunning seeds,
   O million-murdering Death.

I know this little thing
   A myriad men will save.
O Death, where is thy sting,
   Thy victory, O Grave!

Before Thy feet I fall,
   Lord, who made high my fate;
For in the mighty small
   Is shown the mighty great.

> —Lines written by Sir Ronald Ross on finding himself in possession, after infinite toil, of conclusive proof of the causal relation of the mosquito to malaria.

Malaria is an infectious disease caused by three species of plasmodia: *Plasmodium falciparum, P. vivax* and *P. malariae,* which cause the subtertian (estivo-autumnal), tertian and quartan fevers, respectively. The organisms are conveyed from infected to healthy persons by the bite of certain mosquitoes of the subfamily *Anophelinae,* in whose stomach the organism passes a part of its life cycle. Once prevalent throughout the world, the disease is rapidly declining in the more northern civilized countries, its incidence and virulence increasing as the equator is approached. In such warm temperate regions as Macedonia, Italy, the southern United States, etc., it remains a major health problem, and in moist tropical regions it is the greatest of the decimators of man.

The disease was well known to the ancients. Garrison, quoting Sir Harry Blake, says that the theory of the conveyance of malarial fever by mosquitoes was indicated even in the Sanskrit Susruta, while another author holds the disease responsible for the vacillation of the Greeks before Troy. Hippocrates gave classical descriptions of malaria; and it has been learnedly held that this ailment, by driving the population cityward, was a pronounced causal force in the final decline of the Greek civilization, and that the later Roman Empire must sooner have succumbed to attacks from the north, had not the barbarian hordes been decimated by the ague. The

Middle Ages knew its ravages, while in many a military campaign of the eighteenth and nineteenth centuries more men fell victims to this disease than succumbed to the havoc wrought by shot and shell. What part it (and yellow fever plus bad financiering) played in the French failure to construct the Panama Canal is too well known to require comment, but the fact is often overlooked that at Santiago, in the late Spanish-American War (I quote Col. C. C. McCulloch, U. S. A.): "Malaria struck about half our force at the same time; the parasites were of the malignant variety and the infections all severe. If military conditions had not permitted the return of the expedition to the United States when it did return our Army would most probably have been practically annihilated; and if the Spanish had put up a stronger resistance than they did the whole course of the history of that conflict might readily have been changed." In the recent World War the sanitary measures which had been so brilliantly employed by Ross in Egypt and Gorgas in the Canal Zone were extensively utilized for the protection of the armies, despite which malaria remained one of the chief causes of disability at concentration areas lying within the "malaria zone."

The disease is characterized by regularly intermittent paroxysms of chill, fever, and sweating in the order named. If the disease is caused by the *tertian* type of organism these paroxysms occur every third day, if by the *quartan* type every fourth day, if by the *estivo-autumnal* type the fever is continued or remittent and the paroxysms irregular in occurrence. Many cases of mixed, or double, infection occur in which developmental cycles of the organisms are superimposed with consequent alterations in the periodicity of the paroxysms. In the typical case of moderate severity the patient presents a swollen spleen (and often liver also), herpes simplex about the mouth, and the organisms in the blood; he is a weary, worn, anemic individual, appetiteless, spiritless, with oftentimes headache and backache and a host of other ailments in addition to his "chills and fever." There are a number of pernicious and atypical forms of the disease.

In infancy and up to three years of age malaria presents a different clinical picture from that seen in the adult, as was emphasized in the paper of Mulherin and Mulherin, in 1922. The younger the patient, the more decided is the difference. Periodicity in subjective and objective symptoms is more frequently absent than present, and fever is oftener remittent, irregularly intermittent or absent, than regularly intermittent. Enlargement of the spleen is absent in perhaps 30 per cent of cases of malaria in infancy. A few cases of fetal infection through the placenta are on record.

THERAPY

In quinine we have the specific remedy *par excellence*, for if given early enough and in sufficient doses and long enough it will cure all cases—a blythe statement, indeed, so I shall add two modifications: (*a*) *Plasmodium falciparum* cases are influenced by the drug more readily than *P. vivax* cases, and the infrequently seen quartan type of infection is slowest of all in its response; (*b*) cases which have already become chronic before therapy is instituted respond much slower than do acute cases. I think that, with the exception of a few cases that are real rarities in the literature, all reported cases of *quinine-resistance* may fairly be construed as criticism of the physician and not of the drug (see p. 104 for further discussion). Witness the following editorial which appeared in the Journal of the American Medical Association, April 5, 1924:

"In 1917, reports began to appear that English soldiers in the tropics were being attacked by malaria that quinine would not cure. Pratt-Johnson and Gilchrist found that relapses were reported in 23 per cent of 18,000 soldiers in Africa while quinine was being administered; Phear reported in Macedonia that quinine was ineffective in malaria that was complicated by dysentery; Wilcox in Mesopotamia encountered cases that did not improve under quinine by mouth for ten days; Mackie found quinine ineffective in malaria in northern Persia, and the accumulation of invalids in Saloniki was constantly increasing. Such contradiction and disappointment concerning quinine led to an extensive experimental and clinical inquiry into the treatment of malaria at the Liverpool School of Tropical Medicine, the results of which, unfortunately, did not entirely restore confidence in quinine.

"Many soldiers were sent back to England from Macedonia in 1918, and Sir Ronald Ross arranged to treat the malaria patients in special wards at Southampton. In recently published notes, Fletcher says that 1150 patients were admitted to these wards in twelve months, and that on landing parasites were found in the peripheral blood in 487. Although many had documentary evidence of treatment with quinine in various hospitals, they were placed on 10 grains of quinine by mouth twice a day. There was strict supervision of these patients, and special interest in relapses that might occur. In every instance the routine treatment prescribed at Southampton caused both fever and parasites to disappear.

"Fletcher emphasizes the Southampton experience by a report of his observations in the Federated Malay States since the war. The patients seen there were little more than skeletons, and dysentery was a complication in 53 per cent. Forty-four difficult cases in which quinine had been disappointing were selected, and 10 grains (0.65 Gm.) of quinine by mouth twice a day was given for four weeks. The drug was placed in the patient's mouth by the physician, and, after it had been swallowed, the mouth was inspected. Not one of these coolies in Kuala Lumpur failed to improve. There was in one a small number of parasites that persisted in the blood in spite of quinine, but in every other case, both fever and parasites disappeared. Dysentery did not make any difference. When quinine was actually swallowed and retained, malaria in dysentery patients was as easily controlled as in patients who did not have dysentery. The conclusion of this study was the same as among soldiers in Southampton: that the so-called resistance to quinine vanished when the quinine was actually swallowed and retained."

However, quinine is not the only valuable drug in the treatment of the disease, for the arsenicals and plasmochin have also proved their worth. In the first edition of this book, I presented as the basic article on the treatment of malaria the treatise of Fernan-Nuñez, who had at that time just published his excellent résumé of the essentials of success in the treatment of the malady, based upon the close observation of over 8000 cases in tropical South America (the Lebrija River valley in Colombia), in the proportions of quartan, 6 per cent, tertian, 44 per cent, and estivo-autumnal, 50 per cent, as determined by microscopical blood examinations. His treatise, to my mind, still remains the best practical presentation of the subject for the busy practitioner, and so I retain it—of course, by the exercise of certain editorial liberties and the free use of interpolations and addenda, it has been brought up to date.

Acute Malaria.—"Malaria is the diagnosis in 90 per cent of all sickness beginning with high fever in the tropical hot lands, except during the frequent mild influenza epidemics which invade the lowlands from the mountain districts where the latter disease is endemo-epidemic.

"Paludism presents a wonderful variety of forms, and may at times closely simulate practically all other known diseases. For instance there may be malarial pneumonia, meningitis, pleurisy, neuralgias, rheumatism, otitis media, coryza, stomach disorders resembling ulcer, appendicitis, diarrhea, typhoid, disturbances of vision, lumbago, pseudo-angina pectoris, heart murmurs, hepatitis suggesting gallstones, severe pains in the spleen, pyelitis and kidney pains, cystitis or hematuria, generalized lymphadenitis, skin eruptions, extensive furunculosis, etc.

"As a general rule in the malarial belt every patient, regardless of his presenting symptoms, should have his temperature taken. Malaria patients in the beginning of the disease will often be unaware of the presence of fever, although the thermometer may show at that very minute a temperature of 104 or 105 F.—they do not feel it. The tongue should be scrutinized for the heavy, dirty-white, furred coating, an almost pathognomonic symptom, and the complexion examined for the peculiar faded-out color, very characteristic of paludism, and a careful history elicited concerning past malarial attacks.

"If in doubt of the correct diagnosis, try the therapeutic test, viz., the treatment of malaria. It is surprising to see the great majority of cases clear up even after having resisted all other lines of treatment. One of our axioms is that in any case of obscure pain occurring in a patient in the malarial district, quinine in full doses is to be made the basis of treatment.

"*Treatment.*—1. As soon as a diagnosis is made, give calomel 5 grains (0.32 Gm.) together with quinine 15 grains (1.0). No other purgative seems to clear up the coated tongue, cleanse the catarrhal stomach, stimulate the torpid liver, and facilitate the absorption of quinine like *calomel in large doses.* Give four compound cathartic pills (vegetable), or podophyllin 0.5 grain (0.032), if calomel can not be used.

"2. If the patient presents a chill, fever, sweat, or complains of pain, administer phenacetin 5 grains (0.32) or aspirin 15 grains (1.0). This often shortens a paroxysm and brings on a sweat sooner than without these drugs. Repeat at end of two hours if symptoms indicate the need of it.

"3. If patient is strong, and nausea is not troublesome, Warburg's tincture with aloes [Antiperiodic Tincture of the N.F.] 0.5 ounce (15 cc.), repeated in three hours, is preferable to the aspirin or phenacetin. The drug should not be diluted or followed by other drink. The patient can remove the bitter taste by merely rinsing the mouth with water. The second dose of this remedy usually brings on a profuse perspiration after which all the symptoms of the attack rapidly disappear.

"4. A full dose of magnesium sulphate or other saline should invariably be given within eight to twelve hours after the calomel.

"5. Of course, ice-bags and sponge temperature baths are very gratifying to the patient when the fever is troublesome.

"6. Neoarsphenamine (neosalvarsan) 0.45 to 0.75 Gm. intravenously as soon as convenient. It can be given at practically any time, even during the fever or sweating stages, except when Warburg's tincture is being administered. It should then be given on the following day.

"7. Ten grains (0.65) of quinine three times daily after meals for one week.

"8. Thereafter 10 grains (0.65) of quinine daily, preferably after evening meal, for *seven weeks longer.* This is absolutely necessary to sterilize the patient of his infection and prevent relapses in the estivo-autumnal infestations, but should be the routine in all cases of malaria regardless of type.

"If the patient neglects to take quinine daily, it would probably be easier for the physician to supervise this part of the treatment by having the quinine taken only on two successive days in the week. For convenience on Sundays and Mondays, when 10 grains (0.65) should be taken after each meal, a course of 60 grains (4.0) every week-end." The interval between these drenchings with quinine should not be "about a week," as so frequently stated, but actually not more than six days.

"A great variety of individual symptoms naturally occur in malaria. They usually are of fleeting character and disappear with the fever. If persistent they may be treated symptomatically as indicated. The loss of appetite complained of by nearly all malaria patients is but a symptom of the disease, and will correct itself upon overcoming the ague. Stomachic treatment is rarely necessary, as calomel and salts is the best treatment. In case the anorexia persists for a week or more the course of calomel may be repeated. Pain in the splenic area practically never requires special medication."

Chronic Malaria.—"This is usually associated with relapses occurring at intervals which are multiples of a week (septenary periods), *i. e.*, four, five or six weeks after acute attacks of malaria.

"*Treatment.*—Same as for acute malaria, with following suggestions: In longstanding cases with history of other relapses, (1) give injection of neo-arsphenamine 0.45 every week for two to six injections; (2) quinine 10 grains (0.65) daily, *plus* 30 grains daily on two successive days each week, *for two months.*"

Malarial Cachexia.—"This state is characterized chiefly by severe anemia, lemon-colored complexion, weakness, loss of weight, enlarged spleen, often enlarged liver, and marked digestive disturbances.

"*Treatment.*—1. The same as for chronic malaria.

"2. It is important to add a good chalybeate tonic, such as Aiken's tonic [Mild Pills of Iron Quinine, Strychnine, and Arsenic, N.F.—dose 1 pill], Blaud's pill [Pills of Ferrous Carbonate, U.S.P.—dose 2 pills], Elixir I. Q. & S. [Elixir of Iron, Quinine and Strychnine, N.F.—dose 1 drachm (4 cc.)], or Tincture of Ferric Chloride [U.S.P.—dose 10 minims (0.6 cc.)]. The last mentioned is especially effective and may be conveniently given in ordinary gelatin capsules, prepared by the patient with aid of a medicine dropper immediately before taking, thus avoiding the astringent taste and damage to the teeth.

"3. A mild saline purge every three or four days.

"4. Ingestion of large quantities of water constantly.

"Such a large percentage of malaria patients, particularly malarial cachectics, suffer with hookworms, ascarids (lumbricoids), trichocephalae, and other intestinal parasites as a complication, that it is a good general rule to give a vermifuge in practically all cases. Thirty minims (2.0) of oil of chenopodium mixed in an ounce of castor oil and taken at a single dose, or 1 drachm (4 cc.) of carbon tetrachloride in an ounce of water. Oil of chenopodium or carbon tetrachloride given in this simple manner usually does not require any subsequent purgation or dietary regulation, and they seem equally as safe and efficient as by any other method of administering these drugs."

Pernicious Malaria.—"The treatment of every case of pernicious malaria is heroic. There is no scene more spectacular in medical practice than the recovery of such a patient; it is one of the few instances in which a physician can truly feel that he has saved a life. The problem is to get into the victim's system a sufficient quantity of quinine *without one minute of unnecessary delay.*"

(*a*) *Comatose and Delirious Forms.*—"Remember that the temperature may be normal or *subnormal* when these patients are first seen.

"In the tropics every comatose or delirious patient who comes under the supervision of the physician should be regarded first as a victim of pernicious malaria. Sunstroke is exceedingly rare in the tropics, and comatose malaria is the diagnosis nine times out of ten. In coma with acute alcoholism, a history of injury—even a blow on the head—you can not go far wrong in applying the treatment outlined below, as very frequently the intoxication or the traumatism has merely flared up a latent malaria which produces the symptoms of coma. Too often patients have died in the tropics as a result of the physician's failure to recognize these facts.

"Delirious cases should receive the same treatment.

"*Treatment.*—1. Quinine hydrochloride, dihydrochloride or bisulphate, 15 grains (1.0 sterilized in 10 cc. or more of water) *by vein immediately*. Hurry!

"2. Spinal puncture.

"3. Calomel 5 grains (0.32) sprinkled under patient's tongue. Or, 1 drop of croton oil on back of tongue.

"4. If temperature is subnormal, apply blankets and hot-water bottles.

"5. Quinine 15 grains (1.0) intramuscularly within one hour of the above intravenous injection, and every twelve hours thereafter until patient is able to take medicine by mouth.

"6. Then begin treatment outlined under 'acute malaria,' and continue as there directed."

Umansky (1931) has obtained good results in these cases by the intravenous injection of methenamine (urotropin). His belief is that the "purification" of the blood capillaries in the brain is brought about by the fixing power of the formaldehyde produced from the methenamine, this explanation completely lacks experimental support and is probably untrue, but the important point is that Umansky claims that all the symptoms of the comatose or convulsive states disappeared in three to six hours after a single injection of 3 cc. of a 40 per cent solution of the drug (sterilized by boiling) in the 10 treated cases. The pyrexia, presence of the organism in the blood, etc., were not affected.

(*b*) *Bilious Pernicious Malaria* (*Vomiting Type*).—"1. Calomel 5 grains (0.32). Calomel is soothing to the stomach and will often be retained when all other laxatives would be immediately rejected. One-half ounce (15.0) of sodium hypophosphite, a full dose of magnesium citrate, or other effervescent salts should be given, in divided doses, beginning eight hours after the calomel. If the saline is rejected, small amounts should be continuously repeated at fifteen-minute intervals until the patient has retained a full dose.

"2. Due to the lessened coagulation time of the blood resulting from its large content of bile, and the fact that these patients are greatly weakened, intravenous injections are contraindicated. Intramuscular injections of quinine, 15 grains (1.0) in 10 cc. or more of solution, every twelve hours until fever is controlled are recommended.

"3. The weakness of these patients makes it dangerous to use the stomach tube. If gastric lavage is desired it usually suffices to administer a couple of glasses of water, which will soon be vomited and thus cleanse the stomach.

"4. To control the vomiting, morphine by hypodermic is efficient. Do not torture the weak sufferer with chloroform water, chloral, iodine, or other supposed gastric sedatives. Even if they might take the edge off the retching, they are dangerously depressing."

Sinton (1930), in his vast experience has found that the oral administration of 20 minims (1.3 cc.) of the 1: 1000 solution of epinephrine hydrochloride (adrenalin) is remarkably effective in controlling the vomiting.

"5. The vomiting in these cases, which is Nature's effort at elimination, soon dehydrates the tissues, and it is a problem to supply such patients with a sufficient amount of fluids. Large quantities can be given by enema and by *subcutaneous injections*. Rectal feeding may be necessary where the vomiting continues several days.

"6. When the fever is controlled, and the patient can retain medicines by mouth administer an iron tonic as suggested for malarial cachexia; 30 grains (2.0) of quinine daily for one week; and 10 grains (0.65) daily thereafter, at the evening meal, for seven weeks longer.

"7. When jaundice begins to disappear a rectal injection of neoarsphenamine 0.9 will greatly aid convalescence."

Remittent Ardent Fever.—"Cases in which the temperature does not fall to normal, and often remains dangerously high.

"*Treatment.*—1. Quinine 15 grains (1.0), in 10 cc. or more solution, intravenously at once.

"2. Neoarsphenamine 0.9 by rectum.

"3. Temperature baths at frequent intervals.

"4. Within one hour of above intravenous injection of quinine, administer quinine 15 grains (1.0), in 10 cc. or more of solution, intramuscularly. Repeat every twelve hours until fever has been controlled.

"5. Quinine 10 grains (0.65) by mouth, three times daily, beginning on afternoon of first day, and continuing for one full week after fever has been controlled.

"6. On second day of treatment give calomel 5 grains (0.32), followed at end of eight to twelve hours by a saline purge.

"7. Quinine 10 grains (0.65) daily, after evening meal, for seven weeks longer."

Other Pernicious Types.—The four forms of malignant malaria described are those most frequently seen. Treatment for the other types does not differ materially from that of remittent ardent fever.

Quinine Intramuscularly.—"No injection of quinine should be given in less than a 1:10 or greater dilution. The contents of the small quinine ampules should always, if possible, be diluted with sterile water to the proper proportion. A 10 cc. Luer syringe filled to capacity will hold enough solution for an injection of 15 grains (1.0) of quinine. Due to the almost certain tendency to produce a slough quinine ought never be given subcutaneously. Intramuscular injection is the method of choice, the injections being made into the gluteal muscles 1 or 2 inches below the iliac crest. Rigid asepsis is imperative. Quinine in concentrations of 1.5 per cent are anesthetic, and a dilution of 15 grains (1.0) in 10 cc. does not need the addition of novocain, urethane, or other local anesthetics, to prevent pain.

"In spite of all precautions indurations and abscesses sometimes result, although but rarely when a 1:10 or higher dilution is employed. A 30 per cent ichthyol ointment and a hot-water bottle if applied early will usually abort an abscess. A short rubber tube connection between the needle and syringe is of great service in preventing a struggling patient from breaking off the needle during the injection."

It seems to me that Fernan-Nuñez states the case rather mildly when he says that abscesses "sometimes result" from intramuscular injections. Most observers find them occurring very frequently; Sinton (1930) probably expresses the consensus when he states that "there seems only one indication, and that is in those very rare comatose cases, usually children, where oral administration, or intravenous injections, are found impossible."

Quinine Intravenously.—The patient's blood is no more effectively sterilized by placing the quinine directly into the blood stream than when it is given by mouth, but something is gained in the rapidity with which this is accomplished; it is therefore the method of choice in grave cases. Strict asepsis should be observed, of course, and the injection made very slowly to lessen the probability of inducing a fall in blood pressure, a reaction which is counteracted by the immediate injection of 1 cc. of epinephrine hydrochloride (adrenalin) solution. In Cantlie and Moubarak's series of 2484 intravenous injections, there was slight acceleration of the pulse and fainting only twice—however, I repeat, inject slowly!

Fernan-Nuñez says that 15 grains (1 Gm.) of the salt—hydrochloride, dihydrochloride or bisulphate—should be dissolved in 10 cc., or more, of water. The higher dilution is usually preferred, and physiologic saline solution used as solvent if it is at hand; Fantus (1930) directs that the solution be made in the proportions of 10 grains (0.65 Gm.) of the salt to 100 cc. of the saline solution; filtered and sterilized then by boiling. To obtain the 15-grain (1 Gm.) dose recommended by Fernan-Nuñez, 150 cc. of such solution would have to be given.

Quinine by Rectum.—It is usually considered that quinine is absorbed very unreliably from a retention enema and that the drug is quite irritant to the rectal mucosa. Some physicians deny these things, however. Rigby and Rigby (1929) advocate the rectal drip method of administration, dissolving 30 grains (2 Gm.) of the salt in 1 quart (1000 cc.) of physiologic saline solution, and injecting this during the course of twenty-four hours. They have also dissolved the drug in distilled water and added glucose, thus giving fluid and nourishment to a patient dehydrated by continuous vomiting, and at the same time providing a medium through which quinine may be administered.

Disguising Quinine.—"Many people of the malarial districts, especially in Spanish-America, have little faith in quinine. During their attacks of malaria they have been accustomed to take only enough of the drug to relieve the acute symptoms without continuing its use until they were sterilized of the plasmodia, and as a consequence have suffered repeated relapses. Commonly they will not take quinine for malaria, but are strong believers in 'tonics for the liver,' readily accepting almost any liquid medicine recommended to them as such. The following formulas have been used in our practice with success, many of the people even using daily doses as a prophylactic:

℞. Quinine hydrochloride (or bisulphate)................. ℥v	20.0	
Antiperiodic tincture without aloe (N.F.) to make..... ℥viij	250.0	
Label: Each teaspoonful contains the therapeutic equivalent of 5 grains of quinine.		

or

℞. Quinine hydrochloride (or bisulphate)................. ℥v	20.0	
Strychnine sulphate.............................. gr. j	.065	
Glycerin....................................... ℥j	32.0	
Water to make.................................. ℥viij	250.0	
Label: Each teaspoonful contains approximately 5 grains of quinine.		

Idiosyncrasy to Quinine; Desensitization.—The most usual symptoms in individuals who are hypersensitive to quinine are skin rashes, gastro-intestinal disturbances, pseudo-asthmatic and anginal phenomena. Occasionally a patient dies quite dramatically during such a reaction, but in most instances the prognosis is good.

Desensitization to Quinine.—Method of Héran and Saint-Girons, quoted by Castellani and Chalmers: The first day a "defensive dose," or ⅛ grain of quinine sulphate mixed with 8 grains of sodium bicarbonate, is given, and two hours later, 1½ grains. The second day, two hours after the "defensive dose," 3 grains are administered. The third day 6 grains, and so on, gradually increasing the amount of quinine.

Method of O'Malley and Richey: One-twelfth grain of quinine sulphate is given as a "desensitizing dose" by mouth plus 7½ grains sodium bicarbonate. One and one-half hours later, an additional 1½ grains of quinine sulphate and 7½ grains sodium bicarbonate are given. The "desensitizing dose" remains constant each day, while in the second dose the amount of quinine is increased 1½ grains each day, the quantity of sodium bicarbonate remaining the same. Two other methods have been used by these authors. One was the administration of quinine bisulphate by mouth in increasing doses once each day, beginning with ½ grain and increasing by as much each day. The other method consisted in giving a "desensitizing dose" of ⅙ grain of quinine bisulphate in 5 cc. of sterile water intravenously, and after thirty to forty-five minutes giving a second dose, starting with 3 grains of the same drug and increasing 1½ grains a day.

Menoussakis (1931) is attempting to show and apparently successfully, that the indispensable condition of tolerance is the presence of quinine in the system, and that one can prevent the symptoms of idiosyncrasy by giving each dose before the previous one has been excreted. In a typical case he gave 1½ grains (0.1 Gm.) on September 19th, producing rash, fever, vomiting and faintness; but, beginning the next day, and continuing each day thereafter until September 29th the patient took 15 grains (1 Gm.) in three daily injections without symptoms. On October 4th after a period of five days without the drug, the injection of 4 grains (0.25 Gm.) provoked a severe reaction, but the same dose was well tolerated on the following two days. After another interruption, the reactions recurred.

Substitution of Alkaloids.—Fletcher and Travers (1923), and others, have reported cases in which cinchonine was successfully substituted for quinine in persons sensitive to the latter drug; Dawson and Garbade (1930); Sanders (1932), and others, have successfully substituted quinidine for quinine. This is, therefore, one way of avoiding the troublesome process of desensitization.

Quinine in Menstruation and Pregnancy.—Other things being equal, it is probably well not to use quinine during menstruation as it tends to cause uterine contractions which may either diminish bleeding or increase it if there is a tendency toward menorrhagia. This is usually not taken into account when the drug is imperatively needed.

Pregnancy.—It is established by very definite proofs that extensive infection of the placenta with the subtertian malaria parasite is very likely to cause the death and premature expulsion of the fetus; Blacklock and Gordon (1925) have stated that more than a third of the placentae of West African native women examined by them contained large numbers of organisms, and that, of the children born of these placenta-infected mothers, 25 per cent died within seven days. It is agreed by all observers also that the disease may lie dormant in a woman's blood until awakened during labor, at which time the first typical pyrexial attack may occur. So much for the undoubted effect of the disease upon the pregnant woman, but of the effect of quinine upon her we do not know so much with certainty. In the Far East the opinion is widespread, and apparently fostered by European practitioners, that periodical dosage with quinine predisposes to abortion. Thus Manson-Bahr (1932) states that he has treated pregnant patients at term who were suffering from advanced malarial cachexia but had been strictly forbidden by their medical attendants to take quinine in any form in order to check the ravages of the disease. Many observers are wondering whether the abortion so often induced by the disease is not wrongly ascribed to the drug in at least some instances. Certainly, if given to promote labor at full term in nonmalaria-infected women, it has been shown to have practically no effect upon the well-being of the baby—Dilling and Gemmell (1929) have collected a series of 9765 cases so treated and have concluded that in only 8 stillbirths can the drug have been responsible. Unfortunately the prejudice against the drug—perhaps well-founded, I do not say that it is not—makes it impossible to present an equally impressive statistical study of the use of the drug in full doses throughout term in malarial women. One can only cite isolated instances: Yorke and Murgatroyd (1931) treated a seven months' pregnant West African, who had a moderate subtertian infection, with 15 grains (1 Gm.) of quinine daily for nine days, at which time the parasites had disappeared. Subsequently she was given 15 grains every Saturday and Sunday up to full term; during this period there were several mild relapses. The maternal sinuses of the placenta were shown to be massively infected, but the blood in the fetal vessels of the chorionic villi was free from infection, and the child was healthy.

The malaria inoculation treatment of paresis, with its concomitant use of quinine (see p. 187), is successfully administered to pregnant women.

7

Dosage of Various Salts of Quinine.—The question of the actual amount of quinine alkaloid in the various salts is often raised. The following table gives direct comparison of dosage on the basis of a 10-grain dose of official quinine (Table 8).

TABLE 8.—DOSAGE OF VARIOUS QUININE SALTS

	Quinine, per cent.	If dose of U.S.P. quinine is 10 grains.
Quinine, U.S.P. (contains 3H$_2$O)...............	85.71	10.00
Quinine hydrochloride, U.S.P..................	81.72	10.49
Quinine dihydrochloride, U.S.P..............	81.63	10.50
Quinine bisulphate, U.S.P....................	59.12	14.50
Quinine sulphate, U.S.P.....................	74.33	11.54

Dosage for Children.—The dose of quinine in children of various ages, equivalent to the 10-grain dose in adults, is given as follows by the National (U. S.) Malaria Committee, in 1920: under one year, ½ grain; one year, 1 grain; two years, 2 grains; three and four years, 3 grains; five, six and seven years, 4 grains; eight, nine and ten years, 6 grains; eleven, twelve, thirteen and fourteen years, 8 grains; fifteen years and older, 10 grains. It is now generally agreed that infants can stand, and should be given, much larger doses than recommended by this Committee. Also, the frequent remittent rather than intermittent type of the disease in these young individuals, which is possibly due to an asynchronous sporulation of the malarial parasite, would seem to call for a more frequent administration of the drug during the course of the day than is the rule in the treatment of adults.

Quinine Prophylaxis.—"To prevent infection with malaria is possible in the great majority of cases, provided a sufficient dose of the drug is taken. Practically all authorities in the tropics now agree that 10 grains (0.65) of quinine daily is the required amount. A lesser quantity, while giving a certain measure of protection, is not adequate. We have seen no ill results from the above amount daily over long periods of time."

In this matter of prophylaxis there is considerable difference of opinion. Deaderick prefers the method of giving 15 grains on each of two successive days in each week. The following appeared in the Journal of the American Medical Association, October 24, 1925, in reply to a query addressed to the editor: "The value of quinine prophylaxis is doubtful. Krauss and Mitchell, in a recent treatise on malaria in children, say that in very malarious regions it is practically impossible to prevent malarial infection, though it may keep symptoms in abeyance. Of a group that had been given 15 grains of quinine three times weekly for five months and 10 grains daily during the remainder of the year, 43.3 per thousand showed active malarial symptoms in spite of the prophylactic use of quinine. Another group of persons who were exposed to malaria were not given quinine and 45.8 per thousand fell ill with the disease. Quinine prophylaxis was used among 2000 coolies, with discouraging results. Stitt thinks that the quinine acts as a slow poison without compensating results. Experience also shows that as soon as the quinine is stopped, very often in less than a week, the symptoms of the disease begin to appear.

"In contradistinction of these views, Bass believes that the prophylactic use of quinine should be carefully employed. He advises the following doses: children under one year, ½ grain (0.03 Gm.) daily; one year, 1 grain (0.06 Gm.); two years, 2 grains (0.13 Gm.); three and four years, 3 grains (0.2

Gm.) ; five, six and seven years, 4 grains (0.23 Gm.) ; eight, nine and ten years, 6 grains (0.4 Gm.) ; eleven, twelve, thirteen and fourteen years, 8 grains (0.5 Gm.) daily. The doses should be taken at night before retiring, as in the treatment for disinfection of carriers. Bass also says that the disease is prevented as long as the treatment is continued."

Individuals Returning from Malarial Regions.—I quote Mühlens (1932): "After the War, it became customary among German residents of West Africa, as well as those in other lands, to employ a daily prophylactic régime with quinine—0.2, 0.3 or 0.4 Gm. (4, 5 or 6 grains), or alternating one day with the other 0.2 to 0.4 Gm. (4 to 6 grains). This was preferred to the so-called intermittent method with larger doses, about 1 Gm. (15 grains) every sixth and seventh day. According to my experience with a large number of private patients from East and West Africa in recent years, the results are satisfactory when the régime is persisted in until the return home. When attacks or relapses occur in spite of the prophylaxis, they usually run a relatively light and short course. Usually the attack of fever occurs during the vacation at home when the prophylactic, or 'postphylactic,' practice is given up to soon—about the eighth to fourteenth day after leaving the malarial region. Many Germans on the way home from West Africa now put themselves through a regular malaria cure, even if they do not have, or have not had, fever."

Arsphenamines in Malaria.—"The employment of the arsphenamines in malaria has received but passing attention, most writers only referring to it as a last resort when quinine fails, to be used in the later or chronic stages of the disease. Some men of authority do not even mention it in their works. We desire to call particular attention to these drugs in the *early treatment of malaria,* as it has been constantly demonstrated that they will abort the symptoms in practically every attack of malarial fever. The principal value of neoarsphenamine is that it immediately cuts short the tertian, quartan or estivo-autumnal seizures before the repeated fever can have time to severely debilitate the patient, thus his convalescence is markedly shortened and the chances of recovery correspondingly enhanced.

"There usually succeed no other paroxysms after the injection; although only one more single attack may occur the same or following day. Reactions from neoarsphenamine, when given in concentrated solution, are very few in malaria—the chill, fever and sweat which rarely follow within a few hours constitute merely the typical malaria picture which has been precipitated by the injection, a sort of malarial Herxheimer. It would have come tomorrow anyway.

"The utility of neoarsphenamine in malaria, then, is (a) it stops the attacks promptly before the patient is greatly weakened by the fever and plasmodial toxins, (b) through its excellent tonic value it rapidly builds up the patient, (c) patients recover their strength quickly and return to work considerably sooner than with quinine treatment alone, (d) it is effective when even quinine in enormous doses fails, *i. e.,* where quinine-fast organisms are present, or for some reason the quinine is not properly assimilated.

"Neoarsphenamine alone is specific in tertian malaria. Estivo-autumnal constitutes 50 per cent of all malaria in the river valleys of Colombia, and this type requires quinine in addition to neoarsphenamine, but in much smaller quantities than would be necessary without the arsenical. As estivo-autumnal (subtertian) may very closely simulate true tertian malaria, presenting quotidian or tertian recurrences, it is advisable to combine neoarsphenamine and quinine in all cases of malaria regardless of type.

"Malaria is often complicated by other constitutional diseases, such as yaws, syphilis, trypanosomiasis, filariasis, uncinariasis, amebiasis, etc., which usually are greatly aggravated by the fever, and may quickly carry a patient to his death. As neoarsphenamine has a specific effect in the first three and is a distinct help in combating the anemia of the other diseases mentioned, its routine use in malaria will correct a large number of complications arising from other sources.

"American relapsing fever (the spirochetal fever of Dutton and Novy) is increasing in frequency. The clinical symptoms at the beginning resemble malaria so that it is very readily confused with the latter. Quinine has practically no effect upon relapsing fever, but the arsphenamines are specific, so that their use as a routine in malaria also 'catches' the case of relapsing fever.

"All brands of neoarsphenamine, American and foreign, have been given a thorough trial in our medical service, and we are partial to the product of the Dermatological Research Institute, Philadelphia. It is rapidly soluble (very important where many injections are given in a busy clinic), makes a beautifully clear solution, is remarkably free from anaphylactic or nitritoid reactions, and gives distinctive clinical results in malaria. Each ampule is packed in an individual sealed wooden box which eliminates breakage, but more important still protects the drug from rapid temperature changes (wood being a poor conductor of heat) and thus reduces almost to zero the number of tubes which so frequently are prone to go bad. Only physicians living in warm climates who have had a large percentage of organic arsenicals damaged by the heat, with the consequent financial loss, and the very grave danger to their patients in the use of a partially deteriorated drug, can fully appreciate the genuine value of the above apparently insignificant matter of packing. In the tropics, all supplies of neoarsphenamine or arsphenamine should be kept in a refrigerator, but such advantages are available to only a relatively small number of tropical practitioners.

"*Intravenous Method.*—Contraindications: Albuminuria, severe jaundice, organic heart disease, marked anemia or debility, idiosyncrasy to arsenic.

"1. Sterilize syringes (2 cc. size) by boiling in filtered river water for two minutes. Double-distilled water is good but not necessary where river, rain, or other nonimpregnated water is available.

"2. Pour off all water but an ounce or two and set boiler in a basin of cold water. This will quickly cool the syringes and the sterilized water to room temperature. Hot water should never be used for dissolving the neo-arsphenamine.

"3. Sterilize the points of a hemostat or other forceps by dipping in alcohol, or passing through a flame. With forceps take out (*a*) barrel of syringe; (*b*) then needle, attaching it to barrel; (*c*) next plunger of syringe, inserting into barrel. All of this can be done with fingers sterilized in alcohol.

"4. Draw into the syringe 2 cc. of the water in which the syringes were sterilized.

"5. File off the small tip of the neoarsphenamine ampule.

"6. Inject the 2 cc. of water into the ampule. Dissolve the neoarsphenamine by drawing the solution back into the syringe and reinjecting it into the ampule several times, or better by sterilizing the tip of the index finger in alcohol, clamping it over the opening in the ampule and shaking. This dissolves the drug at once, and replaces the air-tight, glass-stoppered bottle formerly used for effecting the solution.

"7. Draw up required dose of solution in the syringe. Next fill the syringe completely by drawing in more sterilized water.

"8. Sterilize site over vein with tincture of iodine.

"9. Have an assistant, or the patient himself, grip the arm tightly with the hand above site of injection (no need to bother with a tourniquet). When vein is distended, insert needle (with bevel on under side), watch for column of blood to rise in the syringe, indicating that the needle is in lumen of the vein. Release grip on arm, and begin injection.

"10. Inject very slowly, *being extremely careful that none of the solution gets into the tissues outside the vein.* It will cause severe pain and indurations. Should this happen, give the patient a dose of codeine or morphine to relieve his discomfort, and do not irritate the painful area with local applications. The indurated spot will be absorbed within a couple of weeks.

"11. If the plunger should stick in the syringe, twist it to loosen. If at any time in doubt as to whether point of needle is in the lumen of the vein, slightly withdraw the plunger. A column of blood appearing in the syringe will set you right. If no blood appears upon careful backward manipulation of the plunger, withdraw needle, eject a few drops of the solution to clear it out, and begin injection in another vein.

"The little syringe filtering adapter for administration of neoarsphenamine, described by Dr. Schamberg (Jour. Amer. Med. Assoc., July 15, 1922, p. 216, Becton, Dickinson & Co., Rutherford, N. J.) is an excellent improvement which refilters the solution while being injected.

"While it may appear that the operation just described does not show the necessary refinement of the intravenous method, yet it has been proved in over 3000 injections given in this medical service that there is probably no more practical, efficient, or less dangerous way of administering neoarsphenamine, and we would not consider returning to the elaborate artillery in common use. The advantages claimed for the method are that it is very simple, requires but little time, and renders the application of neoarsphenamine possible in practically any case, a thing of real importance to the general practitioner. With the little pocket sterilizing hypodermic outfit marketed by Becton, Dickinson & Co. the injections may be given anywhere and under almost any circumstances. This means that neoarsphenamine can thus be made available to the greater number of people who suffer with malaria, the country population. One of the practical advantages of the small syringe and needle is that the injections are almost painless and patients do not resent them any more than other hypodermic medication; many submitting when otherwise it would be difficult or impossible to get them to take it. With the small needle it is frequently possible to enter a very small vein, which could not be done with the large needles or cannulas usually employed in arsenical injections. It is never necessary, even in children, to dissect out a vein for an injection.

"*Rectal Method.*—Neoarsphenamine administered in this manner is not attended with bowel irritation, reactions, or other uncomfortable symptoms, and there seems to be practically no contraindications to its use by rectum, except possibly arsenic idiosyncrasy. Apparently it equals the intravenous method in efficiency, but is somewhat slower in action, requiring two or three days to check the fever. The rectal dose is double the intravenous dose.

"1. Boil 4 ounces (128 cc.) of water and allow to cool until lukewarm.

"2. Dissolve in the water neoarsphenamine 0.9 Gm.

"3. Inject in rectum, with or without previous cleansing enema.

"4. Require patient to remain in reclining position from six to eight hours."

Substitute for Neoarsphenamine.—"If inadvisable for any reason, except idiosyncrasy to arsenic, to administer neoarsphenamine by vein, it may be substituted by sodium cacodylate 5 grains (0.32), or di-sodium methylarsenate [(Arrhenal)—a French proprietary—H. B.] 5 grains (0.32). Either of these may be dissolved in 10 cc. of water, sterilized, and given intravenously or intramuscularly. The dosage may appear to be large, but large doses of all drugs are required in malaria. We have seen no reactions or bad effects from such quantities. An injection on two successive days each week, for two weeks in acute malaria; for five weeks in chronic malaria.

"*Sulpharsphenamine* (Sulfarsenol), 0.3 to 0.5 Gm., subcutaneously or intramuscularly, is convenient and satisfactory. It has relatively the same value as neoarsphenamine given by rectum. It must be given with much care in algid malaria due to the deficient superficial circulation.

"If injections of any kind are impracticable, saturate the patient quickly with Fowler's solution or arsenous acid, observing the usual precautions.

"Some doubt has been expressed by certain writers as to the value of arsenic in malaria. Without going into theoretical discussion, we wish to express our absolute faith in the genuine clinical value of the drug, as demonstrated in our practice on hundreds of occasions."

Stovarsol (*Acetarsone, N.N.R.*).—This drug has been used quite a bit since Marchoux's investigations of it, in 1925, and it has now been definitely established that, although malignant tertian and quartan parasites are unaffected by it, the simple tertian parasites are effectively removed from the peripheral blood stream in nearly all cases. Indeed, claims have been made that a clinical cure can be accomplished with this drug alone, but enthusiastic reports of freedom from relapse have not been substantiated to a sufficient extent to warrant us in concluding that we have here a new specific in malaria. The best place for the drug is as an arsenical adjuvant to quinine, in the place of neoarsphenamine, in benign tertian cases. It is given usually as stovarsol in the form of tablets by mouth, or as the sodium salt intravenously; in either case, the dose most often employed is 15 grains (1 Gm.), sometimes repeated on the second and third days. Diarrhea, colic, tachycardia, collapse, skin and eye disturbances, severe rigors, urinary signs of acute nephritis, have been many times reported. Sinton's (1927) cases escaped these sequelae, perhaps because the kidneys and liver were "protected" by the glucose and alkalis which his patients also received. Bass (1930) believes that all of the arsenicals have a damaging effect upon the blood cells and tend to make them an unfavorable soil for the malarial parasites to grow in, and that it is in this way that they exercise whatever beneficent effect they have in malaria. If this is true, then it would seem that the patient who experiencs a reaction after being given an arsenical can expect the best results from the use of the drug in supplementing quinine.

Quinine stovarsol, a salt which contains about equal quantities of quinine and stovarsol, has been tried in malignant tertian and quartan cases; the preliminary reports are upon the whole favorable. Raynal (1927) gave his case 7½ grains (0.5 Gm.) twice a day for ten days, a rest period of five days, and then another course; the routine was continued for two months.

Other Drugs in Malaria.—"Quinine is the king of antiperiodics, but in persons who suffer from quinine allergy, quinine neuritis (particularly optic neuritis), or who are greatly nauseated by the drug, it may be advisable to try some of the remedies presently to be described . . . where a substitute for oral quinine is desired, selection may be made from the following, each of which we have found efficient:

15 grains euquinine (quinine ethyl-carbonate)	= 8 grains quinine sulphate
15 grains methylene blue	= 25 grains quinine sulphate
15 mm. oil of eucalyptus, or eucalyptol	= 10 grains quinine sulphate
60 mm. Warburg's tincture	= 5 grains quinine sulphate

"A very pure product of methylene blue must be used, accompanied by large quantities of water, and if the drug shows a tendency to produce strangury equal parts of powdered nutmeg should be added. [Pitschugin (1925) advocates ⅙ grain (0.01) methylene blue for every year of age three times daily for a week.—H. B.] It is advisable to give equal parts of sodium bicarbonate with each dose of oil of eucalyptus or eucalyptol. Most drug houses-put on the market Warburg's tincture in tablet form, a tablet representing 1 drachm of the solution. While these are efficacious and convenient, yet the solution is probably more active.

"Splenic extract has been extolled in malaria. After giving it a thorough clinical trial we failed to note any antiperiodic value from it, even the results of extremely large doses of a fresh product being almost nil. Possibly there resulted a transient tonic effect through the nucleins it contained."

It has been frequently stated that some of the other alkaloids of cinchona—cinchonine, cinchonidine, quinidine and cinchona febrifuge, or quinetum—are more effective than quinine in preventing relapses, but the testimony is quite conflicting. The opinion of the Malaria Commission of the League of Nations (1927) was that, if given in the same doses, quinine, quinidine and quinetum were equally efficient, though the circulatory depressant action of quinidine must be borne in mind; it was considered necessary to give cinchonine in half again as large doses. Sanders and Dawson (1932) have successfully controlled a small series of benign tertian and estivo-autumnal cases with quinidine sulphate in a single daily dose of only 10 grains (0.6 Gm.).

Relapses.—"It is our practice to forbid alcohol in any form to persons suffering with malaria. We recognize the excellent value of alcohol properly used in fevers due to pneumonia, tuberculosis, influenza and sepsis, but are confident that it is all wrong in malaria. We have often seen acute paroxysms of fever precipitated in latent malaria by very ordinary quantities of alcoholics. The old popular 'whisky and quinine' prescription produced more chronic cases of malaria than it ever cured. The small amount of alcohol in Warburg's tincture can be classed as a necessary evil.

"If possible to prevent it, malaria patients should never be given iodides, adrenalin, serums or vaccines, treated with ultraviolet rays or therapeutic lamps, and should avoid the sunlight, as all these are peculiarly prone to produce relapses. Excessive heat of any kind is contraindicated, malarial relapses among cooks, firemen, laundry workers, and the like, being notoriously frequent.

"Cold or prolonged baths are to be avoided, except during the fever stages, until the patient is thoroughly convalesced.

"Many patients with chronic malaria or severe acute malaria can only be cured in bed. Rest is a most important part of the treatment in every case of the disease. The patient who is up and around throws off a great part of the effective value of the drugs he is taking.

"Do not be too quick to decide that a patient requires to go to a colder climate or to the seashore to be cured. While this is always desirable, if practicable, yet by following faithfully the line of treatment given in the preceding pages and demanding that your patient rest at home just the same as he would on a vacation elsewhere, every case of malaria can be cured right in the hot lands. We have seen dozens of patients, even among North Americans and Europeans, suffering with chronic or pernicious malaria, recover completely and show a gain in weight over that enjoyed upon arrival in the torrid areas of the tropics. The invaliding rate for the above class, once a serious problem for our medical department, has been reduced to practically zero. In fact, in this most pestilential of regions, malaria is but little feared now. Neoarsphenamine applied early in all instances, and, if necessary, throughout the course of the chronic cases, has largely made this possible."

Nevertheless, the removal of the patient to a temperate climate increases his bodily resistance and shortens the life of the parasite. In a temperate climate the subtertian organism lives about one year, the benign tertian about three years, and the quartan somewhat longer than three years.

De Buys has emphasized the advisability of examining the blood of all members of the household in which there is a cured case which persists in relapsing. In his experience in Louisiana such examinations have exposed nonclinical carriers who were reinfecting the supposed "relapsing" cases.

THE NEW SPECIFICS IN MALARIA

(Plasmoquin and Atebrin)

In order to understand the tremendous readjustment which is taking place in the field of malarial therapy and prophylaxis, a brief review must be made of the following factors having to do with the disease, with quinine, and with the new drugs: (a) The stages in the life of the causative organism; (b) the several types of the disease; (c) the relapse rate; (d) the world supply of cinchona; and (e) the matter of quinine idiosyncrasy.

The Stages in the Life of the Organism.—When the mosquito bites a malaria-infected individual she takes into her stomach two forms of the plasmodium: schizonts and gametes, the latter called "crescents" in the case of malignant, estivo-autumnal infections. The schizonts are destroyed just as any other food substance, but the gametes, which are sexual forms, survive, fertilize, and eventually give rise to active sporozoites, which make their way into the salivary glands and are then injected into the blood of an individual subsequently bitten by the mosquito. These sporozoites enter red blood cells, undergo developmental changes (the so-called "ring forms"), and finally erupt into the blood stream as a shower of schizonts (asexual forms) and gametes (sexual forms). The gametes cause no symptoms and finally die if not taken out of the blood again by a mosquito, but the schizonts reenter fresh red corpuscles and repeat the cycle, giving rise to the fever and all the other symptoms of the disease. Now we do not know in what manner, or exactly when in the course of the asexual cycle within man, quinine strikes—but that the schizonts are pretty generally destroyed by the drug in effective doses is a fact established beyond all doubt. That is to say, other things being equal, quinine cures the disease, but it does not kill the sporozoites or the gametes (indeed, it even seems to stimulate the development of these latter), and so it does not prevent reinfection of the patient, on the one hand, or infection of mosquitoes, on the other.

The Several Types of the Disease.—So-called "benign" tertian malaria is caused by *Plasmodium vivax*, subtertian (malignant or estivo-autumnal) malaria is caused by *P. falciparum*, and the quartan form of the disease is caused by *P. malariae*. These three types of the disease not only vary typically in their symptomatology, but the virulence of the organisms themselves varies with the different geographical strains of the same species, as shown by James (1931) and his associates, who have found within the same species of subtertian parasites various geographical races which, while not morphologically different, can be recognized as distinct by their clinical virulence, immunological reactions, and other biological properties. Quinine cures very slowly in *P. malariae* cases, exerts its action somewhat more rapidly and effectively in *P. vivax*, but is far more truly "specific" in *P. falciparum* infections—though the above-mentioned workers have found wide variations in its action against strains of the latter from India, West Africa, Rome and Sardinia. Undoubtedly, temperate zone cases respond somewhat more rapidly and thoroughly to quinine than do cases in the tropical malaria belt, which is very likely due to the heavier load of infection which the latter have to sustain; and again, the greater ease with which severe cases are cured in such nonmalarial countries as England is no doubt in many instances attributable to the fact that the English cases are seen in persons who have experienced their earlier attacks in the tropics and have already acquired a certain amount of immunity to their particular infection. Watson's (1932) experience in Malaya causes him to think that the virulence of a strain, and hence to some extent its resistance to quinine, might vary. Nonimmune people entering an area where malaria is mild frequently become infected, and in turn infect the Malay population, with malaria which decimates both the new-comers and the residents; the virulence of the local strain had been increased by passage, would be his assumption.

The Relapse Rate.—In malaria the word "cure" must unfortunately be accepted as having two meanings: one which applies to the immediate response to therapy, which is practically always very excellent; and a second, which is a measure of the permanence of that response. In the second sense of the word, the cure of malaria is rarely accomplished in a short time, for although quinine will cause the complete subsidence of clinical symptoms and the disappearance of the parasites from the blood stream in all cases, the occurrence of one or more relapses—within a few days to weeks or months— is to be expected in a discouragingly large number of patients. The statistical evidence is difficult to cite comprehensibly because in all instances the quinine regimen employed by the patients must be very carefully taken into account; but it is evident in a general way that relapse occurs in 20 to 100 per cent of cases, the average being perhaps about 50 per cent if tropical and temperate zone cases are considered together; the rate in subtertian fever is much lower, but perhaps fully as high in quartan infections. The faith of Bass, and some others in the southern States, in the curative power (as evidenced by nonappearance of relapses) of an eight weeks' course of continuous quinine in practically 100 per cent of subtertian cases and just under 90 per cent of benign tertian and quartan cases, is certainly not shared by observers in other malarious regions—but it must be borne in mind that adverse conditions of many sorts have made practically impossible the institution of such a rigorous therapeutic regimen in any of the very heavily infected regions where mass measures must be employed. Whatever it is that causes these relapses in individuals clinically and parasitologically cured remains still a mystery—one of the most fascinating in the whole of medicine, by the way —but, be it what it may, quinine is quite ineffective in combating it.

The World Supply of Cinchona.—Ninety-five per cent of all the quinine produced in the world comes from cinchona bark raised in Dutch-owned Java. Upon the political and strategic import of this fact who could more feelingly speak than a German; I quote Mühlens (1932): "One who went through the World War on one of the malaria fronts (for instance in Macedonia) knows well what a great danger to health the shortage of quinine in the fight against malaria caused to our troops and those of our allies in the last years of the war. Whole army organizations were put out of commission by malaria. At times there was not even enough quinine for the thorough treatment of active cases at hand, to say nothing of prophylaxis! Our German chemical works could not supply enough quinine because of the lack of cinchona bark."

The Matter of Quinine Idiosyncrasy.—Quinine idiosyncrasy is encountered quite frequently, and though perhaps the majority of cases can be desensitized, the process is one requiring greater care and more intelligent cooperation than can be hoped for in most instances.

The Development of the New Drugs.—Since quinine consists of a quinoline ring bound to a basic heterocyclic group, it has generally been assumed that any synthetic substitute for it must be built upon some such conformation, and attempts to fashion such a compound had for some time been under way when, in 1925, it was the good fortune of the I.G.F., in Elberfeld, Germany, to put a stop temporarily at least to the search by their production of plasmoquin. The development by Roehl of a technic by which

many groups of drugs could be assayed upon canaries under controlled experimental conditions, and the treatment of general paralytics with malaria
inoculated through the mosquito, made possible the carrying out of tests in a
northern climate which ultimately brought success to this research; the
immediately responsible chemists were Hörlein, Schulemann, Schönhöfer and
Wingler.   The new drug (N-diethylamine-isopentyl-8-amino-6-methoxy-
quinoline) has a group formula and molecular weight very close to those of
quinine, but it is made entirely independently of cinchona bark—a purely
synthetic substance it is.   Studies in this field quickly showed that alone it is
not so destructive of schizonts in the subtertian form of the disease as is
quinine, and is therefore not of equal curative value, but that it has the
peculiar ability (possessed by no other drug hitherto employed) of rapidly
destroying gametes and thus rendering the patient noninfective, and also
that in combination with quinine it apparently increases the schizont-destroy-
ing power of the older drug.   More recently (1930), the same German dye
industry—Mietzsch and Mauss and Kikuth being the fortunate investigators
this time—has produced the second of the two new specifics: atebrin, an
alkylamino-acridine derivative, whose exact formula has not yet been
divulged.   This second product has been shown to have a destructive effect
upon schizonts and, for that reason, to be curative in the same sense that
quinine is.   It is therefore apparent that in these two drugs we have synthetic
substances of the first importance; their place in practical therapeutics, in
so far as it is already established, I shall attempt to set forth in what follows.

   The Use of Plasmoquin Alone; Therapeutic Effects.—The first to use
plasmoquin alone in the treatment of human malaria was Sioli (1926), who
successfully cured his 40 cases of paresis that had been inoculated with the
benign tertian organisms; not so very remarkable this, however, since quinine
will do the same thing.   But soon Mühlens (1927), and Mühlens and Fischer
(1927), reported on the treatment of 172 naturally acquired cases—either
acute relapsing or chronic cases treated in hospital in Hamburg.   With daily
doses of 0.05 to 0.1 Gm., and occasionally up to 0.15 Gm. (approximately
1 to 2 and 2½ grains), they conquered the fever after the second or third
day and caused disappearance of the parasites from the blood stream in five to
seven days; also the relapse rate was appreciably lower than would probably
have followed the use of quinine.   But these fine results could be obtained only
in benign tertian and quartan cases.   The failure in subtertian cases was evidenced not only by the fact that subtertian schizonts were very little reduced
but also by an excessively high relapse rate—in Mühlens' series, 34 relapses in
49 infections.   Roehl (1927), in Spain, cured 3 benign tertian and failed in 3
subtertian cases.   In Italy, Schulemann and Memmi (1927) put the drug to a
good test in over 100 cases, their dosage being 0.02 Gm. (⅓ grain) three
times daily for a week, a rest period of four days, the same doses three times
daily for three days, a rest period of four days, and then the three- and four-
day periods of alternating treatment and rest continued for six weeks.
Among the 24 benign tertian and the 4 quartan cases there occurred but one
relapse; in the remaining 60 odd subtertian cases the drug was a complete
failure.   This continued to be the tenor of all the reports that were made during the succeeding two years in which the drug was still being tried alone,
Hasselmann and Hasselmann-Kahlert (1928), in the Philippines, adding the
observation that in double infections in which only benign tertian parasites
appeared in the beginning, after the administration of plasmoquin subtertian
schizonts and gametes appeared in the blood stream.   The final verdict, then,
upon plasmoquin alone, so far as its therapeutic properties went, was that
it was at least equally as effective as quinine (and probably even more effective) in benign tertian and quartan cases, but that it was almost completely
ineffective in subtertian cases; and, furthermore, that whenever it was prob-

able that a subtertian infection had been superimposed upon a benign tertian or quartan infection, the drug should not be used alone.

Toxicity.—During the period in which plasmoquin was being used alone in the large dosage described above, cases of quite severe poisoning were included in practically all the reports—cyanosis of lips, face, fingers, toes; cardiac arrhythmias; gastro-intestinal pain and vomiting; pronounced disturbances in the proportions of the formed elements of the blood, usually lymphocytosis or leukocytosis being noted when looked for; jaundice; methemoglobinuria and methemoglobinemia. Orachowatz (1928) found that, in man, one third of the oxygen-carrying power of the blood may be lost through conversion of hemoglobin into methemoglobin. Sinton and Bird (1928) had to discontinue treatment in 22 of their 29 patients because of serious symptoms of poisoning. A number of fatal cases were reported, the principal finding at autopsy being an early central necrosis of the liver. The drug is better tolerated by children than by adults. It is neither necessary nor desirable to give it intravenously, since it is not effective in coma, and it has been shown experimentally to act upon the bundle of His to cause heart block.

The Effect on Gametes.—Almost from the first it became apparent that the outstanding characteristic of this drug, in addition to its ineffectiveness against the schizonts of subtertian cases, was its ability to destroy the infectiveness of the gametes of all three types of fever, thus enabling us to render malaria-infected individuals noninfective for mosquitoes, and therefore noninfective for man. Investigators in the Medical Department of the United Fruit Company (Barber, Komp and Newman; Whitmore; and Whitmore, Roberts and Jantzen) have established the fact that a single dose of 0.3 mg. per kilo body weight (approximately ¼ grain per hundred pounds) is sufficient to render the gametes noninfective for mosquitoes and to maintain this noninfectivity for a probable period of four to seven days.

Plasmoquin Combined with Quinine (Plasmoquin Compound).—Because of the limitation of the usefulness of plasmoquin when given alone, Schulemann and Memmi, in 1927, strongly advocated its combination with quinine. Now such a compound—to be referred to hereafter as "plasmoquin compound"—if it is to establish a place for itself must satisfy the following requirements: (*a*) Since it comprises the use of large amounts of quinine, as well as small amounts of plasmoquin, it must accomplish either quicker cures or more permanent cures (lower relapse rate) than quinine when used alone; (*b*) it must be fully as effective, and preferably more effective, than quinine in these same doses in subtertian cases (in which plasmoquin alone is not effective), and it must be more effective in rendering gametes noninfective for mosquitoes than quinine in the same doses alone (that is to say, by combining plasmoquin with quinine it must not lose the antigamete effect which it is known to have when given alone).

The reports of the usefulness of the compound in benign cases (tertian and quartan) have been favorable from the beginning. Manson-Bahr (1927–28) gave tablets containing 0.01 Gm. (⅙ grain) plasmoquin and 0.125 Gm. (2 grains) quinine; two such tablets three times daily for seven days, an interval of four days, then alternating seven-day dosage periods and four-day rest periods until the entire treatment had comprised a term of fifty-one days —that is to say, about the seven to eight weeks that it is usually considered necessary to give quinine alone to accomplish permanent cure. The parasites disappeared from the peripheral blood stream in two or three days and the relapse rate was very low. Sinton (1930) and his associates, among many others, agreed as to the efficacy of the compound but felt that the plasmoquin dosage was too large and the quinine too small; they advocated not more than 0.04 Gm. (⅔ grain) of plasmoquin daily, preferably 0.03 Gm. (½ grain), and 0.2 Gm. (20 grains) of quinine. There is now general agreement that the lesser dosage of plasmoquin is just as effective and should be employed. Deeks and Connor (United Fruit Company, 1930) believe that in the chronic, quinine-resisting cases in which the drug acts so well, it should be given in dosage of 0.01 to 0.03 Gm. ($\frac{1}{6}$ to $\frac{1}{2}$ grain) daily for five or six days, then suspended for three days, and again given for five or six days— always in combination with quinine, of course. Of the many other reports essentially in agreement with those already cited, I can consider only one more—the recent exhaustive trial of the compound in the Indian army, as reported by Manifold (1931). In the treatment of all cases of benign tertian malaria, a tablet was used which contained 0.02 Gm. ($\frac{1}{3}$ grain) of plasmoquin and 0.6 Gm. (10 grains) of quinine, one such tablet being given morning and evening uninterruptedly for twenty-one days. In all, 3187 (1286 British, 1901 Indian) completed the course. It was not possible under the conditions to vary the dosage in accordance with individual requirements, and any fresh attack within six months of completion of the treatment was considered a relapse. As regards the pyrexia, it was found that upon the whole the patients responded more rapidly than they would have done under quinine alone, and in no case was it necessary to administer quinine intravenously, or intramuscularly. The average relapse rate was astonishingly low—5.2 per cent. If cases relapsing after what could be roughly considered the end of the malaria season at the various stations only were accepted as relapses, then the relapse rate would be as low as 2.4 per cent.

Other dosage schemes than the above have been used; such as 0.04 Gm. ($\frac{2}{3}$ grain) plasmoquin and 1.2 Gm. (20 grains) of quinine daily for one week, followed by four days' rest and three days' treatment alternately for the next five weeks; or with the plasmoquin reduced to 0.03 Gm. ($\frac{1}{2}$ grain) throughout the course; indeed, Bustillo (1930), who carries his patients on quinine for two months, combines only 0.01 Gm. ($\frac{1}{6}$ grain) of plasmoquin with it for the first four days, and reports excellent results (in children under five years of age he gives 0.005 Gm. ($\frac{1}{12}$ grain) daily for eight days). Practically all observers are agreed, then, that the addition of small amounts of plasmoquin to the quinine regimen increases both the rapidity and the permanence of cure in benign cases.

In subtertian (malignant or estivo-autumnal) cases the compound has not been a brilliant success; that is to say, such increase in rate and permanence of cure as has resulted from adding plasmoquin to quinine in handling these cases can probably be ascribed to its rendering the quinine somewhat more effective, plasmoquin itself being not deadly to the schizonts in this type of the disease. It is of interest to refer here to Bass's belief that the injury to the blood cells which might be assumed to occur as a result of the methemoglobinemia, would tend to make unfavorable the soil in which the plasmodia live, and thus aid quinine indirectly in its attack upon them. Schulemann and Memmi treated 63 cases thrice daily with 0.02 Gm. ($\frac{1}{3}$ grain) of plasmoquin and 0.25 Gm. (4 grains) of quinine, with the elimination of parasites after the eighth day; the relapses were 20 per cent. Polychroniades (1927) employed the same dosage in 139 cases; the gametes (crescents) had disappeared by the eighth day, schizonts (ring form) by the tenth; the relapse rate was 10.8 per cent. Sliwensky (1927), in Bulgaria, gave 0.06 Gm. (1 grain) and 0.75 Gm. (12 grains) per day for from five to twelve days; relapses 30.4 per cent. I believe that the compound is not well thought of at all in regions, such as West Africa, where the cases are almost exclusively of the subtertian variety.

Effect of Plasmoquin Compound on Gametes.—I have earlier referred to the publications of Col. Whitmore, Dr. Barber, Mr. Komp and their associates, in which the devitalizing effect upon gametes of a very small dose of plasmoquin was shown. In Bustillo's series of cases, also previously mentioned, the very small dose of 0.01 Gm. (⅙ grain) plasmoquin, plus 1.2 Gm. (20 grains) quinine, for four days caused the crescents to disappear from the blood in 31 of 34 cases in from one to eight days, and in the remaining cases by the twelfth day. Macphial (1930), summarizing the results of the administration of 1,388,000 tablets in the United Fruit Company service, states that the gametes of all forms of malaria are destroyed by doses of 0.03 to 0.04 Gm. (½ to ⅔ grain) daily for one week—all observers all over the world are in agreement with this, so that there can be no doubt that the drug *does* render the infected individual noninfective for mosquitoes.

Toxicity of Plasmoquin Compound.—In the Indian army experiment, in which, it will be recalled, 3187 cases were treated uninterruptedly for twenty-one days, a careful study of the toxicity of the compound was made. The outstanding feature of this aspect of the report is that there could not have been any great amount of seriously unpleasant symptoms, since the above large number of patients, all of whom completed the full course, represents 99 per cent of the original number at the outset of the experiment. The one constant complaint was abdominal pain, which occurred with less frequency when the drug was taken on a full stomach or with a large draught of water. It began usually quite early and increased in severity during the first weeks but disappeared very quickly on temporary cessation of the plasmoquin administration. Cyanosis was recorded in 4.3 per cent of the British and probably occurred in a like proportion of the Indians; it became clinically evident about the seventh day and appears to have been greater in frequency among anemic individuals. Many patients lost their pink complexion during the treatment without becoming actually cyanosed. In the average case continuance of the treatment did not increase the methemoglobinemia and apparently did no harm. There were two deaths among the Indian cases; one was thought to have been ascribable to the plasmoquin and the other was probably a blackwater fever fatality. Whether or not such symptoms indicate an idiosyncrasy toward the drug, corresponding to such occurrences under quinine, is not as yet definitely known. It is of considerable importance to note that this large series of cases was at all times under careful medical scrutiny, since there are many physicians both in and out of the tropics who believe that the drug should be administered only under these circumstances. Such experienced physicians as Deeks and Connor, however, believe that in the small daily doses of 0.01 to 0.03 Gm. (⅙ to ½ grain) it is practically nontoxic and may be safely left in the hands of the layman to administer. It will be extremely interesting to watch the development of opinion upon this point.

Plasmoquin Compound in Pregnancy.—Several papers have appeared upon the successful administration of plasmoquin to pregnant women in both the tropical and temperate zones. The most recent to come to my attention is that of Manson-Bahr (1932), who has treated 5 cases of malaria of all three types in women in the third to eighth month of pregnancy. All were given full therapeutic doses of the compound over a period of five separate weeks. There were no further relapses either during pregnancy or postpartum, and all the children were born at full term, there having been one stillbirth due to instrumentation. He writes, "I consider that the appropriate therapeutic dose of plasmoquin compound in this condition is four tablets of the standardized product daily—0.04 Gm. (⅔ grain) of plasmoquin plus 0.5 Gm. (8 grains) of quinine sulphate—for five separate weeks with a pause of three days interval between each weekly course."

Plasmoquin Compound in Quinine Idiosyncrasy.—The compound in the usual doses, has a number of times been successfully used in individuals with a pronounced idiosyncrasy to quinine. In a recent discussion of the usefulness of plasmoquin in malaria at a meeting of the Royal Society of Tropical Medicine and Hygiene, in London, Castellani stated his belief that one of the special advantages of the drug is to be found just here.

Plasmoquin Compound in Blackwater Fever.—The compound has been used with apparent success in a small number of cases of blackwater fever, but since the recovery rate is 75 to 80 per cent normally in this disease, the part that any new remedial agent plays in promoting recovery is extremely difficult to determine except upon a prodigiously large series of cases under perfectly controlled conditions. There are a few observers who believe that the drug may play a part in precipitating the attack, as quinine is alleged to do, but they have not yet been able to establish the worth of their thesis.

Plasmoquin Compound in the Prophylaxis of Malaria.—So far as measures which may be applied to the mosquito-bitten individual are concerned, the only ones by which malaria can be prevented are the administration to him of a drug which will kill the active sporozoites injected by the mosquito, or the more indirect one of employing in the treatment of active cases a drug which will kill the gametes and thus prevent infection of mosquitoes. Quinine will do neither of these things but apparently plasmoquin will under the circumstances which I shall attempt to set down here. James, Nicol and Shute (1931) performed the classical experiments by which the prophylactic properties of the drug were demonstrated. Under conditions of absolute control in the Horton Mental Hospital, in England, they proceeded as follows: (*a*) Mosquitoes were infected from a case of benign tertian; (*b*) ten volunteers were bitten by these mosquitoes on the second day after instituting a prophylactic régime consisting of one tablet of 0.02 Gm. ($\frac{1}{3}$ grain) of plain plasmoquin three times a day (after breakfast, after lunch and at bedtime) for six days; (*c*) four persons who took no prophylactic and one who took quinine as a prophylactic were also bitten. Result: Malaria developed in all of the unprotected individuals within the usual fourteen days, but it did not develop in any of the individuals taking the plasmoquin as prophylactic. This work was accepted as establishing the prophylactic value of the drug beyond doubt, and it was felt that, though the dosage employed was certainly too high to be continuously used by persons resident in malarial regions, it could nevertheless be at once accepted as a great boon to the large population of merchant ships who could easily take the drug during the few days of their stay in infected tropical ports. Then unfortunately James was obliged to report that 50 per cent of the plasmoquin-protected individuals developed clinical malaria between seven and nine months later. And Swellengrebel and de Buck (1931), reducing the daily dose of plasmoquin from 0.06 to 0.03 Gm. (1 to $\frac{1}{2}$ grain), failed to prevent the appearance of the disease in practically all cases a few days after the conclusion of the six-day prophylactic drugging. Thus it is apparent that a more satisfactory method of using the drug must be sought, and has quite likely already been found, for it is known that many persons in regions of heavy malarial infestation are successfully using it in small prophylactic doses. Ronnefeldt (1931) reports the cases of six adult European residents of West Africa who have successfully protected themselves against all forms of the disease— malignant tertian has its principal stronghold in this region—by a daily régime as follows: 2 cases, plasmoquin 0.01 Gm. ($\frac{1}{6}$ grain) once daily for over three years; 4 cases, one tablet of the same twice daily for more than one year. There have been no side-effects noted. Two children have successfully received a single dose every second day during one year and eight months, respectively. Mass prophylactic measures, too, employing smaller dosage, are beginning to appear in the literature. The most valuable of these field experiments so far is that of Kingsbury and Amies (1931), who have given 0.04 Gm. ($\frac{2}{3}$ grain) plasmoquin twice weekly to 330 people on a rubber estate in the Straits Settlements, using the populations of two contiguous estates as controls. The experiment was continued for a period of twelve months. In the preceding twelve months the case incidence of subtertian and benign tertian respectively had been 30.4 and 52.5 per cent of the population. In the experimental year the incidence was respectively 7 and 8.7 per cent. The improvement in the general physical condition of the laborers was marked; on the experimental estate the general sickness rate fell 51 per cent during the year, as against a fall of only 11 per cent on one of the two control estates and a rise of 21 per cent on the other. The cost of this method of prophylaxis, in the Straits Settlements, was about $600 per annum per 100 laborers, including treatment of the average number of dependents. By a different mode of attack, namely, the thorough treatment of all active cases with plasmoquin compound Clemesha and Moore (1931) have practically eliminated malaria from a number of large tea estates in Ceylon that had previously been very heavily burdened with the disease; but unfortunately a controversy has arisen between Col. Clemesha and Sir Malcolm Watson, of the Ross Institute, regarding the part antilarval measures played in this fine achievement. However, I feel that plasmoquin is undoubtedly of tremendous value as a prophylactic agent; only the proper methods of utilizing it to best advantage are still to be developed.

Atebrin.—It seems now to be definitely established that the newer of these two new drugs, atebrin, has a powerful destructive action upon schizonts in all three types of the disease but practically no effect upon gametes. It would therefore be in no wise superior to quinine and would have its only field as a substitute for that drug when such substitution was financially advantageous or was forced by political necessity—I say this would be true were it not for the fact that it is beginning to appear that atebrin is oftentimes effective in curing cases in which quinine has acted only very sluggishly. In the 17 cases of this sort recently reported by James, Nicol and Shute (1932), it seems that the drug has wrought what appears to be a permanent cure in all save 1 case—these were all subtertian infections, atebrin being given alone in a daily dose of 0.3 Gm. (5 grains) for five days. Greene (1932) has published his notes on 50 cases of all three types treated in Malaya against 46 controls that were quinine treated. The atebrin rid the blood of schizonts fully as well as quinine but was not effective against gametes, particularly those of *P. falciparum* (subtertian parasite). In relief of symptoms it seemed superior to quinine in that it had more effectively prevented relapses up to the time of the report. He feels that the optimum dosage in all forms of malaria is probably 0.1 Gm. per 15 Kg. (approximately 5 grains per 100 pounds) body weight per day for six or seven days, the treatment to be preceded by a purge just as in the use of quinine. The drug is yellow and causes the urine to assume the same color on about the third or fourth day; if it has not appeared by that time Greene believes that medication should be stopped, for the drug will then cause a yellow discoloration of the skin which persists for one to two weeks and is regarded by him as an indication that it is accumulating in the body in greater concentration than is desirable. This yellow discoloration of the skin is due to the acridine dye nature of the drug and not to jaundice as the result of injury to the liver.

Atebrin in Combination with Plasmoquin.—Mühlens (1932), who has had probably more experience with atebrin, both in Hamburg and in tropical Central and South America and Mexico, than anyone else, has tried it in various dosages and combinations and now favors, for tropical practice at least, and especially in subtertian cases, a dosage of 0.1 Gm. (approximately 2 grains) atebrin plus 0.01 Gm. (⅙ grain) plasmoquin three times daily for seven to ten days. In very severe cases he advises in addition the intramuscular administration of quinine on the first two days. The combination of atebrin, as powerful schizont-destroyer, and plasmoquin, as powerful gamete-destroyer, he regards an ideal two-pointed weapon with which to attack malaria, especially the malignant (subtertian) cases.

Atebrin in Quinine Idiosyncrasy, in Blackwater Fever, and in the Prophylaxis of Malaria.—A single isolated instance of the successful use of atebrin in each of the first two above-listed conditions is mentioned in passing by Mühlens; of it as a prophylactic little is probably to be expected— but this is only my own personal surmise from the nature of the drug's reported action, and may easily be refuted by experience in the future.

Atebrin Toxicity.—In Greene's series of 50 cases, two complained of headache and three of severe, and one of mild, abdominal pain unaccompanied by vomiting. These symptoms appeared either during the administration of the drug or several days after the cessation of same; they lasted only for some hours. The atebrin did not appear to give rise to albuminuria, and in 2 cases an initial albuminuria disappeared during its administration.

MEASLES
(Rubeola, Morbilli)

Measles is an acute infectious disease more than 95 per cent of whose victims are under fifteen and more than 50 per cent under five years of age. It is so highly contagious that practically every child who is exposed contracts the disease, with the exception of infants under four months. Adults also are susceptible, as was distressingly shown during the late World War when severe epidemics prevailed in the American mobilization camps among recruits from rural districts who had escaped the disease, and the immunity a single attack confers, in their childhood. The disease is endemic in large cities and often becomes epidemic. In London these epidemics occur regularly at intervals of two years, attacking no less than 50,000 children each time. In New York City in recent even-numbered years the cases have averaged about 35,000, while in the odd-numbered years there have been only about 3000 cases. The incubation period may be as short as seven days but is never longer than fifteen days. The early symptoms are catarrhal inflammation of the eyes, nose and upper respiratory tract, fever, and the malaise, chilliness, loss of appetite, vomiting, etc., which characterize many of the acute infectious diseases in their incipiency. In addition there is an eruption (Koplik's spots) on the buccal mucous membrane which, together with an early reduction in the number of lymphocytes, is of very great diagnostic importance. Then, on about the fourth day and often after the fever has entirely disappeared, the typical dusky, crescentic, blotchy, maculopapular rash appears, principally on the face and back, and is accompanied by a recrudescence of all the symptoms. After the eruption reaches its height, which occurs in from thirty-six hours to three days, the patient begins rapidly to improve, though the skin usually retains for a week or more a brownish stain where the eruption has faded. The branny desquamation is complete within ten days.

Measles respects neither climate nor race. In early days it was confused with scarlet fever, but Sydenham clearly differentiated the two diseases in the seventeenth century. Of the two, measles has become in recent years the more serious menace to young life. In a London letter to the Journal of the American Medical Association, of date November 13, 1926, it was stated that the annual death rate due to measles in that metropolis had become 251 per million, as compared with 42 per million from scarlet fever. Herrman has said that measles is responsible for 2.4 per cent of all deaths in children under ten years of age. The disease itself is practically never fatal, but the complications, bronchopneumonia, laryngitis and enteritis, bring the mortality up to 6 per cent among children in good hygienic and nutritional surroundings, 15 per cent among children in institutions, and as high as 35 per cent among adults living under barrack conditions. Complicating encephalitis and other clinical types of nervous sequelae do not very much contribute to increase the mortality.

Caronis and others, in Italy, claim to have isolated the causative organism, propagated it and produced a protective vaccine from it, but attempts to confirm their findings have failed in both England and the United States. The researches of Tunnicliff and her co-workers, also of Ferry and Fisher, and of Cary and Day with a green producing diplococcus obtained from the nose, throat and eye secretions and the blood of early measles patients, are interesting, but before we look with too great enthusiasm upon this work it is well to recall that the Dicks, in their early scarlet fever investigations, were forced to conclude that in the acute stages of scarlatinal angina, organisms from the throat, regardless of their identity, often enter the blood stream in considerable numbers. The production of immune goat serum with this organism (p. 116) is, of course, a point strongly in its favor. The preliminary investigations of Degkwitz seem to show that the measles virus, whatever it may be, has the ability to grow outside the human body.

THERAPY

The general treatment of measles is that of catarrhal fever (see p. 24), for there is no specific remedy. Especial care *must* be taken to prevent cross infection as death rides jauntily in the wake of complications here. Complete isolation with the nurse is the ideal to be approximated as closely as is possible. Keep the patient warm in an airy room, protected from direct drafts. Admit all the sunlight possible, but protect the eyes, either by the use of dark glasses or improvised screens, and irrigate them frequently with boric acid solution; the application of petrolatum (vaselin) may prevent adhesion of the lids. Placing the child for a few minutes in a warm pack will often "bring out" a delayed rash. The irritation of the skin which is sometimes annoying during the period of the rash will usually yield to sponging with a dilute sodium bicarbonate solution; if excessive, 1 per cent phenol may be substituted. The daily bath should be continued during the desquamation period, but it is well to follow it at this time with an application of albolene or petrolatum. Petrolatum to soften crusts, and sprays (see Catarrhal Fever, p. 30) for whatever they may be worth, are available for keeping the nose clean and comfortable, but their application in a way that will suit the young patient will tax the ingenuity of any nurse.

Watch the ears, watch the throat, watch the temperature and respirations: in a word, *watch for complications*.

Amidopyrine.—In 1924, Loewenthal published an account of the use of amidopyrine (pyramidon), and a number of physicians have since reported its successful use. Ronaldson and Collier (1930) have surveyed their results in 150 cases, which they carefully point out were treated in a year in which the measles prevalent in London was milder than usual. The dosage adopted was 1 grain (0.06 Gm.) for every year of age, with a maximum of 5 grains (0.3 Gm.), administered in aqueous solution of 1 grain to the drachm (0.06 to 4.0) every four hours until the temperature had settled. In addition to the antipyretic effect, the tendency to bronchopneumonia and some of the other complications was lessened, but not laryngitis and enteritis. On the other hand, in Attle's record of a school epidemic of 129 cases among boys of twelve and one-half to sixteen and one-half years of age, the 9 cases treated with 5 grains (0.3 Gm.) per four hours, as above, were more uncomfortable than the others, they vomited frequently, their rashes took longer to mature, their fever was more prolonged, and they suffered a higher percentage of complications. Likewise, in Borovsky and Steigmann's (1933) study of 194 cases, in which alternate patients were given the drug, they found nothing that would indicate a special therapeutic value for it.

PROPHYLAXIS

Measles spreads so rapidly because it is most infectious in the period prior to the appearance of the eruption. After the eruption has reached its height the contagiousness is practically nil; indeed, many municipal health departments permit the release of a child from quarantine five days after this time, provided, of course, that it is well and that the acute rash has disappeared. The bounden duty of physicians toward the individual and the community is to quarantine all susceptible exposed persons, preferably in a separate house from the sick individual, for a period of two weeks from the date of exposure.

Several methods of preventative inoculation have recently won a place for themselves and must be considered here.

Convalescent Serum or Plasma.—More than thirty years ago a German physician is said to have successfully employed large amounts of serum from convalescents in the treatment of several cases of measles in which the symptoms were just beginning, but Nicolle and Conseil, in France, 1918, were the first to publish on the method. Since that time the efficacy of convalescent serum in preventing or modifying the disease has been established by many well-qualified observers; full references to the work of the following investigators will be found in the Bibliography: Park and Freeman; Zingher; Haas and Blum; Richardson and Connor; Degkwitz; Zimmermann; Spencer; Reitschel; Blackfan, Peterson and Conroy; Davis; Brügger; Weaver and Crooks; Debré and Ravina; Nabarro and Signay; Bang; Morales and Mandry; Warwick; Siegel and Ermann; Burn. I shall not attempt here a detailed analysis of these reports for the reason that it would occupy too much space. The practical facts which have already emerged lend themselves to very simple statement.

(a) Convalescent serum may safely be collected five days after defervescence of the fever, or any time thereafter, but the more recent the attack, the more potent the serum. The dose of such serum is 5 to 15 cc., according to the age of the child; it is best given intramuscularly. If administered prior to the fifth, or at most the seventh, day after exposure it will entirely prevent the occurrence of the disease in about 90 per cent of individuals. The immunity it confers is passive and lasts for only two to six weeks. If, however, it is administered in the same dose after the seventh day, though it fails to prevent the attack it does so modify it that complications are very little to be feared, and the child has a lasting active immunity conferred upon him by this light attack. Also, if one half the above dose, i. e., 2.5 to 7.5 cc., is given before the fifth day after exposure it will cause the appearance of this modified form of the disease. The incubation period in these modified cases is usually abnormally long.

(b) The serum of grown children, or adults who have had the disease some years previously, is also to a considerable extent effective in causing the occurrence of modified cases. It must be given in a dose of 25 to 100 cc. if the attempt is to be made to completely prevent the attack, or in a dose of 10 to 20 cc. if it is desired to permit the disease to appear in the attenuated form which brings life-long immunity with it.

(c) Park and Freeman have described a method of using plasma instead of serum because of the greater yield for the amount of blood drawn and the greater ease of handling; their method is described as follows:

"At the Willard Parker Hospital, blood was drawn on the ninth day after the defervescence of fever up to the twenty-first day, but at the Southern University the time was more varied, and some was drawn as late as five months after the disease. In the case of adults, all the blood was drawn through a 16 gage Luer needle into a 500 cc. bottle containing 20 cc. of 25 per cent sodium citrate solution and 0.3 Gm. of oxyquinolin sulphate (chinosol) as a preservative. This preparation was used because it was found that in the dilution in which it was used it was an efficient bactericidal agent; the red cells were not destroyed, and it was not irritating when injected intramuscularly. The bottles were then put in the icebox and the cells allowed to settle, or were centrifugalized, and the plasma pipetted off. Blood for a Wassermann test was taken at the time of bleeding, and a sterility test was done at the time the plasma was put up in small bottles. . . . All the blood drawn within six days of the same period of convalescence was pooled. Thus far, the figures indicate that the efficiency of the plasma is not markedly diminished by postponing bleeding for three months after the occurrence of the disease, and that storage in the icebox for six months does not appreciably alter its usefulness."

The plasma is used in the same dose as is the serum. Haas and Blum have confirmed Park and Freeman as to the efficiency of the plasma thus prepared and stored.

(*d*) Lichtenstein (1931) has described the preparation of dried serum. Serums that have been Wassermann and sterility tested are pooled, 0.5 per cent phenol is added, the mixture divided into 5-cc. portions in wide-necked flasks, and completely dried in an exsiccator with a suction pump—a procedure that takes one to three days. The flasks are then corked and sealed with paraffin and stored in the refrigerator, specimens being tested for sterility from time to time. Such dried serum, even after several years of storage, can be dissolved in one or two hours; its efficiency seems to be somewhat diminished after two or three years, so that slightly larger doses than of the fresh serum must be employed.

(*e*) Finkelstein (1931) has employed pooled placental serum: 5 per cent phenol was added, the serum was inactivated for one-half to one hour at 56 C., and the sterility was subsequently tested. The results—using doses of 40 to 60 cc.—were equally as good as with fresh adult serum; Jorge (1932), Dulitskiy (1932), and de Souza (1932) have also reported favorably. McKhann and Chu (1933) are studying a concentrated preparation of the globulins from placental blood and tissues; the standardization of the extract and its dosage are still to be worked out, but the preliminary observations indicate that it has high protective value.

Convalescent Blood from a "Family Donor."—Except in child-caring institutions, donors for convalescent blood are difficult to find as the parents of the convalescent school child are usually unwilling that their child should contribute his blood for the sake of others in the community. A number of cities are following the example of the New York City Board of Health in obtaining measles serum for distribution, but most physicians in private practice still face a real problem in their responsibility toward their young patients at the beginning of a measles epidemic. However, if the blood is needed to protect a sister or brother, no objections are raised by parents, a fact which can be turned to good account while waiting for a supply of convalescent serum to become available, as was recently pointed out by Forbes and Green. They write: "The family epidemic of measles is almost invariably inaugurated by the oldest child, who is, as a rule, attending school. . . . Measles contacts are probably exposed from one to two days before the rash appears on the patient, and the patient's febrile period is usually terminated about three days after the rash appears unless complications develop. Thus, immune blood is available to the contacts in most cases about five to six days after exposure. The titer of immune bodies at this time is presumably less than will develop later, according to the work of Degkwitz, but a reasonably high titer of immune bodies must be present at the termination of fever." They therefore withdrew blood on the first or second day of normal temperature and injected this whole blood into the gluteal muscles of the younger children; the dose varied from 6 to 12 cc. At the time of their report (1927) they had a series of only 7 cases, ranging from nine months to eight years, but it is worth noting that they modified the measles attack in 6 of the 7 and that in the other case, the nine-month old infant, the disease did not appear at all.

Adult Whole Blood.—Following the results reported by Degkwitz (1920), in Germany, the use of adult whole blood gained wide recognition on the Continent, but in America no great amount of interest in the method was shown until Park urged its more general adoption in 1930. The thing is simplicity itself. About 30 cc. of blood is drawn from a vein at the elbow into a sterile syringe and then half of it is immediately injected into the child's right buttock, the other half into the left. There are no ill effects, and it is not necessary to type the blood of the child or of the parent, who is usually the donor. Indeed, it would seem to be scarcely necessary to inquire whether the donor has had measles, since most adults in large cities have had the disease in childhood; at least one of the parents will probably have had it anywhere. It is probable that in children above five years of age double the amount of blood should be injected, but it is well to remember that the principal object of the procedure is to insure a mild attack rather than to prevent the disease altogether.

Bader (1931), who was one of the pioneers in employing prophylaxis of this type in the United States, now advocates discrimination in the choice of donors: "older children in the family who have had measles, or adults who have had measles not more than ten to fifteen years previously, or persons (interns and nurses) who have had measles and are in frequent contact with the disease." Such blood (*i. e.*, not obtained from the parents) should, of course, preferably be Wassermann tested; but even it does not have to be typed since the injections are again intramuscularly.

All observers have found this method (particularly if parents' blood is employed) the least objectionable and most practical means of preventing or modifying measles particularly at the onset of an epidemic before convalescent serum becomes available—all, that is, except Blauner and Goldstein (1931), who failed in their attempt to immunize a group of 117 children, in 112 of whom citrated whole blood from professional donors was employed, and in 5 cases whole blood from parents with a positive history of measles.

Immune Goat Serum.—Tunnicliff has showed that the serum of a goat convalescing from the reaction produced by inoculation of her green producing diplococcus is capable of protecting rabbits against a subsequent injection of infective material from measles, though it should be pointed out that the susceptibility of rabbits to the same virus that produces measles in man has not been proved. However this may be, it seems that the repeated inoculation of goats with this diplococcus and the filtrate of dextrose broth cultures of the organism is capable of producing an antiserum which has protective value against measles in man. Hoyne and Gasul used this immune goat serum in 39 children over six months of age, and concluded that if the serum was administered not later than the fifth day of exposure protection seemed assured in about 90 per cent of cases. There were no deaths or complications in any of the patients who developed measles after getting the serum, while among the nine contacts who received no serum, eight contracted measles and two of these died. Peterman (1928) reported that 31 of 34 children inoculated on or before the fifth day after exposure did not develop measles; and he later (1930) added 61 children and 6 adults (with reliable negative histories) to his series, obtaining protection in 74.6 per cent of this last 77 persons. Favorable results have also been published by Tunnicliff and Hoyne (1926), Halpern (1928), and Hoyne and Peacock (1928). Barenberg, Lewis and Messer (1930) have failed completely to obtain any protection—either against the disease, its severity or its complications—in 38 children, 20 of whom were given the serum during the first three days of the incubation period, 12 from one to six days, and 6 from eight to eighteen days prior to infection.

The dosage of this serum is from 5 to 8 cc., given intramuscularly. Serum reactions are to be expected in about 12 per cent of cases, though in Halpern's series of 50 cases there were no reactions. The passive immunity conferred persists for only a few weeks.

Active Immunization of Infants.—In 1914, Herrman inoculated a group of healthy babies between four and five months old by swabbing the fresh nasal mucus of patients just coming down with measles on the nasal mucosa of his subjects. His purpose was to introduce the virus at a time when some degree of inherited immunity would be present, but with the object of producing an active immunity. Seventy-five of his subjects were watched from four to eight years; 70 of them remained free from measles, 62 of the number having been directly or indirectly exposed to the disease. The method is scientifically sound, though probably considered impracticable for use by most physicians in private practice.

German Measles (Rubella, Rötheln).—This highly contagious disease resembles measles and scarlet fever but is distinct from both. It is probably caused by a filtrable virus present in the nasal secretions. The differential points in its diagnosis will not be gone into here; suffice it to say that an outstanding feature of the disease is an adenitis of the mastoid, occipital, cervical, and often the inguinal and axillary glands. An attack of measles seems to predispose to infection with German measles. Complications are very rare and when they do occur are usually not severe.

MILIARY FEVER

This is a disease of unknown etiology that occurs in limited epidemics of not more than a week or two. There is high fever, great sweating, profound prostration, and an erythematous rash with miliary vesicles. Between 1718 (when it was first described, though it had probably existed before) and 1861 there were about 175 epidemics recorded in France alone; Italy and southern Germany have also known the disease, but not, I believe, Great Britain. The last reported outbreak occurred in France, in 1926. The mortality is usually low.

It is very doubtful if this disease is the same as that "sweating sickness" which devastated England and the Continent several times in the fifteenth and sixteenth centuries, for John Kaye, or Caius, an eminent London physician who described the outbreaks of 1552, had nothing to say about an eruption of any sort.

THERAPY

I do not know of any treatment that warrants particular description.

MILK SICKNESS

This is a very old disease in the United States, having been known apparently to the Indians, but it has never appeared anywhere else. In the early frontier days, cattle browsing in uncleared land and wild pastures were often attacked by a peculiar disease known as "trembles," from which they died, and from which birds and beasts of carrion that fed upon their carcasses died also. Man was attacked if he drank the milk or ate the flesh of affected cattle even though these products were thoroughly cooked. The symptoms are: Violent vomiting, extreme weakness, obstinate constipation, swollen tongue, subnormal temperature, and a characteristic odor of the body emanations. The mortality is extremely high. It is described here among the infectious diseases because a distinctive micro-organism has been found more or less constantly upon the vegetation eaten by affected animals; it is most probably caused, however, by the ingestion by the cattle of poisonous snake-root and rayless goldenrod plants, irrespective of their contamination with the micro-organism.

Although the disease has practically disappeared with the bringing of most of the land in the country under cultivation, an outbreak is recorded in Illinois as late as 1904. It is a fact of no little interest that many of the apparently purposeless peregrinations of the Lincoln family during the boyhood of the Emancipator were in reality flights from this blighting disease. Abraham's mother, and at least three of his close kin, died of it.

THERAPY

I know of nothing to record, except that the studies of Bulger, Smith and Steinmeyer (1928), in animals poisoned by white snake-root, indicated that some of the symptoms of milk sickness might be caused by the marked ketosis, lipemia and profound hypoglycemia which they observed. This would, of course, call for the prompt administration of glucose.

MUMPS
(Epidemic Parotitis)

Mumps is an acute infectious disease of goats, dogs, cats and man. It occurs all over the world and tends to become epidemic during the winter months. The greatest age frequency has been thought to be between five and fifteen years in man, but in Meyer and Reifenberg's series (1926) of 136 cases, 66 were between two and six, and 35 between six and fifteen years old. The disease is also of frequent occurrence among young men in their twenties and early thirties if they are crowded together as in barracks or aboard ship. The Surgeon General of the United States Army reports that in 1918 mumps accounted for 7.15 per cent of admissions to army hospitals, the total number of cases of this disease being 166,370. It was the fourth disease on the list of admissions, both in America and abroad, according to Wollstein, but it was the second largest cause of loss of time. Attacks in early infancy and in the years beyond forty are rare but not unknown. Well-authenticated second, third and even fourth attacks are on record. Moore (1931) has recorded a case complicating pregnancy in which the symptoms were so severe as to jeopardize the patient's life.

The chief symptom of mumps is a swelling of one of the parotid glands, accompanied by stiffness of the jaws and pain which is accentuated upon opening the mouth or attempting to swallow. There is usually a slight rise in temperature. In some cases the opposite parotid swells also but involvement of the other salivary glands is infrequent. Only in the more severe cases do the constitutional symptoms progress beyond slight prodromata, such as headache, chilliness and loss of appetite. A slowed pulse rate and a lymphocytosis are observable in practically all cases. The attack is usually terminated within a week of its inception; a quarantine period of two weeks is sufficient in average cases. Orchitis of the affected side occurs in 15 to 30 per cent of boys past puberty and young men who are attacked by mumps. It is frequently preceded by epididymitis, is accompanied by a considerable degree of prostration, and results in atrophy of the testicle in about half the cases. A similar involvement of the ovaries is less common in women. Other complications are rare and mild, except that in some epidemics a benign type of meningitis occurs in about a fourth of the cases. Deafness, unassociated with meningeal involvement, occasionally occurs and is usually permanent.

Wollstein has shown that the virus of mumps is present in the mouth secretions of individuals having the disease. Droplet infection is therefore probably the rule, since transmission can take place before the swelling appears, but the possibility of human and cat and dog carriers has not been investigated. Kermorgant believes that the filtrable virus is a finely granular spirochete; Tang (1931) has more recently offered a virus of his own— neither investigator has substantiated his claims.

THERAPY

Very little treatment is indicated save for relief of the pain. The patient usually is somewhat relieved by the prolonged use of hot or cold applications. The U.S.P. belladonna ointment sometimes eases the pain also if applied over the swelling. The attempt is sometimes made to have an antiseptic mouth wash used to prevent secondary infection, but this measure, if properly employed, adds greatly to the pain in most cases and is of very doubtful value. However, when the mouth must be kept artificially moistened, as is necessary in those cases in which the salivary ducts have become occluded by swelling, there is no reason why the fluid used should not be some such antiseptic as diluted Dobell's solution.

It is generally believed that the incidence of orchitis will be greatly lessened if absolute bed rest is enjoined in boys and young men, but there are observers who doubt the possibility of statistically proving the point. The usual practice when the complication develops is to support the inflamed scrotum (do all medical students know how to accomplish this?) and make use of cold applications in a fluffy light manner so as not to increase the discomfort by their weight. A local application of 50 per cent methyl salicylate in lanolin is said to be serviceable. In severe cases, Wesselhoeft informs me that he still very successfully employs the treatment which he advocated a number of years ago: incision through the tunica vaginalis and multiple incisions of the tunica albuginea to bring about relief of pain through permitting escape of the serous fluid imprisoned under pressure. The operation takes about one minute under gas.

The organic arsenicals are beginning to be used since Kermorgant has advanced his belief that the causative organism is a spirochete; I know as yet of no careful studies of their efficacy.

PROPHYLAXIS

It has been shown that convalescent mumps serum possesses considerable value as a prophylactic. Regan (1925) collected the serum from adults in the fourteenth to sixteenth day of the disease and injected 2 to 4 cc. intramuscularly in 81 children. Eleven individuals disappeared from observation before the expiration of the incubation period, but of the remaining 70 only 1 developed the disease. Skrotskiy (1929) used 5 to 15 cc. according to the age of the child; mumps was observed in a light form in only 2 of the 179 children. Barenberg and Ostroff (1931), giving a routine dose of 12 cc. of serum obtained both from convalescents and from adults who had had the disease in childhood, found that, in a study employing 180 children between one and one-half and three years of age, the adult serum was not as effective as that obtained from recent convalescents.

The use of serum after the attack of mumps has developed does not alter its general course though it seems to lessen the incidence of orchitis. Teissier reports 172 treated cases, with an orchitis incidence of 8.13 per cent, while among 176 untreated control cases the incidence was 23.29 per cent. He gave 12 to 20 cc. in the beginning but later increased this dose to 40 cc. and found that the higher dose was more effective. The treatment was given before the fifth day of the attack. In Lavergne and Florentin's series of 113 treated cases the incidence was 4.4 per cent; in the 107 control cases it was 23.3 per cent.

MYCOSES

ACTINOMYCOSIS

Actinomycosis is a chronic infectious disease caused by the ray fungus, *Actinomyces bovis*, which probably exists normally among the abundant flora of the alimentary tract and gains access to the tissues through microscopical lesions, carious teeth, wounds made by penetrating foreign bodies, or reaches the respiratory tract by aspiration from the mouth and pharynx. The disease occurs quite commonly in cattle ("lumpy jaw"), but there is no good evidence that it can be conveyed from cattle to man, or, indeed, from man to man. Though looked upon as a rare disease, recent statistical studies tend to show that it occurs with much greater frequency than has heretofore been believed. Most of the cases in the United States have been in the upper Mississippi valley and the northwestern States.

The essential lesions of the disease are multiple, more or less painless, abscesses, usually surrounded by a considerable area of proliferative tissue. Discharging sinuses develop from the abscesses, and the process extends by continuity of tissue or sometimes by metastasis. Fifty per cent of reported cases have been in the region of the head and neck, usually beginning about the jaw, and here the diagnosis is not difficult. In 20 to 30 per cent of cases some abdominal organ is primarily affected; here the diagnosis is more difficult until the lumpy process extends to the abdominal wall and a characteristic sinus appears. In approximately 15 per cent of cases the involvement is thoracic with physical signs usually indistinguishable from pulmonary tuberculosis until perforation of the external wall takes place.

Under proper treatment the prognosis may be considered fair in the head and neck cases, but if ultimate cure is to be accomplished the iodides must be continued for a long period after the patient is apparently well. In the pulmonary type the prognosis is absolutely bad; it is slightly better in abdominal cases.

THERAPY

Sodium and potassium iodide are considered specific in a limited way in actinomycosis. They are doubtfully effective in cases in which the diagnosis is made late, and even in early cases must be given in larger doses than is customary in the treatment of other diseases, such as syphilis. Fortunately, these patients seem to be rather exceptionally tolerant to the iodides. I recall one case in which I gave 640 grains (42.6 Gm.) of sodium iodide daily for a period of many months, 60 grains (4 Gm.) intravenously and the remainder by mouth. During this time the patient was delivered of a normal baby and neither the mother nor the child showed any signs of iodism.

While the iodides are the sheet anchor in treatment, surgery is also indicated, but only if, as in jaw and neck cases, the involved tissues can be widely excised. Surgery would seem to be essential where softening and abscess formation have occurred, but the hard inflammatory nodules before the stage of softening has been reached usually respond well to the iodides alone. Radium and x-ray are of value only as adjuncts to medical and surgical treatment.

I believe it to be the consensus of opinion among surgeons that abdominal actinomycosis yields but poorly to the iodides, and that bold and persistent surgical attack offers the patient his best chance.

BLASTOMYCOSIS AND BRONCHOMYCOSIS

Blastomycosis is an infectious but apparently noncontagious disease caused by a number of closely allied species of fungi, which may be called here the *Blastomycetes*. Most of the cases have been reported from the vicinity of Chicago, but the disease is known elsewhere in both hemispheres. Many of the milder pulmonary cases are not strictly blastomycoses but are due to yeasts of the genus Monilia or related genera.

The disease affects usually the skin only, but deep-seated involvement of the long bones and of internal organs, especially the lungs, occurs not infrequently. The cutaneous lesions take the form of papules, pustules, nodes, abscesses, or ulcers, and this form of the disease runs a course of many years during which active and quiescent periods alternate. In the systemic cases the symptoms are those of pyemia with ultimate evidence of pulmonary involvement.

THERAPY

Here, as in actinomycosis, the iodides if given in large doses are effective. Most skin cases will yield to this treatment if it is begun before there is involvement of the deeper structures, and if it is persisted in for a sufficiently long time. In those rare cases where it is possible, total excision of the affected part is the ideal treatment, but it must be excision and not merely curettement, for this latter procedure is thought to have been responsible at times for a spread of the disease. Copper sulphate has also been used effectively in some cases in doses of $\frac{1}{4}$ to 1 grain (0.015 to 0.06 Gm.) three times daily by mouth. Recently, radiotherapy and diathermy seem to have proved themselves definitely useful. Hedge has reported (1928) 2 cases in which complete cure without any sign of recurrence in more than a year was accomplished by the application to the lesions of carbon dioxide snow under moderate pressure for ten to fifteen seconds. Pupo's (1928) 4 cases were successfully treated with intravenous injections of 10 cc. of 1 per cent methylene blue, or alternated with injections of 5 cc. of 0.5 per cent trypoflavine, according to the seriousness and obstinacy of the case. Steinfield (1931) says that the use of a vaccine prepared from yeast cultures is helpful in pulmonary cases; autogenous vaccines have also been used.

Where there is involvement of the internal organs the mortality reaches about 90 per cent, though there is apparently a mild pulmonary form of the disease.

SPOROTRICHOSIS

Sporotrichosis is an infectious disease caused by a fungus of the genus *Sporotrichium*. It is possible that it may be conveyed from man to man, and from the lower animals to man, as it is known to occur in the rat, the dog and the horse. Cases have been reported all over the world but the disease is most frequent, or is most frequently recognized, in rural France and in the upper Mississippi valley in the United States. Foerster (1926) has presented it in the light of an occupational disease, since many of the cases reviewed by him have occurred among farmers and horticulturists; he suggests the barberry bush as the source of infection.

The disease is characterized by the appearance of a subcutaneous nodule which attaches to the skin, breaks down in the center, and becomes chronic as a cold abscess whose periphery remains well defined and indurated. A number of these lesions may appear on widely scattered portions of the body, but it is more usual for an ascending lymphangitis to develop from the primary nodule (the "chancre"), with numerous lesions appearing along its course. The disease is usually chronic and in the United States the inflammation is of so low an order that there is little pain and practically no disturbance in the general health, but in France it would seem that radical amputations are often necessary and that visceral involvement is frequent.

THERAPY

Here again, as in the two fungus diseases previously considered, the iodides in large doses are usually curative. Their use must be persisted in for a considerable time after apparent cure to prevent recurrence. Such tempting surgical procedures as radical incision or curettement should be avoided as they only prolong the process. However, abscesses which show no tendency to resorption are sometimes aspirated with advantage; it is the practice usually to refill the cavity with a weak iodide solution (1 per cent). Exposure to x-ray sometimes hastens the disappearance of the lesions.

STREPTOTHRICOSIS

This is a very rare disease caused by a fungus-like organism called, perhaps erroneously, *Streptothrix*. In the something less than 40 cases that have been reported the lungs were principally involved, though in a few cases there was implication of other organs as well. The symptoms are those of pulmonary tuberculosis, abscess and bronchopneumonia—a confusing picture. I believe that all proved cases of *Streptothrix* infection have died.

THERAPY

I know of nothing to describe.

COCCIDIOIDAL GRANULOMA

This disease is caused by the fungus, *Coccidioides immitis*. First reported in South America in 1892, the vast majority of the 218 proved cases (up to 1931) have been contracted in the San Joaquin Valley in California. The symptoms very closely resemble those of blastomycosis with, in addition, the appearances of a fulminating pulmonary tuberculosis.

THERAPY

The best hope, such as it is, for these unfortunates lies in early and radical amputations where possible. Iodides, tartar emetic, colloidal copper, intravenous dyes, colloidal lead, x-rays, have occasionally been of some value.

MADUROMYCOSIS (MADURA FOOT, MYCETOMA)

Maduromycosis is a chronic affection of the foot caused by fungi of a number of different genera and species. It has been known since time out of mind in India, where it was first scientifically described, and is reported rather frequently from many other tropical countries. However, its occurrence is by no means confined to these warm regions for it has been recorded all over the world. Brindley and Howell (1932) have reviewed 28 cases reported in North America.

The disease usually follows a penetrating wound, most frequently in a bare-footed person. Following its implantation in this way the fungus grows within the deep tissues and causes necrosis which eventually reaches the surface. The typical lesion is a deep sinus that is discharging a foul-smelling fluid containing certain characteristic grains. The whole foot may be riddled with a network of intercommunicating sinuses of this sort and is much swollen and characteristically deformed. Pain is usually of a dull aching sort and constitutional symptoms are slight and inconstant. The disease may last many years; there is no tendency to heal.

THERAPY

Internal medication is a failure. Local measures are of no avail. Amputation is the only treatment of value.

OROYA FEVER AND VERRUGA PERUVIANA

(Carrion's Disease)

"Oroya peruviana" is a disease peculiar to certain clefted valleys on the western slopes of the Peruvian Andes, where it manifests itself in two forms: One, Oroya fever, a constitutional and fatal malady, and the other, verruga peruviana, a cutaneous and nonfatal affection. It has been endemic in this region since early historic times. Many of Pizarro's invading troops perished of the disease, and in more recent times it has taken a heavy toll in all the heroic railway building ventures that have taken place in these cruel mountains. A Harvard Commission, formed to study the matter in 1913, cast considerable doubt upon the common causative factor in the two conditions, but this has been dispelled by the work of Noguchi, Battistini and Hercelles, in 1926, who have cultured the *Bartonella bacilliformis* from the blood of an Oroya fever patient, and have produced Oroya fever or verruga peruviana in monkeys by inoculating them with this culture, the particular manifestation produced being entirely dependent upon whether the intravenous or the intradermal method was used. They have also produced Oroya fever by inoculation of material taken from a verruga nodule, and have obtained a pure culture of the organism from the blood of the inoculated animal.

It is considered extremely likely that some blood-sucking insect is the transmitter of the disease but *Phlebotomus* is not yet completely convicted. It is certain, however, that if the stranger leaves the endemic valley before nightfall his liability to contract the disease is much lessened. The incubation period is from two to three or more weeks.

Oroya Fever.—This type of the disease is characterized by a rather abrupt onset with weakness, malaise, slight rigors, moderate irregular fever, and a rapid pernicious anemia with the parasites present in the red blood corpuscles. The mortality is variously estimated at from 40 to 80 per cent, but as many of these patients are affected with other chronic tropical diseases at the same time it is perhaps unfair to ascribe all the deaths to uncomplicated Oroya fever. The recent study of Ribeyro (1932) indicates, indeed, that the prognosis is favorable in simple uncomplicated Oroya fever and that the only complication which makes death almost certain is due to paratyphoid B bacillus. The fatal cases run their course in a few weeks.

Verruga Peruviana.—This type is characterized in the beginning by joint pains and a moderate fever of short duration, after which the eruption appears. This eruption is at first miliary and is usually confined to the arms and legs, but it may occur elsewhere on the body and even on the mucous membranes. In most cases the rash becomes papular and sub-cutaneous nodules appear. Some of these nodules, attaching to the skin and ulcerating, are called "verrugas" and have given the disease its name. The mortality is also high in this type, but individuals who are not harboring other malicious tropical diseases at the same time nearly always recover. Only the ulcerated lesions leave any scars.

THERAPY

Despite the havoc which "Oroya peruviana" has wrought and the interest it has aroused in the modern scientific mind, no effective treatment has been devised. In view of Ribeyro's recent report (see above), the imperative necessity for protective vaccination against typhoid-paratyphoid organisms of all persons who are obliged to visit Oroya-infested regions, is quite evident.

PAPPATACI FEVER
(Three-day Fever, Sandfly Fever)

This disease, which is caused by a filtrable virus conveyed by the bite of the sandfly *Phlebotomus papatassii*, is common in the Mediterranean basin and is also encountered, though less frequently, in many other parts of the world. It is characterized by abrupt onset with a fairly high fever, severe joint and muscle pains, and a characteristic flush of the face and neck. The fever usually drops by crisis on the third day and the other symptoms abate, but the flush persists for ten to fifteen days in about half of the cases. Convalescence is oftentimes slow but all cases recover.

THERAPY

There is nothing to describe.

PLAGUE

1. And the Philistines took the ark of God, and brought it from Ebenezer unto Ashdod.

6. But the hand of the Lord was heavy upon them of Ashdod, and he destroyed them, and smote them with emerods, even Ashdod and the coasts thereof.

7. And when the men of Ashdod saw that it was so, they said, The ark of the God of Israel shall not abide with us: for his hand is sore upon us, and upon Dagon our god.

8. They sent therefore and gathered all the lords of the Philistines unto them, and said, What shall we do with the ark of the God of Israel? And they answered, Let the ark of the God of Israel be carried about unto Gath. And they carried the ark of the God of Israel about thither.

9. And it was so, that, after they had carried it about, the hand of the lord was against the city with a great destruction: and he smote the men of the city, both small and great, and they had emerods in their secret parts.

10. Therefore they sent the ark of God to Ekron. And it came to pass, as the ark of God came to Ekron, that the Ekronites cried out, saying, They have brought about the ark of the God of Israel to us, to slay us and our people.

11. So they sent and gathered together all the lords of the Philistines, and said, Send away the ark of the God of Israel, and let it go again to his own place, that it slay us not, and our people: for there was a deadly destruction throughout all the city; the hand of God was very heavy there.

2. And the Philistines called for the priests and the diviners, saying, What shall we do to the ark of the Lord? Tell us wherewith we shall send it to his place.

3. And they said, If ye send away the ark of the God of Israel, send it not empty; but in any wise return him a trespass offering: then ye shall be healed, and it shall be known to you why his hand is not removed from you.

4. Then said they, What shall be the trespass offering which we shall return to him? They answered, Five golden emerods, and five golden mice, according to the number of the lords of the Philistines: for one plague was on you all, and on your lords.

5. Wherefore ye shall make images of your emerods, and images of your mice that mar the land; and ye shall give glory unto the God of Israel: peradventure he will lighten his hand from off you, and from off your gods, and from off your land. I Samuel, v–vi.

Plague has ever been the arch-enemy of man. Indeed, so great have been the ravages of this disease in the past and so threatening is its present menace, that I own to a certain quiver of fear as I sit to the task of describing the thing. Accounts of epidemics believed to have been plague occur in some of the earliest preserved writings. It is customary to recognize four pandemics in historical times: That of the Mediterranean basin in the second century A. D., that of the same region in the sixth century; that of the fourteenth century, and the one of the present time. The one which began in the fourteenth century lasted for several hundred years and is estimated to have killed twenty-five million persons. This disease has certainly wiped out whole peoples in its time, and I quite agree with certain gentlemen of the Ohio Archeological and Historical Association that the disappearance of the race of American mound builders could be accounted for in this way. This people vanished very quickly and might have been plague stricken in such great numbers, and in so short a time, that burial was impossible. In the London visitation of 1665 ("black death"), the burial difficulty was very great, some churchyards being so overcrowded as to raise their level several feet above that of the surrounding streets—as may still be seen— and becoming finally entirely inadequate, after which the bodies were thrown into great dug pits. The present pandemic began in 1894, probably on the border of Thibet and Yunnan, and has worked great havoc in Manchuria, China, Japan, India and Java. Smaller outbreaks have also occurred during this time in many other places. Endemic cases occur infrequently in practically all the ports of the world, though the North Atlantic United States have been singularly free. The two persistent foci in California and Louisiana constitute a present serious American menace. More than fifteen million deaths has been the toll in the present century. In the first three months of 1924 there were 38,000 (estimated) plague deaths in British India, and during one week, April 12th to 19th, of that year, there were 12,393 deaths —in an epidemic which is stated to have been less severe than in 1902, 1904, 1905, 1907, and 1915! The latest available League of Nations reports show a marked decline in Egypt, East Africa, Senegal and India, and complete disappearance of the disease from Algeria, Tunis, Tripolitania and Nigeria; but on the other hand fresh territory has been invaded in Southwest Africa and Angola and the cases have increased in Madagascar. The disease is on the decline in Ecuador and Peru, but fresh small foci have appeared in Bolivia and Argentina. In the Netherlands East Indies plague has spread to the mountainous area in the west but declined in the center and east; in Iraq it has been localized in Bagdad. At the moment of writing (early November, 1933) both the pulmonary and bubonic forms of the malady are raging in Manchuria and due to the political-military situation there constitute a serious world menace.

Plague is caused by *Bacillus pestis* and is primarily an enzootic of rats, ground squirrels, marmots, and perhaps other rodents. What causes it to become epizootic at times in these animals is unknown, but it is definitely established that the great epidemics in man follow immediately upon these periods, the bite of the infected rat flea conveying the disease from rat to man. With Lethem, I think that the human flea (and the bedbug) have been ruled out as vectors on very little evidence.

Bubonic Plague.—The attack is very sudden with chilliness, rise in temperature, pulse and respiration; pains in head and body; nausea and vomiting; a dusky appearance of the skin ("black death") ; enlarged spleen; a staggering gait, mental sluggishness and extreme anxiety. The characteristic buboes of the groin, less frequently of the neck and axilla, usually appear the first day. There is always great toxic involvement of the internal organs and, in most cases, septicemic invasion as well. The glands slowly suppurate and slough, but death occurs in many cases before this takes place. The average duration of a case is perhaps three to five days, but in the more virulent epidemics death sometimes occurs almost without any prodromal symptoms. Deaths occurring a week or two after the onset of the disease are usually from sudden myocardial failure or by hemorrhage from a large vessel involved in the sloughing of a bubo.

Pneumonic Plague.—With the advent of sepsis in bubonic plague, focal lesions occur in all organs, including the lungs. These lung lesions quickly become necrotic, and the unfortunate victim sprays the room with virulent bacilli each time he coughs. Attendants then acquire the disease by droplet infection, the type of the attack being pulmonary in them from the very beginning. In some epidemics the pneumonic form is singularly late in appearing, while in others it predominates almost from the beginning.

The mortality in bubonic plague is about 75 per cent, in the pneumonic form it is very little under 100 per cent.

THERAPY

Antiplague Serum.—The use of this serum offers us our best means at present of combating this dread disease. It is prepared by immunizing horses with cultures of dead and living bacilli by several methods, all of which are difficult. In the days soon after Yersin's introduction of the serum, in 1896, it was employed in small doses subcutaneously. Nowadays it is realized that large doses must be used, preferably intravenously, if good results are to be obtained.

Dosage and Administration.—The following plan of serum treatment is Kolmer's slight modification of Choksy's method: (1) The intravenous injection of 80 to 100 cc. of serum as soon as the diagnosis is made. For children under twelve years the dose may be 50 cc. If an intravenous injection cannot be given a child, the serum may be injected intramuscularly or intraperitoneally. (2) Repeat the injection six hours later if the temperature has not fallen. If this has occurred the second injection may be given twelve to eighteen hours later. (3) The amount of serum to be injected subsequently will depend upon the rise of the temperature the previous evening, and the general condition of the patient. If the temperature be the same as on the first evening the same amount may be injected; if it be lower, 30 cc. or less should be injected. (4) The quantity of serum injected should be lessened gradually until the temperature falls to normal in the morning. (5) A sudden fall of the temperature between the second and the seventh day should not indicate a suspension of the treatment. (6) The injections are given every twelve hours if secondary buboes present themselves, or if the temperature rises rapidly one or two degrees. (7) If the evening temperature be lower than that of the morning, the dose is reduced on the following day. (8) From six to eight injections are generally sufficient to complete the treatment. (9) The total quantity of serum required varies between 150 and 300 cc., according to the gravity of the symptoms and the condition of the serum.

Administration to Children.—Fontes, quoted by Kolmer, has given the serum intraperitoneally to children and has published the following table of results (Table 9):

TABLE 9.—USE OF ANTIPLAGUE SERUM IN CHILDREN

Method.	Cases treated.	Died.	Death rate, per cent.
Subcutaneous	21	8	38.0
Intraperitoneal	11	2	18.0
Intravenous	69	5	7.2

Value of the Treatment.—It is difficult to truly evaluate the serum treatment for the reason that so many factors have to be taken into account. It has its enthusiastic advocates and its detractors. For instance, Johns, of Louisiana, states that when given soon after the onset of symptoms it is "in every way comparable to the results attained by the use of antidiphtheritic sera"; while Wu, according to Nicoll, looks upon the serum as of very doubtful value. I fancy that Dr. Johns would find very few persons willing to follow him quite so far, while Dr. Wu's pessimism may arise from the fact that his extensive experience in Manchuria is usually with the notoriously resistant pneumonic type of the disease. The average experience with the serum probably lies between these two extremes. Burnett, quoted by Kolmer, reported in Queensland a mortality of 29.7 per cent among serum-treated cases as against a mortality of 73.9 per cent treated without serum. The same author quotes Penna, in the Argentine, who reports that among 664 cases treated with Yersin's serum during the period 1905 to 1912, the mortality ranged from 23 per cent in 1906 to 7.3 per cent in 1912, with an average mortality of 12.5. From 1914 to the middle of 1919 Kraus' serum was used with an average mortality of 7.8 per cent. Lloyd analyzes the results in 1491 cases of the bubonic type treated under his supervision in Guayaquil, Ecuador, in 1908 and 1909, as follows: (1) Mortality among the untreated, about 60 per cent, (2) mortality among the treated, about 33 per cent, (3) mortality among those treated within twenty-four to thirty-six hours of the onset, 18 to 20 per cent. The preliminary trial of the new Haffkine Institute serum, developed by Naidu and Mackie (1931), which is made from cattle instead of horses indicates that it may be much more potent than serum of the Yersin type.

It would seem that the following factors are of considerable importance in limiting the effectiveness of the serum treatment:

Time of Administration.—The importance of early treatment was shown by Choksy in Bombay; I quote his table as published by Kolmer (Table 10):

TABLE 10.—VALUE OF ANTIPLAGUE SERUM ACCORDING TO TIME OF ITS USE

Day of the disease.	Number of cases.	Died.	Recovered.	Mortality, per cent.
First	323	98	225	30.3
Second	311	164	147	52.7
Third	248	155	93	62.5
Fourth	106	60	46	56.6
Fifth	52	32	20	61.5
Sixth	14	8	6	57.1
Seventh	4	4	0	100.0

Age of the Serum.—I am not aware of the performance of any experiments designed to determine the age-potency of the serum, but numerous men experienced in its use feel that it deteriorates rather rapidly, especially if it has been exposed to extremes of temperature. Lloyd writes as follows of his experience in Guayaquil:

"On one occasion I received a consignment of serum that had been kept for about six months on the Isthmus, under what conditions I do not know. I questioned the advisability of using this serum when it arrived, but as serum was scarce and somewhat hard to obtain at the time in quantities required, I decided to use it. After losing several patients, who I thought should have recovered, I discontinued its use and returned the quantity remaining to the Isthmus, saying that it was of no value."

Specificity of the Serum.—It is now becoming apparent that the particular strain of *Bacillus pestis* responsible for the various outbreaks of the disease varies somewhat with locality. In certain epidemics the "stock" serum has been of little value, whereas serum made on the spot by immunizing with organisms taken from the then present buboes was very efficacious. I believe that we will make a closer approach to victory over the disease when this fact is more generally taken into account, though of course the delay incident upon making the serum is of serious moment; when made, however, it combines the two desirable qualities of high specificity and absolute freshness.

Bacteriophage.—D'Herelle asserts that bacteriophage therapy should constitute the specific treatment for plague. From 1 to 2 cc. of a very virulent bacteriophage culture should be injected as soon as possible. Since the treatment is harmless, it can be given as soon as the diagnosis becomes clinically probable, without waiting for bacteriological verification. A single injection is indicated if the temperature falls steadily; otherwise, a second, or even a third, injection may be given. A dose of 1 cc. is injected in one bubo; or two injections, each of 0.5 cc. in two buboes. In the absence of buboes, in septic and pneumonic cases, he believes that intravenous injections should be tried; local or general reactions do not need to be feared.

Preparation of the Bacteriophage.—To 1 cc. of a culture of *Bacillus pestis* (cultivated in bouillon for twenty-four hours) is added 3 cc. of fresh bouillon inoculated with 0.02 cc. of a previously prepared bacteriophage culture of high virulence for the plague bacillus. After being heated in an autoclave for twenty hours at a temperature of 37 C., bacteriophagia being then complete, the clear fluid is filtered and is ready for use.

D'Herelle, in Egypt, and Couvy, in Senegal, have each used this treatment successfully in a small number of cases, but when subjected to a careful trial in India it proved ineffective.

The Use of Drugs.—Obviously, to review here all the drugs which have been employed in the treatment of plague would be neither possible nor profitable, for their number is legion and their effectiveness almost nil. Occasionally results are claimed from some particular drug—iodine, a dye, Bayer-205, or what not—but it should be borne in mind that the entity known as *Pestis minor* recovers without any treatment at all, though the organism can be recovered from the glands.

PROPHYLAXIS

To write that all rats should be exterminated about the wharves of seaport towns and cities is, of course, banal, since any second-year medical student will gladly, may pompously and quite gratuitously indeed, supply one with that information; but what of our inland cities? In the rear premises of a grocer's shop which my laboratory windows overlook in a huge middle-west city, two rats are this moment grubbing about in the murky light of approaching night. I cannot but recall in contrast the fact that in the harbor of Colon one is forbidden to throw the least article overboard (even an empty match-box, as well I know!), lest the carcass of a rat be thus secretly disposed of. Do we sit on the lid of a cauldron? The brown rat which in northern Europe and much of North America has displaced the black fellow has lessened the menace, I know; and we are certainly "building them out"—but what of the low unhygienic shacks which are tolerated, of all places, about the railway terminals in most American cities?

> Across the market-place 'neath dawn-hush'd skies
>   Slinking, one of the million-horded pest
> Of rats would seek it's vermin festered nest,
>   But falters—then in sudden frenzy tries
> To mount the reeking curb that shadowed lies
>   Athwart it's stricken path—and fails, it's best
> By much too death-blown now to meet the test
>   Of scourge indifferent to puny cries.
>
> What ancient ghostly veil is this withdrawn?
>   These unseen lips that pest'lent curses pour
> From belly belching of a rot long gone—
>   Is Black Death then upon us, blight of yore?
> What loathsome Presence shudders through this dawn?
>   Awake, O Town!—of men who will wake no more.

On with the campaign of rat extermination, both coastal and inland—and especially more power to the search for a specific remedy in the disease!

The Protective Hood.—All physicians and others should be carefully hooded when attending a case of plague, whether of the bubonic or pneumonic type. For a description of the special costume worn by Chun and his associates during the terrible pneumonic outbreak in Harbin, China, in 1921, the reader is referred to the Journal of the American Medical Association, November 8, 1924.

Prophylactic Vaccine.—The Haffkine vaccine, introduced in 1897, is composed essentially of the intact bacilli and autolytic products of a heat killed culture of *Bacillus pestis* in neutral bouillon. The ordinary subcutaneous dose of this vaccine for adult males is 3 to 3.5 cc., for females 2 to 2.5 cc. A second injection is given after eight to ten days. The local and constitutional effects are more severe than those following typhoid vaccination.

The duration of immunity is only a few weeks, so that in times of epidemic the inoculations should be repeated several times a year. This necessity for repetition, plus the fact that protection is not conferred until several days after inoculation, has often produced strenuous opposition to its use among ignorant native populations. The Indian Plague Commission reported a few years ago as follows (Kolmer): (1) Inoculation sensibly diminishes the incidence of attacks of plague. It is, however, not an absolute protection against the disease. (2) The death rate is markedly diminished by its means, not only the incidence of the disease, but also the fatality, being reduced. (3) The protection is not conferred on those inoculated for the first few days after the injection. (4) The duration of the immunity is uncertain, but it seems to last for a number of weeks, if not for months.

Col. Taylor, director of the Haffkine Institute in Bombay, has concluded, in 1933, from all the available statistical evidence that prophylactic inoculation with Haffkine's vaccine gives a fourfold protection against attacks and an eightfold protection against death. He also believes that none of the numerous modifications of this vaccine have shown themselves to be in any wise superior to the original preparation.

PNEUMONIA

Lobar Pneumonia.—Lobar pneumonia is one of the most widespread and dangerous of all the infectious diseases of the temperate zones. Its occurrence in the tropics in relatively rare. The disease is caused in about 90 per cent of cases by *Diplococcus pneumoniae,* of which 32 types are now recognized. During ordinary times (*i. e.,* nonpandemic times) about one third of all cases are caused by Type I, the other cases being scattered principally but rather irregularly between Types II, III, and IV. The old belief has been that pneumonia is auto-infectious; that is, that when resistance becomes lowered the organisms always harbored in the mouth are able to establish themselves on a pathogenic basis in the lungs. Recent studies, however, have shown that the type of organism present in the mouth of most individuals is not the one responsible for most cases of the disease; present knowledge therefore inclines toward the position that the disease is contracted by actual droplet infection from an active case or from a recovered case still harboring the causative organism, or from an individual who has become a temporary carrier following such contact, and that the number of chronic carriers is small. The point is not definitely decided. Recent catarrhal fever, exposure to wet and cold, and excessive fatigue are frequent precursors of the disease; the incidence is decidedly higher among blacks than whites. The average mortality range is as follows: Private practice, 15 (!) to 25 per cent; good general hospitals, 25 to 35 per cent; public institutions treating the lowest classes, including many alcoholics, 50 to 60 per cent.

Lobar pneumonia is characterized by the suddenness of its onset, typically by a chill, stabbing pain in the side, high rise of temperature and pulse rate, rapid respiration often with dyspnea, cough and rusty sputum, and involvement of the nervous system, ranging from mere anxiety to active delirium. Herpes simplex, jaundice, and initial vomiting are frequently seen. There are typical physical "findings" in the chest, whose description has no place here. Cyanosis, varying in degree with the respiratory and circulatory involvement, always makes its appearance later. In the average case the symptoms last for from five to ten days with very little remission, and then the attack terminates by a gradual lessening in severity of all symptoms, or, in perhaps not more than 20 per cent of cases, by a "crisis" in which the defervescence occurs within twenty-four hours.

Bronchopneumonia.—Bronchopneumonia is a diffuse lobular inflammation of the lungs in which several organisms can be identified as the causative factor. There are three types: (1) The primary bronchopneumonia occurring in children under four years of age. This type is not directly associated with any other disease, is usually mild, and is nearly always caused by *Pneumococcus;* the symptoms are much like those of lobar pneumonia except for the difference in the distribution of the pulmonary lesions. (2) Secondary bronchopneumonia is caused by *Staphylococcus, Streptococcus, Pfeiffer's bacillus,* and only rarely *Pneumococcus.* It is the most dreaded complication of the infectious diseases in children and of the infectious and chronic debilitating diseases of middle and old age. The symptomatology of bronchopneumonia is too diverse and complicated to warrant description here; suffice it to say that the occurrence of this complication is usually marked by a change in the severity, and finally the type, of the symptoms which the patient is manifesting, until ultimately the picture of bronchopneumonia, with its diffuse chest involvement, cyanosis, respiratory and circulatory embarrassment, and general toxemia, completely supersede or overshadow the symptoms of the original condition. (3) Primary epidemic bronchopneumonia. This type is caused by *Streptococcus hemolyticus,* and is seen when this organism at intervals acquires an unwonted virulence. The mortality is very great in these cases, as witness the epidemic during the late World War. Most of the postinfluenzal pneumonias of that dark period were caused by *Streptococcus hemolyticus,* with or without the accompaniment of other organisms whose virulence had been temporarily raised to a high pitch.

THERAPY

The treatment of lobar and bronchopneumonia can be described together with such exceptions as will be noted later. I shall employ the three heads: general measures, symptomatic treatment, and specific treatment.

General Measures.—The patient should be at rest in a well-ventilated room, but I do not see the sanity of forcing upon him and his nurse the extreme exposure advocated by some. Many physicians of long experience insist that, whether exposed or not, the arms, shoulders and chest should be continuously swathed in a flannel jacket, which can be easily made extemporaneously. The diet should be sufficient to sustain the patient in the fight he is making, but one should be ever on guard against the digestive disturbances which are so frequent in this disease. External hydrotherapy should not be employed, save for the daily, quietly given, tepid sponge bath; the cold pack is a valuable circulatory stimulant, but it disturbs the patient far more than is advisable in this disease.

SYMPTOMATIC TREATMENT

Cough.—Though this is a beneficent measure, designed to rid the bronchi of foreign material which is choking them, it is sometimes excessive. Whenever cough is in the least degree exhausting the patient, attempt should be made to control it by such measures as have been described in the discussion of Catarrhal Fever (see p. 26).

Pain.—The pain in the side is often satisfactorily controlled by a judicious employment of adhesive plaster. If very severe and causing considerable restlessness, the opiates must be used for its relief. I believe that all the former objections to the use of opiates in this disease have been swept away; it is well to bear in mind, however, that some individuals are made quite ill, even to the point of vomiting several times, a few hours after taking morphine; codeine does not share many of the objectionable attributes of morphine and often suffices to control the pain here. Diathermy is said to be analgesic (see p. 134).

Restlessness.—Restlessness and sleeplessness must be overcome since peace of mind and body are of the utmost importance to the patient. If opiates are not being employed for the control of cough or pain, they will often be required to secure bodily quiet. It is well, however, first to try a milder sedative, such as veronal (barbital), 5 to 10 grains (0.3 to 0.6 Gm.); or amytal, 1½ to 5 grains (0.1 to 0.3 Gm.). The value of glucose in controlling restlessness is described a few pages further on.

Tympanites.—Distention of the abdomen with gas is a symptom which is frequent, distressing and serious, for it oftentimes adds to the respiratory embarrassment. It is best treated by prevention; that is to say, by cleaning out the lower intestinal tract by a 1 per cent sodium bicarbonate enema as soon as the case comes under observation. This enema should be repeated at least every twenty-four hours, a rectal tube being used during the interim. When the distention persists despite these enemas, turpentine stupes may be employed as in the following method which I have seen Curran Pope demonstrate.

First place a blanket under the patient in such manner that it can be drawn across the abdomen in "double-breasted" fashion. Anoint the abdomen with vaselin. Then spread a Turkish towel over a small pan and place in the center of it another Turkish towel folded to the size of the abdomen. Now pour over this second towel boiling water, to which has been added 1 teaspoonful of turpentine to the quart, take up the two ends of the first towel, and quickly wring the stupe nearly dry by twisting these ends in opposite directions. Then remove this stupe, which is so hot that you can only hold it by rapidly shifting hands, from the wringing towel and place it upon the abdomen—and lift and replace, lift and replace, until the patient can bear the heat; then draw a layer of the blanket tightly across the abdomen from each side—and you have done it! The stupes must be applied every five minutes until relief is obtained.

The following carminative enemas are of value: (1) ½ to 1 drachm (2 to 4 cc.) of turpentine, emulsified by beating with the white of an egg, and added to a quart of water. (2) One to 3 drachms (4 to 12 cc.) of the emulsion of asafetida added to a quart of water; this latter preparation is esthetically very objectionable.

In very obstinate cases it may be necessary to give surgical pituitrin in intramuscular injections of ½ to 1 cc.—in addition to stupes and enemas. Every effort must be made to keep the abdomen flat, for persistent tympanites adds greatly to the respiratory and circulatory difficulty. In a considerable number of cases we have to deal with dilatation of the stomach also. It is my opinion that whenever we shall have placed at our disposal a quick means of relieving this symptom the mortality in pneumonia will at once be considerably reduced. Of course the stomach tube is indicated, but the very nature of things usually makes its passage out of the question.

Cyanosis.—The fact is now definitely established that anoxemia, *i. e.*, deficiency of oxygen in the arterial blood, occurs in some degree in practically all cases of pneumonia. Except in anemic individuals, who may be anoxemic without showing blueness of the skin, this unsaturation of the blood with oxygen is manifested clinically as "cyanosis." The pertinent inquiry, "What harm is there in a lessened amount of oxygen in the arterial blood?" is easily answered. I quote Barach: "In summary, it might be said that the disturbance of the gastro-intestinal system is manifested by nausea, vomiting and diarrhea; the respiratory system by increased rate and depth of respiration or by periodic respiration, and later by rapid, shallow respiration; the circulatory system by a constant and progressive increase in pulse rate, and in the end by a fall in diastolic pressure and cardiac failure; the central nervous system by headache, visual disturbances, irrational states and delirium, and finally, coma and death." That is to say, any of these symptoms, when occurring in pneumonia, may be due wholly or in part to anoxemia. Now let us examine the three most plausible causes of anoxemia, as manifested by cyanosis, in pneumonia.

1. TOXEMIA.—What direct part the general toxemia characteristic of the disease, with its alteration of metabolism and poisoning of the medullary centers, plays in regard to the lessened amount of oxygen in the blood we can only surmise and attempt to treat by such specific measures as will be described at a later time.

2. ALTERATIONS IN THE BLOOD.—It has been possible to demonstrate a lessened oxygen-combining power of the blood in only a very few cases of pneumonia, and in these cases only by inference can the presence of methemoglobin be stated as the cause. We are certainly not warranted at the present time in directing our therapy toward the overcoming of methemoglobinemia.

3. ALTERATIONS IN THE RESPIRATORY SYSTEM (Oxygen Administration). —Rapid and shallow breathing is the rule in pneumonia. Haldane, Meakins and Priestley have shown that shallow breathing tends to produce anoxemia,

and, on the other hand, that anoxemia tends to cause rapid, shallow breathing. I believe that it is permissible to hold that the local changes in the lungs are to some extent guilty of perpetuating this vicious circle. If this is so, the fault must lie in one of two things: (*a*) the amount of consolidation prevents the free access to the blood of sufficient oxygen to maintain its normal content of that element; or (*b*) there is an alteration in the permeability of the alveolar walls which renders them relatively impervious to the oxygen which reaches them in the inspired air. If the former, one is perhaps justified in saying, "Well, there you are!"—but if the latter, this nonchalance is entirely inexcusable *until it has been finally proved that oxygen of a higher concentration than that of the atmosphere cannot be forced into the blood.* At the present time we have the following facts fairly well established by the careful observations of a number of workers, chief among whom are Haldane in England and Barach in the United States.

1. The old method of discharging the oxygen through a funnel held before the patient's nose and mouth is practically useless.

2. The method in which the oxygen is discharged through a nasal catheter (conceived at the front during the World War by Prof. Adrian Stokes, who died in 1927, at the early age of forty-one, from yellow fever while investigating the disease at Lagos) is of limited value provided the catheter has several openings and is introduced well back into the posterior nares; provided also that the patient does not breathe through the mouth at the same time; and provided also that the oxygen is delivered at the vigorous rate of 2 liters per minute, which is about all that the average patient will tolerate without being made extremely uncomfortable. (N.B. The necessity for this rapid delivery adds two serious objections to the employment of the method; first, the low-pressure tanks in universal use will require almost constant regulation to make it possible; and second, the cost is excessive since from four to ten tanks, depending upon their size, will be used per day by one patient.)

3. Barach has shown that the optimum concentration of oxygen is 40 to 60 per cent, and he and others have described a rebreathing apparatus and a tent that make steady delivery of this concentration possible. In view of the many variables which must be taken into account in evaluating such therapy as this, precise statistical proof of its benefit is still lacking, but I think that both theory and general experience continue to favor its extended trial. Many observers believe that oxygen administration should begin before there is actually any cyanosis. This much can be looked upon as established: that the prognosis is extremely grave in a case which does not respond to oxygen therapy by a marked slowing of the pulse rate and decided reduction in the degree of the cyanosis; the dyspnea itself is not always relieved. The following are well-known tents: Barach-Davidson; Cecil-Plummer; Oxygenaire; Barach-Roth; Henderson-Haggard; McKesson. The chief difficulty in operating tents is to maintain the temperature and humidity inside adequate on hot summer days. Rosenblüth and Block (1932) claim that with ordinary nursing care the oxygen content of a tent cannot be maintained at a desirable level with the flow of oxygen less than 8 liters per minute. With a rate of 8 to 10 liters the carbon dioxide will not rise above 1.5 per cent; since this gives rise to no subjective symptoms, the use of soda lime may be dispensed with, probably at a saving despite the increased use of oxygen. Henderson (1931) believes that the most effective way of inflating or clearing an occluded lobe or lung is the increased depth of breathing induced by inhalation of carbon dioxide; he therefore maintains 4.5 to 5 per cent of this gas in his tent. The carbonic acid may also promote the solution of pneumonic exudate as well as having some bactericidal power upon the pneumococcus.

Diathermy.—Those who use diathermy in pneumonia commonly record the disappearance of cyanosis, but Binger and Christie, finding no significant changes in oxygen content or capacity of the blood, concluded that the change in the patient's color had perhaps best be explained on the basis of an accelerated rate of blood flow through the peripheral capillaries. Coulter (1932) says that it has not been proved that the duration of the disease has been affected by the use of diathermy, but that symptomatically the results are good. The one fairly constant response seems to be the relief of pain in some degree.

Circulatory Disturbances.—In many cases of pneumonia of moderate severity from which the patient recovers after seven to ten days of fever, the pulse is throughout no more rapid than is consonant with the elevation of temperature. Also, it not infrequently occurs in fatal cases that the failure seems to be entirely respiratory, the pulse rate and force remaining quite good almost to the end. Again, we have to date no blood pressure studies which can be accepted as proof positive that early primary circulatory failure is typical of this disease. However, these facts which I have just stated are but the half; now let us examine the reverse of the coin. What are the evidences that some degree of circulatory failure and especially damage to the heart muscle itself, is to be very much feared in all cases of pneumonia?

First, the frequent occurrence of pulse irregularities. I wonder if it is a matter of common knowledge just how often the pulse shows irregularities at some time during the course of the disease. In Cole's series of 489 cases at the Hospital of the Rockefeller Institute, this phenomenon was remarked in over 10 per cent of the cases, and in Chatard's 658 cases at the Johns Hopkins Hospital, in almost 15 per cent. Cole states that *complete* irregularity, with fibrillation or flutter of the auricles, undoubtedly occurs in from 3 to 5 per cent of all cases.

Second, dilatation of the right heart. I know that at present students of the disease are inclined to believe that the right heart is not so much overworked as it was formerly thought to be, for it may be that very little effort is made to maintain the circulation in the affected areas in the lungs. However, until this fact is *proved,* I believe that we are well advised to look upon the heart as pumping harder than is its wont because of these consolidated areas in the capillary bed.

Third, the poisoning of the heart muscle by the toxin. The work of Newburgh, Means and Porter, some years ago, was generally hailed as showing that the heart is not "poisoned" in pneumonia; but this was a hasty judgment, as will be realized if the work performed by Newburgh and Porter at the same time is also examined. The sum of what was added to our knowledge by these studies, and a valuable accretion it is, was just this: that in dogs, at least, the pneumonic heart muscle contracts well when fed with pneumonic blood, but the contractions of the *normal* heart muscle are very much impaired if suddenly fed with pneumonic blood. Now, by analogy, we may assume that the human heart is able to adjust itself to the relatively gradual increase in toxins in the blood, but that it will fail if, and whenever, these additions of toxin are rapidly made. As to clinical support for this contention? I think the evidence is quite unmistakable, for the gravity of a given patient's condition depends upon the rapidity and extent of the successive involvement of the several lobes of the lungs and not upon the total involvement when the diagnosis is first made. In other words, each time a new focus for the dissemination of toxin is established, there follows an increase in the symptomatic signs of the disease, *including an augmentation of the evidences of cardiac weakening.*

Very well. Granting, then, that we have in some cases of pneumonia, and potentially in all cases, pulse irregularities, dilatation of the right heart, and poisoning of the heart muscle by the toxins, what shall we do about it? Let us see: (*a*) Pulse irregularities? Time, at least, has hallowed the use of digitalis in such instances. (*b*) Dilatation of the heart? A dilated heart is one that is doing much more work than the normal heart with much less nourishment, for the reason that the coronary vessels are stretched and thus made narrower, which means a lessened blood supply to the organ. Surely digitalis will afford these coronaries a longer time in which to fill. (*c*) A poisoned heart muscle? If we have any drug in our armamentarium which will help this heart to function more efficiently with a lessened number of contractions, shall we not use it? And so digitalis again!

And so much for theorizing, which—I confess it reluctantly in this instance—is beginning to be mightily assailed by actual bedside observation. Just the needed sort of steadfast study of this subject over a period of years has been undertaken by the committee for the study of digitalis in pneumonia, at Bellevue Hospital. Their preliminary findings (published by Niles and Wyckoff; Wyckoff, DuBois and Woodruff) are: (*a*) One cannot safely give digitalis to pneumonia patients until the appearance of slight evidences of the toxic effects of the drug, as in heart failure (see p. 530), but must rather arbitrarily limit the total dosage to an amount considerably less than would be used routinely in heart cases *per se;* (*b*) the mortality in 338 digitalis-treated cases was 41.4 per cent, in 404 control cases, 33.7 per cent. These most valuable studies are being continued.

STRYCHNINE AND METRAZOL.—Warfield, of Milwaukee, among others, is stoutly championing the position that the circulatory disturbance in pneumonia is due primarily to peripheral vascular dilatation rather than to failure of the heart itself; in his view there is withdrawal of much blood into the "depots" of the spleen, liver, splanchnic area and the subpapillary capillary skin plexus. Of course, instead of giving digitalis he would make every effort to force the blood out of these depots in order to increase the venous return to the right ventricle. Unfortunately, there is no known drug which will reliably accomplish this; however, in his own practice he has used hypodermic injections of strychnine sulphate, $\frac{1}{20}$ to $\frac{1}{10}$ grain (0.003 to 0.006 Gm.) every one to three hours, with good effect. Parenthetically, I would remark that strychnine is one of those remedial agents which my friend Bernard Fantus likes to call "doctors' drugs"; *i. e.*, one of those drugs to which experienced physicians cling despite all "proof" of its nonefficacy emanating from the laboratories of pharmacology.

Caffeine and camphor are unreliable but it seems that metrazol (Cardiazol), a synthetic drug which is like camphor in its action, may make a place for itself. It is given intramuscularly or intravenously in a dose of $1\frac{1}{2}$ grains (0.1 Gm.) every one to three hours; orally, from $1\frac{1}{2}$ to 3 grains (0.1 to 0.2 Gm.), several times daily as required.

ALCOHOL.—To the habitual hard drinker alcohol must be given in fairly large doses throughout the attack, else we add to the onslaught of the disease the additional insult of withdrawing a substance to which the organism has made some sort of pathologic-physiologic adjustment. And there is another valuable use for the drug in pneumonia, namely, the induction of a state of mild euphoria. If, in the beginning of a case, the patient can be freed of apprehension and given ease of mind and body by small doses of alcohol, then the drug should be judiciously continued. Unfortunately, the pneumonia patient is very often quite resistant to the inebriating effects of alcohol, and this condition of very mild intoxication which is desirable can only be attained by the use of large doses of the drug; I believe these large doses to be contraindicated.

Alterations in the Blood.—It has been known and variously commented upon for some time that the blood chemistry in pneumonia is characterized typically by a considerable decrease in chlorides and increase in nonprotein nitrogen and urea nitrogen; also that there is not an acidosis, as in other infectious diseases, but indeed oftentimes an actual alkalosis. Underhill and Ringer have also shown that in fulminating cases of influenzal pneumonia the blood becomes greatly concentrated.

1. CHLORIDES.—Haden has supplemented the food chloride by 6 to 24 Gm. salt daily; Sunderman, 15 to 30 Gm.; Wilder and Drake give 2 ounces of the following per pound body weight: 1 part physiologic saline, 2 parts orange juice, 3 parts 10 per cent glucose.

2. BLOOD CONCENTRATION.—(a) Venesection. Underhill and Ringer studied a series of 43 cases of influenzal pneumonia from the standpoint of blood concentration, and were able to show a distinct relationship between the gravity of a given case and the extent of the abnormal concentration of the blood. Upon theoretical grounds they advocated the withdrawal of blood by venesection and the introduction of fluid into the body, but were unable to carry out the treatment in many cases. It may be surprising to some to learn that a definite and logical basis exists for the letting of blood in pneumonia, a procedure which was at once the darling of our forefathers' hearts and the object of their greatest therapeutic abuse. A number of independent investigations, in pointing out the reactive leukocytosis, the coagulation changes, the hyperglycemia, and the mobilization of antibodies, indicate that it may be considered as a form of protein therapy. Also, Petersen and Levinson, in reviewing the work of Lord and Nye and others, by which it was shown that a ferment-antiferment balance exists in the pneumonic exudate, have very well reasoned that following venesection there may occur an alteration in this balance by reason of the withdrawal of some of the antiferment when fluid is rushed from the tissues into the vascular bed. To understand the logic of this it must be borne in mind that the ferments which are looked upon as overcoming the organisms are believed to be shed by the dying leukocytes at the focus of the infection.

(b) Glucose. Bloodletting will probably not become popular again, but I believe that we will find it profitable to look upon the good result which often follows the intravenous introduction of glucose as springing from the same causes, namely, a nonspecific protein effect and especially a tidal wave of antiferment away from the infected site. I am aware that hyperglycemia does not follow the introduction of concentrated solutions of glucose into the circulation, but I look upon this as an indication that the volume of fluid that is quickly drawn from the tissues into the vascular bed is sufficient to keep the percentage concentration of the glucose per cubic centimeter of the blood at normal, though the total volume of the blood is for a short time increased. The alternative assumption to account for the failure of hyper-glycemia to make its appearance is that the glucose does not pause at all in the blood stream but instantly makes its way into the tissues, a position which makes necessary the corollary assumption that it saturates the tissues with the fluids which it draws after it from the blood. I find it very difficult to account for the relief often afforded the patient by timely intravenous glucose medication if we are really flooding the tissues in this fashion. The subject is most interesting. Lusk believed that cell activity is stimulated to a certain extent by glucose. The most obvious advantage of glucose therapy is, of course, that it supplies in a short time a large quantity of food material which does not have to undergo preliminary digestive processes, which must be a very pleasing thing to the overworked, undernourished heart muscle.

The use of intravenous glucose solution in the treatment of pneumonia has become very popular since the experience with it in several of the army camps during the pandemic of influenzal pneumonia in 1918. Severe reactions sometimes follow its use, but Titus and Dodds have shown that these are almost invariably due to faulty technic and can be avoided. (For methods and dosage, see p. 776.) The following description of the effect of a glucose injection is that of Litchfield, one of the pioneers in this field of therapy, and its truth has been many times attested by other writers:

"The general appearance improves at once. The features are less pinched. The patient looks brighter and less 'toxic.' The respiration becomes slower. The pulse becomes slower and fuller. The blood pressure rises. The pulse amplitude is markedly and persistently increased. . . . The tongue becomes moist. The patient asks for water and food. The kidneys and bowels become active. If the patient was restless or delirious, he becomes quiet and often goes to sleep while the injection is being given." The effect upon mortality has not been studied sufficiently to make a comprehensive presentation possible at this time; that many practitioners look upon it as a life-saving measure, however, can be easily understood if the picture drawn by Litchfield is a true one. In my own experience I have several times seen it accomplish a degree of improvement which was little short of marvelous.

In cases of pulmonary edema occurring in the course of pneumonia, Bullowa (1932) administers 100 to 150 cc. of 50 per cent glucose solution intravenously at intervals of several hours, attempting to force the lungs to give up their fluids in order to dilute this concentrated solution. The excessive loss of fluid into the urine he overcomes by giving insulin to help metabolize the glucose; a little less than 1 unit for each 2 Gm. of glucose, subcutaneously at the conclusion of the intravenous injection.

(c) Fluids. A good rough rule for fluid administration to the adult is to have the amounts of fluid given by mouth and vein total $2\frac{1}{2}$ to 3 quarts (liters) in the twenty-four hours.

SPECIFIC THERAPY

(A) TREATMENT WITH BIOLOGICALS

Type I Serum.—In 1917 Cole and his co-workers at the Rockefeller Institute introduced the use of specific serum in the treatment of Type I pneumococcus pneumonia. The serum is prepared by the repeated injection of horses, first with dead, then with living, cultures of pneumococci, Type I. In treating the disease the amount of this immune serum injected intravenously at the first dose is 90 to 100 cc., diluted with an equal quantity of physiologic saline, and this dose is repeated, very slowly and at body temperature, at eight-hour intervals until the infection seems to be overcome. Cole states that the blood of the patient becomes sterile following the injection of the serum, the progression of the local lesion in the lung is arrested, the subjective and objective symptoms of the disease are ameliorated, and the mortality is reduced. Unfortunately, the results obtained at the Hospital of the Rockefeller Institute have not been susceptible of general duplication throughout the country, and the use of the serum has fallen into disuse because (a) its low titer makes necessary the giving of unreasonably large amounts; (b) the technical difficulties of its administration are a real obstacle; and (c) very severe reactions, especially serum sickness, are of frequent occurrence.

Huntoon's Antibody Solution.—This is a practically serum-free, aqueous solution of specific pneumococcus antibodies, designed to give the protection of the earlier serum of Cole without the danger of causing immediate or late horse-serum reactions. Unfortunately, the preparation has the ability to cause quite regularly a severe reaction of the foreign protein type, which sometimes causes the patient to become delirious and to which several deaths are directly ascribed; it is therefore no longer used.

Felton's Antibody Solution.—This solution of pneumococcus antibodies is much more concentrated than that of Huntoon and is apparently making a place for itself by satisfying the very requirements in which the original serum of Cole has failed; namely, reduction of mortality in the controlled series of several independent investigators, relative freedom from serious reactions, and a simple technic of administration. The greatest objection to its use is its almost prohibitive price.

Effect Upon Mortality in Type I Cases.—This can be best indicated by a table (Table 11):

TABLE 11.—MORTALITY OF TYPE I LOBAR PNEUMONIA TREATED WITH FELTON ANTIBODY SOLUTION IN SEVERAL CONTROLLED SERIES

Observers.	Specifically treated.			Controls.		
	Number of cases.	Deaths.	Per cent.	Number of cases.	Deaths.	Per cent.
Park, Bullowa and Rosenblüth (1928).................	58	13	22.0	54	19	35.0
Cases of less than three days' duration.................	29	6	21.0	28	10	36.0
Finland (1930)...............	80	17	21.3	70	22	31.4
Cases of less than three days' duration.................	42	4	9.5	16	6	37.5
Cecil and Plummer (1930)......	239	48	20.1	234	73	31.2
Cases of less than three days' duration.................	103	12	11.7	97	26	26.8
Sutliff and Finland (1931)......	28	7	25.0	31	10	32.2
Heffron and Anderson (1933)...	188	20	10.6	85	22	25.9

It would seem that there can be little doubt about the marked reduction in mortality induced by the use of this Felton solution in Type I cases. The preparation is described in N.N.R., but the Type II solution is not yet accepted (1933) by the Council on Pharmacy and Chemistry, and hence does not as yet appear in N.N.R., because of the belief of most students of serotherapy in pneumonia that only Type I can be successfully treated. However, I place here a table (Table 12) compiled from the reports of several independent investigators who have used the Type II solution.

TABLE 12.—MORTALITY OF TYPE II LOBAR PNEUMONIA TREATED WITH FELTON ANTIBODY SOLUTION IN SEVERAL CONTROLLED SERIES

Observers.	Specifically treated.			Controls.		
	Number of cases.	Deaths.	Per cent.	Number of cases.	Deaths.	Per cent.
Park, Bullowa, and Rosenblüth (1928).....................	56	13	23.0	61	18	30.0
Finland (1930)...............	39	11	28.2	32	11	34.4
Baldwin (1931)...............	35	9	25.7	29	15	51.7
Cecil and Plummer (1932)......	252	102	40.5	253	116	45.8
Finland and Sutliff (1933)......	46	9	20.0	81	32	40.0

It seems that even in this very deadly Type II pneumonia something is to be expected from the specific solution of Felton. It is noteworthy, however, that in Cecil and Plummer's series, which is the sum of all cases so treated by them since 1924, the reduction in mortality is least.

Effect upon Clinical Course.—In the Type I series of Sutliff and Finland (see Table 11), the duration of the disease was shortened on the average from one to two days in patients treated on or before the fourth day; the blood culture became negative after treatment and no patients developed positive cultures during treatment; and extension of the infection to new portions of the lungs did not occur in treated patients, though occurring among the untreated.

Reactions.—If care is taken to rule out patients who manifest marked sensitivity to horse serum, the number and severity of immediate reactions of the circulatory, asthmatic or urticarial types is very small; they are controlled by the immediate subcutaneous administration of 1 cc. of 1:1000 epinephrine (adrenalin) solution. The thermal reaction (chill and rise of fever about one hour after the injection) occurs in a mild form in from 12 to 15 per cent of cases. Serum sickness has been reported by the various observers as occurring in about 30 per cent of cases; this is to be compared with the incidence of 93 per cent in Mackenzie and Hanger's (1930) series of cases treated at the Bellevue with the Cole serum.

Dosage.—"After a preliminary test for sensitiveness to horse serum [for such test and method of desensitization, see p. 780], 5 cc. of the concentrated serum is slowly injected intravenously. From one to two hours later, from 10 to 20 cc. is given intravenously, the dose depending on the potency of the lot and the severity of the case. In general we have tried to administer from 100,000 to 200,000 units (from 40 to 100 cc.) during the first twenty-four hours of treatment. It is our present conviction that in most cases serum treatment should be completed in forty-eight hours; that is, if results are to be obtained at all, they will usually be obtained within that time" (Cecil and Plummer). The giving of these small doses is a much simpler matter than the administration of the large quantities of fluid that was necessary when the serum of Cole was being used.

Kyes' Chicken Serum.—Chickens possess a high degree of natural immunity to pneumococcus infection. Kyes increases this immunity by massive intraperitoneal injections of virulent pneumococci, and then injects the serum of these chickens intravenously in the human irrespective of the type of pneumonia. He usually gives one, but sometimes two, daily injections of 2.5 cc. until the temperature remains below 100 F. (37.8 C.). In his series of 115 cases the mortality was 20.8 per cent, while in 538 control cases under identical conditions the mortality was 45.3 per cent. Gray has also used this serum in an army camp. In two groups of typical lobar pneumonia cases, one of 322 cases and one of 118 cases, the mortality was 7.7 per cent and 4.3 per cent, respectively. In another group of 234 cases of epidemic pneumococcus bronchopneumonia, the mortality was 16.7 per cent as compared with a mortality of 53.6 per cent among 1684 control cases. Gray increased the dose to 5 to 10 cc. and gave it twice daily, in some cases giving as much as 30 cc. in a single day.

These figures are fully as impressive as were those of the Rockefeller group with the original Type I serum, but, bearing in mind the failure of most subsequent workers to verify those findings, at present one can only accept these chicken serum figures with certain reservations.

Vaccines and Convalescent Serum.—Both of these agents have been failures in the treatment of pneumonia.

(B) TREATMENT WITH DRUGS

Mercurochrome-220-soluble.—This dye has been used quite extensively in adult pneumonia by scattered practitioners, results in individual cases varying from "no good" to "marvelous"; an entirely satisfactory study of it has not been made. Hoppe, Goldsmith and Freeman (1926) recorded their results with the drug in children, as summarized in the following table (Table 13), there being 90 cases treated with mercurochrome and 90 used as controls.

TABLE 13.—MERCUROCHROME IN PNEUMONIA IN CHILDREN

	Lobar pneumonias.		Bronchopneumonias.	
	Control cases.	Mercuro-chrome.	Control cases.	Mercuro-chrome.
Number of cases..................	29 cases	35 cases	61 cases	55 cases
Average duration of illness..........	12 days	5.1 days	13:8 days	6.4 days
Days sick after treatment began.....	6.9 days	....	8.4 days	....
Days sick after mercurochrome......	....	2.4 days	....	3.3 days
Mortality........................	10.3 per cent	5.7 per cent	42.6 per cent	10.9 per cent

	All types of pneumonia.	
	Control cases.	Mercurochrome cases.
Average total duration of illness.................	13.3 days	5.9 days
Mortality.......................................	32.2 per cent	8.9 per cent

Hoppe *et al.* believe that most of the severe reactions and untoward results can be avoided if the dose of mercurochrome is not more than 5 mg. per kilogram (2.2 pounds) up to 19 Kg., and beyond that 4 or even 3 mg. per kilogram in severe cases. They advise strongly against the use of mercurochrome if calomel or any other mercurial has been recently given. For the mercurochrome technic, see page 163.

Quinine.—(*a*) *The Alkaloid Itself.*—Quinine is highly bactericidal for the pneumococcus in the test tube, but the extent of its bactericidal action in the body is as yet undetermined. Solis-Cohen, who is probably the foremost present advocate of its use, believes that its action *in vivo* is not only bactericidal but definitely antitoxic. It is well known that enormous doses of the drug are tolerated by the pneumonia patient, doses which would deafen or blind or perhaps even kill the normal individual, and from this Solis-Cohen reasons that some of the quinine is neutralized (*i. e.*, rendered harmless) by some of the toxin; or, stated the other way about, some of the toxin is neutralized (*i. e.*, rendered harmless) by some of the quinine. However this may be, Solis-Cohen has for many years used the drug as part of a definite plan of treatment which he claims has given good results. (A large number of patients of approximately the same economic status have never been treated by this plan at the same time, at the same place, and under the same conditions. I therefore use the word *claims* advisedly, but by no means in a derogatory sense.) This definite plan of treatment, which also includes the use of digitalis and pituitrin, is as follows:

1. Quinine dihydrobromide is given in the following initial dose for an

average adult: 10 to 15 grains (0.6 to 1 Gm.) by vein; or 15 to 25 grains (1 to 1.6 Gm.) by muscle; or 25 to 30 grains (1.6 to 2 Gm.) by mouth. (See p. 95 for methods of giving quinine.) The second dose is given three to six hours later and is equal to or less than the first, according to the temperature index. The third dose follows after another three to six hours and is commonly two thirds or only one half the amount of the first dose, again depending upon the temperature. In general, the attempt is made to bring the temperature to normal and keep it there, but Solis-Cohen would have the point especially stressed that he is using quinine as a specific and not as an antipyretic; this fall in temperature is looked upon as merely a gauge or index of this specific action. After the temperature has become normal, 10 grains by mouth every four to six hours may be enough to keep it there; but the effect must be maintained even should repeated intravenous or intramuscular injection be necessary.

If the subject has a quinine idiosyncrasy, a small tentative dose of 3 grains by vein or muscle, or 5 grains by mouth, may be given at first and the quantity gradually increased. Solis-Cohen says: "I have treated six cases of acute pneumonia in subjects of quinine idiosyncrasy, with six recoveries. The doses used were not materially less than in other cases. There was no untoward action—not even tinnitus. The immunity to quinine lasted from three to six months after recovery; then the susceptibility recurred."

2. Surgical pituitrin is given in a dose of 1 cc., intramuscularly or even intravenously, every three hours so long as the systolic pressure (in millimeters of Hg) remains below the pulse frequency (in beats per minute)—"or preferably until there is a safe interval, say 10 points, between them."

Two to 4 grains of caffeine sodium benzoate is preferred to the pituitrin if there is threat or presence of pulmonary edema.

3. Tincture of digitalis, 5 minims three times daily, is given as a routine in all cases "in order to 'digitalize' the organism to a point at which it will readily and quickly respond to the larger doses when these become necessary." This point of necessity is taken to be a fall of the diastolic pressure to 60 mm. of Hg, or less, or an approach of diastolic pressure and respiration frequency to within 10 points of one another—tincture of digitalis is then given in doses of 15 to 30 minims every three or four hours until full effect is obtained.

I hope that I am not misinterpreting Solis-Cohen's attitude when I say that he looks upon these relationships between systolic and diastolic pressures, and pulse and respiration frequencies, as not in themselves phenomena of very great constancy, but that they do become of great importance when they are made the guide-posts in a definite plan of therapy. It will be quite evident from a perusal of the above that this plan is not adequately described in the phrase "the treatment of pneumonia with quinine."

(b) *Optochin Hydrochloride.*—This substance, which was introduced some years ago by Morgenroth as ethyl-hydrocuprein hydrochloride, is a modification of the quinine molecule as it occurs in cinchona bark. It has been shown to be highly effective against the pneumococcus in conjunctival and other external infections with this organism, but as far too toxic to use systemically in the treatment of pneumonia. Blindness has occurred in practically all cases in which effective amounts have been used and some degree of permanent visual impairment has been very frequent.

(c) *Optochin Base (Numoquin Base).*—This drug is given by mouth in the treatment of pneumonia and is said to be less toxic than the above. Perhaps the outstanding report of its use is that of Cross (1927), who tried it in a series of 126 cases in the Methodist Episcopal Hospital in Brooklyn, using 100 untreated cases as controls. His routine follows: (1) One capsule of

4 grains (0.25 Gm.) with 6 ounces (180 cc.) of milk every four hours, five doses in twenty-four hours, until fifteen such doses have been given—then stop this medication.   (2) During these three days additional milk may be given freely, but beyond small amounts of water nothing else by mouth, either food or drugs, is permitted.   (3) Careful watch must be kept for ringing in the ears, deafness, dizziness, blurring of vision, headache, nausea or vomiting. Cross felt that his statistical findings were inconclusive, but his bedside impressions were that the temperature ran a distinctly lower course in the optochin base-treated cases, that the patients were notably comfortable, and that there was a decreased tendency to extension of the lesion.   There were 4 instances of nausea and vomiting, 6 of tinnitus aurium, 1 of profuse diaphoresis, and 1 of headache; the drug was discontinued in all these cases. Cross had no visual disturbances in his series, but Scales (1932) has reported the case of a patient who developed a severe amblyopia during the course of the treatment and had not recovered useful vision at the time of the report, three months later.

Leitner (1932), in Germany, has reported very good results with the drug in treating primary pneumonias in children, giving it mostly in the form of suppositories which must be retained for at least ten to fifteen minutes. Dosage: Under one year, $\frac{1}{6}$ to $\frac{1}{2}$ grain (0.02 to 0.03 Gm.) three or four times daily; one to two years, $\frac{1}{2}$ to $\frac{2}{3}$ grain (0.03 to 0.04 Gm.) ; two to five years, $\frac{2}{3}$ to $\frac{5}{6}$ grain (0.04 to 0.05 Gm.) ; older children, $\frac{5}{6}$ to $1\frac{2}{3}$ grains (0.05 to 0.1 Gm.).   He feels that the drug should not be given longer than three or four days, and that if care is taken not to give it in the presence of inflammation of the kidneys, no toxic effects need be feared.

PROPHYLAXIS OF PNEUMONIA

The Use of Vaccine.—Since 1914 large scale vaccination trials have been going on in the mining population of the Rand, South Africa.   After an early period of good promise, recent reports (Orenstein, 1931) have shown that the disease has not really been effectively prevented.

The experience of Cecil and Austin at Camp Upton, New York, in 1918, is usually referred to as being favorable to vaccination.   However, for my own part, I am not convinced that this is so.   They vaccinated 12,519 men against Types I, II and III of the Rockefeller classification.   Three or four doses were given at intervals of five to seven days with a total dosage of 6 to 9 billion of Types I and II and 4½ to 6 billion of Type III.   Incidence and severity of reaction were comparable to those occurring during typhoid inoculation.   The 20,000 uninoculated men in the camp were used as controls. During the ten weeks over which the observation extended, no cases of Types I, II and III occurred among the men who had received two or more injections, while during the same period 26 cases of these types occurred among the uninoculated group.   So far, so good.   But why do those who advance this experience as proof of the efficacy of prophylactic vaccination overlook the disparity in size of the treated and control groups, and especially why is the fact never mentioned that the incidence of Type IV and streptococcus pneumonias was much lower among the vaccinated than among the unvaccinated—though the troops had not been inoculated against these two organisms?   Cecil and Austin certainly stated the fact very plainly.

Lipovaccines.—The experiment of Cecil and Vaughan with single doses of lipovaccine at another army camp was very much obscured by the influenza epidemic, but, in 1922, McCoy, Hasseltine, Wadsworth and Kirkbride made a careful study of the methods among the 38,958 inmates of certain New York institutions, with findings that can only be looked upon as indicating the present worthlessness of this type of vaccination.

POLIOMYELITIS

(Acute Anterior Poliomyelitis; Infantile Paralysis)

Poliomyelitis is an acute infectious disease which typically attacks young children only, though adult cases are reported less rarely now than formerly. The attack is a generalized one which affects all the parenchymatous organs, the most dreaded symptom, paralysis, being caused by both a toxic and a hyperplastic assault upon the anterior horn cells in the cord. The causative organism seems to go through avirulent and virulent periods; during the former, many mild, so-called "abortive," cases occur in which there is little or no paralysis, though immunity is conferred by such an attack; during the latter periods the disease tends to become epidemic— pandemic too, at least to this extent that a large number of local epidemics may occur at about the same time scattered throughout the world. Burrows (1931) avers that in the great mass of cases there is no involvement of the nervous system proper. I shall go no deeper into the subject of etiology than to say that a filtrable virus is beyond cavil the cause of the disease, and that one school of investigators holds a certain globoid body, and another school a streptococcus capable of becoming globoid, to be the specific agent in this filtrate; into which controversy Eberson (1933) has tossed the claim that he has isolated an extremely minute organism from infected monkeys, with which Koch's postulates are said already to have been satisfied. Transmission is probably by human contact, but I believe that we are too lightly passing over the housefly as a possible vector. The great preponderance of the disease in the summer months is well known; nor do I look upon the recent increase in winter epidemics as proof positive that the fly can be ruled out, for is it not worthy of note that this increase coincides with the increased installation of heating plants which enable the fly to survive far into the winter in our homes and schools? It would seem that at times the causative agent is milk-borne.

The early symptoms of poliomyelitis are "cold in the head," cough, more or less vomiting and diarrhea, fever, and extreme irritability with coincident malaise and restlessness. Reluctance to lower the chin, and also the assumption of a peculiar position in the bed, may be seen at this stage. Then, in severe cases, and either with or without a remission of several hours to several days, the more severe headache and typical flaccid paralysis of some portion of the body appear. The bulbar type of the disease has of late been growing commoner relative to the spinal form. The case is now usually afebrile, but the child experiences so much pain on being moved that it frequently manifests excessive apprehension when any person approaches the bed. The approach of fatal respiratory paralysis is often very horribly foreshadowed by the way in which the little sufferer, with prescient alertness, marshals his forces for the final agony. It is felt to be usually true that the higher the cell count in the spinal fluid, the more severe the attack; in the prodromal stage the fluid is clear but under increased pressure.

Poliomyelitis is a very ancient disease; it is thought to be represented on one of the stelae of the eighteenth Dynasty (1580 B. C.) in Egypt. The first modern account of the predominating infantile type was that of Michael Underwood (1784). It was the great Duchenne who, in 1855, first pointed out that the paralysis is due to definite lesions in the anterior horns of the cord.

THERAPY

The importance of complete rest from the very beginning is universally recognized, but the advisability of early splinting in all cases is considered to be still debatable.   After the disappearance of pain, massage of the affected muscle groups may be begun, though very little is accomplished by this procedure unless performed by a trained masseur; under-water massage in recovered cases sometimes accomplishes a great deal.   Orthopedic corrective measures of course cannot be discussed here.   The value of x-ray therapy has been both affirmed and denied on the Continent; I know of no studies as yet (1933) in America.   The independent work of Burnham, McGuigan, Voit, de Eds, and others, must be accepted as conclusive proof that nothing is to be expected from urotropin in this disease.   To be sure, it does appear in many of the body juices, but sufficient formaldehyde to be antiseptic is not liberated elsewhere than in the urine.   The recently perfected Drinker respirator has apparently saved some lives in cases of respiratory paralysis.

Convalescent Serum.—The blood serum of individuals who have recovered from an attack of poliomyelitis contains antibodies which will protect an animal that has been artificially inoculated with the virus.   These protective bodies are probably at their point of greatest potency about three months after recovery, but they are present earlier, of course, and seem to persist to some extent for many years.   This convalescent serum has been used in treatment since 1911, often with success, perhaps less often with failure; unfortunately there has not been published a statistical survey on a large scale in which alternate cases were used for controls.   This fact, however, is certain: its effectiveness is very much less after signs of meningeal involvement have appeared.   Therefore to gain the really tremendous advantage which many times accrues from the use of the serum in the preparalytic stage, the watchword should be, "Early diagnosis!"

The serum was formerly used intraspinally exclusively, but, since the recognition of the general nature of the attack, it is now felt to be advisable to give it intravenously as well.   The dose for children is 10 to 30 cc. intraspinally (after the withdrawal of an equivalent amount of fluid) plus 40 to 100 cc. intravenously; adults should be given even larger doses.   In the treatment of early paralyzed cases, or if some degree of paralysis develops, it is advisable to repeat at least the intravenous injection in twelve to twenty-four hours, and perhaps several times after that.   Bear in mind that the intraspinal injection should be given *very slowly,* and fluid shown be withdrawn at once upon the appearance of respiratory symptoms during the injection.   Sometimes the injection by either route causes a brief exacerbation of the symptoms, or a thermal (chill and fever) reaction.   The interesting suggestion of Montgomery and Cole that spinal drainage is in itself enough to forestall paralysis has not been as yet thoroughly put to the test.

Blood should be taken from the donor under aseptic precautions, twice centrifuged to entirely free the serum from red cells, and this serum stored in a cool place.   It is best to culture it for sterility, but the addition of 0.2 per cent of tricresol does not impair the curative power.   Healthy adults can give from 500 to 750 cc., and children of twelve to fifteen from 200 to 250 cc., of blood; 500 cc. of blood will yield about 200 cc. of serum.   The potency of the serum is not appreciably diminished in one year if stored at 4 C. Warm the serum somewhat before injecting it.

The intramuscular injection of the serum or of citrated whole blood (for method of citrating, see p. 115) has been reported by Shaw, Thelander and Fleischner (1925–28), using average doses of 40 to 70 cc.   Results were satisfactory in their 43 patients.   The method—if these findings are confirmed—will have the advantage of simple technic and will thus promote injection without having to wait for spinal puncture.

The preliminary studies of Shaughnessy, Harmon and Gordon (1930) indicate that immunity to poliomyelitis increases with advancing years, as in the case of diphtheria, and that the serum of any adult may be as effective against the disease as that of a person known to be convalescing therefrom.

Antistreptococcus Serum.—Rosenow, of the Mayo Clinic, has for some years been studying a pleomorphic streptococcus which he isolates from the throat, spinal fluid, brain and cord in cases of poliomyelitis. This streptococcus tends to produce flaccid paralysis in the rabbit but does not produce typical poliomyelitis in the monkey, which is just the reverse of what occurs with the virus of Landsteiner and Leviditi—all of which leads to much scepticism in both camps. The Rockefeller Institute group (Olitsky, Rhoads and Long) has completely failed to confirm Rosenow's findings. However, Rosenow prepares a serum by the immunization of horses with increasing amounts of dead, and later living, cultures of his organism; and he claims curative properties for this serum when it is properly used in the treatment of human poliomyelitis.

Several intravenous or intramuscular injections are given at twelve to twenty-four hour intervals. Dosage in general has been: up to two years, 15 to 25 cc.; two to five years, 20 to 30 cc.; six to twelve years, 25 to 50 cc.; over thirteen years, 50 to 75 cc. Serum reactions are very prone to follow the injections.

In his latest report (1930), Rosenow expresses himself still confident that the results of all workers with this serum are as good as those obtained with convalescent serum, but there seem to be very few physicians who feel that he is justified in this belief.

French Antiserum.—Pettit, of the Pasteur Institute of Paris, has been working for several years with a serum which he produces by the immunization of horses to the filtrable virus of poliomyelitis, apparently using the method devised by Neustaedter and Banzhaf, in New York. In America, Weyer, Park and Banzhaf, and Schultz and Gebhardt, and in England, Fairbrother and Morgan, have succeeded in producing the antiviral substances in horses but not with any predictable regularity. Howitt has also succeeded with goats and sheep. In France, the serum is now being produced from monkeys in a shorter time than from horses. In the 1930 outbreak of poliomyelitis in that country there was division of opinion regarding the efficacy of these new serums; they are not yet available for general use.

PROPHYLAXIS

Moro (1930), in Germany, argues that since it is very difficult to diagnose the preparalytic stage of poliomyelitis, all children under five years of age should be inoculated with 20 cc. of their parent's blood during an epidemic, repeating the injection after four weeks. This simple prophylactic measure is deserving of trial, it seems to me.

PSITTACOSIS
(Parrot Fever)

This is an acute infectious disease of parrots, parrakeets, love birds and canaries living in captivity. Experimentally the disease, which is caused by an ultramicroscopical virus, can be transmitted to many other birds and to some of the smaller rodents. In man the disease occurs in rare house epidemics among persons handling infected birds. The two greatest outbreaks have been that in Paris in 1892–95, in which there were 78 cases with 24 deaths, and the present pandemic, which is apparently the result of a large shipment of sick parrots from Paraguay and Brazil to Hamburg, whence the survivors were distributed all over the world. At its height, in 1930, there were reported more than 500 cases on the Continent, in England, North and South America, and the Hawaiian Islands. Cases are still being reported, though with lessening frequency. The mortality in this outbreak has probably averaged 35 per cent. It is of interest to note that in some cases occurring in Breslau, in 1932, the parrots had been reared in Germany and had not been for many years in contact with imported birds.

In man, after an incubation period of eight to fifteen days, there is a chill with subsequent rise of temperature, sometimes to 103 F., and a pulse rate that is not commensurate with the fever; headache, loss of apetite, white-coated tongue with red edges, abdominal distention; there may be vomiting and either diarrhea or constipation; sometimes, but not invariably, there is leukopenia. Upon this typhoid-like picture is engrafted a pneumonia which is atypical in that there is practically no cough, sputum or pain in the chest despite pronounced physical signs of pulmonary involvement. Nervous symptoms as well as albuminuria are often in evidence. The attack may run a course of many weeks, the pulmonary symptoms frequently continuing long after the temperature has subsided.

THERAPY

The treatment is the symptomatic treatment of typhoid and pneumonia. In the present pandemic, convalescent serum has been tried in doses of 50 to 100 cc. daily, mixed with an equal quantity of physiologic saline at time of injection intravenously; smaller doses have been given undiluted intramuscularly. Such evidence as there is in favor of this serum therapy is very inconclusive.

PSOROSPERMIASIS
(Coccidiosis)

This is a very rare protozoan disease (perhaps more correctly called "Coccidiosis") in which all of the parenchymatous organs, but especially the liver and spleen, are riddled with nodular lesions caused by the parasite *Coccidium oviforme.*. The symptoms are too diverse to warrant description here.

THERAPY

All of the 6 reported cases have died within two weeks of the onset of symptoms.

RAT-BITE FEVER
(Sodoku)

This is an infectious disease which follows the bite of a rat. It has long been known, and principally studied, in Japan; a few authentic, and a number of probably spurious cases, have been reported from various other parts of the world. Kenzo Futaki and Kikutaro Ishiwara discovered the causative spirochete in 1915. After an incubation period of ten days to several weeks, the wound site becomes secondarily inflamed, with accompanying adenitis, and the patient experiences a paroxysm characterized by gastrointestinal symptoms, fever, and an exanthematous rash. The symptoms last about two days and disappear by crisis, reappearing again in a few days, however, and continuing a relapsing course for several months. The disease is characterized by progressive anemia. Mortality is about 10 per cent in untreated cases.

THERAPY

Any one of the arsphenamines is curative in from one to three intravenous doses.

RELAPSING FEVER

(Spirillum Fever, African Tick Fever)

Relapsing fever is a remarkable disease which is caused by several closely related varieties of spirochetes that are transferred from man to man by insects. It is not conveyed by the bite of the insect but by crushing the body of the same into the bite wound or the excoriation made by scratching. The so-called "European" variety of the disease, which is conveyed by the body and head louse, and perhaps also exceptionally by flies, mosquitoes and bedbugs, is endemic in European Russia and Poland (it was one of the "natural forces" which helped to decimate Napoleon's army in the retreat from Moscow), the Balkan States, and the whole of the Mediterranean basin. It has also frequently appeared in epidemic form in the Far East and in Central and South America. Europe suffered considerably from it during and subsequent to the World War; in the United States, 6 cases were reported from one locality in 1916–18. The African variety, which is conveyed by ticks, is endemic in the ex-German East Africa, whence it spreads along the caravan routes to many of the other colonial possessions in "native" parts of Africa; it also occurs in Palestine, Persia, Central and South America, and sporadically in Mexico and the Southwestern United States. Fernan-Nuñez (1931) has reported a case in Milwaukee in an individual who had just flown there from Panama. The causative organism of the European variety was discovered by Obermeier, in 1873; of the African variety, independently in 1904 by Ross, Nabarro and Milne, in Uganda, and Dutton and Todd in the Congo. Dutton succumbed to the disease in proving its transmission by a tick.

The onset is typically very sudden, with chilliness, severe headache and pains all over the body, dizziness, gastro-intestinal symptoms, and a high fever. These symptoms last for an average period of seven days and then disappear by crisis, following which the patient seems to be in quite normal health for about a week; then comes a relapse which is usually somewhat milder than the first attack. In the European variety, a second relapse is uncommon, a third very rare; as many as eleven relapses have been observed in African cases. The organism is with difficulty detected in the blood during a paroxysm.

THERAPY

The disease tends to be self-limiting, but any of the arsphenamines will cut short an attack and prevent the relapses. St. John says that eradication of the infection follows one intravenous injection of 0.3 Gm. arsphenamine or 0.45 Gm. neoarsphenamine in about 80 per cent of cases. The mortality is very low in European cases, even though untreated, though it would appear to be invariably fatal to infants under one year. The African cases seem to be uniformly more malignant, and these cases do not all respond to the arsphenamines as well as might be wished. Atkey (1932) has found that the intramuscular injection of 1 cc. of gray oil (see preparations of mercury, p. 205) gives slightly better results than do the arsenicals. He had also previously found such injections to have some value in prophylaxis.

PROPHYLAXIS

For a description of delousing measures, see page 685.

RHEUMATIC FEVER

(Acute Articular Rheumatism)

Rheumatic fever is an acute disease characterized pathologically by the appearance of minute, focal, proliferative lesions in certain tissues of the body, and clinically by fever, pronounced toxemia, a proliferative and exudative arthritis, oftentimes a proliferative valvulitis (endocarditis), and sometimes pericarditis and pleuritis. There are three explanations of its etiology currently offered: (a) it is caused by some one strain of the hemolytic *Streptococcus rheumaticus;* (b) the lesions are those of "chronic anaphylaxis" (the allergic theory); and (c) it is caused by a protozoan or spirochete carried by the rat flea. The disease occurs most frequently in children of school age and is disposed to return many times, but a first attack may also appear when the individual is well along in years. Sometimes, but by no means invariably, the removal of a plausible focus of infection will prevent recurrence of the attacks. There is some evidence that rheumatic fever may be a "house disease" and also that the tendency to contract it is inherited. It is from fifteen to twenty times more prevalent among the poorer classes than in persons better housed and fed; in the tropics it is almost unknown.

Following a sore throat or an attack of catarrhal fever, or symptoms resembling those of acute appendicitis, or without any prodromata at all, the bout of rheumatic fever becomes suddenly established with high fever, sweating, prostration and very painful and tender polyarthritis. The successive involvement of two or three sets of joints may be completely recovered from in ten days to two weeks, but more often several sets of joints are simultaneously involved and the attack lasts much longer. The physician should be ever on the watch for signs of cardiac involvement, not because there is much that he can do to forestall or limit it during the acute attack, but for the important reason that accurate knowledge of the time of its appearance and the extent of its existence will dictate his ordering of the convalescence. One school of observers calls those cases in which the heart is affected only slightly, if at all, "rheumatoid (infectious) arthritis."

De Baillou (1538–1616), whom Crookshank declared to be "the first epidemiologist of modern times," introduced the term "rheumatism." So late as 1836, Jean-Baptiste Bonilland established what he chose to call a "law of coincidence" between the occurrence of heart disease and this malady.

THERAPY

The patient's comfort can be much increased by transferring him to a blanketed bed and wrapping the affected joints in many layers of cotton. He should be carefully protected from the chilling to which he is liable by reason of the excessive sweating; this sweating also calls for the ingestion of large quantities of water, even more than is given as a routine in other acute infectious diseases. Nutrition should be maintained at as high a point as possible, bearing in mind that the patient may be in for a long siege of pain which is exhausting to both mind and body.

The Salicylates.—That the salicylates, given in full doses, act in some sort of specific fashion in rheumatic fever is too well known to require definite statistical affirmation. The fever promptly subsides and there is a considerable and sometimes a complete reduction of the pain, heat, redness and swelling in the joints. We do not know how this is accomplished. Morphine will accomplish an equal reduction in pain but will not reduce the inflammation; likewise the other antipyretics, such as quinine, will reduce the fever but are not equally as effective as the salicylates in ameliorating the other symptoms. This much we do know: (1) Unlike the specific drugs and biologicals that are used in other diseases, the salicylates do not shorten the duration of an attack of rheumatic fever, nor do they lessen the incidence of valvulitis, etc. (2) Careful research has failed to show the salicylates responsible for antibody increase. (3) Salicylic acid is bactericidal in the test tube, but it is extremely improbable that it can accumulate in the tissues in sufficient quantity, under the conditions existing in the living body, to be bactericidal there during life. (4) Both the salicylates and the cinchophens—the two effective classes of antirheumatics—lower the renal threshold for urates, thus materially lessening the concentration of uric acid in the blood. (It will be observed, please, that I only state this as a known fact and one that is worthy of note.)

The synthetic are fully as good as the "natural" products, as was amply shown by the independent laboratory and clinical studies of Waddell and Hewlett. Not a whit more toxic either—and the "natural" are several hundred per cent more expensive.

(a) *Sodium Salicylate.*—This is perhaps the most used preparation. It should be given in a dose of 15 to 20 grains (1 to 1.3 Gm.) every hour for eight or ten doses, then stopped for twelve to twenty-four hours, depending upon the gravity of the case; upon resuming, the same dose should be given every four hours until a week or ten days after the disappearance of all symptoms, when it may be discontinued by a gradual diminution of the dose. In perhaps the majority of cases the patient will not tolerate as much as eight hourly doses, in which event the drug should be given at this time interval only until the first signs of saturation appear (tinnitus, deafness, slight visual disturbances, nausea, vomiting, and perhaps diarrhea).

The gastric irritation manifested by nearly all patients can be lessened by prescribing the same or double the amount of sodium bicarbonate with the salicylate. These may be placed in solution in peppermint water, which will somewhat disguise the mawkish taste; or, as preferred by some physicians, in capsules. When the gastric irritation limits the dosage to less than is necessary to obtain the therapeutic effect, the drug may be given by the rectum. Heyn has reported a series of 125 cases in which he satisfactorily used the salicylates intrarectally. His technic follows:

"A cleansing soap-suds enema is given [I believe 1 per cent sodium bicarbonate would be better—see p. 434—H. B.] and as soon as effective is followed by the salicylate enema given by means of a Davidson syringe and a rectal tube inserted 6 to 8 inches. The dose varies according to the size and sex of the patient and also according to the severity of the case. The first adult dose in men is usually 8 to 10 Gm. [120 to 150 grains], in women 6 Gm. [90 grains], women being apparently more susceptible to salicylism than men. . . . The amount of salicylate to be given is incorporated in 120 to 180 cc. of plain or starch water with the addition of 1.0 to 1.5 Gm. [15 to 23 minims] of the tincture of opium. The dose of salicylate may be repeated in twelve hours, when it can usually be determined whether symptoms of salicylism will appear. Usually, however, a daily enema suffices with doses increasing perhaps from 30 to 50 per cent daily until the limit of tolerance is reached. The largest daily dose which has been given has been 24 Gm. [360 grains] and the only symptoms of salicylism which have usually appeared have been tinnitus and excessive perspiration. Once or twice there has been vomiting present, which might occur in the administration of even a simple enema. Where salicylism has been excessive, it usually appears within from three to six hours and the remaining unabsorbed portion of salicylate may be washed out of the bowel by subsequent enema. This has been resorted to very infrequently indeed, and it is rare also that the rectum is intolerant of the drug."

It is doubtful whether intravenous salicylate medication possesses any advantages over the administration of the drug by mouth or rectum; however, when neither the stomach nor rectum is sufficiently tolerant, it must be resorted to. Mendel, quoted by Fantus, gives the following formula:

R. Sodium salicylate... 8.0 Gm.
    Caffeine sodium salicylate.............................. 2.5 Gm.
    Sterilized water to make................................ 50.0 cc.

Inject 2 Gm. (one fourth of this solution) every twelve hours.

(b) *Strontium Salicylate.*—The studies of Blankenhorn, in 1916, would seem to have cast considerable doubt upon the vaunted superiority of strontium to sodium salicylate. However, in a patient whose stomach is revolting against the sodium salicylate, equivalent doses of strontium salicylate may sometimes be substituted with advantage.

(c) *Acetylsalicylic Acid (Aspirin).*—This drug perhaps causes less anorexia and nausea than sodium salicylate, but there are several cases of violent idiosyncrasy on record. It is used in the same doses and at the same intervals as the sodium salicylate. Acetylsalicylic acid is too insoluble and unstable to be prescribed in water. Assertions have been made, however, that it may be dispensed in water by the aid of sodium citrate and that the acetylsalicylic acid is not decomposed in such a solution. Leech has shown that this is not true; decomposition does take place, and after several days the ingredients of such a solution are just the same as if sodium acetate and sodium salicylate had been used in the first place.

Acetylsalicylic acid should not be prescribed in combination with alkalis, such as sodium bicarbonate, for the gastric irritation due to the formation of alkali salicylates will be greater than if the acetylsalicylic acid is given alone. Under the conditions in which the drug is used in rheumatic fever it is not a heart depressant.

(d) *Methyl Salicylate (Oil of Wintergreen, Oil of Gaultheria).*—This drug is sometimes used in about the same doses as sodium salicylate, but as it is no more efficient and is capable of causing profound poisoning, as recently attested by Wetzel and Nourse, it is perhaps well to confine its use to external application. When given by mouth the prescribed dose is usually dropped from a medicine dropper into capsules just before use. For external application it is mixed with one or two parts of olive oil and painted on the joints.

The Cinchophens.—Cinchophen is phenyl-quinoline-carboxylic acid, of which the official U.S.P. preparation, or any Council-accepted brand, is just as good as that marketed under the trade name of Atophan. Neocinchophen is ethyl-methyl-phenyl-quinoline-carboxylic acid, and any Council-accepted brand is just as good as that marketed under the trade name of Tolysin. These two substances were introduced with the hope, and at first the rather extravagant claims, that they would be superior to the salicylates in the treatment of rheumatic fever and gout. Regarding their use in gout, more later (see p. 388). In rheumatism, they have not been a failure, but the work of Hanzlik and Scott (1921), Chase, Myers and Killian (1921), and Boots and Miller (1924), together with the unpublished experience of numerous practitioners, lead me to believe that the following is a true summary of their present status:

(*a*) In order to accomplish comparable results in the symptomatic relief of rheumatic fever, they must be given at the same intervals and in the same doses as the salicylates, or even slightly larger.

(*b*) In effective doses they produce toxic symptoms about as often as the salicylates, but these toxic symptoms are as a rule less severe than those induced by the salicylates—see, however, below!

(*c*) They are both capable of causing renal irritation, but perhaps not as often, certainly no more often, than the salicylates.

(*d*) There are perhaps no more cases of idiosyncrasy toward the cinchophens than toward the salicylates.

(*e*) Cinchophen often causes a burning irritation in the throat and stomach. In the average case, neocinchophen causes less gastric disturbance than either cinchophen or the salicylates.

A liberal quantity of water should always be given with these drugs to prevent the precipitation of uric acid; sodium bicarbonate in large doses (given separately and not mixed with the drug) is an additional safeguard. Cinchophen may be suspended in water, neocinchophen must be given in tablet form. Tolstoi and Corke (1932) are trying to reduce the amount of cinchophen given by employing it in tablets containing magnesium cinchophen and magnesium oxide; 15-grain (1 Gm.) doses, 75 to 90 grains (5 to 6 Gm.) daily. Their studies are based on the experimental observation of Barbour and Winter (1929) that magnesium potentiates the action of cinchophen. So far only a few cases have been treated, but they were relieved with smaller total quantities of cinchophen than are often required and without the appearance of toxic symptoms.

I believe that these drugs are a valuable addition to our armamentarium, but they have not replaced the salicylates. Some cases will respond to them when the salicylates have given no relief, but the reverse is also true. The wise practitioner will avail himself of the one or the other, or perhaps alternately the one and the other, as seems to be indicated in the individual case.

Cinchophen Cirrhosis.—Since Cabot described the first serious case of cinchophen disturbance of the liver, in 1925, the danger of this unfortunate occurrence has been most astonishingly emphasized. Weis has collected the reports of 92 cases between 1925 and July, 1932; 40 of the patients died, and the diagnosis was confirmed in 33 instances at autopsy. The following is a brief résumé of the subject:

(*a*) The usual signs of idiosyncrasy to cinchophen are purpuric, urticarial or scarlatinal eruptions, with or without edema; gastro-intestinal disturbances; circulatory disturbances; and occasionally general malaise, headache and even fever. The first definite symptom of liver poisoning is loss of appetite, followed by sleepiness and jaundice, and then the symptoms of acute atrophy of the liver develop progressively.

(*b*) The evidences of this type of poisoning may appear during the time that the drug is being taken or not until several weeks or months after it has been discontinued.

(*c*) It is pretty generally believed now that under certain conditions the liver becomes sensitized to the toxic action of the drug; for there is great variability in toxic dosage in the reported cases. For instance, Evans' (1926) patient took only 15 grains (1 Gm.), one of De Rezende's (1927) 45 grains (3 Gm.), and the patient of Lind (1932) about 75 grains (5 Gm.); whereas, Hench and Rowntree (1930) report a patient who took 40 to 90 grains (2.6 to 6 Gm.) daily for eighteen years without any untoward symptoms at all. Rabinowitz (1930) believes that the following conditions are predisposing:

gallbladder disease, cirrhosis of the liver, pregnancy, chronic alcoholism, chronic nephritis, a past history of jaundice. Many observers feel that the occurrence of any of the usual signs of idiosyncrasy indicate high susceptibility to this serious type of liver injury; theoretically, at least, the drug would be particularly dangerous in conditions favoring decreased glycogen content of the liver cells, such as malnutrition, cachexia, chronic infection and acute fevers. It might also be that sensitization of the liver to protein, as by surgical trauma or the parenteral injection of milk or vaccines, would increase the danger.

(d) The treatment as outlined by Rabinowitz is followed in most cases: "With the earliest appearance of toxic phenomena, the drug should be stopped and the patient hospitalized. Dextrose by mouth or rectal drips in large amounts should be given, and from 5 to 10 units of insulin, three times daily ordered. If the symptoms are at all severe, intravenous dextrose in large amounts as well. Proteins in the diet should be reduced to minimal amounts, as the liver is no longer capable of detoxicating the products of protein metabolism."

Cinchophen cirrhosis, then, is a very dangerous affair, and would seem to call for the desertion of the drug by the profession, even though the cases are not of frequent occurrence relatively to the large number of persons who take the drug. Intermittent use to avoid retention of dangerous amounts is probably of little avail. Neocinchophen has a cleaner slate probably only because it is not so widely used by either laity or profession.

Miscellaneous Drugs and Biologicals.—*Mercurochrome.*—Young (1926) reported 10 cases of nongonorrheal rheumatic fever treated by the intravenous administration of mercurochrome; seven were cured or improved, one was only temporarily relieved, and in two the treatment failed entirely. For the mercurochrome technic, see page 163.

Amidopyrine (Pyramidon).—During the latter years of the nineteenth century, the use of this drug was several times enthusiastically advocated by Continental physicians, but in neither hemisphere did it find a secure place and was forgotton in this connection until Schottmüller rediscovered its value, in 1927. Schultz (1931) has given it a very careful trial in a series of 32 patients at the Hospital of the Rockefeller Institute, New York City. He finds it fully as effective as the salicylates or neocinchophen in the reduction of fever, relief of pain, and lessening of exudation; but, also like the other two drugs, it did not influence either the incidence of complications or the tendency toward relapse. The drug was given in single doses of 5 grains (0.3 Gm.), and acute cases were relieved by the astonishingly small total daily amount of 10 to 20 grains (0.6 to 1.2 Gm.), which was often reduced or discontinued within a week. Cases in a chronic or subacute phase of the disease required from 15 to 30 grains (0.9 to 2 Gm.) daily, and the administration had to be continued over a longer period. There was complete absence of side actions and apparently a wide margin between the effective therapeutic dose and a probable toxic quantity. Schultz found these features particularly valuable in patients in whom cardiac decompensation developed, for the entire absence of gastric irritation from amidopyrine permitted the certain identification of the visceral congestive signs of cardiac insufficiency: epigastric discomfort and tenderness, nausea and loss of apetite. Furthermore, when digitalis and amidopyrine were both being given it was always possible to be sure that when gastric symptoms appeared they were caused by the digitalis.

Nirvanol.—There is no doubt that this drug, which is quite effective in many cases of chorea (see p. 627), has a definite antirheumatic effect in some patients; but it fails in many instances and I see no reason for ever preferring it to the salicylates.

Sulphur and Iodine.—In Germany, various proprietary combinations of these two drugs are being employed by a few clinicians, but I have not as yet found a carefully controlled study of their effectiveness.

Antistreptococcus Preparations.—Swift (1931) and his associates in this country, and Collis and Sheldon in England, have been studying the effect of serums and vaccines variously prepared in their laboratories, and believe that they have at times been able to induce a state of resistance in patients with a continuing low-grade infection or in those at the time free from symptoms but reasonably sure to have relapses. Of course satisfactory evidence of this sort would be very difficult to adduce; many physicians believe that the whole attempt has no rationale since we do not know with certainty whether the streptococcus is the etiologic agent in rheumatic fever. The preparations are not commercially available.

Milk Injections.—The advocates of this method of therapy at least do not claim any specificity for it, but I am unable to unearth any evidence that these injections accomplish anything that the salicylates or cinchophens will not; the reactions they cause are more disagreeable than the side actions of the drugs.

Effect of Tonsillectomy on Rheumatic Fever.—Here is a tremendously important question, which, so far as I am aware, has not yet been satisfactorily answered. Kaiser's (1927) investigations among 48,000 school children indicated that the procedure was distinctly valuable in influencing the course of the disease and the incidence of cardiac complications, though the actual incidence of rheumatism was practically unaltered. Upon the other hand, the smaller but carefully studied series of Wilson, Lingg and Croxford (1928) yielded no evidence in favor of the operation and even showed that the incidence of sore throat was not lessened by it. All unprejudiced reviewers of the subject reach some such conclusion as this: until someone produces incontrovertible evidence that children without tonsils are definitely protected against rheumatism, routine tonsillectomy is not justified; but when the tonsils are large, ragged and septic, or small and accompanied by enlarged glands, the removal of tonsils and adenoids is probably well worth while.

Salicylates in Prophylaxis.—Leech (1930) gave 20 grains (1.3 Gm.) of acetylsalicylic acid daily for six months to 67 children with potential heart disease and inactive rheumatic heart disease, controlling the series with 79 similar children untreated. The daily salicylate ration seemed to be the factor which enabled a number of the children to gain weight, and presumably an increase in general resistance, but the study was inconclusive with regard to protection against cardiac complications. Perry's (1933) findings, in England, were also of an indefinite nature.

ROCKY MOUNTAIN SPOTTED FEVER
(Tick-bite Fever)

This is an infectious disease which, in its worst form, is peculiar to certain discrete localities in all the States traversed by the Rocky Mountains; it is most frequent in Idaho and Montana. The causative organism is closely related to that which causes typhus fever and is transmitted to man through the feeding upon his person of several varieties of wood tick. The disease is most frequent in spring and early summer. The symptoms are initial chill, high fever, very severe headache and pains all over the body, a generalized petechial rash of the skin and buccal mucosa (usually appearing first on the wrists and ankles), and extreme restlessness and insomnia. The average duration of nonfatal cases of the disease is about three weeks; when death occurs it is usually between the sixth and twelfth days. The mortality varies with the locality; in certain parts of Idaho it is 3 to 4 per cent, elsewhere in the state it is 10 to 20 per cent; in the Bitter Root Valley of western Montana it is regularly as high as 90 per cent. Parker (1933) gives the following percentage mortality (inclusive of all ages and localities) in some of the Western States over a series of years: Montana, 26.91; Wyoming, 21.44; Colorado, 20; Oregon, 18.94; Nevada, 16.42; Washington, 11.90; California, 11.59; Utah, 6.89, and Idaho, 4.16. Many experienced physicians believe that there is a very mild form which usually escapes diagnosis and thus is not reported.

Isolated case reports, in 1931–33, have shown that the disease is also endemic east of the Appalachian Mountains, in the Middle West, and as far north as Montreal and south as Texas. According to Dyer, Rumreich and Badger (1931), the vector of this virus is the common tick of the dog; the mortality is stated to be about 25 per cent.

THERAPY

All attempts at specific drug therapy have failed. Wolbach says that the arsphenamines and atoxyl are not only useless but are in addition decidedly deleterious. This author, who has had much experience both laboratory and clinical with the disease, advocates the use of hypnotics, though I believe it is not the usual custom to employ them. He also advises that the patient be digitalized as in pneumonia. A liberal diet should be given, even to the point of pushing food in the beginning, and both external and internal hydrotherapeutic measures should be employed.

At Hamilton, Montana, the U. S. P. H. S. prepares a vaccine, which, according to Perry (1928) and Parker (1933), has been of distinct value; the latter writes: "The vaccine affords complete protection in the average person against the milder strains and against the highly fatal strains to ameliorate greatly the course of infection and to insure recovery."

PROPHYLAXIS

When tick-infested areas must be visited in spring and summer, such clothing should be worn as will force the tick to crawl up the outside, when he can be detected as he makes contact with the short hairs of the neck. Rough white socks, worn on the outside of the leggings, will impede the progress of the tick and enable him to be readily seen. The entire body should be examined once during the day and again upon retiring. After removal of the attached tick it is the custom, in the West, to cauterize the spot with the silver nitrate stick or nitric acid; Parker (1933) believes this to be a good practice.

SCARLET FEVER

Scarlet fever is an acute infectious disease caused by *Streptococcus scarlatinae*. It is very much more common during the first decade of life than during any other period, and, though occurring sporadically, has a strong tendency to become epidemic, the seasonal incidence being greatest in the school period of September to June. The virulence of the disease varies, mortality among children in the various epidemics being from 3 up to as high as 90 per cent; after the eighth year, mortality rarely runs above 3 to 4 per cent.

The typical case is characterized by the sudden onset with nausea and vomiting, high fever, sore throat, and the appearance within twenty-four hours of a generalized, scarlet, maculopapular ("goose flesh") rash on the body and a punctate eruption on the roof of the mouth. The "strawberry" appearance of the tongue is regarded as characteristic of the disease. The temperature and other symptoms usually begin to subside gradually within five to seven days, and a few days after the disappearance of the rash the period of desquamation begins. It is during this period of desquamation, which lasts for several weeks, that the secondary symptoms may arise; of these the most severe are peritonsillar and retropharyngeal abscess, cellulitis of the neck, otitis media and mastoiditis, nephritis, and arthritis.

There are several atypical types of the disease and two definitely recognized malignant types: the fulminating type in which death occurs from acute failure of the heart almost before the symptoms of the disease have appeared, and the septic type in which the anginal process in the throat quickly involves the nose and the larynx and trachea, with death from general sepsis.

Scarlet fever is one of the diseases of which the great Sydenham (1624–89) has left a first-hand account, separating it from measles and giving it its present name; its confusion with measles, however, persisted for a long time after his day. Following the period which corresponds roughly with the American War for Independence (late eighteenth century), scarlet fever spread rapidly over both hemispheres, and now occurs all over the world but is extremely rare among natives of Africa and India. In our own times the study of the disease is remarkable for being enriched by the contributions of two women: Ruth Tunnicliff, who separated the causative hemolytic streptococcus from that of erysipelas (1920–27), and Gladys Dick, who worked most profitably on both the bacteriology and serology of the disease (1921–27).

THERAPY

Mild cases of scarlet fever require practically no treatment, though the physician often experiences difficulty in keeping the little patients in bed until the danger of the establishing of secondary symptoms has passed. Children will usually take large quantities of fluid quite readily if offered in the form of lemonade. Diet is usually maintained in the beginning on the liquid basis, with milk predominating, but I believe that the causal relationship of a full diet to nephritis in this disease has not been established. After desquamation begins, the patient is much relieved by the application of ordinary petrolatum to which a small amount of phenol has been added, but it is well to keep the proportion of phenol below 0.5 per cent if the entire body is to be anointed; I have seen a case of mild nephritis caused by one application over the entire skin surface of an ointment containing 2 per cent of phenol. The complications must be treated as such when they make their appearance. Of course most rigid quarantine of patient and nurse is to be maintained throughout and is not to be lifted until desquamation is completed, and then only if there are no discharges from the mouth, nose or ears.

Prophylaxis and Treatment with Specific Antitoxin.—This matter has been revived during the last few years and, thanks to the indefatigable efforts of the Dicks, has been accorded its deserved place in therapeutics. Moser (1902) in Austria, and Savchenko (1905) and Gabritschewsky (1907) in Russia, had advanced far in the utilization of antitoxin in scarlet fever, but they were very much handicapped in their work by the fact that their product lacked uniformity for the reason that no test reactions had been devised by which it could be standardized. Leaving aside, for others to argue, the question of whether or not Gabritschewsky fully identified the specific hemolytic streptococcus as the cause of scarlet fever, the fact undeniably before us is that we are in present possession of an antitoxin of uniform quality—1 cc. of which is just like any other cubic centimeter. The names of Schultz and Charlton, in Germany (1918), and Mair, in England (1923), must be associated with this triumph, but I believe that the chief credit is due the Dicks, in the United States (1923), who have succeeded in causing scarlet fever in the human and have not only devised a skin test that is of great value in the diagnosis and in the identification of those who are susceptible to the disease, but have also utilized this test in the standardization of the antitoxin. Dochez, in the United States (1924), had also devised a method of producing an antitoxin of uniform quality, in which he utilized the Schultz-Charlton test for standardization, but, since his early product was not entirely satisfactory, the palm of priority would seem by right to belong to the Dicks.

The intensive studies that have been made since 1923 in attempting to fix the value of this new antitoxin in both the prevention and treatment of scarlet fever do not, unfortunately, lend themselves to such brevity of discussion as would be suitable here. I shall therefore write below a list of authors whom the reader will find it profitable to consult in regard to the various phases of the subject, and shall then offer a summary of the facts that are already established.

Authors.—Dick and Dick; Dochez *et al.*; Lindsay *et al.*; Nesbit; Rosen *et al.* (Russia); Graham; Park; Henry *et al.* (England); Blake *et al.*; Musser; Friedemann *et al.* (Germany); Toomey *et al.*; Perkins; Okell (England); Blatt and Dale; Place; Hunt. (See Bibliography for complete references.)

Summary.—1. The Council-passed products which are at present (end of 1933) available in the United States are prepared (*a*) after the method of the Dicks by immunizing horses by injecting the soluble toxin of strains of hemolytic streptococci that have produced experimental scarlet fever in human beings, and (*b*) by the method of Dochez in which horses are immunized against the specific scarlet fever organism by the localization of the living streptococci in a subcutaneous agar nodule which grows and stimulates the production of antitoxic and antibacterial substances. Certain modifications of these methods are employed by some producers.

The product is available in three forms: (1) a vial containing sufficient antitoxin to perform several diagnostic skin blanching tests, (2) a syringe containing a single prophylactic dose of antitoxin (the quantity of which varies with the different manufacturers), and (3) a syringe containing a single therapeutic dose of antitoxin (the quantity of which varies with the different manufacturers).

2. The antitoxin is given intramuscularly, only in extreme cases intravenously. When given early in the disease (preferably as soon as the rash appears) it almost invariably causes a marked reduction in the temperature within twenty-four hours and also a very distinct lessening in the severity of the sore throat and the other toxic symptoms. In the majority of cases the rash also disappears within twenty-four hours. Though the severity of the initial febrile stage of the attack is thus lessened, the total duration of this phase may or may not be reduced.

3. The period of desquamation is much shorter, so that uncomplicated cases can be released from quarantine much sooner than was formerly the case.

4. When given very early, the incidence of complications is probably reduced—certainly the patient is placed in a better position to cope with any septic state which may arise.

5. When given after the rash has disappeared it is of little or perhaps no value, and when used solely against the late septic complications it is worthless.

6. There is a growing feeling that the size of the present therapeutic dose should be increased. Immediate reactions and serum sickness occur just as they do whenever horse serum is used for any purpose—that is to say, with the same frequency and severity.

7. It seems that a brief but almost immediate passive immunity is conferred upon a majority of individuals by the use of a prophylactic dose of the antitoxin. This passive immunization is not much employed, however, for the following reasons: (a) its duration is relatively brief, leaving the child then in greater danger of anaphylactic reactions should it be necessary to inject horse serum on any subsequent occasion; (b) only about 9 per cent of children exposed to scarlet fever will contract the disease; and (c) in view of the foregoing the liability to serum sickness following the injection is felt to contraindicate it.

8. It appears that active immunity can be conferred upon an individual by the use of smaller doses at sufficient intervals. The immunity is established in from a few days to eight weeks, depending upon the age of the child among other things. Regarding duration of the immunity, Bull (1933) has recently made a very valuable contribution: after the lapse of eight years only ten of twenty-two children who had received three doses remained negative, whereas of twenty-eight who had received five or six doses twenty-two were still negative. The accepted method is to inject hypodermically the contents of a prophylactic vial once each week for five weeks; two weeks after the last dose repeat the skin test and inject an extra dose if the result of the test indicates it. Both the three-week injection method and the use of ricinoleated antigen yield inferior results, the latter causing at times particularly severe reactions; indeed, I believe that this preparation is no longer commercially distributed. A toxoid preparation, similar to that employed in diphtheria immunization (see p. 43) is also used; it has the advantage of relative freedom from severe reactions because of containing no horse serum, and is apparently challenging the antitoxin also upon the head of simplicity, since it need be given only three times at weekly intervals.

Convalescent Serum.—Interest in the new, standardized antitoxin should not blind us to the fact that good results have been obtained by the injection of convalescent serum. This form of treatment was much used in Germany during the latter years of the nineteenth century and was revived in that country by Reiss and Jungmann in 1912, since which time it has been employed by a few individuals in nearly every country. Like the antitoxin, it is most effective when given very early; apparently the immunity does not last longer than three or four weeks. In Meader's (1930) study, 450 contacts were given 7.5 cc. each, intramuscularly, of the pooled serum of donors who had had scarlet fever within a year or a little later; none of the serum was more than six months old when injected. Of the cases, 2.9 per cent developed the disease as compared with an incidence of 12.8 per cent in a similar group of contacts not injected. Reactions do not follow the use of convalescent serum; for method of preparation, see page 114.

Immunotransfusion.—Gordon (1933) has been trying the transfusion of whole unaltered blood from recently recovered patients, which is believed to have value for its nutritive effect, its benefit to the secondary anemia, its transfer of large numbers of phagocytic leukocytes, and also for the passive immunity which it confers. No person has been used as donor before the fifteenth day of the illness and he prefers that convalescence shall not have exceeded three or four months as the other extreme. For infants and small children usually 100 to 150 cc. has been given, for older children about 300 cc., and for adults 500 cc. Sometimes two or three transfusions were given, much less often a larger number. From his experience in 246 cases, Gordon believes that immunotransfusion has its most important indication in acute septic scarlet fever (so-called "scarlatina anginosa" or "scarlatina necroticans"), in the late septic complications of the ear, nose and paranasal sinuses, and in postscarlatinal bacterial endocarditis; in malignant toxic scarlet fever he feels that less favorable results are to be expected than with scarlet fever streptococcus antitoxin.

The blood of several individuals can be mixed; indeed, this is perhaps advisable as the efficiency of some sera is greater than others, irrespective of the severity of the attack through which the donor has passed.

Mercurochrome and Acriflavine.—Young has treated 4 cases of the severe type of scarlet fever, all of which appear to have been saved by the intravenous use of mercurochrome. (For technic, etc., see p. 163.) One of these cases has been recorded in great detail by Young and Birkhaug.

Gurevich (1930) has used acriflavine hydrochloride intravenously in 11 septic cases, giving 10 cc. of a 0.5 to 2 per cent solution, repeated in two or three days. The course was not shortened but the patients were notably relieved symptomatically.

SEPSIS

(Septicemia)

Following the example of Herrick and the frequent Continental usage, I am employing the term "sepsis" for the description of a syndrome which it is more usual to designate "septicemia" in the United States. This departure is made for the reason that the term "septicemia" places too great stress upon the presence of the causative organism in the blood stream and tends to foster the misconception that this disease entity is characterized by a state of affairs in which large numbers of the organisms are constantly floating about and multiplying in the circulating fluids of the body. To be sure, eruption of the causative micro-organism into the blood stream, and perhaps a succession of such eruptions, is a *sine qua non* for the development of sepsis, but the mere presence therein of these organisms is not in itself enough to justify the diagnosis—as witness typhoid fever, in which there is a more or less persistent bacteremia, despite which we do not refer to the case as one of "septicemia." From first to last sepsis is a clinically recognizable entity, which has at some time in its course the laboratory-demonstrable feature of organisms in the blood stream; but, as Churchman so well pointed out, it is not the fact of their presence there that is of importance, but rather that "they have come somewhence and are going somewhither." He goes on to say: "Their source is the focus of infection; their destiny, other organs, in which they may set up lesions, or the filtering organs (lymph glands, etc.) where those of them which have escaped the antibacterial defensive mechanism of the circulating blood are either in part or in whole destroyed or eliminated. Eliminate their source, as by complete excision of the focus, and you cut off the supply. They will then fairly soon disappear from the blood stream, provided they have not already produced secondary foci elsewhere, and provided the defensive mechanism of the body has not already completely broken down. . . . The mere presence of the bacteria in the blood stream is not, therefore, the most serious feature. The most serious feature is the fact that they are being transmitted by the blood stream, that a barrier has given way, and that a local disease is becoming general." The term "pyemia" should be dropped, for it serves to elevate to the rank of an independent entity what is really only an incident of a state of sepsis, namely, the development of metastatic abscesses at points remote from the original nidus of infection.

Most cases of sepsis follow a surgical operation, an abortion or child-birth, an acute or chronic sinus infection or an infection of the same sort in the male genitals or the female pelvis, a sore throat, otitis media, or an apparently trivial superficial external wound; in a minority of cases the original focus cannot be determined. The onset is usually sudden, with chill and high rise of temperature (the type of which varies somewhat with the organism involved) and rapid pulse and respiration, frequent gastro-intestinal symptoms, leukocytosis, multiform skin lesions, and a nervous involvement which varies between the extremes of wild delirium and coma. What organic involvements are to supervene cannot be pre-dicted in the beginning; endocarditis, suppurative arthritis, and embolic phenomena are frequent. Some patients die very quickly from an over whelming toxemia, others linger only to succumb after several weeks or even months. Tileston places the general mortality at 60 to 80 per cent, Herrick at 70 to 90 per cent; the latter states that if cases with meningitis, endocarditis, general peritonitis, or pylephlebitis (all of which are almost uniformly fatal) are eliminated, the average death rate is only 50 per cent.

It was principally sepsis, of course, that made the hospitals of old the shambles that they were. So late as the eighteenth century even physicians declined hospital service "as equivalent to a sentence of death." Reforms followed the independent reports, in 1777-89, of Tenon with regard to the deplorable state of affairs in the Hôtel Dieu in Paris, and John Howard on numerous institutions on the Continent. However, real cleanliness only came into effect after Florence Nightingale began her labors in 1854. Lister, in 1867, inaugurated the era of surgical antisepsis which finally led to the aseptic technic.

THERAPY

The esteemed mentor of my student days, Professor G. A. Hendon, used eloquently to maintain that the outcome in a given case of sepsis depends upon the interrelationship of the "four big V's," which were the following:

1. Variety of the organism.
2. Volume of the organism.
3. Virulence of the organism.
4. Vital resistance of the patient.

In what follows I have attempted to exhibit a therapy that is directed toward an adjustment of these four factors.

1. **Variety of the Organism.**—There is nothing to do about this. In the majority of cases the invader will be one of the streptococci, or it may be a staphylococcus, or one of the colon group, or what not. I do not believe that the proposers of any of the sera and vaccines have proved the specific value of their products in the treatment of acute sepsis. Antistreptococcus serum has been before the profession since 1895 and is still waging a fight to hold what little good opinion it may have gained, and there is no convincing evidence as yet that the use of scarlet fever antitoxin will be crowned with any greater success (Bibliography: Sanderson *et al.*; Burt-White; Lord and Holmes; Rosher; Comber; Cadman; Burton and Balmain; Benson and Rankin).

2. **Volume of the Organism.**—Every reasonable attempt should be made to halt the influx of organisms into the blood stream by eliminating the primary or secondary foci. Sometimes this is relatively easy, as in the

case of carbuncle or sinus thrombosis following a mastoid operation; but the inaccessibility of the focus, or the gravity of the patient's condition, oftentimes makes radical interference impossible. In puerperal sepsis, especially if it follows incomplete abortion, some practitioners believe that an attempt should be made to evacuate remnants of the placenta from the uterus, if this can be done without anesthetic; following this an antiseptic douche should be used (Hirst recommends tincture of iodine 2 drachms, 95 per cent alcohol 8 ounces, sterile water to make 2 quarts; Hobbs introduces a catheter into the uterus in the morning and irrigates with 100 cc. of warm glycerin every hour for from three to six hours, then removes the catheter), but if the temperature continues high, or drops and soon again rises high, no further manipulations should be performed and even the douche or glycerin irrigation should be discontinued. Perhaps the majority of obstetricians, however, disagree with this plan of treatment and prefer a radical policy of "hands-off!" from the very beginning in *all* cases; the only interference they employ is the draining of accessible pelvic pus collections as soon as they develop.

Placing the patient in the well-known Fowler position is of great advantage in these pelvic cases; walling off of the local process is thus facilitated and its spread to other parts of the peritoneal cavity, as well as the access of organisms and toxins to the general circulation, is made much more difficult.

3. **Virulence of the Organism.**—We cannot avoid a discussion here of the intravenous use of dyes in the treatment of sepsis, of which mercurochrome is the chief. In his most recent (1926) complete review of the clinical results obtained with the drug, Young includes the following table (Table 14), which I have slightly simplified:

TABLE 14.—RESULTS IN ONE-HUNDRED-AND-SEVENTY-THREE CASES OF SEPSIS TREATED WITH MERCUROCHROME-220-SOLUBLE INTRAVENOUSLY

Origin of sepsis.	Total number of cases.	Cured or permanently improved.	Action M-220 doubtful.	Improvement only temporary.	Failed.
Genito-urinary...............	22	16 (72.7 per cent)	0	1 (4.5 per cent)	5 (22.7 per cent)
Traumatic or postoperative....	31	21 (67.7 per cent)	1 (3.2 per cent)	3 (9.7 per cent)	6 (19.4 per cent)
From throat infection........	8	6 (75.0 per cent)	0	2 (25.0 per cent)	0
From ear or lateral sinuses...	14	11 (78.6 per cent)	0	1 (7.1 per cent)	2 (14.2 per cent)
From osteomyelitis or abscess.	10	7 (70.0 per cent)	0	0	3 (30.0 per cent)
Puerperal....................	66	41 (62.2 per cent)	8 (12.1 per cent)	1 (1.5 per cent)	16 (24.0 per cent)
Endocarditis................	18	4 (22.2 per cent)	0	4 (22.2 per cent)	10 (55.5 per cent)
Focus unknown.............	4	3 (75.0 per cent)	0	0	1 (25.0 per cent)
Grand Total.............	173	109 (63.0 per cent)	9 (5.2 per cent)	12 (6.9 per cent)	43 (24.8 per cent)

Here then we have 173 cases of sepsis treated by mercurochrome, in which, counting all the cases in the last three columns as deaths, there was a total mortality of 37 per cent—the average mortality, according to the authorities quoted above, being from 60 to 90 per cent in all types of cases.

Of course if this were the whole of the evidence there could be no doubt about the advisability of using mercurochrome as a routine in all cases of sepsis; but I am aware that it is not and that many adverse reports have appeared in the literature. But in attempting to make a fair survey of the subject one is struck by the fact that all of these reports are upon a much smaller number of cases than is offered by Young, and that in many of the cases the drug was not used until the patient was quite evidently preparing for exitus. Young has published many of his cases in great detail (see Young, Hill and Scott in Bibliography); so too have the adverse writers (see Brill and Myers in Bibliography), but if their cases have all been failures, it cannot be said that Young has not also published failures; indeed, he says: "In many cases I admit a complete inability to explain why the drug, often amazingly effective in many cases, is utterly futile in others." It is also freely stated that among the nonpublishing majority of the profession only the successful cases are talked about. I wonder how true this is; in my own small acquaintance I know two physicians who have many times used mercurochrome successfully in sepsis and have neither communicated their results to Dr. Young nor published them in any form, and I know a third man who has dedicated the rest of his life to the uncritical condemnation of the drug because he had two failures in the 2 cases in which he used it.

The reader will kindly note that I am not writing of the unfortunate advocacy of mercurochrome as a panacea, but only of its use in the treatment of sepsis; nor do I wish to be read as stating that its place is secured as yet even here. But that the drug is gaining rather than losing as time goes on, I do believe—though this is contrary to the prevailing popular opinion. Regarding the danger of injecting this mercury-carrying dye into the blood stream, if we accept the report of St. George, who found mercurochrome responsible for severe kidney and intestinal lesions in 5 cases coming to autopsy, must we not also accept that of Young, who says:

"It has been asserted that mercurochrome is dangerous, particularly to the kidneys. By analysis of all the cases that we have treated at the Brady Urological Institute, the general falsity of this assertion was definitely proved. While we admit that in many instances a mild albuminuria, sometimes accompanied by casts, persisted for a few days or sometimes as long as a week, I have not seen a single case among the 100 or more which I have personally treated in which a definite permanent injury to the kidney has resulted, from even repeated injections of mercurochrome."

Thus it would seem that if the kidneys are sometimes injured, as in St. George's cases, this is certainly the exception and not the rule; and so it is in animal experiments also—for every bit of evidence that the kidneys are damaged there is much more that they are not. One is tempted to believe that occasionally the drug, for reasons unknown, is capable of producing mercury injury to the kidney—which would be in line with experience in the case of other potent drugs, all of which are capable at times of causing violent poisoning of their own peculiar sort.

Mercurochrome is the brightest exemplar of the new chemotherapy, but a number of other substances are also being used, notably gentian violet and acriflavine base; metaphen is perhaps also conveniently included here. That this type of therapy will ultimately be approved or rejected solely upon the record of its use in the clinic is most highly to be desired, for the charge that our medical science is decadent can never be sustained so long as the laboratory is dominated by the clinic. I would therefore wish to consider briefly in this place, at the risk of a seeming pedantry, a few of our preconceived theoretical notions which I believe are militating against the freer trial of a promising innovation in therapeutic tactics.

11

(*a*) First, our belief that only the protozoan infections can be successfully treated by the use of specific chemical agents. That is to say, when we review the list of "specifics" we find no warrant for the belief that bacteria will succumb to such agents—as witness: quinine in malaria, tartar emetic or the arsenicals in trypanosomiasis, emetine in amebic dysentery, tartar emetic in kala-azar, the arsenicals in yaws, syphilis and relapsing fever. All protozoan affairs, yes; but what will happen if we take certain liberties with the arbitrary bacteriological classification now in vogue—if, for instance, the spirillae are lifted bodily out of the protozoa group and placed among the bacteria, a readjustment which is claimed to be long overdue by a number of observers? Simply this, that we shall then have to acknowledge quite a number of bacterial maladies that succumb to specific chemical agents; to wit, syphilis, yaws, relapsing fever, a number of spirilloses in the lower animals, etc. And, furthermore, it is not true that there is no specific chemical agent for an organism that is beyond cavil a bacterium, for the fact is overlooked that in optochin hydrochloride we already have such an agent. The pneumococcus does succumb to this drug, but—and this is wholly incidental—its use happens to cause blindness in the human.

(*b*) Second, the conception that the agent is effective only if it accomplished a total destruction of all the organisms at one fell swoop. I would throw out all of the contradictory rabbit and human experimental work on the *therapia sterilisans magna* idea as unnecessary and cumbersome baggage, since it occupies room which might be utilized to much better purpose by investigations into the matter of bacteriostasis. We know that in diseases other than sepsis recovery can take place without a preliminary disappearance of all organisms from the tissues, in which cases we assume that those remaining are no longer effective in prolonging the attack of the disease because the antibody barrier is raised against them. But the raising of this barrier takes time even in ideal cases, and it would seem to be an especially laborious process in sepsis; would it not therefore be a tremendous help to the patient if the attacking forces could be lamed in some way though they were not actually killed—that is to say, may not an effective bacteriostasis be worth almost as much as bacteriolysis? That dye therapy can best be evaluated upon bacteriostatic grounds is a possibility distinctly worthy of exhaustive investigation. On this point Churchman says: "The dye may only stop motility, it may check sporulation, it may prevent fission, it may produce a curious condition of the bacteria which can only be described as suspended animation, a condition in which they lie dormant for long periods of time, finally becoming active and virulent again. . . . If the blood stream and through it the tissues could be kept in a condition inimical to the growth of bacteria (and very small amounts of dye might accomplish this purpose) a state of affairs might well be produced in which with this slight aid, though no organisms have actually been killed, the patient might turn defeat into victory. Such a generalized bacteriostasis has never been proved to exist after dyes have been injected, but it is quite likely that it does exist, at least for a short time."

(*c*) Third, that the effective contact of destructive agent and infective organism can take place only in the blood stream. The notable example here is quinine, of which we say that it destroys the parasites in the blood stream as they erupt from the erythrocytes, which presupposes of course the constant presence in the stream of a considerable amount of quinine. It may be done in this way, but I believe the evidence is equally strong that the drug is rapidly pocketed in certain organs—probably the spleen principally—where it accomplishes its benevolent purpose when the parasites are in due course served to it by the circulation. The work of Ramsden, Lipkin and Whitley, in 1918, indicated that about 90 per cent of the quinine injected intravenously in man disappears from the blood stream in one minute, and is stored in the tissues. By analogy, the facts with regard to Type I serum in pneumonia are of value here. Whatever curative properties this serum exhibits are not possessed in the form of antitoxic substances but as directly antibacterial substances such as agglutinins, precipitins, etc.—yet the good effects of the use of the serum are best seen if it is used early, *i. e.*, before there is a septicemia. This would seem to show that a specific remedy can accomplish the destruction (or destroy the virulence) of organisms when it is injected even though the organisms are not in the blood at the time.

Mercurochrome Technic.—Mercurochrome is most frequently used in 1 per cent solution, 23 cc. of which are to be given per hundred pounds body weight (this is sometimes expressed as 5 mg. of the drug per kilogram body weight, in 1 per cent solution). One of the standard tablets per ounce of water makes a 1 per cent solution, or the granular form of the drug may be used; this latter form is put up in tubes which contain 7.5 grains (0.5 Gm.), and the contents of one such tube dissolved in 50 cc. of water will make the 1 per cent solution. The water should be freshly distilled, if possible, and should be warmed to body temperature either before or after making the solution; this solution is of course sterile and does not require boiling—indeed, boiling makes its use much more dangerous.

Evidence is accumulating that there may be considerable danger inherent in the liberation of large quantities of bacterial poisons at one time, as is thought to sometimes occur when the dyes are injected in the above dosage, and that it might therefore be a safer procedure to abandon the routine use of large doses at twelve to twenty-four or thirty-six-hour intervals in favor of a smaller dose more frequently repeated. Kilduffe's experience with a very severe case of sepsis in an adult lends support to this belief. He gave in all a total of 0.11 Gm. of mercurochrome as follows: first dose, 5 cc. of 1 per cent solution; twenty-one hours later, 5 cc. of 0.5 per cent solution; four days later, 3.5 cc. of 0.5 per cent solution; two weeks later, 3.5 cc. of 0.5 per cent solution. These doses were small but they certainly were not frequently given; however, Kilduffe used the leukocyte count and the general clinical picture to determine when he should repeat his dose, and he believes that he was thus enabled to avail himself of the bacteriostatic properties of the remedy while still avoiding such large doses as might have caused a fatal termination in his very ill patient.

Reaction.—The type of reaction which follows full doses of the drug in perhaps more than half of the cases is certainly the greatest objection to its use. This reaction is characterized by a chill, which may be slight but often lasts several hours, nausea, vomiting and diarrhea, and a high rise followed by a sharp drop in temperature. In a smaller number of cases there is more or less salivation and sometimes a quite severe stomatitis. This matter of the reaction is additional reason for testing the efficacy of the smaller dose, though it should be pointed out, in passing, that the belief is current among some observers that in the reaction itself lies the greatest therapeutic worth of the dye.

Metaphen Technic.—Bernstine (1933) gives an initial intravenous injection of metaphen 1: 1000; the usual adult dose is 10 cc. with appropriate reductions for children and for elderly individuals—an initial dose of 20 cc. is said to be followed only infrequently by reactions. Bernstine states that the injections may be safely repeated every other day and that some of his patients have received injections daily without any untoward effects (*i. e.*, renal irritation, jaundice or gastro-intestinal disturbances); he points out, however, the necessity of using a small gauge needle and injecting very slowly.

Gentian Violet Technic.—This dye has most frequently been used at the rate of 5 mg. per kilogram body weight, which would seem to be the maximum safe dose. The usual concentration is 0.5 per cent, though some writers recommend a dilution as high as 0.25 per cent. Shallenberger remarks that a concentration of 1 per cent sometimes causes localized thrombosis of veins at the site of injection. After injection of all concentrations the skin and mucous membranes take on a deep cyanotic appearance which persists for four hours or more. There is sometimes nausea but rarely the violent reactions which so frequently follow the use of mercurochrome. Preparation: Dissolve the dye in physiologic salt solution, mark the height of the solution on the flasks and then add distilled water slightly in excess of this; boil down to the mark again. Discard solution in which particles form upon cooling.

Acriflavine Base (Neutral Acriflavine) Technic.—The average dose is 5 mg. per kilogram body weight. Prepare the solution (1 per cent) as in the case of gentian violet. Store in amber bottle and discard all solution more than one week old.

4. Vital Resistance of the Patient.—The diet should be as nutritious and as full as possible. Where nutrition is not being maintained the advantages of an intravenous injection of glucose should not be overlooked. As in all infectious diseases, fluids are to be pushed; indeed, it is usually felt to be necessary in sepsis to resort to hypodermoclysis or proctoclysis.

Blood transfusion is often resorted to, sometimes with a considerable measure of success. In the cases of pronounced anemia, which are many times a part of the picture in streptococcic sepsis, they would seem to be especially indicated. Brody and Crocker (1932) have employed "specific immunotransfusion" with good results in a case in which five ordinary transfusions had been productive of no improvement. The donor was "immunized" by four weekly injections of a vaccine prepared from the hemolytic streptococcus isolated from the patient's blood stream—doses increasing from 50 to 250 million killed organisms one week after the last injection, 150 cc. of his blood was tranfused into the patient by the citrate method. Stephenson (1933) also reports favorably.

The production of a local abscess in the hope of thus stimulating a general production of antibodies is a practice regularly followed by a few practitioners. The procedure is to inject about 10 minims (0.6 cc.) of the oil of turpentine into one of the buttocks and then drain the abscess when it is fully formed.

Protein Therapy.—Since 1914 the nonspecific foreign proteins have been much used in the treatment of infectious diseases but unfortunately we have no extensive statistical studies of their efficacy. Typhoid vaccine intravenously, or milk intramuscularly, will probably accomplish all that can be expected from any of these proteins. The milk is boiled for ten minutes, cooled to body temperature, and 5 to 10 cc. injected into the gluteal region. From 25 to 100 million of the typhoid bacilli, in the ordinary vaccine, are slowly introduced into a vein. It is thought that the good results follow upon the more or less violent reactions which succeed these injections.

Bacteriophage.—There is much talk of 'phage, but I am unable, either in the literature or the experience of my acquaintance, to find a study of it in sepsis that is really worthy of the name. It is used intravenously in doses of 1 to 5 cc.; attempts are now being made to free the suspensions of disturbing ingredients from the culture media.

Venoclysis.—This is the term employed by Hendon to designate the method, introduced by him in 1924, of administering glucose solution by the vein continuously during many hours or days. Among other conditions (see Index), he has used it successfully in several very severe cases of sepsis. In Germany, where the method was independently introduced by Kirstein in 1925, it is being particularly favored in puerperal cases, according to Melzner (1932). This slow, uninterrupted administration of nutriment-containing fluid seems to favorably influence the whole circulatory apparatus as well as to dilute and wash out toxic substances from the blood and organs. Ten per cent glucose solution in physiologic saline, or in Ringer's solution, is employed by means and apparatus described on page 777. Experience has shown that a rate of 200 cc. of fluid per hour, or a range of between 4000 and 6000 cc. per twenty-four hours, is optimum for the adult. McConnell (1930) studied the blood sugar level in 15 of his cases: the first reading by the Folin-Wu method one-half hour before starting the veno-clysis averaged 120 mg. per 100 cc.; first half-hour after beginning venoclysis, 200; second, 175; third, 150; fourth, 135; fifth, 130; sixth, seventh and eighth half-hour readings, 120 each. The urine output is in most cases approximately one half the amount of fluid administered. Increased lacrimal secretion or edema of the eyelids is regarded as evidence of saturation, but is rarely seen. Hendon watches the urine, disregards the trace of sugar, but when it reaches 1 per cent reduces the concentration of the glucose in the fluid "because there is no useful purpose accomplished by allowing an excess of sugar to circulate in the economy." Cases of continuous venoclysis for sixteen and twenty-one days are on record. Küstner (1932) criticizes what he considers an abuse of the method as employed in some quarters, which con-sists in injecting the first 300 to 500 cc. in a few minutes only. Hendon, too, has emphasized the danger of this, for he was always able to produce chills by squeezing the tube to cause a sudden delivery of the fluid into the circula-tion; reactions do not accompany or follow the slower administration.

SMALLPOX
(Variola)

"Since my Lady Mary Wortley Montagu brought home the custom of inoculation from Turkey (a perilous practice many deem it, and only a useless rushing into the jaws of danger), I think the severity of the smallpox, that dreadful scourge of the world, has somewhat been abated in our part of it; and remember in my time hundreds of the young and beautiful who have been carried to the grave, or have only risen from their pillows frightfully scarred and disfigured by this malady. Many a sweet face hath left its roses on the bed, on which this dreadful and withering blight has laid them. In my early days this pestilence would enter a village and destroy half its inhabitants: at its approach it may well be imagined not only that the beautiful but the strongest were alarmed, and those fled who could. One day, in the year 1694 (I have good reason to remember it), Doctor Tusher ran into Castlewood House, with a face of consternation, saying that the malady had made its appearance at the black-smith's house in the village, and that one of the maids there was down in the smallpox."

—W. M. Thackeray: "The History of Henry Esmond"

Smallpox has doubtless existed since the earliest times in China, India, Africa and the Mediterranean littoral, though there is considerable doubt whether it was described by the Greeks or even the early Romans. It did not reach England until the tenth century. Cortez brought it to the western hemisphere (Mexico) shortly after the discovery of the New World. The disease is now held in check by vaccination throughout the civilized world but still holds ravaging sway in the hinterland of the less enlightened countries. It tends to assume a very mild form (varioloid) where com-pulsory vaccination is rigidly enforced, but whenever a community becomes lax in the matter there it appears in the old malignant form; this was very conclusively shown in the several severe epidemics on the American conti-nent during 1922-23-24.

The black race is much more susceptible than the white. The disease is caused by an unidentified virus and is contagious by contact during any time that there are symptoms; it is probably also air-borne to some extent, at least such dissemination has not been disproved. It is more frequent during the colder months of the year. The average period of incubation is from ten to twelve days, but it may be from five to twenty-one days.

In most cases the onset is abrupt with a chill or chilliness, headache and severe backache, rapid and high rise in temperature and accompanying rise in pulse and respiratory rates, generalized body pains and nausea, and many times persistent and violent vomiting. Menstrual flow often appears out of its due order and abortion is frequent in pregnant women. About three days after the onset of the disease a macular eruption appears (on the face and wrists first) which soon becomes papular, and in another three days this has become vesicular; some of the vesicles become umbilicated and multilocular. About the ninth day of the disease the pocks will have become pustular. Schamberg has estimated that in a case of moderate severity there may be as much as 5 quarts of pus contained in the pocks all over the body. At this stage the patient is often very odorous. Lesions, which stop short of vesiculation, are frequent on the mucous membrane of the mouth, nose and tongue; usually also there is enough involvement of the pharynx and larynx to make for extreme discomfort and hoarseness. At the appearance of the eruption the fever and other symptoms usually sharply subside, but this is not invariable; at this time also the patient may manifest signs of cerebral disturbance, which is usually more truly a dementia than a delirium. Following the afebrile period there is a second rise in temperature which coincides with the pustular stage of the eruption. This second period of fever terminates with the beginning of desiccation, about the twelfth day of the eruption, but may continue for a long time if the case has become one of secondary sepsis.

It is not in order to describe here the various types of smallpox, such as the confluent, the purpuric and the hemorrhagic. The African "alastrim" (South American "amaas") is probably, but not certainly, identical with the very mild form of the disease which has been described in various other parts of the world.

THERAPY

There is little to offer in the way of drug or biological therapy in smallpox. In severe cases, the treatment must frequently become that of sepsis (see p. 158). In mild cases, a nutritious diet and plenty of fluids are indicated as in all of the infectious diseases. In the beginning it is desirable to relieve the severe pains by the use of such remedies as acetylsalicylic acid, 10 grains (0.6 Gm.) every three or four hours, phenacetin, in the same dose and at the same intervals, or amidopyrine in a single dose of 5 grains (0.3 Gm.). Sometimes these milder remedies will not suffice and ⅛ grain (0.008 Gm.) morphine sulphate must be given. The vomiting is perhaps best controlled by gastric lavage with 1 per cent sodium bicarbonate solution. Cowie states that severe uncontrollable vomiting is quite regularly controlled by the slow intravenous injection of glucose solution. (For technic, etc., see p. 776.)

The severe itching that often occurs is much relieved by the following lotion, which has the objection, however, that it dries into a thin crust that may aggravate the condition unless it is frequently washed off with olive oil, not with water.

℞.	Phenol	℥ss	2.0
	Prepared calamine	℥iiss	10.0
	Zinc oxide	℥iiss	10.0
	Glycerin	♏xl	2.4
	Solution of calcium hydroxide to make	℥iv	120.0

Twenty per cent argyrol solution should be dropped into the eyes twice daily from the beginning, and one should be especially attentive to the possibility of scarring from conjunctival lesions if the face is so much swollen as to close the eyes.

It would seem that all measures directed toward limiting the amount of scarring are unavailing. If scratching were the chief factor, then it would seem that children should be the most afflicted in this regard; the fact is, however, that the cosmetic result is very much better in children than in adults. Scratching is of course to be resisted as much as possible for it certainly increases the liability to secondary infection.

Removal of Scars.—The use of trichloracetic acid is said to be sometimes successful in removing smallpox scars. (See Wise, F., in the Bibliography.)

Preventive Vaccination.—It is said that the Chinese have for many centuries practiced a crude kind of vaccination by thrusting human smallpox scabs up the nose. The Turks had refined upon this somewhat in that they introduced some of the pus from such a scab into a small incised wound of the arm; after an incubation period of a week or so the patient experienced a mild attack of the disease and was then immune. This was the practice which Lady Mary Wortley Montagu brought home to England in 1727, where, after some preliminary opposition, it was much used until supplanted by the Jenner method. Schamberg says that the custom never enjoyed much popularity on the Continent; certainly by all accounts these induced cases were by no means always mild. Jenner, the English physician, conferred upon the world the great boon of vaccination with the virus of cowpox in 1798. I shall not describe here the technic of a procedure which, through its faithful practice by the profession during the last one hundred years, has brought the enlightened world to regard a person who permits himself to contract smallpox, through a neglect of this simple preventive measure, as a most reprehensible individual. Parenthetically, I would recommend that every physician send to the U. S. Government Printing Office for Reprint No. 1137, P. H. Reports, the authoritative paper of Leake: "Questions and Answers on Smallpox and Vaccination." Women may be vaccinated at any time during their pregnancy without fear of obstetrical complications, but successful vaccination of the mother does not convey specific immunity to the infant. Children should be vaccinated at about six months, again on entering school, and again at puberty; all children and all adults should be revaccinated whenever an epidemic threatens.

Postvaccinal Nervous Disorders.—The recent (1931) British statistical study, which may be accepted as a reliable gauge of conditions obtaining throughout the western world, reveals that for each million persons vaccinated for the first time there are nineteen disorders of the nervous system, with six or seven deaths, and for each million persons revaccinated there is one such disorder, with a fatal issue. Clearly, there is no cause for anxiety here. Since the great majority of the cases are in children primarily vaccinated between the ages of three and thirteen, the well-established precept of vaccinating in early infancy is roundly confirmed. Jorge's (1932) study is most exhaustive.

SPRUE

Sprue is a chronic wasting disease of the tropics with endemic foci in the Malayan Archipeligo, China, India, Australia, all the Island groups of the tropical Pacific, Japan, tropical Africa, and the West Indies. It has probably occurred in the southern United States since very early times; indigenous English and German cases have also been reported. The Panama Canal Zone and Brazil (according to Ashford) are singularly free from the disease.

Sprue, which tends to progress in a series of exacerbations, is character-ized by a sore and excoriated tongue, excessive intestinal fermentation, light colored, frothy, fetid stools, and a blood picture much like that of pernicious anemia. There is usually very little abdominal pain, but the patient often complains of being "sore from mouth to anus." Except in the terminal stages, the diarrhea is not so frequent as it is exhausting. Tetany is occasionally an outstanding symptom. In long-standing cases the victims become very cachectic and die from inanition or intercurrent disease. I have placed this interesting malady among the infectious diseases because Ashford and other investigators believe the fungus, *Monilia psilosis*, to be responsible for the production of the disease, though the etiologic rôle of this organism is far from being universally accepted.

THERAPY

Diet.—Ashford believes that the disease supervenes upon a period of previous ill health due to the excessive consumption of cereals, sweets and greasy foods. This dietary imbalance establishes an acid state of affairs in the digestive tract which enables *Monilia* to colonize there. In his series of cases, of the 976 not diagnosed as sprue, only 1.2 per cent were found to be carriers of the organism, while 85.5 per cent of the 740 clinical diagnoses of sprue were confirmed by serological and mycological examination. However this may be, a strict regulation of the diet seems essential in the treatment of the disease after it is fully established. Ashford says that the majority of patients recover if fed on a diet with a low fat content and free from cereals and the sugar of commerce, but all students of the disease are not so sanguine. Sir Leonard Rogers reported a series of 45 cases from India, in 1921, among which there was a probable cure in only 1 case and material improvement in only 18. All are agreed, however, that in cases of long standing the patient's only hope is to go upon a rigid milk diet, and that in all cases the treatment is best begun with this diet, other foods being added very cautiously after all symptoms have disappeared; in addition, it would seem best to permanently exclude sugar, and perhaps cereals, from the diet. For individuals who cannot tolerate milk, finely chopped beef, as little cooked as possible, may be substituted.

In a few cases, strawberries would appear to act almost as a specific remedy in the disease. In New Orleans the banana treatment, which seems to have originated with Bastedo in New York, is much used: 10 to 15 bananas and nothing else per day for several days; very good results are claimed.

Tetany.—In 1923, Scott propounded the theory that sprue is caused by a diet with excess fat or protein, which is supposed to stimulate a gastric hyper-acidity. This in turn, by overstimulating the pancreas, causes an excess liberation of fatty acids in the intestinal tract, with a resulting toxemia and an increased loss of calcium from the body because much of this element is utilized to form calcium soaps from these fatty acids. Finally, it is assumed that there arises a parathyroid deficiency as well. Ashford (1928), and Starr and Gardner (1930), have confirmed the low blood calcium finding but are inclined to ascribe it entirely to a functional failure of the para-thyroid gland. Linder and Harris (1929) attribute the poor absorption of calcium to failure on the part of the organism to absorb vitamin D. The treatment is that of tetany (see p. 347), but it would seem from the work of Shepard and Fleming (1926) that the use of remedies against tetany does not preclude the necessity of giving the dietary factor the foremost place in therapy. It is, however, of interest to note that Batavia powder, the ancient "Peter Sys's Cure," extensively used in Singapore in the old days and still much employed in the East generally, is a proprietary preparation of ordinary lime.

HCl and Pancreatin.—The concomitant use of these two substances was suggested by Brown, in 1916, but his work does not seem to have attracted very general attention. That the agents are of value is shown in the paper of Lambert, who described his personal experience with sprue in 1923; I quote, in part, as follows:

"I obtained a supply of the acid and pancreatin, and determined to give them a thorough trial. That night I took a dose of the acid and then, for the first time in two months, ate a hearty dinner. This included deviled crab and beef-steak. Half an hour later, I took 10 grains (0.65 Gm.) of pancreatin, and passed a tranquil evening and night, though I had some distention with gas.

"I continued the treatment until September [having begun in March —H. B.], taking 15 minims (1 cc.) of 0.2 per cent hydrochloric acid before, and 10 grains of pancreatin after, each meal without dietary precaution. During this period I modified the method by sipping the acid in a large glass of water with my food. One day in May, I forgot my medicine and was forced to eat a meal without it; the next day I was awake from very early morning with sprue stools. Fasting one meal and resuming treatment corrected the difficulty. In July, I tried to discontinue the medication, but after five days I was forced to resume it, as this time I had a sore mouth as well as sprue stools. My tongue still shows the effects of this experience. By September, I found that I could do without the medicine, and I remained in Australia in endemic centers for another year without the recurrence of symptoms.

"The hydrochloric acid-pancreatin treatment spread into general use along the Queensland coast, and was found quite satisfactory in the treatment of many early cases. We cannot expect it to be effective in cases of long standing when we remember the extreme destruction of tissue occurring in such cases." Castellani (1930) has used with good effect raw minced pancreas from sheep or calves: a teaspoonful built up to a tablespoonful including juice once or twice a day, best taken in milk.

Santonin.—This drug is recommended to be given in olive oil in doses of 5 grains (0.3 Gm.), night and morning, for six to twelve days. Wood says: "Remembering how much of a poison santonin is supposed to be, the writer has never felt safe in continuing its use more than three days. In a long-standing case now under observation the patient insists that the result with yellow santonin [the ordinary colorless crystals turn yellow on exposure to light—H. B.] is much better than anything yet tried. It is to be remembered, however, that he is in bed, on a strict milk diet at the time. In spite of this, the writer believes that the drug deserves a more thorough trial than has yet been accorded it."

Emetine Hydrochloride.—In 1915, Schmitter reported 12 cases that showed marked improvement under treatment with emetine hydrochloride; the drug is given hypodermically in ½ to 1 grain (0.03 to 0.06 Gm.) doses daily for five days. There is a transient increase in the diarrhea, due to the emetine. He was unfortunately unable to follow more than 1 case long enough to note permanent results, which were certainly quite remarkable in this 1 case. I do not know of a later, more extensive, trial of the drug.

Vaccine.—The monilia psilosis vaccine of Ashford is a 1 per cent emulsion of killed and iodized cultures. It is given in weekly subcutaneous injections, gradually increasing from the initial dose of 0.1 cc. It is of very doubtful value.

Liver Treatment.—The use of liver in sprue goes back for a good many years; Castellani says that it is an old native remedy in Ceylon. Sir Patrick Manson and many of his distinguished successors have been employing liver soup for more than thirty years. Recently, the reiteration of the many points of similarity between sprue and pernicious anemia has caused the liver preparations as well as the fresh organ itself to be much used in sprue in the same ways as in pernicious anemia; the results are excellent in many cases but not so brilliant as in the latter disease. The sprue diet is not interfered with during the period of liver diet.

Blood Transfusion.—Law and Cooke (1927), Manson-Bahr (1929), and others of similar wide experience are convinced of the great value of blood transfusion in sprue anemia. Immediate and oftentimes apparently permanent benefit is conferred upon patients who appeared to be moribund. It would seem that iron and arsenic therapy, as employed in secondary anemia (see p. 480), is a valuable adjunct to this treatment.

SYPHILIS

Syphilis is a venereal and general constitutional disease, caused by *Spiro-chaeta pallida,* and unknown in the civilized world prior to the first return of Columbus from Haiti in 1493. None of the ancient or medieval bones— and all the collections have been examined by many of the world's most eminent pathologists—bear incontrovertible evidence of the prior existence of the disease either in Europe or Asia, while, on the other hand, there is some evidence of syphilis in pre-Columbian bones in America; this latter must always remain only presumptive, however, because of the insuperable difficulty in fixing the antiquity of American anthropological relics. The following facts are definitely established by documentary evidence: (*a*) The disease was of great antiquity in Haiti, where it ran a comparatively mild course among the Indians, who nevertheless treated it according to a definite plan. (*b*) The disease was contracted by some of the members of Columbus' crew, at least one of the brothers Pinzon being treated for it upon the first return to Barcelona. (*c*) Spaniards from this port soon thereafter joined the army of Charles VIII of France, who, with his band of mercenaries, was at that time established in Naples. (*d*) The army blamed its sudden infection upon these soldiers. (*e*) With the break-up of this force in 1495 the malady quickly spread over all of Europe—and everywhere that it went it was capped with a new name because neither physicians nor laymen had ever seen anything like it before. (*f*) During this first epidemic the course was very severe and acute death was frequent, but within fifty years the clinical picture had assumed very much its present appearance. (*g*) Contrary to the oft-repeated statement that the venereal nature of the disease was not recognized for a long time, we know that it *was* so recognized both by the Spaniards returning from Haiti and the European physicians. Oviedo, who was in Barcelona in 1493 and knew Columbus and some of the members of his crew, wrote, in an official report drawn up for Charles V of Spain, that the disease was contracted from Indian women; while on April 21, 1497, the town council of Aberdeen, Scotland, ordered that (I quote Pusey): "For protection from the disease which had come out of France and strange parts, all light women desist from their vice and sin of venery and work for their support, on pain, else, of being branded with a hot iron on their cheek and banished from the town." (*h*)

Its subsequent spread to all the rest of the world was characterized in each instance by a preliminary violent epidemic before the disease settled down to its permanent more chronic status; which is what occurs always when a people is attacked by a new disease for which it has built up no immunity.

It is estimated that at the present time approximately 10 per cent of the world's population is afflicted with syphilis, either in the acquired or congenital form. For my own part, I believe that this estimate is based too largely upon statistical studies among urban populations only, and that an exhaustive study of the incidence in rural mankind would considerably reduce this figure. (It is of interest to note in passing that McLester states, upon what authority I do not know, that there are villages in Russia in which the whole population is infected and in which the disease has completely lost its venereal character.)

Syphilis is usually acquired by sexual intercourse with an infected person, and is characterized by the following: (*a*) The appearance of the primary sore (chancre) after an average incubation period of three weeks. (*b*) The appearance of secondary symptoms at an average time of six weeks after the appearance of the chancre: skin rashes of such varied sorts as to make description impossible here, mucous patches in the mouth, anal region, etc., plus the symptoms which accompany all general infections in greater or less degree, such as malaise, fever, anorexia, headache and joint pains, and nervous manifestations. (*c*) A so-called "latent period" during which the infection is apparently quiescent for a variable term of years. (*d*) The appearance of the so-called "tertiary period" of the disease, which is characterized by protean and serious symptoms which are due to gummatous, or more diffuse, pathologic disturbances that may occur in any portion of the body.

The above classification into primary, secondary and tertiary stages is largely arbitrary and is by no means clearly demarcated in all cases. The symptoms in congenital syphilis are the same as those in the acquired variety except that the primary sore is lacking and that the type of damage peculiar to the tertiary period is usually caused early in the life of the patient. The fetus is infected *in utero* by the mother, who must herself be first infected.

THERAPY

I shall treat of the use of drugs and biologicals in the management of syphilis under the following heads:

1. Treatment of early syphilis.
2. Treatment of visceral syphilis.
3. Treatment of neurosyphilis.
4. Treatment of congenital syphilis.
5. Discussion of the arsenicals, the iodides, and the various preparations of mercury and bismuth.
6. Prophylaxis.

TREATMENT OF EARLY SYPHILIS

While it is universally agreed that syphilitic tragedies in later life can be prevented to a very large extent, and of course should be, by prompt and proper treatment of primary and secondary syphilis, it is a surprising fact that the enormous modern literature on the subject is very full of detail as to the proper method of applying this early treatment but very vague as to the actual results, and, it would seem, rather easily satisfied that a case is "cured." Hitherto the European and American systems of attacking early syphilis have differed essentially in that the former has sought to overwhelm the invading organisms with massive doses of the drug, used over a short period; whereas the latter has contented itself with smaller doses continued over a longer period. Of course there have been overlappings of the two systems, but for sake of convenience they will be described here as though they had remained totally distinct entities.

European System.—This is the so-called "abortive" method of treatment and in the hands of its chief exponents apparently has been eminently successful. It consists in the early use of one dose, to two or three courses, of an arsphenamine product, with simultaneous or interim mercury. I say "in the hands of its chief exponents" because in the hands of others, and especially in America, it has largely failed. Nor is the reason for this difficult to ferret out, though it seems to have escaped many observers altogether. The abortive treatment, as practiced abroad, *is based upon a very much larger dosage than we are accustomed to use.* For instance, in most of the large clinics in the United States the average maximum adult dose of arsphenamine is 0.4 Gm., rarely raised to 0.5 Gm. for some burly fellow, and not infrequently reduced to 0.3 Gm. for "small" people. In Europe, however, the average dose is more often 0.5 or 0.6 Gm. (I am speaking, it is to be remembered of the "abortive" method only), since the body weight of the individual entirely determines the size of the dose. Therefore, while we in this country would give to a man of 5 feet, 9 inches, who strips at 125 pounds (certainly a "skinny" fellow) but 0.4 Gm., abroad he would get 0.5 Gm. on their dose-determination basis of 0.1 Gm. per 25 pounds. Likewise, the individual of 150 pounds receives 0.6 Gm., and the one of 175 pounds, 0.7 Gm. When we consider to what extent the 175 to 200 pounder abounds among us, especially in the North and West, it is easily understood that the "abortive" treatment as applied by our average clinician with his "0.4 Gm. maximum" training is not comparable to the European method, and that its failure in our hands is therefore really not a just commentary on that method. Those interested should study Boas, Müllern-Aspegren, Rost, Silberstein, and Feldmann. (See Bibliography.)

There is, however, one valid basis for criticism of the method as practiced abroad; it has already been mentioned above—the too great readiness to enroll a case among those "cured." Witness Rost (*loc. cit.*), who reports on 2993 cases treated in various clinics, with clinical and serological cure in 85 per cent of the seronegative primary, and in 68.5 per cent of the seropositive primary cases; *but none of the workers had employed spinal fluid examinations as a routine.* One wonders whether there is entire justification in looking upon cases as cured unless the routine examination of spinal fluid is one of the criteria of such cures.

American System.—It is not to be understood that I would wish to indicate a rigid continental adherence to a method of treatment, as implied in the term "American," but rather that it is my desire to describe here the system that I believe to represent the ideal in this country. This is most difficult to do, since Americans and Europeans have been equal offenders in the matter of their readiness to accept evidence of "cure," and is rendered additionally complex by the fact that in our less intensive (*i. e.*, smaller doses) but more extended methods there is much room for controversy over such matters as timing the initial dose, the alternate or simultaneous employment of arsphenamine, mercury and bismuth, the place of iodides in the therapeutic regimen, and the length and number of the rest periods. I have therefore chosen to present here a summary—based upon the admirable series of papers of Moore, Keidel and Kemp—of the treatment of early syphilis in Johns Hopkins Hospital in Baltimore, where a definite plan had been followed for more than a decade preceding the reports. In defence of this choice I will only mention that, though the system of treatment employed is, in most of its essential features, quite typical of that which is at least aimed at throughout the country, the criteria of cure are more severe than those generally employed—at least so far as is revealed by a fairly comprehensive review of the literature up to the end of 1933.

Drugs Used.—Arsphenamine, mercury by inunction, and potassium iodide, the latter in the belief that its probable ability to promote dissolution of granulomatous tissue would enhance the penetrability of arsphenamine and mercury even in the comparatively slight lesions of early syphilis. The place of bismuth in such a scheme of treatment is discussed on page 210, bismarsen on page 215, and the substitution of other arsenicals and mercurials on pages 198 and 205, respectively.

Intermittent Versus Continuous Treatment.—The decision to adopt a type of continuous treatment with alternating courses of arsenic and mercury was based upon the following considerations:

(A) There is a limit of tolerance for vasculotoxic arsphenamine and nephrotoxic mercury, past which it is unwise to push even such healthy young adults as early syphilitics; if the drugs are given simultaneously then there must follow a simultaneous rest period without either drug, but if given alternately the patient is resting from arsphenamine while taking mercury, and *vice versa.*

(B) There is an abundance of experimental and clinical evidence that the spirochete acquires a tolerance, or "fastness," for both arsphenamine and mercury, and that this tolerance, which is specific for each of the drugs, is promptly lost when contact between the parasite and the drug ceases. By alternating the drugs the spirochete is at all times being attacked by that one of them toward which at the time it has the least resistance.

(C) There is no satisfactory concrete evidence that the simultaneous use of the two drugs in the first course accomplishes any more than arsphenamine alone in rapidly healing the lesions, reducing the Wassermann, and destroying the parasites.

(D) In untreated cases the patient builds up a considerable amount of resistance, as shown by the spontaneous disappearance of the secondary outbreak, the destruction of large numbers of spirochetae, and the development of latency. The elaboration of these immune reactions, which is sharply interrupted by treatment in the primary or early secondary stages, is resumed if an early rest period is allowed—the result may be a delayed or recurrent secondary syphilis, or "that bugbear of early syphilis," a neurorecurrence.

Dose of Arsphenamine.—First three injections, 0.1 Gm. for each 25 pounds body weight; thereafter, 0.4 Gm. total for men, 0.3 Gm. for women. Eight injections in the first course, six in subsequent courses. The interval between injections one week in order to allow time for resolution of lesions after each dose, thus ensuring the maximal tissue penetration of the next dose. The chief theoretical objection to the so-called "Pollitzer method" of giving maximal arsphenamine doses on three successive days is that it does not facilitate full tissue penetrability.

Dose of Mercury.—The length of the interim mercury courses early in the study averaged about three months, but this was gradually modified in early syphilis in the direction of more arsphenamine and less mercury, especially in the first few months of treatment, the modification being based on the idea of utilizing to the utmost the treponemicidal effect of arsphenamine. At present, the first mercury course is four weeks, gradually lengthened to six, eight, and ten weeks in subsequent courses.

Length of Treatment.—The standard set was one year's continuous treatment after the blood Wassermann *and spinal fluid* had become, and had remained, completely negative.

Criteria of Cure.—A patient was considered probably cured when he satisfied the following requirements: (*a*) A full year of probation during which he received no treatment, developed no lesions of syphilis, and maintained a steadily negative blood Wassermann as shown by frequent tests. (*b*) At the end of the year a complete examination, which must be negative for evidences of progress in the disease, especially in the nervous system or cardiovascular apparatus evidenced in the former by freedom from neurological signs with a negative spinal fluid, and in the latter by negative findings upon both physical and roentgenological cardiovascular examinations. (*c*) The lutein test or the provocative Wassermann procedure not employed because of their unreliability.

"When a patient has completed the requisite amount of treatment, and has fulfilled these fairly rigid criteria during his probationary period, he is regarded as probably cured, and, if he desires, is allowed to marry. It is nevertheless explained to him that while cure is probable, it is not certain, and that the price of continued good health is eternal vigilance. He is urged to keep himself under observation indefinitely, and to return for periodic physical and serological examinations for the balance of his life. No patient is ever finally told that he is cured and need not return to the clinic. It is only by following up of this type, carried on for an indefinite period of years, that ultimate success or failure can be recognized."

Serological Control of Treatment.—During the arsphenamine courses the blood Wassermann was tested each week at the time of the injection, also at frequent intervals during the interim mercury courses and the subsequent probationary period. Routine study of the spinal fluid was begun preferably during the second course of mercury (about five months after starting treatment); before this time all the cytobiological changes in the fluid will not have had time to appear, but if the studies are begun much later certain minor abnormalities may have been cleared up by the treatment. Positive findings necessitate classifying the patient as a neurosyphilitic and treating him accordingly (see p. 179); negative findings indicate that no change in the routine treatment need be made.

This Johns Hopkins plan of treatment, as applied in the average uncomplicated case of primary or secondary syphilis, is here presented in tabular form (Table 15).

Results of Treatment.—The plan of treatment described here is of course looked upon as the ideal which can be carried out from start to finish in only the comparatively rare exceptionally cooperative patient. From the standpoint of its contribution to our knowledge of the essentials of successful treatment of early syphilis, however, this fact is perhaps a fortunate one since this very lack of ideal cooperation on the part of a large number of their patients has enabled the Hopkins observers to answer quite convincingly the two supremely important questions: (1) In early syphilis should treatment be continuous or intermittent? and (2) How long must it be continued in order to attain the maximal probability of cure? This they have done by carefully studying the clinical and serological results attained in the 402 patients with complete records out of a total of 2500 treated cases. This group of 402 patients included those who received varying amounts of treatment, ranging from a single injection of arsphenamine to the completion of the ideal plan, with many who lapsed on one or numerous occasions and whose progress, therefore, consisted of courses of treatment alternating with periods of rest.

The findings may be summarized as follows:

1. A report of the clinical results of treatment in 402 patients with early syphilis, of whom 42 had seronegative primary, 61 seropositive primary, and 299 early secondary syphilis.

A patient was regarded as probably cured if he became reinfected; or, if a complete survey, including physical examination and tests of the blood

TABLE 15.—PLAN OF TREATMENT FOR UNCOMPLICATED PRIMARY AND EARLY SECONDARY
SYPHILIS

1. *Early diagnosis* and *immediate treatment.* To establish diagnosis, laboratory
procedures as necessary (dark-field examination, gland puncture, local Wassermann
reaction, blood Wassermann reaction).
2. Complete physical and neurological examination, accurately recorded, before
treatment is begun.
3. Treatment.

Week.	Arsphen-amine, Gm	Mercury.	Blood WaR.	Remarks.
1	0.4	....	1	Recently dosage for first 3 injections has been raised to
2	0.4	....	1	level of 0.1 Gm. for each 25 lbs. of body weight, subse-
3	0.4	....	1	quent injections at dosage of 0.4 Gm. for men, 0.3 Gm.
4	0.4	....	1	for women.
5	0.4	....	1	In average patient all lesions heal rapidly and blood WaR
6	0.4	....	1	becomes negative during first arsphenamine course.
7	0.4	....	1	
8	0.4	Ung. Hg and KI	1	Mercury overlaps one week at end of first and beginning
9–12	....	Ung. Hg and KI	..	of second arsphenamine course. At this point, a few days without treatment may be dangerous. Neurorecurrence!
13	0.4	Ung. Hg and KI	1	Arsphenamine starts, mercury stops. Watch for provoca-
14	0.4	....	1	tive Wassermann after first dose of arsphenamine.
15	0.4	....	1	Try to prevent even short lapses in treatment, especially
16	0.4	....	1	at this early stage.
17	0.4	....	1	
18	0.4	....	1	
19–24	....	Ung. Hg and KI	..	Bismuth intramuscularly may be substituted for mercury, especially if patient is uncooperative with rubs. *Examine cerebrospinal fluid routinely at about this point.*
25	0.4	....	1	Do not substitute neoarsphenamine unless absolutely neces-
26	0.4	....	1	sary. If this is done, dose of neo ought to be maximum
27	0.4	....	1	(0.9 Gm.), and number of injections in a series 8 to 10
28	0.4	....	1	instead of 6.
29	0.4	....	1	
31–38	....	Ung. Hg and KI		
39	0.4	....	1	
40	0.4	....	1	
41	0.4	....	1	
42	0.4	....	1	
43	0.4	....	1	
44	0.4	....	1	Patients with seronegative primary syphilis may cease treat- ment here, if blood WaR has always been negative.
45–54	....	Ung. Hg and KI	..	Note that courses of mercury are gradually getting longer —4, 6, 8, and now 10 weeks.
55	0.4	....	1	
56	0.4	....	1	
57	0.4	....	1	The average seropositive primary or early secondary patient
58	0.4	....	1	should have at least 5 courses of arsphenamine.
59	0.4	....	1	
60	0.4	....	1	
61–70	....	Ung. Hg and KI	..	It is wise to finish treatment with mercury, rather than
71–123	Probation.		..	with arsphenamine.
	No treatment.		12	Blood WaR tested once a month.
124	Complete physical and neurological examination, spinal puncture, fluoroscopical examinaton of cardiovascular stripe. Thereafter, yearly physical examination, blood WaR every 6 to 12 months. If two spinal fluid examinations have been negative, this need not be repeated.			

and spinal fluid, carried out at least one year after the date of the last
treatment, showed no evidence of syphilis. About half of the presumably cured patients were followed for more than three years of probation.
A patient with a clinical or serological recurrence of any type occurring
during or subsequent to treatment was classified only with treatment failures.

2. Under a system of continuous treatment with alternating courses of
arsphenamine and mercury, the probability of cure was shown to be in
direct proportion to the duration and regularity of treatment. Only 10
per cent of those patients receiving eight or less doses of arsphenamine
without mercury were cured; when two courses of arsphenamine plus interim
mercury were given, 37 per cent were cured; after three courses, 56 per cent,
and after four or more courses, 78.8 per cent of probable cures were obtained.

3. The optimal amount of treatment for early syphilis with the plan
advocated appeared to be a full year of treatment after the serology of
blood and spinal fluid had become and remained negative, excepting only

seronegative primary syphilis, in which a three-course treatment, lasting nine months, apparently produced satisfactory results.

4. Grouping together cooperative and uncooperative patients, without regard to the character or duration of treatment, it was shown that if treatment can be begun within the first two weeks of the infection (seronegative primary syphilis), the chance of ultimate cure is almost twice as great as when it is delayed until the appearance of secondary manifestations. The incidence of reinfection in the groups of seronegative and seropositive primary and early secondary syphilis was 11.9, 8.1, and 3.0 per cent respectively. The extreme importance of early and accurate diagnosis was thus emphasized.

5. With the utmost cooperation on the part of the patient, and painstaking treatment and follow-up on the part of the physician, it appears possible to cure 100 per cent of patients with seronegative primary syphilis, but only 80 to 95 per cent of those with seropositive primary or early secondary syphilis. The refractory 5 to 20 per cent seem likely, in spite of the utmost efforts of therapy, to develop late syphilis, especially neurosyphilis.

6. Recurrences seriously impairing efficiency or endangering life (neurorecurrences, tertiary syphilis, neurosyphilis) occurred in almost half the patients receiving eight or less injections of arsphenamine; in a third of those receiving from one to two courses of arsphenamine plus mercury; in a quarter of those receiving three-treatment courses; but in only 3 per cent of those patients receiving four or more arsphenamine courses plus mercury. The necessity of long-continued treatment was thus emphasized.

7. The tendency of inadequately treated syphilis to repeated relapses in the same patient was shown.

8. The short average time interval (2.1 months) between the date of the last treatment and the onset of neurorecurrences emphasized the necessity of continuous treatment in early syphilis.

9. Cardiovascular syphilis, especially aortitis, was the most common type of tertiary recurrence observed.

10. Twenty-seven patients developed neurosyphilis, usually of the diffuse meningovascular type. The relative infrequency of general paresis (4 cases) and of tabes dorsalis (no cases) is explainable on the basis of the short period of years covered by the study.

11. The evidence of repeated routine spinal punctures in 54 patients permitted the general statement that in early syphilis, if the spinal fluid is normal after six months' treatment, the patient will not develop clinical neurosyphilis or a subsequently positive spinal fluid unless a second dissemination of organisms (clinically manifest by recurrent secondary syphilis or a recurrent positive blood Wassermann) occurs.

12. Periodic reexaminations from physical and serological standpoints are absolute essentials in the evaluation of treatment results. Even though prolonged observation makes cure seem almost certain, a syphilitic patient should never be released from the obligation of periodic reexamination throughout his life-time.

13. Composite Wassermann curves of patients treated continuously with arsphenamine and interim mercury were compared with those of a similar group treated intermittently, periods of treatment alternating with periods of rest. It was shown that from this standpoint continuous treatment is productive of greatly superior results.

14. An attempt was made to correlate the serological data with the ultimate clinical outcome. From this standpoint, also, continuous treatment produced better results than intermittent treatment.

15. An analysis of the material suggests that frequent repetition of the Wassermann test during treatment is of considerable prognostic value.

Nonspecific Measures (Including Fever).—Engman, Jorstad and Engman (1931) have treated a small series of primary and secondary cases with such nonspecific agents as typhoid vaccine, ultraviolet light applications, thyroid substance, etc. There was some serological improvement shown in most of the cases, but the clinical improvement lagged behind. Upon the whole, it seems to me that nothing developed from the study that might cast favor upon this type of therapy. Surprisingly, however, Hashimoto and Iwakiri (1932) have obtained some evidences that primary syphilis may be cured by the inoculation of rat-bite fever without other treatment. They feel that it is the antagonistic effect of the one spirochete upon the other, rather than the mere induction of fever, which is responsible for the result. This will be an interesting therapeutic experiment to watch.

TREATMENT OF VISCERAL SYPHILIS

The physician who is treating syphilis should ever be on the watch for early evidences of an involvement of the kidneys or the liver, which will manifest itself in the first instance as an acute nephritis and in the second as jaundice, with or without some indication of an acute hepatitis. Either of these occurrences, though comparatively rare, is to be looked upon always as very unfortunate since they necessitate such a drastic modification in the treatment with both mercury and arsphenamine, and to some extent also with bismuth, as to make it extremely doubtful whether the disease in this particular individual can ever be attacked in that massive fashion which the above review indicates is necessary for the eradication of early syphilis. Other than this, however, there are practically no visceral disturbances in first and second stage syphilis. By visceral disturbances is meant actual syphilitic disease of the thoracic, mediastinal, abdominal or pelvic viscera. Doubtless the organs within these cavities are more or less affected during the period of invasion—indeed, there are direct evidences of this in many cases—but these disturbances never demand attention in and for themselves since they always disappear promptly under the general antisyphilitic treatment; therefore the term "visceral syphilis" is taken to indicate an essential syphilitic attack upon organs that occurs during the tertiary phase of the disease. Let us consider these disturbances under the following heads: (1) Circulatory, (2) liver, (3) general.

1. **Circulatory.**—(*a*) *Aortitis.*—It is generally agreed that syphilitic aortitis does not indicate a modification in the treatment and that the fullest use should be made of arsphenamine, mercury, bismuth and the iodides. The Hopkins group followed thirty-six such cases for at least one year after the cessation of treatment; the results are summarized in Table 16, in which the advantage of prolonged and continuous treatment is made sharply apparent. Stokes, Miller and Beerman (1931) have reported very favorably upon the use of bismarsen in these cases (see p. 215), as have Blacksford and Boland (1932) upon the use of bismuth (see p. 213).

(*b*) *Aneurysm.*—Without treatment, one may safely assume that the aneurysmal process is seldom arrested; with treatment, though the size of the aneurysm is rarely affected, symptomatic improvement is frequently seen. Hypertension may be relieved, as in one case in the Hopkins series in which the blood pressure dropped from 220 systolic and 100 diastolic to 110 systolic and 70 diastolic. These patients usually do not tolerate arsphenamine well; small, cautiously given doses of neoarsphenamine should be preferred combined with the metals and iodides. Pressure symptoms in patients with large aneurysms are not much influenced. For the relief of the intense suffering, sympathetic ganglionectomy is nowadays preferred to other operative procedures; White (1932) has shown that in inoperable

TABLE 16.—RESULTS OF TREATMENT IN SYPHILITIC AORTITIS (UNCOMPLICATED)

Amount of treatment.	Number of cases.	Improved (Symptoms relieved; no progress in disease).	Stationary (Condition no worse than before treatment).	Worse (Increase in symptoms or physical signs).	Dead.
One year or more............	10	10	..	..	..
From six to twelve months or very irregular...........	8	3	5	..	..
From one to six months......	8	..	..	6	2
None....................	10	..	1	9	..

cases paravertebral injections of procaine or alcohol may be successfully made.

(c) *Cardiac Syphilis.*—In the case of syphilitic heart disease, the general condition of the patient will, of course, often improve more rapidly under intensive treatment with the arsphenamines and bismuth than under mercury and the iodides, but his general improvement will very frequently be followed by a rapid deterioration of the heart itself, with evidence of accentuation of the original cardiac defect. Wile offers two possible explanations of this: (1) that the syphilitic products have been too rapidly replaced by scar tissue; or (2) that their rapid disintegration had produced a chemical change deleterious in its effect on the local lesion. Regarding their experience with these cases, the Johns Hopkins observers write:

"In the group of cardiac syphilis we have placed all patients with aortic insufficiency or with manifest myocardial disease. Of 14 patients, 4 were too ill for ambulatory treatment, and did badly under medical care. Ten patients were treated in the clinic, 3 with arsphenamine, 6 with mercury and potassium iodide, and 1 with tryparsamide. Two of the patients treated with arsphenamine died, apparently as a result of treatment, one immediately after a third injection, and the other a few days after an injection. Both deaths were preceded by signs of cardiac failure. Severe reactions prompted discontinuance of arsphenamine in the third case. . . .

"With mercury and potassium iodide as the only therapy, very little can be accomplished. Only 1 of the 6 patients so treated showed improvement symptomatically, but no change in physical signs. One is no worse after two and one-half years of treatment; one is worse after one year of treatment; two have become too ill to return to the clinic, and one has died. All patients in this subgroup remained seropositive."

2. **Liver.**—Not infrequently in tertiary syphilitic involvement of the liver, the patient gets well of his syphilis under arsphenamine, but grows much worse in respect of his hepatitis symptoms—though occasionally a brilliant cleaning up of the hepatitis occurs as well. In these latter cases, Wile believes that the lesion has been a gummatous hepatitis, hepar lobatum, or perhaps the interstitial type. On the whole, this very competent observer agrees with the vast majority of syphilographers in their preference for mercury and the iodides, which is based on the belief that they permit more gradual cicatrization, during which time compensatory hypertrophy might possibly occur in unaffected portions of the organ. McCrae and Caven, in a treatise on tertiary syphilis of the liver, say:

"There is only one statement to be made in regard to these [arsenic preparations—H. B.], and that is that they are absolutely contraindicated in the great majority of cases. There is no possible excuse of administering arsphenamine or any other arsenic preparation to a patient who has syphilitic disease of the liver."

It is very likely that intensive treatment with the aqueous bismuth solutions would also be objectionable but that the oily suspensions carefully adjusted as to dosage, might be of more value than mercury; not enough clinical evidence has accumulated as yet to make possible any assured statements.

3. **General.**—As for lesions of the internal organs, other than the heart and large vessels and the liver, one cannot be quite so explicit as to the remedy of choice. Many of the older practitioners prefer to omit arsphenamine and use only mercury and the iodides in these cases, and nowadays bismuth as well. However, given an individual who is tolerant toward all four drugs, it would seem of advantage to use arsphenamine also. One rarely, practically never, fails to accomplish a very great degree of resolution and scar formation by either method, but in the average case this is certainly brought about more rapidly when all the drugs are used than when the metals and iodides are alone employed; also, the use of arsphenamine frequently makes possible a reduction in the Wassermann plusage that is impossible without it. These things are also true of bone and skin lesions.

In the presence of a complicating nephritis, one must proceed very warily, and, contrary to the opinion sometimes expressed, this caution is enjoined quite as much in the use of arsphenamine as of mercury and bismuth.

TREATMENT OF NEUROSYPHILIS

The period 1924–27 was marked in the field of neurosyphilis by the appearance of three notable papers on systematic drug treatment and results—I refer to the studies of Fordyce in New York, Stokes and Shaffer at the Mayo Clinic, and Moore at the Johns Hopkins Hospital. Again I am selecting for presentation here a summary of the Hopkins report, this time for two reasons: first, that it is the more recent and actually contains a comparison of results with those obtained by the two previous workers; and second, that it is a report of observations made entirely upon cases of the ambulatory clinic type, whereas the results reported by Fordyce, and Stokes and Shaffer, were obtained largely upon private, and therefore more generally cooperative and tractable, cases.

Classification of Clinical Material.—Since it is of the utmost importance to the patient that he have the type of neurosyphilis from which he is suffering properly classified before treatment is begun, the cases were divided, chiefly on the basis of pathologic anatomy, into the following groups:

1. Purely meningeal neurosyphilis, including acute syphilitic meningitis, neurorecurrences, and early asymptomatic neurosyphilis. These are almost always early manifestations, occurring within the first two years.

2. Neurosyphilis with predominant meningeal or vascular involvement, or both, either with or without minimal parenchymatous changes which rarely enter into the clinical picture. The general catch basket, including diffuse cerebrospinal syphilis and such widely separated entities as transverse myelitis, syphilitic epilepsy, brain gumma, syphilitic hemiplegia, combined symptom disease, and late asymptomatic neurosyphilis.

3. Predominantly parenchymatous neurosyphilis, including tabes and general paralysis.

4. Syphilitic optic atrophy.

Classification of Treatment Systems.—The four treatment systems employed were the following:

1. When the evidence of neurosyphilis was minimal, that is, in early or late syphilis with minor spinal fluid changes, or in late syphilis with minor neurological signs and a negative spinal fluid, the treatment was essentially that employed in early syphilis (see p. 171).

2. In patients with early meningeal neurosyphilis and in the majority of patients with diffuse meningovascular neurosyphilis, the treatment was that of early syphilis intensified in the direction of more arsphenamine—larger doses, longer courses, and shorter intervals between doses. The treatment was usually continuous, but except in cases of early meningeal neurosyphilis, a rest period was not regarded as an almost irreparable calamity as it was in primary or secondary syphilis. Individualization is essential in this group, often to the extent that treatment proceeds by a system of trial and error. Such intensive treatment as that recommended by Stokes and Shaffer, including daily intramuscular injections of soluble mercurials and sodium iodide intravenously, could not be employed because most of the patients were ambulatory.

3. In two restricted groups of cases—in tabes, especially those patients with lightning pains, sphincter disturbances and ataxia; and in primary optic atrophy, whether or not tabetic in origin—intraspinal treatment was added to the scheme, employing the original Swift-Ellis method, with only minor modifications (technic, p. 185), and the Fordyce technic of injection (p. 186). Lower cord reactions were practically eliminated by spacing treatments two weeks apart, giving six or less to a series, and avoiding the giving of more than 20 cc. of serum at one treatment. Such proposed alterations as the Ogilvie method of reinforcing the serum, or its administration, by the intracisternal or intraventricular routes were tried and abandoned as too risky.

4. In general paralysis, in asymptomatic neurosyphilis with group III (paretic formula) spinal fluid, and in certain cases of tabes or diffuse meningovascular neurosyphilis with spinal fluid changes of the paretic type, tryparsamide was used for a prolonged period, either with mercury or bismuth alone, or in combination with an arsphenamine.

Results.—Of the 261 neurosyphilitic patients followed for an average period of four years, 54 had early meningeal neurosyphilis, 88 late diffuse meningovascular involvement, 64 tabes, 35 general paralysis, and 20 primary optic atrophy, tabetic and otherwise.

In an attempted correlation between the clinical and serological results, such as that of Stokes and Shaffer, an estimate of combined results was made in terms of excellent, good, fair and poor, the term "excellent" applying only to those patients who were freed of symptoms or left with only trifling residuals, and in whom also the blood and spinal fluid was rendered serologically negative, with this condition maintained for from one to thirteen years. The percentage of excellent and good combined results used throughout the several tables was estimated from the total number falling into these two classifications as to both clinical and serological results. In a final table (Table 24) is shown a comparison of the results in this Johns Hopkins series with those obtained by Fordyce and by Stokes and Shaffer.

Early Meningeal Neurosyphilis.—Of the 54 patients with early meningeal neurosyphilis, 32 had frank neurorecurrences or acute syphilitic meningitis, while 22 had early asymptomatic neurosyphilis discovered by routine spinal fluid examination. For the whole group, treatment was practically continuous for an average of twenty months, and the probation period without treatment averaged eighteen months. In 83 per cent of the group an excellent clinical result was obtained, and it appeared to make little difference whether the original diagnosis was clinically evident or asymptomatic neurosyphilis. Two patients from the latter group subsequently developed late meningovascular neurosyphilis, in spite of eighteen and thirty months of treatment, and one other, a year after the completion of thirty months' treatment, developed general paralysis.

In only 62 per cent of the whole group was an excellent combined result obtained (Table 17).

TABLE 17.—RESULTS OF TREATMENT IN EARLY MENINGEAL NEUROSYPHILIS

Clinical result.	Serological result.				
	Excellent.*	Good.	Fair.	Poor.	Total.
Excellent*..........................	32	2	3	7	44
Good...............................	..	..		1	1
Fair...............................	..	..	..	1	1
Poor...............................	..	..	..	8	8
Total.............................	32	2	3	17	54

In 83 per cent an excellent or good clinical result was obtained.
In 62 per cent an excellent or good serological result was obtained.
In 62 per cent an excellent or good combined result was obtained.

* In this and subsequent tables, in only those patients included within the box was an excellent or good combined clinical or serological result obtained.
An "excellent" clinical result means complete relief from all symptoms, or only trifling residuals, with ability to resume ordinary activities; "good" indicates marked improvement; "fair," moderate improvement; "poor," slight or no improvement.
An "excellent" serological result indicates that the blood and spinal fluid have become normal and remained so for the period of observation; "good," tests almost but not quite negative; "fair," moderate improvement; "poor," little or no change.

As Table 24 shows, this compares unfavorably with Fordyce's 100 per cent and with Stokes and Shaffer's 90.9 per cent. Two factors might explain this discrepancy as well as that noted for late meningovascular neurosyphilis. (a) Fourteen of the 22 patients with early asymptomatic neurosyphilis had group III (paretic formula) spinal fluids, and would probably have been classified by the other observers as paresis sine paresi. (b) The results in this series were those obtainable in an ambulatory clinic with the majority of the patients of the clinic level of intelligence and cooperation, as contrasted with the almost exclusively private patient class of both Fordyce, and Stokes and Shaffer. Intraspinal treatment was used in only 3 patients with early meningeal neurosyphilis.

Late Meningovascular Neurosyphilis.—Here, excellent or good clinical and combined results were obtained in only a slightly less proportion of patients: 76 and 59 per cent, respectively, though treatment had to be prolonged to an average of twenty-seven months (Table 18). The average period of subsequent observation was twenty-one months, and ranged as high as ten years. These figures are compared with the 84.6 per cent of excellent and good combined results from Fordyce's series, and the 74 per cent of Stokes and Shaffer's cases, the same two factors as before making the figures not quite comparable. Five patients of the group subsequently developed general paralysis. The material is too small to permit analysis of the end-results of subdivided clinical types.

Twenty-six of the 88 patients with late meningovascular neurosyphilis were treated intraspinally. The end-results, indicated in Table 20, were no better than when intraspinal treatment was omitted, though in certain patients treatment was appreciably shortened by its use. This fact, together with the eminently satisfactory results obtained from tryparsamide, led the Hopkins group practically to abandon intraspinal treatment in this type of neurosyphilis.

Tabes.—The results for tabes as a group, presented in Table 19, afford a less evident parallelism between clinical and serological results than in the two preceding groups. An excellent or good serological result was more often obtained in tabetic patients than was a similar clinical result, and

TABLE 18.—RESULTS OF TREATMENT IN LATE MENINGOVASCULAR NEUROSYPHILIS

Clinical result.	Serological result.				Total.
	Excellent.	Good.	Fair.	Poor.	
Excellent............................	42	5	1	9	57
Good................................	4	1	2	3	10
Fair................................	2	..	..	..	2
Poor................................	3	..	2	8	13
Dead................................	..	..	..	6	6
Total............................	51	6	5	26	88

In 76 per cent an excellent or good clinical result was obtained.
In 67 per cent an excellent or good serological result was obtained.
In 59 per cent an excellent or good combined result was obtained.

in only 31 per cent was a satisfactory combined result obtained. Of the 33 patients in whom the clinical outcome was regarded as unsatisfactory, 12 had either gastric crises or charcot joints, lesions notoriously resistant to treatment.

Here in tabes the situation as regards intraspinal treatment is quite different from that pointed out for meningovascular neurosyphilis. The 64 tabetic patients were almost equally divided into two groups. Thirty were treated intraspinally, 34 were not. Of the former group, the result was excellent in 43 per cent. Of the latter group, only 20 per cent, less than half as many, were equally fortunate. Moreover, the length of time under treatment was perceptibly shortened when the intraspinal route was used (seventeen as compared to twenty-six months). The period of post-treatment observation averaged thirty-five months for the group treated intraspinally, and eighteen months for the remainder. The advantage of intraspinal treatment is particularly striking because the tendency was to use it chiefly in those patients who did badly, either from clinical or from serological standpoints, on other forms of treatment. The results from intraspinal treatment in tabes are almost identical with the 50 per cent excellent results reported by Fordyce and the 48 per cent by Stokes and Shaffer.

TABLE 19.—RESULTS OF TREATMENT IN TABETIC NEUROSYPHILIS

Clinical result.	Serological result.				Total.
	Excellent.	Good.	Fair.	Poor.	
Excellent............................	17	1	3	4	25
Good................................	2	..	2	2	6
Fair................................	3	..	..	2	5
Poor................................	7	1	..	11	19
Dead................................	5	..	..	4	9
Total............................	34	2	5	23	64

In 48 per cent an excellent or good clinical result was obtained.
In 56 per cent an excellent or good serological result was obtained.
In 31 per cent an excellent or good combined result was obtained.

General Paralytic Neurosyphilis.—The value of tryparsamide is clearly indicated here, for it was possible to report twenty complete remissions, or 57 per cent, among 35 patients. In the patients with remissions, treatment was continued for an average of two and one-half years; in 12 of these patients, remission had lasted three or more years at the time of the report (2 of seven years, 1 of nine years), and in 8 from one to three years.

TABLE 20.—VALUE OF THE ADDITION OF INTRASPINAL THERAPY TO TREATMENT IN TABETIC AND LATE MENINGOVASCULAR NEUROSYPHILIS

	No. of cases.	Per cent of cases showing.					
		Clinical results.		Serological results.		Combined results.	
		Excellent or good.	Fair or poor.	Excellent or good.	Fair or poor.	Excellent or good.	Fair or poor.
Tabes:							
No instraspinal treatment.........	34	47	53	44*	56	20	80
Intraspinal treatment used........	30	50	50	70	30	43	57
Meningovascular:							
No intraspinal treatment..........	63	76	24	66	34	60	40
Intraspinal treatment used........	26	76	24	61	39	57	43

* Includes 4 patients with negative spinal fluids at start of treatment.

Fordyce also reports 54 per cent remissions in a series of 118 cases. The reader should remember, however, that all of these Hopkins cases were ambulatory, and therefore *early* cases of general paralysis; it is recognized that equally good results cannot be obtained in patients sufficiently advanced to require psychiatric care (Table 21).

The "Paretic" Spinal Fluid.—Upon separating the tabetic cases into two groups, those who showed group III fluids and those who did not, it was seen that an excellent therapeutic result had been obtained in only 18 per cent of the former as against 41 per cent in the latter. For early meningeal neurosyphilis, the corresponding figures were 47 and 65 per cent, and for the late diffuse meningovascular type, 40 and 74 per cent. These findings were interpreted to mean that a neurosyphilitic patient with a paretic fluid is an ultimate candidate for tryparsamide, malaria, or both, and possibly, though not necessarily, for general paralysis (Table 22).

TABLE 21.—RESULTS OF THE TREATMENT OF GENERAL PARALYSIS

Clinical result.	Serological result.				Total.
	Excellent.	Good.	Fair.	Poor.	
Remission, 1–3 years....................	1	..	4	3	8
Remission, 3 years......................	4	5	1	2	12
Total remissions.....................	5	5	5	5	20
No improvement or worse................	1	..	..	6	7
Dead...................................	..	..	..	8	8
Total all cases......................	6	5	5	19	35

In 57 per cent a satisfactory clinical result was obtained.
In 31 per cent an excellent or good serological result was obtained.
In 28 per cent an excellent or good combined result was obtained.

Optic Atrophy.—I quote Moore, of the Johns Hopkins group: "No class of neurosyphilitic patients is so tragic a group as those with primary optic atrophies. Without attempting an ophthalmological classification of our material, or a differentiation of tabetic atrophy from that due to basilar meningitis, I wish to emphasize what I believe to be an important point in

TABLE 22.—THE PROGNOSTIC IMPORT OF THE PARETIC FORMULA IN THE
CEREBROSPINAL FLUID

	No. of cases.	Clinical results.		Serological results.		Combined results.	
		Excellent or good.	Fair or poor.	Excellent or good.	Fair or poor.	Excellent or good.	Fair or poor.
Tabes:							
Cerebrospinal fluid paretic.........	27	44	56	33	66	18	82
Cerebrospinal fluid not paretic.....	29	48	52	84	16	41	59
Early meningeal:							
Cerebrospinal fluid paretic.........	21	76	24	47	53	47	53
Cerebrospinal fluid not paretic.....	26	84	16	65	35	65	35
Late meningovascular:							
Cerebrospinal fluid paretic.........	27	77	23	51	49	40	60
Cerebrospinal fluid not paretic.....	47	78	22	74	26	74	26

treatment. I do not agree with the frequently expressed opinion that arsphenamine is contraindicated in primary optic atrophy. Given a patient with early but rapidly advancing optic atrophy, I am convinced that blindness can be prevented only in one way, namely, by the prompt and energetic use of arsphenamine intravenously *plus intraspinal treatment,* the combination being more important than the arsphenamine alone. It must be pointed out that in the group here reported the atrophy was recognized in every instance but one while visual acuity in at least one eye was as good as $20/60$. If visual acuity in the better eye is less than $20/200$ when treatment is begun, little can be hoped for from any form of therapy. In 14 of 20 patients with early syphilitic primary optic atrophy, this system of treatment arrested the rapid visual failure. In 5, visual acuity and fields were improved over the admission examination, and in 9 the process remained stationary. The serological results were also excellent in 7 of these 14 patients. In a much larger series of cases treated with arsphenamine intravenously without intraspinal treatment, or with mercury, bismuth or potassium iodide, every case has progressed inexorably to blindness. To us intraspinal treatment offers the only avenue of hope for the unfortunate victim of optic atrophy, and we feel confident of at least 50 per cent good results in early cases. Our opinion is borne out by Fordyce's 55 per cent successes in 39 patients" (Table 23).

TABLE 23.—RESULTS OF TREATMENT IN PRIMARY OPTIC ATROPHY

Clinical result.	Serological result.				Total.
	Excellent.	Good.	Fair.	Poor.	
Improved............................	3	..	..	2	5
Stationary..........................	4	1	2	2	9
Worse..............................	1	..	..	5	6
Total.............................	8	1	2	9	20

In 70 per cent a satisfactory clinical result was obtained.
In 40 per cent an excellent or good serological result was obtained.
In 40 per cent an excellent or good combined result was obtained.

Length of Treatment.—All patients in the series were repeatedly reexamined from the physical and laboratory standpoints during and after treatment. In general the attempt was made to apply to neurosyphilis the standard for early syphilis—one year of continuous treatment after the blood and spinal fluid have become and have remained completely negative. The average length of treatment in the whole series was a little over two years. Thereafter observation is continued for a lifetime. The results cannot be duplicated by short nonintensive treatment; the physician must persuade himself and his patient that persistence is justified.

Comparison of the Johns Hopkins Hospital Series with Those of Fordyce and of Stokes and Shaffer.—In Table 24 is offered a comparison of the results obtained in these 3 series, in which there was a total of 1108 patients.

TABLE 24.—COMPARISON OF THE JOHNS HOPKINS HOSPITAL SERIES WITH THAT OF FORDYCE AND OF STOKES AND SHAFFER

Type of neurosyphilis.	Per cent of excellent and good combined clinical and serological results obtained by		
	Moore (Johns Hopkins), 261 cases.	Fordyce, 442 cases.	Stokes and Shaffer, 405 cases.
Meningeal...............................	62.9	100.0	90.9
Late meningovascular..................	59.0	84.6	69.6*
Tabes....................................	31.2	51.3	48.3
Optic atrophy...........................	40.0	55.5	
General paralysis (remissions).............	57.0	55.0†	1.8‡

* Recalculated from Stokes' tables to include vascular neurosyphilis.

† Sixty-five of 118 patients, of whom 24 had a relapse and died, had remissions of various lengths, usually short.

‡ It must be pointed out that this figure of 1.8 per cent in Stokes and Shaffer's series represents, not clinical remissions as in the Moore and Fordyce series, but excellent combined clinical and serological results. Further, Stokes and Shaffer's results antedate the use of tryparsamide.

Swift-Ellis Technic.—"One hour after the intravenous injection of salvarsan (arsphenamine) 40 cc. of blood is withdrawn directly into bottle-shaped centrifuge tubes, and allowed to coagulate, after which it is centrifugalized. The following day 12 cc. of serum is pipetted off and diluted with 18 cc. of normal saline. This 40 per cent serum is then heated at 56 C. for one-half hour. After lumbar puncture the cerebrospinal fluid is withdrawn until the pressure is reduced to 30 mm. cerebrospinal fluid pressure. The barrel of a 20 cc. Luer syringe (which has a capacity of about 30 cc.), is connected to the needle by means of a rubber·tube about 40 cm. long. The tubing is then allowed to fill with cerebrospinal fluid so that no air will be injected. The serum is then poured into the syringe and allowed to flow slowly into the subarachnoid space by means of gravity. At times it is necessary to insert the plunger of the syringe to inject the last 5 cc. of fluid. It is important that the larger part of the serum should be injected by gravity and if the rubber tubing is not more than 40 cm. long the pressure cannot be higher than 400 mm. Usually the serum flows in easily under even a lower pressure. By the gravity method the danger of suddenly increasing the intraspinous pressure to the danger point, such as might occur with rapid injection with a syringe, is avoided. Frequently there is a certain amount of pain in the legs, commencing a few hours after the injection. The pain is more often noticed in tabetics than in patients with cerebrospinal syphilis. It can usually be controlled by means of phenacetin and codeine. Occasionally morphine is required."

Fordyce Technic.—"A preliminary drainage is not necessary, and only a quantity of fluid required for the tests is removed. Into the receptacle attached to the spinal puncture needle 30 to 40 cc. of fluid are permitted to accumulate, and to this is added the inactivated serum. The mixture is then allowed slowly to reenter the subarachnoid space by gravity. In this manner about one third of the entire quantity of spinal fluid is mixed with salvarsinized serum before its reinjection. We have found half an hour after the preliminary intravenous injection the best time for removing the blood. This is permitted to clot over night in the ice-box. The next morning it is centrifugalized and the serum pipetted into a sterile tube. After a repetition of this procedure to ensure the removal of all red cells, the clear serum is pipetted into another tube and heated for half an hour at a temperature of 56 C."

Arsphenamines and the Increase in Neurosyphilis.—Whatever the factors may be that cause the apparent scarcity of neurosyphilis among certain of the Central African aborigenes, it is now fairly certain that abstaining from the use of arsenic in early syphilis has nothing to do with it, for the investigation, in 1930, of a Russo-German commission, which studied syphilis in the Mongolian republic Burjato at Lake Baikal, proved beyond a reasonable doubt that in this primitive untreated people neurosyphilis is just as prevalent as in our own world with its arsphenamine-metals-iodide intensive antisyphilitic measures. Out at the Mayo Clinic, O'Leary and Rogin (1932) have also disposed of the question for the civilized minority of mankind. In a series of 500 cases of neurosyphilis, the more severe types made up the largest percentage of cases in the groups in which arsphenamine had not been given during the acute phase of infection, whereas the less severe types formed the largest percentage in the group which received some form of arsphenamine.

Tryparsamide Therapy.—Lorenz, Loevenhart, Blackwenn and Hodges (1923) were the first to report on the use of tryparsamide in the treatment of neurosyphilis. Their results were very good and stimulated others to use the drug, but the perhaps exaggerated fear of causing blindness with it has kept it from becoming popular. Lichtenstein (1931) has succinctly suggested another reason: "It can and may be easily forgotten because it has no dramatic moments like those attained with malarial therapy to fascinate the physician and the public." The present status of tryparsamide therapy, as ascertained from the studies of Moore, Robinson and Lyman, Woods and Moore, Schwab and Cady, Hadden and Wilson, Cady and Alvis, Fong, Tennent, Lichtenstein, and many others, may be summarized as follows:

1. Tryparsamide's power to destroy spirochetes in ordinary doses is much less than that of the other arsenicals in general use, but it does seem to have a quite astounding ability to stimulate the body of the host toward the accomplishment of a spontaneous cure. Its use was soon abandoned in the treatment of early syphilis, and of late syphilis other than neurosyphilis; but in this latter condition it has won a very high place. In the matter of clinical improvement alone, the drug is perhaps of greater value than any other at present available for the treatment of early general paralysis, meningovascular neurosyphilis, and tabes; in advanced general paralysis the results have not been very brilliant. It is now believed that in order to accomplish as much serological as clinical improvement, mercury or bismuth, or even arsphenamine, should be given also. Perhaps it is safe to say that roughly 60 per cent of paretics, 50 per cent of tabetics, and 80 per cent of meningovascular cases can be arrested by a judicious use of

tryparsamide, and that restoration to a position of more or less satisfactory economic usefulness can be accomplished for many of these patients.

2. The drug is usually given intravenously in a dose of 30 to 50 mg. per kilogram of body weight (approximately 1.5 to 2.5 Gm. per 100 pounds); the average adult dose is about 3 Gm. in 10 cc. of sterile, distilled water, given at weekly intervals for eight to sixteen weeks, followed by a rest period of about six weeks. Many such courses are usually necessary to accomplish full results. The drug may also be given intramuscularly or subcutaneously, though it is often quite irritating under these conditions. Tryparsamide solutions should not be sterilized as this will cause an increase in toxicity. In the practice of many specialists it is usual to give mercury, bismuth or arsphenamine during the rest period. A fact which is being somewhat overlooked at present is that Lorenz *et al.* pointed out that their results were better when they gave 1 cc. of mercuric salicylate intramuscularly three days before each tryparsamide injection; some physicians are now giving full doses of either mercury or bismuth throughout the tryparsamide courses.

3. Nearly all patients gain considerably in weight and well-being while taking the drug. The most frequent complaint is of ringing in the ears and a feeling of being dizzy and dazed. Nitritoid reactions, nausea, vomiting and headache are comparatively rare; urticarial reactions, dermatitis and jaundice have been reported a few times. It appears that the drug occasionally activates mental and physical signs and symptoms in a most objectionable way.

4. Visual disturbances occur with sufficient frequency under tryparsamide therapy that the drug should be used only with the greatest care. Patients with preexisting optic involvement, such as contracted fields or abnormal fundi, are more liable to injury than normal patients; but since some of these patients experience a great improvement in their vision under treatment with the drug, its routine withholding in these cases is not warranted. The most important signs of adverse action of the drug on the optic tract are subjective dimness of vision, flickering or shimmering sensations, or flashes of light; also objective diminution in the visual acuity, contraction of the visual fields and changes in the fundi. The occurrence of subjective symptoms should be thoroughly investigated for an objective basis. If no objective signs are found, tryparsamide may be continued with caution. The presence of objective findings, traceable to the drug, is a contraindication to its further use for at least a month, after which it may be very cautiously resumed.

FEVER THERAPY IN NEUROSYPHILIS[1]

I. MALARIA

Since 1918, when Wagner-Jauregg, in Vienna, and Weygandt and his associates in Hamburg, began the malaria treatment of neurosyphilis on a large scale, this original form of fever therapy has been used extensively throughout the world. I shall attempt to summarize its present status before discussing the newer methods.

Method of Inoculation.—From 2 to 10 cc. of whole blood taken from an individual suffering with tertian malaria is inoculated into the neurosyphilitic patient. Of course, the original inoculation must be made from an individual who has a naturally acquired case of malaria, but, as such material is rare in many parts of the world, most inoculations are made

[1] Beckman, H.: Fever Therapy in Neurosyphilis, Arch. Dermat. and Syph., 28, 309, September, 1933. Brought up to date, the article is included here with the kind permission of the Editor of the journal in which it appeared.

from donors who have the artificially acquired disease; these inoculations seem to be just as successful whether the blood is taken at the time of a paroxysm or during the interval between chills—nor does there seem to be any necessity for hesitancy in using the blood of general paretics in inoculating cases of tabes or cerebrospinal syphilis, since no evidence of superinfection has been reported. Also, no attention is usually paid to ascertaining the blood group of donor or recipient, and no ill effects from this practice have so far been noted other than an occasional slight rise in temperature a few hours after the inoculation. When the injection is made intravenously, the average incubation period is five days, with extremes of one to seventeen; intramuscularly, nine, with extremes of four and twenty; and subcutaneously, twelve, with extremes of five and thirty. The frequency of successful induction of malaria, and its therapeutic effect upon the paresis, are the same with the three methods of injection. In a few cases, due most probably to recovery from a previous attack of malaria, there is failure to "take"; sometimes a second attempt is successful.

The use of the quartan parasite is being advocated by some students of the matter because of the high fever, unaccompanied by severe symptoms, caused by this organism; this would probably permit a longer course of malaria with greater safety in most cases. In England, the malignant subtertian parasite is beginning to be tentatively used in patients who have not benefited greatly from a course with one of the benign types; so far with a surprisingly low mortality (see James, Nicol and Shute, 1932). Another method being experimented with (Caldwell, 1931) at the Horton Mental Hospital is the transmission of malaria by the bite of several mosquitoes, applied in a glass cylinder to the thigh; the average incubation period is fourteen days, with a range of eleven to eighteen. The advantages of this method would be that it would insure a pure infection, eliminate the risk of anaphylactic phenomena, and reduce the chances of successful litigation arising from the injection of syphilitic blood; its outstanding disadvantage is that special breeding, feeding and infecting laboratories would be necessary, since the mosquito cannot transmit the disease from paretic to paretic.

The organism does not seem to lose its power no matter how many passages it makes. By the use of a solution containing 5 per cent sodium citrate and 0.2 cc. of 50 per cent dextrose solution, into which 20 cc. of defibrinated (by agitation) malarial blood is injected, O'Leary's strain at the Mayo Clinic has been transported from Rochester, Minnesota, to Los Angeles, California, and Portland, Oregon, and successful inoculations made seventy-two hours after the blood was drawn. It is transported in vacuum bottles at body temperature.

Course of the Malaria.—The paroxysms do not occur with the precise regularity which characterizes the naturally acquired disease, but the chill, headache, vomiting, dyspnea, back and leg pains may be alarmingly violent. Cyanosis with a hard small pulse, rapid rise of blood pressure, incontinence, delirium and even convulsions are not infrequent symptoms; with the beginning of the sweat the temperature falls and the patient is comfortable in a few hours. The spleen is usually palpable within ten days and may become very large; spontaneous rupture of the organ is certainly a more frequent complication than in natural malaria—enlargement, coupled with collapse, tender abdomen and signs of hemorrhage call for immediate surgical intervention. Driver *et al.* list the following indications for prompt termination of the malaria infection; (*a*) urea increase to 70 mg. or over per 100 cc. of blood, with or without other signs of renal disease; (*b*) systolic blood pressure below 95 mm. during the interval between chills; (*c*) severe icterus with index above 50; (*d*) red blood cell count below 2,000,000;

(e) progressive rapid anemia associated with a spontaneous cessation of chills; (f) profuse diarrhea accompanied by vomiting and dehydration. As was to be expected (see p. 90), cases of congenital malaria following the inoculation therapy are beginning to be reported; the effect of the disease and the subsequent course of quinine upon the pregnant woman herself is not yet definitely determined, though perhaps most observers believe that abortion is the exception and not the rule.

All of the above only means, of course, that as yet the treatment should be attempted only in institutions thoroughly equipped in the details of both materials and trained staff. It seems that the average mortality is 10 to 14 per cent.

Termination of the Malaria.—It has been the general practice to allow the patient to experience from 12 to 16 chills, though Wagner-Jauregg, according to Wile and Davenport (1931), now favors 8 as the optimum; termination of the malaria is then effected by the use of quinine. This artificial form of the disease succumbs with surprising ease to the drug; 10 grains (0.6 Gm.) of quinine sulphate three times daily for three days, followed by 5 grains (0.3 Gm.) three times daily for four more days (or 10 grains once a day for ten days), practically always suffices, though the use of quinine should be continued if the blood continues to show the presence of *Plasmodia*. In patients whose strength is not great it is sometimes possible to check the course of the disease for a few days by a single 2- to 5-grain (0.12 to 0.3 Gm.) dose, thus allowing for a marshalling of forces to withstand the subsequent paroxysms—to gauge the dosage just right and not stop the chills for good and all, is difficult. In patients that have experienced a satisfactory malarial bout but that have not shown as much clinical improvement as was hoped for, the attempt to reinoculate usually fails. In patients in whom the disease is clinically spontaneously aborted, that is to say, those in whom the chills and fever disappear too soon while the plasmodia are still retained in the blood stream, the intramuscular injection of whole milk, typhoid vaccine or plasmodia-free whole blood, or the intravenous injection of 2 to 3 cc. of malarial blood, will very often provoke a return of the chills and fever within twenty-four hours. In England, according to James, one of the important modifications of the technic now being practiced is to allow the disease to continue, modified by quinine if necessary, until the patient acquires a tolerance for the parasite and the symptoms are not very marked. This is based upon the assumption that the curative action of malaria is chiefly dependent upon the presence of the parasites and their toxins in the body and not upon the fever alone; it will be of great interest to watch for comparisons of results obtained thus with those obtained from the universally used method of sharply terminating the attack, particularly as Bunker's (1929) finding that patients having the highest temperature showed the greatest improvement could not be substantiated by Caldwell (1931) in a careful review of 579 cases.

Relapses of the malaria occur very rarely.

Results of Malaria Therapy.—(a) *Paresis.*—Driver, Gammel and Karnosh, in the United States, published a summary of the results of malaria treatment of general paralysis, as reported in the literature prior to April 1, 1926, to which I have added the principal reports appearing up to the end of 1933 (Table 25).

By full remission is usually meant the return to an economic status practically equal to that enjoyed before the onset of paresis, and the maintenance of such status up to the time of the author's report; incomplete remission, the return to some sort of economic and social status, though lower than that previously enjoyed. In the table, the number of cases obtaining complete or incomplete remission is approximately 40 per cent of

TABLE 25.—STATUS of MALARIA TREATMENT of GENERAL PARALYSIS at END of YEAR 1933

	Cases.	Greatly improved (full remissions).	Moderately improved (incomplete remissions).
Driver, Gammel, and Karnosh (total cases in summary to April 1, 1926)	2312	635	607
Caldwell (England)	579	30	14
Ebaugh (Denver)	171	23	30
Haskins (New York)	100	33	
Bennet, Polozker, and Altshuler (Detroit).	441	11	31
Dattner (Germany)	129	44	12
Neymann and Koenig (Chicago)	50	22	22
Johnson and Jefferson (Colorado)	130	32	22
O'Leary and Welsh (Mayo Clinic)—Advanced cases	186	35	35
Early cases	249	46	35
Total	4347	911 (20.9 per cent)	808 (18.5 per cent)

the total, about equally distributed between the two groups; but I doubt if this distribution represents the true state of affairs, since an examination of the more recent reports—from Caldwell on to the end of the table—indicates that the majority of the observers are obtaining complete remission in 30 per cent or more of their cases. In round numbers, then, I think that one may say that 33 per cent of advanced paretics have been "cured"—if one may dare as yet to use the word. Granting that spontaneous remissions occur in 10 per cent of cases, this means that the paretic's chance of a complete recovery so far as his economic status is concerned has been about trebled by the advent of malaria therapy. Enthusiastic readers are respectfully requested, at this point, to turn back to the section dealing with the use of tryparsamide, and, after carefully rereading it, to turn back further still to the summary of the treatise of the Johns Hopkins group on the general principles of the modern treatment of neurosyphilis—when the real truth will emerge, which is *that all things combined, better classification, better diagnosis, better therapy (both drug and fever) and earlier application of the same, and not any one factor alone makes the chapter on paresis much pleasanter reading today than it was a very few years ago.*

The cerebrospinal fluid improves after malaria, sometimes becoming completely normal; this occurred in almost half of O'Leary and Welsh's (1933) cases. In Nicole and Fitzgerald's (1931) studies, this serological improvement, which was most marked on an average four or more years after the beginning of treatment, bore no relation to the clinical condition.

(b) *Other Types of Neurosyphilis.*—A number of reports from various countries have appeared in the literature, showing unequivocally that malaria therapy is of great value in neurosyphilis other than paresis. In a large percentage of Wile and Davenport's (1931) 96 cases immediate improvement was noted: (a) 53 per cent of the tabetics showed immediate improvement amounting in many to complete symptomatic remission; later observation increased the group to 67 per cent; there was one relapse; (b) in paresis plus tabes, 40 per cent immediate improvement later increased to 67 per cent; 13 per cent arrested, 13 per cent made worse; (c) in diffuse neurosyphilis complicating secondary syphilis and in later occurring diffuse neurosyphilis, excellent immediate and lasting results were also obtained. Serological reversal occurred more often in spinal fluid than in blood.

The report of O'Leary and Welsh (1933) may be summarized as follows: (a) In a series of 85 cases of asymptomatic paresis they obtained excellent results in 78 per cent; this group included cases exhibiting the spinal fluid changes characteristic of paresis but failing to show satisfactory serological response to routine antisyphilitic therapy, though not yet progressed far enough to permit of a clinical diagnosis of dementia paralytica; (b) in 65 cases of the tabetic form of paresis excellent results were obtained in 55 per cent and fair results in 39 per cent; (c) in 116 cases of tabes dorsalis with positive tests of spinal fluid, excellent results in 42 per cent, fair results in 41 per cent (serological results were excellent in 43 per cent, fair in 27 per cent); (d) in 25 cases of gastric crises with negative tests of spinal fluid, excellent results in 31 per cent, fair results in 56 per cent; (e) in 12 cases of lightning pains with negative tests of spinal fluid, excellent results in 11 per cent, fair results in 22 per cent; (f) in 48 cases of optic atrophy excellent results in 14 per cent, fair results in 22 per cent; (g) in 74 cases of asymptomatic neurosyphilis serological results were excellent in 42 per cent, fair in 37 per cent; (h) in 17 cases of congenital neurosyphilis of all types excellent results in 8 per cent, fair results in 66 per cent (serological results were excellent in 25 per cent, fair in 75 per cent); (i) in 12 cases of miscellaneous types of neurosyphilis results were excellent in 28 per cent, fair in 71 per cent.

Postmalarial Treatment.—The best results with malaria therapy have followed in those cases in which treatment with all the antisyphilis drugs was resumed and persisted in immediately following the termination of the malaria.

Modus Operandi.—Wagner-Jauregg's pioneer endeavors were purely empirical and, indeed, the work has remained upon that unsatisfactory basis until just recently. Now, in the period 1925–27, Gerstmann, Sträussler and Koskinas, and Freeman have given us at least a morphological foundation for the improvement observed clinically. It seems that the inflammatory exudate in the meninges and about the blood vessels undergoes organization, and that the exudates are resorbed and regression of glia and vascular tissue takes place, and that, finally, there is reconstruction of the architecture of the cortex. The histologic observations of Bahr and Breutsch (1929–30) indicate that the high temperature stimulates a phagocytic attack of the reticulo-endothelial system upon the spirochetes. Of theories, unsubstantiated, there are plenty.

II. RELAPSING FEVER AND RAT-BITE FEVER

The spirochete of relapsing fever has been used instead of the malaria parasite by Mühlens, Weygandt and Kirschbaum, Plant and Steiner; more recently, by Sagel (1931), Marie (1931), and Claude and Coste (1931). It is much less reliably effective than malaria therapy. According to Gerstmann and others the infection is sometimes prolonged over several months and cannot be checked as quickly with arsphenamine as can malaria with quinine. The disease is hard to transmit, and has to be passed through mice which causes further difficulties. Solomon has also proposed the use of rat-bite fever (sodoku), but it is apparent from the studies of Hershfield *et al.* (1929), and Neymann and Koenig (1931), that the therapy is not nearly so effective as malaria therapy, that grave intercurrent effects may develop, and that such remissions as occur are often short-lived.

III. NONSPECIFIC PROTEINS

In 1927, Kunde, Hall and Gerty, in the United States, reported upon the use of mixed typhoid-paratyphoid vaccine for the production of therapeutic pyrexia in neurosyphilis. Their results (twenty-one good remissions in 49 unselected cases of paresis) are certainly of good promise when one remembers that this type of treatment is free from the objectionable feature of the deliberate inoculation of patients with a disease-producing organism. Schelm (1930), O'Leary and Brunsting (1930), and Nelson (1931) have also reported favorably.

Method.—The vaccine is diluted with physiologic saline solution so that each cc. of the dilution contains 200 million dead bacilli. The injections are given intravenously every second or third day, a course consisting of eighteen to twenty-four injections sufficient in quantity to produce a chill followed by fever with a fastigium of 103 to 104 F. (by rectum). The initial dose is usually 50 million dead bacilli, and subsequent increments of 100 million usually suffice to elicit the desired effect, so that at the eighteenth injection the patient receives 1800 million; however, individual differences in reaction are very marked and each patient will have to be carefully studied in order to determine the amount of increase necessary in each dose. The course is usually repeated once after a two months' interval and the same reactions are obtained.

Typical Reaction.—(a) Blood pressure rises within half an hour to a maximum at time of chill, then falls below normal, and returns to normal within twenty-four hours. (b) First chill, of which there may be one to three, between two and three hours after injection; if it lasts longer than twenty minutes there should be suspicion of cardiac collapse, though as long as the blood pressure remains high there is no danger. (c) Average duration of maximum temperature, one and one-half hours in early injections, thirty minutes later; average time above normal, eight to ten hours, later four to five hours. (d) Nausea and vomiting after the chill in most patients. (e) Back pains and headache, controllable with sodium salicylate or acetylsalicylic acid. (f) Excitement sometimes, controllable with paraldehyde or barbital. (g) Rise in blood sugar after each injection; first leukopenia and then leukocytosis—all three returning to normal day after injection. (h) Often a secondary rise of temperature may occur on the day following treatment.

Decidedly, I think this is the fever therapy method of choice for the average general practitioner, even though the remissions are perhaps not as frequent, as long-lasting or as complete as with the much more complex malaria therapy. It would seem that the mortality directly due to this treatment is about 2 per cent, though the number of cases is still too small to make this worth much more than a guess. Absolute contraindications, according to Kemp and Stokes, are myocardial and advanced cardiovascular disease; in arteriosclerosis, pulmonary disease and marked grades of focal infection one must be very careful.

Nelson has successfully produced temperatures of 105 to 107 F. by giving a second injection at the height of the fever.

IV. DIATHERMY, ELECTRIC BLANKET, HOT BATHS, HOT AIR

Neymann and Osborne (1931), Neymann and Koenig (1931), Perkins (1931), Neymann (1933), and others have reported upon the successful treatment of paresis with the diathermy apparatus. Apparently there are no contraindications to the employment of this method, except acute arthritic and pelvic infections and peptic ulcer with tendency toward bleeding, and if these early reports are confirmed (Freeman, Fong and Rosenberg, 1933, were able to observe no case of improvement among the 50 patients treated by them at St. Elizabeth's Hospital in Washington) it will probably replace malaria therapy in institutions, since it seems to produce an even larger number of remissions, even among the depressive types that are so much more resistant to malaria than the expansive patients. The successful treatment depends upon certain mechanical factors necessary to produce elevation of temperature, maintain it, and prevent burns to the patient. The prime requisites are properly constructed electrodes, a machine powerful enough to give sufficient energy, and proper insulation of the patient—things which obviously call for the services of an expert physiotherapist. The technic is changing as the method develops, but Neymann and his associates, who have had probably the most extensive experience, have given from six to forty-nine treatments, the average being fifteen; they look upon a temperature above 103.5 F. for at least five hours as optimal. Wilgus and Lurie (1931) have asserted that the electric blanket is the simplest and safest form of fever-producing agent, and they propose to substitute it for diathermy in their future work at the Illinois State Psychopathic Institute. Mehrtens and Pouppirt (1929) employed hot baths, but gave up the method when they found that it was even more complicated than the malaria treatment as it required greater cooperation from the patient; the hot-air method of Kahler and Knollmayer (1929) has the same disadvantage.

V. SULPHUR

There are many clinical reports available on the use of sulphur for the production of fever since it was introduced for this purpose by Schroeder in 1927 (Marcuse and Kallmann; Harris; Patterson and Switzer; Winkler; McCowan and Northcote; Read; Mackay; Schlesinger; Laptain; Power). One to 2 cc. of 1 to 2 per cent sublimated sulphur in olive oil is injected into the lateral aspect of the thigh (beneath the fascia lata to avoid severe local reaction), every four or five days, increasing each dose by 1 cc. until ten injections have been given. Temperature rises after six to eighteen hours to 103 to 105 F., falls several degrees within three or four hours, and rises several times again within the next day or two; result is a significant elevation of temperature for longer perhaps than with any of the other methods. As with typhoid vaccine therapy, however, the optimum dosage has to be determined for each patient. Chills, or even chilliness, rarely occur. The respiratory rate is very little affected, and the pulse rate is very variable, though there is usually a definite rise. Neither the blood pressure, vasomotor nor diaphoretic responses are very marked; some patients, however, are made quite uncomfortable by the local reaction. Leukocytosis occurs promptly after all injections. Considerable weight is lost by most patients during the course of treatment.

The results with this type of therapy are very good and I should say that, equally with typhoid inoculations, it is the method of choice for the average general practitioner.

Gastric Crisis.—The vomiting in syphilitic gastric crisis is central in origin and the administration of cracked ice, carbonated waters, etc., has usually no effect upon it. The physician is quite helpless in the presence of an abjectly miserable patient, therefore, unless he turns to the sovereign remedy, morphine, which he often does. It controls both the pain and the vomiting, but not infrequently must be used several times with the result that the patient sometimes has his tabes complicated by morphinism, a most difficult combination to treat. It is therefore of interest to note that McFarland has reported favorably upon the rectal use of chloral hydrate and sodium bromide in these cases. In a series of forty-nine injections given to 12 patients he obtained in 76 per cent of the administrations fully as great relief as is obtained with morphine. He gives a retention enema containing in 15 cc. of fluid from 40 to 60 grains (2.6 to 4 Gm.) of each drug, depending upon the size of the patient. Unfortunately it would seem that this method is not readily applicable to all cases, since most of them get their several injections of morphine during their first few attacks while a puzzled physician is trying to rule out gallstone colic, etc.

Marinesco, Sager and Façon have reported upon the use of 1 to 2 cc. of a 25 per cent sterilized magnesium sulphate solution intraspinally in this condition. In the 8 patients thus treated, pain and vomiting disappeared entirely in from thirty to fifty minutes after the injection. Some patients needed another injection after two or three days; in others the interval was lengthened to several months. Alajovanine and Horowitz (1932) have used successfully intravenous injections of 1 to 3 mg. of atropine sulphate, once or twice daily, for several days.

The reader is also referred to page 191, where the results obtained with malaria therapy are stated.

TREATMENT OF CONGENITAL SYPHILIS

The mortality from congenital syphilis in early infancy is very high. This mortality can be very considerably reduced by prompt and proper treatment, but I believe that it is only the excessively sanguine physician who will maintain that the result of such treatment, from the standpoint of clinical and serological eradication of the disease, is as good in early congenital syphilis as it is in early acquired syphilis. However, the addition of arsphenamine to the armamentarium has certainly definitely raised the curability—or I should perhaps more correctly say the arrestability—of the disease, for the discouraging appearance of new symptoms in a child under vigorous treatment is no longer so frequent as it was in the days when mercury was used alone. It is difficult to make a satisfactory statement of the prognosis and amenability to treatment of those cases which are latent in infancy and early childhood only to develop symptoms later in life. They are so variable; occasionally a congenital syphilitic goes through life with few or no symptoms other than a persistently positive Wassermann, while many others develop symptoms which respond very sluggishly to the most vigorous treatment. Most cases can be brought to some degree of clinical arrest, at least, and perhaps a very few can even be cured—insofar as it is permissible to speak of cure at all in this disease. Eye and bone lesions resist the longest. In congenital neurosyphilis, arrest is a thing more often spoken of than accomplished.

To prevent the occurrence of congenital syphilis, or to so modify the disease in the fetus as to make it more amenable to treatment in the child after birth, is now clearly recognized as a possibility. Antisyphilitic treatment of the mother, begun as early in the pregnancy as possible, should be vigorously pushed up to the time of full term; the drugs are well borne by pregnant women. McCord's (1932) studies show that the maximum of safety for the baby is offered by not less than ten treatments during pregnancy; a "treatment" consisting in an injection of 0.45 Gm. neoarsphenamine and an inunction of mercury. Neurosyphilis of the congenital form is treated like acquired neurosyphilis; reports of the use of tryparsamide and malaria therapy in infants are still conspicuously lacking, though the latter is being used with excellent results in older children.

The treatment of late congenital syphilis is that of late acquired syphilis; the treatment of the early congenital form is that of the early acquired form, save that there must be modification of dosage for size of the individual, and especial care must be exercised in the beginning since it is quite possible to cause the death of one of these frail wizened little things by a too vigorous attack. In interstitial keratitis, Carvill (1931) has supplied two excellent reports of the results in 100 cases intensively treated and 100 untreated; I present the results in Table 26.

TABLE 26.—RESULTS OF INTENSIVE TREATMENT IN INTERSTITIAL KERATITIS

Vision.	Treated (100 cases).	Untreated (100 cases).
20/30 or better..........................	58 per cent	28 per cent
20/60 or better..........................	75 per cent	56 per cent
20/70 or worse...........................	24 per cent	42 per cent
Less than 20/100.........................	15 of 178 eyes; 1 eye, light only	45 of 179 eyes; 5 eyes, light only; 5 eyes blind

A check-up 5 years later on 67 of the 100 treated cases: in 23 vision had improved, in 32 it had not changed, in 9 it was worse, and in 3 the data were not obtained.

The consensus of opinion is that even intensive treatment at the beginning of inflammation in one eye does not prevent the involvement of the second eye, usually in a few weeks to months, rarely several years.

Use of Mercury, Arsenic and Iodides.—(*a*) Fordyce and Rosen (1924): The arsphenamine course comprises six to eight injections; the initial dose is 0.1 Gm. for infants two to twelve weeks old; 0.15 Gm. from three to nine months; 0.2 Gm. from one to two years; and 0.25 to 0.3 Gm. for children three years old. The mercuric chloride course is ten to twelve injections at intervals of one week; 1/10 grain for children from two weeks to six months old; 1/8 grain from six months to one year; 1/7 grain from one to two years; 1/5 grain from two to three years; and 1/4 grain for those more than three years old.

(*b*) Veeder and Jeans (1924): The arsphenamine dose is 0.01 Gm. per kilogram of body weight. In this clinic it is given in such concentration that 4 cc. of the solution contain 0.1 Gm. of the drug—a much more concentrated solution than is usually used. The use of the syringe instead of the gravity method is thus made possible; in approximately ten thousand injections no ill effects have been noted which could be attributed to the concentration. The neoarsphenamine dose is 0.015 Gm. per kilogram of body weight, given in such concentration that each 2 cc. of the solution contain 0.1 Gm. The mercuric chloride dose for intramuscular injection is 0.033 cc. (0.5 minim) of a 1 per cent solution per kilogram (2.2 pounds) of body weight, given twice a week, or given once a week and supplemented by daily mercury by mouth; for this latter purpose mercury with chalk (gray powder) is used in tablet form, the dose ranging from 1/5 grain twice daily for young infants to 2 grains or more three times daily for larger children. In young infants of precarious nutrition this mercury by mouth is often objectionable on the score of its excessive cathartic effect. Or mercury ointment (full strength) is used by inunction in daily doses of 1 to 4 Gm., depending upon the size of the child. When prolonged inunction is contraindicated by the delicacy of the child, this ointment may be spread over the inner surface of an abdominal binder. Iodides are also sometimes used in a dose of 3 to 7½ grains (0.2 to 0.5 Gm.) three times daily according to the size of the child. Intraspinal treatment is employed in cases of neurosyphilis that do not otherwise respond. The blood is withdrawn one-half hour after an intravenous injection of arsphenamine; the amount of serum injected later varies from 10 to 25 or 30 cc., according to the size of the child. Three to five such injections, at an interval of five to ten days, are given as a series.

(*c*) Cannon (1927): The plan of treatment is one of continuous treatment. The dose of neoarsphenamine is 0.1 to 0.25 Gm. up to one year; 0.15 to 0.3 Gm. from one to five years; 0.2 to 0.45 Gm. from five to ten years. The first four injections are given twice a week, after that once a week. Each course consists of ten injections of neoarsphenamine and fifteen injections of mercuric chloride, the latter drug being continued after the termination of the neoarsphenamine until the full number of injections has been given. The injection of neoarsphenamine is then continued, this time without the mercury, which is resumed only after the completion of the course of neoarsphenamine. Potassium iodide is given at intervals during the mercury injections. This plan of treatment is continued for three or four courses, or from one to one and one-half years. When an interruption of the injections is necessary, barring physical ailment, the patient is put on mixed treatment. Intraspinal injections are employed in neurosyphilis in the usual way, except that the blood is taken from an adult receiving not more than 0.3 Gm. of neoarsphenamine intravenously one-half to one hour previously. Not more than 10 cc. of serum has been injected.

(d) Cooke: "A course consists of eight weeks' treatment, in which mercury is given by mouth three times daily, as well as by intramuscular injection once weekly; and an arsenical once weekly by intravenous or intramuscular injection during the first three successive weeks of this period. One such course is immediately followed by the next, and a vacation of two months at the end of the year is given when the treatment has been faithful and continuous." Dosage of the drugs corresponds closely to that of Veeder and Jeans above cited.

Sulpharsphenamine.—This drug seems to have won a distinct place for itself in the treatment of early congenital syphilis. Durham (1925) summarized her study of the drug in 28 cases, as follows:

"Compared with neoarsphenamine, sulpharsphenamine seems to have the following advantages: (1) It can be given subcutaneously with slight discomfort during the injection. Following the injection there is little pain or induration. Neoarsphenamine, on the other hand, cannot be given subcutaneously and, if given intramuscularly, indurated areas often result which may remain and cause discomfort for some time. (2) Sulpharsphenamine can be given in larger doses and higher concentration than neoarsphenamine. (3) It clears up active lesions (condyloma and gumma) very rapidly but probably acts no more rapidly than neoarsphenamine. (4) As only two patients with syphilis of the central nervous system have been treated, no conclusions can be drawn as to its efficacy in the treatment of this type of the disease. (5) It does not seem to have any more effect than neoarsphenamine in changing the so-called 'fixed Wassermann reaction.' Possibly a change from neoarsphenamine to sulpharsphenamine may be advantageous. (6) It does not seem to cure early or late congenital syphilis any more rapidly than may be expected with neoarsphenamine. (7) There is probably no advantage in subcutaneous injections of sulpharsphenamine in older children or adults whose veins are accessible. The majority of the children actually prefer intravenous treatment.[!] In fat children or small babies with inaccessible veins, the subcutaneous route has a great advantage. There are a certain number of parents who refuse to have their children treated intravenously and there is a great advantage in having an efficient drug that can be injected subcutaneously."

Durham's routine was as follows: First, daily inunctions of 30 per cent mercury ointment (U.S.P.) or intramuscular injections of mercuric chloride in oil, $\frac{1}{10}$ grain (0.006 Gm.) for infants or $\frac{1}{4}$ grain (0.015 Gm.) for children over five years, once a week for six weeks; then six weekly injections of sulpharsphenamine. After a rest of four weeks, the whole course was repeated. The sulpharsphenamine was given in a dose of 0.02 Gm. per kilogram of body weight (0.6 Gm. maximum), and was made up in a 25 per cent aqueous solution so that with the maximum dose only 2.5 cc. of the solution was injected. The injection was made subcutaneously in the back, between the lower angle of the scapula and the spinal column where the skin is loose. At the site of injection there was seen occasionally the following week a small indurated nonpainful area, which had usually disappeared by the next week.

Boone and Weech, Ähmen, and Sylvester have also reported satisfactory results with the drug. I place below a table (Table 27), taken from the paper of the latter, which shows a striking superiority of the arsenicals to mercury when either of the drugs is used alone in the treatment of congenital syphilis. Sixty-seven sulpharsphenamine cases are included in this table; the number in the neoarsphenamine and mercury series I do not know.

TABLE 27.—COMPARATIVE EFFECTIVENESS OF MERCURY, NEOARSPHENAMINE AND SULPHARSPHENAMINE AS SHOWN BY THE TIME OF DISAPPEARANCE OF LESIONS

	Early.			Late.		
	Skin.	Viscera.	Bones.	Skin.	Viscera.	Bones.
Mercury..............	6 weeks to 6 months	3 months to 6 months	3 months to 6 months+	3 weeks to 6 months	6 months+	Years +
Neoarsphenamine.......	1 to 2 weeks	2 to 3 weeks	2 to 4 months	3 weeks	5 to 8 weeks	Years +
Sulpharsphenamine......	1 to 3 weeks	2 to 4 weeks	3 weeks to 2 months	2 to 4 weeks	2 to 4 months	Years +

Sylvester gave twelve weekly injections of 10 to 20 mg. of sulpharsphenamine per pound body weight in 10 per cent concentration; then a month's vacation followed by a Wassermann. If this was negative, the series was repeated at one half of the original dose, if positive, at one and one-half times the original dose.

Acetarsone (Stovarsol).—This pentavalent arsenical compound, which is available in soluble tablets of 4 grains (0.25 Gm.) for administration by mouth, has been much used in the treatment of congenital syphilis on the Continent, particularly in Germany. Spiethof (1925) gives half a tablet to babies less than nine months old, three quarters of a tablet to those between ten and twelve months, and a whole tablet to children over a year, each day for six months to a year with rest periods. Von den Steinen (1927) gives as much as two tablets per day for seven days to children of two years with rest periods of seven days. Bamberger (1931) begins with one-fourth tablet three times daily and slowly increases until one tablet—in 2 cases, two and one-half tablets—are given three times daily on an empty stomach. Good clinical, not so good serological results, are reported by all of these observers, but I feel that we should be on our guard here, for there is at least a *chance* that the ease of administration, and therefore the ready cooperation of parents, will lead us into an unwarranted enthusiasm. In the United States, Maxwell and Gloser (1932) have used the drug with clinical and serological success in 12 infants syphilitic or from syphilitic mothers; their course was: One tablet once, twice, three and four times daily for one week each, one-half tablet three and four times daily for a week more each respectively, and one tablet twice a day for a week, followed by a six weeks' rest period. Abt and Traisman (1932) were also pleased with the results in a series of 22 patients. Mettel (1931) has used it with clinical but not serological success in a series of periostitis cases with bone manifestations. The toxic effects noted have been chills, fever, aching, sore throat, coryza, abdominal pain, vomiting and diarrhea, malaise, albuminuria, edema, leucopenia, eosinophilia, dermatitis, urticaria and pruritic anal eczema.

Bismuth.—See page 214.

Bismarsen.—See page 218.

Malaria Therapy.—See page 191.

Arsphenamine by Rectum.—Littman and Hutton have shown that the clinical results obtained by the use of arsphenamine by rectum in children with acute manifestations of congenital syphilis are too feeble to warrant the consideration of this method of administering the drug.

Neoarsphenamine Intraperitoneally.—Sanford has reported the intraperitoneal injection of neoarsphenamine in ten infants with satisfactory clinical results and without any evidence that the drug had a deleterious effect within the abdomen. Necropsies were performed on two of the patients who died from other causes, one after six injections and the other after two; in both cases no signs were found of abdominal pathologic disturbance. The usual treatment consisted of four injections at three-day intervals, followed by four injections at seven-day intervals. This was usually sufficient to clear whatever syphilitic pathology existed, including the Wassermann reaction. Sanford's technic follows:

"Our method consisted in washing the whole abdomen with green soap and water, then once with alcohol. The ideal site for entrance of the needle is located in the middle of the left rectus sheath, slightly below the level of the umbilicus. This spot was chosen because in many children the liver on the right side will be at the level of the umbilicus, and it is necessary to go below any possible limit of the omentum, and a site too far below the umbilicus will endanger the bladder. This spot was painted with tincture of iodine, which was then washed off with alcohol. The needle, preferably a small gauge one, was inserted as for an ordinary intraperitoneal injection. The solution consisted of 150 mg. of neoarsphenamine dissolved in approximately 15 cc. of warm, sterile water. The average weight child of 10 pounds (4.5 Kg.) should receive 50 mg., or 5 cc. of the solution. The substance was injected as fast as the plunger would fall in the syringe, and was best sprayed over the peritoneal contents."

DISCUSSION OF THE VARIOUS ARSENICALS, THE IODIDES, AND THE VARIOUS PREPARATIONS OF MERCURY AND BISMUTH (INCLUDING BISMARSEN)

1. THE ARSENICALS

(a) **Arsphenamine versus Neoarsphenamine.**—So far as I am aware, all save one of the leading syphilologists of this country are thoroughly convinced of the therapeutic superiority of arsphenamine (old salvarsan) to neoarsphenamine (new salvarsan) in the routine general treatment of syphilis. Nevertheless, perhaps as much as 90 per cent of the arsenic administered intravenously in private practice is in the form of neoarsphenamine, the reasons being of course that this drug is freer from reactions and is much easier to administer. The ease of administration no one can deny, but whether it is less toxic is really open to reasonable doubt; Cannon and Karelitz (1931), as a result of their study of the rich material afforded by the Vanderbilt Clinic, do not find in favor of a lower toxicity for neo and the similar studies of Cole *et al.* have supported them. However, as Schamberg (1931) well points out, under the conditions of preparation by the average general practitioner with relatively poor facilities and little time, arsphenamine has been and probably will continue to be, considerably more toxic. A very great difficulty in arriving at an accurate estimate of the clinical value of neoarsphenamine lies in the marked variability between different lots of the drug even from the same manufacturer.

(*b*) **Arsphenamine.**—*Dosage.*—It has been shown that small doses are less than useless, since the spirochetes are thus enabled to acquire a tolerance for the drug and become so-called "arsenic fast." Therefore the initial dose and all subsequent doses should be as large as possible consistently with safety. In the United States, adults are usually given 0.2 Gm. the first dose, 0.3 Gm. the next, 0.4 Gm. the next, and either 0.4 or 0.5 Gm. for each of the remaining doses of the course. Women are usually not carried above 0.3 Gm. Children are started on 0.05 to 0.1 Gm. and built up to 0.2, or possibly 0.3 Gm., depending upon age and size. Some practitioners use larger initial doses, both in adults and children, than those just listed.

Preparation of Arsphenamine for Administration.—Arsphenamine is a hydrochloride and its solution in water—it is freely soluble—is acid. This solution must be neutralized with NaOH and then injected slowly at or about body temperature.

STEPS.—1. Have all receptacles absolutely sterile.

2. Immerse the tube in alcohol to see that it is not leaking. An open tube is very dangerous for the reason that the drug oxidizes rapidly into a highly toxic product. Arsphenamine does not undergo toxic deterioration in the sealed tube at ordinary temperatures.

3. Pour contents of tube into fresh, double-distilled water, in such amount that there is 20 cc. for each 0.1 Gm. of the drug. Dissolve with slow rotation to prevent contact with the air as much as possible.

4. Slowly add sterile 15 per cent solution of NaOH, drop by drop, until the flocculent precipitate which forms is entirely redissolved—this usually requires 4 drops per 0.1 Gm. Filter through sterile gauze.

5. Then dilute with fresh, double-distilled water up to 30 cc. per 0.1 Gm. of the drug. Let stand for at least thirty minutes for completion of chemical reactions which greatly diminish the toxicity.

6. Slowly inject into a vein of the arm by the gravity method, allowing at least ten minutes for the full dose to run in.

The water used in the various steps should be warm but not very hot. Chemically pure sodium chloride, 0.5 to 0.85 per cent, or sterile glucose, 5 per cent, may have been added before sterilizing, but the opinion that this is an advantage is not unanimously held. The injection should be made at body temperature.

(*c*) **Neoarsphenamine** (**New Salvarsan**).—While in the sealed ampule neoarsphenamine may undergo a change in color, solubility, mobility in the ampule, odor and toxicity. These changes may either render the particular lot of the drug useless, or, more rarely, dangerous to life. Age of the product is a factor of less importance than the temperature at which it is stored. It should be kept at ice-box temperature and not used if it has changed in color or is not readily soluble. I know from my own experience that physicians in the tropics are partial to those brands which are marketed each ampule in a separate wooden box since the wood is a poor conductor of heat.

Dosage.—Neoarsphenamine is given in doses one half again as large as arsphenamine, *i. e.*, a patient getting 0.4 Gm. of arsphenamine would get 0.6 Gm. of neoarsphenamine, etc.

Preparation of Neoarsphenamine for Administration.—One of the undoubted advantages of this product is its ease of preparation. The powder is simply sprinkled on the surface of fresh double-distilled water—12.5 cc. for each 0.1 Gm.—and permitted to dissolve without much agitation; the flask, which should be tall and of small caliber, is to be stoppered after adding the powder. Water used should be at room temperature as neoarsphenamine solution increases in toxicity above 71 F. (21.7 C.). Also, it should be injected at once after it is prepared for the reason that the solution becomes much more toxic while standing.

Since the World War it has become the custom to prepare the solution directly in the original ampule and to inject this concentrated solution. See the section on arsphenamines in the treatment of malaria for a full exposition of this method (p. 100). When given intramuscularly, a method of administration which is now little employed, the drug is dissolved in the ratio of 3 cc. of water per 0.15 Gm., which furnishes an approximately isotonic solution.

(*d*) **Silver Arsphenamine.**—This drug was introduced with quite a flourish in 1918, being especially highly lauded in Germany (Galewsky, Gennerich, Hahn, Müller, Houck, Favry—see Bibliography). Kolle and Ritz attributed the superiority of the new drug to the fact that when the arsenical molecule is combined with the silver molecule there is a combined action of the two metals, silver being spirochetostatic and arsenic spirocheticidal. In America also it was well received; Parounagian, for instance, after giving 4290 injections at Bellevue Hospital in New York City (1921), stated his belief that clinical manifestations in all stages of syphilis responded more promptly to this drug than to any of the other arsenicals. Strauss, Sidlick, Mallas and Crawford, however, shortly thereafter showed that the spirocheticidal power of silver arsphenamine, as judged by its ability to lower the Wassermann reaction, was far inferior to that of arsphenamine and neoarsphenamine. One does not hear of this drug having replaced either of the older products for routine use in many of the American clinics. In the matter of immediate reactions, the drug probably occupies a place intermediate between that of old arsphenamine and neoarsphenamine. Argyria, which is a theoretic possibility, has occurred with extreme rarity; according to Becker and Ritchie (1931), it is apt to follow the administration of a total quantity above 15 Gm.; Spiegel (1931) places the maximum at 8 Gm.

Dosage and Technic.—Silver arsphenamine is prepared and injected just as is arsphenamine except that neutralization with NaOH is unnecessary; the solution must be very promptly but slowly injected. Parounagian's dosage:

"The patients receive 0.15 Gm. as an initial dose, and this is followed by an injection of from 0.2 to 0.25 Gm. for each succeeding dose, unless smaller doses are indicated by the character of the case. Injections are given every third or fourth day. Eight injections have constituted a course; a rest of four weeks without treatment has been routine, followed by a further rest or continued treatment (mainly with neoarsphenamine) as the serology or history indicate."

(*e*) **Sulpharsphenamine.**—The use of this drug (as Sulfarsenol, the French product) was first described by Lévy-Bing, Lehnhoff-Wyld and Gerbay in 1919. It was rather extensively employed in various European clinics during the next three years and its usefulness reported upon by Yernaux and Bernard (France), Doble (England), Papegaaij and Rinsema (Holland), and many others. The consensus of opinion of these European observers was that an arsenical compound had been found which could be administered subcutaneously or intramuscularly without pain, and yet was equal, if not superior to, the older arsenicals in therapeutic value; very little mention was made of the toxicity of the drug. In America, Voegtlin and his co-workers ascribe to it a higher spirocheticidal value than arsphenamine in experimental syphilis and also, under certain special conditions, a higher trypanocidal value as well; but Myers and Corbitt, and later Raiziss, Severac and Moetsch, found it distinctly less effective as a trypanocide than arsphenamine or neoarsphenamine. The first Americans to report on its clinical employment, Hewins and Acre, 1922, agreed in substance with the early European observers—but since that time considerable doubt has been raised in the minds of syphilologists in this country as to its relative effectiveness in the eradication of syphilis and also its freedom from toxicity. Indeed, further careful studies have shown this latter contention to be a myth. The intramuscular injection of the drug (the subcutaneous and intravenous routes have been practically abandoned) is not always painless; furthermore, hemorrhagic purpura, meningovascular reactions, peripheral neuritis, dermatitis and aplastic anemias, some even taking the form of fatal agranulocytosis, occur after this drug more often than after any of the other arsenicals. I quote Fox (1925) in what seems still to be a fair statement of the position of sulpharsphenamine in the treatment of acquired syphilis; its use in congenital syphilis has been described elsewhere (p. 196):

"A new arsenical must fulfill at least one of four requirements to be awarded a real place in the treatment of syphilis: (1) A therapeutic value, in the tolerated dose, superior to that possessed by the older arsphenamines in the attempted cure of the disease; (2) a particular quality in arresting and healing certain of the later manifestations of the disease resistant to other forms of treatment; (3) a decided usefulness in those cases unable to receive arsenic in the older forms because of toxic reaction of one kind or another; (4) superior availability because of simplification of administration by other than the intravenous method, without, of course, loss of therapeutic value, or increase of toxicity.

"Even the most enthusiastic advocates of sulpharsphenamine can hardly claim a superior curative power for the drug as compared with arsphenamine or neoarsphenamine. Whether it is equal to them in this regard is an open question. The clinical study here presented revealed no inferiority for sulpharsphenamine as far as end-results were concerned. In the matter of control of some of the later more resistant manifestations of syphilis, especially those of the nervous system, proof has not been obtained that sulpharsphenamine has superior value. Certainly on the basis of clinical data now available, one would not be justified in using this drug in preference to tryparsamide, or even intraspinal therapy, in the treatment of resistant neurosyphilis. In that limited number of cases unable to receive the other arsenicals intravenously because of the development of the 'nitritoid' reaction, sulpharsphenamine is of value. However, if one admits that sulpharsphenamine has equal or nearly equal therapeutic value, the fact that it can be administered intramuscularly is a great boon for the patient with small or inaccessible veins. Many of these patients have been deprived in the past of sufficient arsenic for the cure of their disease, unless they happened to fall into the hands of one skilled in intravenous technic.

"The fourth requirement, then, remains the only one in which the drug possesses any important advantage over the other arsphenamines. Because of the higher incidence of systematic reactions following the use of this drug, it seems desirable to confine its employment solely to those cases in which intravenous therapy cannot be used. Further study is especially indicated to determine the nature of this toxic factor in its composition and whether it can be eliminated. In the meantime sulpharsphenamine must occupy a restricted but nevertheless very useful place in the treatment of syphilis."

Sulpharsphenamine is given at the same time intervals as arsphenamine. The intramuscular dose varies from 0.2 to 0.6 Gm., depending on the weight and tolerance of the patient. It should be dissolved in freshly distilled water just before administration. The concentration of 33 per cent (0.33 cc. of water for each 0.1 Gm. of the drug) has been found to cause the least local irritation.

(*f*) **Stovarsol.**—This drug has been used rather much of late in Germany when the arsphenamines are contraindicated, or as "follow-up" therapy after intravenous or intramuscular therapy. The dosage is somewhat larger than that employed in congenital syphilis (p. 197). In going about on the Continent in 1930, I was by no means convinced that there is much to recommend this use of stovarsol save its ease of administration; certainly there are not yet in the literature any controlled clinical studies.

Arsenical Reactions.—These group themselves clinically into early and late reactions.

(*a*) **Early.**—1. Immediate ("nitritoid"): This, the most frequent type of reaction, begins shortly after the injection has been started. Oftentimes the first symptom is a sudden intense pain in the back, though this is by no means invariable. Always, however, there is a quick flushing of the face and injection of the eyes, dyspnea and cough and nausea; sometimes, though unusually, the patient vomits at this point; usually the pulse becomes very weak and deep cyanosis develops. Sometimes there is loss of consciousness with suspended respiration for a few seconds. The symptoms usually persist for half an hour in some degree, sometimes longer. Though frightening to witness, these reactions seldom result in death, their most objectionable feature being that the patient often refuses to take the subsequent treatments in the course—which is easy enough to understand as their sensations are described as being those of impending death.

This type of reaction is ascribed to so many different causes that analysis of the possibilities cannot be gone into here. The most probable cause is simply an idiosyncrasy for the drug, for when a patient has once experienced this reaction he is almost certain to have a recurrence in some degree at each subsequent injection. Sometimes, however, it is due to faulty technic: either to the use of a mixture that is "stale," or failure to sufficiently alkalinize during the process of preparing the solution. Occasionally, also, one particular batch of the drug, however carefully prepared, seems to produce reactions by reason of some unavoidable impurity contained; such a batch must be thrown away as its use is dangerous. Larsen (1931) has maintained that there are two kinds of arsphenamine distributed, a methylated and a nonmethylated type, and that the former is the more toxic; his interesting contention still lacks experimental substantiation.

Treatment.—About the only effective drug is epinephrine (adrenalin), which should be injected intramuscularly at once when the symptoms appear (the injection of the arsenical having been immediately stopped, of course). It is usual to use 1 cc. of the 1:1000 solution. Since the symptoms closely resemble those of the overaction of nitrites, this use of epinephrine is not entirely empirical.

A sudden and intense pain which often makes its appearance in the arm or shoulder during the course of the arsenical injection need not be regarded as a sign of impending reaction; it is usually fleeting though very excruciating. One is usually able to continue the injection without interruption.

Prophylaxis.—It is sometimes possible to prevent the recurrence of this reaction by the injection subcutaneously of atropine sulphate fifteen minutes before the arsenical injection; less than $\frac{1}{50}$ grain is usualy ineffective; epinephrine administered before the arsphenamine, instead of waiting for first symptoms is also occasionally of value. Ephedrine is sometimes given, several doses on the day before and the day of the injection.

2. Other Early Reactions.—1. Skin eruptions sometimes appear several hours after the injection. These are usually of only short duration and do not require any treatment other than for the local relief of the itching, and perhaps the changing to another arsphenamine, such as the silver preparation. A more severe type, which may go on to a true exfoliative dermatitis, is fortunately extremely rare; it is now generally believed to be the result of direct sensitization to the arsphenamines, or to the products of their metabolism, or to a state of general allergic instability. According to Moore and associates (1931), the intradermal skin test for sensitivity is not reliable, since negatively reacting patients often in their experience developed rashes on the subsequent administration of therapeutic doses of the drugs. For the treatment of this latter type, two forms of sulphur have been proposed:

(*a*) *Sodium Thiosulphate.*—Dennie and McBride showed, in 1924, that the use of this drug will often terminate these cases very quickly; most syphilologists, I believe, are no longer particularly enthusiastic about it. The drug is given intravenously in 20 cc. of distilled water every day for four days, and then every other day for as often as is necessary to complete the cure. An ascending dosage is used, as follows: 0.3, 0.45, 0.6, 0.75, 0.9, 1.2, and 1.8 Gm. In fulminating cases the dose may be started higher and be given several times in the first twenty-four hours. Chemically pure and not the ordinary sodium thiosulphate should be used.

(*b*) *Thiosinamine.*—Greenbaum has reported the use of thiosinamine very successfully in a number of cases. He says: "Our method is to put the drug up in ampules containing 3 grains of the drug dissolved in 6 cc. of distilled water, to which is added 1 or 2 drops of a 2 per cent solution of glycerin, which insures permanent dissolution. The ampules are sterilized in the autoclave."

The patient is given the contents of one of these ampules intravenously every twenty-four hours. Many individuals complain of the objectionable taste and odor of the drug during the injection.

2. Chills and fever with violent headache and perhaps legache, nausea and vomiting, perhaps diarrhea, may appear a few hours after the arsenical injection. The suffering is sometimes very severe, but at present I know of no effective treatment other than the use of symptomatic remedies. The reaction usually disappears in twenty-four hours, but many patients of the clinic type never return for treatment after an experience of this sort. This type of reaction often occurs in "epidemics," and Stokes and Busman have perhaps conclusively shown that it is due to the use of new rubber tubing. Whatever the toxic principle may be, it is removable by soaking the tubing for six hours in normal sodium hydroxide solution; as an extra precaution it is thus soaked on a number of a successive days in some clinics. The toxic substance is not destroyed by boiling, is not soluble in water, and is not contained in the washings and mechanically removable débris from the inside of new tubes.

(*b*) **Late Reactions.**—1. *"Herxheimer" Reaction.*—This consists in a lighting up of all the syphilitic lesions, of whatever stage and location, which comes on a day or so after the treatment and lasts several days. All the visible lesions become violently erythematous, but this is usually of little moment in early syphilis; in late syphilis, on the other hand, where there are numerous visceral lesions, very grave symptoms may accompany or follow such a reaction. "Herxheimer" usually subsides in a few days without any special treatment. As yet there is no entirely satisfactory explanation for the occurrence of this reaction.

2. *Jaundice.*—Occasionally a patient who has had a number of treatments—most often in the second or later courses—will suddenly develop a

most intense jaundice, which becomes progressively worse with death resulting from acute yellow atrophy of the liver plus hemorrhages in the other viscera. Those who survive will continue to be jaundiced and sick for many months. The cause is still very much a matter for discussion; suffice it to say that many careful syphilologists feel that any patient who shows even the slightest tendency toward jaundice during arsenical treatment should never be given another injection. Craven's (1931) studies in animals, which are as yet unconfirmed, indicated that high protein and particularly high fat diets afford the maximum protection against this arsphenamine injury to the liver; a most surprising piece of work since it has hitherto been believed that carbohydrates—shown to be deleterious in his experiments— were of the greatest value.

3. *Cerebral Reaction ("Arsphenamine Encephalitis")*.—A certain number of fatal cases have occurred following large doses. The symptoms are severe headache, gastro-intestinal symptoms, convulsions, coma and death. These cases are fortunately rare. Treatment is unsatisfactory. Beeson has collected the reports of three cases in which recovery occurred possibly as the result of the administration of epinephrine. McBride has reported a case of recovery following the use of sodium thiosulphate, but this result would seem to be nullified by Lasersohn's failure with the drug in another case.

4. *Neuritis*.—A mild degree of nerve irritation, usually going no further than the development of numbness and formication in the extremities, is not rare during the administration of a series of doses of an arsenical, neoarsphenamine being perhaps the most frequent offender in this respect. Severe cases of true multiple neuritis are, however, extremely rare; sodium thiosulphate is given in these cases, and the arsphenamines omitted when antisyphilitic therapy is resumed.

5. *Aplastic Anemia*.—This has been considered a very rare but extremely serious complication of treatment, but the number of cases in the literature in recent years, prompts Bronfin and Singerman (1932) to strongly recommend frequent blood examinations in the patient under arsphenamine treatment even in the absence of any untoward manifestations, and the immediate discontinuance of the drug as soon as such symptoms as malaise, pallor, itching of the skin and purpuric signs are noted. Blood transfusions are given; Loveman (1932) believes that sodium thiosulphate is of some value.

Odor.—A great many individuals are much disturbed by an "ether-like" odor and disgusting taste which develop while the arsenical solution is passing into the vein. This may be counteracted by causing the patient to smell bay-rum or a perfume during the operation; the cheaper perfumes are preferable because of their greater pungency. The perfume should be placed on a pledget of cotton and not on the clothing for this latter procedure might cause later embarrassment to the patient. There are some who derive equal comfort from the rapid mastication in quick succession of several pieces of fresh wintergreen chewing-gum.

Diet During Treatment.—It is the usual custom to place the patient on a high carbohydrate and low protein and fat diet during a course of any of the arsenicals (but see p. 203 under "jaundice"). He should be advised to keep the bowels functioning well during the course and should never eat anything whatsoever during the three hours immediately preceding an injection.

Arsenic Resistance.—The German literature indicates that early syphilis is reacting less favorably to the arsphenamines now than in the years before the World War, but there is no evidence as yet of an increase in arsenic-resistant syphilis in the United States.

2. MERCURY

The use of arsenic and mercury has been discussed in the preceding pages with sufficient detail to make it apparent that no direct comparison of the therapeutic virtues of these two drugs will be offered here. In routine treatment it is undoubtedly best to alternate the drugs, departing from this standard in individual cases when it is seen that the patient responds better to the one or the other or is precluded from taking either one because of an especially low tolerance. What follows, then, is but a list of mercurial preparations that have been found of value in the treatment of the disease—indeed, the list is not even complete for their number is legion.

By Mouth.—1. *Yellow Mercurous Iodide* (Protoiodide, Hydrargyri Iodidum Flavum).—The adult dose ranges from ⅙ to 1 grain (0.01 to 0.06 Gm.), three times daily; the average tolerated dose is perhaps about ¼ grain (0.015 Gm.).

2. *Mercury with Chalk* (Gray powder, Hydrargyri cum Creta).—Dose 1 to 4 grains (0.06 to 0.24 Gm.), three times daily.

The above two preparations have the advantage that they can be easily taken by the patient and are very little irritating to the gastro-intestinal tract. The protoiodide is usually prescribed in tablet form, the mercury with chalk as powder; this latter, being sweet—the U.S.P. preparation contains honey—is well taken by children. The very decided disadvantage of these preparations is that the absorption of the mercury is very uneven, thus making it quite difficult to determine or to predict the degree of the patient's saturation.

3. *Mercuric Chloride* (Bichloride, Hydrargyri Chloridum Corrosivum).—Dose 1/20 to ¼ grain (0.003 to 0.015 Gm.), three times daily. This salt is much more evenly absorbed than the two above described, but it has the disadvantage of being quite irritating to the stomach. This irritation is largely overcome by giving it in combination with the iodides. Old chronic cases, which must be shifted about from one to the other type of treatment through many years, are often put upon "mixed treatment" for awhile. The following formula has been satisfactorily used for this purpose at the former New York Skin and Cancer Hospital (now the Stuyvesant Square) for many years; the iron and strychnine are present in the hope of combating the anemia and anorexia that are frequently very prominent features in these cases.

℞.	Mercuric chloride	gr. iss	0.09
	Potassium iodide	℥iv	16.0
	Ferric and ammonium citrate	℥ij	8.0
	Tincture of nux vomica	℥ij	8.0
	Water to make	℥iv	128.0

This preparation, which contains approximately 1/20 grain (0.003 Gm.) of mercuric chloride and 8 grains (0.5 Gm.) of potassium iodide to the teaspoonful, may be given in 1, or cautiously 2, teaspoonful doses three or four times daily.

4. *Red Mercuric Iodide* (Biniodide, Hydrargyri Iodidum Rubrum).—This preparation is also acceptable for prescribing in a form that may be dispensed in a bottle; it is practically insoluble in water but may be rendered soluble by adding an equal quantity of sodium or potassium iodide. The tolerated dose ranges between 1/20 and ⅓ grain (0.003 to 0.02 Gm.); most patients can be safely started on 1/10 grain (0.006 Gm.).

By Inunction.—1. *Stronger Mercurial Ointment* (Unguentum Hydrargyri Fortius).—A dose of about 1 drachm (4 Gm.) is rubbed for thirty minutes into a different hairless portion of the body on each of six consecutive days with a bath and no treatment on the seventh; on the next day the second course of rubs begins. This is a very effective way of mercurializing an individual, perhaps the most effective of all the methods, but is open to the objection that it is difficult to get the patient to persist for long in timed twenty-minute rubs; also it is a very dirty procedure. In regard to the last point, Cole, Hutton and Sollmann have conclusively shown that the excess of ointment remaining upon the skin after an inunction can be easily removed with cotton and benzine and that such removal does not in the least degree lessen the effectiveness of the treatment from the standpoint of mercury absorption; their work has been confirmed by the investigations of Zwick. Practitioners should more often avail themselves of this clean inunction method than they customarily do.

2. *Mild Mercurial Ointment* (Unguentum Hydrargyri Mite).—This preparation is very little used in the treatment of syphilis in the United States, but is much used for this purpose in Great Britain and on the Continent. American physicians have the deplorable habit of many times speaking and writing of "blue ointment"—this preparation—when they really have in mind the stronger preparation, described above.

3. *Calomel Ointment.*—As calomel is more cleanly than the metallic mercury, the following formula was proposed a few years ago for inunction purposes:

℞.	Mild mercurous chloride	gr. xlv	3.0
	Lanolin	gr. xv	1.0
	Benzoinated lard	gr. xxx	2.0

Its use quickly spread thoughout the United States and the fad was only stopped by the careful clinical investigations of Cole and Littman (1919), *who showed that this ointment is almost totally ineffective in the treatment of syphilis.*

Intramuscular Injection.—1. *Mercuric Salicylate* (Hydrargyri Salicylas).—This salt is given suspended in oil once a week, sometimes as often as every four days. The amount of irritation which follows such an injection depends upon the individual—indeed, I believe this whole matter of intramuscular irritation is one of idiosyncrasy. The commercial ampules, containing a single dose, all contain camphor or phenol or quinine and urea hydrochloride as an anesthetic. The dose is from 1 to 2 grains (0.06 to 0.12 Gm.), usually contained in 1 cc. of the commercial preparations.

Sollmann gives the following formula for a permanent and anesthetic suspension of mercuric salicylate:

	Gm. or cc.
Anhydrous lanolin	40
Distilled water	10
Sweet almond oil	150
Mercuric salicylate	29
Phenol or creosote	20
Camphor	40

Each cubic centimeter of this suspension contains 1½ grains (0.09 Gm.) of mercuric salicylate. Cole, Littman and Sollmann, in their x-ray studies of the absorption of insoluble mercurials when injected deep into the buttocks, have shown that mercuric salicylate in oil is absorbed in an average time of four days, with extremes of four to ten days. This means that the customary practice of injecting once in every four to seven days is a safe one from the standpoint of avoiding accumulation.

2. *Gray Oil* (Oleum Cinereum).—This is a 40 per cent suspension of metallic mercury in oil. It was formerly much used, and seems to have been the preparation preferred in the British Army during the World War. It is most capricious in its absorption. Cole *et al.*, cited above, injected the

drug into 27 patients; in no case did they find the oil completely absorbed at the end of their period of observation, which ranged in the various individuals from sixteen to one hundred and twenty-five days, with an average of forty-three days. The usual practice is to inject ¼ cc. of the oil at intervals of one week for five injections and then allow a rest period of five weeks, or the dose is split into two doses per week of ⅛ cc. each. The drug is both dangerous and inefficient and its use should be abandoned.

3. *Mild Mercurous Chloride* (Calomel).—This drug is injected in a 10 per cent suspension in oil, the dose ranging from ½ to 1 cc. once or twice weekly. The average absorption rate of Cole *et al.*, cited above, was two weeks, but in some cases absorption was not completed under five weeks. Though an efficient method of injecting mercury, cases of cumulative poisoning are by no means unknown. The pain of these injections, which is quite extreme, can be considerably lessened by substituting calomel for mercuric salicylate in the formula on the preceding page.

4. *Mercuric Benzoate* (Hydrargyri Benzoas).—Solution of this drug for intramuscular injection may be accomplished as follows:

	Gm. or cc.
Mercuric benzoate	0.3
Ammonium benzoate	1.5
Water to make	30.0

Twenty-four minims of such a preparation contains the average dose of ¼ grain (0.015 Gm.).

	Gm. or cc.
Mercuric benzoate	0.6
Sodium chloride	0.75
Water to make	30.0

Twelve minims of such a preparation contains the average dose of ¼ grain (0.015 Gm.).

Commercial ampules are available containing an individual dose ready for injection. The drug is usually injected every other day.

5. *Red Mercuric Iodide.*—The biniodide is also used for intramuscular injection (see p. 205 for oral use). Commercial ampules are available containing ⅙ grain (0.01 Gm.) suspended in oil. The drug is usually injected daily, or every second day.

6. *Mercuric Succinimide* (Hydrargyri Succinimidum).—This drug is relatively nonirritating when injected. Commercial ampules are available containing the drug in solution. The average dose, ⅙ to ⅓ grain (0.01 to 0.02 Gm.), is given daily.

7. *Mercurosal.*—This is a comparatively nontoxic, and comparatively nonirritating, salt. The usual intramuscular dose is 0.05 Gm. dissolved in 2 cc. of sterile water every four days for ten to twelve doses. There is commercially available a solution containing 0.025 Gm. of the drug per cubic centimeter; also an ampule containing 0.05 Gm. as a powder. Mercurosal is very high in mercury content, but, despite this fact, Cole, Driver and Hutton (1922) were unable to obtain satisfactory results with it in the treatment of syphilis, though they employed full doses every second day. Further investigation of this discrepancy is desirable, for the drug seems to be no more irritating locally than biniodide.

8. *Colloidal Mercuric Sulphide* (*Hille*).—Recently this preparation has been making a strong bid for first place among mercurials, particularly in so-called "Wassermann-fast" cases. Gennerich's (1932) review of its use in Germany indicates that it even challenges arsphenamine, however, in accomplishing with rapidity the suppression of objective clinical signs of the

disease. Of course much water must pass under the bridges before we can be very sure of these things. In the United States, Freeman, Taylor and White (1931) have given 25,000 injections, intramuscularly, to more than 1000 patients of the latent and Wassermann-fast types, and, are convinced of the value of the preparation—especially as to its efficacy in rendering the Wassermann negative and improving the subjective manifestations. They gave 2 or 3 cc. of a 2 per cent solution semiweekly; twelve to twenty injections comprised a course. The injections were practically painless, there were no local reactions, and the incidence of mercurialism was unusually low.

Intravenous Injection.—The French and Italians have always been fond of the intravenous use of mercury, but elsewhere this type of therapy has never become very popular. In the United States, the three preparations most used are mercuric chloride, mercuric oxycyanide and mercuric benzoate—the two former in a dose of $\frac{1}{6}$ to $\frac{1}{3}$ grain (0.01 to 0.02 Gm.) in distilled water, and the latter as a 1 per cent solution, of which 2 to 8 cc. constitute the dose. Now, in the last few years, a number of new preparations have been introduced for intravenous use in this country, three of which—flumerin, mercurosal and mercodel—must be considered here. (It is of interest to note, in passing, that in the Acta Philosophica of the British Royal Society, published in 1674, there is an account of the intravenous injection of a mercurial solution, performed in 1668. An English translation of the Latin original of this document is in the library of the St. Louis Medical Society.)

1. *Flumerin.*—This drug, which is the disodium salt of hydroxymercurifluorescein, was developed by the Johns Hopkins investigators in 1922, who showed by animal experimentation that it has a higher therapeutic index than any of the other mercurials, which would seem to indicate for it a field of considerable usefulness complementary to the arsphenamines in primary or secondary syphilis. Moore and Wassermann, of the Johns Hopkins group, write:

"In early syphilis, then, we would advise a course of treatment somewhat as follows: arsphenamine for eight doses at the usual intervals of five to seven days, followed a week after the last dose of arsphenamine by a series of flumerin injections given every other day, the first two doses of 3 mg. per kilogram, then two of 4 mg. and then eight of 5 mg. per kilogram. Immediately at the completion of flumerin treatment, a second series of six injections of arsphenamine must be given, again followed in one week by a second series of sixteen injections of flumerin. This type of alternating treatment with arsphenamine and flumerin should be continued until the usual criteria of cure are fulfilled" (see p. 173).

In some instances they obtained almost as good results without going above the 3 mg. per kilogram dosage. The drug should not be used simultaneously with the iodides because of the theoretical possibility of increasing its toxicity by the formation of a halogen mercurial compound in the body. In late syphilis, neurosyphilis or resistant syphilis in general, the advantages of the drug would probably not outweigh its costliness. In arsphenamine-intolerant patients, or those with low tolerance for the more usual mercurials, there are some indications that this drug might have especial value.

FLUMERIN REACTIONS.—In general, in Moore and Wassermann's cases, subjective symptoms were mild, but in 8 cases, immediate vomiting, bloody diarrhea or stomatitis were of such severity as to interfere with further flumerin therapy. Of the entire 95 treated cases, about one third became salivated and developed mild stomatitis, usually after eight or ten injections of the drug. So far as could be judged from repeated urine examinations and phenolsulphonephthalein tests, no permanent kidney damage was done, though in patients receiving doses of 4 or 5 mg. per kilogram transient albuminuria or cylindruria was slightly more frequent than in patients receiving doses of 3 mg. per kilogram. There was complete absence of thrombosis and of all other signs of an irritating effect upon the veins.

PREPARATION OF SOLUTION.—Flumerin is a dark red, odorless powder, It is used in a 2 per cent solution in sterile water (*not* in physiologic saline, because of the drug's numerous incompatibilities). It is soluble in 1 to 10 parts of hot water. If solutions are made with sterile water they may be used during three days if kept in well-stoppered bottles in the dark.

2. *Mercurosal.*—The intravenous dose of this drug is 0.1 Gm. dissolved in 5 cc. of sterile water and injected very slowly. It should be repeated every second or third day for ten or twelve doses. Cole, Driver and Hutton found that mercurosal did not compare any more favorably with other mercurials when given intravenously than it did when given intramuscularly (see p. 207).

Sclerosis of the vein developed in 4 of the 23 patients treated.

3. *Mercodel.*—This substance is a finely divided trituration· of mercury with glucose, a grayish-blue powder which is added to, and shaken with, water in a glass mixing container (the contents of one ampule with 50 cc. of sterile, distilled water). After shaking, the mixture is drawn into a glass syringe through filtering cotton in a suitable glass adapter and then injected through a No. 19 (or smaller) gauge needle. It must be quickly injected because the mercury rapidly settles out of the suspension. The manufacturers originally advised that the drug be injected twice weekly, beginning with 20 cc. and increasing 5 cc. with each injection until the full 50 cc. is injected; this point would be reached at the seventh injection, and the dose was to be kept at this size until the full course of ten injections had been given.

This product was studied, in 1924, by Cole, Hutton, Rauschkolb, and Sollmann. I give below the summary of their findings, as reported by the Council on Pharmacy and Chemistry in the Journal of the American Medical Association, May 2, 1925.

"From this work, Cole and his collaborators conclude that intravenous injections of Mercodel produce marked therapeutic response as manifested by the rapid disappearance of spirochetes from the primary lesions, prompt clearing of the secondary lesions and improvement of the spinal fluid. They call attention to the fact that the quantity of mercury introduced in a 'course' is very much greater than that introduced by any other method, and that a large quantity of mercury will remain in the body for a long time. They found that the injections did not provoke anaphylactoid reactions and appeared to have relatively little effect in the kidney and intestines, but that they are likely to cause stomatitis, which may flare up suddenly in severe and even fatal form.

"Contrary to the claim of the manufacturer, it was found that inflammatory reactions were set up in the vein by repeated injections. Intramuscular injections were found to present the same objections and uncertainties as the intravenous administration. As a result of their study, the investigators conclude that, until the conditions that influence the toxicity are better known and controlled, the risks are too great to justify the use of Mercodel."

Rothwell and Maloney, at the Bellevue, found that by reducing the initial dose to 5 cc., and rarely going beyond 10 cc. in later doses, such cases of stomatitis as occurred were controllable by simple mouth washes and sometimes temporary reduction in dosage. The drug has not (1933) been accepted by the Council.

14

Inhalation and Fumigation.—Despite the fact that inhalations, as well as fumigations, of mercury have been tested at various times since very early in the history of syphilis in Europe, the verve with which interested propagandists now and again reintroduce the procedure to the profession (*with* a patented device for accomplishing the necessary volatilization) would lead the unwary to believe that there is something essentially novel in the principles concerned. But it is not so. Mercury can certainly be gotten into the system in this way, but in such irregular, uncertain dosage, and with such likelihood of causing pulmonary irritation, that the method deserves no place in therapy with this drug. Let those who doubt the truth of this statement study the work of Cole, Gericke and Sollmann (1922).

3. BISMUTH[1]

The extensive use of this drug in the treatment of syphilis dates from the work of Sazerac and Levaditi, in 1921, but the experience of the first few years was gained exclusively with French "patent" and "proprietary" preparations which were very diverse in their composition. Even now, at the end of 1933, there is still so much to learn about bismuth that I offer the following as merely a tentative statement of its status.

Method of Administration.—This is simple: the drug is not effective when given by mouth, is very likely to cause severe reactions and even death when given intravenously, and therefore is administered safely and with good effect only intramuscularly. The preparation should be drawn into the syringe through a short thick needle, which is then to be discarded for a longer and slenderer one with a clean lumen. Insert the needle to point down and slightly in from a point in the inner part of the upper outer quadrant of the buttock. After carefully aspirating (important!) to be sure that the point is not in a blood vessel, inject slowly and finish with a bubble of air to prevent drawing some bismuth out toward the surface as the needle is withdrawn, which might later cause a painful button of induration. Sometimes such buttons last for a week or more.

Soluble and Insoluble Preparations.—Early attempts to compare the absorbability of aqueous solutions of soluble salts and suspensions of insoluble salts in oils by x-ray studies of intramuscularly injected compounds were not successful; but the recent studies of numerous investigators (Hanzlik, Mehrtens *et al.*, Von Oettingen, Lomholt, and others) of the rate of excretion in the urine and feces, coupled with accumulating clinical experience, have fixed the status of these two classes of preparations with reasonable certainty.

Water-soluble Salts.—These preparations are more rapidly and more regularly absorbed than the oily suspensions, which is both an advantage and a disadvantage. Advantageous, in that it enables quick results to be attained, so quick indeed that some observers feel that bismuth is challenging the place of arsphenamine in early syphilis (see p. 212), disadvantageous, in that they must be administered twice or thrice in the week, and are thus made quite impracticable for routine clinic use and even for office practice except in unusual instances. Furthermore, these aqueous solutions are very apt to cause a troublesome stomatitis if they are pushed too rapidly. An advantage, on the other hand, is that there is no danger of embolism or infarction following these injections—which, however, are much more painful than are those of the oily suspensions. The following

---

[1] Beckman, H.: Bismuth in the Treatment of Syphilis, Jour. Lab. and Clin. Med., 18, 1136, 1933. Brought up to date, the article is included here with the kind permission of the Editor of the journal in which it appeared.

are perhaps the best of the aqueous preparations; the dosage given is for a single course, which may be repeated one or more times after an intermission of one month.

(a) *Bismuth Sodium Tartrate (N.N.R.)*.—The initial dose is 0.015 Gm. (¼ grain), which is doubled usually with the second dose and continued in two or three doses weekly for six to ten weeks.

(b) *Bismosol (N.N.R.)*.—Administered usually twice a week in 1-cc. doses until twenty doses have been given.

(c) *Thiobismol (N.N.R.)*.—The average dose, 0.2 Gm. (3 grains), is injected twice weekly for a series of twelve to fifteen doses.

(d) *Iodobismitol*.—This preparation is not really an aqueous solution but is included here because it contains an active bismuth salt dissolved in ethylene glycol and has for all practical purposes the above-enumerated advantages and disadvantages of the solutions of salts in water. Ten injections of 2 cc. each are given in about three weeks.

Suspensions in Oil.—These preparations are much more slowly and irregularly absorbed than the solutions and are not generally felt to be as well suited for treatment of early syphilis as are the latter. If this prolonged absorption were regular in rate the advantages would be obvious in late syphilis, but unfortunately during a period of very slow absorption a pocket of bismuth seems at times to be emptied into the circulation with a resultant attack of stomatitis of an explosive type. The injection of these suspensions causes much less pain than the injection of aqueous solutions—sometimes none at all—and the injections need be made only once a week. But to counterbalance these great advantages there are the following disadvantages: (a) Sterile abscesses of rather large proportions may occur even a long time after the injections have been stopped; either they must be opened or they will spontaneously rupture; (b) though embolism has occurred with perhaps no greater frequency than in the use of insoluble mercury, infarction following injection into an artery has been noted in a rather distressingly large number of instances—there is immediately great pain and nearly always ultimately gangrene and sloughing out of the affected area. From the standpoint of clinic administration there is another serious disadvantage of the oily suspensions, as shown by Cole, Henderson *et al.* (1931): syringefuls taken from oily bismuth suspensions in bulk will contain very variable amounts of the metal; this objection does not, of course, apply in office practice where individual-dose ampules are used.

The following are perhaps the best preparations:

(a) *Mesurol (N.N.R.)*.—The initial dose of ½ cc. is increased to 1 cc. at the second dose and injected eight to twelve times at intervals of one week.

(b) *Olio-Bi-Roche (N.N.R.)*.—Weekly injections of 2 cc. are given in a course of twelve to twenty.

(c) *Potassium Bismuth Tartrate (N.N.R.)*.—This preparation is unfortunately commercially available in a rather confusing form: if used in bulk, 1 cc. is injected once (or twice) weekly for twenty-four (or twelve) weeks; or, preferably, in the larger but usually well-tolerated dose of 2 cc. once weekly for twelve weeks. There is also available an ampule containing this larger dose, and another containing half the amount.

(d) *Tartroquiniobine (N.N.R.)*.—Bulk dosage of this drug is perhaps more inexact than that of the other suspensions listed above. The ampule commercially available contains 2 cc.; one-half, or the entire, contents of such an ampule should be injected twice a week for six to ten weeks. It is claimed that this preparation is superior in that its content of water-soluble sodium potassium bismuthyl tartrate effects early action, and the insoluble bismuth iodide prolonged action—which has not yet been conclusively shown to be the case.

(e) *Bismuth Salicylate (N.N.R.).*—One cc. of the commercial suspension is usually given once each week for ten weeks.

Liposoluble Preparations.—In the presence of certain lipoid-soluble substances, such as lecithin, matter may be satisfactorily dispersed in media in which it is otherwise insoluble. The first to make practical application of this fact to obtain optimal dispersion of bismuth were Hermann and Nathan (1925), whose studies have been continued by many other investigators. One of the chief advantages urged in favor of these liposoluble preparations is that they become effective, through rapid absorption, almost as quickly as the water-soluble salts, and that their absorption continues almost but not quite as long as that of the insoluble salts. These claims seem to be borne out by careful excretion studies. The injections are, furthermore, relatively painless and rarely lead to induration. Stomatitis probably occurs more often with these than with the water-soluble preparations, but most of the cases are not severe. At the dedication of the new Dermatological Clinic in Strasbourg, in July, 1930, the subject of bismuth therapy in syphilis was discussed by many of the leading Continental syphilologists, and it was evident that the liposoluble preparations are gaining favor in Europe because of their dosage being more exact than that of the oily suspensions and because they do not cause the late abscesses of these latter, and also because the therapeutic results obtainable with them approach closely those obtained by the use of water-soluble preparations. The greatest objection to their use is the necessity of injecting twice a week.

Perhaps the two best preparations available in this country, where experience with them has not yet been very extensive, are:

(a) *Quiniobine (N.N.R.).*—Used in a dose of 1 to 2 cc. twice weekly for twelve to fourteen injections.

(b) *Bismocymol.*—Injected twice weekly, in doses of 2 cc., for twelve to sixteen injections.

Bismuth in Early Syphilis.—Levy (1930) divided a series of 66 cases into two parts; 41 he treated with various bismuth preparations, 25 with neoarsphenamine. With liposoluble preparations he caused the disappearance of spirochetes from the chancre as follows: in four days in 1 case, six days in 11 cases, eight days in 1 case, and twelve days in 2 cases. With a soluble preparation the disappearance was accomplished in three days in 1 case, six days in nine cases, and eight days in 1 case. With insoluble preparations the results were: six days in 1 case, seven days in 1 case, eight days in 1 case, eleven to twelve days in 8 cases, and sixteen to seventeen days in 3 cases. In the neoarsphenamine-treated cases the same result was accomplished in one day in 8 cases with a dose of 0.3 Gm., and in two days in 6 cases; 2 cases required a second injection of 0.45 Gm. In 9 cases he used the very small dose of 0.15 Gm. neoarsphenamine and accomplished the desired result in one day in 3 cases; in the other 6 the disappearance was completed on the third day by a dose of 0.3 Gm.

Of course the total number of Levy's cases is admittedly small and the two groups are not of comparable size so that statistically the study has no value, but I think that the results may nevertheless be fairly looked upon as fixing the status of bismuth very high in the treatment of primary syphilis but still below that of the arsphenamines. That the drug can quite satisfactorily replace mercury has been many times shown, perhaps no more conclusively than in Lomholt's report of several years ago. He used neoarsphenamine in a series of five or six injections, and insoluble bismuth eight to ten injections, to the total number of about eighteen neoarsphenamine injections and sixty of bismuth in a period of about two years. In 152 patients thus handled there were no clinical relapses during or after treatment, no births of children with congenital syphilis, and only 2 positive,

7 doubtful and 143 negative blood Wassermanns at the end of the treatment. Excellent results beyond doubt, but still there are those who maintain (Cole, in Cleveland, Moore, in Baltimore, O'Leary, at the Mayo Clinic, Parran, in New York, Stokes, in Philadelphia, Wile, in Ann Arbor), and rightly, I think, that the great service of bismuth in early syphilis is as adjunct to or alternate drug with mercury, and not in displacing the older drug altogether. The well-known syphilologists listed just above alternate the three drugs through a course as follows: arsphenamine, bismuth, arsphenamine, mercury, arsphenamine, bismuth, arsphenamine, mercury, and still feel that final judgment on the relative merits of the two heavy metals is premature. That the profession is virtually abandoning mercury in favor of bismuth in early syphilis on the basis of individual results rather than long-time statistical studies, seems to me most unfortunate.

A few men of great experience, particularly in France (Schwartz, Emery, Raisis, Morin), are using bismuth to the exclusion of all other drugs in all stages of syphilis, but they are certainly in the minority.

Bismuth in Late or Tertiary Syphilis.—In this ubiquitous type of syphilis there can be no doubt of the great value of bismuth in rendering the use of the arsphenamines often unnecessary; that is to say, since these cases can now be attacked by two metals—bismuth and mercury—as well as the iodides, it seems the part of wisdom to many syphilologists to employ the more dangerous and in many ways more objectionable arsenicals as little as possible. Since sterilization is very difficult here and holding the disease in check is the most to be hoped for, bismuth had best be used for all it is worth, taking care only, as Cole, Moore, O'Leary *et al.* particularly stress, to keep the doses moderate in size. Quite remarkable results are sometimes obtained. McCafferty and MacGregor gave sixteen injections, then no treatment for a month, then a blood Wassermann, in 25 patients who were asymptomatic with positive blood but negative spinal fluid, all of whom had had many courses of arsenic and mercury. Result after three full courses of the bismuth: percentage of patients improved as to Wassermann test, 64.7 (many rendered entirely negative from 4 plus); percentage unchanged, 22.9; percentage of reversions after second and third courses, 13.8.

Bismuth in Neurosyphilis.—All the preparations are used and with such excellent results at times that enthusiasm runs high in favor of displacing the arsphenamines entirely by the new drug. But the more conservative syphilologists here again favor merely adding the bismuth to the list of remedies—arsphenamines, tryparsamide, mercury, iodides, hyperpyretic measures—which comprise the antineurosyphilitic armamentarium of today.

Iodobismitol may perhaps have some special virtues among the preparations; at least, Mehrtens and Pouppirt (1931), and Hanzlik, Mehrtens *et al.* (1932), have shown that it penetrates well into the brain of experimental animals and that it also penetrates into the spinal fluid in the human much better than control mercury preparations. About 50 per cent of their series of 100 patients of the several usual types of neurosyphilitics were definitely improved clinically and serologically after one year's treatment, although many were in an advanced stage and proved intractable to other antisyphilitic medication. The earlier the treatment was initiated, the more satisfactory was the result.

Bismuth in Cardiovascular Syphilis.—Blackford and Boland (1932) found that pain, the most common symptom in their 100 cases of aortic syphilis, was relieved in all but one case by the intramuscular injection of bismuth sodium tartrate, and that the drug could be administered over long periods with good results. Marked clinical improvement was also noted in 50 patients with heart disease associated with syphilis. These observers feel that congestive heart failure in cardiovascular syphilis urgently demands the immediate administration of bismuth in addition to general measures for the treatment of the failing heart.

Bismuth in Congenital Syphilis.—Unfortunately, bismuth is being too often tried to the exclusion of all other drugs, as was also the case when arsphenamine was first introduced. Still, there is some warrant for this practice in the case of bismuth, for when intravenous arsphenamine therapy is very difficult or impossible, and there are some other reasons for not using sulpharsphenamine intramuscularly, then there are only mercury and bismuth to fall back upon. And of the two, intramuscular injections of bismuth are very much better borne by infants and young children. An evaluation of the drug that is certain to stand long cannot be made yet because no considerable study appeared in the literature before 1925, and even now the reports are all upon small numbers of cases that have not been observed long enough to determine just what the therapy is going to accomplish ultimately. Coppolino's (1930) report will serve to indicate methods and results. Dose: ½ cc. of bismuth salicylate to infants under one year, 1 cc. to older children. Course: Twenty weekly injections, with blood Wassermann at beginning and end of each course; if positive, treatment continued, if negative, a rest period of four weeks allowed; the maximum number of courses was three. Results: Statistically the findings were of no importance, but the observation and impression was that the drug was most efficacious in young infants, rendering them both symptom-free and serologically negative, and that it was useful but not curative in older children. The consensus of opinion is probably that bismuth used alone is a better drug than mercury alone but that it is not so good as the arsphenamines.

There are several reports of the use of bismuth after arsphenamine alone or with mercury had failed to reduce a 4 plus Wassermann in congenital cases. Wright, for instance, used the drug in 47 patients between two and sixteen years, averaging about ten years, nearly all of whom had had considerable arsphenamine and mercury treatment and all but 4 of whom were strongly Wassermann positive. Dose: 5 mg. of potassium bismuth tartrate per kilogram, not to exceed 100 mg. (the bismuth content of the weaker of the two N.N.R. ampules) per week in courses of sixteen injections with a month's rest between courses. Result: Wassermann reversal was obtained in 20 of the cases, or 47 per cent. Stokes has reported a series in which arsphenamine and mercury inunctions, suitably carried out over a period of three to four years, accomplished reversal in 62 per cent of the cases—but of course it is notoriously inaccurate, and perhaps does not even have suggestive value, to compare two different series in this way.

Bismuth in Arsphenamine-intolerant Cases.—Here of course the drug has tremendous value because these patients have a far better chance of having the disease arrested in them with bismuth *and* mercury than they formerly had with mercury alone.

Bismuth in the Prophylaxis of Syphilis.—See page 223.

The Toxicity of Bismuth.—One of the greatest advantages of this drug over both mercury and the arsphenamines is that, though the reactions of a toxic nature which accompany its use are many and varied, they are rarely severe enough to necessitate an interruption of the treatment for longer than a few days. The commonest of the symptoms is the appearance of a thin violaceous gray line on the gums, indicative of saturation. Experience has taught that it is well to examine the urine of patients before beginning the treatments and to use the findings as a quantitative guide to the same. Now and then during the courses the urine even of patients having no pre-existing nephritic disturbances will give evidence of a beginning toxic process in the kidneys, but this does not happen as often as with mercury perhaps and certainly only rarely fails to disappear with adjustment in dosage or after a slight pause in treatment. According to Heimann-Trosien (1928), in most instances the kidneys acquire an increased tolerance for the metal, but the fact is not established and is probably open to considerable doubt (Taralrud, 1931). Very rarely indeed has a severe or long-lasting nephritis been reported.

The single other symptom of a deleterious nature which is relatively often noted (but not nearly so often as with mercury) is stomatitis; it is usually of a mild sort and disappears promptly upon adjustment of the treatment schedule or dosage. Of the local reactions upon injection I have already treated above (see p. 210). Other rare occurrences: loss of ambition, asthenia, etc. (bismuth "grippe"); herpes zoster, purpura hemorrhagica, agranulocytosis, nitritoid crises, polyneuritis, various exanthemata and dermatoses, diarrhea, jaundice, menstrual disturbances, etc. With the more serious reactions of bismuth introduced intravenously we need not concern ourselves, since the introduction of the drug by this route is absolutely contraindicated.

4. BISMARSEN[1]
(Bismuth Arsphenamine Sulphonate)

This new drug is the sodium salt of a bismuth derivative of arsphenamine methylene sulphonic acid with inorganic salts. Its production is the result of a very rational attempt to make available in one compound which may be given intramuscularly the therapeutic properties of arsenic, of which it contains about 13 per cent, and bismuth, in which its content is about 24 per cent. Since late in 1927 certain indications of its usefulness and limitations have been accumulating, so that the following summary of its status may now be offered.

Administration and Dosage.—Bismarsen is a brownish-yellow, readily soluble powder, the single dose of which is dissolved in the ampule just before using in 2 cc. of sterile distilled water to which is added 2 to 4 minims (0.12 to 0.24 cc.) of 2 per cent butyn solution for anesthetic effect. The drug is very stable and uniform. The injections are made intramuscularly just as with bismuth or mercury, taking the same care to avoid entering blood vessels. The usual adult dose at each injection is 0.2 Gm., but Stokes gives only 0.1 Gm. at the first injection. The several experimenters with the drug have been injecting at various intervals and with varying numbers of injections constituting a course: (*a*) Twenty injections twice a week; (*b*) twenty, once a week; (*c*) twenty, more or less, three times a week; (*d*) ten, at five- to seven-day intervals; (*e*) eight, at intervals of four days. The details of these various practices will be developed in what follows, but it can already be seen that the drug is hardly ideally suited to private office practice or even to use on a very large scale in the clinic. There have been administered in the different series from one to five courses with rest periods of two to four weeks, or in some instances with no rest periods at all.

Bismarsen in Early Syphilis.—Stokes, Miller and Beerman believe after their five years' experience with the drug that its ultimate curative effect in early syphilis is equal and even superior to that of other standard treatments with arsphenamines combined with mercury or bismuth. I shall consider their evidence together with that presented in the other outstanding reports.

(*a*) *Spirillicidal Effect.*—In the original report of Stokes and Chambers, in 1927, it was said that spirochetes disappeared from the primary lesions

[1] Beckman, H.: The Present Status of Bismarsen in the Treatment of Syphilis, New England Jour. Med., 208, 487, 1933. Brought up to date, the article is included here with the kind permission of the Editor of the journal in which it appeared.

in twenty-five to thirty-three hours, but subsequent observers have not been able to duplicate these results; all have reported the disappearance to occur more slowly than with arsphenamine or neoarsphenamine.

(b) *Effect on Wassermann Reaction.*—Kolmer gave very thorough treatment (four courses of ten 0.2-Gm. doses at five- to seven-day intervals, length of rest periods not stated) to 4 seronegative primary cases. After periods of eleven months to three and one-half years, all still remain seronegative. Shivers, using courses of twenty weekly 0.2-Gm. doses, was able to keep all of his six seronegative primary cases continuously negative. Of Stokes' 4 cases given twenty injections of 0.2 Gm. (the first, 0.1 Gm.) at the rate of one or two, mostly one, per week, 3 never became seropositive and the other one became seropositive after nine injections. O'Leary and Brunsting treated 6 seronegative primary cases with four courses (four weeks' rest periods) of eight injections of 0.2 Gm. at four-day intervals. All have remained negative for several years. It is therefore apparent that bismarsen is effective in "curing" seronegative primary syphilis. In Shivers' 13 cases of seropositive primary syphilis, an average of twenty injections was required to render the Wassermann negative, and there was one failure; this is about what was accomplished by the other observers, for out of a total of 131 cases reported as seropositive primary, 118 were rendered negative by from eight to forty injections—the average was probably about twenty, though it is not possible to accurately arrive at this figure.

(c) *Effect on Spinal Fluid.*—O'Leary found four abnormal fluids in 30 cases after treatment, Kolmer one in 11, Stokes two in 11. None of O'Leary's 9 patients with asymptomatic neurosyphilis when first seen in acute syphilis showed any improvement in the condition of the spinal fluid under treatment.

(d) *Effect on Healing of Primary and Secondary Lesions.*—All observers are in agreement that healing of the primary sore, and of the condylomas, mucous patches, macular, papular, etc., syphilids of the secondary stage proceeds considerably slower under bismarsen than under arsphenamine or neoarsphenamine. In the series of Stokes, who has probably had the largest experience, healing of the primary lesion occurred between the fifth and thirteenth injections, and involution of the secondary lesions between the second and fifteenth injections according to type, but in 23 of the 25 secondary cases there was healing by the eighth and in 16 cases by the fifth injection. Kolmer believes that it is not the drug of choice unless intravenous medication is impossible, and Shivers favors its use as a second course after twenty injections each of neoarsphenamine and a bismuth preparation.

(e) *Relapse under Treatment.*—The incidence of relapse in patients observed six months or more after treatment was 12 per cent in Stokes' series of 50 cases, but since not all patients had examinations of spinal fluid, these figures are valid only for blood serological findings and clinical evidences. In O'Leary's 30 cases the percentage was 16.6 but when the series was reexamined after a longer period of time the percentage of relapses was found to have risen to 30, and among the 14 patients with seropositive primary syphilis when treatment was begun, 7, or 50 per cent, had relapsed in one form or another. Stokes suggests that shorter intervals between injections (two per week instead of one), and no rest periods until as near forty injections as possible have been given, would increase the effectiveness of the therapy even though the total length of the full treatment would be thus curtailed. Thirty-two of his patients had absolutely continuous treatment (60 per cent received twenty injections or less) and 21 had rests or lapses (86 per cent had twenty-one or more injections, 40 per cent had over forty); the numbers are small for conclusions, yet significantly fewer relapses occurred in the continuously treated group than in the other. However, O'Leary, who was once quite favorably inclined toward the drug, now rejects it on the basis of a higher proportion of relapses, particularly in the nervous system, than under other types of treatment; even the decreasing of the rest period to two weeks and giving a minimum of forty injections has not caused any obvious changes in the results. Apparently, then, bismarsen, in the small number of cases in which it has been used, has not definitely established itself the equal of the arsphenamines and mercury in preventing relapse in seropositive primary and secondary cases, for by the use of the older drugs in some such system as that employed at the Johns Hopkins Hospital, relapse occurs in only from 23 to 40 per cent of cases. Kolmer believes that bismarsen is not the drug of choice in early syphilis.

Bismarsen in Late Syphilis.—In Stokes' 35 cases of cutaneous, mucosal, osseous and rectal gummata, involution of the lesions was accomplished quite slowly in comparison with other methods of treatment. This was Kolmer's experience also. Stokes feels that when rapid healing is desired other drugs should be used, but Kolmer, who favors a combination therapy in chronic syphilis, looks very favorably upon bismarsen as a drug to begin treatment with because, being given intramuscularly, it has enabled him to avoid the acute exacerbations (all observers have remarked upon this absence of Herxheimer reactions) which sometimes follow the intravenous injection of the arsphenamines, and also because with it one is enabled to determine the tolerance for arsenic of a patient who is resuming treatment after a long rest when hypersensitiveness may have been induced by the earlier treatment, or in one who has been previously injured by the drug. Shivers considers it the drug of choice in all patients with late secondary syphilis, and he has been very well pleased with the effect upon late cutaneous syphilids in 60 cases, though he says nothing of the *rate* of involution. He also considers the drug superior to bismuth and much safer than the intravenous administration of arsenicals in cardiovascular syphilis. Stokes' results were also very good in cardiovascular syphilis but the findings were not conclusive in any type except that in aortitis bismarsen was shown to be of equal value when given alone as when used in various combinations with mercury and iodides. Kolmer believes that for the two (at least) courses of treatment per year which he considers necessary in Wassermann-fast cases in order to maintain the latency as long as possible, bismarsen is particularly valuable, and expresses himself as having been frequently surprised by the reduction of serological reactions to negative. However, both Elliott and O'Leary considered their results unsatisfactory in this type of case. Stokes reversed the reaction to negative in 7 of 15 cases, but since it was his observation that if the reversal is going to take place it occurs relatively early after the bismarsen injections have been begun, he is inclined to believe that the result is due more to the change of drug than to the number of injections. Courses: (*a*) Kolmer, ten injections of 0.2 Gm. at five- to seven-day intervals; (*b*) Stokes, twenty injections of 0.2 Gm. (first one, 0.1 Gm.) once, occasionally twice, a week; (*c*) Shivers rarely gave patients over forty years of age more than 0.1 Gm. once a week. All observers have remarked favorably upon the tonic effect of the drug, which is so important in chronic syphilis.

Bismarsen in Neurosyphilis.—In tabes dorsalis it was the experience of Tobias (20 cases), Hadden and Wilson (31 cases), and Stokes (12 cases), that in most instances the lightning pains respond quite favorably to the drug, that there is less response of the ataxia, and no response of the optic atrophy. Shivers, as well as both Stokes and Kolmer, have been especially pleased with the relief of headache in cerebrospinal syphilis of the acute meningeal type. In cases other than those having a paretic formula, the blood and spinal fluid reactions were reduced to normal in about 50 per cent, but the number of patients thus studied is too small to permit the drawing of conclusions.

Bismarsen in Congenital Syphilis.—Chambers and Koetter have recently reported upon the use of the drug in 180 patients ranging in age from birth to fourteen years, the majority being more than three years old. The period of observation was from one and one-half to two and one-half years. Dosage: To a child of two weeks, 10 mg.; six to twelve weeks, 40 to 50 mg.; three to twelve months, 75 mg.; three to five years, 100 to 200 mg.; five to fourteen years, 200 mg. They believe the best treatment to consist in two injections weekly in courses of twenty injections, with rest intervals of two weeks and a total of three courses. The active lesions were healed somewhat more slowly than with the other arsphenamines and the improvement in cases of interstitial keratitis also lagged. Kolmer's and Stokes' experiences were the same in regard to keratitis, but all the observers have found the ultimate results quite as good as those obtained with the older drugs. In 100 cases receiving the full three courses in Chambers and Koetter's series, 65 per cent showed complete reversal of the blood Wassermann, an excellent serological result; of the remainder, 10 per cent belonged to the Wassermann-fast group before the treatment was begun. In the entire series only two abnormal spinal fluids were encountered and these were unaltered by treatment.

Bismarsen Reactions.—The local reactions of pain and stiffness, which are most marked on the second and third days, usually occur with the first five injections and are much reduced by massage. In Stokes' series such reactions occurred in 15.6 per cent of the patients between one and twenty years of age, 35.6 per cent between twenty-one and forty years, 46.3 per cent between forty-one and sixty years, and 57.1 per cent between sixty-one and eighty years. However, they followed only 2 per cent of the total of 7666 injections. In the matter of general reactions in the combined series of Stokes, O'Leary, Chambers and Koetter, Elliott, and Kolmer, with a total of 17,460 injections, the following have been reported: Nitritoid crises, 20; gastro-intestinal reactions, 20; exfoliative dermatitis, 2; miscellaneous skin reactions, 11; jaundice, 3; hemorrhagic purpura, 1 (but Stokes knew of 3 other instances not included in the series); bismuth line or stomatitis, 11; cerebral, neuritic or renal disturbances, none of moment. So far as one can determine from these figures, which still represent a limited experience, the drug has a low systemic toxicity, rather in the supposed range of neo-arsphenamine than of old arsphenamine, but like the other sulphoxylate arsphenamines, including neoarsphenamine and sulpharsphenamine, it is capable of causing grave injury to the hematopoietic system. Furthermore, it cannot apparently safely be substituted for the other arsphenamines in cases in which specific sensitiveness to the arsphenamine radical has already been manifested by the occurrence of an exfoliated dermatitis. In other types of arsphenamine sensitiveness, such as nitritoid reactions, jaundice, skin reactions, pruritus, vomiting, Stokes has substituted it with remarkable success upon the whole. The frequency of exfoliative dermatitis caused *primarily* by bismarsen (once in 8730 injections) compares very favorably with the rather out-of-date statistics of Meirowski for the other drugs: Neoarsphenamine, once in 5260; arsphenamine, once in 1850; sulpharsphenamine (Stokes), once in 700.

5. IODIDES

According to Barker, Biett (1821) first employed iodine combined with mercury in the treatment of syphilis on the Continent, but I believe its extensive employment in the form of potassium iodide since that time is generally accredited to the efforts of Wallace in England (1825). Though in constant use since this latter date, we have as yet no entirely satisfactory explanation for the undoubted effectiveness of the iodides in syphilis. For a presentation of the several interesting and plausible theories the reader is referred to the paper of Barker and Sprunt, from which I quote the following in regard to the clinical employment of the iodides:

"It is in the tertiary and the late secondary stages of syphilis that the iodides have been of the greatest service. It is at this period of the infection that numerous lesions may be found, large or small, on all of which the essential pathologic features are the same, namely, more or less necrosis of tissue, the accumulation of mononuclear leukocytes, and the formation of new fibrous tissue. Since we recognize now the basic similarity of the lesions of syphilis, it is reasonable to suppose that the striking effect of iodides, appreciable in the case of large lesions, the resolution of which may be clinically observed, has its parallel in a similar but less readily recognized change in the smaller lesions, and it is also a reasonable supposition that, with the resorption of lesions, the organism of syphilis is made more accessible to attack by the parasiticidal drugs. This would appear to be the reason for the use of iodides, even in cases that show no gross lesions. To sum up, then, the attitude of most conservative clinicians today, who are actively engaged in the treatment of syphilis, is that the iodides are valuable remedies in the symptomatic treatment of syphilitic lesions and for relieving the pain due to such lesions. There is a general feeling, also, that the iodides contribute, in the way above mentioned, to the efficacy of mercurial and arsenical treatment."

Potassium Iodide.—This is the cheaper salt and the one most frequently used. It is often stated that the sodium salt should be given the preference because of the depressing effect of the potassium ion on the heart, but the fact is overlooked, as Eggleston has pointed out, that potassium is eliminated from the human body with such extreme rapidity that it is almost impossible to poison the heart by the administration of its salts by mouth. Osborne's investigations at the Mayo Clinic suggest that the iodine given in the form of potassium iodide by mouth forms a sodium protein combination, while in the case of sodium iodide by mouth only traces of iodine enter into combination with the proteins—observations which may bear directly on the general clinical impression that, grain for grain, potassium iodide is more effective than sodium iodide.

As to dosage, I again quote Barker and Sprunt: "Potassium iodide is usually prescribed in strong solution, an ounce of the salt being dissolved in an ounce of water, with the direction that the drug shall be greatly diluted as each dose is administered. Since an idiosyncrasy to the drug may be encountered, small doses are usually given at first, say 5 grains [*i. e.*, 5 drops of the solution—H. B.], three times a day, preferably given a half or three quarters of an hour after meals. Even when mild symptoms of iodism occur, they will usually disappear on increase of the dosage to 10 or 15 grains thrice daily. The dose has sometimes been increased, up to 300 grains (20 Gm.) or more a day. Large doses may cause gastric irritation, due to the salt action, symptoms that are quite distinct from those of iodism. This irritation may be obviated to some extent by administering the drug in milk or whey. Engman warns against the use of the excessive doses sometimes employed, especially in certain health resorts where many patients are treated. Fournier was also strongly opposed to what he called 'iodide debauches'; he seldom gave more than from 45 to 60 grains daily. When tolerance for the drug is established, the curative value apparently diminishes and the dose must therefore be increased."

The following prescription is probably as effective as any in disguising the drug; it will contain 15 grains (1 Gm.) in the teaspoonful dose:

R̥. Potassium iodide..................................... ℥j   30.0
    Compound syrup of sarsaparilla..................... ℥j   30.0
    Water to make....................................... ℥iv   120.0
    Label: One or more teaspoonfuls in water as directed.

Iodism.—The symptoms are those of a "common cold" plus any one of a number of types of skin rashes, the latter often appearing some time after the former. Some individuals never manifest these symptoms even on enormous doses, while others do so regularly when a certain dosage is reached. It is usually possible to disregard the iodism, but in some cases the drug must be omitted or greatly reduced for a time. The possibility of an iodide cachexia, in persons who have been taking the drug regularly for a very long time, must always be borne in mind. I think many of these cases pass unrecognized in some clinics.

Organic "Iodides."—More or less complex iodine compounds with proteins and fats, and one with methenamine (urotropin), have been introduced with claims that they are less irritating to the digestive tract than the metallic iodides and that they are less inclined to cause iodism. When given in the doses advised by the manufacturers they are usually distinctly less irritating to the stomach, but it is not quite certainly known whether these nonirritating doses are therapeutically as effective as the doses of metallic iodides that do cause irritation. Regarding the occurrence of iodism, it is doubtful if a susceptible individual will escape this symptom complex if these newer preparations are used in doses comparable with those employed in the treatment with the older simple iodides. The following preparations are contained in New and Nonofficial Remedies, for 1933:

1. *Iodalbin.*—A compound of iodine and blood albumin, which is said to be dissolved in the intestines after passing practically unchanged through the stomach. Dosage: 5 to 10 grains (0.3 to 0.6 Gm.), as indicated. It is supplied in 5-grain (0.3 Gm.) capsules.

2. *Iodo-casein.*—A compound of iodine and milk casein, which is said to be dissolved in the intestines after passing practically unchanged through the stomach. Dosage: 5 to 20 grains (0.3 to 1.3 Gm.), as indicated. It is supplied in 5-grain (0.3 Gm.) tablets.

3. *Iodostarine-Roche.*—A product of iodine and tariric acid, which is claimed to be longer retained and therefore better utilized than the inorganic iodides. Dosage: The same as that of potassium iodide. It is supplied in 4-grain (0.25 Gm.) tablets.

4. *Lipoiodine-Ciba.*—The ethyl ester of diiodobrassidic acid, which is claimed to be longer retained and therefore better utilized than the inorganic iodides. Dosage: 5 to 30 grains (0.3 to 1.8 Gm.), as indicated. It is supplied in 5-grain (0.3 Gm.) tablets, which should be masticated before swallowing.

5. *Riodine.*—A product of iodine and castor oil, which is claimed to be longer retained and therefore better utilized than the inorganic iodides. Dosage: 6 to 18 grains (0.4 to 1.2 Gm.) per day, taken after meals. It is supplied in 3-grain (0.2 Gm.) capsules.

6. *Calcium Iodobehenate* (Sajodin).—A salt which is claimed to be longer retained and therefore better utilized than the inorganic iodides. Dosage: 15 to 45 grains (1 to 3 Gm.) daily. It is supplied in 8-grain (0.5 Gm.) tablets.

7. *Ferro-Sajodin.*—A basic ferric iodobehenate, which is claimed to be easily absorbed but slowly eliminated, thus assuring a more prolonged effect than that obtained from inorganic iodides and iron compounds.

Dosage: 8 to 15 grains (0.5 to 1 Gm.), three times daily. It is supplied in 8-grain (0.5 Gm.) tablets, which should be masticated before swallowing.

8. *Siomine.*—Methenamine tetraiodide, which is claimed to be decomposed in the intestine into methenamine and iodide, the latter being absorbed essentially the same as the inorganic iodides. No therapeutic claims are made for the methenamine, which is present only to render the substance insoluble. Dosage: The same as that of potassium iodide. It is supplied in 5-grain (0.3 Gm.) capsules.

6. COMBINED DRUG AND PROTEIN THERAPY

Some years ago, Kyrle, in Austria, emphasized the value of combined protein and antisyphilitic drug therapy. More recently (1926), Herrold, in the United States, has published an interesting study of the effect of this sort of treatment in Wassermann-fast cases. The serological reduction is shown in the following table (Table 28), which is of course only suggestive in value because of the small number of patients.

The first three courses consisted in the routine use of neoarsphenamine, mercuric chloride and potassium iodide. Regarding the protein course, Herrold writes:

TABLE 28.—WASSERMANN READINGS BEFORE AND AFTER THE USE OF PROTEIN

Case.	Duration of infection.	Stage of syphilis.	W before treatment.	W after one course.	W after two courses.	W after three courses.	W one month after course with protein.	W seven months after course with protein.
1	18 yr.	tertiary	4+	4+	4+	4+	±	0
2	8 mo.	late secondary	4+	4+	4+	2+	0	0
3	unknown	tertiary	4+	4+	4+	4+	0	0
4	10 yr.	tertiary	4+	4+	4+	4+	0	...
5	15 yr.	tertiary	4+	4+	4+	4+	2+	...
6	7 yr.	tertiary	4+	...	...	4+	0	0
7	6 yr.	tertiary	4+	...	...	4+	...	...
8	8 yr.	tertiary	4+	...	...	2+	0	...

"One lot of gonococcus protein was used throughout these observations. It consisted of a clear extract of the gonococcus in physiologic sodium chloride solution in strength of 500 million per cubic centimeter. From 15 to 20 minims (0.9 to 1.25 cc.) was given intramuscularly in the gluteal region with very little local reaction and no unusual general disturbance when followed by neoarsphenamine intravenously. Four injections were given at intervals of three days and five days; after the last injection the combination therapy of neoarsphenamine intravenously and protein intramuscularly was begun and was continued twice a week during a course of eight treatments."

THE PROPHYLAXIS OF SYPHILIS

1. **Calomel Ointment** (Unguentum Hydrargyri Subchloridi, B.P.).—It has long been felt that the thorough inunction of this ointment into the parts exposed in a suspicious contact will effectively prevent the contraction of syphilis. Certainly its successful use on a large scale during the World War has lent support to the belief, but the limitations of the method should be clearly recognized. In the first place, it is more or less positively effective only if applied within four or five hours after the contact, and

only doubtfully so up to eight hours; after twelve hours its use probably does more harm than good, for it does not prevent the development of the disease though it does make the diagnostic search for spirochetes much more difficult. Also its thorough use by women is very difficult, if not impossible. Formula on page 206.

2. Soap.—Reasoner showed, in 1917, that a soap lather, such as that used in shaving, or a "good" lather as produced in the vigorous washing of the hands, is quite effective in killing the spirochete. There is of course no way of knowing to what extent this measure, as employed merely for the sake of personal cleanliness, is effective in preventing the disease among those addicted to promiscuous intercourse, but it is extremely probable that the careful washing of hands is accountable for the great rarity of extragenital chancres among the professional attendants at syphilis clinics.

3. Weak Acids.—A number of years ago, Goodman stated his belief that weak acetic acid might be effectively used in prophylaxis and showed that it is spirocheticidal in a degree comparable with soap. I know of no further contribution on the subject.

4. Arsphenamine.—In 1919, Taege, in Germany, proposed the use of arsphenamine during the incubation period of syphilis when there are no lesions present, if exposure to a known case of syphilis is proved. He gave three intravenous injections of an arsenical within twenty-four hours. I quote the following from the excellent paper of Michel and Goodman:

"Fournier and Guenot (1919) report on the abortion of syphilis by arsphenamine used during the incubation period. Forty women were exposed to infection by sexual congress with syphilitics having genital lesions. The men were all examined, and the presence of *Spirochaeta pallida* was demonstrated by the dark field. The Wassermann reaction was positive in all except five, who had had the chancre less than ten days. The period since exposure for the women was from a few days to three weeks. The women were free from all suspicious lesions, the history did not lead to the suspecting of a previous infection, and the Wassermann reaction was negative in all. Not one had exercised any preventive measures. Five women who refused all treatment, of the group that were similarly exposed, were later attacked by syphilis.

"The forty women were treated by injections of arsphenamine (a total of from 1 to 1.2 Gm.), of neoarsphenamine (a total of 1.2 to 2 Gm.), or of an arsphenamine substitute. Not one of the forty ever showed any syphilitic lesion, and the Wassermann reactions of all have remained negative. Twenty of the women have been under observation over three years. One of the women, who after this treatment continued to receive her lover, who had mucous patches for which he did not take treatment, contracted a chancre of the face.

"Lacapère and Laurent (1919) are able to report four interesting observations on the preventive treatment of the syphilitic chancre:

"Of three officers who had intercourse with one woman who presented a pigmentary syphilid, and numerous mucous patches of the mouth and vulva, two received a dose of neoarsphenamine (the amount not mentioned) intravenously and remained unscathed. The third preferred to take his chances with infection; he refused the injection, and after the usual incubation period, he presented the primary sore of syphilis.

"The wife of an officer, who had connection with her despite his having a chancre and a positive Wassermann reaction, was given three injections of neoarsphenamine, in doses of 1.5, 3 and 4.5 Gm. [?], at intervals of six days. She never presented any lesions, and her Wassermann reaction remained persistently negative.

"A young man with erosive syphilitic lesions of the glans and prepuce had repeated contacts each night for fifteen days with a young woman who presented no lesion, no history of antecedent syphilis, and a negative Wassermann reaction. She was given eight injections (dosage not mentioned) of neoarsphenamine, and she has remained free of lesions, and Wassermann negative.

"A nursing heredosyphilitic had exposed two wetnurses to infection. One of the two later nursed another infant. About eleven days after the last nursing of the first infant she presented a lesion of the nipple, from which spirochetes were demonstrated by the dark field. The child she was then nursing was certainly not a heredosyphilitic, and the possibility of infection was certain. At intervals of five days, neoarsphenamine, in doses of 0.01, 0.015, 0.02, 0.04 and 0.05 Gm., was given intravenously. Eighty-five days after the last feeding from the affected breast, no lesions had appeared in the child."

Michel and Goodman have used this method in 30 individuals in most of whom it was definitely possible to make the diagnosis of active syphilis in the opposing partner. They give not less than three doses of arsphenamine, averaging 0.3 Gm., at varying intervals of every second to fifth day. They believe, as does Spence following his experience in 11 cases, that they have successfully prevented the development of the disease, but I know of no reported series in which the severe criteria of prevention propounded by Moore (1929) have been satisfied: negative monthly Wassermanns for the first year, every two or three months for the second year, and thereafter every six to twelve months for two or three years; and at least one negative spinal fluid examination at the end of the first year. Moore also insists that the prophylactic treatment must consist of at least one full course with arsphenamines followed by a course with mercury or bismuth. Wirz (1932) has reported the case of a young man who acquired a second chancre at the height of the neoarsphenamine-bismuth treatment which had cured his first infection—four hours, indeed, after taking the last combined injections!

We must not forget, what is so well known to every syphilologist, that of all persons exposed with certainty to syphilis only a small proportion contract the disease.

Theoretically there are two strong arguments against this method of prophylaxis: first, it is unnecessary since, as early contended by Riecke, diagnosis of the disease can be made readily enough in the chancre stage to make possible the vigorous institution of "abortive" treatment—which is true to a large extent for men but by no means always true for women; and second, that a patient so treated never knows positively whether he or she has syphilis or not. I think this second objection could be answered by the persistent absence of clinical evidences of the disease and the satisfying of Moore's serological criteria. Pardo-Castelló's suggestion that this is not prophylaxis at all but really the accomplishment of the *therapia sterilisans magna* of Ehrlich, at the only time when this desired result can be attained, is interesting and, I believe, very near to the truth.

5. **Bismuth.**—Kolle's animal experimentation caused him in the early period to champion bismuth in prophylaxis, but he later became more conservative in his attitude. Sonnenberg (1925) gave bismuth prophylactically to 60 prostitutes, of whom 5 contracted the disease; in the control, unprotected group of 50, syphilis infection appeared in 20. But there is much lacking here: were they all equally active, etc.? Pinard (1930), Hofmann (1931) and Wirz (1932) have recorded failures in individual instances. In America, the following authorities, among others, do not believe that bismuth has proved its prophylactic worth: Cole, Moore, O'Leary, Stokes, Wile (1931).

TETANUS
(Lockjaw)

"Another receiv'd an insignificant wound to speak of (for it was not deep) a little below his neck behind from a sharp dart; which being taken out not long after, he was drawn and distorted backwards, as in the opisthotonus. His jaws were also fasten'd; and, if anything moist was put into his mouth, and he attempted to swallow it, it returned again thro' the nose. In other respects he grew worse immediately. The second day he dy'd."

—Hippocrates. Upon Epidemics. Book V, The Cases at Salamis—No. 15.
(Translated by Clifton, London, 1734.)

Tetanus is an acute infectious disease caused by the infection of a wound with the spores of *Bacillus tetani*. The wound is usually an accidental one, but numerous cases of tetanus following peritoneal operations are on record; tetanus neonatorum is becoming very rare now that the umbilical cord is properly cared for as a matter of routine. Wainwright's (1926) compilation of 760 cases showed that 80 per cent were due to injuries on the street, on the farm, in homes, gardens, stables, etc., and only 20 per cent to industrial accidents. It is perhaps not a matter of common knowledge that the organism is harbored to a very considerable extent in the human intestinal tract; Bauer and Meyer found spores of definitely toxic strains in 24.6 per cent of 487 specimens of feces from residents of California. The tetanus organism grows best under the completely anaerobic conditions prevailing in deep wounds and its growth is also aided by the concomitant presence of pus-producing organisms; the retention of a foreign body in a fresh wound also increases the chances of tetanus developing. The toxin reaches the central nervous system by passing directly from the seat of the developing organisms along the axis-cylinders of the nerves or by way of the perineural lymphatics; it is also absorbed into the general circulation in large amounts, whence it reaches the central nervous system by traveling up the nerves from their motor end-plates.

The prodromal symptoms, which it is important to recognize, are restlessness and hyperirritability, perhaps chilliness and headache with some general stiffness of the body, and, the most important symptom, a stiffness of the neck and difficulty in chewing and swallowing. A boardlike rigidity of the abdomen makes its appearance very early. The later, more typical, symptoms are frequent convulsions from which the patient does not at any time completely relax, the characteristic lockjaw (trismus), a sardonic facial expression, several degrees of fever with proportional leukocytosis, spinal fluid that is clear but under increased pressure, and great pain from the severe muscular contractions; the consciousness is usually retained until the end. Death usually occurs on the fourth or fifth day; it is said that if a patient survives the eighth day his chances of recovery are very good.

The incubation period of the disease is from three days to several weeks. Statistics, gathered from civil as well as military practice, show that most cases develop within from ten to fourteen days after the wound is suffered; it is axiomatic that the shorter the incubation period the higher the mortality. Since the prophylactic use of tetanus antitoxin has become more frequent, a local type of the disease, with symptoms confined to the neighborhood of the wound, is rather often seen; the mistaken tendency is to recognize this as a new entity, despite the fact that a case of this sort was seen now and then before the introduction of antitoxin.

THERAPY

Miller, in his study of the 116 cases of tetanus occurring at the Massachusetts General Hospital in the period 1872–1922, writes:

"Given a hundred cases of tetanus, a certain number, perhaps twenty, will get well anyway, with ordinary symptomatic treatment, and without antitoxin. A certain number, to which the author will not attempt to give a figure, will, in spite of the best treatment which our present knowledge enables us to give, die. Between these two groups lies the middle class of those who will die or get well according to their treatment, and by that treatment we mean the proper care of the wound, the intelligent use of sedatives, and the prompt well-directed, and repeated use of large doses of antitoxin."

Local Treatment.—Miller lays down the principles of local treatment as follows:

"1. Sterilization of the part.

"2. Thorough opening of the wound in its whole breadth and depth.

"3. Débridement—complete excision of every scrap of dead or infected tissue.

"4. Sterilization of the wound.

"5. Measures to keep it open. It must not be 'packed,' though gauze, preferably soaked in hydrogen peroxide, may be laid gently in it. It must not be tightly bandaged. Anything tending to close the wound, and shut out the air, must be avoided. The dressing should be renewed very frequently."

In writing of the sterilization of the wound, one should perhaps specifically mention the tincture of iodine, for it not only tends to prevent secondary infection, but seems to have a local specific effect against the toxin. Mac-Conkey and Silva have shown that mixing iodine with toxin definitely lessens the strength of the toxin. There are no data known to me to show whether or not this property is common to all the penetrating disinfectants, such, for instance, as the dyes which have recently become so popular for local use.

In regard to the matter of thorough incision and excision of the wound, it is of interest to note that Sir David Bruce has stated that surgeons were slow to realize the importance of this method during the World War, but that, had the war lasted longer, tetanus would probably have been extinguished. He showed that before incision and excision were practiced, the incidence of tetanus was 103 per hundred thousand; by February, 1918, the incidence had dropped to 24; by May, 1918, to 12; and by June, 1918, to 8 per hundred thousand.

All surgeons are in agreement that the wound should under no circumstances be cauterized, for the resulting area of necrosis is altogether to the taste of the tetanus organism.

Sedatives.—Certainly the judicious employment of all available sedative measures is indicated in these cases, for, even though we do not lessen the mortality thereby, it would seem to be our bounden duty to lessen the suffering of the unfortunate victim of tetanus as much as lies in our power. Morphine is valuable, but must sometimes be given in doses so large as to be dangerous; then, too, the menace of habit formation must be taken into account. A drug which is enjoying considerable popularity for all types of sedation nowadays is phenobarbital (luminal). Here it must be given in a dose of 3 to 5 grains (0.2 to 0.3 Gm.), repeated every three to six hours. If the dose cannot be gotten into the mouth or be swallowed, as is usually the case, the soluble form of the drug must be used, phenobarbital sodium (luminal sodium), which is given hypodermically in a 20 per cent solution in boiled and cooled water; 2 cc. of this solution will contain 6 grains (0.4 Gm.) of the drug—a permissible dose. This soluble salt may also be given by the rectum. Chloral hydrate is well absorbed from the rectum; 30 to 45 grains (2 to 3 Gm.) in olive oil or water every four hours is permissible dosage.

15

General Anesthetics.—Light general anesthesia will induce relaxation, but the prolonged use of chloroform is impossible because of its toxicity; ether is of course out of the question. Cruchet (1932) is advising that at least the patient be anesthetized with chloroform at the time of each injection of the antiserum, maintaining that the drug will release toxins bound to the lipoids of the nerve cells (the "phylactic" theory of Billard) and thus make possible the maximum of antitoxic effect from each injection; the proposition lacks substantiation by adequate clinical trials. The new anesthetic for rectal use, avertin, was first employed in tetanus by Löwen, in 1927. From that time until the present writing (late 1933) I find reports of its employment in 23 cases, apparently very satisfactorily in all instances from the standpoint of symptomatic relief. The average dosage is 0.1 Gm. per kilogram (2.2 pounds) body weight, dissolved in 100 to 200 cc. of water. The patient usually goes to sleep at once and is sufficiently depressed and relaxed to permit of catheterization and the intraspinal, intravenous and intramuscular injection of antiserum without muscular spasm being induced. The period of deep depression usually lasts for eight to ten hours and is followed by several hours of drowsiness, during which, however, the patient is able to take food. One, more rarely two, such enemas has been the rule in the course of the day, but Teichmann (1932) reports a very severe case treated, as regards avertin, as follows: First dose, 0.1 Gm. per kilogram; two hours later, 2 Gm. total dose; eight hours later, 0.05 Gm. per kilogram; six hours later, 0.07 Gm. per kilogram; five hours later, 0.07 Gm. per kilogram. Second day, 0.07 Gm. per kilogram, in the evening, was effective until next morning. Third to tenth days, two doses of 0.07 to 0.1 Gm. per kilogram daily. Eleventh to sixteenth days, one dose of 0.07 Gm. per kilogram daily. Small doses of morphine have been given in a number of instances to prolong the secondary periods of drowsiness. No deleterious effects of the avertin have been reported by any of the observers. Thonnard-Neumann (1931) expresses the belief of many when he predicts that this use of the drug will outlast its employment in surgical procedures.

Magnesium Sulphate.—Following the preliminary work of Meltzer and Auer on monkeys, Blake used magnesium sulphate in the first case of human tetanus in 1906. Since that time it has won many staunch advocates, both in this country and abroad, but it is passed over very lightly in most of the text-books. I wonder why? Perhaps it is the fear that it may encroach upon the partial victory that the antitoxin has won; otherwise, I am at a loss to account for this reticence, for surely no physician who has once seen the remarkable relaxing power of this salt upon an agonized tetanus patient can seriously doubt its value even though it be not in itself curative. Properly employed, rest and comfort and the taking of food are made possible; *complete* relaxation should not be sought. The following is a summary of the dosage which serves Smith and Leighton as a working basis.

Subcutaneous.—One and two-tenths to 2 cc. of a 25 per cent solution for each 20 pounds of body weight, four times in twenty-four hours. Should be continued until disappearance of symptoms. Less dangerous than other methods.

Intramuscular.—To be used only in severe spasms, as the drug is more dangerous thus (respiratory arrest). Lightly anesthetize with ether and deposit intramuscularly 2 cc. of a 25 per cent solution for each 20 pounds of body weight; effect in less than half an hour and lasts two or three hours.

Intravenous.—Most prompt but fleeting; effect may disappear in thirty minutes. Most dangerous of all. Dose: 6 per cent solution, at rate of 2 to 3 cc. per minute until relaxation begins.

Intraspinal.—Effect in less than half an hour and relief lasts twelve to thirty hours. Anesthetize with ether and inject 1 cc. of a 25 per cent solution for each 20 pounds; second dose, 0.8 cc. for each 20 pounds; only 0.5 cc. per 20 pounds in a child.

To combat excessive depression of the respiration by magnesium sulphate, inject 2.5 cc. of calcium chloride in physiologic saline intravenously (slowly). The antidotal effect is seen almost at once.

Glucose.—In experiments on rabbits it has been found that the glycogen content of the central nervous system is reduced more than 50 per cent in animals injected with tetanus toxin; the intravenous introduction of glucose restores some of this glycogen. Jadassohn and Streit have applied these facts to the treatment of two human cases of tetanus, both of which they believe were saved by the use of intravenous glucose in addition to antitetanic serum and magnesium sulphate. (For technic see p. 776.)

Antitetanic Serum.—In recent years the profession has become increasingly dubious of the value of the antiserum in treatment. Statistically, it has certainly not been possible to attest its worth, but then, of course, the variable factors are several: The severity of the case, the length of the antecedent incubation period, the general condition of the patient (*i. e.*, his ability to withstand attack of any sort), the amount of prophylactic serum that was used, and the coincident employment of other therapeutic measures. Likewise, and for similar reasons, the matter of the preferred route of administration of the serum remains a controversial one. There are those who favor the use of the intraspinal route alone while there are equally strong advocates of the exclusive use of the intravenous route, and all fall back upon supplementary intramuscular injections. The difficulty was shown in Wainwright's report, in 1926, in which he advocated the abandonment of the intraspinal route in favor of the intravenous because of a mortality of 61.7 per cent in a group treated by the former method, as against only 52.2 per cent in a group treated by the latter; but Ashhurst showed that a more careful examination of the statistics indicated that the subcutaneous route was superior to either of the other two! A combination of intravenous, intraspinal and intramuscular injections is perhaps most often employed.

Dosage.—It is agreed that in the average case the patient should receive at least 100,000 units within the first twenty-four hours. This is usually distributed as follows: 60,000 units intravenously in three equal portions throughout the day; 20,000 units intraspinally and 20,000 units intramuscularly, both immediately following the first intravenous injection. The doses are very little reduced for children. It is usual to dilute the intravenous doses with an equal quantity of physiologic saline solution; the intraspinal doses are injected undiluted after the withdrawal of 10 to 25 cc. of spinal fluid. All injections to be made very slowly. If anaphylactic symptoms appear they should be combated with a hypodermic injection of 1 cc. of epinephrine (adrenalin). Time permitting, it is well to precede the first injection by a trial subcutaneous injection of 0.5 cc. of the serum. Should this give rise to a painful urticarial wheal, desensitization may be performed as follows: Dilute 0.1 cc. of serum up to 1 cc. with physiologic saline; inject subcutaneously ¼ cc. of this dilution; after fifteen minutes, ½ cc.; fifteen minutes later inject 0.1 cc. of undiluted serum; fifteen minutes later, 0.5 cc. of undiluted serum; fifteen minutes later, 1 cc. of undiluted serum; thirty to forty-five minutes later, the remainder of the first full dose of the serum may be given by any route. A bovine serum is now commercially available.

It is usual to continue the injections on the second and third days in such dosage and at such time intervals as seem indicated; then, oftentimes, if the injections have been discontinued, a "safety" dose of 10,000 to 20,000 units is given on the eighth or ninth day. In severe cases, however, very large doses are given by all routes daily so long as appears necessary; Nabarro (1932) gave 633,000 units in ten days to a child of ten years. Many observers are favorably impressed with the better showing made by the serum since the use of larger doses continued over a longer time has become customary, but one cannot lightly pass by the trenchant statement of Calvin and Goldberg (1930) in discussing the Cook County (Chicago) Hospital cases: "The diminishing mortality with increasing amounts of serum given is misleading, because those that died succumbed within one or two days after the onset, before enough time had elapsed for enormous doses of serum to be given."

And the serum is very costly!

Local Use.—There can certainly be no objection to the injection into the tissues about the wound of several thousand units of antitoxin. Many observers believe the procedure is a valuable one.

Reactions.—Serum sickness in eight to ten days may be expected in half, or more, of those receiving the antitoxin (see p. 335). The thermal reaction (a chill and fever within several hours) may occur as after the use of any serum. It was formerly thought that anaphylactic shock occurred with sufficient frequency after the use of the serum intravenously to contraindicate this method, but experience in and after the World War has disproved this belief. The injection should be given very slowly and stopped at once on the appearance of symptoms; 1 cc. of epinephrine hydrochloride (1 : 1000 solution) will practically always counteract these symptoms.

PROPHYLAXIS

Ample opportunity arose during the World War for the study of the efficacy of antitetanic serum in the prevention of tetanus, and as a result even those who were formerly most sceptical are now convinced of its very great value.

Effect upon Incidence.—Bazy observed 200 French wounded from the same sector. Among the 100 who received the serum, but 1 case of tetanus developed—and that on the day following the injection of the serum, showing that the period of incubation had nearly expired when the injection was given. Among the 100 who did not receive antitoxin, 18 developed tetanus. There were many such observations. The British war statistics were thoroughly presented by Sir David Bruce, who showed that prior to the routine use of the prophylactic antitoxin injection there were from 15 to 32 cases of tetanus per thousand of wounded, while after the injections became routine this figure never rose above 2 or 3 per thousand. Perhaps because the value of débridement had already been established, the routine injection of the antitoxin appeared to be even more effective in the American army; among the 224,089 wounded there developed 36 cases of tetanus, an incidence of only 0.16 per thousand.

Effect upon Mortality.—Among the British wounded who received no prophylactic treatment, 53.3 per cent of those who contracted tetanus died of it; among those who did receive such treatment, only 22.5 per cent of those who contracted the disease came to their death by it.

Effect upon Incubation Time.—Again the British statistics: Before preventive injection became routine, the average incubation period was 10.9 days; after the measure became routine, the period was lengthened to 45.5 days.

Dose.—According to Stone, the British in the earlier days of the World War used 500 units as the prophylactic dose. In June, 1917, it was ordered that four such inoculations should be given at intervals of seven days. In August, 1916, this order was changed and one dose of 1500 units was given. In the United States Army the dose was 1500 units, to be repeated in ten days; this is the dose usually employed in civilian practice also. Stone well advises that the dose be repeated several times at intervals of eight to ten days, especially "if a lacerated wound contains dead spaces, a foreign body or necrotic tissue . . . since in such instances tetanus may not develop for a number of weeks after the injury."

Reactions.—In the more than two million prophylactic injections given by the British during the war there were only eleven instances of anaphylactic shock; all the cases recovered.

Active Immunization with Toxoid.—The preliminary studies of Lincoln and Greenwald (1933) indicate that it may soon be possible to immunize with toxoid in tetanus just as is being so splendidly done in diphtheria.

TONSILLITIS

Acute tonsillitis is characterized by a rather sudden onset with aching pains throughout the body, very sore throat, high fever and rapid pulse, and considerable prostration. Susceptible individuals often have an annual attack some time during the inclement months; the usual duration is three to eight days. The possibility of diphtheria is usually easily ruled out by a careful examination of the throat. *Streptococcus* is the organism most frequently cultured from these throats.

THERAPY

Tonsillitis *per se* is rarely, perhaps never, fatal, but as an attack often ushers in a bout of rheumatic fever, and as endocarditis and acute otitis media are not infrequent complications, the disease merits serious attention. Unfortunately there is practically nothing to say on the head of treatment; we have no specific drug or biological. For the general principles of "fever" treatment, the reader is referred to the article on Catarrhal Fever (see p. 25).

TRENCH FEVER
(Shin-bone Fever)

Trench fever is a nonfatal but extremely debilitating infectious disease caused by a virus that is transmitted in the excreta of the body louse. When this virus is rubbed into the skin, either by scratching or by the normal friction of the clothing against the body, the disease is contracted; the louse can also transmit the disease in the act of biting, though it is not definitely known whether the parasite actually regurgitates and injects the virus from its mouth parts. The prodromal symptoms are not characteristic, but the onset is sudden, *i. e.*, all of the symptoms have usually developed in twelve to twenty-four hours from the first appearance of any one of them. There is chilliness or a definite chill, prostration of varying intensity, rise of temperature to 103 F. or more, anorexia and sometimes vomiting, frontal headache and severe pain "behind the eyes," and generalized pain and tenderness in both muscle and bone; the especial severity of this latter symptom in the lower legs, particularly at night, has given the affection its popular name of "shin-bone fever." A macular rash on the chest and abdomen is typical of the disease. It is impossible to predict the course of a particular case; there may be but one bout of fever which is over in a few days, or the attack may occur regularly at three- to seven-day intervals, or the case may run a protracted typhoid-like course. The tendency to relapse months or even years after the initial attack is typical of the disease. A too early return to active work is almost certain to cause a recrudescence of symptoms. The bronchitis which is present in some cases is not of serious moment, but we do not know as much as might be desired of the extent of the circulatory involvement during the earlier stages of the attack. Certainly many cases of "effort syndrome" have had their inception in a bout of trench fever.

Graham, of the British Expeditionary Force, first described trench fever as a new disease in 1915, though it may have existed as an unrecognized entity long before that time in various parts of the world. Swift says that the condition was probably endemic in Russia and was disseminated to all the fighting fronts by the movement of German and Austrian troops. Recently, Braslawsky (1933), of Kieff, has stated his belief that trench fever (which he prefers to call five-day fever) exists endemically in the form of occasional and unrecognized cases in certain parts of Eastern Europe, thus forming a reservoir from which a great epidemic may again arise in time of war. From 1920 to 1933 he has seen 32 cases; 2 cases were also recorded in Japan in 1927. The reports of the American Red Cross Trench Fever Commission and the British War Office Investigation Committee established the body louse as vector. In 1917, Grieveson stated that at one time 60 per cent of all patients in British military hospitals had trench fever. It is an interesting speculation how much sooner (and in whose favor) the war might have terminated had it been possible quickly to control this debilitating malady.

THERAPY

A great many remedial agents, both drug and biological, were tried in the management of trench fever during its period of great prevalence, but none of them, with the possible exception of collargol, were of very much value. Some such "fever treatment" as is described in this book under the head of Catarrhal Fever was most frequently employed.

Collargol.—In 1917, Richter reported the intravenous injection of collargol to be a specific measure comparable to the employment of quinine in malaria. Sweet and Wilmer's excellent results in all of their 35 cases lends considerable substantiation to this position, but these observers prefer to view their findings with a certain amount of scepticism: "There has been no question in the minds of the clinicians who have followed these cases that the collargol was immediately followed by marked improvement and recovery; it has only been difficult to decide in some cases whether the collargol was merely an incident in the course of the spontaneous recovery from the disease. Some cases do so recover, though of the cases reaching the base by no means the 90 per cent reported by the British Trench Fever Committee. We have learned of no method of distinguishing between a case which will spontaneously recover and one which will spend the next six months in hospital."

Ten cc. of a 1 per cent solution of the drug is injected intravenously at two- or three-day intervals. Care must be exercised to prevent infiltration as the solution is very irritating when placed in the extravascular tissues. A pronounced febrile reaction follows the injection.

PROPHYLAXIS

This is entirely a matter of ridding and maintaining the body free of lice. For a description of delousing procedures see page 685.

TRYPANOSOMIASIS

(Sleeping Sickness)

AFRICAN TYPE

African sleeping sickness is an infectious disease which is conveyed to man by the bite of the tsetse fly, in whose body the causative organism undergoes a part of its developmental cycle. There are in all probability at least two varieties of this organism, *Trypanosoma gambiense* and *T. rhodesiense,* which are carried by separate species of the fly. *Gambiense* is carried by a fly that inhabits the dry scrub land of central Africa and shuns water and the scorching sun; *rhodesiense,* which is the more virulent organism, develops in a fly that frequents water courses and holes in the areas of dense jungle. It has long been the consensus of opinion that the blood of African game animals is the reservoir from which the fly derives trypanosomes for the infection of domestic animals and man, from which has resulted naturally the agitation for destruction of all wild life. Latterly, however, evidence is accumulating that such action does not lessen the incidence of the disease very markedly; Warren's (1932) announcement of Davidson's discovery that the trypanosome may be derived from the latex of certain plants on which the fly normally feeds has added an additional point for controversial departure in this tremendously interesting and important subject. The disease, which is at the present time a great scourge throughout equatorial Africa, was probably first described by John Atkins, a British naval surgeon, who gave the following description (quoted from Strong) on his return from a cruise to West Africa in 1734: "The Sleepy Distemper (common among the Negroes) gives no other previous Notice, than a want of Appetite two or three days before; their sleeps are sound, and Sense and Feeling very little, for pulling, drubbing or whipping will scarce stir up Sense and Power enough to move; and the Moment you cease beating the smart is forgot, and down they fall again into a state of Insensibility, drivling constantly from the Mouth as if in deep salivation; breathe slowly, but not unequally nor snort. Young people are more subject to it than the old; and the Judgement generally pronounced is Death, the Prognostick seldom failing. If now and then one of them recovers, he certainly loses the little Reason he had, and turns Ideot. . . ."

We now know that the disease passes through two stages, which are summarized by Blacklock and Yorke (1922) as follows: "The first is characterized principally by irregular attacks of fever, chronic polyadenitis, exanthemata, frequency of the pulse and respiration, and asthenia; the second, by exaggeration of the symptoms of the first stage, marked emaciation, and by the appearance of nervous symptoms, tremors, incoordination of movements, paralyses, mental disturbances, apathy, somnolence, coma, and death. These two stages are, as a rule, not clearly delimited, but merge into one another, the second stage gradually manifesting itself as the nervous symptoms develop following injury to the nervous tissue from the inflammatory changes in the lymphatics of the brain and spinal cord." Demonstration of the organism is usually required for definite diagnosis in the early stage, the material being taken from the blood, spinal fluid, or the enlarged glands of the posterior triangle of the neck; the organisms are very few and their demonstration often difficult. The incubation period is between seven and fourteen days; cases are seen with extreme rarity among infants.

THERAPY

One sees the statement made in text-books of medicine that first stage trypanosomiasis responds more or less well to treatment but that treatment of the second (cerebral) stage of the disease is practically useless. I believe that the facts of the case do not wholly warrant this glib pronunciamento. The principal drugs in use at the present time are atoxyl, tartar emetic, tryparsamide, Bayer-205, and Fourneau-309 and -270. Biologicals have failed entirely so far.

Atoxyl (Sodium Aminophenylarsenate).—The use of this drug in sleeping sickness was first reported in any detail by Koch (1889). The early reports were very enthusiastic, but we know now that there are two objectionable features which attend its use: First, the parasites become gradually resistant; and second, permanent blindness is not infrequently caused. The incidence of this latter occurrence, however, would seem to be somewhat lessened by increasing the time interval between doses; Blanchard and Laigret have reported excellent results with six subcutaneous injections at two-week intervals, giving ⅓ grain (0.02 Gm.) per kilogram body weight; the drug is much more·toxic when given by mouth. They felt that their results were aided by the employment of tartar emetic (see below) intravenously between the atoxyl treatments.

In 1931, Sicé reported on the treatment of 1118 patients in the Brazzaville district between 1920 and 1928, using approximately the above dosage. Results in the 663 who could be carefully followed: (a) Of 316 with only blood and lymphatic infection, 249 were cured—198 without any other drug and 51 with the ultimate use of tryparsamide (43 dead, 24 disappeared); (b) of 208 with lesions of the cerebrospinal system, 34 were cured—2 without other drug and 32 with the aid of tryparsamide (1 improved, 141 dead, 32 disappeared); (c) of 139 unclassified in absence of spinal puncture, 62 were cured, 45 without other drugs and 17 with the aid of tryparsamide (63 dead, 14 disappeared). Of the total cases, 15.9 per cent exhibited blood relapses; 11.1 per cent of these occurred during the first year of treatment.

Tartar Emetic (Antimony Sodium (or Potassium) Tartrate).—Since 1908 this drug has been used with varying success, the consensus of opinion at present seeming to be that it is of most value when used as adjuvant to arsenic treatment. It is given intravenously in a dose of 1 grain (0.06 Gm.) in a 1 to 2 per cent solution at intervals of two or three days over a long period of time. For the precautions to be observed in using tartar emetic in this way, together with a dosage table, the reader is referred to the article on Kala-azar (see p. 77).

Tryparsamide (Sodium-phenylglycinamide-arsonate).—This drug was first tried in human trypanosomiasis when the Rockefeller Institute sent Miss Pearce to the Belgian Congo, in 1920. Her careful studies of its effects in all stages of *Trypanosoma gambiense* infection have been so amply confirmed (Chesterman, 1922–25; Van den Branden and Van Hoof, 1923; Letonturier, de Marqueissac and Jamot, 1924; Van den Branden, 1925–27; Laigret, 1926; Jamot and Vernon, 1927; Van Hoof, 1928; Pearce, 1930; Vancel and Boisseau, 1931; McClean, 1931) that statistical evidences need not be labored here. Almost all the observers have found that it produces immediate peripheral blood and gland sterilization not only in early cases but also in patients with pronounced nervous involvement. Remarkable recoveries have even been recorded in some cases in the terminal stages. All medical officers at the second international congress on sleeping sickness agreed that this drug should replace all the others in use in *T. gambiense* cases. Great enthusiasm, then, all along the line—but let us wait for *all* the water to flow under the bridges before we throw anything away. In *T. rhodesiense* infections none of these good results are obtained. Keevil, 1926, Maclean, 1926, Corson, 1928, and Lauterburg, 1929, have all failed to accomplish sterilization of either the blood or spinal fluid, nor were they able to bring about much immediate physical improvement in their cases. Whether a certain number of sufferers from either type of the disease suddenly develops a high secondary resistance to the beneficent effects of tryparsamide is still a moot point. The results with tryponarsyl, the Belgian product, are identical with those of tryparsamide.

Dosage.—The larger dosage favored by many is as follows: (*a*) Individual doses range from 0.5 to 3 Gm., according to size and age (in general, 40 mg. per kilogram body weight); (*b*) in early cases, injections once per week until 20 to 40 Gm. have been given; (*c*) in chronic cases, until 50 to 100 Gm. are administered. Latterly, however, Pearce (1930) has recommended an average course of twelve weekly injections, the maximum dose being 2 Gm.; and Lauterburg (1931) urgently recommends that the treatment be begun with doses of 0.5 Gm. and be not raised above 1.5 Gm. per week. Maclean and Fairbairn (1932), who have had vast experience, recommend an individual adult dose of 2 to 4 Gm., the total dosage to be not less than 22 Gm. The injections are usually given intravenously in 20 per cent solution; King (1926) has also used this concentration with success intramuscularly, but the natives usually object to medication by this route. It is of interest to note that in Pearce's 1921 report she stated that the duration of effect of a single dose is longer when given intramuscularly than when given intravenously.

Toxicity.—Visual disturbances, sometimes going on to blindness but usually clearing up if treatment is stopped, occur not infrequently. The smaller dosage is designed to avoid these unfortunate occurrences, since under field conditions careful studies of the visual apparatus (see p. 187) are usually not possible.

Bayer-205 (Germanin) and Fourneau-309 (Moranyl).—In 1920, the German dye industry produced an aniline substance allied to trypan blue which was proposed for use in treating sleeping sickness under the name of Bayer-205. Though the new drug was admitted to contain no mercury, antimony or arsenic, its formula was kept secret until Fourneau, Tréfouel and Valée, by "une voie très detournée," obtained enough of the substance to undertake thorough investigations of its composition, with the result that their product, Fourneau-309, which is the symmetric urea of acid sodium m-amino-benzoyl-m-amino-p-methylbenzoylnaphthylamino-trisulphonate, is now recognized as being identical with Bayer-205. Though most of the clinical studies have been made with Bayer-205, I shall refer to the two drugs as Bayer-Fourneau since the conditions of their use and the results obtained with them are exactly the same.

And rather disappointing are these results, for the bright hopes engendered by the Kleine expedition of 1922–23 have not been fulfilled completely (Hanington, 1923–24; Van den Branden, 1923; Chesterman, 1924; Fontana, 1924; Letonturier, de Marqueissac and Jamot, 1924; Walravens, 1925; Dye, 1926; Kellersberger, 1926; Maclean, 1926; Strada and Lopes, 1927; Corson, 1931). In early cases the response is often excellent and in some instances apparently lasting, but in advanced cases with definite involvement of the nervous system it is agreed by most observers that the drug is not to be favorably compared with tryparsamide in its ability to produce either physical or spinal fluid improvement. Kleine (1931), however, still maintains that of all the drugs he has used in East Africa, none is so good as Bayer-Fourneau, and that the superiority claimed for tryparsamide in West Africa is due to the fact that the virulence of the disease lessens as one travels westward. However this may be, a number of observers feel that Bayer-Fourneau *is* a more valuable drug in early *T. rhodesiense* cases than its rival, tryparsamide.

Bayer-Fourneau "fastness" occurs just as this phenomenon is sometimes manifested against the arsenicals.

Dosage.—The drug is usually given intravenously but may also be given intramuscularly; it is a white powder, easily soluble, and the solution can be sterilized. Perhaps the most usual practice has been to give five or six injections of 1 Gm. each at intervals of one week, but other schemes are latterly being favored in which larger amounts are given in a shorter time; for instance, 1.5 Gm. on the first, second and fourth days, or 2 Gm. on alternate days for three doses. Kleine now advises three to five injections, the first two at intervals of one or two days, the remainder at eight-day intervals. He states that when trypanosomes then reappear and remain in the blood a change to tartar emetic should be made.

Toxicity.—Practically all cases develop albuminuria with casts and sometimes blood; anuria has been observed. These symptoms nearly always disappear when treatment is discontinued. A number of observers have reported an erythematous rash immediately after injection, accompanied by pruritus and later desquamation. Purulent conjunctivitis and stomatitis have also been recorded.

Fourneau-270 (Orsanine).—This arsenical, developed by the French investigators in 1923, is the sodium salt of 4-acetylamino-2-hydroxyphenylarsinic acid. After a number of preliminary studies, its status has now been pretty well determined (Sicé, 1930–31; Vaucel and Boisseau, 1931). Of 106 patients in the first stage of *T. gambiense* infection, 3.7 per cent had relapses, 2.8 per cent progressed to the nervous stage, and 33 per cent could not be followed up. Of 251 patients in the second stage of the disease, 3.5 per cent had blood relapses, 13.1 per cent progressed, 51.3 per cent had prolonged amelioration, in some instances apparently permanent, 14.3 per cent died, and 17.5 per cent were not followed up. These findings have so favorably impressed the physicians of the Pasteur Institute of Brazzaville that they now use Fourneau-270 by preference in all early cases, the relapse rate of 3.5 per cent being far superior to the 18 per cent rate which they have experienced with tryparsamide. In the second stage of the disease the superiority of tryparsamide is acknowledged, the French Sleeping Sickness Commission having recommended a single preliminary "sterilizing" injection of atoxyl.

Dosage.—The drug, which is a white powder, is readily soluble in water and can be given subcutaneously or intravenously (20 per cent solution). Weekly injections are given as with tryparsamide, the dose per injection ranging between 15 and 35 mg. per kilogram; the smaller doses are given in advanced cases where there is much wasting.

Toxicity.—Same as accompanies the use of tryparsamide (see p. 233).

Prophylaxis of Trypanosomiasis.—Fourche and Haveaux (1931) have repeated their earlier studies on prophylaxis and are more than ever persuaded that treatment should be given the healthy while the infected are being treated: Two injections each of either tryparsamide or Bayer-Fourneau are said to protect for six months. On the other hand, Vaucel and Salaün (1931) are still convinced that six injections of atoxyl still remain the best prophylactic treatment, though they are not sure that Fourneau-270 will not prove to be superior.

SOUTH AMERICAN TYPE (CHAGAS' DISEASE)

This type of trypanosomiasis is caused by *Trypanosoma cruzi*, which is conveyed from man to man by the bug, *Triatoma megista*. It is probable that the armadillo is the most frequent intermediate vertebrate host, though the opossum, bat, wood rat, monkey, and pet dog and squirrel are beginning to be incriminated. Whether the bug transmits both by its bite and through its feces is still a moot question; it attacks at night and principally about the face, remaining in hiding in the walls of the native huts during the day. Most of the cases of Chagas' disease have been seen in Brazil, but it has been diagnosed in other South American countries as well; latterly also on the Isthmus of Panama. The preliminary studies of Kofoid and Donat (1933) indicate that the infected insect vector exists in the southwestern United States, though naturally infected mammals have not yet been discovered in this region.

The acute form of the disease is usually seen in children. There is high continuous fever, anemia, enlargement of the thyroid, and a puffiness of the face, accompanied during the several weeks' duration of this stage by a gradual enlargement of the lymphatic glands and the spleen and liver; the organisms can be detected in the blood at this time. The chronic form of the disease, which may persist for many years in those who have survived the acute stage, has a diverse symptomatology. There are various cerebral and neurological manifestations and Chagas and Villela have recently described a type in which death was due to heart block or to cardiac syncope. The picture is doubtless confused in many cases by superimposed infections of the various sorts which abound in this pestilential region.

THERAPY

I know of nothing to describe. All trypanocidal drugs have failed.

TSUTSUGAMUSHI FEVER
(Japanese River Fever)

This disease, which is endemic in Formosa and in the island of Nippon, Japan, is caused by an unknown organism, probably one of the Rickettsia, which is conveyed by the bite of the mite *Trombidium akamushi*. It is characterized by severe headache, a papular eruption, necrosis of the sites of the bites together with surrounding adenitis, and a febrile course of two weeks or more. The mortality is very high, especially in the aged.

THERAPY

All forms of specific therapy, whether chemical or biological, have failed.

TUBERCULOSIS

Tuberculosis in man is caused by both the human and bovine strains of *Bacillus tuberculosis*, cases associated with the bovine organism being usually of the bone and gland rather than of the pulmonary type. Findings with carefully performed tests in recent years have challenged the earlier opinion that nearly 100 per cent of all human beings in civilized communities have been the victims of tuberculous infection by the time they reach adulthood, though incontestibly a large proportion has been so infected. And yet only a relatively small proportion of mankind develops the disease tuberculosis— an anomalous state of affairs for which there is no ready-made explanation at hand. Two rather diametrically opposed views are being principally championed at present: One, that active cases of the disease are due to the "lighting up" of the primary infection of which we have all been the victims; the other that active tuberculosis is the result of successful implantation when the causative organism attacks the body from without for the *second* time. Increasingly, the sharers of this latter viewpoint seem to be carrying the day. They hold that primary infection practically always heals by calcification and leaves as its principal mark an allergic state (positive tuberculin reaction) as evidence that a certain degree of immunity has been lost; reinfection, under proper conditions and dosage, then allows the organisms to produce the typical cavitation which does not calcify. It seems to me that the greatest weakness of this position lies in the rather vexing nonchalance with which the rule is laid down for the initial infection. Postpone your primary infection as long as possible, they say, for then when the organisms strike you in fulminant overwhelming mass at a later date they can never induce more than the allergic state. But suppose that I choose to have my primary infection as *early* as possible, thus insuring myself against that dreadful thing known as galloping consumption, which is probably due to secondary superinfection before the typical resolution of the primary infection has had time to take place, the result being a continuous destructive activity, rapid spread, and an early end? All hope of chronicity—the main hope of the tuberculous individual—is then gone. Perhaps the investigators in recent years have lunged a bit ahead of themselves—which is upon the whole a fine thing, for laggards blaze no trails. Nevertheless, a definite answer to this question must be had as soon as is humanly possible, for most enthusiastic antituberculosis organizations with huge sums of public moneys at their disposal are rather hectically campaigning all over the world for eradication of the disease. That will be a great day in the history of mankind on which we will be able at long last to tell these crusaders against the white plague precisely which of its strongholds they shall concentrate their lances upon. Meanwhile the decline in tuberculosis mortality, which began in the late eighteenth century, steadily continues, uninterrupted even by the present world-wide economic depression. The death rate in the registration area of the United States was about 62 per hundred thousand in 1931, about 60 in 1932; it should be about 30 per hundred thousand in 1940, according to Dublin, the statistician. At the beginning of the twentieth century, tuberculosis led the list of the causes of death, heart disease was third and cancer seventh; at present, heart disease has first place, cancer second and tuberculosis is sixth.

Tuberculosis is characterized clinically by alternating periods of symptomatic activity and quiescence. Rarely does a patient progress to cure or death in an uninterrupted march. All the tissues may be attacked by this disease, but the most usual types are pulmonary, lymphatic, laryngeal, peritoneal, intestinal, pleural, bone and joint, cerebrospinal, genito-urinary, and acute miliary. The pulmonary type of tuberculosis, which comprises the vast majority of cases, is characterized clinically by cough and expectoration, loss of weight and strength, hemoptysis, fever, night-sweats, *B. tuberculosis* in the sputum, and certain evidences of pulmonary disease elicited by physical and *x*-ray examination of the chest. Lymphatic involvement is evidenced by the cervical adenitis of children, adenitis of the bronchial lymph nodes, or adenitis of the mesenteric nodes, in which latter case, in addition the low-grade fever, emaciation and anemia, there will be abdominal distention and watery diarrhea. Peritoneal tuberculosis is characterized by fluid in the peritoneal cavity, often pocketed off by adhesions, or the reaction is fibrous with a resultant matting together of the intestines; cases are also seen in which the patient presents for the first time with an acute surgical abdomen. In ordinary pleurisy tuberculosis should always be suspected, especially if there is effusion. The cerebro-spinal type of the disease generally takes the form of meningitis. Tuberculosis of the kidneys, ureters, bladder or genital organs may sometimes appear to be primary, but careful general examination nearly always reveals a pulmonary involvement as well. In acute miliary tuberculosis there are one or more eruptions of large numbers of organisms into the blood stream, with a consequent establishment of the disease in a fulminating form in various parts of the body; the most frequent forms seen are the meningeal, typhoid and pulmonary; always the prognosis is extremely bad.

I have sought here only to indicate the diverse attacks of this insidious scourge; to attempt more in a work of this sort is unnecessary and would certainly be presumptuous. It is hoped that the reader will set himself to make a deep study of the many symptomatic manifestations of tuberculosis, for without a good working knowledge of this disease no man has a right to practice medicine in any of its branches.

THERAPY

"When we speak of the treatment of tuberculosis, especially pulmonary tuberculosis, we envisage sanatorium regimen, which is the basis of all treatment of the disease; practically every other form of therapy is being applied by its practitioners to patients who are undergoing institutional care or some analogous substitute." Thus Krause in 1926, and I wish the reader to understand that in what follows I am always presupposing "sanatorium regimen," whether it be practiced in the home or in the hospital. Absolute rest in bed during the febrile periods, perhaps to be carried to the point of complete postural rest at times, as advocated by Webb and his associates, and to be followed later by carefully graduated exercises; a sufficient dietary composed of nutritious and palatable foods; the treatment to be carried out as nearly as possible in the open air; such changes of climate and general environment as afford the best opportunity of "building" resistance; and skilled medical supervision at all times; these are the important factors before which the value of such drugs and biologicals as are described below pale into insignificance. Heliotherapy, long recognized to be valuable in the treatment of nonpulmonary types of the disease, now seems to be gaining a place for itself in the pulmonary and intestinal types as well. However, the indiscriminate ordering of patients to expose themselves to the sunlight, or to the artificially produced ultraviolet rays, is certainly to be condemned. Mayer (1932), in his special article under the auspices of the A. M. A. Council on Physical Therapy, says that in most forms of progressive acute tuberculosis light therapy is not indicated, as roentgen therapy is well known not to be; in his experience, intestinal tuberculosis is the exception. In bone and joint tuberculosis, orthopedic treatment with immobilization and traction is felt to be absolutely essential while light exposure is being employed; Lehman and Bartholomew (1932) find heliotherapy for some unexplained reason ineffective in knee joint involvement. Artificial pneumothorax, pneumoperitoneum, the use of massive quantities of antiseptic oil in the pleural cavity, thoracoplasty, and operations on the phrenic nerve have also an assured place, but it is, of course, not in order to describe these methods here; for the interested reader the following names have been added to the Bibliography at the end of the book: Davies, 1932 (all procedures); Irwin, 1931 (phrenic); Trudeau, 1932 (phrenic); Edwards, 1932 (pneumothorax, phrenic, thoracoplasty); Haight, 1932 (thoracoplasty); Dundee, 1932 (pneumothorax); Rubin, 1932 (pneumothorax); Matson, 1932 (oil); Dunham and Asbury, 1932 (thoracoplasty);

Van Allen, 1932 (phrenic); Hawes and Stone, 1932 (all procedures); Leslie, 1933 (all procedures); Wiener and Fishberg, 1933 (thoracoplasty).

I shall describe the use of such remedies as come within the province of this book under the heads of *specific* measures, *symptomatic* measures and *prophylactic* measures.

Specific Measures.—1. *Tuberculin.*—The bright hopes which followed Koch's announcement of this substance as a specific remedy in 1890 were soon followed by disappointment so deep that many men today regard any and all types of tuberculin as absolutely worthless, a position which cannot be so easily defended in view of the fact that *careful* users of the remedy in many lands have shown it to have a definite, if very limited place in therapy. It is certainly in no sense a specific remedy, though usually listed as such, and the number of cases in which it is indicated is certainly very small. Physicians who are not able or willing to make a special study of the treatment should never use tuberculin; the requisite guided experience cannot be gained from the pages of a text-book.

2. *Dreyer's Defatted Antigen.*—This vaccine is prepared by extracting tubercle bacilli with hot acetone after preliminary treatment with formalin. So far as I am aware the original claims which were made for this substance when it was introduced in 1923 have not been substantiated; indeed, the investigations of Bronfenbrenner and Straub, Feinblatt and Eggert, and Nevin, Bittman and Hazen have shown that it is never effective and may even be harmful in the prevention and treatment of tuberculosis in the laboratory. I know of no work showing it to be of value in the human.

3. *Sanocrysin.*—The use of heavy metals as specifics in the treatment of tuberculosis has always met with failure hitherto, nor is it at all certain that gold sodium thiosulphate, introduced as sanocrysin by Møllgaard and his associates in Denmark, is to be the exception. The unfortunate newspaper exploitation of this remedy when it was first introduced is in no wise chargeable to Møllgaard *et al.*, for that sacrosanct modern monstrosity, the "common man," must be served, and it were utopian to expect the public press to defeat its own ends by serving him intelligently even if it could; but I do believe that the following criticism of the work of the Danish scientists is legitimate and admissible:

(*a*) The original claims which were made for sanocrysin were that it is specific for *B. tuberculosis;* that the severe constitutional reactions which follow its use are due to the liberation of toxins from destroyed bacilli; and that these reactions can be combated by the use of an antiserum made by immunizing animals with an antigen of the Dreyer type. I do not think that these contentions have been upheld. Møllgaard claims that the drug inhibits growth of tubercle bacilli in a concentration of 1: 100,000, but five bovine and three human strains grew in a concentration of 1: 5000 in the hands of Bang, while Sweany and Wasick found that organisms that had been exposed to the drug in a concentration of 1: 2000 in bouillon cultures for three months still produced tuberculosis. And what of the reactions? Tuberculosis workers have long been familiar with these reactions which follow the use of all gold salts and have set them down to metal poisoning, to which tuberculous individuals seem particularly prone. At least the burden of proof that this is not so rests upon Møllgaard, who has himself warned against the use of sanocrysin in any individual previously treated with arsphenamine (arsenic). It has been stated, by Elliott, for instance, that this reaction is so specific that it may be employed in the diagnosis of tuberculosis in doubtful cases, but what is to be done with LeBlanc's series of 25 patients, *all* of whom experienced the typical reaction, though 2 of them at subsequent autopsy were found to have inoperable carcinoma without complicating tuberculosis and 4 of them nontuberculous bronchopneumonia? In the laboratory, McCluskey and Eichelberger found the reactions to occur in both normal and tuberculous dogs. Regarding the antiserum, I see no reason for believing that Møllgaard has succeeded in the production of such a substance by measures not essentially differing from those which have always failed in the hands of other investigators. I am not unaware that others in addition to Møllgaard—notably Faber, professor of medicine at the University of Copenhagen—have reported that this serum does specifically counteract the reactions, yet I do not see how we can overlook the assertion of Klemperer, who occupies a position of authority in the treatment of tuberculosis in Germany, that the use of the serum aggravated the condition of his patients who were suffering from reactions. Jessen also failed in his series of 20 cases, and Opitz and Kotzulla obtained no beneficial effects whatsoever in tuberculous guinea-pigs in whom tuberculin reactions had been induced.

(b) The preliminary animal experiments of the Danish workers are not at all convincing. Discussing this phase of Møllgaard's work, the Journal of the American Medical Association said editorially on February 14, 1925, " . . . tests were made of the effect of sanocrysin and serum in calves injected intravenously with bovine tubercle bacilli. Usually the treatment, *i. e.*, the intravenous injection of the drug, was begun in two or three weeks after the injection of the bacilli, and it was found possible 'to save the life of animals affected by even very grave miliary tuberculosis or tuberculous pneumonia and to render them in condition of clinical healing'; but it is only exceptional results that seem to warrant this statement. It is true that there was far less tuberculosis in the treated than in the control animals; but the experiments fall into so many small subgroups, each with only one control, that doubt inevitably rises as to the true significance of the outcome, especially as in some cases the treated animals were killed after a time, while in others they died spontaneously. Two apparently tuberculous monkeys [the diagnosis was based on a positive tuberculin test and the other evidences of their illness were not proved to be the result of infection with the tubercle bacillus—H. B.] were 'cured' by sanocrysin-serum treatment, but the sceptical reader will find himself in doubt as to the true nature of the clinical condition of these monkeys." Futhermore, Møllgaard's work has all been with cultures of *B. tuberculosis* of abnormally low virulence. Certainly a culture, from 50 to 60 mg. of which can be injected intravenously without killing a control animal in two months, cannot be called virulent. Bang, on the other hand, when using fresh cultures or pus from spontaneous tuberculosis of cattle, has never been able to obtain any curative action from sanocrysin.

Clinical Use.—Practically all of the workers, following the example of Permin, have deserted the use of the large doses originally advocated by Møllgaard, and are now bending their efforts, it seems, to the prevention of reactions—thus eliminating the necessity of using the antiserum which in the beginning was declared to be of so much importance in the treatment. Amberson, McMahon and Pinner (1931), who have reported the most carefully controlled and unbiased study to date, used the following dosage: Each patient was started with 0.1 Gm. of the drug, dissolved in 2 cc. of distilled water and injected intravenously; the drug was increased by 0.1 Gm. at each injection (four-day intervals) up to 0.3 Gm., then increased to 0.5 Gm., the larger doses being dissolved in 5 cc. of water. The 0.5-Gm. dose was then repeated until nine to fourteen injections had been given, reducing, postponing or omitting an injection when there was a suspicion of dangerous reaction. The total amounts per patient varied between 3.1 and 6.1 Gm. Bothersome, sometimes very serious, toxic effects are of frequent occurrence: skin rashes, neuritis, stomatitis and a variety of gastro-intestinal disturbances, ocular irritation, various evidences of liver and kidney damage.

I shall not make a statistical review of the results of this treatment, in the hands of many workers, because they do not convince one that the drug has any merit not possessed by tuberculin and obtainable by the use of tuberculin with far less risk of grave results to the patient; the especially interested reader will find a good working bibliography in the Lancet of December 19, 1931.

4. *Calcium.*—I know of no reason for the persistent belief of many physicians that calcium is of value in the treatment of tuberculosis. Like Maver and Wells, my search of the literature has failed to uncover any controlled experiments, whether performed in the clinic or laboratory, which offer any warrant for a continuance of this belief. It is true that Wersen fed calcium lactate to 20 children with tuberculous peribronchial lymph nodes, and believed that they showed greater general improvement and more fluoroscopical evidence of calcification of the nodes than did 20 untreated controls; but Gordon and Cantarow (1929), using parathyroid extract in 60 patients for from one to four months, were unable to confirm this finding. The latter workers gave 20 units of the extract every forty-eight hours, and 30 grains (2 Gm.) calcium lactate three times daily, to 14 of the patients for from one to six months; in some instances certain relief of signs and symptoms resulted, but constipation frequently became troublesome and patients with nonproductive cough were made worse. The old belief that the blood calcium of tuberculars is low is now known to have been based upon faulty chemistry of the early observers; in the late cachexia it is of course diminished, but so are many other substances at that time; however, in early and even moderately advanced cases it is no lower than in normal individuals, and since the normal amount of blood calcium is just about as much as the blood can carry, no amount of calcium lactate feeding can be expected to raise it very much. Even when large amounts of calcium chloride are injected intravenously, the blood calcium level is raised for only a relatively brief time. Nor is it apparent that there is an inability upon the part of the tubercular to utilize calcium. Certainly he can mobilize the element, for Kahn has stated, and Maver and Wells amply proved, that tuberculous tissues are much higher in calcium than normal tissues; also, we know that in cattle tuberculous lesions progress despite the fact that they show partial calcification at all stages. And if the checking of a tuberculous lesion depends upon the deposition therein of calcium, how are we to explain the very considerable existence of bone tuberculosis; how would the disease ever get started there? No, I hold with Wells, who believes that a human tubercle first becomes a quiescent mass of colloidal organic material before it becomes calcified—and therefore calcification is a matter of quite secondary importance since arrest of the lesion must first take place. May it not be that the mobilization of calcium which takes place in all tuberculous lesions, whether or not there is any deposition of calcium, is merely an evidence that nature is ready to wall off a process which she must first overcome in some other way? In the animal laboratory it has been shown that calcium does not influence the course of tuberculosis.

It is commonly believed that workers in lime dust are free from pulmonary tuberculosis, but I do not know of any careful investigations tending to show that this tradition is well founded in fact.

The use of calcium chloride in the treatment of intestinal tuberculosis is another matter: this therapeutic measure is discussed elsewhere (see p. 248).

5. *Cod Liver Oil.*—Despite the fact that cod liver oil has been used in the treatment of tuberculosis for about one hundred years, our knowledge

of its value is still largely based on clinical impressions. The reasons for this state of affairs are: (1) that the oil is so objectionable in odor and taste, and often so disturbing to the appetite, that not many patients can be induced to take it faithfully; (2) that such effects as it may have are usually not seen until it has been taken for a period of many months or even years; and (3) the fact that not even its most enthusiastic champions would urge its use to the exclusion of the sanatorium regimen, as adopted either in or out of a sanatorium. Evaluation under these circumstances is very difficult, and it is easy to understand how the drug has come to have its ardent detractors and equally ardent supporters. The former point to the fact that the oil is no longer so much used in sanatoriums as it was some years ago, while the latter point to the "before-and-after-taking" evidence of individual cases. And each side figuratively thumbs its nose at the other. Kirschner has recently set down the factors upon which he believes its value rests, as follows: "(*a*) Its large amount of unsaturated fatty acids permits it to be almost entirely absorbed and thus furnishes a large amount of fat food. (*b*) It promotes the absorption of other fats. (*c*) It limits respiratory ventilation. (*d*) It has a destructive action on the tubercle bacillus. (*e*) It has a large fat-soluble vitamin A content, several hundred times that found in butter. (*f*) It favors the absorption and deposit of calcium in the tissues." The studies of Kramer, Grayzel and Shear (1929), and Pattison (1930) show that it is the whole oil and not the content of vitamins A and D that is of value in the human; cod liver oil concentrates, viosterol, or viosterol-reinforced cod liver oil are therefore not to be used in tuberculosis. Certainly it has been shown by Williams and Forsyth that the oil is capable of destroying the acid-fastness of tubercle bacilli grown in its presence, while Campbell and Kieffer have found (1922) that tubercle bacilli grown on cod liver oil media for six weeks are not able to grow when transplanted or to produce tuberculosis; cotton seed oil, used for control, has not had this effect upon the bacilli. On the other hand, M. I. Smith, in carefully conducted experiments, was unable to observe any good resulting from its employment in the treatment of induced tuberculosis in guinea-pigs.

The oil is best given two hours after a meal in a daily dose of 1 to 3 ounces (32 to 96 cc.). Many individuals who are unable to take the distasteful substance in the beginning may be trained up to it by starting with very small doses. If both the oil and the spoon in which it is taken are kept on ice the odor is much lessened. Block has called attention to the fact that the eating of a banana immediately after swallowing the oil is most effective in overcoming the objectionable taste and odor and in preventing loss by vomiting. The following preparations have been found acceptable for New and Nonofficial Remedies (1933): Borchert's: Malt Extract With Cod Liver Oil. Maltine Co.: Maltine with Cod Liver Oil, Maltine with Cod Liver Oil and Iron Iodide. Squibb: Cod Liver Oil, Mint-Flavored Cod Liver Oil; Meads Newfoundland Cod Liver Oil (Flavored and Unflavored). Nason's Palatable Cod Liver Oil. Parke, Davis: Cod Liver Oil, Malt Extract with Cod Liver Oil, Soluble Gelatine Capsules—contents, 10 minims, 20 minims, 2.5 Gm., 5 Gm. Patch's Flavored Cod Liver Oil. Scott and Bowne: Norwegian Cod Liver Oil (Flavored and Unflavored), Emulsion of Cod Liver Oil. The U.S.P. emulsion, and the emulsions with malt and egg of the N.F., are potent and satisfactorily flavored; the N.F. emulsion with hypophosphites is unnecessary.

The following prescription is a satisfactory working model for the writing of an emulsion, the rules being that there shall be at least one fourth as much acacia as oil to be emulsified and that the flavoring syrup shall not exceed 10 per cent of the total.

16·

℞.   Cod liver oil.. ℥iv   120.0
      Acacia.. ℥j   30.0
      Syrup of thyme... ℥vj   24.0
      Water to make.. ℥viij   240.0
      Label: One or more teaspoonfuls as directed.

Simple syrup might be substituted for syrup of thyme and flavoring accomplished by addition of 0.4 per cent (of the whole) of the oil of peppermint, spearmint, lemon, orange or almond.

The following formula for an aromatic oil is contained in the Pharmaceutical Recipe Book (1929):

      Gluside.. 0.5
      Compound spirit of orange................................... 20.0
      Cod liver oil to make....................................... 1000.0

6. *Iodine.*—In view of the considerable divergence of opinion in regard to the place of iodine in the management of tuberculosis, it is surprising that the past few years, which have been rather more than less productive along specific chemotherapeutic lines, have brought us no nearer a resolution of this question. It is of course generally recognized that iodine is often productive of an increase in the chest signs and in the amount of expectoration, and that it may cause the appearance of tubercle bacilli in a previously negative sputum, but as to the advisability of reserving the drug for use only as a diagnostic aid in doubtful cases, or of employing it in larger doses for whatever therapeutic virtues it may possess, I know of nothing to write. Expressions of opinion, there are many: some to the effect that large doses of iodides are of value, perhaps a larger number that just the reverse is true. I know of no authoritative clinical studies, with controls, that are worth citing. In the treatment of induced tuberculosis in the laboratory the drug has not shown itself to be of any value.

7. *Creosote and Guaiacol.*—Creosote was first recommended for use in tuberculosis in 1830 but did not become popular until the latter part of the century. Here again we have a drug whose use has persisted though there are no controlled clinical studies definitely fixing its value as a specific; the animal work, as reviewed by DeWitt, Suyenaga and Wells, also shows it to have a very low bactericidal power for the tubercle bacillus both *in vivo* and *in vitro.* Those who use it feel that it lessens expectoration, cough, fever and night-sweats, and improves the appetite, physical signs and general condition in early cases. That it definitely checks the associated bronchitis in some cases seems to be undoubted; but unfortunately it oftentimes upsets the digestion, always a serious thing in tuberculosis. The following is the type of prescription in which the drug is given:

℞.   Creosote (beechwood)... gtts. vi   0.4
      Glycerin... ℥j   32.0
      Peppermint water (or plain water) to make.................... ℥iij   96.0
      Label: Two teaspoonfuls every two to four hours, well diluted.

This prescription contains a very small amount of the drug, but when it is finished the next should contain double this quantity, *i. e.,* 12 drops. The creosote should then gradually be increased to the point of tolerance, which means that there is some indigestion, the appetite is lost, or perhaps some intestinal disturbance may occur. The dose is then reduced to the amount that the patient well tolerates, and is then best given directly after meals, three times daily. When the larger doses are being given, the urine should be frequently examined for albumin, or for signs of phenol poisoning, and if the kidneys are at all disturbed or the urine is abnormal, the creosote should be at once stopped. Creosote carbonate is sometimes substituted in doses twice or thrice the size (Creosotal-Winthrop is an N.N.R. brand but the drug is U.S.P.).

Creosote is also sometimes simply administered by dropping it into a half glass of milk or in extemporaneously filled capsules. It is claimed for the proprietary remedy, calcreose, that it does not readily produce gastric distress, nausea and vomiting. New and Nonofficial Remedies (1933) has this to say: "There is some evidence to indicate that by the use of Calcreose, relatively large quantities of creosote may be administered, but it appears probable that such tolerance is due to the slower absorption and excretion and therefore decreased efficiency. That the creosote contained in Calcreose is liberated in the body is evident from the fact that during its elimination by the kidneys it has produced albuminuria and phenol urine." The drug is used in the form of 4-grain (0.25 Gm.) tablets every two to four hours and built up to tolerance, or solution calcreose, the beginning dose of which is 1 drachm (4 cc.), or Compound Syrup of Calcreose, 1 to 2 drachms (4 to 8 cc.). New and Nonofficial Remedies (1933) also includes Proposote (creosote phenylpropionate) capsules, commercially available in 5- and 10-minim sizes; dosage, up to 10 minims (0.6 cc.), one to three times daily.

In advanced cases it is said that the inhalation of creosote will promote expectoration, lessen laryngeal dryness, and thus relieve cough. The inhalant mixture described under Catarrhal Fever (see p. 30) may well be used.

Guaiacol itself is very toxic and very objectionable in taste, also its use in large doses is said to cause the appearance in the urine of a viscous substance thought to be capable of obstructing the uriniferous tubules. The ester, guaiacol carbonate, is free from these objections; it has a maximum dose of 15 grains (1 Gm.); Duotal is an N.N.R. brand. Thiocol-Roche (potassium guaiacol sulphonate) shares the advantages of guaiacol carbonate over guaiacol itself, but "the guaiacol is so firmly bound that almost none is split off when the salt is administered, and it is questionable whether its action is due to small quantities of guaiacol set free or to the guaiacol-sulphonic group as a whole."—N.N.R. (1933). This potassium guaiacol-sulphonate is very similar to sodium phenolsulphonate, which has been omitted from U.S.P. X because of its very slight value. Thiocol-Roche is given in a dose of 5 to 20 grains (0.32 to 1.3 Gm.), either in tablets of 5 grains each or in the form of the syrup which contains 6 grains to the drachm. Guaiacol benzoate (Benzosol of N.N.R.) is also claimed to be nonirritating; it has a dosage of 3 to 10 grains (0.2 to 0.6 Gm.), in powder, capsule or pill, or suspended in liquids or as an emulsion.

8. *Sodium Morrhuate, Spengler Treatment, Spahlinger Treatment.*— The first two of the three methods listed were scientific and open, though unsuccessful and discarded, attempts at specific therapy; the last, that of Spahlinger, does not seem to me to be sponsored by a man who is particularly zealous to share his remedies for the benefit of medicine and mankind. Sir Frederick Menzies, health officer of the London County Council, has said, "From the information available there is no evidence which would at present justify the trial of this vaccine, under the auspices of the Council, on human beings."

9. *The Sauerbruch, Hermannsdorfer, Gerson Diets.*—These diets have been evolved in an effort to change the nature of the soil in which the tubercle bacillus grows, and are so complex as to exclude their use from all save those institutions in which expert dietary supervision is possible. The essentials are the following: (a) Practically complete exclusion of sodium chloride and the substitution therefor of a sodium-poor but calcium-rich salt compound; (b) a large percentage of uncooked fresh vegetables (ex-

tracts by pressing, or salads with added fruit juices similarly prepared); (*c*) vegetables cooked (steamed) in their own juices in waterless cookers; (*d*) marked restriction of meats; (*e*) rich fat and protein but low carbohydrate elements; (*f*) restricted water intake but fairly liberal amounts of freshly expressed juices of fruits and vegetables; (*g*) spices for seasoning. The differences in the diets are shown in Table 29 (Mayer, 1931).

TABLE 29.—COMPARISON OF SUGGESTED DIETS FOR TUBERCULOUS PATIENTS

	Gerson diet.	Hermannsdorfer-Sauerbruch diet.
Proteins.....................	About 55 to 67 Gm. daily	About 90 to 120 Gm. daily
80 per cent Animal	Meat.....100 Gm. weekly	600 Gm. weekly
20 per cent Vegetable	Fish...... 70 Gm. weekly	About the same
	Viscera....None	Rather freely permitted
	(sweetbreads, etc.)	
	Legumes..None	Permitted
Fats.......................	About 170 Gm. daily	About 170 Gm. daily
	Cream....None	About 250 cc.
	Eggs......Yolks only	Whole egg
Carbohydrates..............	Total—250 Gm. carbohydrates given daily	
	Sugar..... 20 Gm. weekly	About the same amount
	Honey.... 50 Gm. weekly	About the same amount
Fluids.....................	1400 cc. vegetable juices; fruit juices 600 cc.	Restricted vegetable and fruit juices; about 2½ pints in form of milk, cream, soup, juices, etc.
	Milk......250 cc.	About 1000 cc.
	Soup......None	
Sodium chloride............	About 1.56 Gm. in food	
	About 1.15 Gm. in juices	
	About 2.7 Gm. of sodium chloride intake daily	
	Ratio of protein to fat to carbohydrate is about 1 to 5.6 to 3.4	Ratio of protein to fat to carbohydrate is about 1.5 to 2.7 to 3.7
Aim.......................	Dehydration of tissues and altering body's mineral metabolism. Rich in fat, vitamins, and minerals (perhaps protein). Poor in salt and carbohydrate. Vegetables steamed; much raw food given, with cod liver oil with phosphorus, and mineral compound (chiefly calcium). Calories: 21 to 22 calories per pound of body weight; 2770 or 3030 if patient weighs 132 pounds (60 Kg.). In Hermannsdorfer diet, calories furnished are 15 per cent by protein, 53 per cent by fat, and 32 per cent by carbohydrates.	

I think that there is considerable reason to wonder whether the great stir that has been made by these diets on the Continent, particularly that of Gerson which has been very well publicized, is not really a tempest in a teapot. Certainly not even the most enthusiastic supporters of this therapy are in agreement as to which particular factor is the important one: we hear that such diets acidify, and also that they alkalize; that they desiccate the tissues, and also that the tissues undergo hydration. Can one disregard the temptation to reject altogether the existence of a scientific basis for the employment of the method? So far as I can gain any disinterested understanding of the many German reports, a large number of which are quite violent in support or denunciation, it seems that in lupus vulgaris, and occasionally in bone and joint tuberculosis, the treatment is to some extent effective, but that in pulmonary cases its value is by no means determined. Hermannsdorfer includes among his successes patients who did not respond favorably under one and one-half to two and one-half years—what of those other elements in modern treatment, rest and fresh air.

which they were also enjoying? Ziegler (1931) asserts most emphatically that the treatment is being given up in the sanatoriums almost without exception, apparently, in some instances at least, because Gerson's findings are more convincing to himself than to others. Certainly it requires active imagination to find any very valuable supporting evidences in the three American reports: Mayer and Kugelmass, 1929; Mayer, 1931; Banyai, 1931.

Symptomatic Measures.—1. *Fever and Night-sweats.*—Under the sanatorium regimen which is being presupposed throughout this entire discussion, these two symptoms usually do not persist in aggravated form long enough to warrant a resort to drugs in their correction. However, when the former is felt to be excessively wasting the patient by its daily high rise it is nearly always possible to forestall it by the use of 5 to 10 grains (0.32 to 0.65 Gm.) of aspirin or phenacetin, or 5 grains (0.32 Gm.) of pyramidon. The latter symptom is more difficult to treat. The sweating can oftentimes be prevented by the use of atropine sulphate in a dose of 1/200 to 1/100 grain (0.00032 to 0.00065 Gm.), but frequently at the price of an increase in cough and restlessness; also agaricin may be used in ½-grain (0.032 Gm.) doses in pill or capsule, not to exceed three of which should be given in the twenty-four hours, but this drug is extremely unreliable in its action. Hare wrote enthusiastically of camphoric acid, as follows:

"In a large number of cases suffering from night-sweats the author has found this drug to act very favorably indeed where other remedies failed, and he has never seen it produce unfavorable symptoms.

"It may be given in a dose of from 20 to 30 grains (1.3 to 2 Gm.), taken an hour or two before the sweat is expected. In very obstinate cases as much as 60 grains (4 Gm.) should be given, but under these circumstances it should be used in two separate doses of 30 grains (2 Gm.) each, two hours apart, to avoid irritating the stomach. It is best given in capsule or cachet, as it is insoluble in water. In other instances camphoric acid may be given in the following formula [which is transposed into the English form of prescription writing used in this book—H. B.]:

"℞. Camphoric acid.................................... ℥iv   16.0
     Alcohol... ℥ij   60.0
     Mucilage of acacia................................ ℥iij   90.0
     Syrup of orange to make.......................... ℥vj   180.0
     Label: Dessertspoonful (8.0) to a tablespoonful (16.0) one hour before
        sweat is expected."

An alcohol rub at bedtime, or a sponge bath with tepid water to which has been added 15 grains (1 Gm.) of alum per ounce, is also sometimes effective in preventing mild sweats.

2. *Cough.*—Here again, as in the case of fever and night-sweats, the rest, which is so important a part of the sanatorium regimen, is the most valuable remedy of all. Many patients succeed in training themselves to control this symptom remarkably well, only permitting themselves to indulge in a thorough "cleaning-out" cough in the morning; but when a wracking cough is disturbing the rest of the patient both night and day, some attempt must be made to check it. The reader is referred to the discussion of cough in the article on Catarrhal Fever (see p. 26), and also to the use of creosote in tuberculosis (see p. 242) in this present article.

3. *Hemorrhage.*—The patient must of course be kept as quiet as possible with the head propped in such way that the blood will easily flow out of the mouth. It is a time-honored custom to place an ice-bag on the chest over the suspected site of the hemorrhage and to restrict the diet to cold dishes and drinks. The use of sandbags on the chest and against the side is sometimes resorted to in an attempt to accomplish partial immobilization.

It is certainly well to prevent straining at stool by giving a cathartic and to insure easy passage of the feces on several succeeding days by the use of enemas or rectal instillations of oil. The attempt to lower the blood pressure by the use of amyl nitrite or nitroglycerin (see p. 562) is occasionally successful, but should be resorted to only if the patient is not in shock.

For a full discussion of the treatment of gross hemorrhage, see page 425; the necessary modifications required here will suggest themselves. In patients who have a long period of blood-spitting after the subsidence of the acute hemorrhage, Gordon, Roark and Lewis have found it of advantage to inject 10 units of parathyroid extract every second day for two or three weeks. In similar conditions, Solis-Cohen and Githens recommend hydrastis. The dose of hydrastimine hydrochloride, the preferred preparation, is ½ grain (0.03 Gm.) in pill or capsule three times daily; hypodermically ¼ grain in 10 per cent solution.

In instances of seriously persisting bleeding, a tourniquet may be applied on the thigh—near the inguinal region and gradually released after thirty to sixty minutes; sometimes blood transfusion, artifical pneumothorax, or the major surgical procedures must be resorted to.

4. *Care of the Digestion.*—This is extremely important for the majority of sufferers from pulmonary tuberculosis have some form of indigestion; it is best accomplished by enjoining slow and thorough mastication and complete rest both before and after meals. Sodium bicarbonate in a dose of 15 grains (1 Gm.), or ½ drachm (2 cc.) of the aromatic spirits of ammonia, the former dissolved in warm but not hot water and the latter to be well diluted before taking, will usually dispose of postprandial distress; or, if these fail, the opposite treatment with dilute hydrochloric acid in a dose of 15 minims (1 cc.) may be indicated. It is extremely doubtful whether pepsin or pancreatin are of any value here. Such simple remedies as the drinking of a little hot water before meals or placing an ice-bag on the abdomen will often relieve nausea. If there is vomiting and much distress during the day an evening lavage of the stomach using preferably the duodenal tube, may give relief for the night. To stimulate a lagging appetite any one of the following excellent U.S.P. stomachic mixtures, with a dose of one teaspoonful before meals, is of value: Compound Tincure of Cardamom, Compound Tincture of Gentian, Compound Tincture of Cinchona; or the Tincture of Nux Vomica in a dose of 15 minims (1 cc.). Also "tonic" mixtures should not be overlooked; arsenic is of especial value as an appetite stimulator. Some such capsule as the following may be used for a short time:

℞.   Arsenic trioxide....................................... gr. ½   0.03
     Extract of nux vomica............................. gr. v   0.32
     Quinine sulphate.................................... ℥ ½   2.0
     Make 40 capsules.
     Label: One, later two, capsules three times daily after meals.

The full tonic dose is contained in two capsules, but the precaution of giving only one for the first day will make possible early detection of quinine idiosyncrasy.

5. *Pleuritic Pain.*—The pain accompanying pleuritic inflammation is oftentimes very severe and greatly retards the patient's progress. A few cases will respond favorably to counterirritants: two of the small mustard plasters obtainable at drug stores should be used end to end under the arm, so that one extends toward the nipple region in front and the other over the lower part of the scapula behind. In an unfortunately large number of cases, however, it is necessary to resort to opiates. Swetlow, in 1926, reported in detail on 5 cases in which he had succeeded in relieving the pain

by the injection of 80 per cent alcohol into the intercostal nerves close to where they emerge.

6. *Laryngeal Pain.*—For the relief of the excruciating pain which often accompanies deglutition in tuberculosis of the larynx, cocaine is used in a spray of 1 to 4 per cent; this is always to be considered dangerous, however. Orthoform, which is an insoluble anesthetic, may be blown into the larynx, but Lockard prefers to use it in the form of an emulsion. He gives the following formula:

Orthoform	12 parts
Menthol	1 part
Almond oil	30 parts
Yolk of egg	25 parts
Water to make	100 parts

This emulsion is too heavy for use in an atomizer, but it can be self-administered by the patient using a Yankauer laryngeal medicator. Iodoform is also frequently used by insufflation, but a small amount of talcum must be added to give weight to the otherwise too light powder. The drug seems to be antiseptic in its own peculiar way and somewhat anesthetic, though it is wise to precede the insufflation with a spray of cocaine to prevent coughing. A number of writers advise the addition of morphine to the powder mixture; Hare used $\frac{1}{16}$ grain (0.004 Gm.) to each drachm of iodoform. Another mixture sometimes successfully used is known as Lake's pigment, the formula of which is:

Lactic acid	50.0
Solution of formaldehyde	7.0
Phenol	10.0
Water to make	100.0

The phenol in this preparation acts as an anodyne but it is usually necessary to precede the first few applications with cocaine. Ulcers and granulations may also be touched with 5 to 10 per cent formalin in glycerin, preceded with a cocaine spray.

Lukens (1922) has stated that the local application of chaulmoogra oil, without preliminary cocainization, exerts an analgesic action on the larynx which becomes more complete after repeated treatments. His report was based on the study of 60 cases over a period of eight months; the final method is here quoted:

"Chaulmoogra oil works best by intratracheal and intralaryngeal injection. One cubic centimeter of the oil, of the strength desired, usually 10 or 20 per cent in liquid petrolatum or olive oil, is drawn up in a Luer syringe armed with a metal eustachian catheter. While the patient holds the tip of the tongue, wrapped in a paper napkin, between the index finger and the thumb of the right hand, the syringe tip is introduced, guided by the throat mirror, into the pharynx (not the larynx) above and behind the epiglottis, care being taken not to touch any portion of the mouth or throat. Two thirds of the contents of the syringe is discharged, drop by drop, into the trachea while the patient breathes quietly. The remainder is then dropped on the cords while the patient phonates. In this way, cough following injection is very slight and often absent. When present, it occurs within five minutes after the injection and lasts for a minute or two."

Alloway and Lebensohn have in some measure confirmed Lukens in their series of 40 cases, and Van Poole had excellent results in 21 of 28 cases, but Peers and Shipman warn that the general condition of a febrile patient may possibly be made worse by these treatments. In experimental tuberculosis in animals, Voegtlin, Smith and Johnson found chaulmoogra oil to have no value, as did also Kolmer, Davis and Jager.

Galvanocautery and various surgical measures sometimes give gratifying results in the hands of qualified experts.

Here is a tremendously practical point which Dundas-Grant (1932) has called to the attention of the profession: "I wish, however, to indicate a cause of what patients call 'pain,' the relief from which is anxiously desired. In reality it is a painful 'burning' stiffness of the pharynx caused by the drying and inspissation of mucus on the back wall, and is experienced chiefly on waking. Patients have frequently described the discomfort as severe pain and have been delighted to have it removed by gargling with a little bicarbonate of soda in water, warm if possible, otherwise cold. Such a solution can be put into a thermos-flask at night so as to be ready for use when the patient wakes up. I am sure that this condition is overlooked while deeper-lying sources of pain are being sought for. It seems a trifling method of treatment, but it gives great relief and is, of course, available to any practitioner if he only keeps the condition in mind and looks for it."

7. *Intestinal Symptoms.*—Until the appearance of Saxtorph's report, in 1918, on the use of calcium chloride as a palliative agent in the treatment of intestinal tuberculosis, we were practically helpless in the presence of the severe abdominal pain, exhausting diarrhea and tenesmus suffered by patients who are the victims of this type of the disease—whose number, by the way, would seem to be between 30 and 50 per cent of all those having advanced active tuberculosis. The value of light therapy, more recently recognized, has been pointed out on page 237. The various astringents are of little or no value, and dietetic treatment, even when faithfully persisted in, succeeds only exceptionally—unless the excellent results reported by McConkey, 1929, are to be confirmed: ½ ounce (15 cc.) of cod liver oil is floated on 3 ounces (90 cc.) tomato juice in a small glass, the dose taken ice cold immediately after each of the regular full hospital meals. The opiates are, of course, somewhat effective, but they must be used in very large doses and when they are intermitted the symptoms are oftentimes much aggravated. In calcium chloride, however, we have a really valuable addition to our armamentarium. It is usually given intravenously in a dose of 5 cc. of a 5 per cent solution (sterilized in the autoclave) at intervals of three to seven days; this dose may be repeated as long as necessary, it would seem. In Robert's series of 70 cases, published in the United States in 1924, there was relief of symptoms in 80 per cent; not complete relief, but "sufficient to make life much more bearable and cheerful for these men." Fishberg has this to say of the treatment:

"When the diarrhea in a tuberculous patient is due to dietetic indiscretions, to the catarrhal condition of the intestinal mucous membrane, or to slight intestinal ulceration, an intravenous injection of 5 cc. of a 5 per cent solution of calcium chloride will give prompt relief. When, however, the intestinal symptoms are due to extensive ulcerations—especially to amyloid infiltration of the intestine—the chances of attaining relief of the pain and annoying diarrhea are remote. Similarly, when the abdominal pains are due to irritation of the intestinal mucous membrane by the contents of the intestine, relief may be attained by intravenous injection of calcium chloride. When, however, the pains are due to localized peritonitis over deep intestinal ulcers, or to peritoneal adhesions, which are not uncommon in tuberculous subjects, calcium chloride is impotent to give relief."

Cantarow says that good results may be obtained in less urgent cases by giving calcium by the mouth, avoiding the irritating chloride: calcium gluconate, 60 grains (4 Gm.), calcium lactate, 30 grains (2 Gm.), or aromatic chalk powder, 30 to 60 grains (2 to 4 Gm.), three or four times daily.

8. *Terminal Opiates.*—In the terminal stages of many cases the suffering is very severe. Here the opiates in full doses are oftentimes truly a godsend for they enable us to make the last days of these poor unfortunates much less terrible than they would otherwise be. However, the question of expediency often arises, for opium many times prolongs life in such patients.

Psychotherapy.—There is so much talk nowadays of the great value of this method—as though it were *new*, indeed!—that I fear some of us are beginning to believe all of it. For my own part, I know not a few persons who revolt temperamentally against the sort of planned cheerfulness that is current. Perhaps the reader may feel that they are then almost certain to die if they come down with tuberculosis—and it may be that they are!

PROPHYLAXIS

Calmette's BCG.—During the past few years the medical world has been much interested in the attempt of Calmette and his associates at the Pasteur Institute of Paris to prevent the development of tuberculosis in the newborn by inoculating them by the mouth with cultures of living bovine bacilli that have been attenuated by growing them for years on bile potato media, it being claimed that these organisms are still capable of stimulating antibody production though they have lost their power to produce the disease either in a general or local form. The aim is not to produce permanent immunity but only to support the child's reactions during the period when natural immunization is taking place. Calmette says that in France the tuberculosis mortality between one month and the end of the fourth year is 15.9 per cent in unvaccinated children born to tuberculous mothers or raised in tuberculous environment, while it is only 3.4 per cent among a similar group vaccinated with BCG. There have now been about 400,000 infants vaccinated in France and over a million in the entire world. However, even such an array of figures is not entirely satisfactory, for the difficulty of obtaining absolutely satisfactory control conditions is very great. Bernard; Biraud; Blanc; Keller; Malvoz and Van Beneden; Moine; Ott; Rougebief; and Weill-Halle and Turpin have supported Calmette's position, but such competent statisticians as Greenwood; Rosenfeld; Báron; Götzl; von Berghaus; and Blümel have sharply attacked it not only upon technical statistical grounds but also by pointing out the inherent dangers of fallacy lying in the fact that infants receiving any special prophylactic treatment are likely, even though unwittingly, to be given better care than they would otherwise have received. Calmette admits that his organism is capable of producing lesions in the animal body and that it can be recovered from these lesions, but denies that it can develop into active centers of tuberculosis or that it is capable of setting up progressive tuberculosis on reinoculation into fresh animals. The chief supporters here are Lange and Clauberg; Kühn; Okell and Parish; Jensen, Morch and Orskov; Remlinger and Bailly; King and Park; Wilbert; Gerlach and Kraus; and Griffith. The chief opponent, and a most able one, has been Petroff of the Trudeau Sanatorium, whose results have been checked by Park. He has differentiated "rough" (avirulent) and "smooth" (virulent) colonies in cultures, which strongly indicates that a return to virulence on the part of the BCG strain is not impossible; Watson; Nohlen; Schlossmann; Armengol; Chiari, Nobel and Sole; Galli-Valeria; Hutyra; Moti Malkini; Petroff, Branch and Steenken; Lignières; Löwenstein; Dreyer and Vollum; Begbie; and Much have in the main supported these findings. Wallgren observes that the amount of BCG absorbed by the oral route is uncertain, and that a tuberculin reaction is the only evidence that vaccination has taken place. Disregarding the Lübeck disaster, fatalities among BCG-vaccinated children have been reported by Baigue; Chennard and Ferrier; Girod and Debarge; Heynsius van den Bergh; Munoverro; Nobecourt; Pirquet; Saye, Domingo and Miralbell; Taillens; Weill-Halle and Turpin; and Jaso. It now seems to be established that the culture sent from Paris to Lübeck, where during three months in 1930–31 there were 68 fatalities in vaccinated infants, was not virulent; however, something happened to the culture in Lübeck, and whether or not that something was that it was merely subjected to careless handling in the laboratory, is not yet definitely determined, and probably never will be.

In France, and in portions of some of the other Continental countries, the vaccination continues to be performed upon a large scale, but in England and America we shall probably persist in an attitude of reticence in the matter until we can somehow assure ourselves (*a*) that there are no risks in this method which cannot be guarded against by such precautions as are possible under the conditions of preparation and administration of the vaccine; (*b*) that the danger of tuberculous infection in infants is great enough to justify the taking of certain risks in attempting to combat it; and (*c*) that the BCG vaccine, under proper safeguards (whatever they may finally prove to be), does actually accomplish what is claimed for it by Calmette. The especially interested physician should read the late Prof. Calmette's reply to Sir George Buchanan, in the Lancet of March 25, 1933, in which both sides of the question are aired.

TULAREMIA

(Rabbit Fever)

Tularemia is an infectious disease of wild rabbits, squirrels, mice, rats, muskrats, woodchucks, opossums, game birds and doubtless many other animals; cats, coyotes, cattle and sheep are already partially convicted. Originally considered to be confined to the United States, it is now recognized that tularemia is probably world-wide in its distribution. Human beings sometimes contract this malady while dressing the carcass of infected animals, or through the bite of one of the several flies, ticks and mites which act as vectors, and perhaps also through ingestion of the insufficiently cooked flesh of infected animals. The causative organism, *Bacillus tularense,* was discovered by McCoy and Chapin in 1912, but the disease in man has been definitely known to be caused by the same organism only since the work of Francis in 1919. The onset is sudden, with chills and fever, pains all over the body, vomiting and prostration. The fever lasts for two or three weeks and is usually of the septic type, with marked daily remissions. In addition, there is pustulation and finally ulceration at the site of infection, and the glands draining the area become swollen and painful; sometimes they too break down. During the second week the serum agglutinates *B. tularense,* but Foshay (1932) has pointed out that the intradermal test may be positive a week earlier. Death is rare but convalescence is usually a matter of months. In laboratory-contracted cases the local and glandular symptoms are absent, probably because the organism is ingested in these instances; a pulmonary type of the disease, without the other typical signs, is also beginning to be recognized.

THERAPY

There is really nothing to describe as no satisfactory treatment has been evolved as yet, though Foshay's (1932) antiserum, prepared from inoculated goats, is of good promise. His preliminary report described the intravenous injection of 10 cc. on the first and second days; in 9 of the 10 cases, abrupt subsidence of symptoms followed the second injection. Reports of successful treatment with quinine, the intravenously injected dyes, etc., are still very scattered. Convalescent serum has not been of value. The usual palliative measures are of course indicated.

TYPHOID AND PARATYPHOID FEVERS
(Enteric Fever)

Typhoid and paratyphoid fevers are acute infectious diseases caused by *Bacillus typhosus* and *B. paratyphosus A* and *B*. They are unquestionably separate diseases since an attack of any one of the three does not confer immunity against the other two, a fact which is also true in regard to artificial immunization; nevertheless, they will not be considered as separate clinical entities in this book for the reason that in their symptomatology (save for the relative mildness of the paratyphoids) and their therapeutics they are one and the same. Serologically and bacteriologically they can be distinguished the one from the other; at the bedside this differentiation can never be made with certainty. I shall discuss the three under the single designation "typhoid fever."

In typhoid fever the attack is essentially upon the lymphoid tissues of the body, being especially marked by enlargement of the spleen and hyperplasia and ulceration of the Peyer's patches in the intestine. The majority of those who fall ill of this disease are between the ages of fifteen and thirty. There is usually a prodromal period of about a week, during which there is malaise, headache, loss of appetite, and pains all over the body; then the patient goes to bed and the attack is looked upon as definitely established. The fever is considered to be typical in that it rises to its peak—which may be as high as 105 or 106 F.—by the end of the first week, remains at this level for a variable period but usually one to two weeks, and then falls gradually during a length of time which is usually twice as great as that required for it to rise; throughout the entire course of the fever there are daily morning remissions of one or more degrees. It should be remarked that there are many variations from this typical fever picture. The pulse, too, is characteristic in that it is much slower than one would be led to expect by the height of the temperature and nearly always contains at some time a dicrotic wave. At about the end of the first week the so-called "rose spots" appear, usually only on the abdomen, in crops of ten or twelve. Though present at some time during the course of perhaps 95 per cent of cases it is nevertheless certain that true typhoid does occur without the appearance of these spots; I shall never forget a young practitioner who dramatically renounced a medical career because in one of his early cases a consultant overbore him by diagnosing typhoid fever *without* rose spots. The blood pressure is low throughout the attack. The tongue is clean and red around the border, including the tip, and heavily furred in the center. Nosebleed and bronchitis are frequent early symptoms. Distention of the abdomen practically from the beginning is regarded as very characteristic of typhoid, but with the more ample diet now in vogue this symptom is not so regularly seen. Constipation is the rule; when diarrhea occurs it is usually of the "pea-soup" variety. Delirium, usually of a canny rather than a violent type, is frequent. Prostration is always great, and in severe cases progresses to the state of stupor known as the "typhoid state," during which the patient lies in a low muttering delirium, eyes open and staring, and hands ceaselessly pulling at the bedclothes. The progressive secondary anemia, so common in typhoid, is not so severe nowadays as it was during the era of starvation treatment. At the height of the disease there is nearly always a leukopenia. The specific agglutination of the organisms by the patient's serum is of diagnostic importance, but the worth of this Widal reaction is considerably lessened by the frequency with which it is negative until as late as the third week. The bacilli are themselves present in the blood during the first week; after that they appear in the stools and often in the urine as well.

The principal complications of typhoid fever are intestinal hemorrhage and perforation, pneumonia, venous thrombosis, and ulcerative laryngitis. Relapses, in which all the symptoms reappear after a brief asymptomatic period, are frequent; they are usually less severe and of shorter duration than the initial attack. The mortality from typhoid is now about 10 per cent under the best conditions. Perhaps 50 per cent of the fatalities are due to toxemia, 15 per cent to perforation and subsequent peritonitis, 10 per cent to hemorrhage, and 10 per cent to pneumonia.

Although typhoid fever is undoubtedly a very old disease, it was not definitely differentiated from typhus until the early part of the nineteenth century. The belief was formerly held that certain parts of the tropical portions of the globe were free from the disease, but more careful studies of the fevers prevailing in these regions have shown them to be the same typhoid which ravages the rest of the world. The human body is the only natural habitat of the causative organisms and all cases are caused by contact with the feces or urine of an infected individual, whether he be actively infected or a "carrier." This contact may be direct or indirect: through a contaminated water or milk or ice-cream supply, by the ingestion of food over which flies have dragged their infected filth, or the eating of oysters which have been infected in their feeding or fattening beds, or even through the medium of ingested dust—this latter method of infection was held responsible for many of the cases in the British army during the Boer War. Being a filth-borne disease it is to be expected that modern sanitation would have greatly lessened its incidence, and so it has; indeed, the decrease in typhoid in this present century is one of the things of which medical sanitary science has most reason to be proud. But we have still far to go, especially here in North America. Data are available for seventy-eight large cities in the United States, which in 1910 had a population of 22,-573,435 and in 1932 an estimated population of 35,691,815. Despite this population increase of over twelve million, the actual number of typhoid deaths fell from 4637 in 1910 to 442 in 1932, and the rates per hundred thousand of population from 20.54 to 1.24. Many major cities now have rates below 1, but the average for the whole United States is still somewhat below that of England for the reason that typhoid is still a major problem in the South. Some of our most able public health officials are laboring in that section, yet such cities as New Orleans, Atlanta and Memphis had the shockingly high rates of 8.6, 8.8 and 11.4, respectively, in 1932; this, however, marked a considerable improvement over the rates of 35.6, 58.4 and 35.3, respectively, in 1910.

There seem to be certain years in which the disease is more generally prevalent than in other years. In the United States, 1913, 1921, and 1925 were such "typhoid years." The incidence of the disease increases after

June to a peak in late fall and early winter. Typhoid fever is by no means the "thing of the past" that it is unfortunately represented to be in some quarters. How this pestilence is lurking about all great cities, ready to swoop down upon the inhabitants when the guard is the least bit relaxed, was amply shown in the Montreal epidemic of the spring and summer of 1927. In a certain portion of this city of approximately a million inhabitants, during a considerable period of time, and for reasons which need not concern us here, the raw milk from a district outside the city in which sanitary conditions were unsatisfactory was allowed to be distributed without being adequately pasteurized. The result was that there developed in the city, between the approximate dates of March 1st and September 1st, a total of 5014 cases of typhoid, 500 of which terminated in death.

THERAPY

Typhoid fever has greatly changed in my time—which is an astonishing thing since no specific remedy has been added to the typhoid armamentarium. But changed it has, for I well remember that during my childhood, which was spent in a large city in Kentucky, it was quite as usual for a number of relatives and acquaintances to be hovering about the edge of one's consciousness as gaunt and tottering specters who were "recovering" from typhoid, as it was for all of us to be dosed with quinine during a part of each year. I was twice attacked by the disease (typhoid or paratyphoid? Widals were only beginning to be done then) in my youth, and twice, though neither attack was very severe, I had to "learn all over" to walk again. Where are the convalescent ataxics of yesteryear? And why are we so seldom able to show to our students of today the wasted individual with grotesquely protuberant abdomen, exhausting himself in hallucinatory delirium, or worse still, lying in the low distressing "typhoid state"? Perhaps the organism is becoming less virulent or mass immunity is being built up, but I believe that the true answer lies in the changed attitude toward diet in the treatment of this dread disease. All of which is but a verbose preamble to the following statement: *the introduction of the full diet in the therapeutics of typhoid fever is the greatest contribution of all time toward the control of the malady.* The mind at once leaps to the question, how has it affected mortality? This is of course very difficult to answer statistically, though the studies of Warren Coleman and others seem quite convincing, but it is the almost unanimous clinical impression that full feeding has had much to do with the reduction in the death rate which has occurred in the last few years. Certainly the severity of the symptoms is greatly lessened: extreme tympanites is unusual, and when it occurs can often be overcome by a proper adjustment of the diet; diarrhea often yields in the same way and constipation, on the other hand, is less stubborn because there is actually considerable food residue present to be propelled through the bowel; both delirium and stupor are modified; bed sores are practically a thing of the past; anemia is scarcely ever so profound as on the starvation diet; and what is best of all, the patient leaves the bed very little more wasted than he entered it, thus tremendously reducing the period of convalescence. And if it cannot be proved that the high calorie diet has reduced the incidence of hemorrhage and perforation, it certainly cannot be proved that it has increased it either. Relapses seem to be more frequent, however, under the new treatment.

Proper feeding, then, is the most important element in the treatment of typhoid fever. Indeed, the old difficulty of devising means of reconciling the patient to the exclusive milk diet which was imposed under the old régime has given way to a diametrically opposed problem, namely, that of getting as much food into him as it is now considered desirable for him to take. Four thousand calories per day is perhaps the optimum amount if we are entirely to prevent loss of protein from the tissues, but it is almost impossible for any but convalescent patients to accomplish the daily consumption of this much food; 3000 calories, however, should be possible with skilful nursing. While it is certainly not within the province of this book to discuss dietetics in any great detail, I cannot refrain from appending here one of Coleman's diet lists which will furnish this amount of calories in a day (Table 30):

TABLE 30.—TYPHOID DIET WHICH WILL FURNISH 3000 CALORIES

Breakfast.	Calories.
Farina (4 tablespoonfuls, cooked)....	100
Toast (1 slice, 30 Gm. before toasting)	80
Cream, 100 cc. (3½ ounces) 20 per cent which is approximately the same as the top 4 inches from a quart bottle of milk that has stood at least six hours.........................	200
Butter, 8 Gm......................	60
Lactose, 40 Gm. (1⅓ ounces) To add lactose to milk, boil 15 Gm. in 30 cc. of water: cool and add to milk..	160
Sugar, 20 Gm......................	80
Coffee, 1 large cup................	00

10 to 10.30 A. M.	
Milk, 200 cc. (6⅔ ounces)..........	140
Cream, 50 cc. (1⅔ ounces)..........	100

Dinner.	
Eggs, 2...........................	150
Potato, 1 medium, about...........	100
Bread, 1 slice, or roll, 1............	80
Butter, 30 Gm. (1 ounce)..........	234
Apple, 1 medium sized (pared and cored)........................	75
Sugar, 15 Gm. (½ ounce)..........	60
(Potato baked, served with butter. Apple baked with 15 Gm. sugar and about 8 Gm. butter. Some patients will eat more butter if the unsalted is used.)	

3 to 4 P. M.	Calories.
Tea, 150–200 cc....................	00
Lactose, 50 Gm. (1⅔ ounces)........	200
Sugar, 5 Gm......................	20
Cream, 50 cc. (1⅔ ounces).........	100
Crackers, 3 Uneeda or 2 soda, toasted	75
Butter, 8 Gm.....................	62

Supper.	
Rice, 25 Gm. (1 ounce), boiled......	100
Milk, 100 cc. (3⅓ ounces)..........	70
Toast, 30 Gm. (1 slice)............	80
Butter, 8 Gm.....................	62
Sugar, 5 Gm. (for cereal)...........	20
Cream, 60 cc. (2 ounces)...........	120
Orange, 1 sliced...................	100
Sugar, 5 Gm. (with orange).........	20

8 to 9 P. M.	
Cocoa, 5 Gm.....................	25
Sugar, 10 Gm....................	40
Milk, 150 cc. (5 ounces)...........	105
Cream, 30 cc. (1 ounce)..........	60
Lactose, 25 Gm..................	100

Of course it is not necessary to accurately determine the quantity of calories; the idea is to get as many into the patient as possible. Simple diarrheas will usually respond to an adjustment of the amount of cream (fat) allowed; sometimes the lactose has also to be reduced. It is well to bear in mind that if a patient has aversion for particular foods when well he will continue to dislike them when ill. Some patients cannot tolerate milk in any form or amount. For such, Garton has devised a diet which, according to Wisart, Johantgen and Clarke, is used in the University of Michigan Hospital in the form given in Table 31.

Care of Mouth and Skin.—The tongue and mouth tend to become very foul, and the lips cracked and sore, in typhoid fever. The teeth should be kept well brushed and the mouth washed at sufficient intervals with the

TABLE 31.—TYPHOID DIET WITHOUT MILK

6.30 A. M. Cup of hot coffee, sugar, 2 drachms (8 Gm.); 2 slices of zwieback or toast, butter.

8.30 A. M. One portion of oatmeal or Robinson's prepared barley, with six buttered crackers, saltines.

10.30 A. M. 6 ounces of soup, various kinds (180 cc.).

12.30 P. M. 1 medium baked potato, mashed and prepared with butter and salt; two thin slices of buttered toast, hot, and 1 cup of hot weak tea with 2 drachms (8 Gm.) of sugar.

2.30 P. M. 2 teaspoonfuls of pudding, bread or tapioca; six saltines.

4.30 P. M. 2 ounces (60 Gm.) of rice, farina or cream of wheat mixed with 1 ounce (30 Gm.) of butter and 4 drachms (16 Gm.) of sugar.

6.30 P. M. 3 slices buttered toast.

8.30 P. M. 6 ounces (180 cc.) of soup.

N.F. alkaline aromatic solution; it is well to anoint the lips with glycerin and water. A daily cleansing bath with soap and water should be given, to be followed by an alcohol rub; areas especially liable to the development of bed sores should have alcohol applied to them several times daily and be kept well powdered in the interim. These things have a double purpose, first, they make for the greater comfort of the patient and serve the ends of ordinary cleanliness, and second, they serve to keep up the morale of the patient; to this latter end he should be encouraged to actively participate in the daily routine procedures as much as is possible consistently with the avoidance of fatigue.

Control of Temperature.—The new tendency in the therapy of all acute fevers is to look upon the rise in temperature as a physiologic process and to direct no drug treatment toward its reduction, and undoubtedly many lives have been thus saved; but I cannot hold with the extremists who would totally disregard all antipyretic measures. External hydrotherapy seems to me a wholly rational and nondangerous measure; not the Brand bath, nor perhaps even any of its modifications, but tepid sponge baths when the temperature reaches 102.5 to 103 F., and a carefully applied cold pack (the patient to be placed on two blankets which are doubled lengthwise of the bed under his body, then quickly enveloped to include the arms in a sheet which has been wrung out of cold water, and thoroughly wrapped round with the blankets which are brought up from each side and over-lapped) when the temperature becomes excessively high. We were formerly allowed to believe that this shock, with the warm glow which subsequently spreads over the body, acts as a tonic to the circulatory apparatus; now there are those who cavil even at this, but for my own part I still believe that these packs are "stimulant."

Fluids.—As in all acute infectious diseases, fluids should be pushed. Most patients will take lemon- or orangeade when they rebel at plain water. When the patient's interest cannot be sufficiently aroused to ensure the taking of sufficient fluids by mouth resort should be had to hypodermo-clysis or protoclysis with physiologic saline solution.

Care of the Bowels.—If the patient is seen early, *i. e.*, before there is any likelihood of intestinal ulceration having already occurred, there is no reason why a dose of 2 or 3 grains (0.13 or 0.195 Gm.) of calomel should not be given, followed in a few hours by one of the milder salines, such as a Seidlitz powder, but I believe that most students of the disease are nowadays opposed to all dosing with cathartics after this time. Typhoid fever most certainly cannot be "flushed out of the system," and it would therefore seem, with the ever-present danger of perforation, that we are well advised to leave the peristalsis stimulators out of the picture. On the full diet treatment, a small soapsuds, or better still physiologic saline, enema at a regular time each morning accomplishes the daily evacuation of the rectum, and what more is needed? Many men have relinquished the old favorite, castor oil, but use instead cascara sagrada frequently throughout the course of the disease; however, even this mild emodin cathartic may at times violently stimulate peristalsis. Liquid petrolatum has enjoyed some vogue of late, but I believe it will soon be recognized that whatever good may accrue from the employment of this intestinal lubricant is more than counterbalanced by the increased dissemination of the bacilli incident upon the constant leakage of the oil from the rectum.

Diarrhea.—On the full feeding regimen diarrhea is seldom a prominent symptom and when it does occur usually yields to a careful readjustment in the cream and lactose portions of the diet; when it persists, resort is usually had to the tannins or to bismuth. Acetyltannic acid (tannigen) may be given in a dose of 3 to 10 grains (0.2 to 0.6 Gm.), four times per day, taken dry on the tongue followed by a swallow of water, or mixed with food, avoiding warm or alkaline liquids. Protan is given in 5-grain (0.3 Gm.) tablets, from two to six of which may be given at intervals of two hours or more. Albumin tannate (albutannin or tannalbin) must be given in doses of 30 grains (2 Gm.) or more, in capsules or as a powder. For the employment of bismuth the following is a satisfactory prescription:

R. Bismuth subcarbonate............................. ʒj   30.0
    Glycerin.. ʒss   15.0
    Syrup of ginger to make........................... ℥iv   120.0
    Label: 1 teaspoonful every two hours for ten doses.
    "Shake."

It is well to avoid the use of opiates in typhoid if possible for the reason that meteorism is likely to follow their withdrawal.

Tympanites.—When this symptom does not yield to dietary adjustment it should be treated as described in the discussion of Pneumonia (see p. 131), though of course resort must never be had to pituitrin as there mentioned.

Delirium.—Dissuasion is the best sedative in the treatment of typhoid delirium, but it must be painstakingly and tirelessly employed. When resort to drugs becomes necessary the soluble form of diethylbarbituric acid, soluble barbital (veronal sodium) should be used in aqueous solution in a dose of 5 to 10 grains (0.3 to 0.6 Gm.). The following is also a useful sedative prescription, which is not to be used carelessly, however:

R. Sodium bromide.................................... ʒvij   28.0
    Chloral hydrate................................... ʒvij   28.0
    Peppermint water to make.......................... ℥iv   120.0
    Label: 1 teaspoonful in water every three or four hours.

In rare cases nowadays is it necessary to apply a restraining sheet, though its more frequent use in the muttering, restless, but not actively delirious, state of severe cases would doubtless save much of the patient's strength. How many of our doctors know how to effectively restrain a patient's movements in the bed?

Circulation.—There is a firmly entrenched clinical impression (and doubtless a correct one) that there is a certain amount of myocardial degeneration during the height of the attack in a rather large number of cases. When there is an apparent loss of strength in both the pulse wave at the wrist and the first sound of the heart, resort to stimulants would seem to be indicated even though pulse rate and blood pressure changes have not appeared. Digitalis is of little use here and camphor is of very doubtful efficacy; strychnine, in a dose of $\frac{1}{20}$ to $\frac{1}{10}$ grain (0.003 to 0.006 Gm.) of the sulphate in a tablet every three hours, may have some ability to increase the vascular tonus though it does not raise the blood pressure (see p. 135). Caffeine definitely improves the tone of the heart and increases the pulse rate, but the improvement in the circulation, though undeniable, is unfortunately not constant. Caffeine citrate may be used in a dose of 5 grains (0.32 Gm.) in a large amount of water, or caffeine sodium benzoate in a like dose; this latter salt is suitable for hypodermic use. The drug may be repeated several times during the day but the doubtful possibility of a slight irritation of the kidney should be borne in mind. Alcohol has long been felt to be the drug *par excellence* to bolster up the circulation in typhoid fever. There are some dissentient voices but I believe most students of the disease favor its use. Coleman writes as follows:

"The widespread denunciation of the use of alcohol as a circulatory stimulant makes it necessary for the writer to state briefly the reasons for his continued faith in it. The case against alcohol is based mainly, if not entirely, on the fact that it does not raise arterial blood pressure. Therefore, it is concluded, alcohol cannot be a 'cardiac' stimulant. In the writer's opinion such a conclusion is not warranted by the facts. Measurements of the arterial blood pressure effects of a remedy are not a complete test of its action upon the circulation. For example, while digitalis is restoring broken compensation, it may not only fail to raise blood pressure, but may actually lower it. Further, the conclusion with respect to alcohol is vitiated by the fact that it fails entirely to take into consideration the rôle of the vessels, both arteries and veins, in maintaining the circulation. A single illustration of the rôle of the vessels will suffice. Yandell Henderson has shown that a reduction of the CO_2 content of the blood (acapnia) is followed by marked circulatory depression, without impairment of the power of the heart or fall (usually) in arterial pressure. The venous pressure does fall, however (venodepressor effect), the blood stagnates in the capillaries, and the venous return to the heart is diminished, it may be, with fatal results. A remedy which restores the venous pressure (increased CO_2 tension, for example) may not act as a 'cardiac' stimulant and raise arterial pressure, but surely it must be considered a circulatory stimulant under the conditions stated.

"The above-mentioned facts are not intended as an exposition of the physiological action of alcohol on the circulation. They do, however, deprive the argument that alcohol cannot be a circulatory stimulant because it does not raise arterial pressure of its force; they also redistribute the burden of its proof. The writer's opinion is based entirely on clinical observation; he believes that alcohol improves the circulation in typhoid fever, and that a favorable change may be detected in the *quality and often the rate of the pulse after its administration.*

"Alcohol may be administered in the form of whiskey or brandy, though champagne and other wines may be used. Whiskey should be given in doses of ½ to 1 ounce three or four times a day, or as often as every two hours. It may be administered in water, soda-water, lemonade or milk, though generally speaking it is not advisable to add it to foods. Alcohol is not only valuable as a circulatory stimulant but possesses important food value."

Vaccine Treatment.—The subcutaneous or intravenous use of vaccines in the active treatment of typhoid fever has been pretty generally given up because the production of the rather violent foreign protein reaction necessary to obtain a good result was felt to be an unwarrantably severe procedure. Several recent reports have focused attention upon the use of the vaccines by mouth. Melnotte and Farjot report the treatment of a series of cases during a severe epidemic in Fez, Morocco, in 1926. Their vaccine was given in daily adult doses of 200 cc. in water between feedings and appar-

17

ently very favorably influenced the course of the disease. The average mortality in the stricken area was 26 per cent; they had only 10 deaths among their 210 vaccine treated cases, all of which were severe. Alissow and Morozkin treated 50 cases with Besredka's vaccine by mouth during an epidemic in Smolensk in 1925 and 1926. They gave 60 to 100 billion organisms for three or four consecutive days and had a mortality of 4 per cent as compared with 15.2 per cent in those not treated with vaccine.

Bacteriophage.—Use of the bacteriophage by Rutschko and Melnik (1932) in 69 cases did not definitely prove that the course of the disease was essentially altered by this agent.

Hemorrhage.—1. Keep the patient absolutely quiet by the use of morphine sulphate ⅛ to ¼ grain (0.008 to 0.015 Gm.) every three or four hours; this will also splint the bowel.

2. Withhold all food, and nearly all water, until the bleeding has apparently stopped.

3. Apply continuous cold to the abdomen.

4. If it seems desirable to attempt to increase the coagulability of the blood, resort should be had to calcium—see the treatment of gastric hemorrhage, page 425.

Perforation.—Surgical intervention as soon as the diagnosis is made—which is easy to write but difficult of accomplishment for the reason that the diagnosis is oftentimes extremely hard to arrive at and very often a surgeon *with the skill here needed* is not at hand.

Venous Thrombosis.—Keep the leg at rest on a pillow and apply heat or cold.

Tonics.—Iron, arsenic and strychnine are profitably given during convalescence in nearly all cases of typhoid. Some such prescription as the following may be used for a short time:

℞.			
	Arsenic trioxide	gr. ½	0.03
	Extract of nux vomica	gr. v	0.32
	Reduced iron	gr. xxx	2.00
	Make 20 capsules.		
	Label: One capsule three times daily after meals.		

PROPHYLAXIS

The prevention of typhoid fever groups itself into three subdivisions, in addition to those measures in public health sanitation which are so largely responsible for the reduction in the incidence of the disease in recent years: (*a*) The care of the patient, (*b*) treatment of the "carrier," and (*c*) preventive inoculation.

(*a*) **Care of the Patient.**—Everything and everybody coming in contact with the typhoid patient should be considered potentially contaminated. Of course subsequent sterilization of all these objects and persons is a practical impossibility, but it may be approximated by maintaining a state of the most absolute cleanliness in the room or ward, by screening out and exterminating flies, by insisting that the attendants frequently change their clothing and wash and disinfect their hands, and by frequently changing the patient's clothing and bed linen. All clothing and bed linen are to be boiled thoroughly after each use. The patient is to have individual dishes, which are to be boiled after each use. It is doubtful to what extent thorough disinfection of the feces and urine is accomplished, but any one of the following substances should be added to, and thoroughly mixed with, the contents of the bed pan and urinal before it is emptied into the toilet or privy; chloride of lime solution (½ pound to the gallon of water will make a satisfactory solution provided the lime contains enough chlorine to markedly irritate

the eyes when brought near the face; otherwise much more must be used);
5 per cent phenol solution; 5 per cent compound cresol solution; 5 per cent
solution of sodium hypochlorite (antiformin). The odor and irritating
properties of formaldehyde are too great to make its use practicable. When
the urinal and bed pan are not in use one of these solutions, or a 1:1000
solution of bichloride of mercury, should be allowed to stand in it; in
some hospitals it is possible to completely sterilize these articles with live
steam, a thing not possible of course in the home.

(b) **Treatment of the "Carrier."**—This "carrier" problem is a tremendous one which still resists satisfactory solution. About the best that we
can do to date is train the individual in personal hygiene and prevent his
engaging in the food-handling vocations. I know of no drugs or biologicals
worth describing in the treatment of the condition, though the use of tetra-
iodophenolphthalein intravenously as in cholecystography (Onodera, Wa
and Liu, 1931) is interesting. Cholecystectomy, for the removal of "nests"
of bacilli in the gallbladder, is apparently coming into some favor again:
Vogelsong and Haaland (1931) reported 19 definite cures in 25 operated
cases; Senftner and Coughlin (1933) 35 in 53 cases (there were 8 deaths in
the series); Swenson (1933) 9 in 13 cases (3 deaths); Bigelow and Anderson (1933) 12 successes in 12 cases.

(c) **Preventive Inoculation.**—The late World War conclusively proved
the worth of prophylactic vaccination against typhoid and paratyphoid
fevers. During the period of the participation of the United States in the
war, April, 1917, to November, 1919, four million men served in the army.
Regarding the ravages of typhoid fever in this host, the Surgeon General's
report for the year 1919, page 47, contained this statement: "With the
same admission rates for typhoid fever in 1917–1918 as in 1861–1862, there
would have been 226,001 cases and 62,694 deaths; as it was, there were
1083 cases and 158 deaths." Testimony of this sort was unanimous among
the allied armies, but it is strange to note that Germany dissented. A
review of the literature by Banus, however, indicates that German scepticism arose from the inefficiency of the vaccine and the faulty methods
used. Experience in civilian life all over the world since the war has
firmly established typhoid prophylactic inoculation as one of the triumphs
of modern medical science.

The vaccines in use today vary somewhat in the details of their preparation and content, but the following description, from the 1933 N.N.R., of
one of the commercially available preparations is indicative of their general
nature: A suspension in physiologic solution of sodium chloride, containing
0.3 per cent of cresol. Marketed in packages of 5 and 20 cc. vials, each
cubic centimeter containing 500 million each killed paratyphoid A and B,
and 1000 million killed typhoid bacilli; in packages of three 1-cc. vials, one,
containing 250 million each killed paratyphoid A and B, and 500 million
killed typhoid bacilli, two, the second and third doses, containing 500
million each killed paratyphoid A and B, and 1000 million killed typhoid
bacilli; also marketed in hospital size packages of ten complete immuniza-
tions in ten vials, each vial containing a complete immunization.

The injections are made subcutaneously (*not* intramuscularly) in the
deltoid region at intervals of seven to ten days. There is always a local
reaction of some severity; if, for any reason, the abdomen has been chosen
for the injections a more painful reaction must be expected even than that
which occurs in the arm, and the reaction in the thigh is so severe as practically to contraindicate the use of this site. The general reaction, which
follows in six to ten hours after the injection, is characterized by chills and
fever, backache, headache, muscular pains, and in some cases nausea and
vomiting and even diarrhea. Most individuals experience some degree of

this reaction, which, however, lasts usually not more than twenty-four hours and can be minimized by remaining inactive after the injection. The development of a method of immunization by a single injection of a highly concentrated dose would be a welcome innovation; according to Malaret (1931), the thing has been effectively done in the Argentinian and Cuban armies and he is at present studying the possibilities of such inoculation among the natives employed by the United Fruit Company; he is injecting an average dose of 2500 million killed bacilli in the normal adult.

Pregnant women after the fifth month are usually not vaccinated, nor menstruating women, nor infants under two years; the dosage in children older than this should be adjusted accordingly as their weights vary from that of the average adult of twenty-five years. Lopez-Rizal, Arguelles and Lara, in Manila, have shown that nursing infants are immunized by vaccinating the mother. Regarding other contraindications, Russel writes: "No one with a temperature above normal should be vaccinated until the temperature has fallen and a normal state of health has been restored. Endocarditis, and particularly nephritis, are contraindications. Clovis and Mills and Brown, Heise, Petroff and Wilson have shown that patients with inactive tuberculosis may have typhoid fever, or antityphoid vaccination, without any detrimental effects on the pulmonary condition, and that patients with active tuberculosis may have typhoid fever or antityphoid immunization without a more rapid advance in their pulmonary condition than they would have had otherwise. The first authors also note that the pulmonary tuberculosis did not have any appreciable effect on the course of the typhoid fever."

Maximum protection is certainly had within two or at most three months but there is apparently some response within a few days, as indicated by study of the agglutinin titer of the serum. The advantageous use of the vaccine during the period of incubation of the disease has been reported. It is not as yet definitely known how long the immunity lasts, but it is believed to persist for at least two years in average cases. In recent years the oral route has been much used on the Continent and in South America. The results seem generally favorable. Cantacuzène and Panaitescu observed 16,534 persons at Morine, Roumania, from midsummer of 1924 to January 17, 1925. Subcutaneous inoculation was used in 8673, mouth inoculation in 2286, and no preventive treatment in 5575. Ninety-nine cases developed, of which 3 were in the subcutaneous group and 6 in the mouth group. This would seem to show a distinct advantage for the injection method, but other observers have shown a much smaller incidence for the mouth route. Guerner compared 63,000 persons who were vaccinated orally in São Paulo, Brazil, in 1925, with 10,000 vaccinated by injection. Of the 31 cases that developed, 20 were in the subcutaneous group and 10 in the mouth group; one had been vaccinated both ways. Inouye (1932) reports 1 case in 7980 persons vaccinated by mouth, 6 cases in 24,235 vaccinated by injection, and 377 in 328,159 not vaccinated at all.

TYPHUS FEVER

Typhus fever is an age-old decimator of the dirty majority of mankind, though it was not recognized as a clinical entity until the sixteenth century. It is a disease of the cooler portions of the earth, for the body louse, which transmits it from man to man, does not thrive in the tropical regions. The principal endemic foci are in the Balkan States, northern Italy, a number of spots in central Europe, Siberia, northern China, Ireland, and the high plateau lands of Mexico and northern Chile and Peru. Practically all the countries of the north temperate zone have had severe visitations of this disease; the typhus years in the United States were 1812, 1830, 1847, 1865, 1881, and 1893. Whenever large numbers of people, of whatever social status, are gathered together under conditions of poor personal hygiene, there the disease appears. All wars have felt its ravages except, it would seem, the Franco-Prussian and the Russo-Japanese. In the recent World War the French, British and American armies on the western front were practically typhus-free only because the Germans and Austrians, upon whom it laid a heavy hand from Russia, were fiercely fighting to keep it away from their front lines. Eastern Europe suffered heavily after the war, the mortality in the epidemics averaging 20 per cent, with a range of 5 to 70 per cent. The endemic Mexican variety of the disease, known as tabardillo, is perhaps less virulent upon the whole, though occasional local outbreaks in the United States, through importation, have had a high mortality. The unclassified *Rickettsia prowazeki* is probably the causative agent, though that one of Koch's postulates which requires that the organism be cultivated outside the body is not yet satisfied. Typhus is distinctly more prevalent during the winter months and increases in severity with the age of the patient. There is a distinctive microscopical pathology of the skin and central nervous system.

The disease, which usually has few prodromata, is characterized by a sudden chill and rise of temperature which is accompanied by nausea and vomiting and a headache; sometimes there are aching pains throughout the body also. The rise in temperature is accompanied by a proportional increase in pulse rate and in the severity of the headache, but the gastro-intestinal symptoms disappear early. The temperature often reaches 105 F. on the second or third day, where it remains with remarkably little daily remission until the close of the attack. On the fifth day a maculopapular rash appears which changes from pink to red and then purplish-brown, and rapidly involves all of the body except the face. On reaching full efflorescence, some of the spots become hemorrhagic and purpura appears irregularly. The patient experiences sleeplessness from the bginning, which gives way to wild delirium, and, in severe cases, the delirium passes into a state of "coma-vigil," in which the sufferer lies in a relaxed position though the body is usually trembling; the eyes are wide open and staring, there is a low muttering delirium, and a rapid thready pulse. There is usually a loose cough almost from the beginning. Small areas of spontaneous necrosis of the skin are not rare. The crisis is reached on the thirteenth or fourteenth day, after which there is a rapid disappearance of all symptoms. The two complications chiefly to be feared are secondary broncho-pneumonia and thrombosis of the large vessels.

The Weil-Felix agglutination test is of not very great value as a diagnostic aid for the reason that it unfortunately does not become positive until the rash has appeared.

The endemic type of the disease (known as Brill's disease), which prevails in the eastern and southern United States and has its highest incidence in the summer, is a much milder affair having a mortality of less than 1 per cent. The recent final proof, brought by Dyer and his associates of the U. S. Public Health Service, that the rat flee transmits American typhus is a vindication of Brill, who always felt that the louse did not serve as vector of this form of the disease. It is very likely that cases in the tropics, where the louse does not thrive, are also conveyed by flees, mites or ticks.

THERAPY

The patient should be given plenty of easily digestible food and much fluid for he is facing a sledge-hammer type of toxic attack which quickly batters thin his reserve of stored energy. The mouth must be kept clean else it becomes very foul and an easy prey to secondary infection; liquor antisepticus of the N.F. is a good preparation to use for the purpose. Alcohol is just as valuable a stimulant in typhus as it is in typhoid fever; for a discussion of its use see page 257. For treatment of the cough see the article on Catarrhal Fever, page 26. All authorities agree that it is usually necessary and advisable to control the insomnia by the use of morphine. If this latter drug is not being used some less powerful analgesic will be indicated to control the headache: phenacetin (acetphenetidin) or pyramidon (amidopyrin), either one in a dose of 5 grains (0.32 Gm.).

There is no specific remedy in typhus fever, and indeed nothing has been shown to have greater value than simple rudimentary symptomatic treatment and good nursing. Of course the patient must be deloused at the very beginning of the attack and should be given a daily bath thereafter.

PROPHYLAXIS

This is entirely a matter of delousing in the classical form of the disease; for a description of the most effective measures, see page 685. Now that we know the vector of American typhus another reason is given us for unrelenting warfare upon the rat.

UNDULANT FEVER

(Malta Fever, Mediterranean Fever)

Undulant fever is an infectious disease caused by *Brucella melitensis*. This organism is harbored by goats, apparently without being harmful to these animals, is passed out in the urine and by external contamination enters the milk; the milk and milk products then infect the human. The disease is endemic and epidemic in the Mediterranean littoral and also occurs sporadically throughout the world, especially in the warmer climates. Home (1933) contends, very interestingly, that it was unknown in Malta until British troops in 1856, enroute home during the Crimean War brought it there from South Russia. Where prevalent, it is a difficult disease to stamp out for the reason that the goat is a profitable animal in these regions and the sterilization of its milk renders it decidedly objectionable in taste. Besides, the goat-herders in the rural districts refuse to believe that such a disease exists, perhaps because of their own immunity owing to a gradual vaccination.

Due to the increasing prevalence of the disease in the United States and other countries, where goat's milk as the carrier can be practically ruled out, recent search for some other organism capable of causing the disease has been rewarded by the discovery that *Brucella abortus,* the organism responsible for the infectious abortion of cattle, sheep and hogs, is also the etiologic agent in human undulant fever in many parts of the world. The disease is perhaps most frequently conveyed in infected and insufficiently pasteurized cow's milk, and may appear endemically or in epidemics. The extent of the human carrier problem is not yet known but it is recognized that there are many latent infections.

The symptoms closely resemble those of typhoid fever with catarrhal fever (influenza) engrafted upon it, *i. e.*, there are more respiratory and neuralgic symptoms than would be expected in typhoid; tularemia should also not be overlooked in the differential diagnosis. Arthritis and orchitis are frequent complications; undulant fever, spondylitis and also endocarditis have been reported. The mortality is usually low but in rare instances the disease is quite malignant. The course, even of mild cases, is very protracted. There are several laboratory procedures of assistance in making the diagnosis.

THERAPY

The symptomatic treatment at present can only be that of typhoid, catarrhal fever and acute arthritis.

Vaccines.—A number of observers have reported favorable results from the subcutaneous injection of either autgenous or stock vaccines (Bibliography: Goiny, Simpson, Harbinson, Miller, Angle, Helwig, Bassett-Smith, Cumston, deFinis, Guiffrè, Prausnitz, Cambessédès and Garnier, Shilling *et al.*). The stock vaccines (N.N.R.) are given at intervals of three to seven days for 3 or more doses.

Intravenous Dyes.—There are several reports in which the course of the attack seems to have been favorably influenced by the intravenous injection of acriflavine hydrochloride (Izar and Mastroeni, Darré and Laffaille, Hoffman, Thurber). Four doses of 0.1 Gm., 0.2 Gm., 0.3 Gm. and 0.4 Gm., respectively, are given at intervals of two or three days. A reaction of variable degree usually follows. Thurber (1930) starts an intravenous injection of warm saline; when this is running well he adds 20 cc. of saline containing the drug freshly dissolved, and continues the injection of 200 cc. of the solution at the rate of 5 cc. per minute.

None of the other dyes have been impressively reported upon, unless we include the oral and rectal administration of methyl violet and thionin by Leavell *et al.* (1930). One or the other of the dyes was given for a week at a time, from 1 to 8 salol coated pills (each containing 25 mg.) in the twenty-four hours. At the same time, a retention enema of 300 cc. of 1 : 25,000 to 1 : 100,000 of the dye was given daily following a soap suds enema. No untoward results followed and it was thought that improvement was observed in the 3 cases so treated.

Whole Blood Transfusion.—Quelvi and Nelson (1932) were very favorably impressed by their results with one or two transfusions by the usual method in 9 of their 10 cases. The blood was not taken from donors who had had the disease.

VINCENT'S ANGINA

(Fusospirillosis, Trench Mouth)

This is an acute infectious disease which seems to have been endemic throughout the world for a long time but was not forcibly brought to the attention of more than a few physicians and dentists until it became epidemic in the armies during the World War, since which time it has been recognized with increasing frequency among the civilian populations of all countries. It is primarily an affection of the tonsillar area and pharynx, the floor of the mouth, the gums about the teeth, and more rarely of the tongue, lips and cheeks. The mouth lesions are single or multiple small red areas which become gray sloughing patches and finally ulcerate and are covered with a yellowish-gray pseudomembrane; the latter is easily removed and displays a bleeding surface beneath, but it soon becomes covered over again.   The breath has nearly always a fetid odor and the interference with eating may be great due to the pain of chewing and swallowing, and there is often an adenitis, but only in exceptional cases are there any noticeable constitutional symptoms.   Note should be taken, however, of Goldman and Kully's (1933) report of 7 fatal cases in the Cincinnati General Hospital from 1929 through the first six months of 1932; in 6 of the cases there was very extensive ulceration which likely offered a portal of entry for other organisms; in the seventh case edema and sepsis played prominent rôles.

Pulmonary complications, often confused with pulmonary tuberculosis, are being recognized with increasing frequency; they may take the form of pulmonary gangrene or abscess, ulceration of the bronchi, lobar pneumonia, bronchopneumonia, or empyema; apparently the disease may also appear primarily in the lungs.   Infection of mucous membranes other than those of the respiratory passages, and recovery of the organisms from the parenchymatous organs has been reported numerous times.   The disease is caused by a spirillum and a fusiform bacillus, both of which are easily found in stained smears.   Whether these are pleomorphic forms of a single organism, or whether they are really two distinct organisms living in symbiosis, is still a moot point.

THERAPY

Sodium Perborate.—Bloodgood, whose mouth clinic at the Johns Hopkins Hospital has become well known, states that this drug will rapidly cure more than 95 per cent of cases, if properly applied.   He writes: "I would not have any difficulty in presenting at my weekly clinic one or more examples of sore mouth in which the cover slip examination revealed the organism of this disease predominating, and I would be able to present the same patients almost completely well at the next clinic, or within two weeks."   One is inclined to be just a little sceptical of such enthusiasm and to wonder what proportion of those patients would still be "cured" after the expiration of another interclinic period and another still.   However, since the Vincent organism is anaerobic, the use of sodium perborate, which liberates large amounts of oxygen, is rational; indeed, in the hands of all who have used it faithfully it seems to have given better results than anything else.   Bloodgood describes his method as follows:

"A thick paste of the chemically pure salt should be made with water and spread over all the teeth with the clean fingers.   If there are any red or ulcerated areas in spots not around the teeth, they should be treated in the same way.   The patient holds this paste in the mouth for about five minutes.   During this time it foams as a result of oxidation.   Then the mouth should be rinsed with warm water.   It is a mistake for the patients to do this themselves until they are thoroughly trained, and as a rule, by the time they are trained the lesion is cured.   If the treatment is too frequent it produces an irritation.

"When the entire oral cavity is involved, with extension to the fauces and pharynx, there must be, in addition, a gargling with a thinner solution [2 per cent] two or three times a day.   The more extensive the lesion and the more ulcerated the areas, the longer before the expected cure."

Sodium Perborate (or Hydrogen Peroxide) and Arsphenamine.— Barker, whose experience with the disease has been extensive, uses 2 drachms of sodium perborate to a tumblerful of water as a mouth wash, gargle or irrigation in early or slow healing cases, but in more active cases, especially in the throat, he substitutes one-half to full strength hydrogen peroxide.   In addition he applies arsphenamine locally after carefully washing off the oxidizing agent. A cotton-tipped applicator is moistened and dipped into the arsphenamine powder and the adhering particles are rubbed into the lesions, or the drug is applied in 10 per cent solution in glucose; he favors the use of the powder and describes the following method of getting it between the teeth:

"The application of arsphenamine in these spaces is accomplished with facility by taking pieces of coarse knitting wool about 2 inches long, moistening them with water, and dipping them in the powdered salvarsan. These bits of yarns are threaded between the teeth and sawed back and forth after the manner of dental floss, and are then allowed to remain in place for from fifteen minutes to half an hour."

The entire treatment, consisting of the cleansing with an oxidizing agent, the washing out of the oxidizing agent, and the rubbing in of the arsphenamine, should be employed two or three times daily in severe cases. If it is desired to use the arsphenamine in solution instead of powder, and the commercial solution in glucose is not to be had, a 10 per cent solution in glycerin (0.6 Gm. arsphenamine dissolved in 6 cc. glycerin) may be substituted. This solution does not deteriorate. No bad effects will follow swallowing of arsphenamine.

Arsphenamine Alone.—A number of writers have reported favorably on the use of arsphenamine alone, either applied locally or introduced intravenously, but it would not seem to be nearly so effective as when used in conjunction with an oxidizing agent (see above). Arsphenamine, or neoarsphenamine, is usually given intravenously in smaller doses than are employed in the treatment of syphilis. It should be noted that Vincent's angina has been known to appear and become quite severe in persons who were at the time undergoing routine intravenous arsenical treatment for syphilis.

In the pulmonary cases, any of the organic arsenicals are used as in the treatment of syphilis, with excellent results (Kline and Berger, 1925; Smith, 1930; Heffernan, 1932).

Bowman's Solution.—This is a mixture of wine of ipecac, ½ ounce (16 cc.), glycerin, 1 drachm (4 cc.), and solution of potassium arsenite to make 1 ounce (32 cc.). In mild cases this preparation seems to effect a cure if a few drops are used on a soft tooth-brush with thorough scrubbing several times a day, and in more severe cases it is good adjunct treatment. One has to be a bit careful with it, however, for some of the potassium arsenite solution (Fowler's solution) may be swallowed, or it is conceivable that quite large amounts of it might be absorbed through eroded surfaces.

Bismarsen.—Kolmer (1930) found that this drug aided materially in bringing 6 cases of unusual severity under control. He gave 0.2 Gm. (0.1 Gm. for children) intramuscularly every three to five days for a series of seven injections.

Miscellaneous Remedies.—Practically all the antiseptics and disinfectants have at one time or another been advocated for local use in this disease. Those which have had the greatest vogue are tincture of iodine, 10 per cent chromic acid, 10 per cent silver nitrate, 2 per cent zinc chloride, 1 per cent potassium permanganate, 2 per cent methylene blue, ST-37 solution, and potassium chlorate in saturated solution. The results obtained with none of these substances warrant special mention here.

Soap.—The careful studies of Reasoner and Gill (1927) have shown that solutions of ordinary toilet soaps, as well as pure soaps prepared in the laboratory, have a definite spirocheticidal effect, and that their use in dentrifices assists in keeping the oral cavity free from mouth spirochetes, thereby affording a measure of protection against tissue infection with the Vincent organisms.

WHOOPING COUGH
(Pertussis)

Whooping cough is an acute infectious disease which we now believe is possibly caused by the *Bordet-Gengou bacillus,* with which is usually associated large numbers of the *influenza bacillus* of Pfeiffer. It is highly communicable and is therefore principally seen in very young children; nearly 50 per cent of cases are in infants under two years of age. There is no distinctive gross or microscopical pathology and the disease is therefore looked upon as one which remains local throughout its course; but one attack confers lifelong immunity, which, as pointed out by Haynes and St. Lawrence, is a faculty rarely possessed by other than general systemic infections. There are a great many individuals who possess a natural immunity to the disease.

There is an incubation period of one to two weeks and then another week or two during which the symptoms are those of coryza and bronchitis with cough. Gradually during the latter part of this period the paroxysmal nature of this cough becomes apparent and clinical diagnosis becomes possible. The paroxysmal stage is characterized by a very distinctive group of symptoms: the patient usually clutches at something for support and then begins a series of rapid, short, loud coughs, during which the tongue is protruded from the mouth, the eyes water and become injected, and the face is suffused or deeply cyanotic, and at the end of which there is a deep inspiration through the narrowed glottis, which causes the "whooping" sound. In most cases there are several such attacks in quick succession, but they cease at once for the time being when a little mass of glairy mucus is brought up. There is often vomiting during the seizure and many times bleeding from the nose and other mucous membranes. The subconjunctival hemorrhages which occur are usually ascribed to the violence of the coughing. Altogether the attacks are a distressing thing to witness as well as to experience. Between paroxysms the patients, if old enough, are sufficiently undisturbed to engage in their customary amount of mischief making, provided the case is of average severity. The "whooping" period usually lasts from three to six weeks but in many cases it is protracted for a much longer period; it subsides finally into a subacute bronchitis which often persists for many months. The total case mortality is low because it includes those cases contracted by older children and adults, but among very young children, and especially those debilitated by any other cause, it may be as high as 25 to 60 per cent. Bronchopneumonia is the complication that accounts for most of the deaths. Meningeal hemorrhage due to violent coughing is a rare complication but one that is very dire in its results.

The disease is transmissible throughout the prodromal period and up to and including the first part—but just how much of the first part, is not known—of the whooping period. Many departments of health in the United States require that the child be kept out of school until he no longer whoops, but elsewhere, notably in France, he is permitted to return after he has been whooping for four weeks. The presence of a leukocytosis with 50 to 80 per cent of lymphocytes, the finding of the organism, or the obtaining of a positive complement-fixation test, are considered valuable aids in establishing diagnosis before the whoop appears.

Whooping cough was apparently unknown to the ancients nor is it mentioned by physicians of the Middle Ages. De Baillou described the first epidemic in Paris in 1578. By the middle of the eighteenth century it was widespread throughout the civilized world. It reached the Western Hemisphere in 1732, but for some strange reason Australia escaped until 1890. The disease is very mild in the tropics.

THERAPY

There are two measures of paramount importance in the treatment of whooping cough. First, the child should be kept out of doors as much as possible, for in this way far better than any other will the number of paroxysms be reduced. While not denying the influence of fresh air in bringing about this effect, I am inclined to believe that a more important factor is the child's immersion of himself in enjoyable play. Who has not seen a little tot trudging a weary circuit of the park hand in hand with a bored nurse who had to assist him through a cough and vomit at frequent intervals, while a group of nearby children, kept out of school by the same disease, were merrily romping past some of their attacks. Confinement within doors, or attachment to the apron strings without doors, is an irksome thing to the normal robust child; irksomeness makes for irritability, and irritability undoubtedly increases the number of paroxysms in whooping cough. Of course we cannot put very young or very weakly children out of doors, so for them the best we can do is to provide adequate ventilation of the house and change them about from room to room for diversion.

The second matter of great importance is the feeding of the patient, for the frequent vomiting in severe cases often brings about a state of malnutrition almost before we realize it. To adequately treat of this phase of the subject would carry me into the field of infant feeding where I certainly am not qualified to go, nor would such an excursion be fairly within the scope of this book. Suffice it to say, therefore, that a radical reduction in the amount of fluids and the replacing of the regular feeding periods by a number of small feedings at frequent intervals between the paroxysms, is usually provocative of good results in children of all ages.

Of drugs and biologicals I must necessarily have much to say because the subject cannot be summarily dismissed, but I would wish to preface what follows with a tripart statement: (1) There is as yet in whooping cough no remedial agent that even approaches specific value. (2) Other things being equal, turning the child free out of doors in mild cases, and carefully nursing him, *i. e.*, providing comfort and nutrition and diversion and sharply watching for complications and emergencies, in severe cases, are the simple mandates in the handling of the disease. (3) The fewer drugs placed in the stomach the better.

Sedatives.—In mild cases, especially when the weather and other conditions make it possible to turn the patient out of doors, the use of drugs of this class is usually unnecessary, though the night will often be very disturbed unless a sedative is given at bedtime. A teaspoonful of the following mixture (4 grains each of the chloral hydrate and sodium bromide) may be given to a child of five or six if he is robust and of the average weight:

R. Chloral hydrate...................................... ℥j   4.0
    Sodium bromide..................................... ℥j   4.0
    Syrup of orange to make........................... ℥ij   60.0

Or, since belladonna seems to be of some value here (see below), the bromide may be combined with a member of that group, as in the following prescription:

R. Sodium bromide.................................... ℥j   4.0
    Tincture of hyoscyamus............................. ℥j   4.0
    Tincture sweet orange peel to make................ ℥ij   60.0

Epstein (1933) has been very much pleased with the use of gold tribromide in 75 children; the average dose of $\frac{1}{20}$ to $\frac{1}{10}$ grain (0.003 to 0.006 Gm.) was given in solution three times daily ($\frac{1}{30}$ grain, 0.002 Gm., in very young children); a standard, uniform elixir may be obtained from Schieffelin and Co., New York City. Henricke (1930) uses a capsule containing sodium amytal, ½ grain (0.03 Gm.), and amidopyrine, 3½ grains (0.22 Gm.), administering the contents of ¼ to 1 such capsule according to age (one to seven years), one-half hour before bedtime in jelly, followed by a hot drink; or one-half hour before mealtime and at midnight if necessary. Chlorbutanol (chloretone) is said also to be useful as a sedative here. Two grains (0.13) may be dissolved in a little whisky, sweetened and diluted to taste, and given to a child of five or six. Older children may take it in capsules; the adult dose is 5 to 20 grains (0.32 to 1.3).

In severe cases in which it is necessary to make some attempt to control the paroxysms throughout the twenty-four hours, antipyrine is much used. Practically all writers are agreed that it is worth a trial in every case. I am unable to explain the effectiveness of this very mild sedative, nor do I know of a careful study of its use with control cases. Regarding administration, Haynes and St. Lawrence write: "The former, antipyrine, may be used with safety in doses of 1 grain every three hours to an infant of six months. Later it may be increased to 1 grain every two hours. At two years of age 2 grains may be given at four to six hour intervals, gradually increasing the frequency until 2 grains every two hours is reached. The drug is well tolerated in fairly large doses by children. Sodium bromide may be combined with the antipyrine."

Belladonna is also rather universally used. Regarding this drug, the same authors write: "In using belladonna it is important to begin with small doses and to exercise care in increasing their frequency and size. It is well to begin with ⅒ of a minim of the fluid extract three times a day for an infant of six months. At two years ¼ of a minim may be given every four hours, gradually increasing until it is given every two hours." It is claimed that the antipyrine or the belladonna lessens the frequency but does not reduce the violence of the paroxysms.

Ephedrine.—Anderson and Homan have obtained relief from the spasmotic symptoms in 18 of 20 cases in which ephedrine hydrochloride was used: ¼ grain (0.015 Gm.) to children over one year of age, ⅛ grain (0.008 Gm.) to those younger, in solution at bedtime or night and morning, and occasionally three times daily. Some of the usual toxic symptoms (see p. 328) were observed.

Synephrin.—This drug is beginning to have some vogue in doses of 1½ grains (0.1 Gm.), scaled up or down for age. It is said to be accompanied by fewer side-effects than ephedrine.

Inhalants.—Occasionally a patient is benefited by the use of some such preparation for inhalation as is described in the discussion of Catarrhal Fever (see p. 30); Epstein (1933) uses a teaspoonful of his elixir of gold tribromide in this way. However, these inhalants should not be used in children who are running in and out of doors during the colder months, for the mucous membrane seems to be especially susceptible to secondary infection for an hour or more after their use.

Henderson (1932) has administered his well-known mixture of 6 or 7 per cent carbon dioxide and air (or 93 per cent oxygen) to 10 children of nine months to seven years of age, using either the common portable infant inhalator or a specially constructed tent. In all cases, the distressing paroxysms of coughing were much relieved in three or four days and the treatment could be stopped by the end of the eighth day.

Abdominal Binder.—In 1907, Kilmer reported that a general improvement, and especially a reduction in the number of vomiting spells, was noted in 95 per cent of 550 cases treated with an elastic abdominal belt. Since that time this device has come to be employed by a great many practitioners, usually employing Luttinger's modified binder (marketed by Becton, Dickinson and Company). This author says:

"I found these bandages very serviceable in all stages of whooping cough. When applied early, they positively lessen the number of vomiting spells, and thereby contribute to better nourishment and resistance to the infection. The child is comfortable, and the older children often cry for it. They seem to feel a sense of security with it as they have 'something to cough against.'

"I do not think the bandage has any direct influence on the paroxysms. The improvement noticed by Kilmer was probably due to its indirect effect of promoting the general comfort and preventing vomiting. It is possible that this is due to pressure on the vagus, as it has been noticed by ocean travelers that tightening the abdomen often prevents seasickness.

"In view of the decided benefit from the wearing of the abdominal bandage, particularly the almost immediate disappearance of the vomiting, I strongly recommend its use in every case of pertussis."

Whooping Cough Convulsions and Tetany.—The idea that the convulsions often seen in infants who have whooping cough may be due to tetany and not to the effect of the disease itself upon the nervous system has been tossed about among the German investigators for a good many years. In 1925, Powers, in the United States, produced evidence which he thought rather strongly tended to show that this is the case, and many observers seem to have agreed with him (see editorial in the Journal of the American Medical Association, 86, 200, 1926). He advocated the administration of calcium chloride to all infants having convulsions during whooping cough, whether or not the calcium concentration of the blood and the electrical reactions pointed toward the existence of tetany. For my own part, I am still far from convinced by his work. He reports but 5 cases, all of whom had fever, all but one had otitis media, 3 of the 5 had bronchopneumonia; and there are no control cases in his series. Furthermore, according to the accepted standard of Howland and Marriott to the effect that "when there are convulsions and other symptoms due to tetany, the calcium of the serum is 7 mg. or less per hundred cubic centimeters," only 1 of these 5 cases could be diagnosed, at least upon the determination of blood calcium, as manifest tetany. Nor do I find any sort of conclusive evidence in the paper that the calcium chloride which he administered was helpful to his patients. Most decidedly, I believe that the argument in favor of an association of tetany with the convulsions of whooping cough must be based upon sounder work than this if the sceptical among us are to be convinced.

Ether Injections.—The intramuscular injection of commercial anesthesia ether was introduced in France by Audrain, in 1914, and has since been rather extensively employed, especially by the Italians. Castorina is very enthusiastic, Genoese reports good results, Macciotta is conservative in his conclusions. In the United States, Mason treated 26 cases, ranging in age from six months to eight years, during a mild epidemic. Sixty per cent of the patients stopped coughing and were apparently cured; 24 per cent were definitely benefited; 16 per cent failed to respond or became definitely worse. The dosages used were: first day, 0.5 cc., two injections; second day, 1 cc., two injections; third day, 1.5 cc., two injections; fourth day, 2 cc., two injections; fifth day, 2 cc., one injection; each day thereafter, the same amount as on the fifth day. These doses were slightly reduced for children under one year. Of the 16 patients in whom the cough stopped, none had whooped to exceed four days, 6 had whooped for the first time on the day the treatment was instituted, and the other 10 had whooped from two to four days. Of the 6 patients definitely benefited, 2 had vomited but had not whooped (later both of these patients developed a mild whoop), and the other 4 had been whooping for from four to seven days. Three of the 4 who were not benefited had been whooping for more than seven days. Tow reports results of much the same sort; in 82 per cent of 61 cases the number and severity of paroxysms were reduced, vomiting was lessened, and appetite and sleep improved. In Canada, Goldbloom selected 18 severe cases for study. Injections were given on alternate days, the initial dose being 2 cc. to the older children and 1 cc. to the infants, increasing to a maximum of 2, 2.5, or 3 cc. Definite improvement occurred in 10 of the children, the results being described as "dramatic" in 3 of the cases.

The risk of local necrosis is certainly the main objection to this ether treatment, though there is also a certain amount of pain occasioned by the injections which seems to persist for two or three hours. In Tow's series of 385 individual injections there were eight instances of necrosis—a small percentage, to be sure, but, as Goldbloom says, "I imagine it would be difficult to convince a mother that the development of a slough in the buttocks was part of the most modern treatment of whooping cough."

Ether-Oil by Rectum.—This form of therapy was introduced by Elgood (1925). Goldbloom (1925), Magliano (1926), Okutani (1928), Finkelstein (1931), and McGee (1931) have succeeded well with it. The last-named observer obtained as good results with ether-oil alone in 121 cases as he did in a control series in which its use was combined with other measures. A 50-50 mixture was given in dosage of 1 drachm (4 cc.) per year of apparent age, except under one year, when 25 per cent ether was given in double quantities. The mixture was introduced twice daily by gravity through a No. 18 to 20 French rubber catheter, adding 1 or 2 extra drachms in severe cases. If defecation occurred within thirty minutes despite elevation of the hips and pressure upon the anal region, the dose was repeated. The treatments were given for from five to twelve days, marked reduction in severity of symptoms usually being noted within four to six days, and more or less freedom from paroxysms within a week or two.

Vaccines in Prophylaxis and Treatment.—I shall not review the literature of this subject very exhaustively here because I believe it would not be worth while, the vaccine enthusiasts to the contrary notwithstanding. There is no single report to date in favor of the use of vaccines in this disease which is not offset by much more convincing data against their efficacy. More convincing, that is, because the variables have been fully taken into account. In the study of no disease do these variables form a greater stumbling block for the investigator, however well-intentioned and earnest he may be. To an exceptional degree, whooping cough varies in severity according to epidemics and the different periods of a given epidemic, season, environment and age of the patient, and the prevalence at the time of other epidemic diseases to act as secondary invaders. This would indicate that statistics of only an enormous number—many thousands, indeed —of cases would have value; but even here, the amount of grouping and regrouping which would be necessary in the attempt to keep the conditions even fairly comparable throughout the course of the study, would make the task laborious in the extreme and would so complicate the findings that any conclusions ultimately drawn therefrom could be held on only the most precarious tenure. And the controls must be adequate not only in type but in number. Numerous difficulties stand in the way of obtaining these controls; witness Luttinger's statement:

"The number of curative cases tabulated amount to 1101, of which 952 were treated with pertussis vaccine (three or more injections) and the rest (149) with drugs. We had planned at the outset to have an equal number of cases of each class; but we found it difficult to carry out this plan in practice. In the early days of the clinic we had an overwhelming number of drug cases because parents did not trust the 'needle' treatment.

Later on, with the increasing popularity of the vaccine treatment, it became difficult to secure an adequate number of control cases. Guardians could not be persuaded to go home without an injection, and refusal to give it to their charges would invariably result in lack of attendance."

This author, who is reporting studies made by the Department of Health of New York City, makes out a case in favor of the curative value of the vaccine, but I think his conclusions are inadmissible. The great disparity in numbers between the treated group (952) and the untreated group (149) would be quite sufficient to render practically negative the value of any deductions which might be made from this study, even though the two groups had been entirely comparable in all other respects, which was certainly not the case.

Regarding the vaccines employed, Luttinger writes: "It is equally regrettable that no minute comparative study of the various vaccines supplied to the clinic by Dr. Anna W. Williams could be made. The floating clientele of the dispensary and the lack of sufficient time and help to do the necessary follow-up work seemed to combine against a thorough investigation. Besides, it is not always possible to continue the injection of a vaccine which appears to aggravate the condition of the patient, especially when this patient is a child, helpless and poor. A good deal of switching, therefore, from one vaccine to another occurred. A solution of sterile milk, however, which was sent to the clinic having the same appearance as the regular pertussis suspension was promptly recognized, owing to the negative results and to some quite marked reactions. With this exception, all other vaccines seemed to be equally potent, except old strains or old suspensions of new strains of pertussis bacilli. This is merely an impression, as I have no reliable figures on the subject."

Reliable figures on this latter point are to be had, however, in the report of Von Sholly, Blum and Smith, which was made from this same city health department and at the same time. These investigators used pertussis vaccine, influenza vaccine and highly diluted milk, but did not know at the time which was which. Of their 264 cases, those given the pertussis vaccine (136) whooped for an average of thirty-two days, those given the influenza vaccine (94) for an average of thirty-five days, and those given milk injections and terpin hydrate medication (34) for an average of twenty-six days. Bayer (1932) has had a similar experience with distilled water and the vaccine.

Many investigators report the use of the vaccine every other day until they got a response. Bloom, of New Orleans, whose enthusiastic advocacy of pertussis vaccine is well known, writes: "Give injections on alternate days until one of the marked symptoms shows a remission. Then every third or fourth day until the more pronounced symptoms (number of coughing spells, intensive coughing spells, cyanosis, vomiting, loss of appetite and restlessness) are on the wane. Do not limit the number of doses— give as many as are indicated in your particular case." The average number would seem to be between six and ten injections, carried on during a period of two or three or even more weeks. Now assuming that the first injection is not made until the typical whoop has declared itself, which must be the case in the great majority of instances, since it would be highly irrational to begin a series of "curative" treatments until the diagnosis has been positively established, would not this series of injections carry the patient well over into what would ordinarily be the declining stage of the disease; that is to say, would not "one of the marked symptoms show a remission" in most cases after this interval of whooping, even though no treatment whatever had been administered? In Bloom's own series of cases, 286 out of the total 374 were "cured" within twenty days, and 317 out of the total

374 were "discharged" within thirty days. Is this very remarkable in view of the fact that 236 of the cases were declared to have been "mild"?

Bloom's cases were obtained from his office practice, but most of the other reports dealing with large numbers of cases come from public clinics. As to the scientific value of the data obtained in these clinics, I think many questions can be legitimately raised. One needs to have had but a brief experience in the clinics of New York City, or of any large city in the United States, to be made extremely sceptical of the validity of any facts elicited by questioning the untrained and often unintelligent parents or guardians who bring their own children or the children of others into these clinics. Upon this point, Von Sholly *et al.* write:

"As often as not, they try to answer to please the questioner; or exaggerate symptoms, hoping for better treatment; or they lessen symptoms to get a discharge for the child to go to the country or return to school, etc.

"Unless the child coughs in the clinic or presents some corroborative suggestive symptoms, such as subconjunctival hemorrhage, ulcer of the frenum, or puffy eyelids, how can one be sure that the child has whooping cough? It is not unusual for a young mother to say after one or more visits, 'My child does not cough like those I have heard. I do not believe he has whooping cough after all.' During last summer, at least, according to subsequent confession, some mothers brought their children for injections 'because they thought "the needle" would prevent infantile paralysis.' The Italians, particularly, feel that the 'syringa' is wonderful treatment for anything that happens to ail one. It makes weak children strong."

Regarding the prophylactic use of this vaccine, many apparently undeniably successful reports are to be found in the literature, both in America and abroad. Miller, reporting on its employment in the public schools of Akron, Ohio, states that sufficiently large doses will establish positive immunity and check the spread of the disease. It is his belief that the failures are due to insufficient, timid dosage at too long intervals. Bloom has always subscribed to this belief and in addition stresses the point that the vaccine must be freshly prepared. He reports on its use in an orphan asylum having 204 inmates. From the first week in May, 1919, to the first of January, 1920, no case of whooping cough developed in this institution, though in previous years 50 per cent of the children contracted the disease. Davies (1922) used the vaccine in an outbreak in a state institution in which 33 cases developed among 177 girls before prophylaxis was started. Of the 144 persons receiving prophylactic treatment only 4 developed the disease. Of the entire 177 girls only 20 had a history of having had the disease, so it is considered that the vaccine prevented whooping cough in the 124 who were probably susceptible. I must confess myself unconvinced by all of this for it smacks too much of *post hoc ergo propter hoc* reasoning. In the first place, sufficient and unquestionable exposure is a difficult thing to prove even where the unit under observation is a small one, such as a single family. In the second place, a much larger number of individuals is non-susceptible than is commonly believed. In the studies of Von Sholly, Blum and Smith, it is shown that of 243 families, the children of which were exposed to whooping cough, 77 families (31.6 per cent) exhibited a partial immunity—58 per cent of the children escaped the disease after exposure *within the immediate family*, some of them going unscathed through even a second and a third exposure. Therefore I would say that the evidence in favor of the prophylactic value of the vaccine is no more impressive than are the claims brought forward to prove its curative properties. Here in Milwaukee there has been a decided increase in the morbidity rate of the disease during recent years, an increase in which the inmates of the Home for Dependent Children have shared in spite of routinely receiving prophylactic injections (Schowalter, 1930). The successful studies of Madsen and his co-workers in Denmark, and of Sauer (1933) in this country (who uses only recently isolated strains, grows the cultures only on Bordet medium containing human blood, and requires that there shall be no exposure until four months have elapsed) require confirmation; 7 to 8 cc., containing 10 billion bacilli per cubic centimeter, is Sauer's dosage. Whenever a truly valuable prophylactic and curative agent shall appear for use in combating whooping cough it will not be as vulnerable to critical attack after a few weeks as this vaccine is after the lapse of many years.

The x-Ray in Treatment.—In 1923, Bowditch and Leonard reported favorably upon the use of x-rays in the whooping cough clinic of the Boston Floating Hospital, soon to be followed by Kingston and Faber and then by the reports of a number of other investigators, all extolling the latest method of treating this most untreatable disease. The tide of enthusiasm still runs high, but I wonder how critical is the judgment that is being exercised. Sceptics there are aplenty. Dr. Isaac A. Abt, the eminent pediatrician, after listening to the reading of several papers on the subject, said, as quoted by Kay:

"Gentlemen, in many years of practice I have listened to many cures for whooping cough—the use of x-ray is the nine-hundred-and-ninety-ninth. It now remains for someone to find the one-thousandth, for in my opinion we have as yet no cure for the disease."

I think the doubts which persist in the minds of the majority of practitioners are fully justified in view of the consummate ease with which the x-ray enthusiasts dispose of the obstacles imposed by the many variables that characterize the disease (see discussion of *vaccines* above). For instance, the only statement regarding controls in the work of Bowditch and Leonard is as follows: "In addition to the 400 cases treated with the roentgen ray we also followed and tabulated for comparison 200 cases which were not so treated." And Smith, Bowditch, Leonard and their associates, in summarizing the 850 cases treated in this same hospital, say: "The treatment of these cases had fallen into two main groups. First, the series treated by roentgen ray alone, and, second, a group given combined vaccine and roentgen ray therapy. There is a small series of controls which have not received treatment. This has been a difficult group to secure, as our cases have presented themselves very definitely for roentgen ray treatment. It is possible to utilize other reported series of cases, notably those of Herrman and Bell and of Luttinger in New York, and of Bloom in New Orleans for this aspect of the work. These give a definitely longer average duration for the disease than we have noted." That is to say, these investigators, reporting upon a certain type of treatment which they used in Boston in 1923–25, proposed to use as controls cases treated by other investigators in New York in 1915–17, in New Orleans in 1916–21, and again in New York in 1924, finding their justification therefor in the fact that these "control" cases were treated differently than their own. And the disease under consideration is whooping cough, which is never alike in two successive cases, let alone two successive years or two widely separated cities!

Faber and Struble (1925) carefully studied equal numbers of treated and control cases—44 consecutive patients in the Stanford Children's Clinic, divided into two equal groups. Despite the fact that their single and total dosages of x-ray appear to have been larger than those of Bowditch and Leonard, and contrary to their own confessed expectations, their studies in the end only afforded strong evidence against the assumption that roentgen therapy has a curative or even beneficial effect in whooping cough. Sudden remissions did occur in some instances, but they account for these very rationally as follows:

18

"The fact that such remissions have been reported from so many different methods may be accounted for largely by the sudden and frequently unexpected fluctuations in the normal course of the disease and partly (as is well recognized) by the psychic reaction made by a strange or startling procedure on a young and highly impressionable child. The roentgenray treatment is well adapted to produce such a reaction. The patient is laid and held on a table, usually much against his will, while strange lights and sparks and noises play about him. Indeed, it has been reported to us that the mere taking of a roentgenogram has caused a striking, though temporary, diminution in attacks."

YAWS
(Frambesia Tropica; Pian)

Yaws is an infectious disease of the tropics which is acute in its onset but chronic in its course. After a noncharacteristic prodromal period of two to four weeks, there appears a skin lesion known as the "mother yaw," often upon the site of an abrasion of some other origin. From one to three months after the appearance of this primary lesion, during which time the patient has generally been free of systemic symptoms, the secondary stage begins. This stage is characterized by a brief period of headache, rheumatic pains and intermittent fever, and then the appearance of the secondary crop of lesions. The eruption is quite generalized but occurs with greatest frequency on the limbs and face; there may be a ring of lesions around the anus and mouth; the scalp nearly always escapes. Characteristically a "yaw" is a nodule varying in size from a pea to a large nut and covered by a yellow or yellowish-brown crust from beneath which there exudes a thin fluid. If the crust is removed, there is revealed a raw surface the fungoid granulations of which have given the name "frambesia" to the disease (*frambesia:* raspberry). Surrounding this lesion there is a dark area in natives, a reddish area in whites. The lymph glands often enlarge in groups but never become painful or suppurate. Mucous membrane lesions are very rare. Occasionally there is a juxta-articular condition closely resembling acute rheumatic fever, but it does not respond to the salicylates. The lesions, which are usually itchy but never painful, disappear in three to six months in children and six to twelve months in adults, leaving behind apigmented or hyperpigmented areas. Most cases terminate at this point, but when a tertiary stage appears it is characterized by a periostitis or ostitis, or by a gummatous type of nodule or ulceration, which, on healing, accounts for much later deformity. Gangosa, a very destructive condition of the nose and mouth, which often before it subsides has converted the two cavities into one hideous opening in an almost featureless face, is most probably an unusual manifestation of third stage yaws.

The causative organism, *Treponema pertenue* (Castellani, 1905), may be found in abundance within the thickened epidermis in early yaws and also, as shown by Goodpasture, within the perivascular connective tissue of the papillae. This organism can with difficulty be differentiated from *T. pallidum* of syphilis, but the lesions which appear when it is inoculated experimentally in both animals and man differ clinically and histologically from those of the latter disease. In addition, the primary lesion is never venereal, the central nervous system is not attacked, the disease is not hereditary, and an individual may have both yaws and syphilis at the same time. The Wassermann test is positive, however, in practically all cases. Capt. C. S. Butler, (M. C.) U. S. N., is valiantly maintaining his thesis that syphilis and yaws are one and the same disease; the controversy interests me immensely, but I cannot come over to his side—not yet, at least!

Yaws occupies no place in medical literature until after the discovery of America, which does not necessarily mean, however, that like syphilis it was introduced from the Western Hemisphere. Castellani opines that the disease may have had its original home in Africa since epidemics frequently broke out on slave ships and the early planters in the West Indies quarantined the newly arrived slaves in an attempt to hold it in check. At the present time it is unknown in Europe and perhaps has been so at all times, though a few cases developed among white troops quartered near black Africans during the recent World War. It abounds in tropical Africa, in the Federated Malay States and in Java. It is common in southern China and in Burma, but is rare in India. It is very prevalent in the West Indies and the northern parts of South America, in the Philippines, and in all the mid-Pacific islands. Thieme states that yaws is so prevalent in Samoa that practically every native has had it at some time, children usually becoming infected before the age of six, while Collin goes so far as to state that that one of the Loyalty Islands with which he is most familiar, Lifou, is in danger of depopulation by the disease. Cases are not infrequent in subtropical countries, especially around the southern coast of the Mediterranean; a few have been reported from the southern United States. The recent studies of Ramsey among the hill tribes of Assam, and of Lopez-Rizal and Sellards in the mountains of northern Luzon, have completely upset the previous belief that the disease is confined exclusively to the lowlands, though in the highlands it does assume a somewhat different character.

THERAPY

Yaws is definitely and easily curable. The organic arsenicals, potassium iodide and tartar emetic are the most successful drugs. Bismuth is being tried and will probably be shown to have some value; mercury is practically worthless.

Neoarsphenamine.—This is the arsenical which has come to be most used because it is the easiest to prepare and to inject and is productive of just as good results as is the old arsphenamine or any of the newer preparations. It is often stated, and I suppose quite generally believed by non-workers in yaws, that one intravenous injection of this drug suffices to cure any case of the disease. This belief, however, accords but very poorly with the actual facts as they were developed by the excellent studies of Moss and his associates in Santo Domingo. These workers treated 1046 cases in the summer of 1920. About one half of the cases were reexamined from one to six weeks after treatment: of 362 cases given a single injection, only 19.8 per cent were cured or practically cured at this time, while of 169 cases given two injections, 51.5 per cent were cured or practically cured. The final conclusion, however, based upon another examination of 419 of the original 1046 patients, which was made (1925) nearly five years after their treatment, indicated that about 50 per cent of a miscellaneous series of yaws cases may be cured by one injection, that a second injection does not greatly raise this percentage, but that three injections very considerably increase the number of permanent cures. During a brief visit to Haiti a few years since, I gained the definite impression that the one-injection treatment is not looked upon as satisfactory there, but that it is recognized as a necessary compromise with the ideal since most patients are so much improved by the injection that, unless hospitalized, they do not return for subsequent treatment. Castellani writes: "Three to six injections at three to six day intervals are generally sufficient to obtain a clinical cure, though in many cases one injection is sufficient to make all the symptoms disappear." As in syphilis one injection causes the disappearance of the organism from early lesions within forty hours (Goodpasture, 1923).

The dose is usually 0.6 Gm. for adults, scaled down to one half or one third for children. Mixing the drug and water directly in the ampule is usually the preferred technic; for details of this method see page 100.

Tartar Emetic and Potassium Iodide.—These two drugs are usually employed in the following formula, which is known everywhere in the tropics as "Castellani's Yaws Mixture":

℞.			
Tartar emetic	gr. j	0.065
Potassium iodide	ℨj	4.000
Sodium salicylate	gr. x	0.650
Sodium bicarbonate	gr. xv	1.000
Water (or chloroform water) to make	℥j	32.000

This amount (1 ounce of the mixture), diluted to three or four times the volume with water, is given three times daily to adults, counting everyone over fourteen years an adult; half doses are given to children of eight to fourteen, and one third or less to younger children. Only the tartar emetic and the potassium iodide are active against the causative organism, the sodium salicylate being added to hasten the disappearance of the thick crusts and the sodium bicarbonate in the hope of lessening the emetic properties of the mixture. This latter drug renders the preparation cloudy and inelegant, though it becomes clear when diluted with water at the time of administration. If emesis is produced, Castellani advises that the sodium bicarbonate be increased or that a small amount of an opiate be given before each dose. Europeans do not stand the full doses as well as do the natives.

The mixture is given for ten to fifteen days, discontinued for a week and then given again for ten to fifteen days. The use of this formula is said to give very good results, though neoarsphenamine is preferred wherever it can be obtained.

Bismuth and Mercury.—The various preparations of these drugs suitable for intramuscular injection are used very much as in syphilis; that is to say, as an adjunct to the arsenicals (see pp. 210 and 205); but of course no such long courses of treatment are necessary as in the latter disease.

PROPHYLAXIS

In countries in which yaws is endemic all abrasions of the skin should receive immediate and thorough treatment with antiseptics because of the predilection of yaws for a wound site. Regarding insects as vectors of the disease there is very little direct evidence, though there are many who believe that the common housefly will some day be incriminated. Since the disease *is* eradicable, segregation of its victims would seem to be indicated, but such a thing, however rational, is certainly impossible of accomplishment. It is most interesting to note that Sellards and Goodpasture (1923), writing of their experience in Santo Domingo, state that all persons infected with yaws were studiously avoided and were barred from the villages, not by law but by native custom. Within the home, a small outbuilding was erected where the patient lived during the entire granulomatous stage, not being permitted in any of the other buildings. It was their opinion that this primitive quarantine "was apparently of some value in checking the spread of the disease within the family." They further state that even in the Philippines, where no such measures are practiced, one may visit homes in villages where yaws is abundant without seeing any cases until search is instituted or treatment is offered.

YELLOW FEVER

Yellow fever is an acute infectious but not contagious disease which is transmitted from man to man principally by the bite of the mosquito, *Aedes aegypti (Stegomyia fasciatus)*, although recent studies have shown that seven additional African, one other Oriental, and three additional South American species are capable of acting as vectors under laboratory conditions. Following the ingestion of the blood of a patient in the first three days of the disease, the filtrable virus undergoes development in the body of the female *Aedes* for about twelve days in warm countries, after which period and to the end of its life, about three months on the average, this mosquito is capable of transmitting the disease each time it bites. Since the discovery of the availability of several monkeys for experimental purposes due to their proved susceptibility to the disease, the work of Stokes, Bauer, Hudson (1928) and others has conclusively shown that the etiologic agent in yellow fever is not the *Leptospira icteroides,* with which Noguchi worked so tirelessly, nor yet the *Bacillus hepatodystrophicans* of Kuczynski and Hohenadel, but belongs rather to the group of filtrable viruses.

After an incubation period of two to twelve days, with an average of three to six days, the attack comes on suddenly; most cases begin at night. There is malaise, chilliness, nausea and vomiting more frequently than in the prodromal stage of other infectious diseases, nosebleed, a rise in temperature to 102 F. or a little more, and headache, backache and legache out of all proportion to this moderate degree of fever. The patient is very restless, has a congested face and gums and injected eyes, and complains of pain and thirst. Then, either with or without a remission of a few hours, new symptoms appear and the "typical" picture is established: the restlessness and pain, especially that in the head, persist; the temperature rises to 104 F., but the pulse curve not only fails to parallel this rise but actually falls away from the curve of the temperature; a dusky pallor overspreads the face, the mouth becomes parched, and the eyes become dry but still injected; there is intense jaundice over the whole body; the gums bleed, the nose bleeds, the female genitalia bleed, there are ecchymoses here and there about the body, and there is bleeding throughout the gastro-intestinal tract; nausea followed by acid vomiting comes on, there is severe epigastric pain, and finally the belching-hiccup and persistent vomiting of blood ("black vomit") appears; the urine becomes increasingly scant, is colored with bile and full of casts, and contains much more albumin than is ever seen in any other of the infectious diseases. This picture is usually fully established by the fourth day and death does not lag far behind, for the end comes on the sixth or seventh day in most fatal cases. "It is a bad death," writes Carter, "as bad as hydrophobia or smallpox." In recovered cases convalescence is rapid and there are no serious sequelae—which is an astonishing thing in view of the fatty degeneration of the liver and the large amount of tubular damage to the kidney that has occurred during the course of the attack.

The negro is not naturally immune to yellow fever, but the disease is very mild in him; in all other races the severity equals that in the white man. One attack seems to confer lifelong immunity. The mortality rate is shown in Table 32, but it should be remarked that such figures as these

TABLE 32.—MORTALITY IN RECENT YELLOW FEVER

	Cases.	Deaths.	Mortality percentage.
Guayaquil, Oct., 1918–Mar., 1919........	386	217	56.2
Guatemala, July–Sept., 1920..............	16	11	68.7
Salvador, May–Dec., 1920...............	181	91	50.2
Mérida, Dec., 1919–Dec., 1920............	5	4	80.0
Vera Cruz, July–Dec., 1920...............	106	57	53.7
Gutierrez Zamora, 1920..................	3	3	100.0
Tuxpan, Aug. 29–Oct. 7, 1920............	86	59	68.6
Senegal, 1926..........................	27	23	85.1
Senegal, 1927..........................	116	109	93.9
Gold Coast, 1927.......................	107	41	38.3
Rio de Janeiro, 1929....................	738	435	58.9
Total and average mortality...........	1771	1050	59.2

are probably a little higher than the truth for the reason that a few light cases are doubtless not reported during epidemics. A laboratory test is now available for determining whether or not an individual has ever had the disease, the serum from persons who have suffered from it possessing the power of protecting *rhesus* monkeys from the effects of an injection of the yellow fever virus.

Modern medical sanitarians, emboldened by the invaluable support of the International Health Board of the Rockefeller Foundation, have dared to contemplate a world entirely freed from yellow fever. Certainly their record to date is one that may be pointed to with wholesome satisfaction. Such epidemics as formerly occurred as far north as Spain, France, England, and the North Atlantic States are a thing of the past, thanks largely, it is true, to the change from sailing vessels with open water supplies to steamers with closed tanks; but due in no small degree also to the improved sanitation and quarantine facilities of ports. The last outbreak in the United States occurred in New Orleans in 1905. By direct attack of the mosquito problem, the disease has been eliminated from Mexico, Central America and the pestilential west coast of South America as also from the West Indies. Only a few areas still hold out, but the persistence of the disease in northern Brazil, Bolivia and Colombia in spite of extensive control work in the principal coastal cities, the serious setback in Rio de Janeiro in 1929, and the epidemic in the interior of Colombia in the same year, have caused serious apprehension among field workers, for it is recognized, according to such an authority as Sawyer, that a susceptible generation has been growing up in the countries which have been freed from yellow fever and that disastrous reinvasion must be viewed as a possibility. The increasing use of the airplane certainly does not lessen the threat; from South America to North America, or from West Africa to East Africa and then to India, are really not great distances nowadays as measured in flying hours. The outbreak along the west coast of Africa has resisted all efforts directed toward its control since 1926. It extends from Senegal to the Cameroons and has already numbered among its fatalities the internationally known investigators, Adrian Stokes, William A. Young, Hideyo Noguchi, Paul A. Lewis, Theodore B. Hayne and A. Maurice Wakeman. Certainly the warning of Pittaluga, of Spain, that the disease may soon again become a serious problem for Mediterranean countries, where *A. aegypti* prevails almost universally, must be seriously heeded if the period of world depression enforces a curtailment of sanitary precautions.

THERAPY

Principles.—Carter's famous three principles of treatment—rest, no food, water—were described by him as follows:

"1. The patient should be put to bed and stay there. He can be moved, if necessary, during the first twenty-four or forty-eight hours; after this grave risk is incurred. He should exert himself the least possible, use a bed pan, and not lift his head to drink. Too much stress cannot be laid on absolute rest, physical, mental and emotional; it is essential.

"2. No food is needed for the first three days; to withhold it longer *may* harm weak adults and children, though probably not for two days longer. The writer never saw a death from withholding food, but many from giving it; in case of doubt it should not be given. When food is first given, milk is not the best; the stomach is acid and, even with lime water, milk forms curds and causes pain and vomiting. Rice-water, the juice of oysters, chicken soup, the yolk of a hard-boiled egg crumbled are all better than milk. The appetite returns before it is safe to satisfy it.

"3. Drink as much water as can be borne without vomiting, taking small frequent sips. Weakly alkaline water, natural or artificial, is best and should be taken cold. This is grateful to a tender (and acid) stomach. Vichy (Celestins) was much esteemed in New Orleans. What is wanted, however, is water, to prevent the kidney block, and if it cannot be taken in sufficient quantity by mouth, it should be given by enema—plain water, not saline. The writer has not used the continuous drip, but it should be good; the administration of water by hypodermoclysis, so far as observed by the writer, has been followed by death."

Miscellaneous Measures.—Most physicians who have had experience in the disease advocate the giving of calomel, 2 to 3 grains (0.13 to 0.2 Gm.), followed in a few hours by a saline, as soon as the case is seen; it is hoped that the dreaded hiccup-belching will be prevented or postponed by thus giving definite impetus to normal peristalsis; during the continued course of the disease, one or more daily enemas may be administered for the same purpose.

Pain may perhaps be controlled in the early stages by such analgesics as phenacetin, 5 grains (0.32 Gm.), or pyramidon in the same dose, but the later and more severe pains in the head, back and epigastrium call for the use of opiates. Very small doses of morphine suffice here, $\frac{1}{16}$ to $\frac{1}{8}$ grain (0.004 to 0.008 Gm.) hypodermically; of course, after signs of severe kidney involvement appear, the opiates are contraindicated. Writing of epigastric pain, Carter says: "If the tenderness is severe and if the hiccuping-belch comes on—a precursor of black vomit—nothing equals cocaine. A half (or even a whole) grain in a minute capsule, washed down with a minimal amount of water, acts like magic."

Serum Treatment.—Since the recent positive identification of the filtrable nature of the yellow fever virus, and the discountenancing of Noguchi's claims thereby enforced I shall not consider here, as in the first edition of this book, the results obtained by him with the *L. icteroides* prepared serum, for it is now recognized that he and his associates were probably dealing with Weil's disease and certain other jaundices which continue to accompany both the African and South American epidemics of the graver malady.

PROPHYLAXIS

The whole world knows what enormous projects have been made possible, to say nothing of the number of lives that have been saved, by destroying the breeding places of the mosquito vector of yellow fever.

This matter is of relatively easy accomplishment since *Aedes aegypti* is not such a wide-ranging mosquito as are *Anopheles quadrimaculatus*, etc., the malaria mosquitoes. *Aedes* oviposits in artificial containers and collections of clear water near dwelling houses, seldom flying more than 100 feet away from the site of her own hatching; when driven to it, however, she will oviposit in queer nooks and crannies, but always near a human habitation, which is the natural feeding ground. The larvae in these containers may be destroyed by any of the following means: (1) Adding kerosene once a week, (2) completely emptying once a week, (3) screening (18 meshes to the inch), (4) introducing small larva-eating fish. The fourth method is nowadays considered the most satisfactory. Destruction of all *Aedes* is not necessary, and indeed is seldom possible; there seems to be a critical number below which they are no longer capable of continuing an epidemic. Especially is this true in endemic centers where there is a great number of immunes. I certainly saw and was bitten by *Aedes aegypti* in Guayaquil, Ecuador, and in Buenaventura, Colombia, during a brief visit in 1922, though there had been no cases of yellow fever in either place for some time. Indeed, small towns to which sojourners from outside seldom come, may even sterilize themselves in this way, *i. e.*, all inhabitants having died or become immune through recovery, the *Aedes*, even though still present in swarms, has no disease to transmit. However, seaports and frequently visited inland towns cannot allow their mosquito index to rise very high except at their own peril.

Communication with a stricken community only at midday is a rational procedure since this mosquito is principally a morning and evening feeder. Isolation and screening off of patients, without mosquito control, will not stop an epidemic except in very small towns where every case can be seen in the very beginning of an outbreak.

Vaccine Prophylaxis.—Since the announcement of the discovery of the filtrable virus which is the causative agent in the disease, a number of attempts to produce a protective vaccine have been made but none were entirely successful until Sawyer, Kitchen and Lloyd (1931), by utilizing their modification of Theiler's mouse protection test, were enabled to use living virus in the production of an agent of high antigenic power. With this new vaccine persons in the laboratory have been immunized to the extent of having demonstrable antibodies in their blood; the serum of such persons when injected into monkeys protects them from virulent yellow fever virus from monkey source. Aragao (1933), of Brazil, has apparently eliminated the danger inherent in the use of pure virus by his recent modification in the technic of preparing the protecting serum. At the end of 1933 no report has appeared of the use of these new prophylactic measures upon a large scale under field conditions, but it is certain that we are upon the verge of revolutionary developments in the history of yellow fever control.

DISEASES CAUSED BY FLUKES

INTESTINAL FLUKES

The following intestinal flukes have been reported in man: *Fasciolopsis buskii* (India, Assam, Siam, Natal, Borneo, Straits Settlements, Sumatra, Cochin-China, Tonkin, Formosa, and the coasts of China; *F. rathouisi*, *F. goddardi* and *F. fuelleborni* are probably identical with *F. buskii*); *Watsonius watsoni* (Nigeria); *Heterophyes heterophyes* (Egypt, China and Japan); *Metagonimus yokogawai* (Formosa, Japan, Korea and China); *Echinostoma ilocanum* (Philippines); *Echinostoma malayanum* (Malacca); *Artyfechinostonum sufrartyfex* (Assam); and *Euparyphium jassyense* (Roumania). The only one of these flukes that is of sufficient importance to warrant further mention here is *F. buskii*, which gives rise to a syndrome of diarrhea, anemia and edema in a very small proportion of the individuals who harbor it. Those who have studied the disease are agreed that death, when it occurs, is apparently due to exhaustion. The vicious circle responsible for the perpetuation of the malady is as follows: (*a*) The use of human excrement containing the eggs for fertilizer, (*b*) the hatching of the eggs in the water and their penetration into the body of certain snails wherein they pass a portion of their life cycle, (*c*) eruption of metamorphosed forms from the snail and their encystment on aquatic plants, (*d*) the eating, raw, of contaminated water nuts, (*e*) maturation of the fluke in the human intestine where it sows its eggs.

THERAPY

Under proper anthelmintic treatment dead flukes appear in the stools within twelve hours. Thymol, betanaphthol and carbon tetrachloride have all been used successfully (for details of their employment see the section on worms). Barlow (1925) favored carbon tetrachloride. Goddard (1919) pointed out that all anthelmintics must be used with great caution (*i. e.*, small doses) in these cases; his best results were obtained with betanaphthol. Chloroform has also been used with good results but it is certainly much too dangerous for routine employment.

LIVER FLUKES

Liver flukes are common parasites in sheep, cattle, pigs, dogs and cats; the following have been reported in man: *Clonorchis sinensis* (China, Korea, Japan, Formosa, east coast of India, Annam, and the Philippines); *Fasciola hepatica* (scattered cases in Europe); *F. gigantica* (Senegambia); *Distomum sibiricum* (Siberia); *Opisthorcis viverrini* (Siam); *Metorchis truncatus* (Siberia); *Dicrocoelium dendriticum* (scattered cases in Europe and Africa); and *Opisthorcis noverca* (Calcutta). The most important of these flukes is *Clonorchis sinensis*, which passes a portion of its life in the body of a small snail and later penetrates into a certain species of small fish in whose muscles it becomes encysted; when this fish is eaten raw the parasite is introduced into the intestinal tract of man and the other animals which harbor it, whence its eggs finally issue to complete the vicious circle. It seems possible for the majority of individuals to remain apparently healthy though the bile ducts, and occasionally even the pancreas and duodenum, are considerably infested with this fluke. When symptoms arise they are the following: gastro-intestinal pain and tenderness, nosebleed, jaundice and bloody diarrhea; in severe cases edema, ascites, anemia, and death from cachexia.

THERAPY

The anthelmintic drugs have been a complete failure in the treatment of liver flukes. Shattuck (1924) has reported on the treatment of 6 asymptomatic cases with tartar emetic and arsphenamine. In 2 of these cases disappearance of ova took place during a course of intravenous injections of tartar emetic alone (for dosage, see Kala-azar, p. 77). In 1 case the ova disappeared suddenly after the intravenous use of a few doses of arsphenamine which had been preceded by an intensive course of tartar emetic. In another case a like result occurred after a few doses of tartar emetic which had been preceded by an intensive course of sulpharsphenamine intramuscularly. In the other 2 cases treatment was a failure. Shattuck writes: "The facts seem to indicate, first, that both tartar emetic and arsphenamines are somewhat poisonous to Clonorchis; and, second, that it may be advantageous to give them in successive courses."

LUNG FLUKES

The fluke, *Paragonimus westermani* (known also as *P. ringeri* and *P. kellicotti*), infests dogs, cats, pigs and the larger carnivorous animals over a wide range. It is also established as a human parasite in China, Korea, Japan, Formosa, Philippines, Sumatra, Peru, Venezuela and Mexico. No indigenous cases have occurred as yet in the United States, though animals are infested in the Ohio and Mississippi valleys. The fluke passes a part of its life cycle in the body of a snail and finally is taken up by freshwater crab and crayfish. When these mollusks or crustaceans are eaten uncooked, or the water in which they have disintegrated is swallowed, the metacercariaen form of the fluke works its way through the tissues intervening between the intestinal tract and the lungs, in which latter organ it forms a cyst in which it undergoes full development. Not infrequently other organs or tissues, even the brain, are invaded. The pulmonary type of invasion is characterized by cough, frequent hemoptysis, and signs of cavity. The eggs are present in the sputum or feces.

THERAPY

So far as I am aware no successful treatment has been developed for this malady.

BLOOD FLUKES
(Bilharziasis)

The disease which bears the name of Bilharz, who first wrote of it in 1852, is caused by the three flukes, *Schistosoma haematobium*, *S. mansoni* and *S. japonicum*. The cycle of events is as follows: The eggs are discharged in the urine and feces of infested men or animals; in fresh water, motile larvae develop and enter certain specific snails; after about six weeks another form of larvae leave the snails and move about very actively in the water; it is these latter larvae that pierce the skin or buccal mucous membrane of persons or animals during bathing or drinking and set up the disease. The venous system is quickly entered and in the larger portal vessels the flukes mature and become paired. In pairs (male and female) they then travel toward the periphery and become lodged in the submucosal veins of the intestines and bladder, where they deposit enormous numbers of eggs; more rarely the cerebral cortex, lungs and genital organs, especially the latter, are selected as sites for these flukey nuptial couches. The pathologic reactions consist in a cellular response to the general toxemia and a local inflammatory reaction to the presence of the aggregations of eggs.

When the larvae penetrate the skin there is for a short time an intense pruritus and erythema; then, after what may be termed an *incubation* period of three weeks, the toxic symptoms appear: malaise, headache, cough, chills and fever, and abdominal pain and tenderness which finally localizes over the liver region. The symptoms due to the local processes in the bladder and intestine usually do not appear until another three to twelve months have elapsed. In the intestinal cases the symptoms are not clear cut but there are usually recurrent attacks of bloody dysentery and colicky pain and tenesmus; there are palpable papillomata of the rectum and distinctive signs upon sigmoidoscopical examination. In bladder cases there is burning and frequent micturition, suprapubic aching, hematuria and urethral bleeding, and, perhaps in later cases, symptoms of cystitis and vesical calculus; tubercles and papillomata are found upon cystoscopical examination. There is a tendency for malignant growths to engraft themselves upon these local lesions. Laboratory tests are of great assistance in the diagnosis of bilharziasis: marked eosinophilia, the presence of ova in the stools and urine and in sectioned tissue from the bladder and rectum, and a positive complement deviation test as devised by Fairley.

Schistosoma haematobium causes the bladder type of bilharziasis. It prevails in Egypt to an enormous extent and is endemic in Tunis, Nyassaland, South Africa, Mesopotamia, and in foci scattered throughout Asia Minor; sporadically it occurs also in West Africa, the western portion of Australia, Persia, Madagascar and the two neighboring islands of Réunion and Mauritius. *S. mansoni* occurs quite generally in Africa, cases in Egypt, for instance, being often mixed, *i. e.*, caused by infestation with both *S. haematobium* and *S. mansoni*. *S. mansoni* occurs alone also in Brazil, Venezuela and Dutch Guinea in South America, and in Antigua, Guadeloupe, Martinique and Porto Rico in the West Indies. *S. japonicum* occurs to a very considerable extent in rice-growing districts in Japan and in the Yangtze Valley in China; cases are also being reported in the Philippines. I think the eventual spread of bilharziasis to other countries is reasonably certain, for the proper snail host for *S. haematobium* is common in ponds of the Mediterranean region. Recent experiments in Corsica, which is still free from infestation, have shown the ease with which colonial African soldiers coming from regions in which the disease is endemic may infect the mollusks in that island. Of course isolated imported cases are occasionally diagnosed all over the world.

THERAPY

Prior to 1918 there was little that could be done for victims of bilharzial infestation. Then Christopherson introduced the use of tartar emetic, since which time we can legitimately speak of the disease as one in which we have a specific remedy. Davies (1927) treated 2100 cases in the Sudan between 1921 and 1924. In the latter year, 520 of these patients were re-examined and only 28 (5.4 per cent) were found to be still infested. Statistical studies made since that time are all in agreement that the drug is remarkably effective. It is given intravenously, ½ grain (0.032 Gm.) being dissolved in 6 cc. of sterile physiologic salt solution. Injections are given every second day and are increased by ½ grain (0.032 Gm.) on each occasion, though it is considered advisable to give no more than 2½ grains (0.16 Gm.) at any one time; indeed, many patients will show signs of intolerance on much smaller doses than this (see Kala-azar, p. 77, for symptoms of tartar emetic intoxication). A total of 25 to 30 grains (1.63 to 2 Gm.) is needed for complete eradication of the disease. After a few days general clinical improvement begins and the number of ova in the urine or feces is considerably decreased. At the end of the first week there is an increase in the number of ova but many of them appear granular and black, and after two weeks half of them are obviously dead; at the end of the third week all are dead. Christopherson admits that granular ova are passed in cases not undergoing treatment but points out that the number is never so large as in the treated cases. He believes that the tartar emetic kills the ova as well as the embedded flukes. If treatment has not been entirely successful, reexamination will show ova within a month or six weeks, whereas if reinfestation has taken place, the ova will not reappear until three or four months have elapsed.

Bongenault reports a patient who was very intolerant to the drug when given intravenously but who bore it very well when given by the rectum. He states that six daily enemas of 4 grains (0.25 Gm.) of tartar emetic in 50 cc. of water were sufficient to effect clinical and laboratory cure. This is very astonishing in view of the fact that students of kala-azar have not been able to obtain satisfactory rectal absorption of the drug in that disease. I should think that in cases of bilharziasis (other than *Schistosoma japonicum* cases, in which there is ascites) in which the intravenous route proves unsatisfactory, the intraperitoneal route might be utilized as it has been in the treatment of kala-azar (see p. 78).

Fuadin.—This drug, which is one of the newer antimonial preparations, has been in use since 1929. Khalil and his associates (1930) report more rapid "cures" than with tartar emetic. The treatment consists of nine intramuscular injections beginning with 1.5 cc. and increasing, in injections every two days, to 5 cc. at the third injection and finishing the course at that dosage. Where necessary for cure, more injections are given. In 2041 cases, they obtained cure after nine injections in 44.3 per cent, after ten in an added 13.4 per cent, after eleven in an added 2.1 per cent, and after more than eleven in 0.5 per cent. Uncured were 2.1 per cent, 32.8 per cent did not complete treatment and 10.5 per cent refused it. These observers find the drug less toxic than tartar emetic, but a number of experienced men have disagreed with them on this point: Gordon and Hicks (1930), Orenstein (1931), Maciel (1931). It is more expensive than the older drug.

Spontaneous cure is undoubtedly effected in some cases of bilharziasis after a variable length of time, and it is often stated that ova cease to be passed in the urine and feces of an individual after three years of residence outside an endemic center. However, in Cutler's review of the American cases it is clearly shown that both clinical and laboratory evidences of the disease may persist for ten or more years of consecutive residence in a nonbilharzial country.

PROPHYLAXIS

The best method of preventing the occurrence of bilharziasis would be to eradicate the disease in all infested men and animals by the proper employment of tartar emetic, or fuadin, but this is of course a practical impossibility. The next choice among prophylactic measures is to seek the destruction of the snail which serves as intermediate host. Sufficient advances have been already made in this direction to show that it is a practicable means of fighting the disease, but only in some regions. Leiper advocated the periodic emptying and drying out of the irrigation canals in the Nile delta, which is an effective measure for the reason that nonoperculate snails that harbor *Schistosoma haematobium* and *S. mansoni* there are easily killed by drying, but, as he says, the method "is scarcely applicable in the regions (*e. g.*, South Africa) where the rivers are infested"; the plan has been put into very successful operation in the Gezira district of the Sudan since 1925 when the new irrigation project which affected that great area between the Blue and the White Nile went into effect. Still, even where there is river infestation, something may be accomplished by the "drying out" method, as has been shown along the river Guaire in the valley of Caracas, Venezuela, where such draining of the infested areas as was possible was accomplished and in addition cultivation of all lands bordering upon the river was prohibited. Iturbe, who has studied conditions there, believes that these measures are to a considerable extent responsible for the local reduction in bilharzial incidence, though it should be remarked that a vigorous tartar-emetic-treatment campaign was going on at the same time. The use of chemical agents against the snails is probably of better promise. Ammonium sulphate, which kills the snails and their eggs in a dilution of 1:1000, has been advocated as a chemical manure for use in the cotton-growing districts of Egypt, but I do not know to what extent it has been employed. Copper sulphate, however, has proved its worth. Khalil (1927) reports that in an Egyptian oasis where 63.5 per cent of the inhabitants were infested with bilharziasis, copper sulphate was continuously added to the stream supplying the drinking water for four days and nights by an especially devised apparatus, the dilution aimed at being five parts of copper sulphate to a million of water. At the end of the experiment, all specific snails were dead and when the area was revisited after six months there were still no living snails. The copper sulphate, thus used, was not observed to have any deleterious effects on vegetation, animals or man. Another method employed in Egypt is to add to the water of the canals sufficient of a commercial phenol solution to make a dilution of 1:20,-000. Religious propaganda against the fouling of water has also been an effective weapon there. The snails that harbor *S. japonicum* live in the irrigation ditches of rice fields and are very difficult to eradicate for the reason that they withstand drying for a long period and succumb only to such chemical agents as are quite destructive to vegetation also; quick lime, however, is said to eradicate them, though I am unable to describe here the details of its use.

Suspected drinking water may be rendered safe for use by storing it in snail-free tanks for forty-eight hours or more, for most of the larvae perish unless they enter the human host within twenty-four hours after they leave the snail and all of them are dead at the end of forty-eight hours. Sandbed filtration is not effective against them but Berkefeld or Pasteur-Chamberland filters hold them back. The ordinary chlorination of drinking water does *not* destroy Schistosoma larvae. Water for ordinary washing and bathing purposes may be rendered safe (according to Leiper) by the addition of cresol in the proportions of 1:10,000.

DISEASES CAUSED BY WORMS

A very large proportion of all the men, women and children in the world are infested with worms of one sort or another. Physicians who practice among the better class of people in large cities will doubtless find it difficult to accept this statement, but it is nevertheless possible to marshal a considerable bit of presumptive evidence in its support and even to cite a few statistics. We are all quite ready to admit that many types of worms are apparently capable of thriving at one and the same time in individuals who live in the tropics, but are prone to believe that nothing even approximating this state of affairs obtains in the temperate zones. Or perhaps some of us will accept a high incidence "in the country but not in the city." The truth is, I believe, that no one knows accurately just what this incidence is whether in town or country. Falling back upon what little is known, however, the evidence is very much in favor of a considerable degree of infestation. Schloss, in 1910, made consecutive examinations of the stools of 280 children, of whom he found that 28.57 per cent harbored worms. In De Buys and Dwyer's series (1919) of 595 individuals, ranging in age from three weeks to eighteen years, the figure is even higher, namely, 53.2 per cent. McLean, in studies which lead him to the conclusion that worms are of infrequent occurrence in New York City children living under good hygienic conditions, points out that De Buys and Dwyer's cases were studied in institutions treating the poorer classes only. In his own series of 308 children in the out-patient department of the Babies Hospital, which he believes to be patronized by a better class of people, there was an incidence of worms in only 2.27 per cent; but I think that one can legitimately question his findings in view of the fact that, except in a few instances, only one specimen was examined from each child, and that, despite the supervision of the hospital pathologist, there is no evidence of the proper qualification in his clinical microscopists of whom he says only, "The examinations were made by two young women students of Hunter College." The subject needs to be exhaustively studied, especially as to adult incidence. Magath and Brown (1927), of the Mayo Clinic, have written: "A careful study of the symptoms of these patients has revealed the fact that if they are ignorant of infestation they never complain of symptoms, but if they know they harbor the worm almost any kind of symptom may be elicited." Certainly it is high time that the classical tetrad—anemia, eosinophilia, depraved appetite and ova in the feces—should be dethroned as the only syndrome indicative of the presence of worms.

It is my opinion that the investigator who will make a careful study (i. e., several consecutive examinations) of the stools of several thousand individuals of all ages and classes in any city and its suburban environs in the north temperate zone will reveal a state of affairs which, in conjunction with the nearly 100 per cent infestation of natives in many parts of the tropics, will quite amply support the contention that a large proportion of all persons in the world are worm infested. If this is so, then it becomes immediately evident that the treatment of helminthiasis deserves a much more important place than is usually accorded it in our medical schools.

TAPEWORMS

The principal tapeworms infesting man are *Taenia saginata, T. solium, Hymenolepis nana,* and *Diphyllobothrium latum* (*Bothriocephalus latus*). The following have also been occasionally recorded: *Hymenolepis diminuta, H. lanceolata, Diphyllobothrium cordatum, Dipylidium caninum, Diplogonoporus grandis,* and *Davainea madagascariensis. Taenia saginata,* the beef tapeworm, occurs all over the world wherever beef is eaten; it and *Hymenolepis nana* are the two most common tapeworms in the United States and Canada. It attaches itself in the upper part of the intestinal tract of man only, usually but one worm being present at a time. The larvae encyst in the muscular tissues of cattle, and it is the eating of these tissues raw or insufficiently cooked that introduces the parasite into its human host. If beef is solidly frozen the larvae die within six days and they die also in ordinary cold storage of three weeks' duration, but in the latter case their death is due not to the low temperature but to the fact that they are unable to survive the death of their host for a longer period.

Hymenolepis nana, the dwarf tapeworm, is quite common throughout the world though it particularly favors the warmer climates; in the Western Hemisphere it shares the honors with the beef tapeworm. It is acquired by the direct swallowing of the ova from an infested individual and is especially frequent in children. There is some presumptive evidence that the rat flea may act as intermediate host by harboring the larval stage of the worm. *Taenia solium,* the pork tapeworm, on the whole infests man much less frequently than the beef tapeworm but is rather common in parts of South America and also occurs in somewhat circumscribed areas elsewhere in both hemispheres; in North America it is of very infrequent occurrence. The larvae are encysted in the tissues of pigs and pass into the human intestinal tract when this "measly" pork is eaten raw or insufficiently cooked. Infested pork is not rendered safe for human consumption by cold storage or even by freezing. The larvae are also harbored in deer, bear, monkeys, dogs and cats. Man can become infested with the larvae by eating foods contaminated by another infested individual, as it does not seem necessary for the larval stage to be passed in another animal. The larvae sometimes wander about in the tissues and cause a variegated array of symptoms, the brain and the eye being most frequently affected. The adult worm develops only in the intestinal tract. Multiplicity of worms is not the rule but the occurrence of more than one is more frequent than with the beef tapeworm. *Diphyllobothrium latum,* the broad or fish tapeworm, is common in Japan, Turkestan, Roumania, Poland, Switzerland, many parts of Africa, and particularly in the countries bordering upon the Baltic Sea. The eggs of this tapeworm hatch in water and the larvae enter the bodies of certain small crustaceans; fish are infested by swallowing the crustaceans and man by swallowing, uncooked, the fish. Neither smoking nor salting will destroy the larvae; only thorough cooking will do it. The adult worms develop in large numbers in the intestinal tract of man, dogs, cats, foxes, and perhaps all other fish-eating animals; they are very long-lived, a case being on record in which one of these worms was harbored for sixteen years. It is therefore not remarkable that the western portion of the Great Lakes region of the United States and Canada, so largely populated by immigrants from the Baltic region, has finally come to be recognized as an endemic focus for the dissemination of the larvae of this worm. Warthin, in 1897, warned that this might be expected, and his later observations and those of Vergeer have proved how true was the prediction. At least four species of food fishes have been already inculpated. It seems that these are taken commercially in only very small amounts from the contaminated portion of Lake Superior, but Vergeer believes that infestation will spread through the shipping east, for the Jewish trade, of large amounts of fresh fish from Lake Winnipeg, Lake Manitoba, Lake of the Woods and Lake Winnepegosis. To date, the end of 1933, I find the records of 43 indigenous cases (Magath, 1933), and undoubtedly many times this number have not found their way into the literature.

Tapeworm infestation is said to be manifested by any or all of the following symptoms: Abnormal appetite, picking of the nose and scratching of the anus, restlessness at night and a large array of nervous symptoms by day, vertigo and a sinking sensation, anemia, a sensation of weight in the epigastrium, attacks of colicky abdominal pain, nausea and vomiting, and ova in the stools. The ova can always be found if the microscopist is an expert and is not satisfied with a single examination. In the case of *Taenia saginata*, segments often wander out of the anus when the patient is not at stool so that he soon becomes aware of his malady; segments of the other members of the group are usually passed unnoticed with the feces. The anemia is most frequent in individuals harboring *Diphyllobothrium latum*, in whom the blood picture often closely resembles that of pernicious anemia; they often have puffed ankles as well. However, it cannot be too strongly impressed upon the reader that his patient may harbor any of the tapeworms and manifest no symptoms whatever. To examine the stools of any individual whose symptoms are of a vague nature is good practice.

THERAPY

In the treatment of a patient infested with any of the tapeworms several things are essential to success. In the first place, the intestinal tract must be thoroughly cleaned out in order that the vermifuge may have free access to the parasite. The work of Macht and Finesilver has shown that magnesium sulphate is the best cathartic to employ for this purpose since for several hours after its use the absorption of all other drugs is much retarded. Second, the dose of the vermifuge must be large enough to stun the worm but not to kill him, for excessively large doses, and oftentimes even moderate doses, are somewhat dangerous to the patient. Death following the use of these vermifuges is rare, but great depression and even collapse are not infrequent; therefore the patient should be caused to stay quietly in bed throughout the course of the treatment. Third, the dose of the drug must be followed by another saline purge in order to sweep out the worm and the remnants of the drug. Fourth, careful search must be made for the head. If the treatment has been successful it will nearly always be found *if properly searched for by the physician himself*, though it sometimes is discharged separately within the next few days, or it may be digested and not discharged at all; the latter occurrence is probably very rare. In any case, if ova continue to be passed in indication that the treatment has failed, it should not be repeated in less than one month and in weakly individuals not for a much longer time.

For a brief general presentation of the toxicology of vermifuges, see page 312.

Aspidium (Male Fern).—The usual dose of the oleoresin of aspidium as gauged for children is 0.5 Gm. per year of age, but not to exceed 5 Gm. Indeed, even in an adult, it is doubtfully advisable to much exceed this latter dose. The substance is extremely disagreeable in taste and is difficult to disguise. The following prescription, which is for a child of five, is about as satisfactory as any:

R̥. Oleoresin of aspidium............................... gr. xl   2.6
    Fluidextract of glycyrrhiza......................... ℥iss   10.0
    Syrup of orange flowers............................ ℥v   20.0
    Peppermint water to make.......................... ℥ij   64.0
    Label: To be taken in one dose.

Magath and Brown have described the following procedure as employed at the Mayo Clinic:

"Preparation of the Patient.—The patient should not have luncheon or supper the day preceding treatment; black coffee or tea and water may be taken freely. At 6 P. M., from 15 to 30 Gm. of magnesium sulphate is administered, and at 6 A. M. the same dose is again administered.

"Administration of the Drug.—The patient is not given breakfast, and after the bowels have moved, 30 cc. of the following emulsion is administered: oleoresin of aspidium, 6 cc. or Gm.; powdered acacia, 8 Gm.; distilled water sufficient to make 60 cc. One hour later, a second 30 cc. of emulsion of aspidium is administered. Two hours later 30 Gm. of magnesium sulphate is administered; two hours after this a large soapsuds enema is given. The patient then passes the stool into a container, which is sent, together with the stool passed before the administration of the drug, to the laboratory. He is cautioned not to put toilet paper into the specimen.

"Search for the Worm Head.—If the patient has been properly prepared, the stool will consist of practically nothing but water, a few shreds of digested food, and the worm. The top half of the stool, which usually consists of about 2 quarts of water, may be poured off, and the rest of it is poured through a sieve with a 20-mesh bottom. Warm tap water is now run through the sieve, and if the procedure is properly carried out, the sieve will contain nothing but the worm. The contents of the sieve are now emptied into a flat enamel pan measuring about 25 by 30 cm., the bottom of which has been painted black with asphalt paint. The sieve is rinsed out into the pan by running water through the bottom. One may then carefully look for the head, using wooden applicators. . . . If each step has been carefully carried out, the finding of the head will be comparatively simple. The large soapsuds enema given at the end of the treatment is extremely important, for often, when the worm is dislodged, the head breaks off and passes into the colon, where it will remain unless swept out by the large enema. It is also essential to use saline purgatives instead of castor oil as aspidium is highly toxic and soluble in oil. We believe it safer to carry out the treatment in one day rather than to have the patient take the anthelmintic the night before."

Pepo.—Pumpkin seeds not over a year old, and the fresher the better, have definite anthelmintic value. Thirty to 50 Gm., according to the age of the individual, may be given as a dose. They should be reduced to a paste in a mortar and rubbed up with sugar and perhaps a little honey. It is said that children will readily accept this mixture, to which a little milk may be added if desired.

Pomegranate Bark (Granatum).—From 50 to 60 Gm. of fresh bark are thoroughly bruised in 750 cc. of water and allowed to stand for twelve hours; this is then boiled to about 500 cc., cooled, a little syrup added, and administered. An effective remedy but one which is nearly always vomited. Half this dose is sufficient for children.

Pelletierine Tannate.—This is a mixture of several alkaloids of the above bark and is easier to give since the dose is small, being only 4 grains (0.26 Gm.) and it can be easily suspended in simple syrup. This is considered by many practitioners to be the most surely effective of all the vermifuges available for the treatment of tapeworm, but it is too toxic for

19

any but very robust individuals and it should perhaps never be given to children at all.

All the other vermifuges are used, of course, in the treatment of tape-worm, but I believe that none are as uniformly effective as those above described. A word should be said, however, about the "early bird" treat-ment that is still employed in so many hospitals. This concoction is pre-pared as follows:

Pumpkin seed.. 8 Gm.
Cusso... 4 "
Pomegranate.. 4 "

Make an infusion, to which is to be added:

Kamala... 4 "
Oleoresin of aspidium................................ 4 "
Glycerin... 15 cc.
Mucilage of acacia................................... 15 "
Water to make.. 240 "

This quantity is taken in two drafts two hours apart, after the usual preliminary treatment. Bastedo says: "The 'early bird' usually gets the worm," but he has several times seen severe gastro-intestinal irritation with vertigo and prostration result from the use of this mixture.

HYDATID CYST
(Echinococcus Disease)

Taenia echinococcus is a small tapeworm of the dog and his congeners, the jackall, the wolf, etc.; more rarely it is contracted by other carnivorous animals. The ova are spread in the feces of the infested dog and are also deposited upon the objects which he licks with his tongue. Grass-eating animals such as cattle, sheep, pigs and rabbits take up the ova with their food and act as secondary hosts for the parasite; when the dog eats the uncooked viscera of these animals he acquires the larval form of the worm, and so the vicious circle is perpetuated. Man may acquire the ova by too intimate association with infested dogs, or by ingesting uncooked con-taminated vegetables or drinking water. The embryo is freed by the di-gestive juices in the stomach, passes down the intestine, is taken up by the portal vein and passes to the internal organs, where the larvae in developing cause the condition known as echinococcus disease. The liver is the stopping place for the parasite in about 75 per cent of the cases, the lung in about 9 per cent, and all the other organs and tissues combined in about 16 per cent. Since a pathologic description of a hydatid cyst is not within the province of this book, it must suffice here to say that the ultimate form of this cyst is a brood capsule which contains, if not secondarily infected, a crystal-clear fluid and a great many scolices or rudimentary worm heads; there are usually quite similar cysts within the cavity of this primary cyst, and even these secondary cysts may themselves contain cysts. The symptoms are those of a characteristic tumor in an individual not otherwise greatly affected in health. *x*-Ray and the complement deviation test are of great assistance in making the diagnosis. Of course if rupture takes place into any of the body cavities, the symptoms of shock and collapse are to be expected. After such a rupture a new crop of cysts may develop in great number. If a cyst becomes infected, which often takes place through the bile ducts apparently, the picture of sepsis plus jaundice and often urticaria is superimposed. In regions where the disease is frequently encountered it is not often confused with other entities, such as malignancy, tuberculosis, etc., but where it is unusual the diagnosis is rarely made outside the operating or autopsy room.

At the present time echinococcus disease is most prevalent in Australia, the Argentine, Uruguay, Cape Colony, southern Brazil, Mecklenburg, Pomerania, Bavaria, Switzerland, Austria, Yugoslavia, Dalmatia, Bulgaria, Greece, Turkey, Russia, Siberia, and Iceland. In the last-named country it has long been a serious problem, but, according to Matthiasson (1927), its incidence is now rapidly declining as the result of educational propaganda, the increase in number of physicians, and a great decrease in the number of dogs. In North America, Mills' review shows a total of 379 cases to have been reported up to 1927.

THERAPY

I am unable to find any satisfactory evidence that either drugs or biologicals are of the least value in the treatment of hydatid cyst. Direct surgical attack, on the other hand, is often productive of most excellent results. Theoretically, the use of the x-ray would be indicated, but the work of Dévé has conclusively shown that its employment is impractical for the reason that the scolices within the cysts succumb only to a dose of the ray which would be highly injurious to the tissues of the patient.

PROPHYLAXIS

Regarding prevention of this disease, the Argentine Government Commission reported as follows (as quoted by Herrera-Vegas and Cranwell):

"With the knowledge of the cycle which the parasite must make in order to complete its evolution, we can understand that it may be interrupted in two ways; either on its outward passage, from the dog to the ruminant, or on its return from the ruminant to the dog. The first stage is represented by the dissemination of the taenia ova over the herbage of the country, the vegetables of the gardens, and in the drinking water, whence they pass into the organs of man or of other animals. Can this first migration, or first evolutionary hemicycle, as Dévé terms it, be interrupted? As far as the animals are concerned, it is exceedingly difficult, as they cannot be prevented from eating the herbage or drinking the contaminated water. As for men it could only be done by vigorous hygienic measures, such as the boiling of all water and vegetables, which would be difficult to put into practice.

"The second hemicycle is represented by the passage of the cysts contained in the viscera to the intestine of the dog. It is easy to see that it would be practical and easy to prevent the return of the parasite during this migration to the carnivora. As the dog can be infected only by eating contaminated viscera, the destruction of the offal would be sufficient to suppress completely the *Taenia echinococcus*, the common source of hydatid cysts in men and animals. From the above we see that prophylactic measures must be classed in the two following groups:

"1. Those referring to the first evolutionary hemicycle and which would protect man; these measures consist of the hygienic rules: to drink pure water, not to eat raw vegetables, and to avoid contact with dogs.

"2. Those referring to the second evolutionary hemicycle, prophylactic methods 'par excellence,' which are practical in realization and which protect both men and cattle; these measures consist of the reduction of the number of dogs, feeding them with cooked meat, and the burning of the viscera of animals used for food, which may contain cysts."

ROUND-WORMS

(A) THE COMMON ROUND-WORM

Ascaris lumbricoides is the most common of the intestinal worms in-festing man. It is quite ubiquitous, but in cool climates is encountered usually only in children. In the tropics, however, where reside more than half of the inhabitants of the globe, the incidence is very much higher and the worm occurs in individuals of all ages. For instance, the recent studies of Noone, Waltz and Donally (1927), in Philadelphia, showed the worm to be present in only 2.3 per cent of 304 school children, whereas Fernan-Nuñez (1927), in Barranquilla, Colombia, found it present in 33.9 per cent of 1336 adult laborers. In China, and other countries where the Chinese custom of employing night-soil in vegetable gardens prevails, it is also harbored with a frequency which is astonishing to practitioners in Europe and North America. In Morgan's series (1927) of 976 patients in China, 30 per cent showed *Ascaris* infestation; in Ludlow's series (1927) of 454 patients in Korea, 45.5 per cent were infested; and in Walker's examinations of British troops in the Singapore garrison (1927), the infestation varied in the different companies from 65.35 to 79.54 per cent.

This parasite needs no intermediate host for its full development. When the egg is swallowed by man it hatches in the small intestine, migrates to the liver and then to the lungs; from the latter situation it passes up the trachea and down the esophagus and through the stomach to settle down to maturity in the small intestine. An individual usually harbors from four to six of the adult parasites but sometimes the number is much greater than this. Any, many or no symptoms may herald the presence of round-worm; the infestation is most often diagnosed by suspecting its presence, *i. e.*, searching for the ova in *several* stools. When an individual harboring round-worms develops fever, as during the course of one of the infectious diseases, the worms seem to be disturbed and show some tendency to wander from the intestine into the stomach, esophagus, upper air passages, bile ducts, or even more remote parts of the body. Remote wanderings are very rare, however. Christie found only ten instances of migration in a study of 800 postmortem reports of round-worm cases. Their liability to complicate laparotomy cases is of more importance and should be taken into account in all regions of heavy infestation. Ludlow's experience in Korea has shown him the advisability of routine anthelmintic treatment prior to surgical procedures in all cases in which it is not definitely contraindicated.

THERAPY

Santonin.—This drug is the oldest of the remedies used against round-worms and is perhaps the one still most frequently employed. Being in-soluble outside the intestinal tract and practically tasteless, it may be easily administered to children by incorporating the dose with a little sugar. Calomel or castor oil, which are used to lessen the absorption and to sweep out the stunned worms, may conveniently be added to this mixture; the Compound Tablet of Santonin (N.F.), containing ½ grain (0.03 Gm.) of the drug and an equal quantity of calomel, is so pleasing to children that they will eat too many of the tablets if the supply is not carefully guarded. Ransom, in his excellent treatise on the intestinal parasites of man, writes of the use of santonin as follows:

"It may be given in a dose of 1 to 3 grains (0.065 to 0.2 Gm.) to adults, mixed with an equal quantity of calomel, or to children at the rate of ⅙ grain (0.01 Gm.) per year of age, also with calomel. This dose is given two or three days in succession and the treatment repeated in about ten days if eggs are still present in the feces." Castor oil may be substituted for the calomel in a dose of from 1 drachm to 1 ounce (4 to 32 cc.), depending upon the age and size of the patient.

Very large doses of santonin have often been given without untoward results, while small doses have not infrequently caused severe poisoning. It is doubtful if one can with impunity exceed 3 grains as the maximum adult dose. I have so often recounted to my students an astonishing and illustrative experience which befell me during a brief sojourn as ship's surgeon in the tropics, that I would feel quite remiss if I failed to place it on record here. One day, off the coast of Ecuador, a Mexican fireman appeared at my door and announced that he had "borned a bug." Being entirely without understanding of his meaning, and furthermore altogether fearful of the volubility which I knew would greet an attempt to question him in my sorry distortions of his native language, I merely signified a desire to be led to the scene of this delivery. Whereupon he promptly conducted me to the after part of the main deck, where, surrounded by a a gleeful group of his fellow-countrymen, a large round-worm lay in the scuppers. And before I could quite realize the significance of the scene, he began obligingly to cough and retch—and in a moment, with the assistance of two fingers inserted into his throat, he had brought up another! But now for the illustrative part of the tale, so far as it concerns the drug under discussion. This man gave a history of malaria which had been "cured" two years before, and was certainly not suffering from any sort of febrile disturbance at the time of this incident; furthermore, at the examination of the crew six weeks previously, and often in deck encounters since, I had remarked him as an exceptionally robust and hearty fellow. I therefore gave him 5 grains of santonin, 3 grains of calomel and a little sugar—with the result that within the hour he was in convulsions, from which he went into coma, and only escaped foregathering with his Aztec fathers because they seemed not quite ready to call him in. Moral to adorn a dull tale: never give 5 grains of santonin to any man alive *if* it is desired that he continue in that condition.

Oil of Chenopodium.—This drug has latterly won a high place for itself in the treatment of round-worm infestation. All laboratory experiments have shown it to be more effective than santonin, and time will doubtless confirm these findings for the human. It has the additional advantage of being less toxic than santonin. As its use in round-worm is practically the same as in hookworm, the reader is referred to the discussion of the latter infestation (see p. 305) for a description of methods.

Hexylresorcinol.—Lamson (1931–32) and his associates have removed between 90 and 100 per cent of ascarids with this drug. Administered in crystalline form in hard gelatin capsules (the oil in which the drug is dissolved in the commercial caprokol greatly lessens its anthelmintic action) in the following dosage: 0.4 Gm. to very young children; 0.6 to 0.8 Gm. to those from six to twelve years; 1 Gm. above twelve years. The drug is given on an empty stomach in the morning, no food allowed for four to five hours, and then a saline purge the next morning. Occasionally there have been complaints of slight gastric irritation and a few patients have vomited, but nothing of more serious moment has been recorded. The objectionable feature of this new treatment is that the drug, when given thus in crystalline form, reacts with the gelatin of the capsules after a time—almost immediately in warm, moist climates where infestation is heaviest. Brown (1932) has stated that by the substitution of sugar-coated pills practically equally as good results can be obtained: 90 per cent reduction in the 650 persons treated; two doses three weeks apart increased this to 93 per cent. In addition to the above-mentioned gastric irritation, an occasional superficial "burn" of the mucosa of the mouth will be seen if children are allowed to chew the pills. It is hoped that a more satisfactory method of administration will soon be devised.

Carbon Tetrachloride.—This substance, which has been a valuable addition to hookworm therapy, is not nearly so valuable as either santonin or the oil of chenopodium in the treatment of round-worm; it will therefore not be discussed further at this time.

Spigelia.—This drug is a very weak vermifuge. It was formerly much used in the South, where it is known as "pink root," but I believe that it has even there largely given way before the more efficacious santonin or oil of chenopodium. It is used as the fluidextract, the dose of which is 1 to 2 drachms (4 to 8 cc.) according to age. Very young children can tolerate the 1-drachm dose, though there are some cases of poisoning on record. It should be followed after several hours by a cathartic. A popular mixture is that of equal parts of the fluidextract of spigelia and the fluidextract of senna, the dose of this mixture being, according to age, 2 to 4 drachms (8 to 16 cc.). If catharsis has not occurred after a few hours it is well to stimulate peristalsis with a saline enema. I have always thought this a very poor preparation as the senna is almost certain to gripe.

(B) THE PINWORM OR SEATWORM

Oxyuris vermicularis is a frequent infester of the anal region in infants and young children all over the world, but, as in the case of all worms, most frequently in the warmer climates. Adults do not often harbor this worm, and among children it is more commonly encountered in the city than in the country. An intermediate host is unnecessary, the entire life cycle being passed within the infested individual. The vicious circle is as follows: When the eggs are swallowed, the worms hatch and develop in the small intestine and appendix, but when mature they pass down to the lower part of the large intestine; when the females are ready to deposit their eggs they crawl out of the anus and wander about the perineum, even entering at times the vagina; the biting of the worms in the rectum and on the perineum causes intense itching; in the process of scratching many of the females are crushed and their eggs liberated; the hands, contaminated with eggs, are ultimately carried to the mouth, and the whole circle is completed with the reinfestation which thus takes place. The severe anal pruritus is the only definite symptom of pinworms, though it is perhaps not entirely incorrect to ascribe some of the nervous disturbances of young children, especially those with erotic manifestations, to this infestation. Some observers believe that the worm is responsible, directly or indirectly, for many cases of appendicitis, but this is certainly not proved though the worms are many times found in that appendage when it is removed. Diagnosis is made upon finding the eggs in the feces, but this often requires the examination of many specimens; time will be saved if scrapings from the perianal region are searched as well. Serbinow and Schulmann (1927) report that in two children's institutions in the Ukraine a very low *Oxyuris* infestation was made out—only 3.5 per cent of the inmates in one of them—when careful examination of the feces was made by the salt flotation method, but when they examined the material obtained by scraping the anal folds lightly after moistening with caustic soda solution, 52 to 69 per cent of the children were found to be harboring the worm.

THERAPY

The length of the life cycle of *Oxyuris*, from the time the eggs are ingested to the time the females crawl out the anal opening, is a little more than two weeks. If, therefore, the conveyance of eggs from anus to mouth by contaminated fingers can be *absolutely* prevented for a period of two to three weeks, the infestation will be cured. This apparently simple feat is extremely difficult of accomplishment. The treatment should begin with a full bath with soap and water, special attention being paid to the anal region. After this the anal region and perineum are to be anointed with an ointment composed of 2 per cent of ammoniated mercury in equal parts of lanolin and petrolatum, a pad of cotton applied, and the child clothed in heavy drawers that are closed front and back. After each defecation the anal region is to be thoroughly washed with soap and water, the ointment and a fresh pad applied, and the drawers put on again. At night, when the itching is at its worst, the following anesthetic preparation may be substituted for the mercury ointment.

℞.			
Ethyl aminobenzoate (benzocaine)	gr. xlv	3.0
Salicylic acid	gr. xij	0.78
Hydrous wool fat (lanolin)	℥ss	15.0
Petrolatum to make	℥j	30.0

Label: Apply as directed.

It may be necessary to tie the hands, especially at night, so that they cannot be carried to the site of itching. In any case, the cleansing of the hands is of the utmost importance since ordinary washing will not suffice to rid them of the eggs. They must be *thoroughly and frequently* scrubbed with brush, soap and water, and the nails kept scrupulously clean. Daily full baths are desirable. If several children are closely associated, all must be simultaneously treated else mutual reinfection will be certain to take place. Bed sheets should be boiled at least twice weekly.

It is believed that a carbohydrate-free diet, such as would be used in the treatment of diabetes mellitus, is of advantage in these cases, but I know of no careful studies showing that this is true.

Internal Medication.—It is the usual practice to use vermifuges by mouth in the treatment of pinworm but they are of very doubtful value, though of course in obstinate cases all measures must be tried. Santonin, as employed in round-worm infestation (see p. 292), and oil of chenopodium, as employed in the treatment of hookworm (see p. 305), are the two drugs most often used. Recently, Brown (1933) has reported good results in a small series of cases in which he used hexylresorcinol; the following is recommended: (a) No food until noon; (b) the drug in pill form, 1½ grains (0.1 Gm.) per year of age up to ten years, with a maximum dose of 15 grains (1 Gm.); (c) drink plenty of water; (d) after soapsuds enema, an enema of crystalline hexylresorcinol in water in proportions of 1: 1000, the enema to be given high and retained five minutes. Fernan-Nuñez (1927) has claimed that intramuscular and intravenous injections of the oil of chenopodium are specific for *Oxyuris*, and, indeed, has shown that this is true; but Smillie has pointed out that both animal and human experience has proved that the reactions are too severe to justify the employment of this type of medication in a condition which, though bothersome and obstinate, is practically never a real menace to life.

Rectal Medication.—The female *Oxyuris* is difficult to discourage in her egg-laying orgies about the anus. It is certain that the use of rectal irrigations is entirely secondary in importance to the regimen of scrupulous cleanliness already described. Many formulae have been employed, of which I can list but a few here; they are all intended for use every day or every second day over a long period of time. The quantity administered should be sufficiently large that retention is impossible, though the patient should be instructed to resist expulsion as long as possible.

(a) *Saline.*—Six per cent aqueous solution of sodium chloride (approximately 15 teaspoonfuls of salt to the quart of warm water).

(b) *Quassia.*—Two ounces (64 Gm.) of the chips are to be added to 1½ pints (750 cc.) of water and boiled down to 1 pint (500 cc.), strained, and introduced when cooled to body temperature. This infusion may be made in saline, as above, instead of water.

(c) *Salicylic Acid.*—The following formula is used:

℞. Salicylic acid.....................................	℥ss	2.0
Sodium borate...................................	℥ss	2.0
Water to make...................................	Oj	500.0

Introduce warm, using half quantities for young children.

(d) *Soap.*—The ordinary warm soapsuds enema is employed; many of the females are believed to be killed by 1 per cent soap solution.

(e) *Vinegar.*—Ordinary table vinegar in the proportions of 30 to 100 parts to 1000 parts of warm water.

(f) *Quinine.*—Any of the quinine salts may be employed in 1:2500 to 1:1000 aqueous solution. The possibility, which is not at all remote, of inducing cinchonism must always be taken into account.

(C) WHIPWORM

Trichocephalus dispar is a very common worm all over the world, but is most frequently harbored in warm climates. Smillie states that it is probably the most widely distributed worm in the United States except *Ascaris.* In Colombia, South America, Fernan-Nuñez found it present in 41 per cent of 1336 laborers. No intermediate host is required to complete the life cycle of this worm. Infestation takes place when the eggs, which are distributed in human feces, are swallowed in contaminated water or upon uncooked food. The adult worms inhabit the cecum and appendix principally. *Trichocephalus* only very rarely causes symptoms and when these symptoms arise they are too variable to permit of description here. For the most part, however, the worm seems to be harmless—if, as is extremely improbable, one is justified in considering harmless any parasitic invader of the body.

THERAPY

Probably the most effective substance for use against this worm is the fresh sap of a fig tree, *Ficus laurifolia,* peculiar to certain river valleys of Colombia, where it is known as "Leche de Higueron." Fernan-Nuñez states that it has been used for centuries by the South American natives and that he has employed it with very good results but that it is not generally used by physicians there because of the difficulty of obtaining it in sufficiently fresh state. Aside from this substance, which has only recently begun to be investigated, there is no other drug which gives any sort of uniform results. The one most successfully used is the oil of chenopodium (see the discussion of hookworm treatment for details of its employment). Fernan-Nuñez says that it should be repeated three times at intervals of ten days. He has also shown that it is specific for the worm when given intramuscularly or intravenously, but I believe that the toxicity of the drug is far too great to warrant its introduction by either of these two routes except in extreme instances. Hexylresorcinol, used by Lamson *et al.,* as described on p. 311, accomplished an average reduction of 55 per cent in the egg count.

(D) GUINEA OR MEDINA WORM

Dracunculus medinensis is a large worm that requires two hosts for the completion of its life cycle. The free swimming larvae penetrate and develop to a certain stage within the body of a very small crustacean of the genus *Cyclops*. When unboiled water containing this crustacean is swallowed man becomes infested. About a year after the ingestion of the larvae, the adult female worm works her way into the subcutaneous tissues in order to discharge her embryos outside the human body. Her presence is first manifested by the pruritus which is set up, then a cordlike lump can be felt beneath the skin; finally, there is a vesicle and then an ulcer, from an opening in the base of which the embryos are liberated in a milky fluid which exudes when cold water is brought into contact with the ulcerated surface. The infestation of the primary crustacean host is easily accomplished by reason of the fact that most of the ulcers—there may be several in one individual—are upon the feet and ankles and are discharging continuously whenever the patient is wading through fresh water. There is a very pronounced eosinophilia but constitutional symptoms are slight.

Guinea worm is harbored in Arabia, Persia, Turkestan and parts of India; it is present in various parts of Africa, being particularly prevalent in the Nile valley; in South America, it is endemic in the Guianas and in certain districts in Brazil; it seems to be disappearing from the West Indies, which were formerly heavily infested, but latterly a few imported cases have been reported in the United States.

THERAPY

The natives everywhere effect the extraction of the worm by slowly winding it out around a small piece of wood. The process requires about two weeks and is open to the serious objection that if the worm breaks, as very frequently happens, secondary infection and a stubborn type of suppuration is almost certain to take place. The physician's method of attack is to kill the worm first and subsequently remove it. Injecting 1: 1000 solution of the bichloride of mercury into the burrow is said to be the most usual procedure, the worm being taken out on the day following the injection. Ransom states that Macfie has good results with the intravenous injection of tartar emetic, 1 grain being given every second day until a total of 6 grains has been given.

(E) TRICHINOSIS

Trichinosis is a disease which is acquired when the encysted larvae of *Trichinella spiralis* are ingested. The larvae are liberated by the action of the digestive juices, the adult worms quickly develop in the upper part of the intestinal tract, copulation takes place, the males die, and the females burrow into the submucosal tissues whence they discharge the new crop of embryos into the lymph spaces. These embryonal forms are carried into the blood stream, which conveys them to all parts of the body; some of the embryos also undoubtedly penetrate through the tissues by their own motile power. Ultimately they come to rest in the voluntary muscles, principally of the lower extremities, where the developing larvae give rise to an inflammatory reaction and are finally walled off by connective tissue, sometimes with calcification in addition. An individual cyst is barely perceptible to the naked eye. This process goes on in the rat, the pig, and in man. The pig acquires the cysts when he eats the carcass of an infested rat, while man acquires it by eating the uncooked or insufficiently cooked flesh of the pig; but just how the rat acquires it is not so clearly known. Certainly his opportunities are sufficiently great, however, for the larvae have been found in the flesh of twenty-five different mammals; this rodent is also not above eating the flesh of its own kind. That the parasite is transmitted only by the ingestion of infested flesh is practically certain, for all attempts to perpetuate the disease by fecal contamination have failed.

The symptoms in man are caused by the presence of the worms in the intestinal tract, by the presence of larvae in the muscles and elsewhere, and through the action of toxins which are liberated by the worms themselves, and by the extensive destruction of muscle tissue. From three days to three weeks after the ingestion of trichinous pork the patient is seized with nausea, vomiting, intestinal cramps, and usually either diarrhea or constipation and tympanites. There are also chilliness and sweating and a fever which much resembles that seen in typhoid; many times a typhoid-like skin eruption also appears. Edema around the eyes, but often involving the whole face and the lower extremities as well, is a characteristic feature of the disease, as is also tenderness of the muscles near their tendinous attachments. There is usually a pronounced eosinophilia. The encysted larvae may be found in an unstained teased or sectioned bit of muscle tissue that has been removed under local anesthesia; sometimes active embryos are demonstrable in the blood and spinal fluid. There are often symptoms of meningeal involvement, and bronchial and pulmonary signs are present in about 50 per cent of cases. The mortality in trichinosis is usually stated to be about 5 per cent, but bearing in mind that the disease is always mild in children and that many adults undoubtedly have undiagnosed slight attacks, it is very probable that this figure is too high. On the other hand, in family or neighborhood outbreaks in which large quantities of a particularly bad lot of meat have been eaten raw or nearly so, the death rate has frequently been from 50 to 100 per cent. The duration of the disease in nonfatal cases is very variable; an individual may completely recover in a few days, or he may lie in a state much resembling that of typhoid fever for ten weeks or more. Posttrichinal "rheumatism" often persists for many years after recovery from the acute attack.

Trichinosis is undoubtedly more prevalent in certain parts of Germany than elsewhere, but the notion that it is encountered in the Western Hemisphere only in persons of this nationality, is entirely erroneous. In Williams' statistics it is shown that native Canadians and Italian-Americans are more frequently affected than German-Americans; the incidence seems to be particularly high in California. I have heard of many cases among negroes and have myself seen two, both mild and both contracted through the eating of small amounts of raw pork during "hog-killing" time. South of the Rio Grande the disease is very rare, due to the Spanish-American custom of thoroughly cooking all meat.

THERAPY

The specific treatment of trichinosis is in a most unsatisfactory state, or perhaps one should say a negative state, for the truth is that all measures have completely failed. All the vermifuges have had their advocates, but none has been shown to have any consistent value, bearing in mind that results in single cases are not significant in a disease whose severity and mortality are as variable as they are here. Roentgen ray and radium have failed, as have also arsphenamine and neoarsphenamine. Salzer's rather unsubstantiated claims for the efficacy of immune serum were not confirmed by the careful experiments of Schwartz (1927). Grove (1925) advocated the trial of tartar emetic as used in the treatment of kala-azar (see p. 77); his one case was apparently much benefited.

In the beginning, *i. e.*, while gastro-intestinal symptoms are prominent, all writers are agreed that the patient should be thoroughly purged. Three grains (0.2 Gm.) of calomel, or 1 ounce (32 cc.) of castor oil, should be given, to be followed in either case in four hours by ½ to 1 ounce (16 to 32 Gm.) of magnesium sulphate or an equivalent dose of some other saline. The parasites may live for five or seven weeks in the intestine, and it is possible, at least, that such females as have escaped impregnation and have therefore not burrowed into the submucosa at the time of diagnosis, may be swept out of the tract by this violent purgation. If the case is a severe one, the best symptomatic treatment is believed to be that employed in the handling of a case of typhoid fever, without, of course, the stringent aseptic and antiseptic precautions which are necessary to prevent the spread of this latter disease.

(F) FILARIASIS AND ONCHOCERCIASIS

Filaria bancrofti is a small worm that lives in the lymphatic glands and vessels of man. The female worms give birth to living larvae which pass their life in the blood stream; during the day they accumulate in the lungs, the heart and the large thoracic vessels, but at night they come out into the general circulation in large numbers. If the infested individual reverses his diurnal scheme, the embryos accommodate themselves to the reversal and appear in the blood stream during that portion of the twenty-four hours in which the patient is sleeping. When infested individuals are bitten by any one of a number of *Aedes* or *Culex* mosquitoes, the larvae enter the body of the mosquito and undergo certain changes there; the metamorphosed larva, being deposited upon the skin of another individual, which the mosquito bites at a later period, pierces the skin and enters the lymphatics, there to grow to adulthood and send its own shower of larvae into the blood stream. It is the presence of the adult filaria in the lymphatic tissues, and the irritative changes there set up, that give rise to the symptoms of the disease, though secondary infection probably aggravates the condition. An attack is ushered in by a sudden rise of temperature, usually accompanied by rigidity and often by delirium and vomiting, and an acute lymphangitis of a leg or foot. The affected part is enlarged and erythematous and the lymphatics and the regional glands are swollen and tender. The symptoms disappear completely in a few days, but the patient experiences many of these attacks and it is finally noticed that the swelling is not entirely subsiding in the intervals. Ultimately the attacks cease to recur but the chronic deforming enlargement, known as elephantiasis, remains. The establishment of elephantiasis seems to bring about the death of the adult worms and thus to cause the disappearance of larvae from the blood stream. Next in frequency to the legs, the scrotum is involved; elephantiasis of the arms, the penis, the scalp, the breasts, and the subcutaneous tissues have also been reported. Chyluria is usually a symptom of the disease, due to the blocking of the thoracic duct and the bursting of some of the bladder lymphatics. Large boggy swellings in the groin are frequent, and filarial hydrocele and orchitis are not uncommon. Leg abscesses in filariasis patients often contain portions of dead worms. The living larvae are found in the blood and chylous urine, and sometimes in the fluid obtained from involved glands.

Filaria loa spends its larval stage in the blood, with the diurnal periodicity of *F. bancrofti,* but wanders about in the subcutaneous tissues during its adult life. The name "Calabar swelling" has been applied to the fleeting edemas which it causes during the course of these wanderings; areas of localization in the spleen may also react with inflammation and fibrosis. It sometimes crosses the eye, giving rise to conjunctivitis during its passage. A fly of the genus *Chrysops* is the vector of this form of filaria.

Filariasis occurs in the tropical belt all around the world, but the distribution of endemic centers within this belt is a very unequal one; it is not possible to mention, in a work so limited as the present one, all the places where this disease has been diagnosed. Statistics as to incidence and mortality are of doubtful value since many individuals seem to be able to harbor the adult worms and the larvae without ever manifesting any symptoms. Only a few indigenous cases have been reported in subtropical regions; Saurez (1930) has shown, rather surprisingly, that in Porto Rico a hemolytic streptococcus is apparently responsible for many cases of elephantiasis. Filaria loa disease is confined to a very small area on the West Coast of Africa, though the report of Low (1927) indicates that this entity exists much further inland than had been previously suspected.

In some portions of the Congo where *Filaria bancrofti* is said not to occur, practically all cases of elephantiasis are accompanied by infection with *Onchocerca volvulus*. In Guatemala, Strong (1931) and his associates have been investigating the disease characterized by the presence of subcutaneous fibromatous nodules on the head and in some cases disturbances of the eyes and loss of vision. He has found that the tumors contain adult male and female *Onchocerca coecutiens*, and that not mosquitoes but three species of *Eusimulium* flies are concerned in the transmission of the disease.

THERAPY

The symptomatic treatment of early filariasis involves no especial difficulty as the attacks are of short duration. Rest in bed is usually self-imposed but resort to sedative drugs must many times be made in order to control the patient during the early period of cerebral excitement. The involved part is relieved by hot or cold applications. In the lymphangitis of the cord that often accompanies filarial orchitis the pain is so great that large doses of morphine are required to give relief. Chyluria may sometimes be controlled by elevation of the pelvis and reduction of the fat in the diet. In filaria loa disease the parasite may be removed by simple incision when it crosses the eye; its removal from the subcutaneous tissue is sometimes accomplished in the same manner.

Specific therapy has completely failed in filariasis. None of the claims that have been put forward from time to time for tartar emetic, the various organic arsenicals, etc., have been substantiated by later investigators. The parasitotrophic agent that will annihilate the larvae in the blood stream is yet to be found. Cooke (1928) and Dixon (1930) have reported a few cases treated by protein shock (for method see p. 327), but felt that it was too soon to speak with any certainty of the results.

The treatment of elephantiasis is entirely surgical; scrotal cases give the most satisfactory results, but the operative procedures so far evolved still leave much to be desired.

In onchocerciasis, the tumors (and the contained adult parasites) can be easily removed under a local anesthetic, but in some cases the microfilariae continue to circulate in the body for at least several years. Strong's preliminary experiments with plasmoquin and quinine against the parasites have encouraged him to continue his studies.

(G) STRONGYLOIDES INFECTION

Physicians in the southern United States are becoming very familiar with this entity which has long been recognized in other subtropical as well as tropical regions. The life cycle of the causative worm, *Strongyloides stercoralis*, is much like that of its close relative, the hookworm (see p. 301) —with this exception, that during the time in which the larvae are migrating from the capillaries into the bronchioles an acute inflammatory reaction may take place in the lungs. In very light infestations there may be no symptoms, but in moderately heavily infested patients there is diarrhea with distress after meals, alternating at times with constipation; in severe cases there is intractable diarrhea, great emaciation and, occasionally, profound toxic edema. Positive diagnosis can be made only on finding the typical motile larvae in the stools, since the eggs closely resemble those of the hookworm

THERAPY

The drug most often used is thymol in the following regimen: (1) Three days of soft, fat-free diet, with a teaspoonful (4 cc.) of the fluidextract of cascara sagrada in hot water each night; (2) on the morning of the fourth day, without breakfast, the patient is given three 5-grain (0.3 Gm.) salol-coated capsules of thymol, and each hour thereafter for five hours a cup of hot, weak, sweet, black coffee; (3) shortly after the last cup of coffee, 2 drachms (8 Gm.) magnesium sulphate in hot water, the dose to be repeated in one hour; (4) thereafter, for a week, the patient is maintained on a light, low-fat diet while the stool is being studied, and is given also 10 grains (0.6 Gm.) of precipitated sulphur with an equal quantity of lactose, in capsules three times daily; (5) at the end of the week, repeat the procedure for a second course. It is said that this treatment is successful in most instances, but for safety's sake several such courses should be gone through during the succeeding year.

The areas of dermatitis should be scrubbed with soft soap and kept covered with U.S.P. sulphur ointment plus 1 per cent phenol. Stitt advises that the urticarial wheals in the anal region be treated in the same way.

Faust (1932) reports the treatment of about 200 cases in New Orleans with gentian violet, a method first reported by DeLangen, in Java. Two ½-grain (0.03 Gm.) enteric-coated tablets of the dye (National Aniline and Chemical Co.) are given by mouth three times daily before meals for from seven to ten days. In a follow-up examination of 47 patients, all but 2 had been freed of the infection; in 4 cases, two courses of treatment were needed. Two patients reported mild nausea but no other deleterious symptoms were observed. This treatment is said to kill the adult worms but not the larvae or the eggs.

HOOKWORM DISEASE

(Uncinariasis; Ankylostomiasis)

Hookworm disease is caused by two species of intestinal worms, *Ankylostoma duodenale* and *Uncinaria americana* (*Necator americanus*). The life cycle of these worms is very simple, since man is the only host. The eggs are passed in the feces of an infested individual; if the stool is deposited on the soil under suitable conditions of warmth, moisture and shade, larvae capable of infesting man develop in five days; this infestation takes place when soil, thus contaminated, comes into contact with the bare feet or with other naked portions of the body; the larvae then pierce the skin and enter the circulation, which carries them into the lungs, the alveolar walls of which are pierced in turn and the free air spaces entered; in the next stage the larvae pass up the trachea and larynx and then down through the esophagus and stomach into the middle portion of the small intestine, where they attach themselves and attain maturity. From six weeks to two months after the larvae have penetrated through the skin the adult female worms are laying eggs which are passed out with the feces. Individual worms live as long as seven to ten years, during which time they disengage and reengage at many sites in the intestinal mucosa. Each time the head is withdrawn a point is left which bleeds for some time, as the head of the worm secretes an anticoagulant substance; *A. duodenale* also passes much blood through its body but *U. americana* does not. Both worms very probably secrete a hemolytic toxin, for it is the severe anemia in hookworm disease that gives rise to all the other symptoms.

Hookworm disease prevails throughout the tropics and also in many warm, but distinctly subtropical regions; endemic foci also exist in mines in such of the cooler portions of the globe as central Europe and the south of England. Miners contract the disease by contact of their hands, arms, knees, elbows or buttocks with feces-contaminated soil in the mines, but everywhere else it is almost exclusively contracted by those who go about bare-footed in regions where the first principles of decency in the matter of personal and communal hygiene do not obtain. That is to say, in the tropics where poverty forces the native to go bare-footed and custom permits him to defecate where he pleases, there, other things being equal, hookworm disease will prevail. But that very similar conditions obtain in more "enlightened" communities is certainly a blot upon civilization's record. There is no need to labor the point, for valiant and determined efforts are being made to correct the defect, but the truth is that when the Rockefeller Sanitary Commission made a survey of conditions in the rural districts of the southern United States, in the period 1910 to 1915, it was discovered that of the 274,420 homes inspected, 48.8 per cent were entirely without privies of any sort.

Infestation of individuals begins as soon as they are old enough to range very far away from the house door and continues as long as they go about bare-footed in the endemic region. The passage of the larvae through the skin causes in most cases a local vesicopustular lesion known as "ground-itch." After a variable period of time, depending upon the degree of the infestation and the individual's resistance, the symptoms begin gradually to appear. At first there are slight gastric disturbances, which disappear upon the taking of food; then the individual develops a desire for unusual articles of diet, such as clay, chalk and hair. This symptom is often denied by patients but in some regions the craving is openly confessed and pandered to, as in mid-Java, where, according to Darling, a certain lumpy earth of volcanic origin is kept on sale in the shops. Pallor appears, there is dizziness and palpitation and breathlessness on exertion, oftentimes the pulse is erratic and sometimes there is a low-grade intermittent fever, and the patient becomes mentally dull and indifferent and physically less and less suited for the more arduous forms of labor. Examination of the blood reveals an eosinophilia and a reduction in the hemoglobin which is out of proportion to the reduction in the number of erythrocytes; the stools contain many hookworm eggs. If the patient is a child he is often pot-bellied and much below the average in size. Thus stunted, mentally and physically, weak, anemic, shiftless and indifferent, the hookworm victim goes through life, an economic drag upon the region which, in his ignorance, he continues to pollute; but he seldom dies of his malady. In the tropics, however, where infestation is much heavier than in the temperate zones, death primarily due to hookworm disease is not rare; the terminal picture is said to be one of extreme anemia, physical exhaustion, anasarca and cardiac failure. Ashford *et al.* (1933) have recently performed a very great service by placing on record 7 cases acutely and massively infected from the same source; during the first week there was much discomfort from dermatitis and at the end of this period soreness in the throat and a feeling of having caught cold. Within another week great weariness and fleeting epigastric pain had appeared, which was followed by colic, great loss of weight, strength and color, and in all save one case by diarrhea; loss of blood in the stool was alarming in several cases and all had severe secondary anemia.

It is thought the mysterious AAA disease of the Ebers papyrus, dating from the Egypt of about 1550 B. C., might have been hookworm; other intestinal worms are with certainty mentioned and prescribed for in that ancient compilation. As century followed century, from being known as Egyptian disease it came to be called tropical chlorosis, miner's anemia, St. Gothard tunnel disease. In 1843, Dubini described *A. duodenale,* and in 1866 Griesinger showed its causal relation to the disease. *U. americana* was discovered by Stiles in 1902. In 1898 Looss discovered the remarkable route by which the larvae reach the intestine.

THERAPY

It is a fact of tremendous social and economic importance that there are few diseases of as great seriousness as hookworm infestation that yield so readily and surely to medication with drugs. Whether one is justified in using the term "cure" in connection with the results obtained with these drugs is given some consideration at another place (see section on prophylaxis of the disease, p. 311), but certainly the rapid increase of 25 to 50 or 60 per cent in the earning capacity of treated individuals can leave no doubt of the practical effectiveness of the remedies. There is a rather large number of substances capable of killing these worms, but in doses of sufficient size to accomplish this desired result they are all unfortunately destructive of the life of the host as well. In the modern mass attack upon the disease it soon became apparent that the absolutely safe dose of any of these drugs was in all cases a noneffective dose from the standpoint of worm elimination, and the problem soon became one of selecting that drug, or those drugs, which, when administered in sufficient dose to kill a satisfactory proportion of the worms, could be rendered nonlethal for the patient by employing proper safeguarding and fortifying measures before, during and after the treatment. In the early work in the field thymol was almost exclusively employed; then, in some quarters, betanaphthol was much used; both of these were to a considerable extent superseded, after 1914, by the oil of chenopodium; and now, *i. e.,* since 1922, carbon tetrachloride has rapidly advanced to a position of apparent superiority to them all, though what is to be expected of the still newer drugs, hexylresorcinol and tetrachlorethylene, is not yet determinable. To adequately treat of the use of these drugs, and especially to institute satisfactory comparisons between them under varying conditions, is not possible in a book such as this present one. The reader is most strongly urged, therefore, to supplement what follows by his own application to the large literature of the subject.

For a discussion of the toxicology of hookworm remedies see page 312.

Thymol.—During the period when thymol was being used almost exclusively all over the world, Ferrell, of the Rockefeller Sanitary Commission, described the routine methods of administration as follows (1914):

"Hookworm disease is usually treated with Epsom salts, and with powdered thymol given in capsules. The object of the Epsom salts is to free the intestine from mucus or other substances surrounding the hookworms and protecting them from the action of the thymol. The patient should take little or no supper on the evening before the thymol is to be administered. As early at night as is convenient he should take a dose of Epsom salt. The next morning as early as the salt has acted, half the number of capsules of thymol prescribed for the whole treatment should be taken. Two hours later the remaining capsules should be taken. Two hours after the second dose of the thymol, another dose of Epsom salt should be taken, which will expel the hookworms that have been forced to loosen their hold on the intestinal wall by the action of the thymol, and will also get rid of the excess of thymol before it has had time to produce any harmful effects on the patient. Nothing should be eaten on the day the capsules are taken until the final dose of Epsom salt has acted well. A little water or strong coffee, *without* milk, should alone be allowed.

"As alcohol and oils dissolve thymol, making it actively poisonous to the patient, the use of them in any form would be exceedingly dangerous. Gravy, butter, milk, all alcoholic drinks and patent medicines, which generally contain alcohol, should be forbidden on the evening before and on the day of the treatment. Moreover, as many hookworm patients have dilated stomachs which do not readily empty themselves and it is important that the thymol reach the small intestine at once, the patient should lie on the right side for at least half an hour after taking each dose of thymol."

The drug tends to form lumps very readily; therefore, in order to insure adequate distribution and close contact with the worms, it should be powdered and placed in the capsules only a short time before it is to be used. According to Washburn, its efficiency is increased if mixed with equal parts of lactose or, better still, sodium bicarbonate; clinical opinion differs on the point.

A 90-grain (6 Gm.) adult dose of thymol is exceedingly effective in removing hookworms; 97.8 per cent of the worms were removed by one such treatment in the 19 test cases of Darling, Barber and Hacker. However, these writers did not recommend this dose, nor is it felt by any of the workers to be a safe one for routine use; indeed the present maximum adult dose of 60 grains (4 Gm.), which removed only 88.6 per cent of the worms in the studies of Darling *et al.*, is not often given in field work where constant supervision over cases cannot be maintained. Unfortunately the small doses which necessity forces us to use are far less effective even than the 60-grain dose. The following dosage table is taken from Darling's treatise in the Nelson Loose Leaf Medicine (1922); the metric equivalents are added by me. It is important to note that in hookworm infested regions an eighteen-year-old individual can often appear to be no more than twelve or thirteen years of age, and that it is the apparent, not the real, age that is taken as the basis for this table (Table 32*a*).

TABLE 32*a*.—DOSAGE OF THYMOL IN HOOKWORM DISEASE

Apparent age.	Dose in grains.	Dose in grams
1 to 5	3 to 5	0.2 to 0.3
6 to 10	10 to 15	0.6 to 1.0
11 to 15	15 to 30	1.0 to 2.0
16 to 20	30 to 45	2.0 to 3.0
21 to 50	45 to 60	3.0 to 4.0
Over 50	30 to 45	2.0 to 3.0

Thymol is usually given at intervals of one week until the desired result is obtained. Regarding the effectiveness of the drug under field conditions, I think the following statement of Ferrell fairly represents the consensus of opinion:

"In a majority of cases two treatments like the one just described will expel all the worms. In 1518 out of 3630 patients treated in Porto Rico a single treatment effected a cure; a second treatment was sufficient in 1166 cases; 518 required a third; 247 a fourth; 104 a fifth; 47 a sixth, and so on until the last case was freed from hookworms by the eleventh treatment."

In the matter of fatalities directly ascribable to its use, thymol has an exceedingly good record. In 1922, Barnes, of the International Health

Board, was able to find the reports of less than 20 cases, though the number of doses that had been administered in the various antihookworm campaigns up to that time probably surpassed one and a half million. In more than 82,000 treatments in Siam, he states that there were only two fatalities, and in addition to these cases he knew of only one other during six years' experience in Siam, Java and Ceylon; this case occurred in the latter country, when a planter forgot instructions and administered a liberal dose of brandy to a coolie who was weak and dizzy from the absorption of the drug. Of course many more deaths from thymol poisoning have occurred than the records actually show, but even so the mortality is undoubtedly very low; however, it should be remarked that many of these millions of nontoxic doses have been noneffective anthelmintic doses as well. The drug is certainly contraindicated in feeble persons and in those who have chronic cardiac or nephritic disease; also in pregnancy, dysentery, all dropsies, and any of the fevers.

Two more facts require mention: First, that thymol is very little effective against the round-worm, which is so often harbored together with the hookworm in the tropics; and second, that the drug is quite expensive.

Oil of Chenopodium.—This substance is now widely accepted as an efficient drug in the treatment of hookworm disease. In the early days of its use, the maximum adult dose of 3 cc. was found to remove approximately 99 per cent of the worms in one treatment; however, as was the case with thymol, it was soon found necessary to very considerably reduce this dose for routine field work. To review here in detail all the important studies from which our present knowledge of the drug was evolved would be quite impossible; I shall therefore attempt in what follows merely to tersely summarize the present methods of administration and the results obtained therewith, referring the reader who wishes to make an exhaustive study of the subject to the work of Darling, Barber and Hacker, *i. e.*, the International Health Board work in Malaya, Java and the Fiji Islands, and that of Darling and Smillie, in Brazil; the following names also appear in the Bibliography at the end of the book: Bishop and Brosius, Billings and Hickey, Hall and Foster, Salant, Royer, Fernan-Nuñez, Darling, Levy. The following publication will also be found to be of great value: Bibliography of Hookworm Disease, International Health Board, Rockefeller Foundation, Publication No. 11, New York, 1922.

1. The adult dose now most often employed is 1.5 to 2 cc. (24 to 32 minims, *not drops*). This dose, once repeated, results in the elimination of about 99 per cent of the worms in the majority of cases. It is important to delay the second treatment for ten days, or preferably two weeks, to avoid the cumulative effect of the drug. The following table (Darling) indicates the dosages which experience has shown to be safest for use in treating children (Table 33):

TABLE 33.—DOSAGE OF OIL OF CHENOPODIUM FOR CHILDREN

Age.	Dose in cc.
4	0.2
6	0.3
8	0.4
10	0.6
12	0.7
13–14	0.8
15–16	1.0
17–18	1.25
19–20	1.5

The drug is best administered by placing it in dry hard gelatin capsules shortly before using; the soft ready prepared commercial capsules have

20

been shown to be less efficient. The small doses given to young children may be placed on sugar in a spoon, but large amounts are rather difficult to get down in this way. Acacia emulsions separate and are quite unsatisfactory.

2. Preliminary purgation on the evening before treatment does not increase the efficacy of the oil of chenopodium. However, when the preliminary purge is omitted, it is best to divide the dose of the drug into two parts and to give the first half (0.75 cc. for an adult) at 7 A. M. on an empty stomach; two hours later the second half should be given, and after another two hours the purge. The vast majority of field workers are agreed that this purge should consist of a full dose, *i. e.*, 1 to 1½ ounces (32 to 48 cc.), of castor oil, the belief being that the castor oil greatly lessens the absorption of the oil of chenopodium. It is worthy of note, however, that among the dissentient voices is that of Darling, whose very considerable experience in the Orient has convinced him that magnesium sulphate is to be preferred to castor oil.

Because of the difficulty of observing patients under field conditions, it has become customary in some places to give the entire dose of chenopodium at one time, to be followed immediately by the castor oil. Fernan-Nuñez, whose anthelmintic studies in Colombia were very carefully performed, states that quite satisfactory results are thus obtained.

3. A preliminary starvation period is not necessary when treating hookworm disease with oil of chenopodium; indeed, it even seems to lessen the efficiency of the drug. If the diet for several days previous to the treatment contains larger amounts of fats and carbohydrates than usual, the danger of absorption of the drug seems to be lessened. On the other hand, a small amount of whatever kind of food given coincidently with the drug, *i. e.*, at any time before the purgative has thoroughly acted, greatly diminishes the efficiency of the treatment. After purgation has taken place, the patient may eat.

4. Oil of chenopodium is very efficient against the round-worm also, which is of great importance since many hookworm sufferers in the tropics also harbor ascarids.

5. There was a brief period, largely following the publication of Hall and Foster's work on dogs, when a small amount of chloroform was added to the castor oil in the belief that *all* the worms might thus be eliminated in one treatment; the increased amount of vomiting which occurred with this combined therapy, however, soon caused it to be abandoned.

6. Several millions of doses of the oil of chenopodium have been administered with only a few deaths; even the number of cases showing mild or moderate toxic symptoms is very small; this does not mean, however, that there is no danger attendant upon the injudicious use of the drug. As compared with thymol, it may be employed with greater safety in weak, feeble and infirm individuals, and in those suffering with any of the fevers or chronic cardiac or nephritic diseases of a mild order, but the dose must always be modified to suit the conditions, being especially cautious in poorly nourished individuals; in advanced cases of chronic cardiac or nephritic disease, in pregnancy, and in acute or chronic dysentery, the drug is considered to be contraindicated. For a brief discussion of the toxicology, see page 312.

Comparison of Thymol and Chenopodium.—In the Orient, Darling, Barber and Hacker made very carefully controlled studies of the relative efficiency of these two drugs. The following summary of their findings, which is only slightly rearranged for purposes of convenience, is taken from a paper published by them, in 1918, preliminary to their report to the International Health Board of the Rockefeller Foundation.

1. Thymol.—The 90-grain dose produces a very satisfactory removal of worms.

Chenopodium.—Three cc. produced the largest vermifugal effect of any single treatment tried, but the result is only slightly superior to the corresponding dose of thymol.

2. Thymol.—Higher doses, for example 120 grains, removed fewer worms because the vomiting that occurred reduced the amount of drug retained in the stomach to below the amount required for efficient removal of worms; but with 180 grains, though much vomiting occurred, the amount of the drug retained was still sufficient to effect a satisfactory removal of worms.

Chenopodium.—The dose at which the vomiting causes loss of efficiency was not reached at one institution, although 3 cc. were given. At another, 46.9 per cent of vomiting occurred with loss of efficiency at the 15 minims three times, or 2.8 cc. dosage.

3. Thymol.—No serious toxic symptoms were noted even with the highest dose.

Chenopodium.—The highest dose (*i. e.*, 3 cc.) occasionally produced toxic effects on the nervous system, such as nerve deafness and coma. In the lower doses, 1.5 cc. and under, no deafness or coma occurred.

4. Thymol.—Diminution of the dosage produced a rapid falling off of efficiency.

Chenopodium.—The efficiency was well maintained when the dose was reduced even down to a quarter of the maximum dose.

5. Thymol.—Two treatments with a small dose did not produce a good summation in the results.

Chenopodium.—Two half maximum doses produced a better result than the full maximum dose, and the highest percentage of worms removed was obtained by this treatment, *i. e.*, 99.6 per cent of necators and 97.5 per cent of ankylostomes.

6. Thymol was voted, by a great majority of the patients treated, as more unpleasant to take than oil of chenopodium. [One patient refused to differentiate, saying that each was as bad as could be!—H. B.]

7. The comparisons made under 4, 5 and 6 render thymol less suitable for use in the treatment of children than oil of chenopodium, as for children the smaller doses would be required.

8. The effect on the more resistant forms of worm has been shown to be less, dose for dose, with thymol than with oil of chenopodium. This renders chenopodium the drug of choice in treating Chinese, West Indians or any other people with a high percentage of ankylostomes.

9. Thymol, being a relatively insoluble powder, has less opportunity than chenopodium of becoming uniformly distributed throughout the intestinal contents. Chenopodium, being a thin oil, will become more evenly diffused along the intestine.

10. Based on consideration 9, the action of thymol was less uniform than chenopodium, and showed 23.6 per cent of cases in which relative failure of the treatment occurred. Only 7.6 per cent of the patients treated with chenopodium showed relative failure of the treatment.

11. Thymol removes a proportion of the worms of species other than hookworms. Oil of chenopodium has been shown to be more effective in removing all the other species than thymol.

One other fact needs to be stated, namely, that effective mass treatment of hookworm disease with oil of chenopodium is very much cheaper than with thymol.

Carbon Tetrachloride.—This drug was introduced into hookworm therapy in 1921 upon the suggestion of Hall, a veterinarian of the U. S. Department of Agriculture, whose success with it in many carefully controlled experiments on animals led him to strongly urge that it be tried in the human. It is my belief that the first report of its use in the treatment of man was that made by Leach, of Manila, P. I., in the early part of 1922, but shortly after this time reports began to appear detailing the tremendous success with which it was being used in many parts of the world. The ease with which this new drug lends itself to field work has enabled students of hookworm disease to study its effects in astonishingly large numbers of cases in a very short time. In December, 1922, Lambert published observations upon the use of carbon tetrachloride in 20,000 cases in Fiji, and early in 1933 he brought his series up to more than 100,000; the report of O'Brien (1925), in Siam, dealt with 225,000 treated individuals. Since it would be impossible to present here in a brief way a complete consideration of all the clinical and laboratory work that has so rapidly advanced carbon tetrachloride to a position of preeminence among hookworm anthelmintics, I shall content myself, as in the case of chenopodium, with a summary of its present status and modes of administration. References to the work of the following authors appear in the Bibliography: Hall, Hall and Shillinger, Hampton, Nicholls and Hampton, Leach, Lambert, Manalang, Phelps and Hu, Smillie and Pessoa, Meyer and Pessoa, Wells, Insfrán, Soper, Schultz and Marx, Kouwenar, Rice, O'Brien, Strong and Lamson, Minot and Robbins.

1. The adult dose of carbon tetrachloride is 3 to 4 cc. (45 to 60 minims, *not drops*). Much larger doses can be given with impunity, for the occurrence of poisoning bears very little relation to the size of the dose; these larger doses, however, are no more effective than the 3 cc. dose, which has therefore come to be accepted as the adult maximum by most workers. This dose is given to all persons fifteen years or older and apparently does not require modification for the very aged. For children under fifteen, the dosage established by Lambert and used by others in many campaigns since 1922, is 0.2 cc. (3 minims) for each year of age.

2. Preliminary purgation does not increase the efficiency of the treatment unless the patient has been constipated for several days. Preliminary starvation is also unnecessary, but the drug should be given in the morning to an individual who has taken no food since supper the night before, and no food should be taken again until the final purge has thoroughly acted; fatty foods should be avoided for an even longer period.

3. In the early work with carbon tetrachloride it was felt that a final purge would also be unnecessary, as Hall's experimental work showed that the drug does not depress peristalsis and might even at times exert a mild laxative effect. However, it was soon found that if the drug is followed in two hours by 1 ounce (32 Gm.) of magnesium sulphate, the incidence of slight transient symptoms is lowered. The work of Macht and Finesilver, in 1922, indicated that the absorption of carbon tetrachloride would be lessened by the simultaneous administration of the salts, and Hall and Shillinger (1924), and Schultz and Marx (1924), showed respectively that, in lower animals, the anthelmintic properties of the drug are not lessened while its toxicity for the liver is decidedly decreased by this method of administration. During the past few years the drug has been administered in this way very successfully in many thousands of cases. Strong, in 1926, reported upon the successful employment of the drug mixed with ¼ to ½ minim of croton oil; if this method proves entirely satisfactory, it will have the advantage over the magnesium sulphate technic of requiring the transportation into difficultly accessible regions of a much smaller bulk of medicines, but I find no more recent reports.

4. It is believed that the best way to give the drug, whether or not it is followed at once by the salts or incorporated with the croton oil, is in hard

gelatin capsules. The reason for this preference is that when it is swallowed from an open container there is some danger of inhaling a sufficient amount to cause rapidly fatal intoxication. Without wishing to deny the possibility of such intoxications—indeed, there are several on record—I think it is also necessary to point out that the chance of such a thing occurring is extremely slight. At the time of this writing surely more than a million persons must have safely swallowed the drug from an ordinary tumbler in which it had been previously overlaid with a little water or with the magnesium sulphate solution. Carbon tetrachloride has only a faint odor and practically no taste. It is the easiest of all the anthelmintics to administer, even children interposing very little objection to the dose.

5. With all the other anthelmintics it is necessary that the patient go to bed, or at least remain very quiet, during the treatment. Experience with carbon tetrachloride has shown that, though enforced quiet may be desirable in some cases, it is not at all essential either to the success of the treatment or to the lessening of the toxicity of the drug. In many of the large-scale antihookworm campaigns of recent years, workers of all classes have for the most part stopped their activities only long enough to procure and swallow the dose of the medicine.

6. Carbon tetrachloride has usually only an undesirable effect upon round-worms, namely, that of increasing their activities. The possible relationship of this fact and one of the types of poisoning induced by the drug is discussed at another place (see p. 314). The delinquency is easily overcome, it seems, by administering a small amount of oil of chenopodium with the carbon tetrachloride. Lambert (1923) was the first to describe a technic which has been since employed in many parts of the world. "After our experience with the heavy *Ascaris* infection in Navua, it was thought wise to modify the treatment for young children by adding to the carbon tetrachloride a vermifuge more effective for *Ascaris*. Oil of chenopodium is considered such a drug. It was added in the proportion of 1 part of chenopodium to 11 parts of carbon tetrachloride. The dose of the mixture remained at 3 minims (0.2 cc.) for each year of age. This meant 2¾ minims of tetrachloride and ¼ minim of chenopodium for each year. We have now treated with this dosage several hundred persons, many of whom have had fairly severe *Ascaris* infections. The worms have all been removed dead. The mixture is not disagreeable to take, and children have not objected to it. The oil is held in a perfect solution in the tetrachloride. The drugs may quite properly be given in the same proportions to adults in the accepted dosage of from 50 to 60 minims (3 to 4 cc.)."

7. The following facts are the principal ones responsible for the rapid strides with which carbon tetrachloride has overtaken all other anthelmintics in the treatment of hookworm disease: (1) A single dose will remove 95 to 100 per cent of all the hookworms harbored by an individual, whether the infestation be light or heavy; (2) this certainty of action has eliminated the necessity of reexamining the stools after treatment, thus greatly reducing the technical staff needed to conduct a campaign; (3) natives cooperate eagerly in the mass attack with this drug because its administration involves no tedious before-and-after-taking routine, because the substance is not difficult to swallow and causes practically no inconvenience, whether in the matter of objectionable symptoms or great disturbance of the daily round of life, and because the "cure" is certain.

8. Chronic alcoholic addiction is the outstanding contraindication to the use of carbon tetrachloride; the drug should not be given to such an individual nor to a merely casual drinker who has taken any amount of alcohol during the twenty-four hours preceding the day selected for treatment. The taking of a small amount of alcohol before the drug has been fully

purged out of the intestinal tract has also caused death in a number of instances.

9. Pregnancy is not a contraindication to the use of the drug. Lambert first drew attention to the fact in 1923, and its truth has since been attested in many thousands of cases. Insfrán, in 1926, reported the treatment of more than one hundred thousand of the general population of Paraguay without any noticeable effect, other than anthelmintic, upon the pregnant women among their number; 225 of these women were kept under observation for a minimum period of fifteen days after treatment, during which time no abortions occurred that were traceable to the effect of the drug.

10. It is becoming increasingly apparent that carbon tetrachloride is not quite so effective against ankylostomes as it is against necators. Therefore the custom has arisen, in regions where the former worm predominates, of using a mixture of carbon tetrachloride and oil of chenopodium. The toxicities of the two drugs do not reinforce each other, though they seem to be to some extent complementary in their action on the worms. In O'Brien's treatment of 225,000 persons in Siam, the maximum adult dose was 2 cc. of a mixture composed of 60 per cent of carbon tetrachloride and 40 per cent of oil of chenopodium.

The number of fatalities from the use of carbon tetrachloride in the treatment of hookworm disease is extremely small; Lambert (1933) has given more than 100,000 consecutive treatments without a death and with few untoward symptoms. Such cases as have occurred, however, have been quite puzzling in that they are reported from widely separated parts of the world, they occur as isolated instances among thousands of cases not affected adversely, they fall into several types, and they are easily shown to be unassociated with the size of the dose or with any impurities that the drug might contain. For a brief presentation of our present state of knowledge on this subject, the reader is referred to the discussion of the toxicology of vermifuges (p. 312). Excepting for the occurrence of a few deaths in perhaps several million cases, it may be said that almost no symptoms follow the administration of carbon tetrachloride if a full dose of magnesium sulphate (or croton oil, see p. 308) accompanies or follows it; at most there is complaint of drowsiness and headache, with nausea and perhaps vomiting in a very few cases.

One more fact needs to be stated, namely, that carbon tetrachloride is much the cheapest of all anthelmintics available for use against hookworm.

Betanaphthol.—This drug is probably the least effective of those that have been given extensive trial in the treatment of hookworm disease. In a dose of 3 to 7½ grains (0.2 to 0.5 Gm.), which was originally recommended, it is probably only very slightly toxic but only very slightly anthelmintic as well. In 1918, Bayma and Alves, of São Paulo, Brazil, began using much larger doses in patients who were under careful supervision in a hospital. A preliminary saline purge was given, and on the next day a capsule containing 1.5 grains (0.1 Gm.) of betanaphthol was administered every fifteen minutes until 90 grains (6 Gm.) had been given, two hours after which there was another saline purge. They reported 85 per cent of cures and no deleterious effects from the large dose. Gonzaga and Lima, under the direction of Dr. Neiva of the sanitary service of São Paulo, altered this treatment to make it more appropriate for field use by omitting the preliminary purge, giving the entire 90-grain (6 Gm.) dose at one time, and repeating this on three successive mornings, the patient being on a light diet throughout and receiving a dose of salts two hours after the last dose of betanaphthol had been administered. They reported no severe toxic symptoms and 73.5 per cent of cures among 400 heavily infested cases so treated. Smillie, however, in 1920, used this large dosage in 79 cases and observed very severe toxic symptoms in 2 cases and in 2 other cases a pronounced destructive action on the red blood cells similar to that of benzol. He writes: "The type of cases that are most susceptible to the toxic action of betanaphthol has not been determined. In all three of the severe cases of poisoning there was a history of recent malaria. It is probable that those cases in which the red blood cells are rendered more fragile by recent malaria are more susceptible to betanaphthol poisoning." Leach and Hampton, restudying the matter in 1923, did not observe any toxic symptoms though they used doses of 50, 60 and 75 grains (3.25, 3.9 and 4.87 Gm.), without preliminary or later purge, in more than 300 patients. But they also failed to obtain satisfactory anthelmintic action; microscopical cures resulted in only 31.6 per cent of cases after one treatment, while a second dose, administered after an interval of eight days, produced such cures in only 38.1 per cent of those cases remaining positive after the first treatment. One individual was given 50 grains (3.25 Gm.), and two days later another dose of 75 grains (4.87 Gm.): no worms were passed. Upon autopsy two days after the last dose (the drug was not the cause of death), seventeen necators were found in the colon and two still attached in the small intestine; the average worm count from 54 patients had been found to be only eight.

For the symptoms of poisoning with this drug, see the discussion of the toxicology of vermifuges (p. 312).

Hexylresorcinol.—Lamson *et al.* (1932) are highly pleased with their preliminary studies with this drug (for methods and account of the slight toxic effects, see p. 293), for in single doses they found it to remove 80 to 85 per cent of hookworm in over 2500 cases, findings which have been confirmed in Ceylon, Samoa, Mexico and Guatemala. Of course they are as yet unwilling to compare these results with those obtained with the other drugs, which have been given to millions of patients. Because of the action of hexylresorcinol upon both round-worms and hookworms, it would be suitable for use in mixed infections.

Tetrachlorethylene.—This drug is thought to be about as effective against hookworm as carbon tetrachloride, but it is ineffective against round-worm; whether or not it causes the same dangerous migration of these latter is not yet determined. Garin *et al.* (1931) have administered 371 treatments, usually giving 45 grains (3 Gm.) on the first day, 60 grains (4 Gm.) on the second, and 75 grains (5 Gm.) on the third—15 grains (1 Gm.) at a time in capsules at hourly intervals, patients being confined to their rooms, alcohol forbidden and milk encouraged, and the urine tested daily. Albumin was not found but a dark red color showed up with nitric acid. A feeling of drunkenness was described immediately after taking the drug; Kendrick has described a more frightening experience, but Lambert (1933) reports more than 46,000 treatments in the South Pacific without a death and without untoward symptoms.

PROPHYLAXIS

"The spread of hookworm disease is entirely due to neglect of sanitation. If the feces of all infected persons were properly disposed of, no new larvae could gain entrance to the human host, and with the expiration of six to eight years—the usual life of the parasites in the intestines—the hookworms already in the bowel would be expelled and the disease would automatically die out." Thus Darling in his excellent treatise on the prophylaxis of hookworm disease in Nelson Loose Leaf Medicine. The problem is mainly one for sanitarians and public health propagandists, and it is therefore hardly within the province of this book to do more than remark that many zealous workers are slaving in this field and that successes, if only partial, can already be counted; failures, too, unfortunately. To conduct a campaign for eradication of the disease by drugs alone is certainly showing itself not to be worth the enormous expenditure of money always required. In an unsanitated rural area in Porto Rico, Hill (1927) observed 1000 people, of whom 98 per cent were infected; these were treated intensively and 73 per cent were cured, *but in the following year 81 per cent were again positive.* Even where mass attack upon the disease by the proper use of drugs is combined with a well-financed campaign for the erection of sanitary privies, the result is often discouraging, for to erect a privy is one thing but to get it used is another altogether. No group is more deserving of the commendation of the profession than are these public health officers who are laboring at once for health and for decency. The question of what constitutes a "cure," and when an individual may be considered a "carrier" and when a "patient," is being much agitated at present; the reader is referred to the interesting papers of Smillie and Augustine and of Stiles.

It seems to me that Stiles (1933) is fully justified in taking issue with the Rockefeller Foundation for the statement in their Thirteenth Annual Report that "hookworm disease has almost disappeared from the United States."

THE TOXICOLOGY OF VERMIFUGES

1. **Aspidium.**—The milder symptoms consist, according to Sollmann, in colic, diarrhea, headache, dizziness, dyspnea, yellow vision, and sometimes blindness. Any one, or all, of these symptoms are not infrequently seen in slight degree, but more serious manifestations of poisoning, such as violent muscle cramps, jaundice, evidences of renal injury, delirium, convulsions and coma, are very unusual; death is rare.

The stomach should be emptied by the use of a nondepressing emetic, such as powdered mustard (a teaspoonful in a cup of lukewarm water), copper sulphate (4 grains, or 0.25 Gm., in water), or zinc sulphate (15 to 30 grains, or 1 to 2 Gm., in water). A full dose of magnesium sulphate, 1 to 1½ ounces (32 to 48 Gm.), should be given to flush out the bowel. The patient may be stimulated by heat, strychnine, caffeine, digitalis, etc., as indicated by the symptoms. Recovery is slow.

2. **Pepo.**—The toxicology is unimportant.

3. **Pomegranate.**—The toxicology is unimportant.

4. **Pelletierine Tannate.**—Mild toxic symptoms, which are frequent, consist in dimness of vision, dizziness, muscle cramps, formication, weakness and trembling. Overdoses cause partial blindness with dilated pupils in addition to the above symptoms in aggravated form; there is also violent headache, vomiting and diarrhea, sometimes convulsions.

The treatment is the same as for poisoning with aspidium, but when an overdose of pelletierine has been taken one should proceed very cautiously as these patients are profoundly prostrated.

5. **Santonin.**—Overdoses of this drug cause early vomiting, abdominal cramps and sometimes, but not always, diarrhea. The patient is dizzy and very weak and may complain of headache and painful urination; it is said that hematuria may also occur. In severe cases there is an astonishing fall in temperature and the patient may go into violent convulsions; coma usually precedes death (see also p. 293).

The treatment is the same as for poisoning with pelletierine. Every attempt must be made to keep the patient warm, and all available stimulants may be tried. An anesthetic, carried only to a light stage of relaxation, will control the convulsions, but if the patient sinks into coma he is almost certain to die.

Yellow vision often occurs in the routine use of the drug but is of no importance if unaccompanied by other symptoms.

6. **Spigelia.**—The symptoms are much the same as from an overdose of pelletierine; treatment would likewise correspond. The cases are very rare.

7. **Thymol.**—Barnes, whose experience with thymol in the International Health Board campaigns has been very extensive, writes that the majority of patients treated with the drug show some signs of its toxic action, such as flushed face, slight dizziness, and drowsiness. Very rarely more serious symptoms appear; vomiting and gastro-intestinal pain, severe vertigo, headache, tinnitus, and visual disturbances; cyanosis and collapse. There are very few reported deaths.

The treatment is the same as for poisoning with aspidium. *Alcoholic stimulants must not be used.*

8. **Betanaphthol.**—Smillie describes 4 cases of poisoning in 79 patients treated with large doses of this drug. "The toxic action of betanaphthol in these 4 cases was a destruction of the red blood cells. The drug selected the red blood cells and destroyed them in great numbers, with resultant severe anemia, icterus, enlargement of the spleen and liver, enlargement of the gallbladder, and hemoglobinuria. The white blood cells apparently were not destroyed by the drug. The liver, spleen, kidneys and other organs of the body were not affected primarily, but were markedly affected secondarily, because of the anemia, and because of the injurious effects produced by the elimination of large numbers of destroyed red blood cells." One of the patients had no subjective symptoms whatever, and another complained only of thirst and a slight weakness. The other two were very ill; there was nausea, vomiting and diarrhea, headache, exquisite tenderness in the regions of the spleen and gallbladder, a rise in temperature, pulse and respirations, and profound prostration. Both patients recovered.

The treatment consists in promoting elimination and providing stimulation as in the treatment of aspidium poisoning. Blood transfusion would seem to be indicated.

9. **Oil of Chenopodium.**—The symptoms of chenopodium poisoning are referable to the central nervous system and consist in nausea and vomiting, dizziness, internal ear deafness, tingling of the hands and feet, muscular incoordination, and semicoma. The kidneys are also affected as is shown by albuminuria and the appearance of casts.

The treatment is similar to that employed in combating aspidium poisoning. In laboratory experiments, Salant found digitalis especially valuable as a stimulant. To combat the renal irritation, Darling advises the administration of hypotonic salt solution by the Murphy drip.

10. **Carbon Tetrachloride.**—The subject of carbon tetrachloride poisoning has been exhaustively studied by Lamson, Minot and Robbins, who find that the cases fall into several well-defined groups. I shall quote at some length from their (1928) paper.

(a) *Effect of Alcohol.*—"Shortly after the introduction of the drug as an anthelmintic, it became evident that carbon tetrachloride is extremely toxic both for chronic alcoholic addicts and for those who drank alcohol immediately after treatment. In such cases, vomiting comes on within a few hours after the administration of the drug. The signs and symptoms are extremely severe, vomiting is violent and continuous, and there are almost always hemorrhages into the gastro-intestinal tract, which cause the patient to vomit either bright or changed blood and to pass bloody stools.

Jaundice may be very severe after forty-eight hours; the urine scanty and highly bile-stained. This clinical picture can be reproduced easily in dogs by giving alcohol with carbon tetrachloride."

(b) *Ascariasis as a Complicating Factor.*—"In the case reports from several million persons treated with thymol, chenopodium and betanaphthol over a period of from eight to ten years, no mention was made of ascariasis as a complication in cases of intoxication. This may perhaps be due to the fact that in every region where ascariasis is prevalent, large numbers of ascarids are found to migrate in the body after death from any cause, and they are seen so commonly that no clinical importance is attached to their presence or activity in unusual parts of the host. With the introduction of carbon tetrachloride, it was extremely interesting to see the gradual development of the conviction that ascarids play some part in the intoxication. Dr. S. M. Lambert, who treated cases in the Fiji Islands, probably first sponsored this idea. He observed that symptoms were more common in districts in which patients were heavily infested. He later reported having been called to see several young children severely ill after taking carbon tetrachloride. Writhing masses of ascarids could be seen plainly through the abdominal wall. After a dose of chenopodium which caused the patients to pass these worms, all symptoms disappeared. Similar reports began to come in from different countries. Later, cases were described in which definite pharyngeal and intestinal obstruction were found at autopsy. . . . Carbon tetrachloride undoubtedly causes an increase in the activity of these round-worms."

The following cases are cited to illustrate the different types of death in this acute ascariasis:

"Case 4.—A girl, aged six years, was given 0.5 cc. of carbon tetrachloride, followed by 1 ounce of magnesium sulphate. The bowels moved and a few ascarids were passed. She was well and played about until the next noon, when she began to vomit and complained of pain in the liver region. Forty-eight hours after taking the drug, she still complained of pain and was vomiting ascaris worms. Seventy-two hours after, she was lying quiet, vomiting, and still complaining of pain in the same region. Ninety-six hours after, the patient went into coma. Vomitus was black. Death occurred after one hundred and thirty-two hours. Autopsy showed a plug of coiled ascaris worms in the small intestine surrounded by a gangrenous area.

"Case 5.—A girl, aged five years, was given 5 minims (0.3 cc.) of carbon tetrachloride early in the morning followed by magnesium sulphate without result. She was perfectly well until noon of the next day, when she began to vomit. Three days after taking the carbon tetrachloride, she awoke at 2 A. M. shrieking and vomiting and remained in this state of 'despondency and despair' until 6 in the morning, when she died. An incomplete postmortem examination showed the pharynx completely blocked by a plug of ascarids.

"Case 6.—A boy, aged seven years, was given 5 minims (0.3 cc.) of carbon tetrachloride, followed by magnesium sulphate in the morning. He was perfectly well throughout the day and was left alone the next morning, playing about by himself. The mother returned at 2.30 P. M., and found the child lying down and unable to speak. He died one hour later. Autopsy showed the intestine 'literally packed with ascarids.' No mention was made of a pharyngeal examination."

(c) *The Relation of Food to the Intoxication.*—"It has been found that when carbon tetrachloride reaches the brain in sufficiently high concentration, nervous symptoms are manifested." The following case is cited to illustrate this type of intoxication.

"Case 7.—A woman, aged twenty-six, was found to have hookworm disease and was advised to take carbon tetrachloride in the morning on an empty stomach. In spite of this, she took 60 minims (3.7 cc.) at 7.30 P. M. after a hearty evening meal. Thirty minutes later she vomited, and at 10 P. M. had rigors accompanied by nervous symptoms such as restlessness, jerkiness of the arms and head, and intermittent convulsions of the neck and both arms. She later became drowsy and prostrated. The next day she vomited, and remained prostrated and weak. Two days later she appeared much better. Jaundice developed and the urine contained bile. On the third day the jaundice began to disappear, and the urine cleared up. Eight days after treatment, recovery seemed complete.

"When carbon tetrachloride is given to animals by mouth none of these symptoms normally occur, but when it is given by inhalation or by vein, they come on at once. It has been found, however, that if carbon tetrachloride is given orally after the animal has taken food, especially fatty food, symptoms appear as they do after inhalation. On this account it has been suggested that carbon tetrachloride always be given on an empty stomach and not be followed by the ingestion of fatty foods for a considerable period of time. A possible explanation of this intoxication is that the carbon tetrachloride is absorbed by the lymphatics and reaches the general circulation by way of the thoracic duct without passing through the liver, thus coming to the brain in higher concentration than when it is absorbed through the portal system. In the latter case, the liver takes out a considerable amount of the drug. Experiments are under way to determine whether the route of entry is a causative factor in this type of intoxication or whether lipemia in itself favors retention in the blood of carbon tetrachloride in concentrations sufficient to produce intoxication."

(d) *Calcium as a Factor.*—"Besides the deaths in alcoholic addicts, in patients heavily infested with ascarids, and in those who have taken the drug with food, there still remains a considerable number which cannot be accounted for in any of these ways. Most of these have occurred in children, and the doses given were so small that they seemed at first insufficient to cause death. Autopsy showed, however, the central necrosis characteristic of carbon tetrachloride poisoning. Analysis of these case histories shows that there is a considerable latent period before the onset of symptoms, from twenty-four to thirty-six hours being passed in relative comfort. Nausea and vomiting, which is at times perfectly uncontrollable, then begin. The patient may gradually become unconscious and have convulsions toward the end. Some persons develop marked jaundice and excrete a small quantity of highly bile-stained urine; others vomit and may have more or less severe gastro-intestinal hemorrhages. This may occur after carbon tetrachloride has been given, alone or with oil of chenopodium, to persons with or without ascaris infestation, or to alcoholic addicts. In the latter, apparently the only difference is the greater severity of the symptoms. . . ."

The authors quoted studied this type of intoxication for several years at the Johns Hopkins University without being able to reproduce the symptoms in dogs, no matter what doses of carbon tetrachloride were used. Then, upon the transfer of the work to Vanderbilt University, the dogs were accidentally placed on a diet which was very low in calcium, with the result that symptoms such as have just been described in the human quickly made their appearance when the dogs were again given carbon tetrachloride.

"As soon as calcium carbonate or calcium lactate was added to this lean-meat diet, the animals showed the same tolerance to the drug as was found in the early work in Baltimore. After conclusively proving that the tolerance or susceptibility of dogs to carbon tetrachloride is directly dependent on the calcium content of their diet, it was shown that intoxication from calcium deficiency could be relieved at almost any stage by proper calcium therapy. . . .

"Accurate methods for the determination of ionized calcium in the blood are not yet available, and sufficient time has not elapsed for a complete analysis of the part played by calcium in these intoxications. Sufficient data have been accumulated, however, to allow the formulation of an hypothesis that may be of help in the rational treatment of human cases of intoxication. Carbon tetrachloride causes an acute central necrosis of the liver with an increase of bilirubin in the blood. It is well known that bile pigments are precipitated by calcium *in vitro*, and it has been shown that such a combination between bile pigments and calcium occurs within the organism. Though the calcium may not be actually precipitated and removed from the blood, it probably enters into a complex un-ionized molecule with the bilirubin. Thus, although the total calcium content of the blood may be normal or even high, the active or ionized calcium may be decreased in the presence of increased amounts of biliary constituents. In a poorly nourished animal whose calcium reserve has become low, the colemia caused by the giving of carbon tetrachloride may decrease the amount of ionized calcium below the necessary level, and thus cause acute symptoms of calcium ion lack, such as characteristic tetany, tremors, convulsions, and a great tendency toward hemorrhage. When calcium ions are furnished by any of the methods mentioned, the symptoms disappear, but recur as these ions combine with bilirubin or other biliary constituents."

Prevention and Treatment of Carbon Tetrachloride Poisoning.—Care should be taken, especially in children, to administer a drug, such as chenopodium, which will eliminate the ascarids while the carbon tetrachloride is operating against the hookworms. The authors just quoted believe that this chenopodium should be given several days before the administration of the tetrachloride, but I think that field workers have sufficient faith in the ascaris-destroying power of chenopodium to trust it to overcome the stimulating effect of tetrachloride even when the two drugs are given together. To rid a population of ascarids *first* would add very greatly, perhaps even prohibitively, to the cost of a campaign.

The necessary precautions in the particulars of alcohol and food have already been considered (see pp. 313 and 314, respectively).

Regarding the prevention and treatment of calcium lack, the authors above quoted write: "Since toxic symptoms occur very seldom, and then as a rule only in poorly nourished individuals, it seems safe to assume that most normal adults and children have a sufficient calcium reserve to withstand anthelmintic doses of carbon tetrachloride. As a routine procedure a calcium reserve should be built up in poorly nourished children before treatment. Where either whole or skimmed milk is available, the total daily adult requirement of calcium . . . can be furnished by adding to the diet about 1 quart of milk. In the absence of milk, the same result may be obtained by feeding various calcium salts." They regard calcium chloride by mouth as the most rapid and effective method of increasing the calcium ions in the blood of a patient who is actually having symptoms; intravenous injection of this salt is considered too dangerous to be justified except in moribund cases. They also point out the value of ammonium chloride or hydrochloric acid in making stored calcium available, and state that parathyroid extract has been of value in intoxication induced in the laboratory. For discussion of the dosage and precautions to be observed in using these drugs, the reader is referred to the index at the end of this book.

DISEASES OF ALLERGY

There is a small but baffling group of diseases, comprising principally hay fever, asthma, serum sickness, certain gastro-intestinal disturbances, angioneurotic edema and urticaria, to which the general designation "allergic diseases" has recently been applied. They have in common the following characteristics: They are not infectious; single attacks begin quite abruptly but usually decline gradually; between attacks there are no disturbing residual symptoms (chronic asthma is an exception to this by reason of the accompanying chronic bronchitis and chronic emphysema, and for other reasons); an individual may be the victim of several of these diseases at the same time; the attacks continue to occur with their wonted frequency throughout the course of most of the nonfebrile attacks of disease that may incidentally afflict the individual; the predisposition for these diseases is inherited; with or without treatment, the afflicted individual continues to be susceptible to attacks of these diseases throughout life, though the incidence and severity sometimes decline with advancing years; and finally, diseases of the allergic group are rarely fatal though they cause great suffering and inconvenience. Allergic individuals, then, form a relatively small group of persons who over and over throughout their lives suffer from a few diseases to which the great majority of mankind is not susceptible. In explanation of this unique and distressing state of affairs many men have offered many hypotheses throughout the years; but as early as 1905, Dunbar had introduced the specific protein sensitization theory which is now held by the vast majority of workers to be the right and true explanation; this is to the effect that allergic individuals are those who are hypersensitive to certain foreign proteins and that they experience an attack of one or more of the allergic group of diseases each time that a sufficient quantity of the specific foreign protein comes in contact with their sensitive mucous membranes or skin or enters their blood stream. Minute amounts of these proteins, which are contained in foods, pollens, dust, and many other substances, when deliberately introduced intradermally, give rise to typical local lesions which are considered to be of great diagnostic importance. This theory is at present serving us well, though I feel bound to point out the possibility that it may at any time give way to some other explanation. Indeed, the assumption that only proteins cause the allergic symptoms is already disproved, it would seem, by the work of Hanzlik and Karsner (1924), who have induced similar symptoms in guinea-pigs with such substances as copper sulphate, sodium iodide, fullers' earth, etc., and by the well-confirmed findings of Landsteiner and his associates that numerous crystalloids acquire specific antigenic properties when conjugated with protein "carriers." Also, Grove and Coca (1925), and Black and Moore (1926), have obtained positive skin tests and performed satisfactory treatment with ragweed extract from which protein had been excluded. Also, the specificity of the reactions has been questioned and nonspecific protein therapy in some cases satisfactorily substituted. I look upon Freeman's (1932) studies as convincingly showing the *non*specific, *non*antigenic properties of "proteose," for which Oriel and his associates have made certain claims, but it is nevertheless rapidly becoming apparent that the number of alleged specific substances may be legion; indeed, after the work of Feinberg (1927), it is difficult to escape

317

the feeling that it will eventually be possible to demonstrate sensitiveness to all substances under the sun, when the task of desensitizing the world will logically follow unless it be beforehand recognized and freely admitted that many individuals may be convicted by these skin tests who never throughout their lives evince allergic symptoms, even when in environmental contact with the offending substances. These pages are not the place for a searching enquiry into the admissibility of the current hypothesis, and I would urge the reader to accept it since it has undoubtedly much advanced our knowledge of these matters. But an open mind is a most valuable asset at such a juncture as that which has now been reached in the allergy question. Perhaps something of vital importance with regard to the fundamental cellular dyscrasia underlying the bizarre allergic manifestations has been overlooked during these years of skin-testing. To me it has been a source of much pleasure to observe the apparently complete lack of bias with which the recently constituted British Asthma Commission is approaching its investigations.

HAY FEVER

There are two types of hay fever. The more common, or seasonal, type is that which begins every year when the particular pollen by which it is caused begins to be wind-borne, and persists until pollenation ceases. The quite accurately predictable date of initiation of the annual attack, which used very often to bring down upon the heads of the victims of this disease the charge of being hysteriacs, is now known to be due to the fact that the flora of a given region pollenates with astonishing regularity despite the forwardness or backwardness of a particular season. The pollens of the common trees, grasses and ragweeds are the most usual offenders, conferring, respectively, the titles "spring," "summer" and "fall" hay fever. The symptoms are itching and congestion of the eyes, violent paroxysms of sneezing, and a thin irritating discharge from the nose, often very profuse; oftentimes there is also itching inside the mouth and "behind the eyes." The symptoms vary a great deal in severity during the day, being usually worst in the morning. In most cases there are "good" days and "bad" days, though very many individuals are entirely incapacitated for active participation in affairs throughout the entire "season." Perhaps more than one third of the patients experience asthmatic attacks in conjunction with their hay fever. Those who are affected by the ragweeds can entirely escape their attack by annual migration to a region where the wind does not contain these pollens, but escape for spring and summer sufferers is to be had usually only at sea, since the offending trees and grasses are quite ubiquitous upon the land. Perennial hay fever, the so-called "vasomotor rhinitis," is characterized by the persistence throughout the year of such symptoms as have been described above. Animal danders, vegetable powders, house dust, foods, and drugs are held to be principally responsible for this type of the disease. The line between seasonal and perennial hay fever can be by no means always sharply drawn.

I believe that the earliest clear account of this disease was that of John Bostock, in London, in 1819. It is apparently primarily a malady of the temperate zones, being almost entirely absent from the moist, low-lying, torrid portions of the tropics. The American Indian is thought to be much less susceptible to the disease than the members of any other race, at least in the western world.

THERAPY

1. **Specific Desensitization.**—The practice of "desensitizing" hay fever patients by injecting them with increasing amounts of pollen extracts at frequent intervals during the several months preceding their annual attack was initiated by Noon, in 1911, and has since attained a considerable vogue, though the rationale of the procedure is not as yet entirely established.

Methods of Testing Sensitivity.—(a) *Scratch Test.*—After cleansing with alcohol, the skin is scarified with a needle without drawing blood, a small quantity of the suspected protein is lightly rubbed in, and a drop of N/10 sodium hydroxide is added. An urticarial wheal with pseudopods and an erythematous area is considered positive.

(b) *Intradermal Test.*—About 0.01 cc. of a liquid extract of the suspected substance is injected intradermally; this method is probably more clear-cut and reliable than the previous one but the liability to constitutional reactions is greater.

(c) *Patch Test.*—A small area is washed and rubbed lightly with pumice stone; the suspected material, either in solution or rubbed into a paste, is placed on the area and covered with some impermeable material and held in place by adhesive plaster. The reading is after twenty-four hours or longer.

(d) *Indirect Testing (Prausnitz-Küstner Technic).*—One-tenth cc. of the patient's blood serum is injected intradermally in a normal arm, and twenty-four hours later the suspected substance is injected or scratched into this site; the usual urticarial wheal is a positive reaction.

The latter two of these tests (patch and indirect) are being nowadays much employed in dermatological practice (see p. 665).

Technic of Desensitization.—Nearly every person reporting desensitization studies has described a technic differing slightly from that of someone else, usually the person upon whose work he has modeled his own; the result is that we have in the literature a greater number of methods than can possibly be described here and accredited to their proper originators. Therefore I am obliged to give the standard technic of the New and Nonofficial Remedies, quoting from page 26 of the 1933 edition.

"It is regarded as important that the individual dosage be determined by testing each patient's susceptibility to the specific protein extract, as sensitiveness varies greatly and an overdose may cause disagreeable or alarming symptoms or even death. A method used for such test is to make a series of scratches on the patient's skin (it is important that these should be made at some distance from the scratches of the first test) and to apply to these scratches 25 per cent, 10 per cent, 1 per cent, or even weaker dilutions of the protein extract. From 2 to 5 drops of the dilution which fails to produce a definite skin reaction may be injected subcutaneously as the first dose. Injections, increased by a few drops at first, and later by the use of a stronger dilution, may then be given at intervals of a few days or a week."

Timing the Injections.—The usual practice in administering preseasonal treatment is to give about sixteen injections at intervals of five to seven days, the time of the last injection to coincide approximately with the beginning of the patient's "season," or either to antedate or postdate that time by a few days. Of course the immunity conferred by these injections, when successful, is only sufficient to carry the patient through his "season" in the vast majority of instances, and even then only if the "season" is a short one; the whole course of treatments must be gone through with again during the next year. In regions where pollens are in the air continuously, as in the southern United States, recurrence of symptoms is the rule a few weeks after cessation of the injections. Under these conditions Kahn (1927) adopted the practice of giving the maximum protective dose every six or seven days after this dose had been established and had ceased to cause any local reaction. The inadvisability of teaching patients to give this treatment to themselves, as advocated by Kahn and by Stewart (the originator of "perennial" treatment), is indicated in the occurrence of a severe uterine spasm in one of Kahn's cases. Vander Veer, Cooke and Spain have been continuing once a month throughout the year an injection of the maximum dose attained during the season; their patients so treated obtained greater relief from the more intensive treatment when it was resumed for the succeeding season, but their constitutional reactions were considerably increased in incidence. Vaughan (1931) continues the treatments through the season with maximum or somewhat reduced dosage at two or three weeks' intervals (occasionally, at one, two or three days' intervals with much reduced dosage); after the season he continues a dosage of one fifth the quantity of the dilution used at the height of the season, increasing the dosage up to full quantities again for the next season. With intervals of two weeks for these between-seasons injections he has seen no severe reactions. In Figley's (1930) experience with monthly injections of maximal doses, constitutional reactions occurred at the rate of 1 to 200 injections. In recent years, Freeman, in London, is using his "rush" method with increasing satisfaction; *i. e.*, he waits for the onset of symptoms, then hospitalizes the patient and goes through the whole course of injections in a very few days.

Efficacy of the Treatment.—The therapeutic efficiency of the pollen desensitization treatment of hay fever is very difficult to adjudge for the reason that many of its advocates are addicted to the practice of finding the amount of relief afforded by the injections susceptible to a greater number of divisions than most of us believe to be admissible. That any remedy may cause complete or marked or slight relief in the treatment of any condition is self-evident, but to make further divisions than this in a disease so variable as hay fever, and especially to make a number of subheads under the class "slight relief," is certainly not allowable in my opinion. As one who has had more or less intimate knowledge of a number of cases, I must most earnestly state my belief that the best interests of scientific medicine are but subversibly served when fine shades of relief are drawn in order to prove the efficacy of this remedy. Indeed, I am even sceptical of the value of the treatment to all those patients who are placed in the "slight relief" class, even though no attempt to subdivide these cases is made—so tremendously variable from day to day, and particularly from season to season, is this disease.

There is presented here a tabulation of the results obtained by five well-known workers in the treatment of 2185 cases (Table 34).

Piness has stated that the average of complete relief obtained by all workers is about 23 per cent. It will be seen that in this table the average of complete relief is only 19.3 per cent, but the disparity is undoubtedly due to the fact that both Rackemann and Smith preferred to classify cases as "markedly relieved" which the other workers would have placed in the complete relief column. It would seem, then, that the method was successful in the treatment of 70.5 per cent of all the cases, if we consider that marked as well as complete relief from symptoms may be looked upon as evidence of success. On the other hand, the treatment failed in an average of 33.2 per cent of all the cases, if we consider those obtaining only slight relief as failures also (the percentages reported by the authors are only roughly calculated, hence the number of successes and failures does not add to an even 100 per cent). Two facts, not observable in the table, should be

TABLE 34.—RELIEF OBTAINED BY PRESEASONAL DESENSITIZATION IN 2185 CASES of HAY FEVER

Authority.	No. cases.	Complete relief, per cent.	Marked relief, per cent.	Slight relief, per cent.	No relief, per cent.
Rackemann (1920)	91	9.0	62.0	....	28.0
Vander Veer (1922)	1744	23.0	49.0	18.0	10.0
Bernton (1923)	56	25.0	40.0*	24.0*	10.0
Piness (1925)	202	29.6	40.0	21.4	9.1
Smith (1927)	92	10.0	65.0	19.0	6.0
Averages	....	19.3	51.2	20.6	12.6
		Average success 70.5		Average failure 33.2	

* Sixteen per cent were said to have been relieved 50 per cent of their symptoms; I have considered it fair to allot half this number to the "slight" and half to the "marked" relief columns.

noted here. First, that some of those who obtain no relief are actually made worse by the treatment; one writer, Caulfeild, places this number at 2.3 per cent of the total number treated. Second, that both local and constitutional reactions are of frequent occurrence and both types are oftentimes severe; a few deaths have been recorded. Piness reports that in 202 cases, local reactions occurred in 132 patients and that constitutional reactions occurred seventeen times; he further states, "the greatest percentage of reactions occurring in those patients who received the greatest measure of relief, which is in accordance with the experience of others." Duke (1930) mixes each dose of protein solution with the following, and injects the whole: 0.15 cc. of a mixture of ephedrine (3 per cent), 2 parts, and epinephrine (1: 1000 solution), 1 part, plus 0.3 cc. physiologic saline. With this mixture, and by controlling the dissemination of the pollen by the application of a tourniquet above the site of injection, he claims to have very greatly reduced the number and severity of reactions.

In view of the above considerations, I think a fair summary of the present status of this type of therapy would be as follows: Of the total number of hay fever sufferers who will submit to desensitization, approximately two thirds will be very considerably relieved, while only slight or no relief will be obtained by the other third; also, a considerable number of the patients will have to undergo local and constitutional reactions of varying severity; and, finally, as a result of the treatments, from 2 to 3 per cent of the total number of patients will have worse symptoms than they had ever experienced before. These are the results obtained by expert allergists who confine their practice to this class of maladies exclusively; it is quite generally acknowledged that in the hands of the profession at large the results are very poor.

2. **Nonspecific Protein Therapy.**—Nonspecific proteins are much favored in Europe, but in North America they have not given results at all comparable with those obtainable by the use of the specific pollen substances. The method of using them may be found in the paper of Schiff (1926), who reports the employment of a 50 per cent aqueous solution of peptone, administered intracutaneously, beginning with 1 minim as the initial dose and increasing by 1 minim every other day, up to 3 minims; then continuing on 3 minims for twenty days. This author states that in some cases practically all symptoms disappeared after the second or third dose (*i e.*, after

three to five days); unfortunately the number of cases treated and the percentage responding thus favorably are not given. Vaughan (1931) has also experienced some success with the method.

3. **Calcium and Viosterol.**—The successful employment of calcium chloride internally in the treatment of hay fever was first reported by Emmerich and Loew, in 1913, the treatment finding its rationale in the fact that calcium is believed to decrease the permeability of blood and lymph vessels and thereby to lessen exudation, though its possible stimulation of the sympathetic portion of the autonomic nervous system, as pointed out by Pottenger, must not be overlooked. Recently (1929), I have added the hypothesis that the calcium may act favorably by reason of the fact that much of it is converted into the carbonate in the intestinal tract and that the chlorine, thus liberated, is rapidly absorbed and serves to increase the acidity of the tissues. Emmerich and Loew advised the use of the drug daily over a very long period, as much as a year, if possible, before the onset of the "season," but from the experience of those who have tried the remedy faithfully during the past twenty years the fact has emerged that success or failure depends not so much upon the length of the period of calcium ingestion as it does upon the constitution of the individual patient—that is to say, there are some who respond remarkably well to calcium therapy even though the drug be administered during only a relatively short period of time, whereas, there are others, and these seem to be vastly in the majority, who obtain no relief even though they ingest large amounts of calcium each day for a very long time. Wilson treated 22 patients with calcium chloride during one season. In no case did any patient take the drug for more than eight or ten weeks before the time of the expected attack, and in most cases the period was much shorter; yet of this number, 10 were much relieved (6 being practically symptomless during their "season"), while the remaining 12 did not in the least respond to the treatment. In the cases responding favorably, the relief came after taking only a few doses. On the other hand, Criep and McElroy (1928) failed to obtain any relief at all in any of their 43 patients. Wilson's method of administration follows.

"For most patients the calcium chloride was prescribed thus:

"℞. Calcium chloride, crystals................................ 100 Gm.
    Distilled water to make.................................. 500 cc.
    Label: Take 1 teaspoonful in sufficient water during or after each meal.

"This gives the patient about 3 Gm. of calcium daily. The crystalline salt is used in preference to the anhydrous, as making a cleaner and clearer solution. When the anhydrous salt is prescribed, allowance should be made for the water of crystallization, of which in the crystalline salt there are six molecules ($CaCl_2 + 6H_2O$):

"℞. Calcium chloride, anhydrous............................ 50 Gm.
    Distilled water to make.................................. 500 cc.
    Label: Take 1 teaspoonful in sufficient water with or after each meal."

The ingestion of even larger amounts of calcium than this is not harmful. One of Wilson's patients experienced gastric distress until the dose was reduced; another complained of weakness and loss of appetite, and had to use it intermittently in a lessened dose; another thought it caused a diminution in the urinary output, while another thought the flow of urine was increased.

The preliminary studies of Rappaport and Reed (1933) with viosterol are of great interest. In a small group of patients suffering with allergic hay fever and asthma they obtained marked relief from symptoms by the daily administration of viosterol of much greater concentration than that of the preparations at present commercially available. Their promised studies of the effective dose of viosterol that will produce changes in the calcium-potassium ratio within physiologic limits and yet be of therapeutic value in the allergic conditions will be awaited with great interest.

4. **Endocrine.**—Although endocrine therapy is on the whole usually quite satisfactory, it has sometimes been directly responsible for the disappearance of allergic symptoms. The coincidence of one of the classical endocrinopathies is the indication for its use, and not promiscuously in allergy *per se.*

5. **Surgery.**—Despite the allegations of those who hold out for surgery in all conditions, I believe it is now the consensus of opinion among otolaryngologists that little, if anything, is to be hoped for from operative procedures in the treatment of hay fever.

6. **Topical Applications.**—The application of a cocaine solution to the mucous membranes of the nose several times during the day will give considerable relief in many cases, but the remedy is absolutely contraindicated as a routine procedure for very obvious reasons. Butyn or Alypin is sometimes very well substituted, 1 or 2 grains to the ounce (0.06 or 0.12 to 30 cc.) in solution; the latter may be used in alkaline medium. The use of a dilute solution of epinephrine as a nasal spray is often unsatisfactory for two reasons: First, it is in itself sometimes very irritating when used under these conditions; and second, the patient often experiences an attack of hay fever of explosive violence when coming out from under the brief influence of this drug.

Duke (1925) gives the following formula for an epinephrine mixture:

R. Solution epinephrine hydrochloride (1 : 1000)................ 1.0 cc.
Dilute acetic acid... 0.3 "
Resorcin solution (3 per cent) to make..................... 32.0 "
Label: Apply to conjunctiva and nasal mucosa when necessary.

Ephedrine hydrochloride or sulphate, used in a 1 to 3 per cent aqueous solution is relatively free from the objectionable features of epinephrine's action and is effective for a much longer time. Synephrine is used in 5 per cent solution and in many instances with good success, apparently, too, without disagreeable by-effects.

Chandler (1932) inserts a probe covered with cotton saturated with full strength phenol through the nasal speculum into the nasopharynx, thus coating the surface of the anterior portion of the nares and inferior turbinate. He states that the patient is usually much improved on the second day and that the treatment may be repeated in one week, if necessary; coughing caused by acid dropping into the throat is neutralized by an application of alcohol.

7. **Ephedrine, Synephrine.**—The use of these drugs systemically in asthma and hay fever is discussed on page 328.

8. **Nitrohydrochloric Acid.**—In 1893, Bishop proposed the uric acid theory of hay fever in the first prize essay of the United States Hay Fever Association and advocated the theory at the meeting of the American Medical Association the same year. Learning in 1894 that Tyrrel, of Toronto, had published a paper in 1892 advancing the same theory, he readily accorded full credit to Tyrrel for his work. The use of acid upon purely theoretical grounds was advocated by Bishop. However, the excellent results obtained by him were soon lost sight of in the welter of papers then appearing upon the subject of "uric-acid diathesis," to which Bishop himself considerably contributed. Also, the causal relationship of pollens to the disease was beginning to be urged at this time, and further contributed to push the newly advocated drug into the background before it had had

any sort of fair trial. Certainly, I can find no account of its extensive use with a report of the findings anywhere in the literature between 1897 and my own revival of the method, in 1927, though Gleason has always carried a reference to it in the various editions of his well-known text-book of otolaryngology.

In the first few cases I prescribed the acid to be dropped (10 drops) into water just before taking, but soon found this method open to the following objections: (1) Druggists are reluctant to dispense the full-strength acid, looking upon 10 drops of "aqua regia" (the "official" dose is 3 minims) as dangerous; (2) the full-strength acid is so corrosive that its handling in the household is very difficult. Latterly I have, therefore, written the following prescription:

Ŗ. Nitrohydrochloric acid (*not* the dilute)................ ℥ivss   18.0
      Distilled water to make............................ ℥iv   120.0

The patient is directed to take 1 teaspoonful of this in ⅔ glass of water, followed by another glass of water, after each meal and again upon retiring (as near midnight as possible). This is a pleasantly acid but not corrosive tasting mixture, which may be dispensed in the usual bottle with a cork stopper. The midnight dose is very important; when it is omitted the patient will almost invariably have early morning symptoms. The ingestion of the acid, even in this large dose, cannot be looked upon as in any sense dangerous. One precaution, however, I have always taken, namely, that of forbidding the use of any laxatives or purgatives not prescribed by me, as there is perhaps some very slight danger of calomel being converted into corrosive sublimate by the acid. The use of the remedy is begun only with the onset of the individual's season.

Since the publication of the first of my papers on this subject in 1927, I have gathered the accounts of 610 cases in which the acid has been used. Sixty-three per cent of these cases obtained marked or complete relief from symptoms by taking four doses of the acid daily (in some instances the full dose is taken every two hours). None of the patients experienced reactions of a more serious nature than a transient diarrhea or diuresis, and either of these only very rarely, nor did any person who obtained relief object to the "strong" taste of the mixture.

In Table 35 there is offered a comparison of the acid and desensitization types of treatment. In studying this table, it should be borne in mind that

TABLE 35.—COMPARISON OF RESULTS IN ACID AND DESENSITIZATION TREATMENT OF HAY FEVER

	No. cases.	Complete relief, per cent.	Marked relief, per cent.	Successfully treated (Marked plus Complete), per cent.	No relief, per cent.
Acid treatment...................	610	37	26	63	37
Desensitization (see p. 321)........	2185	19	51	70	30

I am comparing here the results obtained by general practitioners using the acid with those of expert allergists using the desensitization method—obviously this is more than fair to desensitization since general practitioners have no such success with it. Only 27 of these acid-treated patients were seen by me personally, the remainder of the cases being reported to me by physicians residing in all parts of the country. Of course statistics compiled in this fashion have no exact value, but I feel that they do clearly show that widely scattered practitioners are using the remedy with some measure of success. Some men report to me large numbers of cases in which they have almost completely failed, others report series of equal size in which success has been phenomenal. I do not understand this, but I am certain that the measure deserves trial in every case. Thommen, in the recent exhaustive treatise on the allergic diseases of Coca, Walzer and Thommen (1931), states his belief that this acid therapy is the most promising of the new departures in the symptomatic treatment of hay fever.

9. **Pollen Filters and Air Conditioning.**—The use of filters for supplying pollen-free air to dwelling rooms has been advocated by a number of observers recently. There seems to be no doubt that hay fever sufferers are greatly, sometimes completely, relieved during their sojourn in a room thus equipped. Apparently "air conditioning" is equally effective.

10. x-**Ray, Ultraviolet Ray, Diathermy.**—See page 330.

ASTHMA

The asthmatic individual is one who is prone to attacks of difficult breathing whose immediate cause has been known, since its first mention by Sir John Floyer (1648), to be spasm of the bronchial muscles plus edema of the bronchial mucous membranes; the fundamental, though the more remote, cause of these spasms still remains unknown. The disease is included by all authors among the allergic group, but I cannot too earnestly repeat (see p. 317) that allergy itself is but a symptom of a hereditary constitutional dyscrasia. The attacks may last for a few minutes to several hours and are very distressing, though death from asthma *per se* is very rare. Characteristically, the patient coughs at the end of each attack and raises sputum which contains Charcot-Leyden crystals and the bodies known as Curschmann's spirals. These attacks may be infrequent or they may occur every day or several times during the night over a long period. In simple uncomplicated asthma relaxation is usually complete between spasms, but most long-standing cases are complicated by emphysema and chronic bronchitis and are therefore "wheezy" and somewhat distressed at all times. Unless complicated by the two diseases just mentioned, pain in the chest and cyanosis are rare during attacks. The studies of Harkavy (1924) strongly indicate that the syndrome hitherto known as "cardiac asthma" is merely the coincidental existence of asthma and cardiovascular disease in the one individual.

THERAPY

When it first became apparent that asthma could best be studied upon an allergic basis, it was felt by investigators that it would ultimately become possible to desensitize and thus cure all individuals suffering from the disease; however, this enthusiasm has now considerably waned, and it is frankly admitted by the more conservative students of the subject that there is need for more than one type of therapeutic approach to the disease. As a result, it has become the fashion to classify the cases as "extrinsic," "intrinsic" and "miscellaneous unclassified" asthma. The extrinsic cases are those that are believed to be caused by hypersensitiveness to some foreign substance outside the body, the individuals having asthma on exposure to, or contact with it. Pollens, animal danders, dusts, and foods are the principal offenders. Of 1074 cases reported by Rackemann, 39.5 per cent were in this class. The intrinsic group comprises cases that are believed to be due to infection in the upper or lower respiratory tract, cases that are reflexly caused by bad teeth, nose and throat pathology, constipation, cholecystitis or other well-defined foci of infection, and cases more or less directly associated with such conditions as pregnancy, obesity, nervousness, and bad hygiene (the latter to include such items as unwise dietary schedule, a lack of proper fresh air and exercise, insufficient intake of fluids, and continued overwork without proper rest periods). In Rackemann's series, 46.6 per cent of the cases were placed in this group. The miscellaneous unclassified cases are, of course, just what the name implies; the remaining 13.9 per cent of Rackemann's cases fell here. In the extrinsic group, treatment consists in attempting to find the offending substance and eliminate it from the environment, perhaps by removing an animal, such as a cat or horse, or deleting a certain type of food from the dietary, or by removing an article, such as the feather pillow or a substance met with in the occupation, or by a more radical procedure, such as a change of climate, residence or work. Where these methods fail, or seem impracticable, attempt is made to desensitize by injection as in hay fever. In the intrinsic group, attempt is made to remove foci of infection, to build up resistance by the employment of bacterial vaccines, and to correct the bodily and mental pathology which is believed to be responsible for the asthmatic condition.

The results attained in the treatment of asthma are extremely variable, but it is becoming more and more apparent that the conservative investigators of the disease are essentially in agreement as to what can be accomplished. In 1927, Rackemann, of the Massachusetts General Hospital, reported a study of 1074 cases that had been followed for two years. In 213, or 20 per cent, of these cases "cure" was claimed, but reviewing the cases again in late 1932, he finds that the number of these cured persons has shrunken to only 12 per cent of the total. Some observers prefer not to recognize a "cured" class, holding that an absolute cure is probably never attained in the treatment of asthma.

1. **Specific Desensitization.**—When indicated, this type of therapy is instituted just as in the treatment of hay fever. For the methods, see page 319. It is generally conceded to be less effective in asthma than in hay fever.

2. **Bacterial Vaccines.**—Despite the many theoretical, and allegedly experimental, arguments against the efficacy of bacterial vaccines in the treatment of asthma, a number of authors have been able to report results with these vaccines that are quite comparable with those obtained by the institution of "specific" desensitization. The usual method is to prepare vaccines from pure cultures of organisms obtained from the thick mucus coughed up from down in the lungs during the breaking-up of an attack. Skin tests are performed with these vaccines and the injections then made with the one, or with a mixture of the several, that gave positive reactions. The first dose averages 50 million killed organisms, but it may be as high as 200 million if the test reaction was very slight. Subsequent doses, at five- to seven-day intervals, are increased by the size of the original dose until 1 to 2 billion (occasionally as high as 4 billion) organisms per dose is reached; it is then sometimes the practice to continue the administration of this maximum dose at intervals of a month for a long period. It is desirable to obtain a local reaction from every treatment, but if this reaction

is very severe or if there is a constitutional reaction, the next dose should be the same in size as the one causing excessive reaction or perhaps even smaller.

It is noteworthy that Rackemann and Graham (1923), and Hooker and Anderson (1929) have obtained just as good results with stock vaccines as with autogenous preparations.

3. **Nonspecific Proteins.**—There is good reason to believe that there is a nonspecific factor in both the specific desensitization and bacterial vaccine types of therapy, as witness the fact that relief is often obtained by these two methods without much alteration in the skin test. Pagniez and Widal, Abrami and Brissaud, Auld, Schiff, Urbach and others have reported the use of peptone. Boyd claimed success with typhoid vaccine; Van Leeuwen, Maxwell, and others with tuberculin. A number of observers have used injections of milk and of whole blood; Nelson and Porter media broth; Van Leeuwen sulphur. All have reported more or less success, but there is no lack of dissentient or at least healthily sceptical voices: Ramirez, Behrman, Irons. Fever therapy is discussed on page 331; methods on page 187.

Peptone.—Schiff prepares a 33 per cent solution in glycerin and water by rubbing Armour's peptone siccum (dry) in the mixture of the other two ingredients, warming to complete solution, and then filtering until clear. This solution may be sterilized and will keep at room temperature. Three minims is a safe initial dose, increased by 1 minim at biweekly or triweekly intervals up to 1 cc. Auld sometimes modifies the mixture as follows: To 1 ounce (30 cc.) of serum, pipetted off the patient's blood drawn from the arm on the day before, is added 1.5 Gm. of Armour's No. 2 peptone, 0.006 Gm. agar which has been well boiled, and about 10 drops of chloroform; the mixture is incubated at 37 to 40 C. for three hours and the clear fluid pipetted off for use the next day. Very slow intravenous injections of this fluid are given twice a week, beginning with about 10 minims (0.6 cc.) and increasing 5 minims (0.3 cc.) each injection until 45 minims (3 cc.) is reached, or continuing at any time with the dose which gives greatest relief.

Whole Blood.—From 5 to 10 cc. of blood is withdrawn from the arm vein and immediately reintroduced intramuscularly into the buttock; injections twice or oftener per week, usually not exceeding a maximum of 20 cc. per dose.

Milk.—Straight whole milk is poured into a 2-ounce (60 cc.) rubber-capped bottle, stood in a water bath up to the neck of the bottle and boiled for one hour. Initial dose of 0.5 to 1 cc. is increased by 0.5 cc. at triweekly intervals up to 2 or at most 3 cc.; the injections are usually given subcutaneously.

Tuberculin.—Old tuberculin is used in dilutions of 1 in 1,000,000; 1 in 100,000; 1 in 10,000; 1 in 1000; and 1 in 100 (rarely). The first dose of 0.1 cc. of the 1: 1,000,000 is increased at weekly intervals to 0.2, 0.4 and 0.6 cc., after which the next dose is 0.1 cc. of the next dilution, and so on. When the 1: 1000 dilution is reached, Maxwell (1930) increases the interval to two weeks and the dose by 0.1 cc. until 0.5 cc. is reached; this dose is repeated monthly as long as necessary.

Broth.—A standard broth such as that used in making artificial culture media is employed in dilutions and dosage much the same as tuberculin (see above).

Sulphur.—Van Leeuwen injects intramuscularly about 1 cc. of a 1 per cent suspension of sulphur in olive oil.

4. **Calcium and Viosterol.**—What has been said of calcium in the treatment of hay fever (see p. 322) applies here equally well. A few patients respond remarkably to its use, while the majority remain unaffected. The

study of viosterol in this disease will be watched with great interest and hope (see p. 322).

5. **Iodides.**—The use of iodides as adjuvants in the treatment of asthma seems to be of such general acceptance that recent medical literature reveals no special studies of its efficacy. The employment of sodium and potassium iodide probably finds its rationale in the well-known ability of these salts to increase the exudation from the respiratory mucous membranes and to liquefy the mucus. Many practitioners feel that the administration of small doses of potassium iodide over a long period of time definitely prolongs the interval between spasmodic attacks. At the Mayo Clinic, 10 per cent solution of sodium iodide in doses up to 10 cc. has been tried, but it is felt (Jour. Amer. Med. Assoc., 84, 698, 1925) that this intravenous method is not superior to the oral method except in a few patients in whom massive doses of iodides by mouth cause an iodism. Some patients, however, are equally intolerant to the intravenous medication; the concentration of iodides in blood and spinal fluid seems to be about the same when given by either route. The Council on Pharmacy and Chemistry of the American Medical Association holds that intravenous medication, generally, is not as safe as oral administration, and, further, that there is little if any justification for the intravenous administration of such an agent as sodium iodide, because its systemic effects are promptly obtained from oral administration.

6. **Epinephrine (Adrenalin).**—It is often tersely stated that a subcutaneous injection of epinephrine will relieve any attack of asthma, but this statement, like so many categorical pronouncements, can be accepted only with certain reservations with regard to dosage and tolerance. The best practice when attempting to relieve an attack with the drug is to give subcutaneously ½ cc. of 1: 1000 solution at five-minute intervals until relief is obtained or tremor appears; the latter more often than not presages the appearance of the former. The amount required to control subsequent attacks varies greatly with individuals but is usually less than used in the first instance. The custom nowadays is to teach patients to administer the injections themselves in the attempt to forestall attacks; such individuals can usually assure themselves a comfortable night by the injection of a few drops in the evening—in the beginning, that is, but as time goes on they nearly always require larger and larger doses. This is true drug tolerance but there is no such thing as addiction in the opium-addiction sense. However, there is a considerable "nervous" element in some allergic individuals and I feel that Lamson's admonition is worth heeding when he points out the psychic dependence upon the drug in the history of several of his patients.

Duke finds that 15 minims (1 cc.) of the drug in a half glass of water by mouth is sometimes as effective as a small dose by needle, but few observers agree with him; one would think the water would have to be held in the mouth to permit sublingual absorption. Rackemann states that in the treatment of children especially, dry epinephrine (1.5 mg.) placed under the tongue is frequently efficacious. Following the animal experiments of Luckhardt and Koppányi, both Lilienthal (1928) and Balyeat (1928) have found that massage of the site of injection of epinephrine one-half to several hours later causes the typical effect to be manifested again to a diminished extent. Epinephrine should be given intravenously in asthma only under circumstances of the direst necessity. No advantage is gained by combining pituitrin with it.

7. **Ephedrine and Synephrine.**—In the treatment of asthma, ephedrine has certainly been shown by Althausen and Schumacher, Piness and Miller, Munns and Aldrich, Middleton and Chen, Thomas and many others, to be (a) very much less reliable than epinephrine in either relieving or pre-

venting the attacks; (*b*) when given by mouth, much slower (ten to thirty minutes) in exerting its effect than the older drug; (*c*) much longer lasting (often many hours) in its effects when they are obtained; (*d*) much more toxic. In severe cases it is usually very little if at all effective, and in moderately severe or mild cases the result seems to depend upon whether or not the patient happens to be susceptible to the drug's action, whereas practically all persons respond favorably to epinephrine given by the needle. The chief advantage of ephedrine is of course the fact that it may be given by the mouth. The average dose is perhaps 25 to 50 mg., but it varies widely; some patients are able to prevent an attack by taking a small dose upon retiring, whereas many others are forced to take 50 to 100 mg. or more at intervals of several hours throughout the day in order to obtain any measure of relief. Both the sulphate and hydrochloride (the asserted superiority of this salt is largely academic) are available commercially in a wide range of tablets, capsules, solutions, elixirs, syrups, etc., and ampules for hypodermic administration. In Munns and Aldrich's experience with children, the minimum and maximum doses were 12 and 50 mg., respectively.

Many physicians have noted that the drug often becomes less and less effective with succeeding doses, but habit-formation or abstinence symptoms have never been reported to my knowledge. The chief objection to ephedrine is the frequency and oftentimes marked though not serious nature of its side-actions, which preclude its use altogether in a large proportion of patients: nausea, vomiting, sweating, bladder irritability, urinary retention (Balyeat and Rinkel, 1932), skin eruptions, dysmenorrhea, palpitation, vertigo, tremor, general nervousness and apprehension, insomnia, etc. Caffeine and nicotine in most instances definitely increase the severity of the symptoms. The greatest possible care should be exercised to avoid giving epinephrine and ephedrine in a way that their effects might overlap. The barbiturates, especially amytal, are much used to counteract the ephedrine effects.

Many observers have reported the successful use of ephedrine by mouth in hay fever, subject to the same qualifications as to dosage and undesirable side-effects that apply in asthma. Thommen's (1931) series comprised 245 patients, more than 70 per cent of whom obtained some measure of relief; 22 per cent could not use the drug at all because of its untoward effects.

Synephrine.—Thommen (1931) was able to successfully terminate several mild attacks of asthma in 8 patients with the oral administration of this drug in 1½- to 3-grain (0.1 to 0.2 Gm.) doses, but he failed to affect the severe attacks. No disagreeable side-effects were observed.

8. Other Drugs.—*Atropine.*—I quote Duke: "Drugs of the atropine series are time-honored remedies in the treatment of asthma. . . . Atropine is effective in some cases even when given in small doses. In others it is ineffective. In can be used either locally or subcutaneously or by inhalation. If given by mouth or subcutaneously it should be pushed to the point of causing dryness of the mouth. It is rarely advisable to push the drug to the point of blurring vision. Some patients can tolerate $\frac{1}{100}$ grain two or three times daily, while others who are more susceptible cannot tolerate this amount. Atropine can frequently be used to advantage in conjunction with adrenalin. Often the appropriate use of atropine in small doses marks the difference between success and failure in the relief of patients who have been treated according to other principles. . . . A patient nearly relieved by other means may often be completely relieved with the help of atropine."

As compared with epinephrine, atropine when used alone is the less valuable drug for two reasons: First, because most patients are not markedly relieved until doses large enough to cause flushing, considerable dryness of mucous membranes, and more or less cerebral excitement are used; and second, because the majority of patients become tolerant to it much sooner than they do to epinephrine.

Depressants.—Because of the chronic nature of the disease, morphine is absolutely contraindicated except when it is imperative that the patient have a respite from the mental and physical distress of extremely severe paroxysms, and then it should be used only if all other drugs have failed. It is by no means a sovereign specific in the treatment of asthma. Maytum (1931) has relieved several extremely severe attacks by the colonic administration of ether.

Inhalants.—In mild cases the inhalation of the smoke from an ignited mixture of stramonium and a nitrate may be resorted to with advantage once or several times during the night; there is available a number of commercial asthma powders and cigarettes, but the following is more economical:

℞.	Sodium nitrate.....................................	℥ss	15.0
	Powdered anise.....................................	℥ss	15.0
	Stramonium..	℥j	30.0

Label: A teaspoonful to be ignited and the smoke inhaled.

A few patients will be helped by the inhalation of a steaming preparation such as described on page 30.

Acetylsalicylic Acid-whisky.—Five to 10 grains (0.3 to 0.6 Gm.) of aspirin, administered together with a hot toddy, is a potent mixture which will oftentimes conquer even severe paroxysms (Duke, 1928). The first dose of the aspirin should be very small, however, because many asthmatics are hypersensitive (*i. e.*, have an allergic reaction) to the drug.

9. Endocrine.—What has been said on this head in discussing the treatment of hay fever (see p. 323) applies here also.

10. x-Ray.—In the beginning of this type of therapy, which originated in Germany, only the chest was exposed anteriorly and posteriorly, but subsequent reports have shown that the treatments need not be confined to this portion of the body as the results are probably due to a constitutional reaction akin to the nonspecific protein reaction. At the present time, either the lung or spleen area, or both, are usually exposed; a symptomatic reaction typically follows each treatment, but this is succeeded by temporary, occasionally permanent, improvement in a variable number of cases; in Waldbott's (1928) series of 81 patients, 21 were apparently permanently, and 25 temporarily, relieved. All observers have not had such good results.

11. Other Types of Physiotherapy and Breathing Exercises.—Various forms of hydrotherapy, baths, spa cures, ultraviolet ray exposures, etc., have been advocated from time to time, but none merit special description here. In hay fever, diathermy is sometimes applied locally to the nasal mucosa, or special quartz rods are used to carry ultraviolet rays to the anterior and posterior nares. Perhaps the best known of the several schemes for inducing forced expiration is that of Hofbauer, in Vienna; I was not at all favorably impressed when I saw him demonstrate his method, in 1931.

12. Special Diets.—Of course the whole gamut of dietary experiments has been run in this disease, but it seems to me that the most rational of these has been the ketogenic regimen, as practiced by Peshkin and Fineman (for methods of inducing ketosis, see p. 641). On the other hand, it is not difficult to see how the glucose-feeding studies of the British Asthma Commission may also succeed, since the liver, which functions best when well supplied with sugar, is known to play a large part in antigen-antibody reactions. Moll's (1932) success with liver diet, as used in pernicious anemia, is worthy of note.

13. **Nitrohydrochloric Acid.**—The acid is also being used with some success in asthma, particularly when complicating hay fever (see p. 323).

14. **Fever Therapy.**—All practitioners of wide experience know that a bout of fever often entirely relieves allergic maladies for the time being and in some instances even for a long period following recovery from the intercurrent acute infectious process. Latterly a number of attempts have been made to accomplish the same thing by fever artificially induced as in the treatment of neurosyphilis (see p. 187). Diathermy is being preferred by a number of the observers (Leopold and Stewart; Vallery-Radot and Mauric; Feinberg, Osborne and Afremow; Bezançon and Jacquelin), but it is still too early to judge of the value of this new therapeutic departure; however, in accord with my view that there is likely an acid-base imbalance in allergy, I find these attempts entirely rational.

15. **Lipiodol.**—A few physicians have with great caution begun the introduction of iodized oil into the tracheobronchial tree in asthma. Cole and Harper (1933) have obtained some relief in all of their 26 patients but they feel that all other measures should be tried before resorting to this method of treatment. This is work only for fully qualified experts, of course.

ANGIONEUROTIC EDEMA AND URTICARIA

Urticaria, or "hives," is characterized by the sudden appearance in the skin of a firm, elevated, whitish patch, which is surrounded by a pink zone and is accompanied by intense itching or stinging sensations. The lesion may be single or multiple and usually resembles in size the wheal caused by the ordinary mosquito bite; in the cases known as "giant" urticaria, however, the individual lesions are much larger than this and several often coalesce to form a relatively enormous patch. The wheals disappear in a few minutes to hours, or, in the more severe cases may persist for several days. It is usual for hives to appear in crops with relatively long asymptomatic periods between, but some individuals are rarely free from these distressing lesions for more than a few days in succession. In angioneurotic edema the subcutaneous tissues as well as the skin participate in the transient swelling, which usually affects the forehead, eyelids or lips, and is only rarely accompanied by pronounced subjective symptoms; when the internal organs are involved also, as is very occasionally the case, the symptoms may of course simulate almost anything. All the recorded fatalities have been due to sudden edema of the larynx.

In Menagh's (1928) analysis of 260 cases, in which urticaria and angioneurotic edema were considered to be the same process involving only different layers of the skin, food or other proteins were found to be causative in 30 per cent, biliary tract involvement in 48.8 per cent, both in 11.2 per cent, and no etiology was discovered in 10 per cent. In a group of 40 patients very carefully studied, Criep and Wechsler (1931) found evidence of increased or decreased thyroid activity in a rather large proportion; the incidence of hypo-acidity and actual achylia was also rather high.

THERAPY

In the matter of specific desensitization, nonspecific protein therapy, and the administration of calcium, what has already been written in regard to hay fever and asthma applies here equally and need not be repeated.

Unfortunately the results of such treatment are usually very unsatisfactory
in the entities at present under consideration. In the group of cases associated with biliary tract disease, Menagh found that therapeutic biliary
drainage often brought striking relief. Some patients are almost at once
relieved by brisk saline catharsis, but they are certainly in the minority;
perhaps it is only those whose symptoms are due to food allergy (see below) who obtain this relief. Brown (1931) has found that the administration of dilute hydrochloric acid as in achlorhydria (see p. 409), or 20 to 30
grains (1.2 to 2 Gm.) of citric acid in a glass of water with each meal, is
sometimes helpful. One-half to 1 cc. of epinephrine hydrochloride (1: 1000
solution) usually gives considerable relief during the attack; it is sometimes possible to lower the subsequent doses. Massage of the site of injection (see p. 328) might be helpful here. The use of splenic extract is discussed on page 664. For local application, nothing perhaps gives as great
relief as "pink lotion" (see p. 166). Fantus recommends the application of
any one of the following solutions, applied as hot as can be borne and followed, without drying, by dusting with talcum: sodium bicarbonate, 1 to 5
per cent; sodium carbonate, ½ to 3 per cent; borax, 1 to 4 per cent.

FOOD ALLERGY

It is not possible in a single small volume of this nature to describe the
host of ailments which investigators nowadays recognize as being in all
probability allergic manifestations to specific food substances; chief among
them, however, are many cases of the following: Urticaria and angioneurotic
edema, migraine, hay fever, asthma, eczema, several other dermatoses, and
gastro-intestinal disturbances which may simulate any of the well-known
acute or chronic syndromes.

THERAPY

Specific desensitization usually fails in these cases; indeed, skin reactions to the offending food are seldom positive. The two principal methods
of treatment are the dietary, whose chief advocate in America is Rowe,
and the use of peptone by mouth, according to the plan of Urbach in Vienna.
Just worthy of mention in passing, however, is the proposal of Richet
(1932) to protect the intestinal mucosa from offending substances by mixing mineral oil with the food. The treatment consists solely of having the
patient take a dessertspoonful of the liquid petrolatum at the beginning and
end of each meal; so far, the results are excellent but still unconfirmed,
and the method is included here only because of its attractive simplicity.

Dietary Treatment.—Rowe has exhaustively exploited the possibilities
of this type of treatment. After eliminating at the beginning such foods as
the patient definitely dislikes or knows to disagree with him, further study
of the case is based upon the use of "elimination" diets (Table 36), consisting of foods which experience has shown rarely cause symptoms. The
diet best suited to the patient is chosen for the start; diet 1, Rowe has
found most generally useful (the menu possibilities of this diet are shown
in Table 37); diet 4 is planned for a possible sensitization to all meats;
diet 5 may be used if the patient does not give any indications of milk
sensitization, other foods being gradually added and the effect of each
watched. In Table 38 there is a cereal-free diet (included here with the
recipes by Dr. Rowe's kind permission). On whatever diet is chosen, the

TABLE 36.—"ELIMINATION DIETS" FOR THE TREATMENT OF FOOD ALLERGY (ROWE)

	Diet 1	Diet 2	Diet 3	Diet 4	Diet 5
Cereal.......	Rice (natural)	Corn	Rice Tapioca	Rice Rye	Milk alone for the test period 2-3 quarts a day
Bread........	None	Corn pone*	None	Rye Rice† Rye Crisp	
Meat or fish...	Lamb	Bacon Chicken	Beef	Cod, halibut and white fish	
Vegetables....	Lettuce Spinach Carrots	Squash Asparagus Peas Artichokes	Tomatoes Celery String beans	Lettuce Carrots Peas Beets	
Fruits and jams and fruit drinks......	Lemon Pears Peaches	Pineapple Apricot Prunes	Grapefruit Pears Peaches	Pineapple Apricots Pears	
Miscellaneous .	Sugar Olive oil Salt Olives (unstuffed) Maple syrup Gelatin	Sugar Mazola oil Salt	Sugar Wesson oil Salt Gelatin Maple syrup	Sugar Olive oil Salt Olives (unstuffed)	

* Corn pone is made with cornmeal, salt, water, and Crisco.

† Rye rice bread: ⅓ cup rye flour, ⅔ cup rice flour, 6 level teaspoonfuls baking powder (Royal), 4 level teaspoonfuls sugar, ¼ teaspoonful salt, ⅔ cup water, ½ teaspoonful shortening. This recipe makes eight small muffins. This recipe doubled can be made into a loaf. Perhaps more palatable if toasted. Royal Baking Powder does not contain egg.

TABLE 37.—MENU FOR DIET 1 OF TABLE 36 (ROWE)

Breakfast:	
Rice	Boiled. natural, served with peach or pear juice and sugar Fried in olive oil and served with sugar or maple syrup
Pears or peaches	Large helping, fresh or canned
Drinks	Lemonade with plenty of sugar
Lunch and Dinner:	
Soup	Lamb broth with rice and carrots
Salad	Lettuce with pears or peaches with olives and olive oil and lemon. Green or ripe olives, unstuffed
Meats	Roast lamb with gravy made with rice flour Broiled lamb chops
Vegetables	Spinach or carrots. Boiled natural rice
Dessert	Lemon gelatin or pears or peaches
Drinks	Lemonade with plenty of sugar

1. Absolutely no foods other than those specified in each diet can be used. Thus, in diet 1 rice must not be fried with butter or lard but only with the fat specified, which is olive oil. Absolutely no bread, milk, cream or other nonspecified foods can be used.

2. Prescribed fruits can be used in drinks, in salads, for desserts and for jams and sauces.

3. Gravies for meats and sauces for vegetables can be thickened only with flour allowable, i. e., rice in diet 1; cornstarch in diet 2, and so on.

4. Olive oil in diet 1, corn oil in diet 2 and cotton seed oil in diet 3 are indicated according to sensitizations to olive, corn or cotton seed antigens. These may be interchanged if necessary.

5. Calories must be increased by plenty of sugar, oil and starch prescribed. Vitamins must be assured by plenty of vegetables and fruits prescribed.

6. In diet 2, baked corn pone made with corn meal and water, or corn meal mush fried in maize oil or bacon fat eaten with prune or apricot juice or plain sugar syrup would be in order.

7. In diet 3, tapioca, baked with peaches and sugar and flavored with orange or orange peel may be suggested.

8. In diet 4, if the patient is sensitive to fish but not to eggs, eggs may be substituted.

9. These diets are models on which other diets composed of foods indicated by history of food sensitizations and skin tests may be formulated if desired by physician Diet 1 has been found especially useful either as it is or with foods substituted for those to which patients were sensitive.

10. The "elimination diet" found to relieve the patient's symptoms can be increased by gradual addition of foods to which the patient is found to be nonsensitive.

TABLE 38.—SUGGESTED MENU FOR CEREAL-FREE DIET (ROWE)

	Amounts.	
	Grams.	Approximate.
Breakfast:		
Grapefruit juice..................................	200	1 large
Tapioca with apricots...........................	....	⅔ cup
Bacon, medium..................................	33	5 slices, thin and long
Peach or apricot preserves......................	48	2½ teaspoonfuls
Lima bean and potato muffin*...................	....	2 small
Lunch:		
Salad:		
Tomato.......................................	100	1 medium
Lettuce......................................	100	¼ medium head
Olive oil....................................	13	1 tablespoonful
Lemon juice for French dressing...............		
Lamb chops....................................	100	2 medium
Baked potato..................................	100	1 medium
Lima bean and potato muffin...................	....	1
Lemonade (lemon juice)........................	30	2 tablespoonfuls
(sugar)..	10	2 teaspoonfuls
Peaches...		
Cookies, lima bean and potato..................	....	3 small
Dinner:		
Lamb broth....................................		
Roast lamb....................................	100	4 slices, 4½ x 2 x ⅛″
Sweet potato..................................	100	1 medium
Carrots.......................................	133	1 cup
Salad:		
Lettuce hearts................................	100	¼ medium head
Olive oil....................................	13	1 tablespoonful
Lemon juice for French dressing...............		
Muffin, lima bean, and potato.................		1
Peach jam.....................................	48	2½ teaspoonfuls
Lemon Jello (whipped).........................		1 serving
Lima bean and potato cup cake†................		1
Lemonade (lemon juice)........................	30	2 tablespoonfuls
(sugar)..	10	2 teaspoonfuls

* Muffins:
   ⅔ cup potato flour   4 teaspoonfuls sugar
   ½ cup lima bean flour   ½ cup water
    3 teaspoonfuls baking powder   2 teaspoonfuls shortening
   ½ teaspoonful salt

Sift dry ingredients together. Melt fat and add to water, add slowly to dry ingredients. Put in greased muffin tins and bake at 400 F. for twenty minutes. Serve hot. Makes ten small muffins.

† Cup cakes:
    6 tablespoonfuls lima bean flour   2½ teaspoonfuls baking powder
   ¾ cup potato flour   ½ teaspoonful vanilla
    5 tablespoonfuls shortening   ½ teaspoonful lemon extract
   ½ cup water   Few grains salt, few drops yellow
   ⅔ cup sugar   coloring

Sift dry ingredients, cream fat and sugar, add dry ingredients and water alternately to creamed mixture. Add flavorings and coloring. Put in greased muffin tins and bake in oven at 430 F. for thirty minutes.

patient should be encouraged to eat enough to prevent loss of weight, the physician substituting similar foods for any causing disturbance. If symptoms are relieved, one or two vegetables or fruits may be added the second week, and during succeeding weeks the other foods, always eliminating any which cause recurrence of symptoms; wheat, eggs and milk should be added last and their effect carefully scrutinized. Rittinger and Dembo (1932) have pointed out the nutritive and biological value of soy-bean milk, which might be tried as a substitute in patients sensitive to cow's milk.

With full cooperation, patients can usually be gotten up to satisfying and nutritionally correct diets in a few weeks. In the hands of Rowe the results are excellent in a wide variety of allergic disturbances, though the psychic effects of "dieting" must not be overlooked. This is a type of specific therapy which, because of its freedom from dangers, its relative simplicity, and its inexpensiveness, deserves a full trial—if only patients were not so prone to snitch forbidden foods!

Peptones by Mouth.—Both the French and English schools had for some time been using peptones by mouth in cases of food allergy with indifferent results, when Luithlen, in 1926, showed that the fault probably lay in the use of preparations that were not truly specific. Urbach, who has been very actively carrying on the clinical investigations in Vienna since the untimely death of Luithlen, has demonstrated that the treatment is worthless unless the exact peptone toward which the patient is sensitive is employed; for example, if an individual cannot eat chicken, the peptone to be used must be made from the flesh of the chicken, and if eggs are the offenders, the peptone must come from the white of eggs. Small doses of these specific peptones are then given by mouth before each meal in which the offending foods are to be included (these foods having been determined by an elimination diet régime much like Rowe's, see above), in the belief that not only can the individual attack be thus prevented but that desensitization will also take place in time. The ingestion of the peptone must occur exactly three-quarters to one hour before the meal and a considerable time after digestion of the last meal has ceased; it is therefore necessary to forbid all between-meals eating, which means of course that cooperation is difficult to obtain in children and that the method is hardly practicable in frequently fed infants. I have been somewhat sceptical of this work, but Urbach, whom I had the pleasure of visiting in 1931, has partially converted me; he, at least, is getting good results, and I feel that it would be well if the peptone tablets were to be made available to a few qualified investigators in this country.

SERUM DISEASE

Serum disease is an allergic reaction caused by the parenteral introduction, by whatever route, of foreign serum. Mackenzie says that if amounts below 10 cc. are used, only about 10 per cent of patients show symptoms. but that when amounts of 100 cc. or more are injected, fully 90 per cent develop the disease. The symptoms are a mixture of urticaria and erythema, fever, arthritis without pronounced objective changes in the joints, swollen and tender lymph nodes, and edema of various portions of the body accompanied by urinary evidences of temporarily impaired renal function. The time elapsing between the giving of the serum and the appearance of the disease is usually one week; in most cases the symptoms disappear in four to six days, but occasionally they persist for as long as two weeks. Recovery is the rule, though relapses are not uncommon.

THERAPY

The disease cannot be prevented nor can it be very satisfactorily treated by any routine methods devised to date, though it is worthy of note that full doses of magnesium sulphate (Epsom salt), perhaps repeated several times in the twenty-four hours, are often provocative of an astonishing degree of relief. One-half to 1 cc. of 1:1000 epinephrine solution, given subcutaneously, is oftentimes temporarily effective in relieving the itching, but it must be frequently repeated; for local treatment of the urticaria, see page 331. The arthritis does not respond to the salicylates or cinchophens.

DEFICIENCY DISEASES

RICKETS

Rickets is a disease of infants which is characterized by a diminution in the inorganic phosphorus of the blood—or, in those cases in which there is an associated tetany, low calcium but approximately normal phosphorus—and a faulty calcification of the newly laid down bone tissue. It is encountered most frequently between the ages of six and eighteen months, its victims being for the most part well nourished and rapidly growing children. The seasonal fluctuation of the disease is one of its most characteristic features, the case incidence rising from October to a peak in March and then falling to June; new cases very rarely develop in the summer. Rickets is most prevalent in the industrial cities of the north temperate zone and is infrequent in the tropics; indeed, in subtropical regions with plenty of winter sunshine it would seem to be very unusual; witness the fact that Torroella has stated, apparently as the result of exhaustive study, that the disease is nonexistent in Mexico. A typical case of rickets shows the following symptoms: restlessness, especially turning of the head from side to side; irritability; sweating of the head; enlargement of the costochondral junctions, giving the rachitic "rosary," and enlargement of the epiphyses at the wrist; an abnormally open fontanel, coupled with a tendency for areas of softening to develop below the occipitoparietal suture. Squareness of the head, protuberant deformity of the chest, knock knees or bowlegs, and curvature of the spine; any or all of these may be present. There is often "pot-belly" and usually some muscular weakness; the blood is deficient in inorganic phosphorus, and a radiograph of the lower end of the ulna shows certain abnormalities which are diagnostic.

Artificially fed infants are more prone to develop rickets than are the breast fed, though the latter are by no means infrequently attacked; prematurely born infants almost invariably become rachitic. It is felt by many pediatricians that the number of demonstrable cases of rickets, i. e., those showing some of the symptoms listed above, is not an accurate index of the prevalence of the disease, for it would seem possible, by careful examination, to elicit one or more signs of its presence in practically all rapidly growing infants; indeed, Eliot has even suggested that this state of affairs might be physiologic. It is felt at present that rickets is caused by deficiency in vitamin D (with associated calcium-phosphorus imbalance), in some other factor not yet determined, and by insufficient exposure to sunlight during the dark months. The prognosis in rickets *per se* is very good; even very pronounced deformities often disappear when the period of most rapid growth is passed and sunny "open" weather comes round again. Tetany is the most frequent and pneumonia the most serious immediate complication. The most serious residual defect is deformed pelvis in the female.

Some historians think that at one place in the second Iliad of Homer (*circa* 950 B. C.) there is a clear description of rickets. In a number of the medieval holy pictures the Christ child is shown as strikingly rachitic. But the classic description of the disease was that of Francis Glisson (1597–1677); indeed, so far as I know, this was the first account to appear in medical literature. In 1908, Finlay produced the disease experimentally for the first time by the use of a deficient diet.

THERAPY

The number of "specific" remedies in this disease has now become so large that I shall have to discuss all of the following here: cod liver oil, halibut oil, viosterol, cod liver oil with viosterol, halibut oil with viosterol, light therapy, irradiated yeast, yeast milk, irradiated milk.

Cod Liver Oil.—Clinicians have used the oil empirically for a long time with excellent results in both the cure and prevention of rickets—unless we wish to apply the most delicate clinical tests to these results, in doing which it will be found to be very doubtful if any of the antirachitic agents is able absolutely to prevent the disease. In addition to readily digestible and assimilable fats, the oil contains vitamin D, which exerts a favorable influence on calcium and phosphorus metabolism and particularly in the prevention of rickets, and vitamin A. This latter vitamin undoubtedly exerts a direct influence over the growth and development of the young, but none of the claims that it is able to prevent respiratory infections have been substantiated. The antirachitic properties of the oil are not raised by ultraviolet irradiation. The administration of the oil to mothers (Weech, 1927) very much lessens the incidence of rickets in breast-fed infants.

It is not possible at the present time to effect a simple correlation of the vitamin potency of different cod liver oil preparations because of the considerable variety of unitage under which they are marketed; indeed, the numerical values are confusing to all save investigators in this field. Hope for clarification, however, lies in the recent adoption of an international unitage by a subcommittee of the League of Nations Health Organization; the proposal of the Vitamin Standardization Committee of the United States Pharmacopoeia XI to distribute to individuals and firms officially standardized samples, labelled with respect to their potency in vitamins A and D, is an excellent one.

In view of the wide differences in recommended dosages of cod liver oil at present, the Council on Pharmacy and Chemistry of the American Medical Association has recently (1932) obtained an expression of their opinion in the matter from seventeen eminent American pediatricians, the gist of which may be presented as follows:

(*a*) It is now the practice to begin the administration when growth begins to accelerate—within two weeks or at least before the end of the first month—and to reach the maximum during the third and rarely later than the fourth month; the maximum dosage then continued up to two years of age.

(*b*) Little attention is paid to vitamin A content of the oil, dosage being determined upon the basis of the vitamin D content, the feeling being that, though it may be difficult to prove that a diet contains the optimum amount of vitamin A, there is probably no suffering from the lack of it if adequate amounts of milk are received.

(*c*) With due allowance for variations in potency (but using only such oils as are Council-accepted and appear in N.N.R.), and for the factors of age, diet, sunlight and climate, and the rôle of intercurrent infections in the production of rickets, the dosage of 3 teaspoonfuls—3 drachms (12 cc.) —daily is considered upon both experimental and empirical grounds to be the optimum for the average infant of three months of age, for both prevention and cure.

Hess (1932) administers this dosage as follows: As a prophylactic, 5 to 10 drops at one month (increasing rapidly to ½ teaspoonful daily); 1½ teaspoonfuls at six weeks; and 3 teaspoonfuls daily at three months, this last dose being continued throughout infancy.

(*d*) The usual daily dose is somewhat augmented in the case of premature and unusually rapid-growing infants. In Negro infants, with their marked predisposition to rickets, 4 to 5 teaspoonfuls should be reached if well tolerated, otherwise the cod liver oil should be fortified with viosterol.

The greatest disadvantage of cod liver oil has always been its objectionable taste and odor. Any one of the N.N.R. concentrates in vegetable oil or in tablets, or the N.N.R. emulsion, may be substituted in such dosage as is stated on the package.

Halibut (Haliver) Oil.—This oil is fishy but has not the rancid odor and taste of cod liver oil, for which it may be substituted in the N.N.R. dosage (standard dropper accompanies package): Infants, 6 to 10 drops daily; premature and rapidly growing infants, 15 drops; severe cases, 20 drops or more. Available also in soft capsules; daily dosage, 1 or 2 capsules.

Viosterol.—Irradiated ergosterol is the most potent of the antirachitic agents in vitamin D content, but it does not contain the growth-promoting vitamin A. For this reason, Prather *et al.* (1931), and other students of the matter, have emphatically maintained that the apparently widespread tendency to substitute viosterol for cod liver oil is not logical and may result in an appreciable decrease of the child's strength and resistance to infections.

The product is standardized as Viosterol in Oil 250D, the N.N.R. dosage being: Average infant and child, 8 to 10 drops daily (standard dropper in package); premature and rapid-growing infant, 15 drops; daily curative dose, 15 to 20 drops. It was earlier believed that the use of larger doses frequently induced a toxic hypercalcemic state, but since the drug has been standardized and has been widely used in the treatment of severe cases, we know from the studies of Hess *et al.* (1930), Grayzel *et al.* (1931), and others, that doses many times as large as those recommended above may be used with safety—though of course it is infrequently necessary to exceed the usual dosage. Jampolis and Londe (1932) have given 20 cc., and Blatt and Saffro (1932) have recorded the administration without untoward symptoms of 6400 drops daily for a period of twenty-one days.

The use of the drug in large dosage certainly enables one to give premature infants large doses of vitamin D without upsetting digestion. May (1931), in his careful studies in the Herman Kiefer Hospital in Detroit, found a gain in weight, increase in appetite and apparent physical well-being, greater resistance to infection, and also a reduction in the percentage of deaths in premature infants when adequate dosage was started within twenty-four hours after birth. His dosage, suggested as a point for departure in the further study of the problem: 1 drop on the tongue before each feeding, increased 1 drop each day up to 10 drops before each feeding; in other words, increased to 60 drops daily. After two or three months, the dose is gradually decreased to 30 drops daily.

Cod Liver Oil with Viosterol.—In this preparation we have oil fortified with viosterol to obtain a ten times greater vitamin D effect than can be obtained from the oil alone in usually tolerated doses. N.N.R. dosage: Infants and young children, 2.5 to 3.3 cc. (53 to 67 minims) daily; adults and in severe cases, up to 7 cc. (140 minims) or more.

Halibut (Haliver) Oil with Viosterol.—This preparation (Council-accepted, November 18, 1933) is less disagreeable than the above and the same vitamin D effect may be obtained with smaller dosage. N.N.R. dosage (standard dropper in package): Infants, 8 to 10 drops daily; premature and rapidly growing infants, 15 drops; older children, 15 to 20 drops; adults, 20 drops or more. Available also in soft capsules; children, 1 or 2 capsules, adults, 2 capsules or more.

Light Therapy.—Rickets may be both prevented and cured when infants are exposed in the light of a good type of ultraviolet-ray-producing apparatus when properly used. It is important, however, to emphasize, what Hess and Lewis (1932) have pointed out, that unless direct ultraviolet irradiation can be provided in an inexpensive and practical form combined with illumination, this method cannot be considered of much value in the protection of the community at large from rickets. The work of Tisdall and Brown (1932) is teaching us much in regard to the antirachitic value of the sun's rays and of the reflected rays from the sky and clouds (skyshine). In the latitude of Toronto, they find that the sun's rays during the latter part of October, all of November, December and January and the first part of February, produces a slight but appreciable antirachitic effect, which sharply increases about February 15th and continues throughout the summer at approximately eight times the winter level. They infer by calculation and a study of the work of Lewis *et al.* (1931) that in such favored places as Switzerland and Denver the sunshine would have a low antirachitic effect only from December 1st to January 15th. The optimum time for exposure to the rays is between 11 A. M. and 1 P. M. Ordinary window glass is impervious to the rays, and Tisdall and Brown believe that in Toronto the use of special glass, the best of which is only partially pervious, is of little value until after March 1st, when the sunshine increases in value before the vagaries of spring weather permit the exposure of patients out of doors.

Irradiated Yeast.—This substance, recommended by Hess (1927), has not become popular because of the great difficulty in disguising its taste.

Yeast Milk.—Hess and his associates began experimenting several years ago with the feeding of viosterol or irradiated yeast to cows and then tested the antirachitic potency of the milk they produced. The yeast proved superior to the viosterol, and it was determined that 1 liter (approximately 1 quart) of such milk was equivalent in protective value to the standard doses of cod liver oil or viosterol. At present the measure is being employed at a number of certified farms throughout the country and is considered to be possibly applicable to grade A farms, which provide a less expensive milk. None of the infants fed through the second year on this milk in Hess's studies developed rickets and all throve excellently.

Irradiated Milk.—This is the latest development of the indefatigable investigators of this disease, the group about A. F. Hess. They have now succeeded in so irradiating both fluid and dried milk that it suffers only an insignificant loss of vitamin A and acquires a vitamin D component which was shown upon adequate clinical trials to render it fully as antirachitic (both for prevention and cure) as any of the other agents already discussed —with the exception that in one premature infant it did not prevent the disease (as even very large doses of viosterol also sometimes fail to do). Irradiated milk will have the advantage of being inexpensive. "It is estimated that the additional cost of the activated milk which we fed this year was but one twenty-fifth of a cent per quart." This new measure is of course by its very nature not adapted for use outside large cities, but it is believed that evaporated milk could be irradiated for use in rural communities. The great advantage of using activated milk of whatever kind would be that it would at once provide calcium and phosphorus as well as the antirachitic factor. Hess and Lewis (1933) have stated that the effective preventive quantity of this milk is only 20 to 24 ounces (600 to 720 cc.) daily.

Phosphorus.—The Council on Pharmacy and Chemistry of the American Medical Association has decided that preparations of cod liver containing phosphorus are unacceptable for New and Nonofficial Remedies. The evidence on which they based this decision (Jour. Amer. Med. Assoc., 91, 97, 1928) constitutes so satisfactory a review of the status of phosphorus therapy in rickets that I am quoting from the report at some length (see the Bibliography for the references contained in the report).

"The use of elementary phosphorus in the treatment of rickets is based on the observations of Wegner, in 1874, that the administration of white phosphorus in minute amounts caused the formation of a dense band at the epiphyses of the long bones. He suggested the use of phosphorus in rickets. Kassowitz, ten years later (1884), reported on the therapeutic use of phosphorus in rickets. At first he used phosphorus dissolved in olive or almond oil, and later in cod liver oil. He reported favorable results. During the succeeding twenty years, many papers were published on the subject, opinions being about equally divided as to the value of the phosphorus. It is also pointed out that death occurred in several instances from excessive doses of phosphorus. Practically all those claiming good results from phosphorus used it in combination with cod liver oil (now known to be specific in rickets). Phemister (1918) and Phemister, Miller and Bonar (1921) showed roentgenologically that the administration of phosphorus leads to the formation of a dense band of calcification at the end of the long bones, and reported two cases of rickets in which this effect was observed when phosphorus was administered without cod liver oil. In both instances, however, treatment was begun in the early summer at a time when rickets ordinarily improves spontaneously. Recently Hess and Weinstock (1926) confirmed the observation that the administration of elementary phosphorus leads to the formation of a dense area of calcification at the epiphyses of the long bones. They considered this a pathologic picture rather than evidence of healing rickets and they showed, in an extensive experimental study, that the administration of phosphorus in either small or large doses did not prevent the occurrence of rickets to any degree whatever. They found, further, that the administration of phosphorus actually led to a diminution of inorganic phosphorus in the blood, thus favoring rather than preventing the occurrence of rickets.

"Since the demonstration of the specific effect of cod liver oil and irradiation in the treatment of rickets, phosphorus has practically fallen into disuse among pediatricians. The accumulated evidence is unconvincing as to the value of phosphorus; furthermore, it is known that phosphorus is a dangerous drug. Certainly the routine administration of phosphorus in combination with cod liver oil is to be discouraged."

SCURVY

Scurvy is a disease which is caused by a deficiency of fresh vegetables and fresh fruits in the diet. In infants it is most frequent between the fifth and fifteenth months of life, being quite rare after the twentieth month. In adults it occurs invariably whenever there is deprivation for as much as six months of foods containing the antiscorbutic factor, now known as vitamin C. The symptoms in adults are loss of vigor, a sallow complexion, pains in the legs principally, shortness of breath, sore, bleeding, spongy gums, foul breath, and ecchymotic spots on the skin, especially of the legs. At the present time diagnosis is usually made before the condition has progressed very far, but when correction of the dietary deficiency is impossible, the patient rapidly becomes a pitiable object; the body becomes edematous, dyspnea and pain are quite agonal, intramuscular and other hemorrhages occur, enormous swelling of the gums and necrosis of the jaw take place, and death, usually by intercurrent pneumonia, finally comes as a blessed release. In infants the symptoms are pallor, arrest of growth and loss of weight, poor appetite, livid, swollen gums which bleed easily, and pain;

this pain is manifested by a worried expression, a whimpering cry, and the eversion of the thighs which are flexed on the abdomen. The tenderest point is at the lower end of the femur. The pain in both infants and adults is caused by subperiosteal hemorrhage; in the former, in addition, there may be separation of the epiphyses and even fractures. A number of cases of intracranial hemorrhage have been reported.

Scurvy was unmistakably described by Jacques de Vitry in the forces of the Crusaders who were besieging Damietta in 1218, but earlier reference to the disease has not been discovered, unless a doubtful passage in Hippocrates be accepted. Always, at least since the Middle Ages, it has ravaged armies and beleaguered cities, and when long sea voyages began to be made it quickly struck at the crews of vessels. It caused severe losses in certain areas during the World War, being especially decimating to the British troops who were besieged at Kut-el-Amara. Now, during the present interim of world peace, the disease seems to be endemic among adults in northern Russia and certain parts of the tropics only. Elsewhere it exists principally as a problem in infant feeding, though cases are beginning to be reported among the underfed during the present wretched period of world-wide unemployment. Muelengracht (1927) has drawn attention to the fact that it is also not to be overlooked in the persons of unmarried individuals who live alone and prepare in their own rooms a diet that is nearly always deficient in the items of meat, fruits and vegetables; a number of recent reports, confirming the contention, have also shown the possibility of scurvy appearing during the course of special dietary regimens enforced during severe gastro-intestinal disturbances.

THERAPY

Drugs and biological agents are of no value whatever in the treatment of scurvy (though Schultzer's report of a case in September, 1933, apparently cured by the use of ascorbic acid, should be noted parenthetically as it marks perhaps a new departure in therapy), which may be easily cured, however, simply and solely by the addition to the diet of a sufficient amount of the antiscorbutic factor. Unpasteurized milk and raw meat contain this factor, but either must be taken in very large quantities in order to suffice; fresh vegetables, especially tomatoes, cabbage and potatoes, best serve the purpose. Orange juice is excellent as is also lime juice, but it should be noted that it is the sweet Mediterranean, and not the sour West Indian lime so well known to us in the Western Hemisphere, that is so highly rated as an antiscorbutic. These fruit juices, *i. e.*, two or three oranges or lemons or limes daily, or the liberal use of fresh vegetables not too long cooked, will very rapidly cure a case of scurvy. Stale vegetables are of less value, and fruits and vegetables preserved by artificially drying them are practically worthless. By new processes it has now become possible to can fruits and vegetables without destroying the antiscorbutic factor; the commercial vogue for quick ripening by ethylene is also not harmful.

The disease is prevented by the same measures which suffice for cure. In the case of infants that are not being nursed by mothers *who are taking liberal amounts of antiscorbutic foods,* the vitamin factor must be artificially supplied after the first month of life. This may be accomplished by the use of either orange, pineapple or tomato juice, the latter being perhaps the most economical. Canned tomatoes should be strained and 2 teaspoonfuls of the juice, uncooked, should be fed daily; the amount must be raised to 5 or 6 teaspoonfuls by the time the baby is three months old. Orange juice need be used in only half these quantities; it may be sweetened and diluted with water to taste. A number of physicians have noticed a febrile reaction during the first few days of antiscorbutic therapy.

In Rhodesia, where he was unable to get scorbutic natives to alter their diet, Dry (1933) successfully injected intravenously the juice pressed from oranges and lemons which had previously been immersed in 5 per cent phenol to sterilize the skins. The juice is filtered aseptically and neutralized with 20 per cent sodium hydroxide. Initial dose, 5 cc.; thereafter from 10 to 15 cc. twice weekly, always using a freshly prepared juice.

Somehow, perhaps by reason of the recent advances in our knowledge of the part that sunshine plays in the causation and cure of rickets, the notion has spread that scurvy, too, is amenable to prevention and cure by the ultraviolet rays, and that irradiation of foods increases their antiscorbutic properties. There is absolutely no warrant for this belief.

PELLAGRA

The four outstanding features of this disease, which will serve to fix the characteristic picture in mind, are dermatitis, diarrhea, dementia and death. All of these symptoms need to be somewhat elaborated upon of course. The dermatitis is sharply defined, is nearly always symmetrical, and is confined to those areas of the skin which are exposed to the light, *i. e.*, the face and neck, the backs of the hands and the lower part of the forearms, the feet and the lower legs. The term "diarrhea" is used to indicate the outstanding feature of the gastro-intestinal involvement; it occurs in at least 75 per cent of the cases, though there is nothing diagnostic in the type of the stool. More or less severe stomatitis and a decrease in the acidity of the gastric contents are also prominent features in many cases. The nervous symptoms which are so serious a part of the pellagra syndrome are so many and varied that they may perhaps best be dismissed with the appellation "neurasthenic manifestations"; true dementias, which simulate any of the well-recognized psychoses, not infrequently develop, however, in advanced cases. Death I have set down as an outstanding feature of the disease, and so it is in all patients who become definitely bedridden, but in those who suffer only from a mild annually recurrent form of the disease the mortality is quite low.

The first published account of pellagra was that of Casal, in Spain, in 1762. Shortly thereafter it was recognized as a widespread malady in northern Italy, where it was exhaustively studied by Strombio in 1786–89. At the present time it is quite prevalent in southern Europe, Egypt, India, the West Indies, Central America, and the southern United States and can doubtless be found elsewhere for the looking, as has already been shown in Germany and Denmark. In the northern United States, sporadic cases had been seen as early as the middle of the nineteenth century, but its existence in epidemic proportions in the South was not recognized until 1907. Between 1907 and 1915, the incidence steadily mounted, then declined for some years, and is apparently during the last few years quite sharply rising again. Pellagra is exclusively a disease of the poor in regions where the habitual diet is faulty; such cases as occur among the well-to-do can almost invariably be traced to some dietary imbalance, whether due to "finickiness" or to gastro-intestinal pathology which interferes with proper nutrition. Cases nearly always make their appearance in the early spring and persist until the middle of the summer; as already stated, some individuals suffer at this season year after year. The disease occurs in persons of all ages, though its greatest incidence is in those who have just come into full maturity. Blacks and whites are equally stricken.

THERAPY

It is impossible to discuss the prevention and treatment of pellagra independently of a brief presentation of our present knowledge of its etiology, since only when we come to a final understanding of the cause of the disease can we hope to completely rationalize its therapy. The three chief theories with which students of the disease have busied themselves are (*a*) that it is caused by some toxin in spoiled food, notably maize, (*b*) that a microbiotic agent is the noxious factor, and (*c*) that it is due to dietary deficiency of one sort or another. Bliss' (1932) recently proposed iron-deficiency theory has been already damagingly criticized by Wheeler. The maize theory, chiefly championed by Lombroso, has not been substantiated and finds few advocates today. Likewise, very little evidence has been brought forward to show that the disease is of infectious origin, though I think I write truly when I say that most physicians in the South still hold to this belief. Certainly there have been many periods in that part of the United States, as, for instance during and after the Civil War, when large numbers of people were partaking of a poorly balanced diet, but it was not until 1907 that the disease appeared, and then it ran a course of a few years closely simulating that of a low-grade infectious disease. I think the explanation that pellagra may have been previously overlooked may be ruled out, for the disease is sufficiently distinctive that *all* cases would not have been missed. I am not qualified, nor have I the wish, to champion the infectious disease origin of the disease, but I would point out to the interested reader that this theory has some points that are not to be lightly passed by, and that at least one piece of experimental work, that of Jobling and Arnold (1923), though incomplete, strongly indicates that a photodynamic intoxication, initiated by an organism which thrives in an intestinal tract overloaded with carbohydrates, might be the true cause of the disease. Smith's (1931) exhaustive preliminary study indicates that biological effects due to solar rays, plus a faulty sulphur metabolism, may play an important rôle. It should be mentioned, also, that from time to time authors have attempted to relate the disease more or less directly with alcoholic addiction, while others refer to the alcoholic "variety" of pellagra, but most physicians in the South scout this idea for they see too many cases in children and in others who have never used alcohol. Thannhauser (1933), in Germany, recently proposed that we explore the possibilities of an underlying endocrine disturbance.

Perhaps the theory which is serving us best today is that of the food-deficiency origin of the disease.. Whatever the secondary factors may be, it would seem that the late Dr. Goldberger and his associates in the U. S. Public Health Service have produced at least partially convincing evidence of the fact that a food deficiency of some sort is of primary importance in the causation of the disease. The missing element has not been positively identified as yet, for the standpoint of these investigators has shifted somewhat from time to time as they have covered the field; that it is the vitamin designated successively as P-P, B_2, and G (a part of the vitamin mixture formerly known as water-soluble B), is their present contention. The subject is still, however, so far from being a closed one that to review here the immense controversial literature would be neither possible nor profitable.

In practice, the diet of the pellagrin will usually be found woefully lacking in fresh milk, fresh meats, and eggs. The addition of these items in liberal quantities often suffices to correct the mild and moderately advanced cases; the therapeutic value of fresh vegetables, though not actually demonstrated experimentally, is also believed to be considerable. Wheeler (1931) has at least tentatively shown that while not all canned foods contain the pellagra-preventive factor, canned spinach is particularly rich in it. When milk is relied upon alone to supply the antipellagra factor, at least a quart a day should be given. It is necessary, also, to reduce the excessive carbohydrate consumption to which victims of this disease are almost invariably addicted whether by habit or circumstance. One cannot be too well forewarned that to lay down the rules for a proper dietary readjustment is one thing and that to get the pellagrin to follow the same is entirely another; no class of patients is so "finicky" as this.

Some authors are sanguine even as to the results to be obtained in severe bedridden cases; the prognosis seems very bad to most observers, however. Of such patients, Wheeler writes, "it is important that the food be administered under competent supervision and in the most easily digested form. Fresh sweet milk, broths made from fresh lean meats, beef juice, soft or raw eggs, and fresh vegetable soups have proved most efficacious. It is often found advisable to conserve the weakened digestive function by reducing the cereals and fats to a minimum in the more severe cases." It is in the treatment of these severe cases that dried brewer's yeast is used; the dose is ½ to 1 ounce (15 to 30 Gm.), three to six times a day. Evidence for and against the efficacy of the use of liver or liver extract, as in the treatment of pernicious anemia, is appearing nowadays (the report of Ramsdell and Magness, 1933, is impressive); likewise in the matter of the use of yeast as a prophylactic agent—many individuals actually develop the disease while ingesting an ounce of the "preventive" a day, but it is equally true that many, certainly the greater number, do not.

As might be expected, since achlorhydria is present in so many cases, the use of hydrochloric acid is often distinctly helpful. The U.S.P. dilute acid should be given in a dose of 1 teaspoonful with each meal. Iron, and perhaps arsenic, are nearly always used as in the other secondary anemias (see p. 480). The treatment of diarrhea is discussed on pages 430 and 60.

BERIBERI

This, perhaps the oldest of the deficiency diseases, is characterized by peripheral neuritis, edema, myocardial weakness, and enlargement of the heart. The attack usually begins slowly with malaise, palpitation and shortness of breath, gastro-intestinal disturbances, and edema, which usually begins in the pretibial region. Then begins the multiple peripheral neuritis, which is associated with soreness of the muscles, with areas of paresthesia and superficial anesthesia, and with diminution or loss of the deep reflexes; the edema spreads up the legs, effusions appear in the serous cavities; ataxia or a marked steppage gait becomes pronounced, or flaccid paralysis with muscular atrophy appears; the heart becomes greatly enlarged, and the patient dies from failure of this organ, usually after an illness of several months, though a number of acute deaths with few or no prodromal symptoms are on record. This is the picture in extremely severe cases only, be it remarked; the vast majority of patients, though manifesting in some degree nearly all of the symptoms mentioned, usually recover. Pathologically the disease is characterized by degenerative changes in the peripheral nerves and also in the anterior and posterior ganglia of the cord. There are also occasional disintegrative changes in the brain cells, though mental symptoms to correspond are very rare.

Recent studies indicate that epidemic dropsy, so troublesome in India, and beriberi are distinct though closely related entities. "War edema," which was so distressingly prevalent in the blockaded countries during the World War, was not a true beriberi since it apparently resulted from living on a diet containing insufficient protein and an excess of fluids and salt; polyneuritis was an infrequent symptom in this malady. Similar cases are beginning to appear in the United States, and doubtless elsewhere, as the economic depression deepens. Strauss and McDonald (1933) very interestingly propose the hypothesis that the polyneuritis of pregnancy is a dietary deficiency disorder similar to beriberi.

It is said that references to this disease are contained in very ancient Chinese and Japanese manuscripts. At present it is endemic in Japan, China, Indo-China, the Straits Settlements, the Dutch East Indies, the Philippines, and here and there in the West Indies and South America and along the coast of West Africa. In Europe and North America, occasional outbreaks occur in faultily managed institutions, but the number of cases is never large. However, in 1903, Young, and more recently, Scott and Herrmann (1928), have called attention to the fact that the "maladie des jambes" of the rice-growers of Louisiana is almost certainly beriberi; and Waring (1929) has pointed out that the disease occurs, perhaps not infrequently, in Negro infants in the South. It was Takaki who, by his dietary readjustment in the Japanese navy, in 1883, first proved that beriberi is caused by a food deficiency. He held that it was protein that was lacking in the diet, but the observation of Eijkman (1896) that a polished rice diet always caused the disease, and the subsequent researches of many investigators have shown that the missing substance is probably the B_1 fraction of the water-soluble vitamin B complex. This substance is concentrated in the outer layers of the cereals that are used for food—rice especially—by the native populations of large portions of the tropical and subtropical portions of the globe; furthermore, it is removed by modern milling processes, and therefore peoples who subsist during certain portions of the year almost exclusively upon this polished rice suffer from the deprivation of vitamin B, that is to say, they develop beriberi. It is a mistaken idea, however, that rice eating alone will cause the disease, for it follows also upon a prolonged period of the monotonous eating of other completely milled cereals, such as wheat or corn, or such a diet as white bread, molasses, sugar and fats. Likewise, too exclusive reliance upon canned foods invites the disease.

In recent years, Matsumura and his associates have been offering interesting evidence that beriberi may after all be an infectious disease, but they have by no means made out a clear case as yet.

THERAPY

The prevention of beriberi is entirely dietary; so also is the treatment except that a few drugs have been shown to be of use. Vedder (quoted by Vanderhoof) summarizes the dietary management as follows: (1) If rice forms the main staple of diet, it should be undermilled. Similarly, when bread is the staple, it should be made of whole wheat flour. (2) Beans, peas, or some similar legume should be served at least once a week. (3) Whole barley should be used in all soups. (4) Fresh meat should be served once daily if possible; eggs and fresh milk as freely as possible, and whenever meat is not provided. (5) The excessive use of canned foods is to be avoided. These dicta can be easily followed of course in institutions, but the problem of preventing and treating the disease among the poverty-stricken masses in the East is very difficult. Coyne, in India, has used the following methods with success: A commercial extract of rice is given in a dose of 20 grains (1.3 Gm.) twice, or preferably thrice, a day; an infusion of rice bran is also used. Rice bran is relatively cheap but the infusion should be made fresh every day. Patients who can afford it are put on a vegetable diet with ground wheat as a cereal, no rice being allowed. Those unable to thus change their diet are instructed to use red or unhulled rice and as much vegetables and fruit as they can manage to procure. He finds it possible to clear mild cases in about ten days, but more severe cases require a month and a half to two months to recover.

The polyneuritis is best treated by keeping the patient in bed and employing heat, massage and passive movements. Strychnine is of some value here also; Walshe states that it is best given in a daily single dose of $\frac{1}{30}$ grain (0.002 Gm.), building up to this point from smaller beginning doses. In rapidly fulminating cardiac cases, digitalis is indicated, and is to be used as described on page 530. Wenckebach (1932) believes that the pitressin (pressor) fraction of pituitrin deserves further study in these cases; it seems able at times to bring about a complete disappearance of the cardiovascular symptoms for awhile but should be used with extreme caution in view of its constrictor action on the coronary arteries. The constipation, which is an almost invariable symptom, usually responds to the saline cathartics.

TETANY

The syndrome to which this name is given is characterized principally by carpopedal spasm, *i. e.*, a tonic spasm in which the hands assume the so-called "obstetrical position" with the fingers and thumb approximated and with contracture at the wrist; the arms are often held against the chest and if the lower extremities are involved there is flexion at the knee joint with the feet in the position of equinovarus. There are also generalized convulsions which start in the eye and face muscles and involve the whole body, with consciousness returning as soon as relaxation takes place. Laryngospasm, giving rise to a peculiar crowing sound, is a characteristic symptom; edema of the dorsal surfaces of the hands and feet is sometimes seen. When the arm above the elbow is constricted in an individual with tetany, the hand assumes the accoucheur position (Trousseau). Tapping the cheek over the facial nerve causes rapid contractions throughout the distribution (Chvostek). Use of the galvanic current elicits signs of hyperexcitability of the peripheral nerves (Erb).

By far the most frequently seen of the tetanies is that so often associated with rickets in young children, a type most likely due to decreased absorption of calcium in the absence of sufficient vitamin D. The tetany of sprue is probably also a result of failure of calcium absorption (see p. 168). Frank tetany during pregnancy and lactation occurs but is rare, though tetanoid manifestations such as irritability, painful cramps in the legs, insomnia, transient paresthesias and edemas are of common occurrence. This type is of course easily assumed to be due to undue loss of calcium, first to the fetus and then in the milk, but it is possible at least that pregnancy and lactation are merely the factors that uncover a latent tendency due to parathyroid deficiency. True postoperative tetany is not often seen nowadays but its occurrence is not reckoned a mark of poor surgery since it is now well known that the parathyroid glands are often eccentrically located and also apparently succumb easily at times though not considerably disturbed. In conditions of persistent vomiting and when too much alkali has either been ingested or injected, there occurs a tetany associated with the state of alkalosis. Another sort of alkalotic tetany is that resulting from the great loss of carbon dioxide through abnormally rapid breathing, as occasionally seen in hysterical or otherwise psychically ill persons. There is recognized a type of "idiopathic" tetany in adults, that is to say, a group of cases in which none of the above etiologic associations seems to apply; however, this group is probably much smaller even than is commonly believed. Leopold and Jonas (1932) think that a critical analysis would show that most of the cases can really be classified with the infantile type due to vitamin D deficiency. It is further worthy of note, perhaps, that among the small number having no other discernible cause than a spontaneous parathyroid deficiency (comparable to the thyroid deficiency in true myxedema), diarrhea is often present though without the other symptoms of a fully developed case of sprue. Unquestionably the syndrome appears transiently at times at the height of serious toxic attacks, such as acute poisoning or a febrile state. Furthermore, the frequently reiterated statement that tetany does not occur in the newborn needs revision, for within one year Bass and Karelitz (1931) saw 3 cases; all were seized in the first days of life with vomiting, fever and the symptoms of tetany (probably as a result of the vomiting). In McGavran's (1932) case the condition had undoubtedly developed *in utero* for the baby was born with every one of the symptoms of tetany and responded dramatically to the therapeutic test. McCarrison has described an adult form of the malady in natives of the Himalayas, in association with goiter; it is probably the dietetic, infantile type, for upon removing to a different locality spontaneous recovery occurs.

In all of the above types of tetany there is a disturbance in calcium metabolism, with a decrease in blood calcium during the period of active symptoms and a rise in the same as improvement takes place; in all, that is, except the gastric, bicarbonate and hyperpneic forms, in which there is a state of alkalosis but normal blood calcium. To explain this discrepancy, we assume that the important matter in tetany is not how much calcium there is in the blood stream but how much of it is ionized; a shift to the alkaline side is thought to decrease ionization. This may be a correct explanation, as it is certainly a serviceable one, but the fact is that there has not yet been devised a method for determining the amount of calcium ion in the blood, and the assumption that it is equivalent to the amount of diffusible calcium can be justified only upon the score of convenience. Since calcium deficiency and the full symptomatology of tetany are not necessarily parallel phenomena, and because chronic cases tend to become less severe (latent), it has become recognized that there are undoubtedly other factors of importance in etiology—certainly the relationship between calcium, phosphorous and carbohydrate metabolism is a close one. Several groups of investigators have shown that the calcium variation can only be properly interpreted in conjunction not only with the inorganic phosphorus but with the serum protein also. Tetany does not occur characteristically in chronic nephritis, though, as pointed out by Meakins (1930), there is often a distinct reduction in serum calcium.

The first empiric use of calcium in tetany was probably that of Walter Harris, of London, who in 1689 "accomplished cure with no other medicines than a few ounces of crabs' eyes mixed with crystals of tartar." Shelling (1932) states that among Negroes of the eastern shore of Maryland the use of shells in the treatment of this disease has been handed down in some instances as a family secret through several generations. The first rational employment of calcium as an anticonvulsant was that of the Italian, Sabbatini, in 1901.

THERAPY

Calcium Alone.—Calcium salts when used alone sometimes induce amelioration of the symptoms but they rarely completely control the condition. However, they should probably be used routinely in connection with the other agents. Calcium chloride is the one most widely employed because, in addition to its calcium content, it increases the hydrogen ion concentration of the tissues and thus aids in the ionization of calcium. It is best given in milk to lessen the gastro-intestinal irritation, in divided doses totalling 90 to 120 grains (6 to 8 Gm.) daily. Calcium gluconate is used in about twice this dosage; it is less irritant. Calcium lactate is usually much less effective even when given in enormous amounts. When the symptoms are very urgent, such as severe convulsions and glottic spasm, 5 to 20 cc. of a 5 per cent solution of calcium chloride, or 10 per cent calcium gluconate, may be given intravenously; for the precautions to be observed in the intravenous administration of calcium salts, see page 714. Subsequently, 10 cc. of the gluconate solution can be given intramuscularly once or twice daily.

Calcium with Acid.—Ammonium chloride is the drug most often used to increase the ionization of calcium, 75 to 105 grains (5 to 7 Gm.) daily in divided doses. Sheer (1922) recommends 260 cc. of N/10 hydrochloric acid (9.5 cc. of full strength acid q. s. 1000 cc. water) made up to 1000 cc. with milk, to be given in small repeated feedings throughout the twenty-four hours.

Calcium with Lactose.—Several years ago, Dragstedt and Peacock showed experimentally that tetany was benefited by a diet of white bread, milk and lactose, findings which were confirmed clinically by others. Dragstedt believed that the diet was helpful through preventing the absorption of toxic substances, but Salvasen presented evidence to show that the calcium content of the milk was the important factor. Others maintained that the beneficial effect was due to the promotion of calcium absorption through the lactic acid acidity in the intestinal tract, but I do not believe that an increase in blood calcium has been demonstrated after lactose administration. Now it would seem that the McCullaghs (1932) have shown that the improvement is associated with a fall in the inorganic phosphates of the blood, though the complete mechanism of the action of lactose on blood phosphates remains obscure. They have demonstrated that symptoms are lessened in severity or completely abolished by lowering the amount of inorganic phosphates in the blood without raising the total calcium content of the blood serum. In 3 cases of chronic postoperative tetany, symptoms continued in spite of the administration of large doses of calcium lactate, but disappeared completely when lactose was added. In another chronic postoperative case, which failed to respond to calcium alone or to large doses of parathyroid extract alone, but did respond to the two together, the addition of lactose to the calcium lactate gave relief without the necessity of employing the parathyroid extract. These are findings of great promise. Two drachms (8 Gm.) of lactose and 1 drachm (4 Gm.) of calcium lactate were given together before meals and, in one of the cases, also before retiring; the effects are slow in appearing.

Parathyroid Extract.—In cases of postoperative tetany, the use of parathyroid extract is the method of choice; in severe cases with serum calcium values as low as 5 mg. per 100 cc. (the normal is 10 to 11 mg.), from 40 to 60 units may be given intravenously and half the dose subcutaneously or intramuscularly four to six hours later. Probably in most cases, 30 to 40 units daily will maintain the serum calcium at normal after this level has been reached, but the action varies markedly in different individuals, and in many cases an immunity develops after a few weeks so that even much increased doses are ineffective in influencing the blood calcium or phosphorus. Aub (1929) points out that this loss of potency is dependent upon a true resistance to the drug, for in his cases increased calcium excretion followed ammonium chloride administration after the parathyroid extract had been discontinued. In infantile tetany the response to parathyroid has been extremely variable and perhaps upon the whole unsatisfactory. Hoak and Rivkin (1926) feel that a safe tentative dose for subcutaneous administration is 5 units per kilogram of body weight for each desired rise of 1 mg. of serum calcium, the total amount to be distributed over a period of twenty-four to thirty-six hours at four- to six-hour intervals. Liu (1928) has reported the effective use of parathyroid extract alone in one case of idiopathic tetany but this is certainly contrary to the usual experience. In maternal cases, small doses of the extract plus calcium salts is satisfactory therapy, but the calcium-lactose combination of McCullagh (see above) would certainly seem worth trying. In 2 of Snell's (1932) 4 cases of sprue tetany the drug was effective but it failed in the other 2; indeed, as he indicates, the fault here is not in parathyroid insufficiency and therefore if the extract is to be used it must be fortified with full doses of calcium. Again I think that the addition of lactose should be made.

Parathyroid extract is a powerful agent and it is extremely important to guard against overdosage. Perhaps the earliest symptom is vomiting, so that when this occurs in an individual taking the drug an immediate check upon the blood calcium should be made. Later there is increasing listlessness, perhaps high fever, and finally coma. Other than immediate cessation of the injections, the treatment rests upon a very insecure foundation. Lowenburg and Ginsburg (1932) employed venoclysis to aid excretion of calcium and possibly also of parathyroid extract and to dilute the blood, which, at least in animals, becomes very viscid and markedly decreased in volume. The administration of calcium at the same time in order to prevent decalcification seems rational.

Cod Liver Oil and Viosterol.—These drugs, the latter preferred because of quicker action, are superior to all others in infantile cases; they are used just as in rickets (see p. 338). In so-called "idiopathic" cases and also in sprue tetany there are enthusiastic reports of its use; Snell has noted that in one of his sprue cases, though the vitamin D acts only through its effect on the absorption of calcium, there has been no excess fat in the stools since the use of viosterol was begun. Brougher (1931) and others have reported favorable results in postoperative cases.

Light Therapy.—It seems that in infantile tetany, as in rickets, the ultraviolet rays have specific value, but according to Cantarow (1931) the treatment should be instituted very gradually in order to avoid the preliminary drop in serum calcium which will only aggravate the symptoms. In Leopold and Jonas' (1932) idiopathic case, light therapy was beneficial. One would expect the method to be worth trying in maternal cases also.

Thyroid Therapy.—Aub et al. (1929) have found that in thyrotoxicosis there is no hypercalcemia but a great increase in calcium excretion; the administration of thyroid substance to normal individuals causes this increase in excretion out of all proportion to the rise in basal metabolic rate. Leopold and Jonas tried for some possible effect from thyroid preparations in their idiopathic tetany patient who had a low basal metabolic rate, but they accomplished nothing beyond the increase in this rate.

Parathyroid Transplant.—This has been a failure in nearly all reported cases, though Borchers (1921) seems to have had partial success for awhile in a few instances.

The Treatment of Alkalotic Cases.—In these cases of course the principal indication is to overcome the alkalosis, which is usually easily accomplished if overdosage of alkalis has been at fault. Where loss of chlorides through vomiting obtains, physiologic solution of sodium chloride must be given in large quantities by all the usual channels. Ammonium chloride may be given by mouth, or intravenously in amounts of 300 to 500 cc. of 0.82 per cent solution, first testing the solution, as recommended by Cantarow, to see whether it causes hemolysis. In the hyperpneic cases there is often difficulty in controlling the causative factor, namely, the hysterical attacks of rapid breathing in psychically disturbed individuals. In one such patient, when an attack had been precipitated by excitement, Meakins (1930) proved that alkalosis was the causative factor by producing instantaneous remission when the patient was caused to inhale a mixture of 5 per cent carbon dioxide and 95 per cent oxygen. The paper-bag method (see p. 629) might be expected to appeal to such patients.

Treatment in the Newborn.—McGavran (1932) handled his case as follows: "Calcium chloride, 7 grains (0.45 Gm.) every hour; viosterol, 3 drops every two hours; phenobarbital, $\frac{1}{12}$ grain (0.005 Gm.) every four hours. Forced feedings, 1 ounce of breast milk, every hour, were administered with a medicine dropper. It took forty-five minutes out of every hour to get the ounce down. In twenty-four hours the calcium chloride was stopped as it produced vomiting. The phenobarbital was stopped in forty-eight hours. In ten days the baby became a simple feeding problem and has developed so far into a perfectly normal healthy twelve months old baby." McGavran feels that many cases of so-called "birth trauma" might well have been diagnosed as tetany and treated as such.

DISEASES OF METABOLISM

DIABETES MELLITUS

The islands of Langerhans in the pancreas normally secrete a hormone, insulin, which promotes in some complex way the oxidation of glucose and its conversion into glycogen and the deposition of this glycogen in the liver and the muscles; in addition it in some way influences the conversion of protein and fat into sugar. When the production of this insulin is markedly decreased, there is an increase in blood sugar above the normal amount, sugar appears in the urine, and we say that the individual has diabetes mellitus. The principal symptoms are a marked increase in the amount of urine voided, water drunk and food eaten, plus a loss in weight and strength which the patient finds difficulty in reconciling with his great increase in food-intake—*plus sugar in the urine*. This latter symptom, or rather laboratory finding, is the most important of all, for it cannot be gainsaid that it is a sound diagnostic principle to regard every person with sugar in the urine as a diabetic until he is proved not to be. Attempts to classify cases as mild, moderate or severe upon the degree of any of the symptoms, and especially with regard to the amount of sugar in the urine or in the blood at the first examination, are usually unsuccessful for two reasons: First, because the patient often presents himself either after a food debauch, and consequently with a high glycosuria, or after a period of severe abstinence designed to impress the new physician with his earnestness as a patient; and, second, because it is by no means infrequent for cases with an astonishingly low carbohydrate tolerance to respond remarkably well to any one of the new types of treatment which utilize insulin as their basis. That most cases of diabetes are actually mild is a truth that is becoming increasingly apparent—which is, however, by no means the same thing as saying that the disease is not a serious one even in the mildest cases. Pruritus, either general or of the pudendal type, is a frequent symptom in diabetes; neuritis is also thought to be quite common, but Joslin, in his vast experience, has seen it associated with the disease only very rarely.

When there is lack of insulin in the tissues—that is to say, in a case of diabetes—not only is carbohydrate oxidation disturbed but there is an interference with fat catabolism as well. The result of this is that beta-oxybutyric acid and its derivatives collect in the tissues and a state of acidosis is set up, which, if allowed to progress, culminates in the most dreaded symptom of all—coma. The presence of these bodies is easily detectable in the urine, but the other symptoms of mild acidosis are too vague to be described here. Indeed, of coma itself the prodromal symptoms are very elusive. Any of the following should arouse suspicion: loss of appetite, nausea and vomiting, restlessness, excitement, unusual fatigue, dizziness, ringing in the ears, and disturbances in breathing. The "coma" itself may range from a state of great drowsiness to deep unconsciousness from which the patient cannot be roused. There is usually Kussmaul breathing, a low plasma CO_2 combining power but a high blood sugar content, a comparatively low percentage of sugar, salt and nitrogen in the urine but a high concentration of acetone and diacetic acid, poor peripheral circulation, leukocytosis, and often a peculiar softness of the eyeball not seen in other types of coma.

The most serious complications of diabetes are gangrene, carbuncle, any of the infections, arteriosclerosis, heart disease, hyperthyroidism, diarrhea, and any syndrome necessitating surgical intervention.

The most frequent time of onset is at about fifty years, but the disease may appear at any age and is distributed about equally in incidence between the sexes. Formerly diabetes in children and in young adults was felt to have a hopeless prognosis, but insulin has now entirely changed the status of these patients. The incidence of the disease is greater in Hebrews than in Gentiles; it is not infrequently seen in Negroes, contrary to earlier belief. The hereditary transmission of a "tendency" for diabetes may tentatively be considered proved, but the contention that obesity predisposes to the disease is still open to doubt. The frequency with which chronic gallbladder disease, and particularly coronary disease, are diagnosed among diabetics is certainly worth remarking. Despite the fact that the literature of diabetes is replete with reports of "acute" cases, we now believe that in practically all instances the onset is gradual. In improperly treated cases, and in noncooperative patients, coma is still the chief cause of death, but in properly treated cases—*i. e.*, patients that have been given a diabetic "education"—arteriosclerosis, chiefly in the form of coronary thrombosis and gangrene of the legs, and the diseases of advancing age, have taken the lead.

In the Sanscrit manuscript of Suśruta (fifth century, A. D.) the principal symptoms of this disease are noted and the entity is given a name which translates into "honey-urine." The observations were several times confirmed by Christian and Mohammedan writers of the medieval period, but it was only in 1776 that Matthew Dobson proved that the sweetness of blood and urine was actually due to the presence of sugar.

THERAPY

I shall discuss the treatment of diabetes here only as that treatment has been remodeled after the discovery of insulin by Banting and Best, in 1922. Not that there was nothing of value in therapy known before 1922; indeed, practically everything was known, even the fact that insulin deficiency probably caused the disease, but it was not until the Toronto group made it possible to supply the missing substance to the patient that the accumulated wealth of dietetic, laboratory and clinical knowledge became completely usable. Evidence that insulin has completely revolutionized treatment is to be found, first, in the fact that the complications of diabetes, once of so little moment, have now leaped into the foreground of importance, for the diabetic, properly treated, may not die of his diabetes; second, that the diabetic child, once given up for lost almost as soon as his case was diagnosed, now needs but to be educated in treatment to become the diabetic adult, though the task is a prodigously difficult one; and third, the fact that arteriosclerosis is replacing coma as a cause of death. But insulin has not simplified treatment; really, it has made it much more complex, for the severe diabetic of today is enabled to live longer and much more comfortably than his fellow sufferers of the Naunyn or Allen periods only if he is able to accomplish in his own case that nice balance between insulin and food intake which is theoretically possible in all cases.

The therapy of diabetes may be conveniently studied under the following topical heads: (1) The essential problem one of dietetics. (2) Hospital *versus* ambulatory treatment. (3) Moderate undernutrition plus small amounts of insulin (Joslin type of treatment). (4) Full nutrition plus large amounts of insulin (Sansum type of treatment). (5) An easy and practical method for the general practitioner (Barach type of treatment). (6) High fat and low protein and carbohydrate diet (Petrén and Newburgh and Marsh

23

type of treatment). (7) Other "cures": oatmeal, etc. (8) Fasting. (9) Levulose (inulin—Jerusalem artichokes). (10) Insulin technic. (11) Insulin reactions. (12) Insulin and exercise. (13) Insulin edema. (14) Insulin-refractory cases. (15) Synthalin. (16) Myrtillin. (17) Treatment of coma. (18) Treatment of complications. (19) Diabetes in children. (20) Diabetes in the aged. (21) Diabetes in pregnancy.

1. **The Essential Problem One of Dietetics.**—The average normal adult individual weighing about 154 pounds (70 Kg.) and performing that moderate amount of daily work well described by the expression "up and about," requires in food the equivalent of 30 to 35 calories per kilogram body weight. Increasing experience has shown that the lower figure is safe and that a diet in which 67 per cent of the calories are obtained from carbohydrate, 16 per cent from protein, and 17 per cent from fat, is physiologically adequate in health and in disease. To obtain these quantities, approximately 350 Gm. of carbohydrate, 84 Gm. of protein and 40 Gm. of fat must be eaten each day—remembering that each gram of protein and each gram of carbohydrate supplies 4 calories and that each gram of fat supplies 9 calories. The diabetic differs from such a normal individual in that, because of the shortage of insulin in the blood, the tissues cannot utilize to the full the principal source of calories in the food, *i. e.*, the carbohydrates. Therefore the chief problem in the treatment of diabetes is the rearrangement of the diet in such fashion that, though only such amount of carbohydrate is employed as can be satisfactorily oxidized by the body, the patient shall nevertheless obtain enough energy-producing food to support life on an endurable plane. The attempt must be made to meet the caloric requirements by increasing either the amount of protein or of fat, or of both, in the diet. To what extent may this be accomplished with the proteins? Only to a very moderate extent for the following reasons: (*a*) The specific dynamic action of protein is so high that, in employing it in sufficient amount to appreciably overcome the shortage in carbohydrate, the total caloric need would be so much increased that the dilemma would become more rather than less trying; (*b*) the amount of protein that would have to be eaten would be so great that the diet would be entirely unpalatable for more than a very short period; (*c*) and finally, this protein in the course of catabolism would yield 58 per cent of itself in the form of carbohydrate to tissues that are already surfeited with carbohydrate which they are unable to use. As compared with protein, fat has three advantages: First, each gram yields 9 rather than 4 calories; second, its specific dynamic action is lower than that of protein, thus enabling it to be used without so greatly increasing the total caloric need; and third, only 10 per cent of it is converted into carbohydrate in the course of catabolism. But its disadvantages are unfortunately grave. Of the two disadvantages of fat the least important, but by no means an *un*important one is the fact that fat, in large enough amount to raise the total calories to a point approaching satisfaction, is very repugnant to the gastro-intestinal tract and often provokes a most undesirable state of indigestion. But the chief disadvantage is this: fat needs carbohydrate for its proper catabolism. Somewhat less than 1 Gm. of carbohydrate must be simultaneously utilized for each gram of fatty acid that is oxidized—"fat burns in the fire of carbohydrate," has been said. But in the diabetic, in whom not much carbohydrate can be burned, what happens to the fat? Simply this, that such amount as cannot "burn in the fire of carbohydrate" is not fully metabolized but stops when the ketone bodies are formed. These ketone bodies are poisonous in that they attach themselves to basic radicals from which they displace the weaker carbonic acid, thus bringing about the presence of CO_2 in excess in the blood. If this goes on in only a small way, the surplus CO_2 is eliminated through the lungs

and some of the ketone bodies are passed out through the kidneys, but if the protein is being kept as high as is thought to be necessary for the body needs, *i. e.*, about 1 Gm. for each kilogram body weight, and the carbohydrate tolerance is very low, then the attempt to completely make up the caloric deficit with fat will finally and inevitably lead to acidosis and coma.

Prior to the advent of insulin for parenteral use in 1922, both horns of this dilemma were grasped firmly, if ineffectually, by simply starving the patient. If his carbohydrate tolerance was very low, and he could not bear large amounts of protein and fat for the reasons which have just been presented, he was merely placed on that amount of carbohydrate, protein and fat which he *could* utilize—and thus was kept alive though hardly of life. The condition of these undernourished patients was, in severe cases, deplorable in the extreme, and they usually died in a short time, either directly or indirectly from the undernutrition, or from coma following the breaking of an intolerable dietary regimen. Then came the discovery of insulin, which made possible the utilization of carbohydrate and thus also the feeding of more fat, and the therapy of severe diabetes was reborn. It is essential for the reader to understand that the new order of things is in the fullest sense only a rebirth of the old. Diet is today, as it was in the Naunyn or Allen period, the bed rock upon which all the structure stands, but, because of insulin, the diet of today is a much more satisfactory diet, and the severe diabetic of today is a living and not a starving, dying diabetic.

Food Chart.—In the brief presentation of the several types of treatment which follows, it will be found that everything depends upon the exact knowledge of the amount of protein, carbohydrate and fat in, and the caloric value of, any and every article of food that the patient eats. I have compiled a chart from several sources (Table 39) showing these values for a number of foods. Many practitioners have found that the weighing of food by the patient at home is greatly facilitated by employing scales which may be set at zero when an empty dish is placed upon them; the weight of food placed in the dish is then read off immediately without counterbalancing.

Diabetic Foods.—Most of the special "diabetic foods" are really very low in carbohydrate but many of them are also quite high in protein, a fact worthy of note since 58 per cent of protein is convertible into carbohydrate. Joslin pertinently points out another disadvantage: "When the patient buys one of these foods, unfortunately he is often given a list of other diabetic foods and a new diabetic diet list, and confusion in the diet frequently results." Joslin does not use any of these special foods at his hospital nor do many of the other practitioners who have blazed the trail in diabetic therapy.

Saccharin.—Benzosulphinide (saccharin) is an antiseptic and tends to hinder slightly the action of the digestive ferments; an excessive quantity of it may, therefore, impair digestion. More than 5 grains (0.32 Gm.) per day has been pronounced harmful by the Government Referee Board of Chemists. In the moderate doses in which it is used for sweetening beverages of diabetics it is not liable to do harm. As a flavored vehicle in which medicines may be administered to the diabetic, the following serves, being similar in taste to aromatic elixir:

℞.	Compound spirit of orange	♏ x	0.60
	Gluside (saccharin)	gr. j	0.06
	Alcohol	℥j	30.00
	Water to make	℥iv	120.00

Glycerin.—This substance may also be used in sweetening the food of diabetics in alternation with saccharin.

Alcohol.—Alcohol is the only food substance of high nutritive value that does not yield glucose or fatty acids when it is burned in the body. One ounce (32 cc.) of whisky, brandy, rum or gin, or ½ pint (250 cc.) of 6 per cent beer (for carbohydrate content, see below), will yield 112 calories; this amount, divided in two equal doses to be taken at lunch and dinner, will replace approximately 12 Gm. of fat per day, and in addition will aid patients, especially elderly persons, in the taking of a monotonous diet. It is much used in this way in all lands not blighted by "prohibition"—and was even so used here during our dry years. A number of authorities do not,

TABLE 39.—FOOD VALUES IMPORTANT IN DIETETIC COMPUTATIONS

100 Gm. contain approximately (Caloric equivalents— 1 Gm. C. = 4 cal.; 1 Gm. P. = 4 cal.; 1 Gm. F. = 9 cal.)	Carbohydrate, Gm.	Protein, Gm.	Fat, Gm.
Meats:			
Fresh meat, cooked (beef, tongue, lamb, mutton, pork)	0	22	19
Ham or sausage (smoked, boiled, fried)	0	22	29
Bacon (too variable for safe use)			
Sweetbreads	0	17	12
Poultry (average)	0	21	16
Broth (thin, clear, skimmed thoroughly)	0	2	0
Fish:			
Fresh fish, cooked (cod, flounder, shad, whitefish, trout, halibut, perch)	1	18	5
Salmon, fresh	1	22	13
Salmon, canned	0	22	13
Sardines	0	23	19
Smoked preserved fish	14	26	16
Shell fish:			
Crabs	1	8	1
Lobster	0	16	2
Oysters (in shell)	4	6	1
Scallops	3	15	0
Milk, cheese, butter, eggs:			
Milk, whole (sweet or lactic acid)	5	3	4
Milk, skimmed	5	3	0
Cream, 20 per cent	5	3	20
Cream, 40 per cent	5	3	40
Buttermilk	5	3	1
Butter	0	0	85
Cheese (American, Camembert, Limburger, Roquefort)	2.5	27	31
Cottage cheese	1.5	21	1
Cream cheese, Crown brand	2	5	58
Swiss cheese	1	28	35
Egg, each	0	6.	6
Egg, white	0	4	0
Egg, yolk	0	2	6
Breads, cereals, and flours:			
Wheat flour	72	14	2
Pure gluten flour	38	42	1
White bread	53	9	2
Whole wheat bread	50	10	1
Rye bread	53	9	6
Brown bread	47	5	2
Crackers	72	11	10
Shreaded wheat	78	10.5	1.5
Cookies	74	7	10
Corn flakes	73	9	1
Oatmeal, dry	67	16	7
Oatmeal, boiled	11.5	3	0.5
Macaroni, cooked	16	3	1.5
Toast	61	11.5	2
Rolled oats	66	17	7
Nuts:			
Nuts (average mixture)	13.5	20.5	59
Chestnuts	42	6	5
Butternuts	3.5	28	61
Brazil nuts	4	17	61
Peanuts	24.5	26	38.5
Miscellany:			
Sugar	100	0	0
Olive oil (or salad oil, lard or crisco)	0	0	100
Mineral oil	0	0	0
Olives, ripe	4	2	26
Gelatin	0	91	0
Chocolate	30	13	49
Cocoa	38	22	29
Beer, ½ pint or 250 cc. (does not include the alcohol)	12.5	0	0
Alcohol (see above)			
Ginger ale, ½ pint or 250 cc.	20	0	0
Horseradish	11	1	0
Tapioca pudding	28	3	3

Vegetables, 3 per cent (sometimes called 5 per cent) and fruits............................	Artichokes (canned) Asparagus Beet greens Broccoli Brussel sprouts Cabbage Cauliflower Celery Cucumbers Dandelion greens Egg plant Endive	Kale Leeks Lettuce Mushrooms Okra Radishes Rhubarb Sorrel Spinach String beans (canned) Swiss chard Tomatoes Watercress	Grapefruit Canteloupe
Vegetables, 6 per cent (sometimes called 10 per cent) and fruits.	Beets Carrots Kohl-rabi Marrow Onions Oyster plant Pumpkin Rutabaga String beans Sour kraut Squash Turnips		Blackberries Cranberries Gooseberries Lemons Muskmelons Oranges Peaches Pineapple Strawberries Watermelon
Vegetables, 15 per cent, and fruits.........................	Artichokes (fresh) Green peas Parsnips Lima beans (canned) Yams		Apples Apricots Blueberries Cherries Currants Grapes Huckleberries Pears Raspberries
Vegetables, 20 per cent or higher, and fruits	Baked beans Shelled beans Green corn Potatoes (baked or boiled) White Sweet		Bananas Plums Prunes

however, approve its use; I quote here Joslin's "reasons" for his opposition: "(1) The pathetic cases, few I will acknowledge, of protracted alcoholic neuritis which I have seen among diabetics, (2) the danger of a patient with a chronic disease contracting a habit, (3) the deliberate and voluntary omission of alcohol by two of my patients as their health improved with insulin, and (4) my personal disapproval of the use of alcohol."

2. Hospital Versus Ambulatory Treatment.—Insulin's great contribution to therapeutics has been that it has returned the diabetic to an active life. There would therefore seem to be no question of hospital *versus* ambulatory treatment since patients *are* ambulatory. This is true, but concerning the advisability of beginning the treatment in a hospital I would wish the reader to have no doubts: only in the hospital can the average patient be taught—by precept, example, harangue and threat, and by observing the results of the mistakes of himself and others—how to live the diabetic life. The sojourn need not be long, but it is certain that nothing else will so repay the diabetic as this initial period in a private room or a ward. It is my belief that Joslin's patients stay on the average only twelve days—surely a short enough period in which to acquire that education which may result in who knows how many years added on to life. After the hospital, who is to treat the case? The answer is implicit in the fact that there are nearly a million and a half diabetics and potential diabetics in the United States. The general practitioner—may his tribe increase!

3. Moderate Undernutrition Plus Small Amounts of Insulin (Joslin Type of Treatment).—The treatment which Joslin employs, and which, with him as preceptor, has been used very extensively throughout the United States, is based upon the belief that as diabetes is slow in its development the disturbed metabolic balance of the body should be corrected slowly, too, always with the purpose in mind to restore pancreatic function rather than to dispel diabetic symptoms. To this end, the islands of Langerhans are spared by restriction of carbohydrate and the acinar tissue by reduction of protein and fat. The successfully treated diabetic under this plan of treatment is considered to be one whose weight is held at about 10 per cent below normal for his age and height, whose urine is sugar-free, and whose diet, restricted though it be especially in carbohydrate, is ample enough to permit him to actively engage in workaday affairs. That is to say, all that is valuable in undernutrition is carried over from an elder day, but the rigors of full undernutrition are softened by the use of enough insulin to make a satisfactory, if not a full, diet possible. The urine is made sugar-free and the blood normal for the following reasons: (1) Because normal values are obviously the best, (2) because a high blood sugar is a stimulus for insulin secretion, which is just the opposite of the rest that is desired, and (3) because disappearance of glycosuria proves utilization of the diet. A fourth reason often given for reducing blood sugar is that a high percentage of sugar in the blood implies the same in the tissues and that this causes degenerative phenomena in arteries and nerves, leads to weakness, weariness and impotence, and conduces to lack of tissue repair and resistance to infection. Joslin doubts the validity of this fourth reason, since sugar in the tissues is not especially high in diabetes, wounds heal well in the presence of a high blood sugar and he believes that there is very little reason for the supposition that high blood sugar causes arteriosclerosis.

After the preliminary partial fast in order to render the patient sugar-free, Joslin's treatment aims to determine his carbohydrate tolerance, to foster this tolerance by feeding as much carbohydrate as can be utilized, and perhaps even to gradually induce an increase in tolerance. The patient first coming for treatment is usually placed on test diet 1 (see Table 40), which, while allowing temporary undernutrition, is considered safe even with acidosis, and within twenty-four hours permits an estimate of the future course of the patient; insulin may be given with it in amounts of 3 to 5 or even more units before a meal, provided its action is adjusted by the results of urine analyses in the morning, afternoon, evening and at night. Blood-sugar estimations are made upon entrance, before breakfast next morning, and subsequently as indicated an hour after a meal, fasting.

"Upon the second day of being sugar-free or nearly so, as shown by the trend of the analyses of the urine for different periods, the diet is changed to a Maintenance Diet with similar quantity of carbohydrate, but protein and fat appropriate to the age, weight, and occupation of the patient. Insulin is reduced and, if the urine is still sugar-free and blood-sugar test favorable, the carbohydrate may be raised by increases of 10 to 25 Gm. daily to a quantity somewhat below that which shows lack of carbohydrate utilization.

"If sugar persists upon the second day, the carbohydrate is decreased by choosing a Maintenance Diet such as C_7PF_7, which contains carbohydrate 74 Gm., protein 52 Gm., and fat 88 Gm. Insulin would be raised to units 5–5–5 (5 units three times a day), because most likely the patient received less on his first day in the hospital, as he may have entered after breakfast.

"Upon the third day if glycosuria is considerable and calories still below 30 per kilogram body weight, the insulin would be raised to 10–5–5 or 10–5–10 or even 10–10–10 and the fat increased by changing the cream from its value of 120 cc. in the C_7PF_7 diet to 180 or 240 cc., the latter quantity (½ pint) being convenient and generally obtainable by diabetics.

"Upon the fourth day, if sugar-free, protein can be brought to 1 Gm. per kilogram body weight by seeking a Maintenance Diet with more protein, such as C_8PF_8 in which the meat is raised from 60 to 90 Gm. The noon

TABLE 40.—TEST AND MAINTENANCE DIETS IN DIABETES (JOSLIN)

		Total diet.				Carbohydrate (C).						Protein and fat (PF).				
		Carbohydrate.	Protein.	Fat.	Calories.	5 per cent vegetables.	Orange.	Oatmeal.	Shredded wheat.	Uneeda.	Potato.	Egg.	Cream, 20 per cent fat.	Bacon.	Butter.	Meat.
Test	T. D. 1	101	35	43	931	300	300	..	1	2	120	3	120	..	..	...
	T. D. 2	66	24	37	693	300	300	..	½	2	...	2	120	..	..	...
	T. D. 3	34	15	30	466	300	200	..	..	..	...	1	120	..	..	...
Maintenance	C4 + PF4	42	29	52	752	600	200	..	..	..	...	2	60	30	15	
	C5 + PF5	52	32	66	930	600	200	15	..	..	...	2	60	30	30	
	C6 + PF6	64	44	84	1179	600	200	30	..	..	...	2	120	30	30	30
	C7 + PF7	74	52	88	1296	600	300	30	..	..	...	2	120	30	30	60
	C8 + PF8	84	61	94	1426	600	300	30	..	2	...	2	120	30	30	90
	C9 + PF9	98	65	106	1606	600	300	30	½	2	...	2	180	30	30	90
	C10 + PF10	109	66	119	1771	600	300	30	1	2	...	2	180	30	45	90
	C11 + PF11	135	80	135	2075	600	300	30	1	2	120	2	240	30	45	120
	C12 + PF12	159	84	135	2187	600	300	30	1	2	240	2	240	30	45	120

insulin may be omitted. Subsequently fat can be raised by addition of butter, oil, or cream, and the fat value of the latter can be doubled, which is rarely indicated, by changing to cream with 40 per cent fat content.

"If glycosuria persists, insulin is usually increased and in addition the diet is changed to C_6, which contains about 60 (actually 64) Gm. carbohydrate as indicated by its digit, the digits of the grams of carbohydrate in the Maintenance Diet being so arranged as to correspond to the C number of the diet. Rarely the patient is placed upon C_5. If not sugar-free with that or with C_6, it is often an indication that an infection or some such complication as hyperthyroidism is present. Cases of considerable severity may require more insulin 15–15–15, or 25–0–20, even 30–0–15, or 25–10–15–10.

"Effort is made by adjustment of diet and insulin to bring the carbohydrate to 100 Gm., the protein to 1 to 1.5 Gm. per kilogram, and the fat sufficient to provide 30 calories per kilogram body weight. He will be a rare diabetic who cannot assimilate such a diet with 45 units of insulin. If such a case is found, the protein can be decreased to ⅔ Gm. per kilogram and if necessary insulin raised. I seldom see such a case.

"Above a diet represented by C_{10} one should seldom go unless very confident that the patient has an adequate tolerance for carbohydrate. The reason for this is that when one reaches 100 Gm. of carbohydrate in the diet, additions in carbohydrate must consist of foods containing high percentages of carbohydrate, and errors, innocently and easily, may creep into the patient's dietetic regimen. Thus a patient cannot readily eat more than 100 Gm. of carbohydrate in the form of 5, 10 and 15 per cent vegetables, oatmeal, grapefruit, strawberries, and orange. Above this level his carbohydrate must begin to be taken in the form of a banana, which to be sure is very useful, because a single banana contains about 20 Gm. of carbohydrate, in potato which is far less easily measured, or in bread which is almost invariably dangerous and therefore does not appear in the diet schedule at all.

"If one wishes to get along with less insulin, more undernutrition and a lower quantity of carbohydrate may be employed, as C_6PF_6, C_5PF_5, or even C_4PF_4. Such diets would be temporary or for an occasional day. One shrinks from forcing a patient to draw too much on his body tissue. However, I cannot escape the conviction that the diabetic who is forced to draw upon his own body tissues for protein and fat will involuntarily reduce his demands upon these to a lower figure, than when they are furnished in food. Ladd and Palmer have stated that in their studies endogenous fat was less likely to give rise to acidosis than exogenous fat.

"The endeavor to develop to the fullest extent the diabetic's power to utilize carbohydrate is the principle underlying the gradation of the Maintenance Diets. In practice it has been found that if undernutrition was maintained to a greater or lesser extent for a few days the quantity of carbohydrate which could be utilized steadily grew. Diabetics are not so bad as painted. They have far more tolerance for carbohydrate than is often supposed. One must give them a chance to demonstrate what they can do, and unless some such scheme is adopted, it is difficult to find out. To follow the schedule of Test and Maintenance Diets in every case would be absurd because of variations in age, weight, and occupation of the patient. It is a very simple matter, however, to modify these. The only aim of the schedule is to simplify orders for the nurse in the hospital, treatment for the doctor in his practice and at the same time to enable patients to become sugar-free, and to acquire the allotment of carbohydrate which their disease deserves with protein and fat sufficient for maintenance."

A small amount of sugar in the urine when the patient is upon a low maintenance diet may often be safely disregarded because it will very likely vanish as the diet progresses. The return of glycosuria during the course of treatment is a very different matter, however; upon this point Joslin writes:

"If the patient is upon Maintenance Diets, the simplest plan is to recede by a day when the restriction of carbohydrate and of calories may immediately clear the urine. If this is not successful still further recession may be tried. However, since the introduction of single specimen days, that is, the testing of each specimen of urine throughout the twenty-four hours, it frequently comes to light that the reason for the appearance of the sugar was simply due to the unbalanced diet. Correcting this by shifting the carbohydrate from the offending meal to another often solves the difficulty. In general less carbohydrate should be given at breakfast than at the other two meals even if the largest dose of insulin is before breakfast. Perhaps the patient should take insulin fifteen to thirty minutes earlier before a meal; perhaps it should be given in a fresh place; perhaps he requires more exercise or there may be an infection or an error in diet. . . .

"The return of sugar demands fasting whenever there is the slightest suspicion that the diet has been broken by design. This was the rule when the treatment by fasting was first adopted. It is a pity now that it is not as strictly enforced, and I confess I seldom enforce it, but it works so advantageously that it should be done. With children confinement to bed for a few hours with a low diet works wonders. In hospitals it simplifies the treatment enormously. So soon as it is understood that the reappearance of sugar means a fast until glycosuria disappears from the twenty-four hour quantity of urine, there is little tendency to break over the diet. Furthermore, most patients are thrifty enough to see the disadvantage of paying their board with no return. The rule must be rigidly enforced with children, because with them disobedience means death."

Mild Cases.—Joslin feels that the mild case is the case which demands the most energetic treatment, for, as in incipient tuberculosis, though a cure may not be accomplished the disease may many times be held in check. He would have these patients taught to take long vacations, secure an abundance of sleep, avoid excess in mental and physical labor, shun obesity, and provide for daily exercise. Their diet does not often work a great actual hardship upon them but such restrictions as are necessary are usually much resented—"with these individuals it is hard to have patience." His plan is to omit butter, cream, or both for a time, and to limit protein to between 1 and 1½ Gm. per kilogram body weight. Combined with these measures, the exclusion of actual sugar from the dietary and the substitution of potato (20 per cent carbohydrate) for bread (60 per cent carbohydrate) frequently secures a sugar-free urine.

The milder cases usually attain a tolerance of 100 Gm. of carbohydrate in a few weeks' time, but they should limit the quantity of carbohydrate in their diet for years, even though sugar does not appear. Many of these patients feel better and have less digestive trouble if the quantity of carbohydrate is held at 125 to 150 Gm. even though they tolerate more. "Such individuals live apparently in perfect health," says Joslin, "and there is always satisfaction in the belief, and I think justification for it, that treatment has prevented progress of the disease." This should not, however, be interpreted as meaning that treatment with diet or insulin singly or together can *cure* diabetes, for apparently nothing of the sort is ever achieved.

Severe Cases.—"What is the ideal diet for a severe diabetic adult? Calories sufficient to maintain weight within 10 per cent of normal, not less than protein ⅔ Gm. per kilogram body weight, and 50 Gm. of carbohydrate. [In a discussion, in 1932, Joslin has said "I have come to believe that much more carbohydrate should be given than is customary."] The carbohydrate would be given largely in vegetables, fruit, and cream, perhaps a little oatmeal. Jonas has demonstrated the advantage of foods with low percentage of carbohydrate. The breakfast would contain one fourth of the carbohydrate and the balance would be divided between noon and night. Additional tolerance can be obtained by giving to these patients so-called 'activating' carbohydrate meals. Two or 3 Gm. of carbohydrate may be given an hour before breakfast and twice as much in the late afternoon and perhaps upon retiring. The stimulus of a little carbohydrate to the utilization of a larger quantity of carbohydrate in a subsequent meal is definite.

"The carbohydrate ration of a severe diabetic without insulin is what he can tolerate, but the protein ration can be more definitely predicated. It should not fall below ⅔ Gm. per kilogram body weight, nor should it rise above 1 Gm. per kilogram body weight. Only by restricting the protein to this minimum was it possible to supply the diabetic with the maximum calories in the form of fat without the production of acidosis. If the severe diabetic was not sugar-free with maintenance calories distributed between carbohydrate, protein, and fat, the only recourse for him was to undergo undernutrition to such an extent that his metabolism was reduced to such a level that a smaller quantity of carbohydrate, protein and fat would hold him in equilibrium.

"What is the ideal amount of insulin for a severe diabetic adult? Enough to make him a happy and useful member of society. Few need over 50 units, and I do not think there are 10 patients among my 2000, more or less, using insulin who are taking 60 units. Additional units give far less return in carbohydrate assimilated. As a rule adjustment of insulin and diet will allow any patients, no matter how severe, to take 100 Gm. carbohydrate. Obviously these remarks do not apply to patients with infections. . . .

"It is not so much the quantity of insulin as it is the intelligence with which it is given. Less is required with good manipulation of the syringe, with variation of the site of injection, with several rather than ,a single dose, with distribution of the dosage and frequency according to the time of day the blood sugar is highest. For these severe cases before breakfast and the evening meal and upon retiring are the choice. Jonas has shown a noon dose is theoretically avoidable, and I have usually found this true. The distribution of quantity of carbohydrate to dose is not as necessary as one would imagine.

"Severe cases of diabetes cause the most worry at the beginning of treatment. An infection, a gastro-intestinal upset, a careless alteration of diet, anxiety, overexertion, a mild intercurrent disease, may favor the outbreak of coma.

"For these severe cases a trained diabetic nurse permanently in charge of the patient is of the greatest assistance to the patient and family. Any diabetic who can afford the luxury of a diabetic nurse is fortunate. It is the best insurance he can take out for his life. Several of my diabetic cases consult me but twice a year because they depend upon their nurses. If a nurse is not available, success in treatment depends upon the thorough education of the patient. The wise live long; the ignorant succumb early."

4. **Full Nutrition Plus Large Amounts of Insulin (Sansum Type of Treatment).**—Some years ago Sansum and his co-workers began carefully studying practically full nutrition diets, especially diets in which carbohydrate was much raised and fat lowered. Except for the omission of sugar and of foods actually sweetened with sugar, their diets were essentially normal, containing white bread, potatoes, milk and large servings of fruit; with some diets sugar was even included. In contradistinction to the older ratio of 2 to 4 Gm. of fat to each gram of carbohydrate, these new diets contained 2 or more grams of carbohydrate to each gram of fat—a very bold dietetic departure, for instead of gradually building up a tolerance for 100 Gm. or more of carbohydrate, Sansum allowed 200 Gm. of carbohydrate from the beginning, giving very large doses of insulin to provide for its utilization. As a routine the total amount of food was divided into equal amounts for each of the three meals of the day, and two doses of insulin were used, five eighths of the total dose being given from fifteen to thirty minutes before breakfast, and three eighths at the same interval before supper, with minor variations as necessary. When the insulin dosage was small, one dose was given daily with the two large meals following it and no insulin preceding the small meal of the day. The patients were kept sugar-free to a subnormal test, *i. e.*, instead of using 8 drops of urine to 5 cc. Benedict's solution, 16 drops of urine were used.

At present, after the passage of a sufficient number of probational years, it is all but universally recognized that this bold experiment of Sansum marks the greatest advance in the therapy of diabetes that has been made since the discovery of insulin (Bibliography: Adlersberg; Barach; Dyke; Geyelin and Mackie; Graham *et al.*; Gray and Sansum; Himsworth; Klemmer; Nixon; Poulton; Rabinowitch). I shall endeavor to set down tersely here the reasons for the favorable tide which is rapidly turning toward the method in practice:

(*a*) Before the discovery of insulin, Allen and his associates had shown that by removing variable proportions of the pancreas in the dog they could cause diabetes of varying severity, which the animal survived if given just that amount of carbohydrate which the reduced amount of islet tissue could handle, but that if he were fed liberally he succumbed because the islet tissue rapidly degenerated. This was the birth of the undernutrition and pancreatic-rest type of treatment.

(*b*) When insulin arrived on the scene its use was merely engrafted upon this treatment, *i. e.*, the "tolerance" of the patient was determined by building up the carbohydrate after starvation to the amount he could utilize, and then insulin was added to enable him to take a little more carbohydrate for a little more comfort.

(c) During this period the proportions which it was felt necessary to maintain between the C, P and F fractions of the diet were dictated by the formula $F=2C+\frac{1}{2}P$, by which Woodyat had made clinically available the laboratory researches of Shaffer. But as time has gone on and experience increased, the following clinical observations have made it apparent that this principle needs considerable revision: (1) Patients so strictly managed are always perilously close to ketosis and therefore at all times in a more or less potentially dangerous condition. (2) Patients who do not take the thing too seriously and now and then moderately indulge in excess carbohydrate often escape acetonuria despite the development of glycosuria. (3) With a little sugar in the urine the patient usually "feels better." (4) The pioneer demonstration of Sansum that, by utilizing to the fullest extent the pancreas-resting function of insulin, carbohydrate can be raised and fat lowered out of all relation to the formula with a tremendous increase in both safety and well-being of the patient.

(d) No very definite relation having been found between insulin and the various types of food when Sansum began the use of his full diets, he assumed that an increase in carbohydrate would necessitate a proportional increase in insulin dosage, and so proposed the injection of 1 unit of insulin for each 2 Gm. of food, *i. e.*, a patient eating 400 Gm. of food was to be given 200 units of insulin. Surprisingly, this proportional insulin increase has not been found to be necessary, all who use the new methods being in agreement that after the first 15 or 20 units the addition of a few more units will take care of astonishingly large increases in carbohydrate. The accompanying chart of Barach (see p. 370) shows this very well. Note that in 1928, with 84 Gm. carbohydrate and 137 Gm. fat, 24 units of insulin were required, whereas in 1931, on 154 Gm. carbohydrate (twice the former amount) and 110 Gm. fat (a reduction of 27 Gm.), 28 units sufficed (an increase of only 3 units). As example, in an individual case the carbohydrate was increased from 95 to 200 Gm. daily from April, 1930, to July, 1931, and the fat reduced from 170 to 115 Gm. At the beginning of treatment the patient required 42 units of insulin daily (25-0-17); at the time of the report, early in 1932, he was taking 40 units (22-0-18). There had also been an increase of 10 Gm. protein, so that he now takes 105 Gm. more carbohydrate, 10 Gm. more protein, 55 Gm. less fat, and 2 units less insulin. "In him and in others I have repeatedly seen an increase in fat followed by glycosuria; at other times he is sugar normal (absence of glycosuria with normal blood sugar)."

A satisfactory experimental explanation for this increase in ability to utilize carbohydrate has yet to be offered. Adlersberg (1932) is inclined to believe that it is due to lower caloric value, but this is not likely since the increase persists even though many more calories are added in carbohydrate than are subtracted through reduction in fat. The suggestion of Graham *et al.* (1932) is interesting; namely, that the presence of ketone bodies in the blood, as was usually the case under the old dietary régime, may cause an increased demand for insulin just as the presence of staphylococcic infection, for instance, will do.

(e) The diets are more palatable, they are cheaper and easier to prepare, they are more nearly normal, and they maintain the patient in a stronger condition—a stoker or plowman *can* stoke or plow—and feeling thoroughly at ease. It has also been remarked that upon the new type of therapy patients who formerly had persistently high blood sugars are seen less frequently and that the "refractory" diabetic becomes a normal diabetic.

(f) Evidence is accumulating that the new diets are to some extent ef-

TABLE 41.—FOR COMPUTATION OF DIABETIC DIET (BARACH)

I

Add or subtract the pounds designated if patient is a female.

Normal Weight—Six Months to Seventeen Years

Height.	Age.	Weight. Male Fem.
26 in.	6 mos.	18 − 2 lbs.
27 in.	8 mos.	20 − 2 lbs.
28 in.	10 mos.	21 − 2 lbs.
29 in.	1 yr.	22 − 2 lbs.
32 in.	1½ yrs.	25 − 2 lbs.
34 in.	2 yrs.	27 − 1 lb.
35 in.	2½ yrs.	30 − 2 lbs.
37 in.	3 yrs.	32 − 2 lbs.
38 in.	3½ yrs.	34 − 2 lbs.
39 in.	4 yrs.	36 − 2 lbs.
40 in.	5– 7 yrs.	38 − 1 lb.
42 in.	5– 8 yrs.	42 − 1 lb.
44 in.	5– 8 yrs.	46 − 1 lb.
46 in.	5– 9 yrs.	50 − 2 lbs.
48 in.	6–11 yrs.	54 − 2 lbs.
50 in.	7–12 yrs.	58 − 1 lb.
52 in.	7–12 yrs.	62 − 2 lbs.
54 in.	8–13 yrs.	70 − 2 lbs.
56 in.	9–14 yrs.	78 − 2 lbs.
58 in.	10–16 yrs.	86 + 2 lbs.
60 in.	10–17 yrs.	96 + 4 lbs.

Normal Weight Seventeen to Thirty-four Years

Ages. Height.	17 to 19 M. F.	20 to 24 M. F.	25 to 29 M. F.	30 to 34 M. F.
4′ 10″	109 − 1	115 − 4	120 − 6	123 − 6
4′ 11″	111 − 1	117 − 4	122 − 6	125 − 6
5′ 0″	113 − 1	119 − 4	124 − 6	127 − 6
5′ 1″	115 − 1	121 − 4	126 − 6	129 − 6
5′ 2″	118 − 1	124 − 4	128 − 6	131 − 6
5′ 3″	121 − 1	127 − 4	131 − 5	134 − 6
5′ 4″	124 − 1	131 − 5	134 − 5	137 − 5
5′ 5″	128 − 2	135 − 6	138 − 6	141 − 5
5′ 6″	132 − 2	139 − 6	142 − 6	145 − 5
5′ 7″	136 − 2	142 − 5	146 − 6	149 − 5
5′ 8″	140 − 2	146 − 5	150 − 6	154 − 6
5′ 9″	144 − 3	150 − 5	154 − 6	158 − 6
5′ 10″	148 − 3	154 − 5	158 − 6	163 − 8
5′ 11″	153 − 3	158 − 5	163 − 8	168 − 10
6′ 0″	158 − 3	163 − 6	169 − 10	174 − 12
6′ 1″	163 − 3	168 − 6	175 − 12	180 − 14

Normal Weight Thirty-four to Fifty-four Years

Ages. Height.	35 to 39 M. F.	40 to 44 M. F.	45 to 49 M. F.	50 to 54 M. F.
4′ 10″	125 − 5	128 − 4	130 − 3	131 − 2
4′ 11″	127 − 5	130 − 4	132 − 3	133 − 2
5′ 0″	129 − 5	132 − 4	134 − 3	135 − 2
5′ 1″	131 − 5	134 − 4	136 − 3	137 − 2
5′ 2″	a133 − 4	136 − 3	138 − 2	139 − 1
5′ 3″	136 − 4	139 − 3	141 − 2	142 − 1
5′ 4″	140 − 4	142 − 3	144 − 2	145 − 1
5′ 5″	144 − 4	146 − 3	148 − 2	149 − 1
5′ 6″	148 − 4	150 − 3	152 − 1	153 − 1
5′ 7″	152 − 4	154 − 3	156 − 1	157 − 0
5′ 8″	157 − 5	159 − 4	161 − 2	162 − 0
5′ 9″	162 − 6	164 − 5	166 − 3	167 − 1
5′ 10″	167 − 8	169 − 7	171 − 5	172 − 2
5′ 11″	172 − 10	175 − 9	177 − 7	178 − 4
6′ 0″	178 − 13	181 − 12	183 − 10	184 − 7
6′ 1″	184 − 16	187 − 15	190 − 13	191 − 10

II
Conversion Table
2.2 lbs. = 1 Kilo

Body weight. Lbs.	Kilo.	Body weight. Lbs.	Kilo.	Body weight. Lbs.	Kilo.
15.4	7	83.6	38	151.8	69
17.6	8	85.8	39	154.0	70
19.8	9	88.0	40	156.2	71
22.0	10	90.2	41	158.4	72
24.2	11	92.4	42	160.6	73
26.4	12	94.6	43	162.8	74
28.6	13	96.8	44	165.0	75
30.8	14	99.0	45	167.2	76
33.0	15	101.2	46	169.4	77
35.2	16	103.4	47	171.6	78
37.4	17	105.6	48	173.8	79
39.6	18	107.8	49	176.0	80
41.8	19	110.0	50	178.2	81
44.0	20	112.2	51	180.4	82
46.2	21	114.4	52	182.6	83
48.4	22	116.6	53	184.8	84
50.6	23	118.8	54	187.0	85
52.8	24	121.0	55	189.2	86
55.0	25	123.2	56	191.4	87
57.2	26	125.4	57	193.6	88
59.4	27	127.6	58	195.8	89
61.6	28	129.8	59	198.0	90
63.8	29	b132.0	60	200.2	91
66.0	30	134.2	61	202.4	92
68.2	31	136.4	62	204.6	93
70.4	32	138.6	63	206.8	94
72.6	33	140.8	64	209.0	95
74.8	34	143.0	65	211.2	96
77.0	35	145.2	66	213.4	97
79.2	36	147.4	67	215.6	98
81.4	37	149.6	68	217.8	99
				220.0	100

III
Diet per Kilo Body Weight in Health

Age.	Gm. carb.	Gm. prot.	Gm. fat.	Calories.
To 4 years	10.0	3.0	3.10	80
4 to 10 years	10.0	1.5	2.66	70
10 to 17 years	7.5	1.5	2.66	60
17 to 25 years	5.0	1.5	2.10	45
Adult	5.0	1.0	0.66	30

Use the table below; the one above is merely for comparison.

Diabetic Diet per Kilo Body Weight
Carbohydrate Approximately One-half Normal

Age.	Gm. carb.	Gm. prot.	Gm. fat.	Calories.
To 4 years	5.0	3.0	2.5	55
4 to 10 years	5.0	1.5	2.6	50
10 to 17 years	3.5	1.5	2.7	45
17 to 25 years	3.0	1.25	2.0	35
c Adult	3.0	1.0	1.5	30

fective in reducing the complication of arteriosclerosis and also in lowering hypertension. Rabinowitch and his associates believe that the fall in blood cholesterol incident to the reduction in fat is responsible for this; Sansum *et al.* attribute it rather to the reduction of general acidity brought about by the large amounts of fruits and vegetables included in the higher carbohydrate diets.

TABLE 42.—CARBOHYDRATE, PROTEIN, AND FAT ALLOWANCES (BARACH)

Carbohydrate Portion

	Carbohydrate. Food.	50 Gm.	60 Gm.	70 Gm.	80 Gm.	90 Gm.	100 Gm.	110 Gm.	120 Gm.	130 Gm.	140 Gm.	150 Gm.	160 Gm.	170 Gm.	180 Gm.	190 Gm.	200 Gm.
Breakfast	6 per cent fruit	100	100	100	100	100	100	100	100	100	100	100	100	100	100	100	100
Breakfast	Cereal (dry weight)	14	20	25	28	34	40	28	34	40	28	34	40	28	32	40	40
Breakfast	Bread	...	...	...	...	...	...	20	20	20	40	40	40	60	60	60	60
Lunch	20 per cent vegetable	50	50	60	70	90	100	70	90	100	120	140	150	170	190	155	170
Lunch	6 per cent fruit	115	165	185	200	200	200	200	200	200	200	200	200	200	200	200	200
Lunch	Bread	...	...	...	...	...	...	20	20	20	20	20	20	20	20	40	40
Dinner	20 per cent vegetable	50	50	50	50	50	50	70	80	100	120	130	150	170	190	145	170
Dinner	6 per cent vegetable	60	80	100	100	135	200	200	200	200	200	200	200	200	200	200	200
Dinner	6 per cent fruit	60	85	130	200	200	200	200	200	200	200	200	200	200	200	200	200
Dinner	Bread	...	...	...	...	...	...	...	...	...	...	...	...	...	...	20	20
	Grams protein to be subtracted from Protein-Fat Portion		5	5	5	5	5	10	10	10	10	10	10	10	10	15	15

Protein and Fat Portion e

Protein.	15	20	25	30	35	40	45	50	55	60	65	70	75	80	85	90
Fat.	15	20	25	30	35	40	45	50	55	60	65	70	75	80	85	90
Breakfast — Grams meat	25	30	40	50	55	65	75	80	90	100	105	115	125	130	140	150
Lunch — Grams meat	25	35	40	50	60	70	75	85	90	100	110	115	125	135	140	150
Dinner — Grams meat	25	35	45	50	60	70	75	85	95	100	110	120	125	135	145	150

Additional Fat Portion f

Additional Fat.	10	15	20	25	30	35	40	45	50	55	60	65	70	75	80	85
Breakfast — Butter	6	6	7	10	12	12	15	17	19	21	22	22	22	22	22	22
Breakfast — Fat, salad or olive oil																
Lunch — Butter or mayonnaise		6	8	10	12	14	15	17	19	21	22	22	22	22	22	22
Lunch — Fat, salad or olive oil												3	2	8	12	14
Dinner — Butter or mayonnaise	6	6	8	10	12	15	17	19	21	23	24	24	24	24	24	24
Dinner — Fat, salad or olive oil											3	5	10	10	14	18

TABLE 43.—QUICK REFERENCE EXCHANGE CHART

Vegetables or Fruit

100 Gm. of 6 per cent for 200 Gm. of 3 per cent or 40 Gm. of 15 per cent or 30 Gm. of 20 per cent.
100 Gm. of 20 per cent for 335 Gm. of 6 per cent or 135 Gm. of 15 per cent.
100 Gm. of 3 per cent for 2 oz. (60 cc.) milk if meat is reduced 9 Gm.
100 Gm. of 6 per cent for 4 oz. (120 cc.) milk if meat is reduced 18 Gm.
100 Gm. of 15 per cent for 10 oz. (300 cc.) milk if meat is reduced 45 Gm.
100 Gm. of 20 per cent for 13 oz. (400 cc.) milk if meat is reduced 60 Gm.
100 Gm. of 20 per cent (or 135 Gm. of 15 per cent or 335 Gm. of 6 per cent) for 40 Gm bread plus 5 Gm. butter if 20 Gm. meat is omitted.
100 Gm. of 3 per cent (or 50 Gm. of 6 per cent or 20 Gm. of 15 per cent or 15 Gm. of 20 per cent) for 2 oz. (60 cc.) cream, omitting 9 Gm. meat and 12 Gm. butter.
100 Gm. of 20 per cent (or 135 Gm. of 15 per cent or 335 Gm. of 6 per cent) for 28 Gm. cereal plus 5 Gm. butter omitting 21 Gm. meat.

Cereals and Bread

14 Gm. cereal for 335 Gm. of 3 per cent vegetable (or 165 Gm. of 6 per cent or 65 Gm. of 15 per cent or 50 Gm. of 20 per cent) if 10 Gm. meat is omitted.
20 Gm. cereal for 465 Gm. of 3 per cent vegetable (or 235 Gm. of 6 per cent or 90 Gm. f 15 per cent or 70 Gm. of 20 per cent) if 15 Gm. meat is omitted and 5 Gm. butter added.
40 Gm. cereal for 465 Gm. of 6 per cent vegetable (or 190 Gm. of 15 per cent or 140 Gm. of 20 per cent) if 30 Gm. meat is omitted and 8 Gm. butter added.
20 Gm. bread for 14 Gm. cereal.
40 Gm. bread for 28 Gm. cereal.

Meat, Poultry, Fish, Cheese, Eggs

100 Gm. fresh cooked meat for:
    70 Gm. chicken or turkey, in either case plus 8 Gm. butter.
    83 Gm. tuna fish (canned) plus 4 Gm. butter.
    86 Gm. sardines (canned) plus 4 Gm. butter.
    90 Gm. salmon (canned) plus 10 Gm. butter.
    70 Gm. fresh fish (shad, white fish, halibut, lake trout) plus 8 Gm. butter.
    69 Gm. American cheese minus 6 Gm. butter.
    96 Gm. cottage cheese plus 24 Gm. butter.
     3 eggs.

5. **An Easy and Practical Method for the General Practitioner (Barach Type of Treatment).**—In employing the words "easy" and "practical" in the title of this section, it is certainly not my intention to imply that the average physician in this or any other land is incapable of understanding, or unwilling to be interested in, any plan of diabetes therapy which does not comply strictly with the meaning of those adjectives. Far from it. But I think the fact needs hardly to be affirmed here that unless a given treatment plan relieves him of the incubus of performing time-consuming calculations from formulae it *is* neither easy nor practical and therefore is of no use to him. The proof of this contention seems to me to be had in the notion going about nowadays that diabetes should really be treated by the specialist—which is of course sheer nonsense! Therefore the methods employed by Barach, of Pittsburgh, are here presented as being quite outstanding in the large lot examined by me, and in the hope that the reader will be convinced by his study of the few succeeding pages that such a thing as an "easy" and "practical" scheme has been evolved. The method is completely in accordance with the newer dictates in treatment; that is to say, it is a high carbohydrate—low fat diet plan (for rationale of which, see p. 362).

(*a*) *The Necessary Tables.*—These are placed on facing pages for convenience, and are to be used in connection with the table of food values on page 356. Table 41 contains age-height-weight tables from six months to fifty-four years, a reference table for quickly converting pounds into kilos, and diets per kilo in health and in diabetes. Table 42 comprises groupings of carbohydrate, protein and fat allowances per meal, and in Table 43 there is a quick reference exchange chart.

(*b*) *The Computation of the Diet.*—On Table 41 find the patient's age column and then the number of pounds it is assumed he should weigh at his height (Part I). Convert this into kilos (Part II). Then with this figure representing his desired weight in kilos, turn to Part III and multiply the grams of carbohydrate, protein and fat for his age by this figure. This will give the grams of each that are to comprise the total for the day, with which to begin the diet. Now, for actually arranging meals from these figures, Table 42 is to be employed. Perhaps a supposititious case had best be used.

J. K., male, aged thirty-seven, height 5 feet, 1½ inches, has been diagnosed as diabetic and requires to be treated. The portions of the several tables indicated by the letters contain the successive steps:. (*a*) At thirty-seven, and measuring 5 feet, 1½ inches, the desired weight would be 132 pounds (127½ had the patient been a woman). (*b*) This is equivalent to 60 kilos. (*c*) Sixty multiplied by the number of grams of carbohydrate, protein and fat for the adult diabetic gives a daily allowance of 180 Gm. carbohydrate, 60 Gm. protein (45 Gm. had the patient been a woman) and 90 Gm. fat. (*d*) With a daily allowance of 180 Gm. carbohydrate, the patient may take 100 Gm. of 6 per cent fruit, 32 Gm. cereal (dry weight), and 60 Gm. white bread for breakfast; 190 Gm. 20 per cent vegetable, 200 Gm. 6 per cent fruit, and 20 Gm. white bread for lunch; 190 Gm. 20 per cent vegetable, 200 Gm. 6 per cent vegetable, 200 Gm. 6 per cent fruit for dinner in the evening. In obtaining this carbohydrate portion he will also have obtained 10 Gm. protein (the lowest figure in the 180 Gm. column). Therefore (*e*) when seeking the protein component, deduct this 10 Gm. from his allowance of 60 Gm. and allow him the amount of protein indicated in the 50 Gm. column, *i. e.*, he will have 80 Gm. meat for breakfast and 85 Gm. for lunch and dinner. Now he was to be given 90 Gm. fat.; but in obtaining the protein he has incidentally obtained 50 Gm. of his fat—therefore, (*f*) the remaining fat is to be derived as shown in the 40 Gm. column in the "Additional Fat Portion" table, this additional fat to be distributed more or less equally between the three meals.

And that is all there is to the computation of the diet; there is not a single formula calculation in it. Table 43 comprises a number of exchanges which can be made. For instance, our supposititious patient may exchange his 100 Gm. of 6 per cent fruit for 40 Gm. 15 per cent fruit, or, if he is a fellow of such poor spirit as not to care for 100 Gm. meat with each meal, he may exchange a portion for 96 Gm. cottage cheese and thus acquire an additional 24 Gm. butter; or he may make the trade for 90 Gm. salmon, plus only 10 Gm. of butter. A number of such permissible exchanges may be worked out from the table of food values on page 356.

(*c*) *The Use of Insulin.*—When the patient has been placed upon the diet computed as above, he is studied for his ability to utilize carbohydrate. If he does not become sugar-free (no sugar in urine and blood sugar not to exceed 125 mg. per 100 cc.), the use of insulin must be considered— 1 unit for each 2 Gm. of glucose output. Barach finds it necessary to employ insulin in 41 per cent of his cases, which is to be contrasted with the report of Speidel (1930) of Louisville, who found it necessary to give the drug to less than 25 per cent of his patients treated upon the Woodyatt formula in general practice. However, there need be no fear in using the drug boldly and freely if necessary in the beginning, for under the new high carbohydrate-low fat plan of treatment it will certainly be possible to very

24

considerably decrease the initial dosage if it has been very high. As shown in the chart, the insulin patients of Barach are now taking an average of 28 units of insulin with an average of 154 Gm. of carbohydrate daily. The patients of Sansum, who initiated the new régime, take much more insulin than this but they are also given larger—some say immoderately large— quantities of carbohydrate. The injection should be made preferably fif- teen to thirty minutes before breakfast, though if this is insufficient another dose must be given before dinner, and occasionally also before lunch; very rarely is a fourth dose necessary. Sansum gives five eighths of the total dose before breakfast and the remaining three eighths before dinner in the evening, or, if three doses are being used, five elevenths before breakfast, three elevenths after lunch, and three elevenths at bedtime. Many prac- titioners give all three doses before the meals. Dyke (1932) states that in his experience it has often been possible to give the full dose for the day before breakfast, provided the total daily requirement is not in excess of 40 units. "In such cases," he says, "it is frequently desirable to arrange

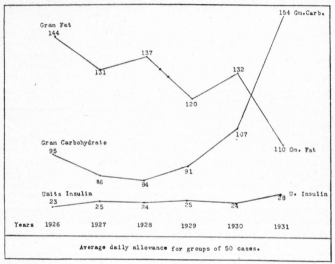

Chart showing C-P-F and insulin relations on the new high carbohydrate-low fat diets (Joseph H. Barach, Jour. Amer. Med. Assoc., April 9, 1932).

the diet so that the patient takes from 10 to 15 Gm. of carbohydrate in the middle of the morning."

Barach finds the following a useful rough guide to insulin dosage: If the urine contains 2 per cent or more of sugar (red color in Benedict test), give 15 to 20 units three times daily. If the urine contains 2 per cent or less of sugar (yellow color in test), 10 to 15 units three times daily. If the test turns green, only a trace of sugar is present.

(d) *Building Up the Diet.*—After the patient has been sugar-free on this initial diet for three days, either with or without insulin, add 10 Gm. carbo- hydrate and deduct 4.5 Gm. fat from the total diet, and repeat this until hyperglycemia or glycosuria appears. In patients who have become sugar- free without insulin, it is sometimes possible to considerably increase the carbohydrate since it was begun at only one half the normal amount; when tolerance is reached it must then be decided whether or not insulin is to be resorted to in these mild cases. After the insulin patient has been sugar- free for one month, try again substituting 10 Gm. carbohydrate for 4.5 Gm. fat without changing the insulin, and continue exchanging toward the normal diet until hyperglycemia or glycosuria appears. Later, if tolerance improves, increase the carbohydrate or reduce the insulin.

Remember that if there is acetone and diacetic acid *without* glycosuria, too little carbohydrate is being given, and both additional carbohydrate and insulin are necessary. If there is acetone and diacetic acid *with* glycosuria, fat and protein must be reduced, and carbohydrate and insulin are imperatively needed.

6. **High Fat and Low Protein and Carbohydrate Diet (Newburgh and Marsh and Petrén Type of Treatment).**—Newburgh and Marsh in the United States, and Petrén in Sweden, have substituted for the preliminary fast a diet of about 900 calories, nearly 90 per cent of which is derived from fat, the protein and carbohydrate being kept very low. The patients are subsequently maintained in a state of undernutrition on a diet high in fat and very low in protein and carbohydrate. This type of treatment would now seem to be completely out-moded.

7. **Other "Cures."**—The oatmeal treatment, the wheat flour treatment, the potato treatment, the banana treatment, the milk treatment—all these "cures" have been reduced to a position of historical interest only by the arrival of insulin upon the scene. It is therefore not desirable, even though space permitted, that they be described in this book.

Liver and Sulphur.—In 1927-30, Murphy and Blotner reported favorable effects from liver therapy in diabetes, but Ralli's (1932) studies failed entirely to confirm their findings. The value of sulphur therapy, as recently proposed in Germany, is still entirely speculative.

8. **Fasting.**—Fasting is a thing of the past, now that we have insulin, and will not be described here.

9. **Levulose (Inulin—Jerusalem Artichokes).**—Levulose seems to cause a different type of metabolism from dextrose (glucose); the mechanisms involved are probably two: The conversion by the diabetic of part of the levulose into fat, and the stimulation by the levulose of a more active production of insulin. It is best used intermittently for its advantages disappear when used continuously. Inulin, the chief carbohydrate constituent of Jerusalem artichokes, yields levulose upon hydrolysis, though the conditions under which this hydrolysis takes place in the body seem to be rather uneven. At times it is possible to render the urine sugar-free by the substitution of carbohydrate in the form of artichokes for carbohydrate in some other form. Joslin states that it is usually possible to substitute 15 Gm. of carbohydrate as contained in artichokes for 5 Gm. of carbohydrate as contained in 5 per cent vegetables. He cites the case of a patient who was able to supplement his usual resting diet with the addition of 100 Gm. of carbohydrate in the form of dried Jerusalem artichokes, it being clearly shown by metabolism experiments that fully 100 Gm. of carbohydrate were absorbed from the artichokes. When an equivalent amount of carbohydrate in the form of potato was substituted for artichokes in this patient's diet, glycosuria and hyperglycemia appeared within two hours and disappeared only after the potato was discontinued and the artichokes resumed. This tuber may be eaten raw but it is best prepared by baking; when it is boiled much of the inulin is lost in the water. A supply for the entire year may be prepared in the season by cutting the tubers into chips and drying in moderate heat, as over a radiator.

I am obliged to report that since the above was written, Soskin *et al.* (1931) in Chicago, and Stein *et al.* (1931) in Denver, have independently published careful studies which it would seem ought to completely prick the artichoke bubble; however, as so many physicians are convinced that they obtain the results described above, I shall retain the paragraph until a little more water has run under the bridges.

10. Insulin Technic.—Joslin writes: "The site of injection is not an indifferent matter. If it is injected into the upper layers of the skin it acts more powerfully, but the pain and the so-called 'insulin burns' make this undesirable. Conversely I have tried giving it before the evening meal deeply into the lower fat layers to delay absorption, but only with indifferent success. It is best injected subcutaneously, distributing the solution so as not to injure any one special area of the skin. But most important of all is to vary the site of injection. For this purpose my nurses have made insulin maps especially for the little children. By this I mean the body forms printed with dots for each dose of insulin during the month so that no two doses will be in the same place, and thus avoid injuring the skin. All my diabetics learn to give insulin on the right side of the body in the morning and the left side at night, and in four longitudinal and parallel lines down the extremities. The Sunday dose begins at the upper end of the line and the Saturday dose is at the lower end. Never give insulin many times in one place. Necrosis of tissue occurs, an abscess may form, failure of absorption is bound to ensue, the dosage in consequence is increased and if by chance the same quantity is given in another part of the body a reaction follows."

In exceptional instances 0.1 cc. of 2 per cent procaine hydrochloride (without epinephrine) may be added to the dose to be injected. If insulin is injected into the muscles necrosis occurs and scar tissue forms. Extensive atrophy of subcutaneous fat following repeated injections has been reported. The compound of insulin with phosphotungstic acid, intended for use by mouth, has not been proved to be of value; indeed, the development of any other means of introducing insulin other than by the needle has been shown my Macleod (1930) to be extremely unlikely.

11. Insulin Reactions.—When an overdose of insulin has been taken the patient experiences a feeling of general muscular weakness, "hollowness" in the stomach accompanied by great hunger, subjective and objective trembling, restlessness and temporary loss of memory, sweating and pallor or flushing of the face, and increased pulse rate. These symptoms may be experienced very suddenly or they may come on gradually during the course of a quarter hour. In the more severe reactions the face assumes a masklike expression, there is diplopia and complete disorientation, and the patient may become unconscious and show a profound fall in temperature and blood pressure; epileptiform convulsions are also seen in some instances. Deaths have been reported but they are rare, though evidence is beginning to accumulate that in older patients these reactions may induce attacks of angina pectoris and even coronary thrombosis. Unquestionably a very few of them are allergic in nature, for they follow the use of one brand of insulin but not the use of another. Other things being equal, the thin, frail, feeble patient is the most likely to develop reactions.

The insulin reaction is commonly ascribed to a sudden hypoglycemia, but it is well not to overlook the fact that some other mechanism may also be involved since not all individuals in whom the blood sugar falls very considerably experience such a reaction; indeed, John has described such reactions with a normal or increased percentage of blood sugar. Foshay believes that not so much the hypoglycemia *per se* as the relatively greater glucose impoverishment within the cell is to be held accountable. Müller and Petersen look upon an acute disturbance of the autonomic nervous system as the cause of the shock, of which hypoglycemia is only one of many symptoms. It is not unlikely also that some disturbance of the circulation in the brain takes place, for a number of cases of hemiplegia have been reported as having occurred during very severe reactions.

Glucose.—Any carbohydrate out of which glucose may be quickly formed in the body is the antidote. Orange juice is usually taken and acts very well; indeed, it would seem to be especially suitable because, as Joslin sagely remarks, while he is peeling the orange the patient has time to reflect as to whether or not he is actually experiencing a reaction due to an overdose of insulin, and thus may sometimes avoid taking the carbohydrate unnecessarily and therefore harmfully. One or two lumps of sugar, depending upon the size of the individual, quickly dissolved in the mouth is also effective in overcoming the symptoms. If the patient is unable to swallow easily, honey or corn syrup may be used. In any case, after a rest, the dose of glucose should be repeated.

Intravenous injection of the glucose may be made if the patient is unconscious; also it must sometimes be resorted to in patients who have not lost consciousness but in whom the hypoglycemia seems to be accompanied by a depression in the absorptive power of the intestinal mucous membrane (or should the failure to respond to the oral administration of glucose be ascribed to acute peristaltic lapse?). Not more than 25 Gm. of glucose should be given in this way in a solution of 5 to 20 per cent strength—500 cc. of 5 per cent, 250 cc. of 10 per cent, 125 cc. of 20 per cent (see p. 776 for the intravenous technic).

The intracardiac injection of glucose has been reported in one case by Imerman: "The pulse was fast failing and the patient was moribund. Because of difficulty experienced previously in entering the veins of this patient, it was not deemed wise to attempt to do so now, as any further delay might be fatal. An intracardiac injection was decided on as the very last resort. This was accordingly done by means of the sterile syringe and the lumbar puncture needle (both of which, together with sterile glucose solution happened to be at hand), and 10 cc. of sterile dextrose was injected. At the end of two minutes, the patient had recovered consciousness." As soon as possible, an additional 80 cc. of the 20 per cent solution was introduced after a vein had been surgically exposed; immediate recovery was complete.

Protein.—Protein, since 58 per cent of it is convertible into carbohydrate, may also serve as antidote; therefore, in the absence of a carbohydrate food, the patient should quickly eat a large amount of some food high in protein content. However, Sherril states that "though hypoglycemia may be prevented by sufficiently large quantities of protein, this influence is surprisingly feeble and by no means proportional to the theoretical value."

Epinephrine.—Epinephrine (adrenalin) is also effective in combating the insulin reaction, but in undernourished individuals carbohydrate should be given with it; indeed, there would seem to be little reason to use this drug when carbohydrate is at hand for in all cases its action is quite transient and must be reinforced by the subsequent taking of glucose. The epinephrine dose is ½ cc. in the child, and 1 cc. in the adult, of the 1:1000 solution, given intramuscularly.

Calcium.—Greiff (1931) has reported 2 cases in which the giving of 1¼ ounces (40 Gm.) of calcium gluconate daily, either by mouth or in enema, has been effective in overcoming insulin hypersensitivity so that a daily injection of 40 units could be resumed; Atchley *et al.* employed 20 to 35 Gm. of calcium chloride.

Myrtillin.—Allen has found this drug of great value in some cases (see p. 376).

12. Insulin and Exercise.—Exercise exerts a very profound effect upon the diabetic. Even before the inauguration of the insulin era it was known that the mild diabetic was improved and the severe diabetic made worse by exercise. In attempting to reconcile these facts, the assumption is made that exercise stimulates the production of insulin. Therefore the mild diabetic, who can at all times burn some carbohydrate because some of his islands are functioning, is enabled to burn more if he exercises, but the patient with a severe case, whose insulin production is practically *nil*, only has his condition aggravated by the extra quantity of endogenous food which is also set free by exercise. Nowadays exercise must always be taken into account in injecting insulin, for, other things being equal, the more exercise the less insulin will be needed. Joslin cites a patient who says a game of golf is worth 5 units; days without golf he takes 20 units in the morning and 5 units at night, but on days with golf he is able to omit the night dose. However, exercise must be indulged in only very cautiously by the insulin-taking diabetic, for the combination of exercise and insulin frequently provokes a hypoglycemic reaction—especially is this likely to occur if the next meal after exercise is postponed.

13. **Insulin Edema.**—Very few cases of insulin edema have been reported in the literature, but there seems to be a clinical impression that this complication occurs not infrequently. The exact nature of this phenomenon, which is not due to impaired renal or cardiac capacity and which clears up when insulin is omitted, is not understood. Joslin feels that it may be accounted for by the fact that 3 Gm. of water are retained for each gram of carbohydrate stored, and also that the alkali set free when insulin is given leads to the retention of water. Other observers believe that insulin edema is a colloidal phenomenon; that insulin increases the hydration capacity of the tissue colloids of the body. Leifer's (1928) patient became edematous and gained 26 pounds in ten days, then lost the edema and 12 pounds during the succeeding ten days apparently as a result of marked reduction in the salt of the diet; insulin dosage had remained practically the same. It is said that the edema can sometimes be made to disappear by dropping down with the insulin dosage and gradually building up again. If alkaline therapy is being employed it should be stopped.

14. **Insulin-refractory Cases.**—There is on record a small number of cases that have failed to respond to insulin by an increase in the ability to utilize carbohydrate. Taussig's case was given as much as 1100 units in one day without becoming sugar-free; after several months, however, the response to insulin showed considerable improvement. Lawrence's nineteen-year-old patient required 400 units per day to reduce his blood sugar to normal and to keep him sugar-free; the patient of Mohler and Goldburgh (1931) suddenly lost his responsiveness and died of diabetes after forty days of 437 units daily insulin dosage; upon the other hand, the patient of Karr *et al.* (1933), in whom over 600 units daily did not keep the blood sugar under 200 mg., suddenly lost her resistance following the injection of a foreign protein (the serum of a rabbit that had been sensitized to a mixture of the patients serum and insulin). Falta's patient, apparently resistant to insulin, was later shown by Basch to be amenable to the substance when placed upon a regimen of high fat and low protein and carbohydrate. Joslin is able to report only 1 case of refractoriness from his large practice; the patient required 850 units day after day, and two days before his death in coma was given 1600 units daily. Hendry (1932) has recorded a case in which great reduction in response to insulin was corrected by the use of thyroid substance; the patient had manifested a slight hypothyroidism.

All explanations of insulin refractoriness upon a single basis, such as the absence of an insulin activator, are still entirely speculative.

15. **Synthaline.**—The discovery of the antidiabetic drug, synthaline, is a forceful illustration of the true internationalism that is being achieved in medical science. Underhill and Blatherwick, in the United States, seek to relate parathyroid tetany to hypoglycemia; Noel Paton and Findley, in

England, had been maintaining that tetany was produced by guanidine; Watanabe, a Japanese investigator, studied the effect of guanidine on blood sugar and found that in truth it does produce a hypoglycemia; and finally, Frank, Nothmann and Wagner, utilizing all of these studies and the even more remote investigations of Kossel, in Heidelberg, were able to announce, in 1926, the production of a dekamethylendiguanidine which, while having the insulin-like effect of lowering blood sugar, is yet strikingly bereft of the toxic properties of guanidine itself. This announcement is not made less interesting by reason of the fact that it comes from the same medical clinic of the University of Breslau whence emanated four decades ago the classic observation of von Mering and Minkowski that the complete removal of the pancreas from animals leads to the appearance of a severe diabetes.

Frank, Nothmann and Wagner reported that the blood sugar was lowered by synthaline in normal and diabetic animals, that *orally the new remedy was nearly as effective as when given subcutaneously*, that in a study of 70 patients the action was slower than that of insulin, and that the patients continued to benefit throughout the day which followed two days of treatment. They also found a reduction of ketone substances in the urine and obtained experimental evidence that glycogen was stored. The toxic symptoms, anorexia, abdominal distress, nausea and diarrhea, could be prevented by omitting all synthaline every third day. Furthermore, they found that its use permitted an increase of 40 to 50 Gm. of carbohydrate, not otherwise tolerated without increasing the insulin; that in severe diabetes it could not replace insulin but was an effective supplement, and that pruritus, infection and gangrene were alleviated by its use. Morawitz (1927) soon confirmed the earlier work with a study of 30 synthaline-treated cases and pointed out that the distaste for fat was a prominent symptom of overdosage and that relief was obtained and a greater synthaline dosage permitted by giving 7½ grains (0.5 Gm.) of decholin (sodium dehydrocholate) with each dose of synthaline. Later, benefit was obtained with 5 grains (0.3 Gm.) of free dehydrocholic acid.

Frank *et al.*, who introduced the remedy, would have it used principally as an insulin sparer, but since the two drugs are about equally expensive, most of the studies have involved attempts to change patients entirely over to synthaline for the sake of greater simplicity—oral rather than injection therapy. I believe it to be very doubtful if the drug will hold what place it has gained, for it cannot be used in patients in whom there is the slightest suspicion of liver disease, it apparently not infrequently initiates a serious liver disturbance where none preexisted, and its use is often accompanied by dyspeptic symptoms of variable severity. Upon this latter account alone, Eismayer (1932) was obliged to give up the use of the drug in 13 per cent of his 68 cases. The experimental work of Karr *et al.*, in the dog, has shown kidney toxicity also.

Duncan (1928) has used synthaline in a few cases in the United States; in 4 of 6 cases he was able to reduce insulin dosage, in 2 instances to eliminate it entirely. Preliminary studies at St. Bartholomew's Hospital, London, yielded the observation that the synthaline action is not so consistent as that of insulin; I have seen no recent report of a continuance of these studies. However, Todd (1932) and his associates at the Bristol Royal Infirmary, which is one of the centers requested to study the drug for the Medical Research Council, is quite enthusiastic about it. They have used synthaline continuously since 1927 and are now able to treat 70 per cent of their patients with it as against only 25 per cent in the beginning of their experience. Their system of treatment consists in the use of a tonic mixture of strychnine, sodium acid phosphate and alcohol three times daily, and the use of sweetbreads in the diet twice weekly and cooked liver once weekly;

the necessity for liberal vitamin B administration is also stressed. The adult patient is started with 10 mg. (⅙ grain) of betasynthaline (two pellets) morning and evening after meals; with every two pellets of synthaline one tablet of decholin is given. The synthaline-decholin combination is always used only two days out of three to prevent cumulation. Synthaline is very slow in action, but if the patient is feeling well the synthaline dosage is increased by two pellets (the decholin by one tablet) every five days or so until either intolerance or diminution of the glycosuria and ketosis is observed. When good clinical and urinary results have been present for some weeks, the synthaline dosage is decreased by one pellet daily in the attempt to find a stabilizing dose. Eismayer, previously cited, says that the daily dose should never exceed 30 mg. (½ grain) and that a rest period of fourteen days is necessary every four to six weeks. The Bristol observers find the transfer from insulin to synthaline usually easy in light or moderately severe cases, especially in elderly individuals. In a 30 to 40 unit case they diminish the insulin by half upon beginning with the synthaline, another half of the remainder when the urine becomes sugar-free, increasing the synthaline if necessary, and gradually the insulin is eliminated altogether. They state that there is no risk in back and forth transfers between insulin and synthaline. Coma and incipient gangrene they feel should be treated with insulin.

16. **Myrtillin.**—In 1925, Professor Durig of the University of Vienna became so much impressed with the benefits of blueberry leaf tea, as used in the treatment of diabetes among the Alpine peasantry, that he suggested an investigation of the subject in his laboratory. The result of this investigation, which was reported by Mark and Wagner, and Eppinger, Mark and Wagner, was the demonstration that blueberry leaves contain two antagonistic ingredients, one tending to raise and the other to lower the blood sugar. To the latter substance, when extracted, was applied the name "myrtillin." This myrtillin is a chemically impure, amorphous substance, whose true nature is as yet unknown, though it may eventually come to be classified with the vitamins. After a considerable amount of animal experimentation, Allen, in the United States, found that the gradual beginning of the drug's effects—a week or perhaps longer—and the gradual wearing off of same made clinical studies difficult in the human. He found it best to use diet restriction, and insulin if necessary, to stop glycosuria and hyperglycemia, and then to begin with myrtillin and look for the results in a gradual rise of tolerance or a gradual diminution or disappearance of the need for insulin. Sixty cases were thus standardized for one year (usually two years or more) before myrtillin was tried. In 24 cases the drug failed but in the remaining 36 it was believed to be beneficial because it became possible rather quickly to make an increase of diet or a decrease of insulin, or both. The insulin decrease, ranging from 6 to 28 units, made possible a welcome reduction in injections. In 6 cases it was possible to stop insulin altogether, though they had previously required the injections for one or more years without any recent signs of a diminishing requirement; the insulin dosage in these cases had ranged from 18 to 54 units. In general the results were best in middle-aged and elderly patients with mild cases, poorest in children.

The effective dose was found to be 15 grains (1 Gm.) daily; even very large doses are nontoxic, the slight indigestion or diarrhea being caused by mineral salts present as impurities. The drug is given on an empty stomach at least one hour before food is taken because absorption is prevented by food, especially protein; it is equally effective when given intravenously. Allen found that trial in each individual case was the only way to determine how long to continue the use of myrtillin before accepting failure. In one child with particularly severe diabetes no change was seen in the usual two-month period, but after a year on the drug it became possible to reduce insulin dosage from 50 to about 30 units, though no such improvement had occurred in the preceding five years' treatment with insulin and diet. The benefit, when obtained, is indefinite in duration, but, because the drug is probably stored in the body, no changes follow its omission for a few doses or a few days. Some patients seem to be able to stop the use of myrtillin after a variable period without losing the food tolerance they had gained.

Myrtillin never causes hypoglycemia, and Allen found that its apparent stabilizing effect upon blood sugar is especially valuable in treating patients, particularly children, who have been subject to troublesome hypoglycemic reactions from insulin. The attacks may be in some instances reduced in number and severity or prevented completely, or they may have their onset sufficiently slowed to make available plenty of time for the giving of protective carbohydrates.

17. Treatment of Coma.—(*a*) *Insulin.*—Insulin has completely revolutionized the treatment of coma, as is well shown in the statistics of Frissell and Hajek: during the period 1920–21, 113 patients with diabetes were admitted to St. Luke's Hospital, New York City, 12 per cent of whom died in diabetic coma; but during 1923–24, *i. e.*, after the institution of routine insulin treatment, 163 patients were admitted with a coma mortality of only 0.7 per cent. Diabetic coma in the total mortality of diabetes has dropped from 60 to 11 per cent (1932).

In Joslin's (1932) experience with 179 cases of coma between January, 1923, and September, 1931, he has found a steady and marked increase in the severity of the cases. In the series 1923–25, the average patient was given 154 units of insulin in the first twenty-four hours, 63 in the second and 58 in the third, whereas in the most recent series, 1929–31, the dosage has been 252 units in the first twenty-four hours, 49 in the second and 41 in the third. He now feels that in the adult, if really unconscious, 100 units should usually be given within the first half hour, and that thereafter— depending of course upon the clinical and laboratory data—20 to 50 units every half hour are necessary until 300 units have been given. Blood-sugar determinations should be made every one to three hours and the insulin discontinued before the normal blood-sugar level is reached in order to avoid hypoglycemia. The extremes of insulin dosage with recovery have been 32 and 840 units. To a child who has never taken insulin before, 5 to 10 units every half hour is given, depending upon age and the severity of the attack. To a child who has had the disease long, much larger doses are given; the average for the first twenty-four hours for all the children in the series was 145 units.

It is the practice nearly everywhere to give the insulin subcutaneously except when death seems very near, for the drug's action is more fleeting when given by vein and less powerful unit for unit.

(*b*) *Glucose.*—Joslin does not fear hypoglycemia in insulin-treated coma cases and therefore does not give glucose to forestall it, employing it only if the insulin administration has been continued too long; but most clinicians feel that it should be routinely used. Thus Mitchell writes: "The amount of glucose used will depend on the symptoms, the age and the weight of the patient and the laboratory examinations, but at least 1 Gm. of it must be employed for each unit of insulin." Five to 50 per cent solution may be given intravenously (see p. 776 for technic), or, if the patient is able to swallow, 1 Gm. of glucose or 10 cc. of orange juice per unit of insulin may be given by mouth. Murphy and Moxon (1931) at the Milwaukee County Hospital, where many of the cases are far advanced before admission, give routinely 1000 cc. of 10 per cent glucose intravenously, adding directly to this 1 unit insulin per 2 Gm. glucose. Foster writes: "I have tried to estimate the available glucose in the blood in some cases, but the blood volume is in question. On the basis that blood is 10 per cent of the body weight, the total glucose in the body varies in different cases from 30 to 75 Gm. More is constantly formed, and the secretion through the kidneys is also continuous. This is insufficient glucose, even if entirely utilized, to correct the disorder in fat oxidation. Therefore it becomes advisable to inject glucose solution, which is easily done into a vein. It has also the added advantage that, if done at intervals, very large doses of insulin may be used without fear of 'insulin shock' (hypoglycemia). When the severity of the case requires it, 20 Gm. of sugar may be injected as a 50 per cent solution every two hours until the patient is able to drink orange juice." Himsworth's (1932) studies have substantiated this position.

(c) *Liquids.*—All patients should be made to take large amounts of fluid to counteract the desiccation of the tissues which almost invariably accompanies beginning coma. While conscious, the fluid may be taken as broth, tea, coffee, oatmeal gruel, etc., at the rate of not more than a glassful (200 cc.)—to be taken in small quantities because of the danger of acute dilatation of the stomach. Ice-cold drinks are agreeable to take but are objectionable for the reason that they may start the undesired vomiting. In unconscious patients, or in very acidotic individuals even though not unconscious, more heroic measures must be employed. On this point Foster writes as follows:

"In this state of affairs, therapeutic indications are definite; water must be restored to the tissues by the methods that will give promptest relief. These are by hypodermoclysis, by intraperitoneal infusion, and, possibly, by intravenous injection. The latter method, however, is not free of danger, since in these cases the heart is always a doubtful factor. Two years ago we were in the habit of depending on the absorption of water given by rectum; but because this absorption is too slow and at best uncertain, the method has been abandoned in treating coma. The rapidity with which absorption occurs in these dehydrated patients when physiologic sodium chloride solution is injected into the tissues is sometimes amazing. The tissue seems to 'drink it up,' and it is a matter of no difficulty to give a liter in an hour. There is also rapid absorption from the peritoneal cavity, and in desperate cases this avenue should not be neglected. A liter of fluid may be injected, slowly, under low gravity, with no danger of distention. The peculiar advantage of these methods is that they throw no sudden tax on the heart. It has happened twice that patients have died suddenly while I was giving saline solution into a vein. Similar unfortunate experiences have been recorded by others, and we are familiar with the degeneration these hearts display postmortem. On that account, while I still give saline solution intravenously in many cases of diabetic coma, I do so only after consideration, and then with every care to make the injection very slowly."

Laurence (1930) is advocating the intravenous injection of 7 to 10 pints (3500 to 5000 cc.) of *hypertonic* saline (1.2 per cent he considers would probably be preferable to the 1.8 per cent which he used) because of evidence that blood chlorides are low. He finds also that to follow this with a pint of 7 per cent gum acacia solution is of value in amplifying and filling up the pulse.

(d) *Lavage and Warmth.*—In most hospitals, lavage of the stomach is employed as a routine nowadays as soon as beginning coma is diagnosed; time has shown the procedure to be of great value, for a dilated or partially filled stomach is a great handicap to one who, during the succeeding twenty-four hours, must grapple catch-as-catch-can with death. Furthermore, the patient should be kept warm by all the usual devices employed in treating a case of shock—nearly all of these patients have a subnormal temperature at the beginning of coma, and an individual with subnormal temperature is not well armed for a fight.

(*e*) *Circulatory Stimulation.*—Joslin writes: "In coma the heart is in jeopardy. The work involved in hyperpnea is considerable and the heart has difficulty in withstanding the demands made upon it. It must be protected and not imperiled by the treatment adopted. A diabetic of ten years duration without coronary sclerosis is the exception which proves the rule. Whatever manipulation of the patient is undertaken must be with this in mind [lavage the stomach gently!]. Therefore, we have made it a rule to use caffeine in the form of caffeine sodiobenzoate freely. The usual subcutaneous does is 0.3 to 0.5 Gm. every two hours, but usually less than 2.3 Gm. have been given in any twenty-four hours. In order to safeguard the heart, fluids are given by the rectum and subcutaneously, cautiously by the mouth, and seldom intravenously [see *Liquids* above]." Latterly (1932) he has stated that the theoretical possibility of caffeine inducing a maximum production of lactic acid from glycogen is beginning to disturb him somewhat.

Strauss observed that during the World War many diabetics died from circulatory failure rather than from the coma *per se*. Von Neergaard recommends epinephrine; the dose is 1 cc. of the 1: 1000 solution given intramuscularly. Csépai and Pinter-Kováts (1927) believe that ephedrine should be preferred because its action is longer lasting and it is not counteracted by insulin as is epinephrine. Joslin reports a case given 50 mg. of ephedrine, with a systolic rise from 80 to 104 mm. within thirty minutes; he does not state how long the rise persisted.

(*f*) *The Use of Alkalis.*—The following statement of Mitchell (1925) may be taken to summarize the position of many practitioners regarding the use of alkalis: "The value of soda in acidosis has been questioned and by some authorities it has been considered harmful. Certainly insulin has rendered it less necessary; but many students of diabetes are not yet ready to discard its use in acidotic states, especially when there is hyperpnea or respiratory distress. In the precomatose stage, a teaspoonful of sodium bicarbonate in 4 or 5 ounces of water may be given every half hour for several doses; if coma is present it may be added in 3 per cent strength to the glucose solution. An alkaline or neutral reaction of the urine is an indication for the cessation of soda medication. Methyl red, rather than litmus, should be used as an indicator, the red changing to yellow in an alkaline medium." Foster has this to say: "Now I have serious doubts whether alkalis *alone* ever prevented coma or saved a patient who had developed coma. . . . The point is that if one relies on soda alone, the patient is doomed. Many of us proved this much to our satisfaction long ago. In the opinion of many, the use of alkalis has its definite but narrow and exceptional indications. For the average case it may be dispensed with; the urgent need is in other directions."

Joslin is opposed to the use of sodium bicarbonate for the reason that it may cause alkalosis or convulsions, both of which occurrences are probably rare, and also because it upsets the stomach, causes renal irritation by virtue of the increase in beta-oxybutyric acid eliminated through the kidneys, and its constant use appears to promote the constant excretion of acid substances. This matter of the excretion of acid substances would seem to be supported by the work of Wigglesworth, and Haldane, Wigglesworth and Woodrow, in the Cambridge Biochemical Laboratory; indeed, it is even indicated that large amounts of alkali have a definitely inhibitory influence on fat metabolism, which must certainly be looked upon as an undesirable interference during the course of diabetic coma. Lemann's (1930) study of 47 cases leads him to the conclusion that soda can do no good and may do harm.

However, Bock, Field and Adair have described a patient in whom a low carbon dioxide tension in the blood persisted in spite of large doses of insulin and the disappearance of large quantities of ketones; a number of similar cases have been described, which lends support to the suggestion of these investigators that some acids other than those of the ketone group account for this persistence of acidosis. Blum, Grabar and Thiers (1927) believe that sodium bicarbonate is definitely indicated, basing their conviction on the chemical analysis of the tissues of a patient dying of diabetic coma, in whom it was found that there was a reduction in the sodium-chlorine ratio in all organs, notably in the gray matter of the brain, which reduction in sodium they attribute to the acidosis. Even Joslin admits that he is giving considerable amounts of sodium ion in the physiologic saline solution which he injects very freely subcutaneously. This controversy over the use of alkalis is not yet at an end; Rupprecht has reported (1927) 3 cases of coma in children who failed to respond to insulin therapy, but in whom the administration of sodium bicarbonate solution was followed by improvement in respiration, return of consciousness, and complete disappearance of coma.

(g) *Diet.*—Foster writes as follows regarding diet: "As soon as the patient is sufficiently conscious to be able to drink, he is given first hot broth or black coffee, 2 or 3 ounces (60 or 90 cc.) at a time, every fifteen minutes. Hot liquids seem less likely to cause vomiting. After a couple of hours we use lemonade, sweetened with glycerin, and as much orange juice as the patient craves. During the first twenty-four hours, milk and orange juice are the only foods permitted, a liter of milk and the juice of six to ten oranges, which amounts to about 100 Gm. of carbohydrate and 1000 calories. . . . After the patient has recovered from clinical acidosis, the further treatment proceeds as in any diabetic case: a matter of diet adjustment and probably the use of insulin."

18. **Treatment of Complications.**—(a) *Intercurrent Infections.*—It is well known that infection makes a diabetic worse, but it does not seem to make him permanently worse. Lawrence has pointed out that the obvious harmful effect of an infection is to be explained by the neutralization of the power of the insulin by the stimulation of the thyroid and suprarenal glands. If the infection is local, prompt surgical drainage is indicated (Rosenthal and Behrendt found that if fresh pus is mixed with insulin and injected into rabbits the influence of the insulin is abolished); if general, it must be recognized that the fever will cause an increase in metabolism and thus bring acidosis nearer. Murphy (1931), in a large public hospital, finds pneumonia particularly disastrous—87.5 per cent mortality as against a general pneumonia mortality for the hospital of 54.5 per cent in the same period. To keep the urine sugar-free with insulin during an intercurrent infection is hardly possible unless heroic doses are employed, a course which Joslin does not advise for the reason that recovery from the infection may begin very suddenly, with the result that the patient will have an attack of hypoglycemia to cope with. He does increase the dosage, however. "The treatment of the patient during an acute infection varies from hour to hour or at least every four hours. If insulin has been given twice a day it is safer to halve each dose and administer it four times a day, increasing the size of the dose if necessary until the total insulin is doubled or more. The urine is tested before each dose and if sugar-free twice in succession the insulin can be omitted for that period. The insulin can be raised to 100 units, but generally I am able to get along with less than this quantity." Regarding diet, he writes: "If the case is doing well, either leave the diet alone or make gradual changes and there will be more chances of having the individual for a patient during years to come than if brilliant dietetic orders are written. It is safer to undernourish than to fan the flame of metabolism by overfeeding, and

better to take an intermediate course and give not over 1 Gm. of protein per kilogram body weight. It is true that the patient may lose weight but so may a nondiabetic in fever, and it is wiser to trust to Nature to draw from the body the requisite stores of protein and fat than to insist upon the taking of food that may be harmful. . . . Carbohydrate in the form of oatmeal gruel, orange juice and even purée vegetables, protein as whites of eggs, oysters, fish and chicken, and fat in the form of cream will tide over many emergencies."

(b) *Gastro-intestinal Disturbances.*—The omission of a dose of insulin is dangerous because the food which has been taken in much larger quantity than would have been possible without insulin is suddenly deprived of the metabolic aid which it derives from this agent—and as a result fat and to some extent protein is incompletely oxidized and acidosis, perhaps even the dreaded coma, appears. In the presence of an acute gastro-intestinal upset which makes the taking of food impossible, insulin should not be omitted, nor should it be omitted because a meal has been vomited. Says Joslin: "Yet these upsets may be complicated by acidosis, so that it requires a clear head to detect what is going on. Bed, nursing, liquids, a little carbohydrate in the form of orange juice or a cracker or two and expectant treatment, will enable one usually to weather the squall. Usually I advise dividing each dose of insulin in half and doubling the number of doses. Then if two urinary specimens remain sugar-free the next dose of insulin may be omitted, but not more than two doses of insulin in succession should be omitted even if the urine does remain free from sugar."

Diarrhea is a serious complication in diabetes. Rest in bed must be enforced and measures instituted for preserving the body warmth. Hot drinks are to be given freely and, if the dehydration is very marked, the subcutaneous injection of physiologic saline solution must be begun. The dose of insulin must of course depend upon the amount of glycosuria, but in general it should be lowered, for Andrews and Schlegel have shown that insulin injected into dehydrated animals has a prolonged and intensified effect. On the other hand, coma is also greatly to be feared for the reason that when absorption of food from the intestinal tract is lessened the body protein and fat begin to be drawn upon.

Regarding diet, Joslin writes that, after a temporary fast, "the carbohydrate of the diet should be continued in the simplest form such as gruels, crackers, toast, rice, macaroni or even grape juice or ginger ale. . . . The return to the diabetic diet is rendered easy by the use of cottage cheese, soft cream cheese, lean meats, oatmeal gruel, milk, cream, biscuits, eggs, purée vegetables. The carefully prepared, tender vegetables are frequently better borne than a diet containing considerable quantities of albuminous and fatty food."

Attempt should be made to clear the bowel of the noxious matter by enema or cathartic just as in any other acute diarrhea, but it should be borne in mind that the diabetic bears castor oil or salts much better than the more drastic purgatives. Bismuth subcarbonate in doses of 10 grains (0.65 Gm.) every two to three hours may be indicated, and in severe cases 1 grain (0.065 Gm.) or more of powdered opium may be given in a pill or capsule.

(c) *Arteriosclerosis and Heart Disease.*—In patients having arteriosclerosis (and the incidence is higher in diabetic than in nondiabetic individuals), whether of the generalized type or expressing itself as angina pectoris or as a peripheral sclerosis, one should be extremely cautious in lowering the blood sugar. Says Joslin: "A sudden lowering of the blood-sugar level even to values still above normal might work disastrously to a heart accustomed for years to work on a much higher blood-sugar plane." All the foremost students of the disease agree with this principle. It is to be expected that the increasing use of high carbohydrate-low fat diets will have some influence upon the incidence and course of these complications (see p. 362). In discussing hemorrhagic retinitis, Grafe writes: "Insulin is to be used here with care. Notable changes for the worse can take place. The more outspoken the alterations in the vessels the more conservatively ought insulin to be given. And what it is possible to observe with the opthalmoscope in the retina ought to hold for other vascular areas."

(*d*) *Pruritus and Furunculosis.*—These two dermatoses are frequent complications in diabetes, the former always very annoying, the latter often very serious. The treatment of pruritus is described on page 450 and on page 679, and of furunculosis on page 672.

(*e*) *Surgery in Diabetes.*—Since the advent of insulin, surgical diabetic mortality has been considerably lowered, but it is still so high that Joslin says (1928): "The surgical diabetic is the serious diabetic, the diabetic who dies"—as is shown by the fact that in his hospital in 1923–26, medical diabetic mortality was 1.7 per cent and surgical diabetic mortality 11.5 per cent. Gangrene and carbuncle are the principal dealers of death. The general practitioner must be ever watchful for early signs of impaired circulation in the extremities: Claudication, coldness, pain, numbness, diminished arterial pulsation, rose spots, blebs, scars. And of course he must enjoin upon his patients the necessity for utmost cleanliness of the body, particularly the feet, and the avoidance of trauma and instant serious attention to local infections, even of the slightest. The treatment of the patient before and after operation, the choice of anesthetic, and the treatment of gangrene and carbuncle: these matters are all more fittingly discussed in text-books of surgery.

19. **Diabetes in Children.**—The treatment varies in no radical way from that of the adult. Boyd, writing in Toronto in 1925, stated that she saw no contraindication to the maintaining of the diabetic child's nutrition at the standard normal level for age and sex, a position which has been strengthened by the experience of many pediatricians. Boyd and Nelson, in the United States, have (1928) recorded a group of carefully managed cases in the majority of which growth would seem to be progressing at an entirely satisfactory rate, so far as can be determined by measurements of height and weight. It has been shown to be advisable to feed for the expected weight, *i. e.*, to work up to a diet such as would be required for a normal child of the patient's age at the normal weight. The proportions of protein to carbohydrate and fat differ from those of the adult, as shown in Table 41. Unless the case is exceptionally mild the child will be almost certain to require insulin, the dosage to be determined for each individual case, just as in the adult.

20. **Diabetes in the Aged.**—The status of these cases is succinctly stated by Joslin in the two short paragraphs which I quote below:

"Diabetes burns out in the old and the tendency of the diabetic is to outgrow the symptoms of his disease. In the care of the elderly patient the physician therefore must not be meddlesome. He must realize that the old man's diabetes is inherently mild. 'No really severe diabetes could have continued as long as this. . . . ' (Woodyatt). Many of these cases eventually become sugar-free, if placed upon a constant diet, with a liberal quantity of carbohydrate, but just sufficient calories to maintain body weight. This may not occur in four days or even four weeks, but ultimately the glycosuria disappears. It is often claimed that such patients need no treatment, and are, in fact, better off without it. With this statement I disagree. Often they are very uncomfortable without medical advice and very grateful to receive it. They are furthermore satisfactory cases to treat, because it is easy to help them acquire a high tolerance. Indeed insulin proves to be a great comfort and, though at first its benefits are not realized and its subcutaneous use disliked, in the course of time patients fully appreciate the benefits it confers and what is more, they may discover in the course of a few weeks that they are able to omit it and yet retain their increased diet.

"Elderly patients are often easily depressed, easily lose their appetite, easily acquire indigestion, and the danger of acidosis is by no means slight. The patient should be considered from a broad standpoint, and the diabetes viewed with a proper perspective."

In so-called "mild diabetes" in the aged, retinitis with a poor prognosis for recovery of good vision even under thorough treatment with insulin may occur; insulin, however, probably prevents the condition from arising in the first place.

21. **Diabetes in Pregnancy.**—In preinsulin days, coma ended the life of most diabetics who became pregnant. It was precipitated by surgical intervention with general anesthesia, and the partial starvation and over-exertion of labor brought it on. Half the babies died *in utero,* and this also was a source of coma. But now all is changed. The diabetic woman of today, if properly treated with insulin and diet, has little more to fear from the ordeal of pregnancy, labor and the puerperium, than has the nondiabetic. The physician must be more on the *qui vive* to detect sudden changes in tolerance and to make the proper dietary and insulin adjustments—but otherwise the treatment hardly varies from that of the nonpregnant diabetic. Peckham's (1931) studies indicate that such aggravation as occurs is likely to be during the first two thirds of the pregnancy, or upon death of the fetus *in utero.* Definite improvement may occur as term approaches, and as this improvement often persists for several weeks or months after delivery and is coincident with lactation, nursing may be safely continued as long as possible.

22. **Diabetes and Angina Pectoris.**—Such reviews as the recent one of Root and Graybiel (1931) are bringing increasingly to our attention the extraordinarily high incidence of angina in diabetes. Recognition of this fact is of particularly great importance from the therapeutic standpoint, for the precipitation of a terrific attack of substernal pain following an injection of insulin is a phenomenon by no means unknown to those who treat much diabetes. Parsonnet and Hyman (1931) have given serious attention to the point and write: "Where diabetes is complicated by known cardiovascular factors we have studiously avoided insulin therapy until all dietary measures have failed to produce results commensurate with safety."

HYPERINSULINISM (HYPOGLYCEMIA) AND DYSINSULINISM

The level of sugar in the blood is regulated principally by two opposing hormones: Insulin from the pancreas and adrenalin (epinephrine) from the suprarenal bodies. The former lowers the level in ways which are not entirely understood though it now seems certain that the promotion of glucose deposition in the liver in the form of glycogen does not take place so simply as was formerly postulated; the latter raises the level by converting the glycogen of the liver into glucose and releasing it into the blood stream. Pituitrin, the internal secretion of the pituitary body, regulates this simple antagonism somewhat in that it abolishes both hypoglycemia and hyperglycemia, though it is apparently without effect on a normal sugar level. The thyroid gland seems to exert an influence in the same direction

as adrenalin, since hyperglycemia accompanies hyperthyroidism, and hypoglycemia is often seen in myxedema. Whether the genital and parathyroid
glands also share in these regulatory processes has not yet been definitely
established. The well-known reaction to the injection of an overdose of
insulin in the treatment of diabetes is due to the induction by this exogenous method of a temporary state of hypoglycemia; latterly, we have come
to recognize an entirely similar condition due to endogenous factors. That
is to say, there are individuals, nondiabetic, who develop spontaneously a
state of hypoglycemia with all the attendant symptoms of insulin shock as
described on page 372. Seale Harris, of Birmingham, Alabama, who first presented the entity in 1924, called it "hyperinsulinism," describing at the same
time a state of "dysinsulinism" in which the condition of hypoglycemia was
at times succeeded by a temporary one of hyperglycemia. In recent years
quite a large number of cases has been reported and it is beginning to be
thought that the incidence of hyperinsulinism (hypoglycemia) is possibly
as great as that of diabetes mellitus (hyperglycemia). The epileptoid
character of the convulsions in some of the severe cases has also given rise
to the opinion that perhaps a surprisingly large number of individuals convicted of idiopathic epilepsy may be in reality sufferers from this newly
recognized metabolic dyscrasia; indeed, Harris (1933) has tentatively
offered the hypothesis that bromides exert their beneficent effect in this
pseudo-epilepsy through the depression of insulin secretion. Cameron
(1930) has also pointed out the ease with which night terrors in children are
sometimes relieved by the administration of glucose; bizarre fatigue states
in youngsters might also be hypoglycemic reflections, since comparable
states of aggravating restlessness, obstinacy and silliness have been noted
at times in adults preceding the onset of unconsciousness. Symptoms usually appear when the blood-sugar level (adult middle-aged normal, Folin-
Wu, 80 to 110 mg. per cent) has reached 70 mg. per cent, but not invariably;
sometimes a patient will be in a serious state at 50 mg., while at another
time he will have only mild symptoms or none at all at the same level.
Apparently the rapidity of the fall is the determining factor in some instances.

Most students of this newly recognized condition have leaped to the quite
obvious conclusion that the syndrome results primarily from the internal
secretion of too much insulin as a result of overstimulation of the islets of
Langerhans in the pancreas. However, Winans (1933) has lately urged
that more consideration be given to the possibility of a loss of the insulin-
inhibiting effect of trypsin, the true external secretion of the gland. Excision of an adenoma or carcinoma of the pancreas, and even of a portion
of the apparently normal organ, has in several instances induced complete
relief from symptoms, but Cammidge and Poulton (1933), who believe
that some sort of interference with glycogenic function of the liver is the
primary causative factor in many cases, find it quite to be expected that an
increased activity of the islets of Langerhans would result as a compensatory process. In the terms of their thesis, such increased activity in the
attempt to keep up the load of glycogen in the liver cells would also deplete
the peripheral circulation of sugar; thus, operation upon the pancreas would
be expected to bring relief in a roundabout way. It is also likely that
more attention will soon be turned to the adrenal, thyroid and pituitary
bodies and to the nervous center in the pons, of which Wauchope (1933)
recently reminds us.

THERAPY

Dietetics.—In cases of mild severity the taking of a little food high in
quickly assimilable carbohydrate between meals and late at night is usually

sufficient to control the symptoms; the frequent drinking of sweetened orange juice or lemonade and the munching of candy is successfully resorted to by many individuals who have recognized the necessity of frequent feeding in their own cases. In going over collected case reports one not infrequently encounters the statement that the patient has for a long time been setting his clock to awaken him in the early morning hours for the snack of food which will prevent his lying helpless in bed, perhaps even in coma, at the time when he should arise for the day.

The dietetic treatment of moderately severe cases at present in vogue consists in the use of a diet low in carbohydrate, high in fats, normal or slightly below normal in proteins, and frequent feedings. Harris, the originator of this régime, believes that there is advantage in using the low percentage fruits and vegetables since their slow digestion yields only small quantities of glucose at a time, by which he believes that the minimum stimulation of insulin secretion is accomplished. Fats, particularly in the form of cream and milk, given with and between meals are believed to delay assimilation of carbohydrate by inducing slow emptying of the stomach. The diet in each case must of course supply the patient's nutritional requirements. For adults of average height and weight, Harris (1933) allows about 2250 calories, 90 Gm. of carbohydrate, 60 Gm. of protein and 180 Gm. of fats, this being divided among five to seven daily feedings. (The reader can easily compute such diets by use of the tables on pp. 356 to 365.) Obesity is a not infrequent accompaniment of hyperinsulinism. In such cases, Harris uses 90 Gm. of carbohydrate, 60 Gm. of protein and only 60 Gm. of fats (1140 calories), with five or six feedings daily. Activities are restricted and the fats increased to 90 or 100 Gm., or even more, if the patient becomes weak or is losing more than 2 pounds (900 Gm.) weight per week. Underweight, asthenic patients are allowed 90 Gm. carbohydrate, 200 to 300 Gm. fats and 60 to 75 Gm. protein, with five or six feedings a day. It will be readily seen that to the diabetics we are now adding another class of patients who must be taught food values.

To bring a patient out of an attack when he cannot cooperate to the extent of swallowing sugar or orange juice, the intravenous injection of glucose must be resorted to: 10 Gm. in 50 to 100 cc. of sterile physiologic salt solution is perhaps the average dosage, but Sigwald (1932), in his comprehensive review, considers it dangerous to give much fluid and recommends instead 10 to 20 cc. of a 20 or 30 per cent solution. Absorption of glucose from the rectum is so slow that much bacterial fermentation takes place, with the result that very little glucose actually gets into the blood stream. Indeed, Pressman's (1930) studies showed that following the introduction of glucose into the rectum there occurs a fall in the blood-sugar level without a significant preliminary rise. Obviously, this method of administration should not be employed in treating hyperinsulinism.

Drugs.—Adrenalin, in the usual dose of 0.5 to 1 cc. of the 1: 1000 solution, is used to rouse the patient from a severe attack; sometimes it fails and always, of course, its effect is only of brief duration. Winans (1933) felt that in one of his cases the frequent use of the drug to mobilize the glycogen reserve would not have been wise in the presence of continued hypoglycemia, a position which increasing experience will probably support. Pituitrin, in injections of 0.5 to 1 cc., is sometimes effective in these emergencies, as is also caffeine in the form of caffeine-sodium-benzoate 5 grains (0.3 Gm.) or more. In a few instances, thyroid substance, administered as in myxedema, has been of some value but of course not as an emergency measure.

Surgery.—Judd *et al.* (1933) of the Mayo Clinic have recently stated the opinion that operation upon the pancreas is justified in all cases in

25

which there is a constant tendency for the blood-sugar level to fall below 50 mg. and severe symptoms of hypoglycemia, keep the patient from earning his living. The experience of the several surgeons who have operated in such severe cases since the first successful removal of a pancreatic tumor associated with the symptoms of hyperinsulinism (Howland *et al.*, in 1929) has been to the effect that there is quite likely to be organic disease in the pancreas. If the new growth is localized, its removal may be curative it seems; where this is not so of course very little can be done. The condition of the patient has usually not been improved by the mere removal of a portion of a normal-appearing gland, but several students of the subject feel that as operative boldness increases the amount of structure to be excised will be definitely determined.

DIABETES INSIPIDUS

Diabetes insipidus is a disease characterized by the excretion of quite enormous amounts of urine and a resultant loss of tissue fluids which has to be compensated by the ingestion of equal quantities of water. The urine is practically colorless, does not contain sugar, is of very low specific gravity, and contains none of the elements suggestive of renal involvement. There is a decrease in the flow of saliva, the mucus becomes thick and tenacious, there is constipation, practically no sweating, and the skin becomes very harsh and dry. The patients are made very miserable by the necessity to urinate so often and to be constantly drinking water. This excessive water drinking usually causes the appetite to become abnormal because of the necessity for a great number of calories in order to bring all the water to body temperature; if, as is often the case, only cold water will be taken, there is in addition shivering, "gooseflesh," weakness and tremor. The disease may occur at all ages but is most frequent in young adults; though formerly considered to be relatively rare in recent years a great many cases have been described. The onset is usually gradual though in some cases it has been quite sudden.

Cranial injuries, brain tumors and other diseases of the central nervous system, especially syphilis, abdominal aneurysm, tuberculous peritonitis, and other disturbances have been associated with diabetes insipidus a number of times, but in many cases it is not possible to trace a connection of this sort. The pituitary body is apparently in some way related to the disease, but the exact nature of this relationship and the mechanism at fault is not clearly understood. There is now conclusive evidence that the disease also exists in an hereditary form which is compatible with the normal length of life in those surviving infancy.

The disease was described by Johann Peter Frank, in 1794. Cushing and his co-workers first drew attention to the apparent hypophyseal relationship in 1912.

THERAPY

Hypodermic injections of pituitrin are practically infallible in controlling the symptoms of this disease; that is to say, the polyuria ceases or is very markedly reduced and there is then a corresponding decrease in the craving for water. The dose necessary to accomplish relief is usually 1 cc. of the obstetrical pituitrin, or of pitressin, but the duration of the relief varies from four to forty-eight hours; in 16 of a series of 26 cases reported by Rowntree, it was twenty-four hours at least. Most patients prefer to take the injection at night in order to have their greatest period of freedom during the sleeping hours, for the necessity to be urinating frequently throughout the night is one of the most distressing features of the disease. Since peristalsis is sometimes markedly increased by pituitrin, it is advisable to have the injection taken about two hours before bedtime in order to permit a visit to the stool before retiring. The continued use of the drug over a long period of time gives rise to no serious untoward effects; however, a case reported by Snell and Rowntree (1927) indicates the wisdom of counseling cessation of water ingestion very soon after taking the injection, for with a sudden decrease in water elimination there is some danger of water "intoxication" if fluid continues to be poured into the system.

Blumgart has reported a series of cases in which intranasal application of the pituitrin was fully as satisfactory as subcutaneous injection. From 0.5 to 5 cc. of obstetrical pituitrin was sprayed into the nose every three to four hours, or a cotton plug soaked in 1 cc. was introduced high up into the nasopharynx of one nostril at a time at intervals of four or more hours. Rowntree also states that he has had good results with this method. Vidgoff (1932) has obtained satisfactory results with freshly desiccated powdered posterior pituitary tissue; $\frac{1}{10}$ grain (0.006 Gm.) was applied to the nasal mucosa by means of the fingertip. Extract incorporated in jelly was found to be less effective and more expensive.

Scherf (1932) has reported 5 cases treated with large doses (30 grains, 2 Gm., daily for five days) of amidopyrine (pyramidon), in 4 of which marked diminution in symptoms was induced. The effect was of only short duration but could be obtained again after a short interruption of the treatment; the effectiveness of pituitrin was not altered by changing for awhile to amidopyrine. In a single case, Bauer and Aschner (1924) obtained, quite to their surprise, astonishingly good results with novasurol (dosage, etc., p. 539).

Treatment of associated diseases, such as syphilis, is of course indicated and will nearly always result in an improvement in the general health; such measures alone rarely bring about any reduction in the polyuria, however. Surgical removal of associated tumors has sometimes corrected the condition. Rowntree says: "Spinal puncture is a desirable procedure in all cases, unless contraindicated by the presence of an intracranial neoplasm," though it is not apparent that it was worth much in his series of cases; cures have followed upon this procedure, but it is well to bear in mind that spontaneous cure is not unknown in this unique disease.

In 1932, Zondek and his associates in Germany demonstrated the presence of what seems to be a new hormone—intermedin—derived from the pars intermedia of the pituitary body. The preliminary studies of Sulzberger (1933) in the United States indicate that this may be the specific hormone regulating water metabolism.

GOUT

A brief description of gout should suffice to differentiate it from all other diseases. An individual, who has apparently been in quite robust health, is suddenly awakened in the night by a severe pain in one of his great toes, a pain that rapidly increases until it reaches almost unbearable proportions; then at about daybreak—at "cock crow," says Sydenham (1683)—great relief is more or less suddenly experienced and the patient usually falls into a heavy sleep. On awaking later in the morning he finds that the affected metatarsophalangeal joint is somewhat swollen, is red and has a glistening appearance, and that the veins around it are peculiarly distended. Throughout the day the swelling increases and the joint becomes very tender but the pain is only slight or may be entirely absent. Then with the night comes a recurrence of the torture. An attack of this sort usually lasts only a few days but is occasionally protracted for a period of several weeks; it is not infrequent for it to shift from one great toe to the other or to some other joint, or for both toes to be affected at the same time. A slight rise in temperature is usually noted. Upon subsidence of the attack, the affected joint is completely restored both in appearance and function. The patient will then be symptomless for a period of months or years—the average time is about one year—and then the second attack is experienced. Thereafter, attacks occur with increasing frequency until a state of chronic gout is reached. This is characterized by marked swelling and deformity of the joints due to the gradual deposition of sodium monourate in the cartilages and ligaments. Strange to relate, it is usually not the toes that are thus involved but the joints of the hands and elbows most frequently; the olecranon and prepatellar bursae may also be distended with nodular masses. In addition, tophi containing urate deposits appear in the skin, most characteristically in the fleshy lobe of one or both ears.

Gout is placed among the diseases of metabolism because it is apparently associated with a faulty uric acid economy, but the exact nature of this association is not understood. Uric acid is a normal constituent of the blood and the urine, but in gout the amount in the blood is abnormally high and in the urine abnormally low; however, this alone is not sufficient to account for the development of the clinical picture, for the same conditions obtain in other diseases, namely, chronic nephritis and leukemia, without gouty symptoms appearing. Furthermore, the substance is not itself highly toxic since it may be quite freely injected intravenously. In favor of the belief in the direct relationship of uric acid to the disease is the fact that a purine-free diet is markedly beneficial in treatment. Most clinicians hold that some other, as yet undiscovered, agent is at work in the causation of the disease. That heredity, overeating and overindulgence in alcohol, especially when taken in the form of red wines and beer, and lack of exercise are factors of great importance has long been recognized. Many cases seem to be in some way associated with lead poisoning. Men are the victims of the disease much more often than women; the proportions are about 40 to 1. The first attack is usually experienced between the thirtieth and fortieth year, which does not mean, however, that gout in children is unknown.

The distribution of the disease, both as to time and place, is very interesting. Gouty deposits have been found in the predynastic mummies of ancient Egypt, and in classical times it was very common in Greece and Rome, but at the present time the Mediterranean lands know it hardly at all. In the tropics of both hemispheres, as well as in China and Japan, it is extremely rare. England has suffered from it for centuries, but it now seems to be quite rapidly decreasing there; on the Continent, too, it is said to have markedly decreased as a consequence of the food privations during and after the World War. But why has it always been extremely rare in the United States, where more people are continuously overfed than anywhere else on the globe? In the answer to this question may lie concealed the key which will unlock the fascinating mystery of this very old disease.

THERAPY

At the height of the acute attack it is usually advisable to give a full dose of morphine in order to bring quick relief from the severe pain. At the same time the first dose of either colchicum or cinchophen should be administered. If colchicum is to be used it may be given either as the tincture or the wine in a dose of 8 minims (0.5 cc.) at three- or four-hour intervals, or in the form of colchicin, the dose of which is $\frac{1}{60}$ grain (0.001 Gm.) in pill or tablet every two hours for four to six doses. Effective doses of any of the preparations of colchicum cause some gastric irritation and usually diarrhea on the second day. Pratt states that he has found the American tinctures and wines quite uncertain in action and he therefore prefers the colchicin. Most physicians have given up all forms of colchicum in favor of the cinchopens from the very beginning of an attack, since in any case the colchicum cannot be used for long because of the gastro-intestinal irritation it causes. Cinchophen, of which any Council-accepted brand is just as good as that marketed under the trade name of Atophan, and neocinchophen, of which any Council-accepted brand is just as good as that marketed under the trade name of Tolysin, are both used. Cinchophen often causes a burning sensation in the throat and stomach which is usually much less marked if neocinchophen is used. A liberal quantity of water should always be given with either of these drugs to prevent the precipitation of uric acid; sodium bicarbonate in large doses is an additional safeguard. Cinchophen may be suspended in water; neocinchophen must be given in tablet form. The usual dose is $7\frac{1}{2}$ grains (0.5 Gm.) every two hours for six or seven doses. The cinchophens increase the uric acid output when first given, but in most cases a decrease takes place after a few days, perhaps to a level lower than the previous one. Pain is greatly relieved by these two drugs. For a discussion of cinchophen toxicity, see page 151.

Local applications and bandages give practically no relief though most patients like to keep the foot swathed in cotton during the attack. The diet should be limited to milk toast, the cereals, potatoes and any of the fruits, while coffee, tea, alcohol and all meats should be strictly interdicted. The patient should be urged to drink a great deal of water.

Dietetics.—Regarding the dietary management of chronic gout, Pratt writes as follows:

"The value of frugal and temperate living in preventing attacks of gout has been recognized since the earliest times. It has been long known that physical labor and the absence of animal food was the best form of insurance against gout. Purines cannot be completely excluded from the diet for a long period, because even the common vegetables are not purine-free. Spinach, green beans and peas contain more than other vegetables, but their use need not be limited. The animal foods that are the most injurious are those that contain the greatest amount of purine substances. These are thymus (sweetbreads), liver, and kidneys. It has been observed repeatedly that an attack of gout has followed the eating of sweetbreads. Roasted or broiled meat increases the uric acid output more than boiled meat, for the purines are extracted by boiling water. Nearly all soups contain meat stock, even creamed soups, and hence are rich in purines. In some hotels no soups are made, except possibly tomato, without meat stock.

"There is no indication that the proteins in the diet should be reduced. Milk, eggs, and cheese may be freely given, and the amount of vegetable protein need not be restricted. The deficiency in calories caused by the withdrawal of meat should be made up by fat and carbohydrates. All kinds of fresh fruits may be taken. Sweets are allowable. The use of alcohol should be forbidden because nuclein metabolism is disturbed by its use. Coffee and tea contain methyl-purines. As it has been shown that coffee may produce an increase in the uric acid output, it is advisable to allow only coffee that has been freed from caffeine.

"After the patient has been on a purine-free diet for three months or a year following an attack of gout, he may be allowed meat or fish once or twice a week at the midday meal. Any kind of meat or fish may be chosen.

The portion, if broiled or roasted, should not weigh over 100 Gm.; if boiled 150 Gm. may be taken. Thymus, liver, kidneys, herrings and sardines should be forbidden. Later the number of purine days per week may be increased. I have sometimes given 3 or 4 Gm. of atophan [cinchophen] on the days purine food is taken. The importance of drinking a large amount of fluid should be emphasized."

The following purine-poor diet is quoted from the same author. It will be noted that in the number of articles permitted such a diet is not very restricted, but the quantities must always be kept small. Indeed, abstemiousness at table cannot be too strongly urged upon the gouty individual.

"Breakfast: Fresh fruit. Caffeine-free coffee with cream, or cocoa. Cereals with cream. One or two eggs. Bacon. Toast or rolls.

"Dinner: Vegetable or cream soups, prepared without meat stock. Meat substitutes made with cheese, such as cheese soufflé and Welsh rarebit (Edam, Swiss and Roquefort cheeses contain less purine than American or cream cheese). Macaroni, rice, potatoes, stewed corn, tomatoes, cauliflower, asparagus, carrots, parsnips, turnips, squash, onions, radishes, celery. Vegetable salads of all kinds; vinegar or lemon juice may be used. White bread or corn bread. Fresh or preserved fruits. Puddings made of rice, sago, tapioca, with cream or fruit sauces. Ice cream. Nuts. Milk.

"Supper: Eggs. Rice or hominy. Buckwheat cakes with maple syrup. Salads. Crackers and cheese. Fresh or preserved fruits. Custards. White bread or toast. Milk or weak tea."

Use of Drugs in Chronic Gout.—It is generally agreed that colchicum is of no value save in the treatment of an acute attack. The cinchophens, however, are employed by many practitioners as a routine in gouty individuals. Apparently these drugs can be given over a long period of time without causing any untoward symptoms (see, however, p. 151), for Graham (1927) has reported the administration of 22 grains (1.5 Gm.) of cinchophen three times a day for three consecutive days in each week for a continuous period of six and a half years, during which time the patient steadily improved in health over the previous five-year period. It is in this way, i. e., full doses during two or three days a week, that most physicians employ the cinchophens, usually continuing the medication, however, for only a few months at a time. Solis-Cohen has stated his belief that the use of smaller doses, i. e., 5 grains (0.32 Gm.) three times a day, for one week in the month over a period of several months is preferable. I think the following words of this eminent physician are worthy of considerable attention: "It is not necessary to reduce the uric acid content of the blood to a theoretically normal standard. Gouty people have a higher normal uric acid index than others. It is only when this is exceeded that symptoms result. This is a natural consequence of evolutionary adaptation affecting every cell in the body. While 7 mg. or even 4 mg. per hundred cubic centimeters of blood is excessive for a normal man, it may not be equally excessive for one of gouty heredity. When the quantity of uric acid has been reduced to the equilibrium-point for the individual one should be satisfied; one does not hope to make the gouty cells of an entire body normal."

It is not proved, indeed not even strongly indicated by results attained, that the routine use of iodides or alkalis is helpful in the treatment of chronic gout. The value of the lithium salts is long ago exploded. Acid, however, is indicated if the patient is on a purine-poor diet since such a diet contains an excessive amount of alkali; the U.S.P. dilute hydrochloric acid may be used in a dose of 15 to 30 minims (1 to 2 cc.) after each meal.

Smith has shown that there is no increase in uric acid excretion following the commonly recommended dose of live baker's yeast; two, three and five times this dose likewise gave negative results. In his studies, live yeast cells appeared in the feces in large numbers, showing that they were not killed to any great extent in the gastro-intestinal tract.

Other Measures.—The value of exercise for the gouty individual has long been recognized. Golf is unfortunately the only form of outdoor exercise that many city men can enjoy, but the fact should not be overlooked that for individuals not too corpulent and whose arteries are not yet markedly sclerosed it is distinctly less valuable than the more vigorous forms of exercise. It is sadly true that the streets of our industrial cities are becoming less and less attractive to the eye and stimulating to the spirit, still a brisk walk is a brisk walk—and as such is worth far more to an individual in need of exercise than is a round of golf as it is played on a crowded city course.

Spa treatment is also endeared to us of old, its value lying not in the ingestion of the mineral constituents of the waters but in the taking of so much water itself, plus the other elements of a complete environmental change which render the resorts so valuable in the treatment of many chronic disorders.

OBESITY

Many hypotheses have been offered to explain the state of overfatness that we call obesity, but I do not think that any of them have been satisfactorily substantiated as yet. Palmer well writes, in discussing the subject in the Nelson Loose Leaf Medicine: "Why one race, family, or individual in other respects normal, should become fat and another be lean, is quite unknown." To Newburgh, however, who has given much thought and study to this matter, the answer is simply that all obesity is caused by overeating, and indeed that obese individuals *do* overeat though they may deny the impeachment, must be granted. Strang and Evans (1930) allowed a group of new patients, who considered themselves small eaters, to take for three or four days exactly what they ordinarily ate at home; 8 of the 13 individuals averaged an intake of 2570 calories, though they were obviously more abstemious than when at home, since they lost an average of 2 pounds each. However, it is argued very forcefully by many observers that obese individuals are not obese because they eat too much, but rather that they eat too much because their metabolism is in some way faulty, so that large quantities of the carbohydrates, etc., are stored as fat in the tissues instead of being utilized. A similar faulty storage of water and salts probably also takes place. Furthermore, the factor of heredity is strongly evident; indeed, it would seem that even the tendency to develop peculiar types of obesity (*i. e.*, fatness of certain portions of the body) is directly transmitted. I recall a case seen recently in Bauer's clinic in Vienna: a woman who had been elsewhere diagnosed as having pituitary disease on the basis of the x-ray finding of some sort of growth in the intrasellar space plus the typical "girdle" distribution of fat, and in which wider investigation showed this type of distribution to have been certainly inherited, since several other members of the family were similarly afflicted. Overweight is a matter deserving serious attention for the following reasons: It predisposes to a number of diseases, particularly diabetes mellitus, gout, cholelithiasis, hypertension and arteriosclerosis; it greatly lowers the resistance against infectious diseases; it greatly increases surgical risk; and its causes considerable inconvenience and even suffering to its victims.

It is a strange fact that in all the prehistortic sculptures, and well up into the definitely historical Sumarian and Egyptian periods, the female figure is always shown as grossly obese and the male as slim and athletic. I wonder if the usual explanation of this, *i. e.*, that it indicates the sedentary life of the woman of those times, is entirely correct; could it not also be that for reasons almost as inscrutable as those obtaining today the canons of art of the time rigidly proscribed all other depiction?

THERAPY

So long as the cause of obesity—metabolic disturbance or simple over-eating—elude us, I do not see how a rational therapy can be evolved which, however, is not in the least preventing dogmatic asseveration in the camps of controversy. What follows in these pages is an attempt to set down the principles and operation of the treatment at present in vogue; it is hoped that the reader has his tongue in his cheek.

Principles.—In obesity, in addition to stored water, the bulk of the excess weight consists in stored fat, which can only be gotten out of the tissues by causing it to burn. That is to say, we must deny food to the patient so that he will live off the surplus in storage. Starvation would be the ideal but for the fact that under such conditions there occurs depression of metabolic activities sufficient to defeat our purpose. The treatment must therefore consist in supplying what one might call a small air-draft of food in order to keep the fat-fire in a good glow of burning.

The Dietary Requirements.—In the dietary approach to all diseases it is considered essential that the nitrogen intake and output will be, and must be, balanced by supplying protein food at the rate of 1 Gm. per kilo body weight for men, 0.75 Gm. for women. In the careful studies of Strang, Evans and McClugage (1929–32), it has been shown that in obese individuals it is practicable to make this calculation upon the basis of the ideal and not the actual weight for an individual of given height and age (the weight and food value tables in the article on diabetes are to be used here); provided a certain amount of carbohydrate is given to prevent diversion of protein for antiketogenic purposes. They have found that the amount of carbohydrate necessary for this protein-sparing action is from ⅓ to ½ Gm. for each gram of protein. Of course no fat is supplied except that which is inseparable from the protein ration. The daily supply of inorganic salts and vitamins must also be adequate.

Strang *et al.*, whose diets are the most severe of any of the principal workers in this field, have been supplying an average of 59 Gm. protein, 7 Gm. unavoidable fat, and 10 Gm. of carbohydrate—though as a result of their most recent studies the carbohydrate has been raised to 40 Gm. in order to increase the palatability of the diet as well as its protein-sparing property. Upon such diets the nitrogen balance fluctuates considerably, and as yet unaccountably, in the beginning, but it finally settles into the normal range. Such a dietary plan supplies approximately only 450 calories daily.

Sansum (1928) considers 60 Gm. protein, 20 Gm. fat, and 100 Gm. carbohydrate (approximately 800 calories) low enough for the start, increasing, as exercise becomes possible, to 60, 27, and 130 Gm., respectively (1100 calories), and finally to 60, 30, and 172 Gm., respectively (1200 calories). Bauman (1928), at the ambulatory obesity clinic of the Presbyterian Hospital in New York City, uses a basic arrangement of 70 Gm. protein, 60 Gm. fat, and 100 Gm. carbohydrate, supplying 1220 calories; Palmer, 70 Gm. protein, 75 Gm. fat, and 85 Gm. carbohydrate, equivalent to 1300 calories.

Actual Diets.—Strang *et al.* meet their protein, fat and carbohydrate relationship, their 450 calorie requirement, and the necessity of supplying salts and vitamins, by allowing about 100 Gm. of lean steak at each of the two largest meals of the day, alternating with fresh fish at intervals, and making up the rest of the protein in egg white and gelatin in order to hold down the fat; the carbohydrate portion is supplied in 5 per cent vegetables. On alternate days, however, the patient receives either 100 cc. whole milk or 100 cc. orange juice and 50 cc. actively growing yeast. One glass of Kalak water three times a day supplies the necessary inorganic salts.

This is of course most stringent dieting and is doubtfully possible except under strictest supervision. Bauman, in his ambulatory clinic which compares more closely with the conditions of general practice, apportions his allowances (1220 calories) as follows:

Breakfast.—One-half grapefruit or one moderate-size orange, or apple or ½ cup of strawberries; two eggs; coffee or tea with ¼ cup of milk; saccharin, and one thin slice of bread.

Lunch.—1. Five per cent vegetables, 2 cups (for a partial list of percentage vegetables, see p. 357); one egg, one medium-size orange or one apple; tea with 2 tablespoonfuls of milk.

2. Five per cent vegetables, 1 cup; 10 per cent vegetables, ½ cup; two eggs or 3⅓ ounces (100 Gm.) of broiler with 2 teaspoonfuls of butter; one medium-size apple or orange or 1 cup of strawberries; tea.

3. Five per cent vegetables, 1 cup; 10 per cent vegetables, ½ cup; bread, one thin slice; meat, 1⅔ ounces or cheese, 1 ounce; ½ cup of milk and custard sweetened with saccharin.

Dinner.—1. Meat or fish, 4⅔ ounces (140 Gm.); 5 per cent vegetables, 1 cup; 10 per cent vegetables, 1 cup; one medium-size orange or 1 cup of strawberries; tea.

2. Meat, 3 ounces (90 Gm.); 5 per cent vegetables, 1 cup; 10 per cent vegetables, ½ cup (some of the vegetables may be used as salad, vinegar and liquid petrolatum being used as dressing); bread, one thin slice; one medium-size apple or orange; tea.

3. Meat, 4 ounces (120 Gm.); 5 per cent vegetables, 1 cup; 10 per cent vegetables, ½ cup; one small baked potato; one-half grapefruit or ½ cup of strawberries; tea.

Acidosis.—The patients of Strang and his associates have never shown more than transient ketonuria and no other evidences of acidosis, but Sansum considers the use of 10 grains (0.6 Gm.) of sodium bicarbonate three times daily advisable.

Water.—The most usual custom is perhaps to restrict somewhat the water allowance below that which is normal, but it is doubtful if this serves any very useful purpose provided the patient is not allowed to gorge herself on water during the periods of greatest weight loss (see below). There are physicians, however, who stoutly maintain that water restriction is of great value in that as water is withdrawn from the tissues the other deposited substances are carried with it. The use of diuretics is even sometimes recommended.

Weight Loss.—Strang *et al.* have determined the basal level in their excessively obese patients to be at most 2400 calories, the estimated total output, 2900 calories. The diet supplying only between 400 and 500 calories, the caloric deficit would therefore be about 2500 calories in the highest cases —supplied by the burning of something less than 300 Gm. of fat. Theoretically, therefore, one week of the most rigid dieting can result, apart from water shifts, in the loss of only about 4½ pounds (about 2 Kg.) of actual tissue. They feel that the much larger weight losses often seen at the beginning of a dietary period are chiefly due to water shifts for which there must inevitably be compensation at a later time, since the early tissue losses are accompanied by considerable dumping of water out of storage. This water is later taken up and at another time let go again; such shifts occur throughout the dietary period, but the steady loss of fat tissue is going on all the while even though, as is so often discouragingly observed, the patient actually gains weight (weight in water, according to this reasoning) though eating the lowest possible quantity of food.

Strang's 133 patients lost an average of 16 pounds in the first month, a total of 30 pounds during the average dieting period of eight and seven-tenths weeks, representing an average weekly loss of $3\frac{1}{2}$ pounds. Sansum's patients lose from 10 to 20 pounds a month, depending upon the amount of exercise they take (see below). Palmer would be more conservative than either of these two observers; he says that in extreme cases a decrease of from 5 to 10 pounds may be safely made in the first month, 5 pounds a month for the next two or three months, and then a gradual decrease to the level of the milder cases, *i. e.*, 2 to 3 pounds a month. Of Bauman's 183 patients, who averaged 54 pounds overweight in the beginning, after an average of about ten months' treatment, 67 had lost 10 pounds or less, 33 from 10 to 15 pounds, 16 from 15 to 20 pounds, 15 from 20 to 25 pounds, and 27 more than 25 pounds.

Subjective Changes.—Strang's experience accords with that of all who have succeeded in gaining the cooperation of obese individuals sufficiently to actually obtain results: "One is astonished at the unanimity with which patients reported a return of vigor, a feeling of well-being and resistance to fatigue which had been lost for months or years. A great variety of obscure symptoms and minor ailments disappeared." Headache and difficulty in breathing usually disappear very rapidly, and as a whole the symptomatic improvement exceeds what can be accounted for by the relief from the mechanical burden of only a relatively few pounds. Menstrual disturbances often strikingly improve.

Exercise.—Sansum gets his patients to walking early but feels that it should begin gradually with a block or so at a time in order to acquire some training; later his patients walk from 5 to 15 miles a day—this latter, or its equivalent in other forms, he considers ample. Tennis, golf and horse-back riding are favored for those who can afford them. Bauman advises the daily walking of 2 miles in forty-five minutes or less, or calisthenics lasting ten minutes morning and night; he finds that ordinary housework does not replace systematic exercise. Strang and his associates are sceptical of the value of exercise, maintaining that routine, spiritless calisthenics are beneficial as mental and circulatory stimulants and possibly have an influence on muscle tone but do not make up for the increased food intake as a result of the stimulation of appetite. They feel that the individuals who most need rapid weight reduction because of impending exhaustion of the circulatory apparatus after years of chronic strain upon it are the very ones in whom the genuine work necessary to accomplish a real loss of 300 to 400 calories cannot be permitted.

Thyroid Therapy.—Sansum does not use thyroid substance unless there is actual depression of the basal metabolic rate, in which cases he employs enteric-coated tablets of desiccated thyroid substance, having found these tablets much more satisfactory than the uncoated form. Bauman writes that thyroid therapy was employed in 34 of his 183 patients, the basis of selection not being stated. He says: "Thyroxin, 0.0008 Gm. daily, was administered to selected patients. No untoward effects were noticeable. The patient was warned to discontinue the hormone in the event of palpitation, cardiac pain, dyspnea or nervousness." He also points out that Von Noorden, in Austria, has used thyroid in the treatment of obesity for the past thirty years. The latter, however, has recently (1931) again indicated his belief that only in cases of thyroid deficiency should it be used. The contention that thyroid substance should be given not in the sense of supplying a deficient internal secretion but rather to speed up metabolism so that the stored materials can be utilized better when food is withheld, has been attacked by Strang as being irrational if not actually dangerous. Though the basal metabolic rates of his obese patients fell within normal limits for their actual size and weight, they were much above normal if computed upon the basis of ideal weight. For instance, a woman, aged forty-one, whose ideal weight was 133 pounds, actually weighed 216 pounds. Her basic metabolic rate was minus 4 in relation to her actual weight but plus 23 in relation to her ideal weight. "In other words, this patient as far as her real self, her active useful tissues, was concerned was operating at a level 27 per cent higher than was normal for her." Such levels of metabolism would normally be associated with thyrotoxic symptoms, and if they really supply an index of the increased work being done by the obese in merely living, the further whipping up of the rate with thyroid substance should certainly be approached with full caution.

Contraindications to Drastic Dieting.—These are felt to be the presence of a tuberculous lesion, myocardial disease, and advanced cardiovascular-renal disease. Some observers feel that nevertheless some effort should be made in all cases of gross obesity to aid the patient to cope with his major disease by at least gradually reducing his weight. Adolescents and the elderly, who are thought to bear reduction measures poorly, have been treated by the drastic diets of Strang and his associates without the occurrence of any untoward incidents.

Dinitrophenol.—The recent report of Cutting *et al.* (1933) that with this substance they were able to so greatly accelerate metabolism in their small series of cases that the patients lost weight without the necessity of dietary restrictions is of very great interest. Daily doses of $\frac{1}{20}$ grain per 2.2 pounds body weight (3 mg. per kilogram) have been given orally for one to ten weeks, but of course much careful study of the subject, particularly with regard to the toxic potentialities of this drug, must be made before the matter can be considered to have reached a practical phase.

Anderson *et al.* (1933) encountered one severe toxic reaction in their 14 cases; Perkins (1919), during the World War, warned of the special susceptibility to this poison (employed in munitions manufacture) of chronic alcoholics, chronic rheumatics, and persons with tuberculosis, renal or hepatic disease.

MALNUTRITION

There are two main types of undernourished individuals: Those who are just "naturally" thin, and those who have lost much weight during a period of excessive physical or mental strain and have subsequently failed to regain it. In both types the difficulty lies in the possession of a subnormal appetite, the person who has always been thin eating just enough to balance his energy requirements, and the other having lost his desire for food during the time of stress. It has often been shown that there is apparently nothing at all to prevent patients of both types from putting on weight if one can only induce them to eat enough. The dietary scheme which has served Ralli and Brown (1933) well is here given in the form of a table (Table 44). Their patients have gained an average of 17 pounds in six weeks on this diet. Once the initial repugnance for these excessive amounts of food is mastered, patients usually eat with relish and after awhile retain an improved appetite without special effort. Ralli and Brown's patients averaged a daily calorie-consumption of 4000 to 4040; the diet provides

TABLE 44.—DIET FOR THE UNDERNOURISHED PATIENT (RALLI AND BROWN)

	Amount.	C.	P.	F.	Cals.
Breakfast					
Cereal	1 oz.	23	3	0	104
Cream	3⅓ oz.	2	2	20	196
1 glass milk	8 oz.	12	8	9	161
Egg	One	0	6	6	78
Bacon (crisp) strips (use fat for egg)	1 oz.	0	3	19	183
Banana or prunes	3⅓ oz.	20	1	0	84
Orange juice	6⅔ oz.	20	1	0	84
Butter	1 oz.	0	0	25	225
Bread	3 slices	54	9	0	252
Jam or jelly (2 heaping tablespoonfuls)	1 oz.	30	0	0	120
Sugar	8 t.	40	0	0	160
Coffee	1 cup	0	0	0	
		201	33	79	1647
At 10 A. M.					
Cocoa malt with 1 egg and cream or 8 oz. milk with 1 egg and cream	1½ glasses	40	19	36	560
Lunch					
Meat-fish-chicken	3⅓ oz.	0	20	20	260
Potatoes-rice-spaghetti	3⅓ oz.	20	2	0	88
Salad {Mayonnaise	1 T.	0	0	15	135
{15 per cent fruit—2 lettuce leaves	3⅓ oz.	15	1	0	64
Bread (1 oz. slices) or 1 large roll	2 slices	36	6	0	168
Vegetables, 5 per cent	3⅓ oz.	3	1	0	16
Butter	1 oz.	0	0	25	225
Dessert {Pie {Puddings or custard {Ice cream	3⅓ oz.	20	4	4	132
		134	53	100	1648
At 4 P. M.					
Cocoa malt with 1 egg and cream (½ glass) or 8 oz. milk with 1 egg and cream	1½ glasses	40	19	36	560
Dinner					
Meat (2 oz. cheese or 3 eggs)	3⅓ oz.	0	20	20	260
Potato-rice or a creamed vegetable	3⅓ oz.	20	2	0	88
Butter	½ oz.	0	0	12.5	112
Bread (2 slices, 1 oz each)	2 slices	36	6	0	168
Vegetables, 10 per cent	3⅓ oz.	6	1	0	28
Dessert (same as noon)	3⅓ oz.	20	4	4	132
		122	57	70.5	1348
Night Meal 10 P. M.					
Vegetables for sand	3⅓ oz.	3	1	0	16
Bread	2 slices	36	6	0	168
Mayonnaise or butter	½ oz.	0	0	8	72
Milk	1 glass	12	8	9	161
		51	15	17	417
or					
Hershey bar (10-cent bar)	One	35.8	5.6	24.5	398
Substitutions					
Noon					
Bread	(4 oz.)	72	12	0	336
Mayonnaise or butter	1 oz.	0	0	30	270
Meat (ham, salmon or chicken)	3⅓ oz.	0	20	20	260
or	or				
Cheese	2 oz.				
Cocoa malt or egg malted milk	1½ glasses	40	19	36	560
Bananas or 20 per cent fruit	Two	40	2	0	168
		152	53	86	1594
Supper					
French toast					
Bread	3 slices	54	9	0	252
Eggs	2	0	12	12	156
Butter	1 oz.	0	0	25	225
Milk	½ c.	5	3	4	68
Sugar	2 T.	30	0	0	120
Jam or jelly	2 T.	30	0	0	120
Cocoa malt or egg malt milk	1½ glasses	40	19	36	560
		159	43	77	1501

Total calories for all meals 5060.

a total of 5060. But not all patients can be induced, or can induce themselves with the best of will, to fully cooperate in this stuffing campaign.

Insulin.—In 1923, Pitfield injected 1 unit of insulin a day in two infants with malnutrition and obtained a considerable gain in weight, Falta, two years later, applying the method with equal success in adults. Subsequently there have been many reports of the beneficial effects of insulin administration in adult malnutrition. The recent study of Blotner (1933) now seems to have placed the treatment on a sound basis. His material comprised a series of 19 physically normal persons who were thin for their age, sex and height. All but one had been chronically underweight for years and had tried unsuccessfully such measures as forced eating, tonics or prolonged vacations and rest cures. In the one case there had been no apparent reason for an acute loss of approximately 45 pounds (20 Kg.) in about five months' time. Most of them were nervous and apprehensive individuals with poor appetites, but there were some who were considered to be hearty eaters; all had been pretty much bandied about among the doctors. Blotner taught them how to measure and inject insulin and how to care for the syringe, and encouraged them to eat a liberal unmeasured diet during the period of observation. The majority were given 10 units of insulin three times daily, twenty to thirty minutes before meals; 4 received 10 units twice daily, and in 3 the dosage was increased to 15 or 20 units three times a day. The red blood cell count, blood sugar level, blood urea and nonprotein nitrogen concentrations, the basal metabolic rate and the phenolsulphonphthalein excretion were studied in 7 cases. The excretion of nitrogen in the urine, the concentration of protein in the plasma, and the total blood, plasma and corpuscular volumes were followed in 6 cases. The fluid intake and output were measured in 7 cases for a period of ten consecutive days during the use of insulin and for a similar period after its omission.

The effect of this treatment upon the weight of these patients is clearly shown in Table 45.

In some of these individuals the weight gain was rapid and fairly continuous and in a few instances continued after the insulin had been omitted; in others the gain became less marked as time went on, and finally the weight remained stationary whether or not insulin was taken. Few lost much of the weight gained, which is not entirely in accord with the observation of Nichol (1932), who found, upon following up 42 of his patients who had gained weight, that 23 maintained their weight for three months or less, while only 19 kept their gained weight for six months or longer. The improvement in appetite (some of the patients became voracious eaters), in the sense of well-being and in physical and nervous strength, was a marked early and persistent effect in all cases. The added fat was distributed as a rule over the face, neck, breasts, abdomen, shoulders, back and buttocks, but in 1 case the deposit of fat was most obvious in the breasts and in another in the abdomen.

The only records of deleterious effects of this kind of treatment which I can find, other than the suggestion above of a perhaps unsightly distribution of fat, are the 3 cases of induced urticaria in Nichol's 63 cases, and the local skin hypersensitiveness to insulin, appearing from one to six weeks after the beginning of treatment, in 6 of Blotner's 19 cases. Tuft's feeling that such reactions are probably due to the protein of a particular insulin is apparently not supported here, for these patients remained sensitive to three different brands of insulin.

Blotner concluded from his laboratory studies that the gain in weight is probably due to an increased food intake and better digestion and assimilation. Lueders and Watson (1932) and others have shown that insulin stimulates the production of gastric juice and also increases the pancreatic and biliary secretions. The increase in weight does not seem to be due to water retention, as may occur sometimes in diabetes. The increase in

TABLE 45.—GAIN IN WEIGHT IN THIN PATIENTS WITH INSULIN*

Case.	Standard normal weight for height, age and sex.	Weight before insulin.	Weekly weights of patients during insulin therapy.								Gain in weight during insulin therapy.	Weight after insulin was omitted.
			1	2	3	4	6	8	10	12		
1	134	97	102	106	112	113	112	112	117	117	20	Same in 8 months
2	137	105	113	116	118	120	120	121	...	...	16	Same in 6½ months
3	141	112	115	118	118	119	121	122	...	...	10	Same in 6 months
4	153	103	108	114	114	119	127½	...	...	...	24½	143 in 12 months
5	102	72	75	78	81	82	83	84	85	...	13	Same in 6 weeks
6	119	90	95½	97	99	101	103	104	105	...	15	Same in 11 weeks
7	135	89	95	98	100	102	104	105	108	...	19	113 in 10 weeks
8	135	98	103	106	107	110	111	114	117	...	19	Same in 7 weeks
9	167	141	146	151	155	159	163	169	171	172	31	183 in 14 months
10	116	97	101	104	107	108	110	...	...	...	13	Same in 6 weeks
11	178	167	172	175	178	179	179	...	...	...	12	Same in 6 weeks
12	154	134	141	145	145	146	...	...	...	...	12	Same in 9 weeks
13	157	132	139	141	143	145	...	...	...	...	13	140 in 10 weeks
14	150	134	137	140	143	...	...	...	...	...	9	Same in 6 weeks
15	133	113	116	119	122	...	...	...	...	...	9	114 in 6 months
16	119	97	97	99	101	104½	107	...	...	...	10	Taking insulin
17	126	100	103	106	108	...	...	...	...	...	8	Taking insulin
18	131	119½	124	...	...	...	...	...	...	...	4½	Taking insulin
19	156	132	136½	...	...	...	...	...	...	...	4½	Discontinued insulin because of local reactions

* Weight is recorded in pounds.

plasma protein concentration, the red cell count and the circulating blood volume all testify to the excellent tonic properties of insulin. Perhaps all the favorable results which are from time to time reported following the use of insulin in very divergent nondiabetic conditions are explainable upon the basis of this tonic action. The basal metabolic rate was either unaffected or tended to show a slight decrease during or after insulin therapy.

DISEASES OF THE GASTRO-INTESTINAL TRACT

STOMATITIS

Catarrhal Stomatitis (Simple Stomatitis).—There is acute diffuse inflammation of the mouth, with tenderness of the gums, lips and cheeks, salivation, coated tongue, bad taste, foul breath; sometimes the neighboring lymph nodes are slightly enlarged. Malnutrition and poor oral and general hygiene predispose to this malady in children; in adults, excessive smoking and chronic constitutional disease. The attack terminates with recovery usually in less than a week. This type of stomatitis may occasionally become epidemic, as was the case in the Ruhr in 1919 and 1920.

Aphthous Stomatitis (Vesicular or Herpetic Stomatitis; Canker Sore). —The onset is sudden. A small inflammatory spot appears at the base of the teeth or under the tongue, or on the inner surface of the lips or cheeks; it goes through a brief vesicular stage, then a whitish pellicle appears and is soon cast off to leave a sharply defined small ulceration which is very painful. There is bad breath and coating of the tongue but usually not pronounced salivation. The lesions may be multiple. The exact cause of this type of stomatitis is not known, though it is very possibly a herpes of the mucous membranes; some individuals seem peculiarly susceptible to frequent recurrences.

Ulcerative Stomatitis.—This is a rare malady among otherwise healthy people, but it may spread in epidemic form among the poor who live under bad hygienic and nutritional surroundings either in or out of institutions. In addition to the symptoms of catarrhal stomatitis there is ulceration of the gums and adjacent portions of the cheeks and under side of the tongue. The lymph glands are of course swollen and tender; in severe cases there may be even loss of teeth and necrosis of the bone.

Gangrenous Stomatitis (Cancrum Oris; Noma).—This type of stomatitis is very horrible, but fortunately occurs rarely and then almost exclusively in young children who have been debilitated by a severe bout of illness; a few institutional epidemics have been reported, however. Beginning as a small ulcer on the mucous membrane of the cheek, lip or gum, a spreading gangrene rapidly destroys a large portion of one side of the face; death nearly always results in from one to five days.

Parasitic Stomatitis (Thrush).—This malady, which is caused by the hyphomycete, *Oidium albicans,* occurs sporadically and sometimes epidemically among nursing infants. It is generally considered that it is due to contamination from imperfectly sterilized nursing bottles or nipples, from the introduction of unsterile cleansing solutions into the mouth, and from the mother's breasts or from the hands of attendants. Premature, weak, athreptic infants, or those suffering from other infectious diseases, are especially predisposed to thrush, but it may also attack otherwise healthy infants. The lesions consist of small white patches, somewhat resembling milk curds, scattered over the cheeks, gums, lips and tongue; their removal, which is difficult, leaves a slightly bleeding area. Examination of one of these crushed "curds" reveals the organism. The attack usually clears up in two or three days, but hospitals fear thrush because an epidemic not infrequently fails to yield even to vigorous treatment, and without treatment may run a course of several weeks.

Mercurial Stomatitis.—The first symptoms are metallic taste and soreness of the teeth upon chewing; then the gums become spongy, swollen, and tender, and they bleed very easily; the breath is quite foul and the salivary glands are swollen and tender. In extreme cases ulceration, loss of teeth, and even necrosis of the bone may take place.

Bismuth Stomatitis.—This type of stomatitis is characterized by a blue-black line along the margin of the gums, soreness of the gums, salivation, and in severe cases ulceration.

THERAPY

Catarrhal.—Attempt should be made to eradicate the predisposing causes of this type of stomatitis. During the attack, the soft foods, such as milk, slightly cooked eggs, soups, custards, etc., are the only foods that adults can take with any sort of comfort; the feeding of infants sometimes becomes a quite difficult problem. Local treatment consists in the use of mouth washes such as the following: tincture of myrrh, 1 part to 25 or 50 parts of water; potassium permanganate, 1 part to 8000 parts of water; or some such mixture as the following, which is a very satisfactory mouth wash:

℞.	Thymol (saturated solution).........................	℥ij	64.0
	Hydrogen dioxide.................................	℥ij	64.0
	Glycerin...	℥ij	64.0
	Potassium chlorate (saturated solution) to make.......	℥viij	250.0
	Label: Use as mouth wash.		

In infants, who cannot of course gargle or rinse the mouth, it is necessary to apply these washes on a cotton swab. The saturated solution of boric acid has long enjoyed a reputation as the ideal mild mouth wash, a reputation entirely undeserved for the reason that it is practically worthless as an antiseptic.

Aphthous.—For general measures and the use of mouth washes, see Catarrhal Stomatitis above. In addition, the silver nitrate stick is almost specific in the eradication of these canker sores. It should be firmly applied to the bottom and sides of each of the ulcers, rinsing the mouth with water afterward if the caustic and metallic taste is very objectionable.

Ulcerative.—For general measures and the use of mouth washes, see Catarrhal Stomatitis above. The ulcers may be either touched directly with the silver nitrate stick or swabbed with a 25 to 50 per cent solution. The use of potassium chlorate to be swallowed is recommended by several physicians of wide experience, despite the well-known ability of this drug to cause methemoglobin poisoning; it is excreted partially through the salivary glands and thus the ulcerated surfaces in the mouth are continuously bathed in a potassium chlorate solution. Bradbury states that the drug is almost a specific when used internally. He recommends for an adult, 10 grains (0.65 Gm.) three times a day, to be taken well diluted; for a child of six years, 3 grains (0.2 Gm.) every four hours. Wise and Parkhurst recommend 20 grains (1.3 Gm.) three times daily for the adult.

Gangrenous.—The only permissible treatment here is early and radical excision of the gangrenous area without consideration of the cosmetic effect.

Parasitic.—Faber and Clark (1927), in a careful report of an epidemic of thrush in newborn infants, write as follows:

"The treatment of a patient who has thrush may follow one of two lines: simple cleansing or the use of antiseptics. For the first, alkaline, but not too alkaline, solutions frequently applied to the mouth may result in cure after a week or two, especially in healthy infants and in infants with mildly virulent strains of *Oidium* [2 per cent sodium bicarbonate solution—H. B.]. The outcome of such treatment is, however, always problematic, and against relatively virulent strains such as we have often seen, is practically certain to be disappointing. Boric acid is not only valueless, but, as the recent experience in Chicago demonstrated, dangerous. We emphasize the point because a recent text in a book on pediatrics recommends the Escherich boric acid sac or teat. This is a small sac of silk or batiste filled with boric acid powder sweetened with saccharin which is placed and left in the infant's mouth, presumably until the thrush is cured. It is possible that boric acid poisoning might result from such treatment. Solution of liquor formaldehydi has never given us satisfactory results, and we believe that the reason is its poor penetration and its rapid dilution by the secretions of the mouth below the point of disinfecting efficiency [1 per cent solution of formalin is usually used—H. B.]. With mercurochrome-220-soluble we have obtained occasional but not constant retrogression of the oral lesions [1 to 2 per cent aqueous solution—Faber and Dickey (1925)]. With gentian violet we have obtained better and more constant results than with any other substance. To obtain them, however, it is necessary to follow certain rules. Treatment should be given at least one hour after feeding. The mouth should be gently cleansed with several cotton swabs to remove the adherent mucus over the affected areas—a most important precaution, since as Churchman has shown, the dye is absorbed and its therapeutic effect on the lesion annulled by overlying secretion. The dye, in 1 per cent aqueous solution, must be freshly prepared (not more than a few days old) and must be applied generously, first to the affected area and then over the tongue and in the buccogingival folds. The treatment must be repeated once or twice daily for at least three successive days, and, if possible, every other day thereafter for from one to two weeks. The mother's breasts should be carefully cleansed with soap and water before each nursing, and the first few drops of milk discarded to prevent reinfection.

"If this technic is followed, the lesions will have nearly disappeared by the second day and entirely so by the third; new ones will not appear. If only one or two treatments are given, recurrences will frequently occur, usually in other areas than the site of the original lesion. In spite of the deep staining of the entire oral cavity, which persists for a day or two after treatment has been stopped, there is no apparent interference with the baby's appetite or ability to feed. Stain on the lips or chin can be easily removed with a little alcohol. The stools during treatment often appear purplish."

Abraham (1926) has reported favorably on the use of ferric chloride. His 33 patients responded to the application of a solution of 2.5 to 3.5 per cent ferric chloride in from two to four days on the average. Higher concentrations produced irritating effects. Animal experiments showed that the virulence of the organism was considerably decreased by the treatment.

Mercurial.—This type of stomatitis will usually not occur in the patient whose oral hygiene is perfect unless the ordinary therapeutic doses of the mercurials are exceeded. After the teeth and gums have been put in as good condition as possible, it is well to employ the potassium chlorate mouth wash (see Catarrhal Stomatitis above) as a routine throughout the period in which the mercury is being given. At the appearance of the first sign of stomatitis the drug should be stopped and then only very carefully resumed upon its subsidence. When the stomatitis is only a part of the general picture of mercury poisoning, one must resort to other measures as well (see Mercury Poisoning, p. 696).

Bismuth.—See page 214.

DYSPEPSIA

(Indigestion)

It is the paramount duty of the physician to approach the diagnosis and treatment of every case of dyspepsia by the purely eliminative process, for though it is undeniably true that the majority of digestive complaints are due to either sensory, secretory or motor disturbances, and are therefore functional rather than organic in origin, yet the gravity of the organic lesions when present it so great that they must all be ruled out before the diagnosis of a purely functional dyspepsia is accepted. Granting, then, that this has been done, *i. e.*, that the patient has been shown not to have gastritis, peptic ulcer or cancer, the functional disturbances remain to be considered—provided that two further possibilities are also eliminated, namely, dyspepsia due to dietary indiscretion, and secondary, so-called "reflex," dyspepsia. *Dietary indiscretion* is usually encountered in those of a fulsome habit, who have regard neither for the quantity nor the quality of their food and drink, and who disdain all the decencies of table deportment; occasionally, however, an individual suffering from this type of indigestion will not be one of the gobblers but merely a person who suffers from the taking of small and even well-masticated quantities of certain foods, such as fried and greasy dishes, heavy hot breads, excessively hot or cold dishes, etc. Any of the symptoms of indigestion may be manifested, and they will all usually disappear if the offending articles are withheld from the diet, or if the individual is made to curb his gluttony—that is to say, if a silk purse is made out of a sow's ear. *Reflex dyspepsia* may indicate the presence of gallbladder disease, chronic appendicitis, peritoneal adhesions, epigastric hernia, intestinal worms, cirrhosis of the liver, etc. It should always be borne in mind, as well, that angina pectoris sometimes simulates an acute gastro-intestinal disease, and that a functional dyspepsia is often associated with disease of the genito-urinary organs, hyperthyroidism, the anemias, and pulmonary tuberculosis.

The functional dyspepsias will be considered under the following heads: (1) Nervous indigestion, (2) pylorospasm, (3) hyperacidity, (4) achylia, (5) atony, (6) intestinal fermentation. There are many other entities, of course, but space does not permit their consideration in this book.

1. NERVOUS INDIGESTION

This type of dyspepsia, whose sufferers are legion, is characterized by the following facts: The gastro-intestinal syndrome changes frequently, so that at one time the picture will be dominated by a gastric symptom of one sort and at another time by a symptom of another sort altogether; there are usually other psychasthenic complaints, such as palpitation, poor circulation, fatigue, peculiar forms of headache, etc.; there is no definite relationship between the quantity or quality of food taken and the type and degree of the gastric disturbance; and the symptoms are very dependent upon the state of mind of the individual at the time he partakes of a given meal. The most usual complaints are of fulness and discomfort in the epigastrium, pain, eructation of gas, nausea, vomiting, and a difficulty in swallowing. Often the appetite is poor, but sometimes a patient, believing that only by forcing himself to eat will he get well, is given to inordinate performances at table. Others attempt to treat themselves by eliminating articles one after another from the diet in the hope of finding the offending food; such individuals not infrequently maintain themselves in a condition of semistarvation—and affect their malady not in the least unless it be to make it worse.

Therapy.—In my opinion, the treatment of this condition has never been so well described as it was by Alvarez, of the Mayo Clinic, in 1927. I am therefore quoting from his paper at some length in the belief that every medical student and young practitioner should be thoroughly familiar with this excellent treatise of a man who has long been well known for his sound laboratory and clinical researches in gastro-enterology.

"The treatment of the functional disorders of digestion may be discussed under four headings: (1) Psychotherapy and instruction in mental and physical hygiene; (2) physical therapy, exercise and massage; (3) diet, and (4) drugs.

"*Psychotherapy and Instruction in Mental and Physical Hygiene.*—The first and often the most important step in the psychic treatment is taken when the physician makes a complete and careful physical, roentgenologic and laboratory examination. If this does not reveal signs of serious disease, many persons immediately lose interest in their symptoms and go away satisfied. Another important factor in the psychic treatment is the taking of a good history, and especially a history that brings out all the details of family and business worries, of domestic infelicity or of the phobias that so often are at the bottom of the trouble. Unless these things are done, it is not only useless but often criminal to tell the patient not to worry. Some consult us simply because they have been shocked by the sudden death of a friend or relative. They fear that they too have cancer or heart disease, but they will not admit it, and come complaining of some minor ailment. Especially when dealing with older patients, it is often well to say at the close of the examination: 'As we examined you we had always in mind the possibility of cancer beginning somewhere, and we are now glad to say that nothing suspicious has been found.'"

It is useless, of course, to tell the patient to simply stop worrying under circumstances that would likely evoke the same reactions in ourselves; in Alvarez's experience the most difficult cases to handle have been in women who are leading a cat-and-dog existence with their husbands, with the usual amount of wrangling at mealtimes.

"Fortunately, much can be done in many of these cases by giving the patient the mental purgation that comes with the pouring out of secret worries into a sympathetic ear. The physician can often help these persons by advising them wisely, and by leading them out of a maze of muddled thought to the point where they can forgive and forget, and acquiesce to things that cannot be cured. For years I have kept in my office a copy of Trudeau's autobiography with a bookmark at page 318 in order that I may turn quickly to his remark that he had learned from his patients that 'the conquest of Fate is not by struggling against it, nor by trying to escape from it, but by acquiescence.' The asthenic person, the person with mucous colitis, or the one to whom nature has given a 'raw deal' can often be made over into a useful and happy member of society if he can be taught this lesson of aquiescence: to stop looking for a cure and instead to settle down to get along as best he can with his handicap.

"The next thing in most cases is to see how a rest can be obtained with the least expense and loss of income. If a vacation is taken, it must be one that will bring the patient back better off than when he left. Too often our vacations are of the type that caused the Irishman to remark plaintively, 'How happy we'd be if it weren't for our pleasures.' If a man cannot well leave his business, he can often, for a month or two, answer his mail and confer with his assistants in the mornings, and can then spend his afternoons at home or on the golf course. I have seen such excellent results from this type of resting that for business men I prefer it to a complete vacation. The mother with several small children and few resources can also be helped tremendously if she is taught to go back to bed after the children are sent off to school. She may have to continue with mending and sewing, but even so, a few weeks of mornings in bed will often work a miracle."

A rest cure in a sanatorium, perhaps with overfeeding, is often helpful if the patient does not have to be greatly concerned about the expense—and provided the hospital practice of awakening the patient at a very early hour does not rob him of his best sleep. Another thing which Alvarez deplores in present-day hospitals in the obsession of many dietitians to force the patient upon a diet containing much spinach, salads, fruit and bran—roughages of which he disapproves—in the mistaken belief that it is dangerous to allow any time at all to elapse without vitamins and iron in full quantities.

"The sick who are so situated that they must either keep at work or starve can often be taught to hoard their small stock of energy and to live within the limits of their nervous strength. Many tire themselves out by putting too much energy and emotion into trivial tasks. Women in particular must be exhorted to break themselves of the habit of getting all stirred up over little things, and of reviewing at great length painful or annoying experiences which a more sensible person would promptly forget. Others must be taught to go to bed earlier at night and some must for a time retire from leadership or active participation in church, civic or social work. Some can get their grip again if they will only rest in bed on Saturday afternoons and Sundays.

"As I have already pointed out, many take their holidays too strenuously: they drive too far in automobiles, they work too hard in their gardens, or they do things that leave them more tired on Monday morning than they were on Saturday night. They must learn the truth of Mosso's statement that all their energies come from one source, and that when mentally tired it is not wise to exercise so strenuously as still further to take away from a small store of strength."

The Securing of Sleep.—Oftentimes the physician overlooks the importance of relieving insomnia, which can often be done by teaching the patient to keep his mind off disturbing thoughts, to avoid mental work or exciting conversation after dinner, to take a warm bath and a little food on retiring, and to go to bed earlier. When these measures fail, Alvarez does not hesitate to use the barbiturates, believing that the opposition of many physicians to sleep-producing "dope" is entirely unjustified.

"These newer synthetics have no relation to morphine; they have none of that 'kick' that makes the taker wish to repeat his experience, and except in the case of the markedly psychopathic person, I am sure they are perfectly safe. I have been prescribing them for twenty years and have yet to see an habitué in my own practice. Actually, in a practice limited largely to the diagnosis and treatment of gastro-intestinal disease, I have found one of the most useful drugs to be not pepsin or bismuth, but carbromal, a sleep producer. Carbromal (bromdiethylacetylurea) is used in doses of from 0.3 to 1 Gm. (5 to 15 grains). In those who are sensitive to drugs, 0.3 Gm. at bedtime will make all the difference between a restless and a restful night. Barbital, or veronal (diethylmalonylurea), produces headache in some persons and a little 'hangover' in the morning, especially if it is taken after midnight. All these drugs are best given early when the patient goes to bed. Phenobarbital (phenylethyl barbituric acid) can be given day or night in doses of from 0.05 to 0.2 Gm. (¾ to 3 grains)." Amytal, in a dose of 1½ to 5 grains (0.1 to 0.3 Gm.) is also being much used as a hypnotic.

"There are a few highly neurotic and psychopathic persons who do not react well to any of these barbituric acid derivatives; instead of becoming quiet they get excited, and if they doze off to sleep they soon awaken with nightmares. They often do better on chloral. The only trouble I have ever had with these drugs has been in trying to get the patients to use them long enough. They are afraid, they are influenced by alarmed relatives, physicians and nurses, and they give up the 'crutch' before they have learned to walk alone.

"Certain nervous and asthenic patients must be guided into less laborious forms of employment, and others must be induced to change their mode of living so that they can get better food and happier surroundings. There is no detail of the patient's life so trivial that it may not play a part in keeping up a neurosis which is expressing itself in some form of indigestion, and the physician must find what it is and if possible correct it.

"*Physical Therapy, Exercise and Massage.*—Many of the weak and partly bedridden patients can be put on their feet, literally and figuratively, only with the help of an intelligent, cheerful and masterful physical therapist who can build their strength until they can stay up all day. Each day the invalid is given something to do, something to think about, something to hope for, and some one with whom to talk. Not all persons, however, are helped by massage. Only those 'pussycats' who love to be stroked will thrive on it; those who are ticklish or who hate to be touched by strangers will be made worse. Stoutly built men who were once athletic but who have since become flabby and fat can often be helped by a course with a trainer. Ultraviolet radiation, in my experience, helps in raising resistance, improving appetite and putting on weight.

"These physical therapeutic measures are invaluable in many cases if only because they keep the patient busy and hopeful and bring him back repeatedly under the influence and guidance of the physical therapist and the physician. They keep him out of mischief and out of the hands of the quacks. One of our biggest mistakes in medicine today is that we have allowed others to monopolize these modes of treatment. One of the great advantages of having the work done under our supervision is that we can be watching the patient, learning more about his troubles, and seeing him on occasions when he has something definite and telltale to show us, like a fever, a point of tenderness, or a tinge of jaundice."

Diet.—Alvarez feels that the most important dietetic considerations are that the patient be taught to eat again, that the diets provided for him be neither too restricted nor monotonous, and that the taking of all unnecessary roughage be forbidden. The virtues of the smooth diet he believes to lie not in the fact that cellulose is so indigestible and by its presence likely to interfere with the action of digestive ferments on starches and other foods, but rather in the assumed existence in the sick individual of areas of reversed peristalsis which fluids will pass but solids will not. To resort in the majority of cases to a milk diet he believes to be unfortunate because milk disagrees with many persons and is bulky and leaves a large residue. If the use of a smooth diet does not bring relief in a few weeks, the case is believed to be one that is not going to be relieved by any form of dietary restriction.

The following are the "smooth diet" instructions often given to patients:

"If you are to give this diet a fair trial, eat no coarse foods with fiber, skins, seeds or gristle. Avoid particularly salads with celery, tomatoes, cucumbers and pineapple, many of the green vegetables, raisins, berries, jams full of seeds, nuts, and many of the raw fruits. Beans, cabbage, onions, green or red peppers, melons, cucumbers and peanuts are notoriously gassy. If you are living in a boarding house you can stick to this diet by simply avoiding the forbidden foods and eating more of the digestible ones which are put before you.

"Avoid sugar in concentrated form and take no candy or other food between meals. Hot cakes and waffles might not be bad if they were not eaten with so much syrup. Fried foods are not bad if they are properly fried, that is, totally immersed in fat at the right temperature. Avoid eating when in a rush and when mentally upset. Family rows should be held away from the table. Chewing gum may cause distress, as much air is swallowed with the saliva. Digestion is greatly helped by a good chewing surface. If there are any gaps in your teeth have your dentist fill them with bridges. Purgatives often cause flatulence and distress in the abdomen.

"The following are suggestions for breakfast: Orange juice, grapefruit (avoid the fiber in the compartments); cantaloupe and melons are inadvisable. Coffee, if desired, is allowed in moderation; it sometimes causes flatulence. If you are sensitive to caffeine try kaffee hag or instant postum. Chocolate, cocoa or tea, one or two eggs with ham or bacon (avoid the tougher part of the bacon), white bread, toast or zwieback with butter, any smooth musk such as farina, germea, cream of wheat, cornmeal or rolled oats (a fine oatmeal can be obtained by calling for Robinson's Scotch Groats), puffed cereals and cornflakes are also allowed. Shredded wheat biscuits and other coarse breakfast foods are not allowed. Bran is particularly harmful. Graham bread is permitted but not the coarser whole wheat bread.

"Suggestions for lunch and dinner: In fruit cocktails avoid the pieces of orange and pineapple. Broths, bouillon, cream soups and chowder are allowed, also meat, fish or chicken, squab or game, excepting duck (avoid the fibrous parts and gristle). Veal may be tried; it is not digested well by many persons. Eat no smoked fish or pork. Crab and lobster had better be left alone. Oysters and sausage may be tried later.

"Bread and butter are allowed, and hot biscuits if they are made small so as to consist mainly of crust. Rice, potatoes, mashed, hashed brown or French fried, are allowed; and later may be added sweet potatoes, hominy, tomatoes stewed, strained and thickened with cracker or bread crumbs, well-cooked cauliflower tops with cream sauce, asparagus tips, Brussels sprouts, squash, beets, turnips, creamed spinach, Italian pastes, noodles, macaroni and spaghetti cooked soft, purées of peas, beans, lentils, lima beans or artichoke hearts. All skins or fiber should be removed by passing the food through a ricer. Sweet corn may be used if passed through a colander. There are practically no other vegetables that can be puréed to advantage. String beans (large tender string beans which can be used as a vegetable or salad can now be obtained in cans) are allowed if they are young and tender.

"No salad should be taken at first. Later you may try a little tender lettuce with apples or bananas, tomato jelly or boiled eggs. Mayonnaise and French dressing are allowed. Potato salad without much onion may be tried.

"Suggestions for dessert are: Simple puddings, custards, ice cream, jello, plain cake and canned or stewed fruits, particularly pears and peaches. Cottage cheese is permissible; other cheeses often cause trouble. Apple, peach, apricot, custard and lemon cream pie may be tried if only the filling is eaten.

"In case of constipation, stewed fruit may be taken once or twice a day. In winter the dried pared fruit may be used for stewing. Prunes are probably the most laxative of fruits and if eaten every other morning they will relieve the average case of constipation. They should be cooked slowly until they almost go to pieces. If the skins are still tough they should be discarded. Apple sauce is much more palatable if made from unpared and uncored apples. The sauce is strained later. It may be mixed with a little tapioca or sago. The apples may be baked. Apples, even when cooked, often cause distress. Blackberries and loganberries can be stewed and strained and the sweetened juice thickened with cornstarch. This makes a delicious dish with the full flavor of the berries. Later you may try fully ripe pears and peaches.

"Make no effort to drink water. Be guided by your thirst. Avoid excessive use of salt or other seasoning. If you wish to gain in weight eat as much cream, butter, fat, and starch as you can. If you wish to lose or to stay thin, live largely on vegetables, fruits and salads, with a moderate amount of lean meat."

Plenty of cream and butter may be added to the diet to correct underweight, and constipation, if present, is regulated by enemas of physiologic saline or small doses of magnesium oxide if the use of prunes is not sufficiently helpful.

Drugs.—The use of hypnotics has already been discussed. Alvarez believes that those patients who are greatly helped by alkalis will be found to be suffering from ulcer or some other organic disease. He has little faith in tonics and bitters and uses them only at times for psychic effect in such instances preferring such high-sounding preparations as "beef, iron and wine." Strychnine he looks upon as the last drug on earth to give to a nervous person and shares with most other gastro-enterologists the justified lack of faith in administered pepsin, pancreatin, etc. Carminatives are sometimes helpful (prescription on p. 412).

2. PYLOROSPASM

Pylorospasm, unassociated with ulcer or other organic lesion, is a spasmodic constriction of the pylorus occurring usually at the height of digestion. There is pain, which is sometimes very intense, eructations and vomiting, sometimes without nausea. A firm protruding mass, indicating the contracted pylorus, may appear in the epigastrium. Vomiting gives great relief, but in many cases the spasms become so frequent that the condition merges into a state of spastic contraction with consequent dilatation of the stomach; the patient can retain no food and of course wastes away rapidly.

Therapy.—Read the treatment of nervous indigestion, page 404.

During the attack, a hypodermic injection of $\frac{1}{120}$ grain (0.0005 Gm.) of atropine sulphate oftentimes gives complete relief, but this drug is not as infallible in its action here as would be expected considering its well-known ability to relax involuntary muscle. In 6 of a group of 16 patients, Beams (1931) obtained relief with the nitrites—amyl nitrite inhaled from the crushed "pearl," or spirits of glyceryl trinitrate (nitroglycerin) 3 drops on the tongue and increasing the dose by 1 drop every two minutes to effect, or sodium nitrite 1 grain (0.06 Gm.) three or four times a day. Eight of the 10 patients who failed to respond to the nitrites responded to atropine given in the form of $\frac{1}{6}$ grain (0.01 Gm.) of extract of belladonna three or four times daily. When an opiate is necessary, morphine should not be used for obvious reasons; combine $\frac{1}{2}$ to 1 grain (0.032 to 0.065 Gm.) of codeine sulphate or phosphate with the atropine.

Dry Diet.—Use of a diet that would be difficult to vomit was advocated by Sauer, in 1921. The following case report of Speidel (1932) is of great interest:

Z. C., female, aged twenty-one, came to my office on September 28, 1925, complaining of general abdominal distress, loss of weight, constipation, poor appetite and vomiting. The onset of these symptoms was gradual and began two years previously, about the time she graduated from high school. There was some emotional upset connected with competing for a medal or honors of some sort. All her symptoms had become gradually worse, vomiting occurs now every time she eats or drinks anything. Upon graduating from high school she weighed 92 pounds. Present weight 69¼ pounds. x-Ray studies revealed that barium left the stomach very slowly and that there was marked ptosis of both the stomach and large bowel. She was sent to the hospital and for the first week received atropine sulphate 1/150 grain hypodermically after each meal, the regular hospital diet and daily gastric lavage. Under this regimen no improvement occurred. On December 3, 1925, the atropine sulphate was increased to 1/100 grain after meals, hypodermically, and she was given a dry diet, which in this case meant the regular hospital diet without fluids and without gravies, sauces, soup, fruit juices, and any other liquid or semiliquid food. She was given water half-way between meals in whatever quantity she desired. Improvement began at once. On December 11th, the atropine was administered by mouth instead of hypodermically and the dry diet was continued.

Dr. Speidel has kindly written me further: "I saw this girl from time to time for the next five years. She was obliged to adhere to the diet and to take atropine tablets by mouth during that entire time. Frequently kindly disposed neighbors would send her soup because of her emaciated appearance, but whenever she took any she vomited immediately. This also applied to any other beverages that she might take, but plain water half-way between meals was retained in sufficient quantities to keep her from becoming dehydrated. When last I saw her on March 11, 1931, she weighed 117¼ pounds and to all appearances was healthy but was still taking the dry diet and atropine tablets—in fact on several occasions, when she inadvertently forgot to have her prescription refilled, she would retain nothing until the tablets were resumed."

In pyloric stenosis in infants it is usually held that immediate operation is indicated, but Sauer believes that thick cereal feedings should be tried for a time to see if improvement will not take place; if the vomiting fails to subside in a week or two and the child to increase in weight and general condition, operation is resorted to, though of course it is advised at once when infants are first seen in a very emaciated unresponsive state. The mixture used is skimmed milk, 9 ounces; water, 12 ounces; farina or rice flour, 6 teaspoonfuls; dextrimaltose, 3 ounces; boil an hour or more in a covered double boiler until thick. From 2 to 6 tablespoonfuls of this is given six to seven times daily, scraped off of a narrow tongue depressor well back in the mouth. Fluid is supplied as 6 per cent glucose in Ringer's solution by rectum. The nutrient enema described on page 427 might well be used here; for an infant, 20 cc. of the mixture per hour, slowly injected from an ear syringe. After an average time of five to eight weeks, Sauer was able to substitute appreciable amounts of ordinary milk mixtures for a part of the cereal feedings. This nonoperative treatment was effective in 28 of his 35 cases.

Lavage.—In an aged patient, in very poor physical condition, Scriver (1931) resorted to the use of the tube and thorough washing out of the stomach twice daily; the patient was saved and became able to retain a diet upon which he gained weight. Subsequent x-ray examination showed disappearance of the previously observed atony.

3. HYPERCHLORHYDRIA

This condition, which is more frequent in young and middle-aged persons than in older individuals, is the most common of all gastric disturbances. The symptoms are caused by a more than normal production of acid (*not* an increase in the relative acidity of the juice) during the digestion of a meal, but it should be borne in mind that a gastric analysis which shows an apparently normal acidity does not necessarily rule out hyperchlorhydria, for the reason that the "normal" acidity of the stomach contents during digestion varies widely, and an individual may actually suffer from the symptoms of hyperacidity though an analysis indicates the presence of an amount of acid that is below the "normal" for the majority of persons. The cycle of events is quite characteristic. Pain comes on an hour or more after eating; it is usually of the mild pressure type but may be very severe and boring and extend into the back and up into the throat. There is heart burn and eructation of acid fluid; occasionally there is also vomiting of very acid stomach contents which burns the throat and mouth as it passes out. Light and starchy repasts are more prone to produce an attack than are heavier meaty meals. The patients are often otherwise in good health, have a good appetite, and are in good flesh.

Therapy.—Read the treatment of nervous indigestion, page 404.

The usual remedy for an attack of this kind is to administer sodium bicarbonate in a dose of 15 grains (1 Gm.) when the pain appears and repeat several times if necessary. The large doses often taken by the layman are not necessary, and it should be pointed out that the drug should be taken in warm, but not very hot, water, for the latter converts bicarbonate into the carbonate which may in itself be irritating. The reader is urged to turn to the discussion of the various antacids as used in the treatment of peptic ulcer, for what is there said applies equally here.

4. HYPOCHLORHYDRIA (ACHYLIA GASTRICA)

Vanzant *et al.* (1932), in the examination of 3746 persons, found a steady increase in the incidence of achlorhydria from youth to old age; 23 to 28 per cent of individuals at the age of 60 failed to show free acid on repeated fractional analysis. The symptoms of the condition are usually few because gastric digestion in these cases is vicariously performed by the intestine. However, there is sometimes loss of appetite and a sense of fulness after eating. Nausea and vomiting are rare. In a few cases there is severe pain, heart burn and eructations just as in hyperacidity; sometimes, too, periods of diarrhea and constipation alternate.

Therapy.—Read the treatment of nervous indigestion, page 404.

Hydrochloric Acid.—Hydrochloric acid may be expected to act in the following ways in cases of hypochlorhydria: (a) As a stomachic, (b) to form acid albuminates and so aid in proteolysis, (c) to release pepsin from the pepsinogen of the glands, (d) to promote an acid medium for the action of pepsin, (e) as an antiseptic, (f) to stimulate pancreatic secretion, (g) to improve tonus and peristalsis, (h) to aid in the solution of insoluble calcium and magnesium salts in the ingesta, and (i) to stimulate secretion of hydrochloric acid. The practice of using acid in these cases has fallen somewhat into disrepute latterly, but I believe the fault has lain in the use of too small and too infrequent doses. Dobson's (1927) studies have demonstrated the undoubted value of the U.S.P. dilute hydrochloric acid when properly administered. He writes:

"1. It should be given in as large amounts as possible consistent with the tolerance of the individual. In the absence of unpleasant sensations a total dosage of 2.5 drachms or more may be given during the digestive period.

"2. A method of fractional administration in which adequate individual doses are given seems preferable to the continuous sipping method. Although it is not well demonstrated in these experiments because of renewed secretion of acid, it is logical to assume and has been shown experimentally [see Crohn, B. B.] that a moderate dose of acid given to a patient with achlorhydria exerts its full effect on intragastric acidity shortly after administration, and that this diminishes until augmented in each instance by subsequent doses. So that, given in this way by a process of 'dumping,' the acid seems to exert its greatest effect in the production of free acid in the stomach. Fractional doses of 30 minims are probably most suitable, considering the necessity for as high dosage as possible in order to produce the desired condition of free acidity and avoid the discomfort sometimes produced by doses that are too large.

"3. Because of its affinity for the protein in the food, acid should be especially given in the early stages of digestion and the frequency of administration determined by the tolerance of the patient. Ordinarily, he should receive 30 minims in the middle of the meal and the same amount at fifteen-minute intervals for an hour or more afterward. If definite unpleasant symptoms are produced the interval may be lengthened and the total number of doses reduced rather than the amount of the individual doses.

"4. Acid should be used in concentration as high as possible consistent with relative comfort in taking it. Two ounces (60 cc.) of water, grape juice, lemonade, or other more potent vehicle of a nonalkaline nature, may be considered the average amount of diluent with each dose of 30 minims. Excessive use of other fluids during the meal should be avoided, the amount being regulated by the nature of the food, and reduced especially when it contains articles of a high water content, such as certain fruits and vegetables. For a meal consisting of relatively dry foods about 6 ounces (180 cc.) of fluid besides that taken with acid is within reasonable limits. The requisite body fluids in excess of this amount may be obtained when digestion is completed.

"5. It may be of advantage to the patient to have one meal in the day consist almost entirely of carbohydrate and to accompany it with the usual doses of acid. By these means a condition of free acidity is much more likely to be produced in the stomach than when protein is contained in the meal, and its possible stimulating effect may be valuable even for only one digestive phase in three. Stimulation due to protein may be obtained with the other meals. The possibility of increasing the total amount and frequency in dosage of the acid given when the meal contains much protein may be mentioned as a corollary.

"6. Patients proved to have complete achlorhydria should be persistently and adequately treated with dilute hydrochloric acid. The fact that symptomatic relief does not always accompany the treatment even with the induction of apparently adequate acidity, is not necessarily a contraindication to the continued use of acid since its digestive, antiseptic, and other influences may still be effective. The value of treatment should be determined by periodically investigating, with the Rehfuss tube and test meal or histamine test, whether a condition of free acidity has been actually produced during digestion or whether there is any indication of reactivation of the secretory mechanism by spontaneous production of free acid. It should be realized, of course, that these suggestions which involve treatment of the local condition primarily should be augmented by such important general measures as adequate diet, rest and the induction of psychic and emotional equilibrium."

Hubbard (1931) has found it worth while to use also an alkali-forming diet in patients who show evidences of systemic acid-base imbalance upon prolonged administration of hydrochloric acid. The addition of citrus fruits and green vegetables to the diet will considerably reduce the excessive acidity of the urine.

Digestive Ferments.—In Dobson's studies, the use of the essence of pepsin and the extract of the gastric mucosa, gastron (the dose of either of which is from 1 to 4 drachms), seemed to be without value, since in the absence of acid the enzymes are not effective and when sufficient acid is placed in the stomach the enzymes appear there.

In 1925, Bastedo reached the following conclusion from a study of the answers to a questionnaire submitted to the members of the American Gastro-enterological Association: "From this report it is seen that among the members of the American Gastro-enterological Association many do not prescribe digestive enzymes at all, while those who do employ such enzymes confine their use almost wholly to cases of demonstrated or believed enzyme deficiency. It is further noticeable that almost all who prescribe them show no great enthusiasm over the results of their use, except possibly in the case of pancreatin in proved pancreatic deficiency. The conclusion is therefore inevitable that they are of minor importance in therapeutics."

5. ATONY

Atony is characterized by a loss of muscular tone, so that the stomach fails to empty itself in the usual time and finally becomes more or less chronically dilated. The victims of this condition are usually nervous individuals who habitually eat inordinate amounts of difficultly digestible foods and drink large quantities of fluids—until the gastric upset occurs, after which they often attempt to subsist on little more than starvation rations. The most common subjective symptom is a feeling of fulness that appears long before the hunger has been satisfied; nausea, eructations, headache and dizziness also frequently occur, but actual pain and vomiting are rare. A characteristic symptom is that food is tasted long after it is eaten. Gastric analysis shows food remnants seven hours or more after a meal, and on roentgenographical examination the stomach is found to be dilated and its peristaltic action impaired.

Therapy.—Read the treatment of nervous indigestion, page 404; indeed, there is little more to do for these patients than to attempt to apply that treatment. The diet should be restricted to easily digestible foods to be taken in small amounts six times a day rather than in three large meals. If either hyperacidity or, what is more usual, hypo-acidity exists it should be corrected as outlined in the discussion of these two entities. The use of strychnine, so long recommended, has never been shown to have any value.

6. INTESTINAL FERMENTATION

The patient troubled with intestinal fermentative dyspepsia complains of distention with gas, abdominal discomfort and pain, and the daily passage of several liquid or semisolid stools accompanied with much gas. The stools are quite acid and show evidence of a marked impairment of starch digestion but a quite normal digestion of fats and proteins; at times there is also an overabundance of fermentative organisms present. The patients are usually otherwise in good health, except for the stigmata of neurasthenia, and are not infrequently asymptomatic for long periods.

Therapy.—Read the treatment of nervous indigestion, page 404.

Occasionally these patients are able to identify the particular food which causes their trouble, and when this is eliminated from their diet they remain free from attacks. In all cases a radical dietary readjustment is necessary to bring about improvement and cure. The diet suitable under the conditions which obtain here is one rich in protein and fat and poor in carbohydrate; indeed, a diet similar to that employed in diabetes mellitus, excepting that vegetables rich in cellulose must also be avoided or at least selected with care—of course the object must be to build back gradually toward a full and normal dietary.

Bacillus Acidophilus.—Attempt is sometimes made in these cases to overcome the excessive fermentation by implanting *Bacillus acidophilus* in the colon. This matter is fully discussed under the treatment of constipation, see page 439.

Intestinal Antiseptics.—The so-called "intestinal antiseptics," salol, betanaphthol, zinc phenosulphonate (zinc sulphocarbonate), etc., are of no value here. However, the decrease in the urinary indoxyl sometimes following the administration of a full dose of calomel indicates that this drug has some antiseptic properties; the recent laboratory investigations of Von Oettingen and Sollmann also point in this direction. It should be given in a dose of 2 to 3 grains (0.13 to 0.2 Gm.) upon retiring, to be followed by a saline in the morning; such therapy may be repeated once or twice a month for long periods.

Carminatives.—The carminative drugs are those which promote the expulsion of gas without in themselves acting as cathartics. They have long been scoffed at by certain therapeutic nihilists, but I believe that many practitioners of long and unprejudiced experience—*i. e.*, the gentlemen who have sponsored more than one empirical remedy that has since been rationalized by scientific experimentation—have considerable faith in their virtues. This group of drugs, whose worth, by the bye, has recently been attested by the careful studies of Plant and Miller (1926), comprises alcohol, capsicum, cardamon, cloves, ginger, mustard, and the volatile oils generally. A very satisfactory carminative prescription is the following:

℞.			
	Tincture of capsicum	℥ss	2.0
	Spirits of peppermint	℥ij	8.0
	Tincture of ginger	℥ij	60.0
	Alcohol to make	℥iv	120.0

Label: One teaspoonful well diluted every half hour until relieved.

GASTRITIS

Acute gastritis is a not infrequent accompaniment of the acute infectious diseases and is one of the outstanding symptoms of poisoning with such substances as the metals, alcohol, acids, alkalis, etc. For the management of this condition reference must be had to these subjects as they are discussed elsewhere in the book; chronic gastritis, however, requires to be separately considered.

Chronic gastritis is caused by persistent overeating, by the prolonged ingestion of foods that are digested only with great difficulty, or are taken too hot or too cold, or by the habitual gobbling of all meals; or by the excessive indulgence in tobacco or alcohol, especially the latter; or by the prolonged taking of such drugs as the iodides, copaiba, etc. It also occurs as a symptom of ulcer and carcinoma, and may be associated with such diseases as leukemia, pernicious anemia, nephritis, tuberculosis, and other constitutional diseases. Heart, kidney and liver affections cause passive congestion of the stomach mucosa and ultimately chronic gastritis. Whatever the cause of the condition, there is always a gradual destruction of the glandular apparatus, though this may be preceded by a period of hyperactivity.

The symptoms are variegated and are such as may occur in any of the dyspepsias. Diagnosis is often difficult, but early morning vomiting of mucus and the finding of large quantities of gastric mucus in the stomach after a test meal, or after a short period of fasting, are very suggestive symptoms.

THERAPY

Diet.—Dietary treatment is essential in these cases. Of course the offending food or drink, if it can be identified, must be absolutely eliminated, and then a very simple dietary regimen must be instituted with the hope of gradually bringing the patient back on to a full and normal diet. A. A. Jones lists the following articles which are usually well borne:

"The foods to be chosen are good milk, thoroughly cooked cereals without husks, milk and eggs, milk and cereal mixtures, malted milk, milk toast, soft boiled, soft poached, soft scrambled eggs, custards (baked and boiled), rice and milk, thoroughly cooked tapioca and sago, light bread, toast and zwieback, crisp light rolls. Clear soups and purées, clam broth, oyster soup, and chicken broth with toasted water crackers may also be allowed. Buttermilk, if well prepared and well kept, and light delicate cottage cheese may be given. Tender meats, preferably ground, fiber and gristle free, or finely minced are advisable. Tender fowl, fresh whitefish, perch, bass, trout, shad, halibut or salmon may be permitted. Bread pudding, rice pudding, blanc mange, light plain cookies, angel cake, sunshine cake, sponge cake, fresh fruit juices, and fruit jellies are permitted. Weak, freshly made English breakfast tea may be taken in moderation. A small quantity of good, mild, freshly prepared coffee is not harmful."

Lavage.—Lavage is very helpful, especially in the beginning of treatment. One to 2 teaspoonfuls of sodium bicarbonate to the quart of water should be used and the washing should be thoroughly done, *i. e.*, persisted in until the fluid comes away absolutely clear; at the end a pint of distilled water should be run in and out. Depending upon the severity of the case, lavage should be practiced morning and evening, or only in the morning, or only two or three times a week.

Drugs.—The use of drugs must depend entirely upon the nature of the symptoms and the findings after a test meal. The treatment of hyperacidity is discussed on page 409 and hypo-acidity on page 410.

PEPTIC ULCER

(Gastric and Duodenal Ulcer)

Gastric and duodenal ulcer are sufficiently alike in their symptoms and treatment that they may be conveniently discussed under the title "peptic ulcer." Gastric ulcer occurs nearly always at a distance of 2 inches or more from the pylorus, and a duodenal ulcer is usually located ½ inch or more away from the landmarks which divide the stomach and duodenum; pyloric ulcer is very rare. It is thought that multiple ulceration occurs in between 20 and 30 per cent of cases. Ulcer incidence is highest in women between twenty and thirty and in men between thirty and fifty; however, it may occur in the infant a few days old or in the centenarian. The vast majority of peptic ulcers occur in the duodenum of the male sex.

The outstanding and characteristic features of peptic ulcer are (a) that the patient is usually actively engaged in the affairs of life, has a normal appetite and is not undernourished, (b) the history is usually of a chronic gastric disturbance of several years' standing, during which time there have been numerous periods without symptoms, (c) there is epigastric pain and tenderness which is extremely variable but not often excruciating and usually not of a radiating type, (d) this pain bears a definite relationship to food intake, which has been described by Moynihan as follows: "In case of gastric ulcer, the pain which, after an interval, follows the taking of a meal, gradually disappears before the next meal. In cases of duodenal ulcer, the pain continues until the next meal, or until food is taken to give ease to a wearisome pain. The rhythm of gastric ulcer is 'food, comfort, pain, comfort'; and then again 'food, comfort, pain, comfort'; of duodenal ulcer it is 'food, comfort, pain'; and then again 'food, comfort, pain'; a quadruple rhythm in the former disease, a triple rhythm in the latter." The location of the pain to the right or left of the midline is probably of no significance in differentiating between gastric and duodenal ulcer. Posture has usually a definite effect upon the pain. Not all cases of peptic ulcer are as easy to diagnose as this very brief description would seem to indicate; indeed, there are many patients with such a multiplicity of dyspeptic symptoms that diagnosis is extremely difficult; in others, again, nocturnal epigastric pain may be the only symptom. Thanks largely to the indefatigable efforts of the late Russell Carman, who himself suffered the ironic fate of an early death from gastric carcinoma, the x-ray has come to play a prominent part in the diagnosis of peptic ulcer. The various motor meals, designed to test the motor sufficiency of the stomach, also yield valuable information at times. Secretory tests are helpful only when they show the presence of hyperacidity; 40 to 50 per cent of ulcer patients show hyperacidity, 20 per cent hypo-acidity, and the remainder is normal. The occult blood test is a very valuable diagnostic aid, for occult blood is unquestionably present at some time in the feces of the great majority of ulcer patients.

Severe hemorrhage and perforation are the two most feared complications of peptic ulcer; the former occurs in perhaps 15 per cent and the latter in from 2 to 5 per cent of clinically recognized cases—I say "clinically recognized" advisedly, for it is the opinion of many physicians that a goodly number of peptic ulcers give rise to only very slight and transient symptoms and are therefore never diagnosed at all.

In the matter of etiology, practically all students of the disease are agreed that the presence of gastric juice, with its ability to digest devitalized tissue, is of foremost importance since ulcer practically never occurs in the entire absence of juice. Also it is granted that, for this digestion to take place, there must exist in the beginning an area of lowered resistance; but as to what brings about this lowering of resistance, there is much dispute. There are many who contend that a general poor nutrition, especially anemia, is of primary importance, and they cite the great increase in ulcer which followed upon the food blockade of the Central Powers during the World War. It is of interest in this connection to note Smith and Mc-Conkey's (1933) production of ulcer in 26 per cent of their guinea-pigs fed a diet deficient in vitamin C, and the prevention of ulcer in all but one instance when this diet was properly supplemented by C, in the controls; Selinger (1932) has also shown an astonishingly high incidence of ulcer—particularly gastric—in infants who have some constitutional disease, especially marasmus. Others again hold that excessive nervous strain and worry cause gastro-intestinal alterations which are in the beginning purely functional, and they also cite the Central Powers statistics; with this position I think most practitioners are at least in partial agreement, for whatever other etiologic factors may obtain it is certain that the ulcer patient is very often nervously and temperamentally unbalanced. A third group would have it that trauma, whether caused by alcohol, tobacco, too hot or too cold foods, or otherwise faulty diets, is the principal offending agent—and they, too, would have cut the World War figures, claiming that the diet in central Europe during the blockade was both too coarse and too difficultly digestible to pass through the upper tract and leave it unharmed. Unfortunately, animal experimentation has been able to throw very little light upon the subject as yet, for it appears that experimental ulcer is so easily produced, and by so many and diverse methods, that direct correlation between these induced ulcers and the spontaneous ulcers of man cannot be made. The work of Kohler, in 1923, strongly suggested that there was present in ulcer cases a decline in "antipepsin" in the blood serum and the gastric secretion, but Hilarowicz and Mozolowski, and, independently, Orator, have failed to confirm the findings. Rosenow believes that the primary cause of peptic ulcer is focal infection in some such remote place as the teeth, the tonsils, the appendix or the gallbladder. It would seem that Reeves has shown that the ulcer-bearing areas of the stomach and duodenum are especially liable to attack by infection because of peculiarities in their blood supply. Many investigators regard Rosenow's theory as already proved. Nakamura would even thus account for the ulcers that occur along the line of closure following gastro-enterostomy, a form of ulceration now generally attributed to suture material. Macrae, in England, has gone so far as to say that "ulcer in either stomach or duodenum is always due to infection from other parts of the body." But the majority of those who have given much thought to the subject—and every member of the profession should be vitally interested in this question!—are still inclined to look upon focal infection as only a part of the etiologic complex. Thus Alvarez, regarding the routine treatment of all patients with ulcer by removing tonsils and dead teeth: "Although striking results occasionally seem to be obtained in this way, and although on general principles the eradication of focal infection is a good thing, until there are statistics to prove that patients so treated do better than others, I do not think this point should be insisted on, especially when it means that a young man or woman will thereby be condemned to the wearing of plates. I would refuse to treat a man if he wanted to go on swallowing pus every day from pyorrhea pockets and carious snags, but in the present state of our knowledge I should not feel justified in promising him any improvement from the removal of dead teeth. I should want him to know that it was a gamble, with the odds probably against him." Von Redwitz (1927) called attention to the fact that, though peptic ulcer at times seems to be an entity, it is in many cases only part of what may be called an ulcer sickness or ulcer tendency, in which case its presence is attributable to a constitutional basis, and recurrence is likely to take place in spite of either medical or surgical treatment; many recent observations have lent strong support to this view.

Undoubtedly carcinoma may develop on top of a chronic ulcer, but recent studies indicate that the occurrence is relatively infrequent. Unfortunately, there seem to be no reliable criteria by which malignancy or nonmalignancy can be determined in a given case until the tissue is subjected to microscopical examination; in 200 proved benign cases reviewed by Bueermann (1930) at the Mayo Clinic, suspicion of malignancy had arisen in the minds of clinician, roentgenologist or surgeon in 34 per cent of instances, and even with the lesion exposed the surgeon diagnosed a carcinomatous ulcer in 12 per cent of the cases.

THERAPY

The treatment of peptic ulcer must be divided for purposes of precise presentation into the following topics: (*a*) Medical *versus* surgical treatment. (*b*) Types of medical treatment. (*c*) Treatment of hemorrhage (*d*) Treatment of perforation.

(*a*) **Medical Versus Surgical Treatment.**—The opinion expressed by Arthur Dean Bevan, himself a most distinguished surgeon, in 1922, has now come to be the opinion of all save a relatively small number of surgical enthusiasts:

"If I attempt to put the question of the medical and surgical treatment of ulcer in figures, I should do so in about this way: Almost all ulcers in their early history should be treated medically. When they persist under good medical management, when they recur in spite of good medical management and the care which the patient can obtain in his or her peculiar station of life, when serious and repeated hemorrhages occur, when pyloric obstruction does not yield to good medical management, when there is a reasonable suspicion of malignancy, in all of these cases medical management should not be too long persisted in but should give way to exploration and surgical therapy as the safer plan and the plan which affords the better prospect of cure. Numerically, I believe that these cases demanding surgical treatment for their best interests would constitute about 10 per cent of the ulcers of the chronic type."

However, an interpretation of the above is necessary with regard to the matter of recurrence. Jordan and Kiefer's (1932) careful studies of the material at the Lahey Clinic show that 46 per cent of patients treated medically may expect one or more recurrences within five years. Many of these are of only short duration, some are due to carelessness on the part of the patient, and some to excessive smoking—but recurrences "in spite of good medical management" (see above) they are, though they by no means in all instances, or even in a large proportion of them, call for surgical intervention.

It is of tremendous importance to note that in Jordan and Kiefer's series, recurrence occurred within five years in 48 per cent of the surgically handled cases, so that the figures stand about even: medical, 46 per cent; surgical, 48 per cent.

(*b*) **Types of Medical Treatment.**—1. *Sippy* (*Bed Rest and Alkalis*).— The principle of this treatment is to keep the patient in bed and to maintain what are considered to be ideal conditions for the healing of the ulcer by the use of frequent small feedings and sufficient alkalis to maintain the gastric juice practically neutral in reaction between 7 A. M. and 10.30 P. M. In cases attended during the first few days by copious secretion during the night, this is removed by aspiration two or three times each night until such time as the amount of juice present in the stomach during the night does not exceed 10 cc.

"Briefly stated, the patient remains in bed for from three to four weeks. Unless some serious complication is present, some or all of his regular work may be done at the end of four or five weeks. A wide variety of soft and palatable foods may be given. The following plan of diet has been found most adaptable: Three ounces of a mixture of equal parts milk and cream are given every hour from 7 A. M. to 7 P. M., after two or three days soft eggs and well-cooked cereals are gradually added, until at the end of about ten days the patient is receiving approximately the following nourishment: 3 ounces of the milk and cream mixture every hour from 7 A. M. to 7 P. M. In addition, three soft eggs, one at a time, and 9 ounces of a cereal, 3 ounces at one feeding, may be given each day. The cereal is measured after it is prepared.

"Cream soups of various kinds, vegetable purées and other soft foods, may be substituted now and then, as desired. The total bulk at any one feeding while food is taken every hour should not exceed 6 ounces. Many of the feedings will not equal that quantity. The patient should be weighed. If desired, a sufficient quantity of food may be given to cause a gain of 2 or 3 pounds each week.

"A large variety of soft and palatable foods may be used, such as jellies, marmalades, custards, creams, etc. The basis of the diet, however, should be milk, cream, eggs, cereals and vegetable purées. Lean meat is not given during the period of accurate observation, since it interferes with the tests for occult blood in the stool and aspirated stomach contents.

"The acidity is more easily controlled by feeding every hour and giving the alkalis midway between feedings. The acidity may, however, be controlled by feeding every two, three and four hours. I have maintained complete control of the free hydrochloric acidity in several cases by feeding three times daily. In most cases, however, the plan of feeding every hour is best. . . . and giving a powder containing 10 grains each of heavy calcined magnesia [the heavy magnesium oxide of the U.S.P.] and sodium bicarbonate, alternating with a powder containing 10 grains of bismuth subcarbonate and 20 or 30 grains of sodium bicarbonate, midway between feedings [at another time Sippy recommended 10 grains of calcium carbonate in place of the bismuth subcarbonate in this second powder—H.B.]. Cases of pyloric and duodenal ulcer that have been associated with stagnation of food and secretion longer than two months almost invariably require larger quantities of alkalis.

"Heavy calcined magnesia has approximately four times the neutralizing power of sodium bicarbonate. Since its neutralizing effect is prolonged compared with that of sodium bicarbonate, and for other reasons, calcined magnesia should be used between as many feedings as possible. An uncomfortable diarrhea usually prevents its exclusive use as a neutralizer. In a few cases of duodenal ulcer with high-grade obstruction it has required the equivalent of 100 grains of sodium bicarbonate every hour, midway between feedings, and three doses with intervals of one-half hour after the last feeding, at 7 or 8 P. M., to neutralize all the free hydrochloric acidity.

"The average length of time that a patient with peptic ulcer should be under the accurate control and observation of the physician is about four weeks. During this period, if observations have been carefully and intelligently conducted, the finer points essential to a complete diagnosis of peptic ulcer, including such conditions and complications that may attend the ulcer, will have been determined, and the patient will have learned how to manage himself accurately. Thus the gratifying results to be obtained by the management advocated are secured."

Alkalosis as an Accompaniment of the Sippy Treatment.—According to the accepted standards for an ideal antacid (*i. e.,* that it is insoluble, does not irritate the stomach and intestines, is neutral in aqueous suspension but capable of neutralizing acid, does not unduly alter the acid-base equilibrium in the body, when taken in any reasonable amount will not alkalize the urine with the attendant danger of precipitating crystalline phosphates in the kidney or ureter, will not cause diarrhea or constipation, and will not seriously alter the mineral metabolism), sodium bicarbonate is far from satisfactory. It is soluble in water; it is irritating in high concentrations; it is absorbed and produces alkalosis when taken in excess; and it alkalizes the urine and occasionally causes the precipitation of crystalline phosphates in the pelvis of the kidney, the ureter or bladder. Lockwood and Chamberlin have reported that sodium bicarbonate in about one half the patients examined caused a rebound in gastric acidity to a point higher than would have been attained had the alkali not been administered. Schrijver has noted a tendency to the formation of renal calculi under the Sippy treatment; and the development of alkalosis in Sippy-treated patients has been reported by a number of observers: Gatewood, Gaebler, Muntwyler and Myers; Jordan; Kast, Myers and Schmitz; Hardt and Rivers; Bockus and Bank; and Rafsky, Schwartz and Kruger. The symptoms of alkalosis most often noted are headache, aversion to food, dry mouth, excessive thirst, lassitude, nausea and sometimes vomiting. With some patients these symptoms appear soon after beginning the alkalis, with others later on. At times they pass away in a few days even though the alkalis are continued in the same amounts, indicating, perhaps, that the organism makes some sort of compensatory adjustment in these cases. Again, the toxic symptoms become so pronounced and persistent that the alkalis have to be stopped for a few days, and sometimes the symptoms return as soon as the alkalis are resumed, so that they have to be abandoned at least in quantities sufficient to continuously neutralize the free hydrochloric acid. Rafsky et al. (1932) have reported a successful attempt, in 61 cases with adequate controls, to build up a tolerance for alkalis, as follows: Daily doses of 50 grains (3.3 Gm.) sodium bicarbonate, 20 grains (1.3 Gm.) calcium carbonate and 12 grains (0.8 Gm.) magnesium oxide, gradually increased by the end of the second week to 160 grains (10.6 Gm.), 35 grains (2.3 Gm.) and from 12 to 20 grains (0.8 to 1.3 Gm.) respectively. In absence of clinical or biochemical evidence of alkalosis, the dosage was further increased until there was a complete cessation of symptoms, for which the average maximum dose necessary was 315 grains (21 Gm.) sodium bicarbonate, 60 grains (4 Gm.) calcium carbonate and from 12 to 35 grains (0.8 to 2.3 Gm.) magnesium oxide.

  Substitutes for Sodium Bicarbonate in the Sippy Treatment.—(a) *Tricalcium Phosphate and Trimagnesium Phosphate.*—Kantor (1923) writes as follows: "The calcium salts being slightly constipating, and the magnesium being laxative in action, the tendency of the patient either to constipation or to diarrhea was used as a guide to the choice of the appropriate drug in the particular case. The dose of either compound was from ⅓ to 2 teaspoonfuls (1 to 6 Gm.) three times a day after meals. No ill results have been observed, nor, indeed, do they seem possible since, in addition to their action on gastric juice and on the bowels, these drugs have no known effect on the economy, it having been definitely shown that they are not excreted through the urine. The salts are tasteless, and may be administered in bulk or in capsules, as preferred. Care should be taken that the neutral (tasteless) and not the acid (sour) phosphates be dispensed by the druggist." Shattuck, Rohdenburg and Booher (1924) write: "The amounts required varied from the equivalent of about 10 grains (0.65 Gm.) each of magnesium phosphate and calcium phosphate every hour, to 25 grains (1.6 Gm.) of each every hour, the average being about 15 grains (1 Gm.) of each every hour. In all cases the urine remained acid. Thus far no toxic symptoms have appeared even when the phosphates were increased to 40 grains (2.6 Gm.) of each every hour. Studies of the urine, blood pressure, and phenolsulphonephthalein excretion have shown no abnormalities arising during the administration of phosphates. For the most part, the phosphates gave the same symptomatic relief as the alkalis to ulcer patients, although in some instances they did not. When they did not give complete relief, alkalis were given for short periods, and later on the phosphates were resumed with satisfactory results. . . . Perhaps it will develop, with greater experience, that the alkalis now commonly used should continue to be used in the usual case, the phosphates being reserved for those patients showing toxic symptoms, alkalosis, etc., with the alkalis, and for patients with damaged liver or kidneys." Kantor, writing again in 1927, says: "My own impression is that although there is a limited field of usefulness for the neutral antacids, they are not sufficiently powerful to displace entirely the alkaline salts in the great majority of cases during the period of active symptoms."

(*b*) *Calcium Carbonate.*—Loevenhart and Crandall (1927) described calcium carbonate administered alone as the ideal antacid for the following reasons: "(1) When suspended in water it is neutral in reaction. (2) It is therefore only a 'potential' alkali, but it neutralizes the gastric acid, forming calcium chloride and carbon dioxide. (3) It can be given almost *ad libitum*. If an excess is taken, it passes out in the feces. (4) It apparently has no effect on the bowel except that, if taken in excess, it increases the bulk of the stool. (5) When taken in excess it will coat over ulcerated areas and may in this manner protect them from the action of irritants." This drug has been in the U.S.P. as Creta Praeparata since the first edition in 1820, but its failure to win popularity as a remedy is probably due to the fact, according to these observers, that it has been offered for sale only as a powder, and if taken into the mouth dry it is easily inhaled, causing coughing. "At our request Hynson, Westcott and Dunning made compressed tablets of calcium carbonate which readily disintegrate in water. The tablets contain 0.7 Gm. of calcium carbonate (10 grains) and 0.0017 cc. ($\frac{1}{40}$ minim) of oil of cinnamon." The cinnamon acts both as a flavoring and a carminative agent.

2. *Alvarez (Ambulatory with Frequent Feedings).*—While admitting that the Sippy treatment is often effective, Alvarez has the following objections to make: (*a*) It requires more training, enthusiasm and faith in this particular type of treatment than can be expected from the average busy practitioner; (*b*) it requires an expensive month in hospital, (*c*) only a very few patients can be expected to come back to the hospital for subsequent Sippy treatments for each recurrence; (*d*) the lack of evidence that the period of relief after a Sippy cure is longer than after little or no treatment; (*e*) the observation that frequent feeding is perhaps the most valuable item in the cure; (*f*) and the fact that, "whether the profession likes it or not," most patients with ulcer will continue to try to worry through their attacks and keep at their work.

In view of the above considerations, Alvarez champions a simple form of ambulant-frequent feeding treatment that has the best prospect of being practicable for the average physician and the average patient.

"If the patients are to stay at work, they must have three good meals a day. Many of them are thin and below par, and any treatment that keeps them that way is undesirable. The three meals are chosen from a 'smooth-diet' list [see p. 406 of this book—H. B.] which is given to them. This is an ample diet in which only the scratchy material, such as is found in raw fruit, bran, many of the green vegetables, celery, salads, nuts, gristle, and berries, is excluded. Such care may perhaps not be necessary, but there is no privation about it, and theoretically it would seem worth taking. Meat is not forbidden as the patients seem to do just as well with as without it, and from a theoretical standpoint one can argue just as well for as against it.

"The essential element of the treatment is the food between meals. In the morning a mixture should be made up which may consist of a quart of milk, two eggs and either a gill or half pint of cream, depending on the patient's need for extra calories. If milk is not well tolerated, a certain amount of thin gruel made from any cereal may be substituted. Robinson's Scotch groats or Robinson's barley flour is very suitable. The patient takes a bottle of this mixture to work with him and drinks a glassful, about 6 ounces, at 10 A. M., and at 2, 4, 8 and 10 P. M. He should have another glassful by his bed in case he should wake during the night. There does not seem to be any theoretical or practical reason for icing it. He takes his breakfast at 7.30 A. M., lunch at 12 M., and dinner at 6 P. M. If he should be traveling or if he should forget to take his bottle with him, he can get a milk-shake or malted milk at a soda fountain. He may also carry around with him a box of crackers of some kind.

"Occasionally I have found cases in which, in addition to the diet, the usual mixture of magnesia, sodium bicarbonate and bismuth was helpful, but in the last thirteen years I have not prescribed it more than five or six times. Much can be said for the theory of alkalization, but the fact remains that in all those years my results with frequent feedings were so satisfactory that rarely did the patients feel the need of going back to their soda.

"In some cases the pain will recur within an hour and a half, and the food must then be taken every hour and a quarter. In my experience, however, cases as severe as this do not do well on medical treatment. In practically all uncomplicated cases the patient gets immediate relief from his distress and begins to gain in weight and strength. He is asked to rest as much as possible on Saturdays and Sundays, and he is forbidden to do any lifting or gardening. He must give up his 'daily dozen' and he probably had better give up his golf. Walking is about the only exercise that is allowable. . . . My experience on this point makes me feel that not enough attention is paid to the dangers of exercise and especially of the movements that cause pulling on the duodenum. One must remember that the first portion of the duodenum serves as a sort of hook from which the stomach swings like a hammock, and I believe that this anatomic arrangement has something to do with the tendency toward ulceration at that point. Men often say that it is the hard work in spring or fall, plowing or pitching hay, which brings their recurrences; and I have seen a number of cases in which, even after operation, the patient could stay well only by avoiding lifting and bending. In fact many persons can obtain permanent relief only by changing to a sedentary occupation.

"He is now comfortable; perhaps he feels that he is cured, and the next question is, how long must he keep up this regimen? I always insist that he keep it up for six months or a year. I think that one of the big advantages of the ambulant treatment is the fact that the patient is started out on a regimen which he can carry on for months. He is advised from the first that he must continue it for a long time, and he therefore has no illusions about a speedy cure. . . . I think it wise for these patients to take food at 9 or 10 A. M. and at 3 or 4 P. M. for months and years after they are apparently cured. I say 'apparently' because I do not know whether a patient with chronic duodenal ulcer is ever permanently cured by medical treatment. Many have relief from pain and indigestion just so long as they persist in being very careful. They cannot exercise as they did before; they cannot drink, they cannot smoke, and they finally get sick and tired of being semi-invalids. They want to be perfectly well and care-free again, and sooner or later they ask for an operation."

3. *Smithies (Physiologic Rest)*.—The plan of treatment with which Smithies has been reporting continuous good results since 1916 is radically opposed to the Sippy method in that it eliminates the use of alkalis and frequent gastric lavage, for which measures an attempt to give the stomach absolute rest is substituted. From the Alvarez treatment it does not perhaps depart so widely as would at first seem apparent, for, after the preliminary period of rectal feeding and bed rest, the most outstanding feature of the Smithies regimen is that the patient is frequently fed.

"*Days 1 to 7* (time varies according to ulcer location, type, and visceral irritation).— The patient begins treatment as a bed patient.

"Feeding: By mouth, ½ ounce (15 cc.) of warm water hourly when awake. Patient chews paraffin wax for fifteen minutes at least once in two hours. Juice of sweet orange or grapefruit occasionally.

"By rectum, nutrient enema consisting of 50 per cent alcohol, 1 ounce; glucose syrup, 1 ounce, and physiologic sodium chloride solution, 6 ounces every four hours. The enemas are preceded by a cleansing irrigation of the colon with physiologic sodium chloride solution. They are given at body temperature by the drop method at the rate of from 30 to 60 drops a minute. During the first two days, tincture of opium, 10 minims (0.6 cc.), may be added if pain and spasm are severe.

"*Days 3 to 14* (case of average severity).—By mouth, from 4 to 6 ounces (120 to 180 cc.) of water gruel at a temperature of 100 F. The gruel is taken slowly through a glass tube. Gruels are made from rice, cream of wheat, oatmeal, sago, corn-meal, cauliflower, beans, peas, and boiled onion. They are strained before feeding. Flavoring with coffee, chocolate, vanilla, caramel, etc., renders the cereal gruels palatable and their administration easier. To the vegetable gruels, small quantities of arrow-root or cornstarch are added to secure a thin emulsion.

"Before each feeding, paraffin wax is chewed for five minutes. Warm water or sweet orange or grapefruit juice are allowed as desired, but never taken in greater quantity than 1 ounce (30 cc.) at a time.

"By rectum, during the first two days of mouth feeding, two alcohol-glucose-saline nutrient enemas are given. During the second two days, one such nutrient enema is administered. After the fourth day of mouth feeding, no rectal feedings are given in the average case.

"*Days 14 to 21*.—6.30 A. M.: A glass of hot water and 1 teaspoonful of noneffervescent sodium phosphate.

"7.30 A. M.: One ounce of sweet orange or grapefruit juice, 2 ounces (60 cc.) of thin cream of wheat, or farina, or well-cooked rice, or corn-meal; 2 ounces of skimmed parboiled milk may be taken with cereal, and if desired a small quantity of powdered sugar used; one zwieback with a thin layer of fresh butter, 4 ounces of parboiled, skimmed milk, containing half volume of lime water, served warm and flavored with coffee, cocoa, caramel or vanilla.

"9.30 A. M.: Six ounces (180 cc.) of thin water gruel from cereals or fresh vegetables, strained and served hot; one rusk or zwieback, or dry toast.

"11.30 A. M.: Four ounces of malted milk, whipped egg, with parboiled milk, corn-starch pudding, simple custard lightly cooked.

"12.30 P. M.: Six ounces of potato, pea, bean, or asparagus purée (strained), or vegetable broth; 4 ounces of salisbury steak (moderately well cooked) to chew; 2 ounces (60 Gm., cooked weight) of thin rice, sago, tapioca, or corn-starch pudding made with parboiled milk and egg yolk; 2 ounces of parboiled milk and a small quantity of pulverized sugar may be eaten with the pudding; one rusk or zwieback, 6 ounces of parboiled milk and quarter volume of lime water flavored to taste.

"4 P. M.: Four ounces of water gruel from cereals, one very soft poached egg, one rusk or zwieback, 4 ounces of hot Vichy water.

"6 P. M.: Four ounces of whipped egg, two rusks or zwieback, 6 ounces of malted milk (thin), flavored to taste, or cereal water gruel or parboiled milk and quarter volume of lime-water gruel.

"9 P. M.: Six ounces of water cereal gruel or 4 ounces of malt marrow, two graham crackers.

"*Days 21 to 42*.—6.30 A. M.: Two teaspoonfuls of sodium phosphate in a glass of hot water.

"8 A. M.: Juice of one sweet orange or half sweet grapefruit, or boiled prunes passed through fine colander; 2 ounces (cooked weight) of thin cereals (cream of wheat, farina, oatmeal, corn-meal); 2 ounces of skimmed milk and small amount of powdered sugar; one soft poached egg; either two zwieback, two rusks or two thin slices of well-toasted graham bread; 1 pint of hot skimmed milk plus a quarter volume of lime water flavored to taste (cocoa, vanilla, etc.).

"10 A. M.: One pint of hot parboiled whole milk and fifth volume of lime water; two rusks or graham crackers.

"12.30 P. M.: Four ounces of creamed soup from vegetables, strained; 6 ounces of rare meat to chew; 4 ounces of well-mashed potato or baked potato (mealy inside), or carrot, peas, beans, cauliflower, Brussels sprouts or asparagus (all vegetables passed through a strainer and served with 15 Gm. of butter); 4 ounces (cooked weight) of pudding from rice, corn-starch, sago, tapioca, cream of wheat or farina, or 4 ounces of custard, pulp of sweet orange, grapefruit or prune whip, or chew 6 ounces of watermelon or cantaloup; half pint of hot skimmed milk.

"3.30 P. M.: One hundred and fifty cubic centimeters of hot whole milk and quarter volume of lime water or 150 cc. of malted milk or weak cocoa.

"6.30 P. M.: Two rusks or zwieback or two slices of well-toasted graham bread; two very soft poached eggs; 100 Gm. of sweet apple sauce or one baked apple (omit skins), or juice of sweet orange or half of grapefruit; or chew 6 ounces of melon; 1 pint of skimmed milk, hot.

"9 P. M.: Two hundred and fifty cubic centimeters of whole parboiled milk and quarter volume of lime water or 250 cc. of malted milk, hot.

"*General Diet for Three Months.*—If distress, patient should go back to seven- to twenty-one-day diet.

"7 A. M.: One pint of skimmed milk and half a gill of cream.

"9 A. M.: Two pieces of toast without butter; juice of one sweet orange or grapefruit or ripe melon or apple sauce or baked apple (do not eat skin) or marmalade; one dish of well-cooked cereal (oatmeal, farina or cream of wheat); two very soft poached eggs; 2 cups of hot, sweetened water. The water may be made more palatable by flavoring with cocoa, coffee or cream.

"11 A. M.: One cup of bouillon (two cubes); two graham crackers.

"1 P. M.: This should be the heavy meal of the day. It may consist of meat (rare beef, rare hamburger steak, lamb or white meat of fowl), fish (never fried), oysters, well-cooked spinach, cauliflower, carrots, squash, peas (hulled), string beans, Brussels sprouts, baked or mashed potatoes (in moderation), rice with gravy, simple puddings made from cereals, corn-starch, gelatin, well-cooked fruit sauces, simple cakes, no white bread (all bread should be made from dark flour and should be at least one day old); 1 pint of skimmed milk taken hot.

"4 P. M.: One glass of hot peppermint water (20 drops of 'essence' of peppermint to the glass), sweeten to taste and drink slowly; two graham crackers.

"7 P. M.: A light lunch consisting of vegetable soup, simple salad, toast, soft eggs, and plain puddings or cake, with or without ripe cooked fruit sauces; 1 pint of hot skimmed milk.

"Bedtime, 1 glass of malt marrow, malted milk or hot skimmed milk.

"*Medicinal Management.*—This consists chiefly in the exhibition of antispasmodics (atropine, tincture of belladonna, bromides) to control hyperperistalsis, orificial spasms, pain or nervous unrest. The average patient receives neither alkalis nor lavage."

4. *Jarotzky* (*Milkless Diet with White of Egg and Butter*).—Based on Pavlov's experiments which demonstrated that the first part of ingested milk, in passing from the stomach into the duodenum, provokes a closure of the pylorus with resulting retention for hours of the rest of the milk in the stomach and that milk, moreover, contains a large amount of substances that cause an abundant secretion of gastric juice, Jarotzky has evolved a milkless diet for the treatment of peptic ulcer. To give the stomach the greatest possible amount of rest, whites of eggs without salt and fresh butter are given alternately during the day. The uncooked whites of eggs, owing to their semiliquid consistency and their neutral reaction, pass quickly through the pylorus and into the duodenum; in addition they have the property of fixing the free hydrochloric acid of the gastric juice. Fresh butter suppresses the secretion of gastric juice and accelerates the emptying of the stomach. In order to diminish the gastric secretion in cases of gastric ulcer with hypersecretion, Jarotzky maintains that the food should have a semiliquid consistency and should consist chiefly of starchy substances and fats; the quantity of proteins should be reduced to a minimum and the diet should never contain either milk or easily digested proteins. On the other hand, it is advisable to give these patients vegetable proteins which resist to a marked degree the digestive action of the gastric juice. The patients

should not be allowed to eat foods producing an abundant secretion of gastric juice, such as the yolk of eggs, bouillons, and, in general, meat and vegetable soups; foods containing a mixture of protein and fat (as beaten eggs and fat meats) are likewise not permissible. The use of milk by all patients with ulcer of the stomach or duodenum is strictly forbidden by this school of investigators, of whom Warren Coleman is the foremost representative in the United States. Not only should fresh milk not be allowed, but the addition of milk to gruels or to purées should be prohibited; the patient should not receive a single drop of milk. The regimen is also said to give good results in cases in which the ulcer is accompanied by gastric hyposecretion.

This diet was proposed by Jarotzky in 1910. It is said to be now widely used in Russia, both at the university clinics and in private practice; Kushelevsky reported its use in 155 cases, in 1931. I quote from Jarotzky's 1925 paper, published in English:

"In applying this diet, I have recourse to two other auxiliary remedies in order to lessen the secretion of stomach juice: (1) I restrain as much as possible the introduction of water into the organism of the patient either by mouth or through subcutaneous injection or through lavage. (2) I cease to introduce into the body of the patient any quantity of sodium chloride.

"When I first adopted this method in or immediately after some cases of hemorrhage of the stomach, I introduced no food at all by mouth and fed the patient exclusively by way of nutrient enemas. But later I saw that, among these difficult patients, those who were fed by mouth with white of egg and fresh butter felt much better than those who were not fed by mouth. This is the reason why I give to the patient on the first day of clinical treatment the raw white of one egg in the morning and 20 Gm. of butter in the afternoon, increasing afterward every day the quantity of butter by 20 Gm.; consequently, on the tenth day the patient will take the white of ten eggs, and 180 Gm. of butter. He must swallow the white of every egg at once, as one swallows an oyster, without salt.

"The main peculiarity of this method is the feeding of the patient with white of eggs and butter separately, at different hours of the day. This is based on the experiments of Pavlov and his followers, who showed that while the raw white of egg is not retained in the stomach and passes through, a mixture of albumins and fats, on the contrary, is retained in the stomach for several hours and provokes abundant secretion of the stomach juice.

"The treatment of peptic ulcer during an acute paroxysm of disease is quite simple. The patient must stay in bed; a gradually increasing quantity of white of eggs in the morning and of butter in the afternoon is given to him. He is allowed no other food, drink or medicaments. I do not prescribe this diet to a patient for more than ten days, for it would cause him unnecessary vexation. After ten days of diet the patient may be fed in the morning by a diminished ration of the white of eggs, and in the afternoon by a watery soup with rice, pearl-barley, semolina, etc., and with some butter; butter may also be given separately; afterward a rubbed purée of potatoes and other vegetables (such as carrots and turnips) boiled in water with butter but without salt may be given. Relying on the works of Pavlov and my clinical experience, I forbid during the treatment any use of milk to all patients suffering from peptic ulcer and hyperchlorhydria."

5. *Continuous Alkalinized Milk Drip.*—As the direct opposite of the Jarotzky treatment (see above), Winkelstein (1933) maintains his patients on a continuous drip of alkalinized milk into the stomach. A Rehfuss tube is passed and connected to a gravity flask with a Murphy drip indicator interposed in the system. The solution employed consists of milk heated sufficiently to remove the chill and containing 5 Gm. of sodium bicarbonate

to the quart. This is allowed to drip into the stomach at the rate of 30 drops per minute day and night, the patient thus receiving 3 quarts of milk and 1 ounce (15 Gm.) of sodium bicarbonate in the twenty-four hours. Theoretically such a solution neutralizes 9 quarts N/10 hydrochloride acid. Sedatives are employed, an occasional sip of the mixture is permitted to relieve dryness of the throat (but this is discouraged) and careful watch is of course maintained for symptoms of alkalosis. The patient seems to tolerate the tube very well as a rule. After two or three weeks, the tube is removed during the day and the patient receives bland feedings every hour or two (with alkalis and atropine) from 8 A. M. to 8 P. M. At 8 P. M. the drip is started again. After four weeks a second night fractional test meal is obtained and a roentgenological check-up, after which the treatment is continued according to indications; several patients have continued, after discharge, to take the milk drip on retiring for a period of several months. Winkelstein's series of cases was small but the results obtained were very good.

6. *The Mucin Treatment.*—Fogelson (1931–32) has found that a neutral mucin prepared from the stomach of the pig meets the requirements of an ideal antacid through its high combining power for free acid, its failure to markedly excite gastric secretion, its soothing and protective action, and its failure to disturb the acid-base balance of the body. In dogs, Kim and Ivy (1931) have shown that mucin has protective value since none of the animals with biliary fistula developed the usual spontaneous experimental ulcers when given the substance. In the human, mucin has already come to be much used, but the reader should distinctly understand that it is not proposed as a new *type* of treatment, but only as a substitute for alkalis in any of the usual dietary treatments; Rosenberg and Bloch (1933) feel that perhaps its demulcent action is also of importance. So far the reports are all very satisfactory and it seems certain that mucin can well be substituted for alkalis in most if not all instances; but whether the proportion and rate of "cures" will be any greater only the passage of much time will tell. Brown *et al.* (1932), in preliminary studies, have found mucin therapy to lower the acid level in healing ulcer; in most instances the acidity rises as healing progresses under alkalis.

The usual dose of mucin is ½ ounce (15 Gm.), a rounded tablespoonful, which is given at such intervals as is found necessary in the individual case. Perhaps the most usual practice is to give doses at intervals of two hours from 8 A. M. to 10 P. M., though in some instances it must be given hourly. In Fogelson's 400 cases treated in two years, the average daily dose for three months has been 80 to 100 Gm., decreased one half for the next three months. Cases in which many times this quantity per day have been given are on record.

Tufts (1932) has combined the mucin with milk and cream to lower viscosity and increase palatability. A mucin paste is made with cold water, forced through a sieve, and cream or milk added plus flavors such as chocolate syrup, malted milk or ovaltine. Eggnog has been similarly used as a vehicle. Atkinson (1932) has found that capsules often pass through the stomach undissolved or remain as a mass of mucin which the acid cannot penetrate.

Rivers *et al.* (1932) have obtained a decided histamine-like secretagogue effect with some specimens of mucin, but it is my belief that the manufacturers are now employing chemical and biological tests to eliminate batches containing this contaminant.

7. *The Pepsin Treatment.*—For several years Glaessner, of Vienna, has been treating ulcer by the subcutaneous injection of pepsin, the hypothesis being that it acts as a hormone to stimulate the production of antipepsin—

which does not seem to me to be proved by any means. He and others—Loeper *et al.;* Buylla *et al.;* Hertzer—have independently reported satisfactory results, but since all of the patients have been on most careful dietary treatment as well, it is at least doubtful what part the pepsin played. Glaessner uses a filtered pepsin solution which he believes to be active in ferment content but sterile and free from albumin. Twice a year the patient receives a series of thirty injections: 0.2 cc. either daily or every other day for three injections; then the same with 0.3 cc., and so on up to 0.5 cc.; twelve injections of the 0.5-cc. dose are given and then the same steps are taken in reverse back to 0.2 cc. If anaphylactic symptoms appear, the practice is to drop back to the next lowest dose and then proceed.

8. *Supplementary Medication.*—For a discussion of the use of atropine, opiates, etc., see the treatment of pylorospasm, page 408. Silver nitrate is no longer in good repute with most practitioners, but the following answer to a query appearing in the Journal of the American Medical Association (88, 1438, 1927) indicates that it is still favorably regarded by some authorities; I do not know the name of the author of this reply.

"Silver nitrate is not in vogue as much at present as it once was and as it probably should be. It has two effects in gastric ulcer; first, a possibly direct healing action on the ulcer as obtained from the application of astringents to ulcers elsewhere; and, second, a lessening of the gastric hyperesthesia, which complicates the ulcer and is responsible for most of the symptoms as well as interfering with the healing of the ulcer. An additional protective action has been suggested, that of stimulating the secretion of gastric mucus, which has been proved to occur in dogs after application of 10 per cent silver nitrate solution.

"The following technic is recommended: The stomach tube is passed, preferably in the morning before breakfast, and the stomach is emptied of its contents. Then, after a brief preliminary washing with a weak alkaline solution (1 teaspoonful of sodium bicarbonate to 1 liter of warm water), about 300 cc. of 1:5000 solution of silver nitrate is introduced into the stomach, evacuated after from a few seconds to one minute, and followed by washing with the alkaline solution, which is less likely to irritate the stomach than the sodium chloride solution usually recommended for the purpose.

"This treatment is repeated daily, the strength of the solution being gradually increased to 1:1000. When improvement has become established, the treatments are given on alternate days and finally once a week, the symptoms of the patient being the best guide for regulating the frequency and duration of the treatment. For stubborn or recurrent cases, when the appearance of argyria is feared, zinc sulphate, in the same strength, may be substituted for the silver nitrate. When the stomach tube cannot be passed, the silver nitrate may be given by mouth in teaspoonful doses of a 1:500 solution, three times daily before meals. This treatment cannot, however, be continued for a very long time because of danger of argyria, which is less with lavage, as the excess of silver is promptly removed."

(c) **Treatment of Hemorrhage.**—The indications here are to combat shock, relieve the thirst, prevent digestion of the edges of the exposed blood vessel, promote clot formation, restore the blood volume, and maintain nourishment.

(a) *Shock.*—Morphine should be given hypodermically in practically all cases not only because of its influence in quieting the patient but because it greatly reduces fear, which is a contributing factor of great importance in shock; the later "splinting" effect upon the bowel is unfortunate but cannot be helped.

(b) *Thirst.*—This symptom is combated by protoclysis or hypodermoclysis with saline or Locke's or Ringer's solutions or by the intravenous injection of glucose; the stimulation of gastric motor activity by the injection of fluid into the rectum, whether for cleansing or retention, has not been proved. It is very important that one or more of these methods be employed to avoid dehydration.

(c) *Protect the Bleeding Area.*—A good many years ago Rodman advocated the immediate lavage of the stomach, using the ordinary stomach tube and water somewhat above body temperature. The measure, designed to rid the stomach of clot which acted as a stimulant, has not remained popular, but Soper (1931) has reintroduced a new kind of lavage: The nasal mucosa is shrunk with 2 per cent cocaine hydrochloride, a Levin tube with a tip finished like that of the ordinary soft rubber catheter is passed by that route—slowly to prevent coiling, the patient swallowing water with each advance of the tube—siphonage to a bottle is established, and the stomach thus kept cleaned out. It is felt that the raw surface is protected from corroding gastric juice by this method, and that nausea and vomiting are prevented and the patient kept remarkably comfortable. The hemostatic agents are injected through the tube directly into the stomach and egg albumin and gelatin water are given by the same route. On the third to fifth day the tube is passed on down into the duodenum, intravenous injections of glucose are discontinued, and a high calorie mixture of raw eggs, milk, cream and lactose is fed through the tube. At the meeting in which Soper read his paper there was adverse criticism of his method on the basis of irritation from constant presence of the tube, but as the essayist pointed out, no one criticized who had used the tube.

(d) *Promote Clot Formation.*—Quiet, of both body and stomach, is of course the chief measure here. Morphine is of great help. The ice-bag applied to the epigastrium, a measure staunchly persisted in by many practitioners of experience, may really quiet the stomach in some indirect way but probably is chiefly effective in aiding the patient to lie motionless. Soper (see above) believes that he promotes stomach rest by frequent siphonage; Andresen (see below) would rest it by keeping food in it; Hendon (see p. 164) has kept the stomach completely empty for several weeks by administering glucose continuously by vein.

The introduction of blood coagulants directly into the stomach by Soper has been mentioned above. It is doubtful whether any of these thromboplastic substances, which are made from the brain tissue of animals, are worth anything when injected subcutaneously, and intravenous introduction is probably dangerous; indeed anaphylactic symptoms must be cautiously watched for when injecting under the skin. Nevertheless, worth or not, these substances are usually injected in doses as stated on the package, in all cases even though blood examinations do not show a reduction in clotting capacity of the blood. Serums are also used, though with what success it is not possible to state in any reliable fashion: normal horse or rabbit serum, 10 cc. or more, intramuscularly at intervals of three or four hours for several doses; anaphylaxis is to be forestalled by determining hypersensitiveness by the usual preliminary tests. Human serum or whole blood, 10 cc. or more, is sometimes injected intramuscularly; one argument advanced in favor of transfusion in hemorrhage is the coagulant property of the injected blood.

Calcium given by mouth is probably worthless in combating hemorrhage. Two or three intravenous injections of calcium chloride or gluconate, 5 to 10 cc. of a 10 per cent solution, at four- to six-hour intervals, or the use of parathyroid extract (parathormone-Lilly and Parathyroid hormone-Squibb are the Council-accepted products to which this dosage applies), 15 to 30 units three times repeated at eighteen- to thirty-six-hour intervals.

will develop all that can be expected from this type of therapy, according to Cantarow (1931). Afenil, N.N.R., is a molecular compound of calcium chloride and urea, which is given intravenously; it is claimed that this compound is less irritating than calcium chloride when given into the vein. The contents of one of the commercial ampules is the dose, which may be repeated after a few hours.

Eason (1932) avails himself of the local styptic action of concentrated glucose by having the patient swallow ½ ounce (15 cc.) of 50 per cent solution hourly during the day and at night also during hours of wakefulness.

(e) *Restore Blood Volume.*—The various methods of introducing fluid into the body have been mentioned under the head of *thirst*. Regarding the advisability of immediate blood transfusion, both for increasing the clotting power of the blood and filling out the vessels, there are two schools of thought. Perhaps most physicians fear the injection of more than 150 to 200 cc. for fear the induced rise in blood pressure will blow out the clots. Some scoff at this diffidence, however, and deny the occurrence of such rises; Smithies (1931) often advises as many as four transfusions of at least 500 cc. of blood in twenty-four hours.

(f) *Diet.*—The vast majority of the profession is in favor of keeping all food out of the stomach for several days, employing glucose intravenously either intermittently or by venoclysis, or feeding by rectum. It must be admitted that not much nutriment can be introduced by the latter route, since we are limited to the giving of glucose, peptones and alcohol. The following is a typical formula, the whole of this mixture being injected slowly from the enema can three or more times in the twenty-four hours.

Witte's peptone	25
Alcohol (50 per cent)	25
Glucose	25
Saline solution to make	250 cc.

Andresen maintains that on the basis of Carlson's showing that an empty stomach is never at rest, the stomach should be kept at least partially filled from the beginning with food substance that combines readily with the gastric juice and does not overstimulate its production. He uses a liquid mixture of gelatin 1 part, lactose 3 parts, water 30 parts, plus the juice of one orange. Beginning with 4 to 6 ounces (120 to 180 cc.) of this every one and one-half to two hours, after two or three days he substitutes a soft gruel of cereal 16 parts, milk 14 parts, cream 4 parts, and lactose 3 parts, for alternate gelatin feedings, and through gradual increase in the milk and on the seventh day adding egg and custard, has his patients on full ulcer diet again in nine days without them having been severely denied food in the interim. The method is said to have been succeeding well for a number of years at the Long Island College Hospital.

(d) **Treatment of Perforation.**—Acute perforation demands immediate surgical intervention. Most patients recover who are operated upon within six hours after the perforation has occurred; for each hour after that time the chances of death are greatly increased.

MUCOUS COLITIS

Individuals suffering from chronic mucous colitis are decidedly neurasthenic; they are invariably constipated and may suffer from any of the dyspepsias elsewhere described; they pass considerable quantities of tenacious mucus either as a coating to hardened fecal masses or in large masses alone; and they may or may not have occasional paroxysms of severe abdominal colic followed by the evacuation of these mucous masses. Abdominal tenderness is oftentimes constantly present especially on the left side. Blood in the stool is very rare in uncomplicated cases.

THERAPY

For some reason many physicians have come to believe that any treatment of this condition is unavailing. Nothing could be farther from the truth, for it is many times not only possible to relieve the colitis but in doing so to actually cure the neurosis as well. Bastedo (1920) very justly holds up for ridicule the flippant statement of a speaker before a state medical society who said that "the prognosis is absolutely hopeless, the treatment is *nil*, and the sole prophylaxis would have been to sterilize the grandfather."

Bastedo approaches the treatment as follows: "In determining the method of treatment, two facts stand out prominently: (1) That retained mucus is harmful mucus, and (2) that the cure requires a long course of treatment. I am wont to tell my patients that a year is the minimum time in which a cure can be effected. The treatment is directed at the prevention of the accumulation of mucus, and at the removal of the associated conditions, such as colic, constipation, intestinal toxemia, disturbed gastric conditions, bad mental states and depressed general health."

Constipation.—The treatment of this symptom is that of any form of constipation; for a full discussion, see page 431.

Removal of Mucus.—It is for this purpose that colon irrigations from a height of 2 feet are principally employed, using either a No. 34 French tube, velvet-eyed with a closed end, inserted about 6 inches, and used for both inflow and outflow of the fluid after the colon has been filled to capacity, or employing the two-tube method in which a 20 to 24 French soft rubber velvet-eyed catheter is inserted 6 inches for inflow, and a 30 or 32 French velvet-eyed closed-end rectal tube (or stomach tube) inserted 3 or 4 inches for outflow. The tubes are inserted about fifteen minutes after an evacuation enema of plain water has cleared the rectum and lessened the chances of disturbances from defecation reflexes. Plain water, slightly above body temperature is used, usually 6 to 10 gallons in the course of an hour, the first gallon with the patient on the left side with knees drawn up in order to clean out the lower colon, then for the remainder of the time on the back in order for the fluid to reach the cecum. Saline would make the patient very thirsty, and it is doubtful if the vaunted ability of sodium bicarbonate to dissolve mucus outweighs the disadvantages of its stimulation of the kidneys, disturbance of acid-base balance and tendency to cause gas and colic.

These irrigations are usually employed every day or two for a week, then every three or four days for several weeks longer, and then once a week for as long as considered necessary. Bastedo is well known as champion of the colon irrigation; it is his technic which is described above. However, a great many physicians do not accept the method as rational— Soper (1932) holds that the more one irrigates the more mucus one gets, and that if continued long enough the "foul-smelling material" described by Bastedo can be secured in persons with normal colons, being, in his opinion, the normal contents of the ileum changed by the treatment. Certainly the commercialized irrigation specialist, who gives "internal baths" for all ailments under the sun, should not be encouraged by the medical profession.

Diet.—The diet described in the treatment of nervous indigestion (see p. 406) suffices excellently here, for there is perhaps no class of patients who profit more, at least in the beginning of their treatment, from the removal of excess "roughage" from the diet. Indeed, these patients should be treated in all particulars as is the nervous dyspeptic.

Treatment of the Attacks of Colic.—Morphine is of course contraindicated here because of the frequent recurrence of the attacks. Bastedo finds that castor oil by mouth and a hypodermic of codeine phosphate, ½ grain (0.03 Gm.), and atropine sulphate, 1⁄65 grain (0.001 Gm.), plus hot applications to the abdomen in the form of a hot-water bag, electric pad, poultice or stupe (method on p. 131), or a hot bath, will be followed by relief and sleep in most instances. If this fails, however, he irrigates, and, if relief is still not obtained, puts the patient in the knee-chest position and slowly injects into the colon ½ to 1 pint (250 to 500 cc.) of warm olive or cotton seed oil, the injection often being followed after a few hours by the passage of an abundance of mucus and the disappearance of the colic.

Nonspecific Proteins.—Rafsky (1931) has had some success with this type of therapy (methods on p. 327), which would seem also the basis upon which to account for the responses sometimes had by Mateer and Baltz (1932) with autogenous vaccines made from the stools.

ULCERATIVE COLITIS

Nonspecific chronic ulcerative colitis is characterized by a chronic inflammation of the mucous membrane and walls of the large intestine, in the pathologic picture of which ulceration predominates. The ulceration usually begins in the rectum and spreads upward eventually to involve the entire colon. It may, however, affect any one part, or several separated parts, of the tube. The course is in most cases a chronic one, extending over months and years, but the symptoms are not usually continuous during this time for there are often long periods of remission between severe attacks of the malady. The symptoms are fever, malaise, prostration, protracted and persistent diarrhea with some tenesmus, and the passage of blood, mucus and pus. Distress from gas, and griping and other sensations along the course of the colon, are often experienced. Much weight is lost, a peculiar gray pallor is common, and varying degrees of anemia exist. In the very severe cases, the body has a peculiar odor and the face a hopeless expression. Bargen, of the Mayo Clinic, has described a diplostreptococcus of definite morphological, cultural and biological properties as the causative agent in the disease, but gastro-enterologists are not unanimously in agreement with him. Many observers hold with Hurst, in England, and Crohn, in this country, who believe that ulcerative colitis is a form of chronic bacillary dysentery. The recent studies of Buttiaux and Sévin (1931), in Lille, indicate that certain organisms ordinarily regarded as saprophytic—such as *Bacillus coli*—may under some circumstances have their virulence enhanced. The rôle of *Endamoeba histolytica* and *Balantidium coli* must also not be overlooked.

THERAPY

Colic.—During the course of a severe attack, hot stupes applied to the abdomen, according to the method described on page 131, often bring relief; morphine, ⅛ to ¼ grain (0.008 to 0.015 Gm.) or, preferably, codeine, 1 grain (0.065 Gm.) may be needed.

Diarrhea.—In all cases some attempt must be made to control the diarrhea, though it is a fact that such success as rewards these efforts is nearly always only temporary. The following drugs are usually tried out in succession:

Bismuth subcarbonate, 20 to 30 grains (1.5 to 2 Gm.) every three hours.

Bismuth betanaphthol, 10 grains (0.6 Gm.) every four hours.

Calcium carbonate, 15 to 30 grains (1 to 2 Gm.) every four hours.

Calcium glycerophosphate, 10 to 15 grains (0.6 to 1 Gm.) every four hours.

Acetyltannic acid (Tannigen), 3 to 10 grains (0.2 to 0.6 Gm.) every four hours.

Protan, 20 to 30 grains (1.3 to 2 Gm.) every two hours.

Local Applications.—Attempt is often made, by means of antiseptic enemas or topical applications, to bring about healing of the ulcers. On this head I shall repeat here what was written on page 61 when discussing the treatment of bacillary dysentery: The silver salts are principally used locally: an enema of 500 cc. of 1:100 argyrol (mild silver protein) solution, or 1:500 protargol (strong silver protein). Copper sulphate is frequently used in 0.5 per cent strength, or 2 per cent tannic acid solution. These solutions, the silver salts especially, stimulate an acute reaction and a reparative process, but the balance between inflammation and repair is not always easy to strike; they should therefore not be repeated too often. Ten per cent silver nitrate, rarely stronger, may be applied directly to the rectal ulcers.

Diet.—These patients profit by a soft diet from which all excess roughage has been removed; such a diet has been fully described by Alvarez (see p. 406). Larimore (1928) has called attention to the fact that there may also be some degree of avitaminosis in ulcerative colitis. Good results followed the addition of tomato juice and cod liver oil to the diet in 4 of his 5 cases. See also discussion of the apple diet, page 60.

Vaccines and Serum.—Bargen has prepared a vaccine with the organism that he considers causative. In his hands its use has seemed to hasten recovery, and Fradkin and Gray (1930) have also reported satisfactory results; however, bearing in mind the variable course of this disease and the fact that other observers have not equalled these successes, it is perhaps too early to adjudge the value of this treatment. Streicher and Kaplan (1930) report favorably upon the use of an autogenous *polyvalent* vaccine and do not accept the Bargen bacillus as the primary etiologic factor. A serum, prepared by immunization of the horse with the organism which Bargen considers specific, has been used by Bargen, Rosenow and Fasting (1930), apparently with some success. I would remind the reader that good results have been obtained in many diseases by simple nonspecific protein therapy.

Mercurochrome.—In his 1926 report, Young collected 7 cases of ulcerative colitis which were apparently rapidly cured by the intravenous administration of mercurochrome. For the methods of using this drug, see page 163.

Intestinal Oxygenation.—For several years, Felsen (1931) has been studying the effects of altering the gaseous tension in the intestines by the rectal introduction of oxygen. Experience has shown that the average acutely ill adult will tolerate 250 cc. (measured by water displacement as it comes from the tank) given alternate hours between 8 A. M. and 8 P. M. Passage through warm water heats the gas, which is then allowed to enter through an ordinary soft rubber catheter introduced only a few inches. There is moderate distention of the bowel as far as the pylorus, but much of the gas is apparently rapidly absorbed since very little is ejected from the rectum. Felsen believes that this treatment leads to the diminution of spore-bearing anaerobes, encourages the superficial growth of obligatory or facultative aerobes, and favors a homogeneity of intestinal flora; the effect of oxygen on the intestinal tissue proper is even more speculative. Forty cases thus treated, with adequate controls, were apparently much benefited.

Calcium and Parathyroid.—Haskell and Cantarow (1931) have used these drugs with satisfaction in 9 of 10 patients. Calcium lactate, 30 grains (2 Gm.) or calcium gluconate, 60 grains (4 Gm.), orally three or four times daily, three and a half to four hours after meals, the patient being cautioned not to eat between meals; 20 to 30 grains (1.2 to 2 Gm.) of ammonium chloride was given with the calcium salt to increase its utilization by raising the hydrogen ion concentration of the tissues. Parathyroid extract was injected intramuscularly, 20 to 30 units, at intervals of forty-eight to seventy-two hours.

Surgery.—Ileostomy is a life-saving measure in severe cases because it puts the bowel at rest, but it is a confession of defeat in a disease for which we should be able to find some specific or at least systemic remedy, and it does not stop the destructive process in the intestinal wall.

Specific Therapy.—See bacillary dysentery, page 57; flagellate dysentery, page 62; amebic dysentery, page 50.

CONSTIPATION

Most adult individuals have a movement of the bowels once every day, though there are some for whom it seems natural to have a movement only every other day or even every three or four days. It is only when the movements become irregular in their occurrence, or require some artificial aid to bring them about at all, that we can speak of the individual as being constipated. That habitual constipation may cause no detectable symptoms is of course well known, but it is equally true that it may give rise to quite a host of ailments. A partial list of these findings, objective and subjective, has been given by Boles: "In my experience these symptoms in the order of their frequency are lack of endurance, disinclination for work or play, headache, irritability, vertigo, anorexia, flatulence, nausea, mental and physical depression, anxiety or fearfulness, and insomnia. Objectively one may find a coated tongue, fetid breath, sallow complexion with pigmentation below the eyes and in the armpits, anemia, malnutrition, poor circulation as shown by cold hands and feet and low blood pressure, brittle hair and nails, and other cutaneous conditions, such as acne, eczema rubrum and seborrheic eczema, erythema multiforme, purpura, lichen planus, and urticaria. Among the neurologic conditions frequently associated with constipation are neurasthenia, neuroses of various sorts, neuritis, neuralgia, loss of memory and lack of concentration. . . . "

A few earnest scientists have modestly stated their conviction that these symptoms are due to the absorption into the circulation of toxins, this absorption taking place by reason of the fact that more time is allowed for putrefactive changes to take place in the colon and also for the products of these changes to make their way through the mucous membrane. This is the so-called "auto-intoxication" about which unbalanced faddists are howling down the highways and byways with such unremitting gusto nowadays. Such intoxications may take place, but it is much more likely, as suggested by Alvarez, that the symptoms derivable from constipation are entirely due to reflexes engendered by distention of the bowel with retained feces; certainly the very quick relief which often follows upon the emptying of the bowel is much in favor of this belief. However, the whole subject is still *sub judice*.

Several types of constipation are to be distinguished. First and foremost, because of their numerical superiority, are the victims of spastic constipation. They are patients who are usually not only of a nervous temperament but are actually neurotic, they are thin, they complain of ill-defined scattered areas of tenderness in the abdomen, and their stools are ribbonlike, pencil-shaped, or are passed in small pieces accompanied perhaps by mucus; this type of individual is almost certain to clamor for the opportunity of giving a minute description of all these things. Examination discloses the fact that the cecum is usually dilated, tender and ptosed; the sigmoid is easily palpable through the abdominal wall as a tender cordlike structure. Spasm of the sphincter, hemorrhoids, fissures, infected crypts, etc., are often associated with these cases. Atonic constipation is the exact opposite of this spastic type. Its victims are persons of the quiet, steady, phlegmatic make-up, usually well up in years; they are often obese and anemic. Their constipation is due to habitual disregard of the call to defecate, to weakness of the voluntary muscles concerned, to anal sphincter spasm, or to unphysiologic posture for defecation. Individuals of this type often take too little food containing the sort of residue that acts as a mechanical excitant to peristalsis; they are eaters of white bread, sweets (sugar, that is), and excessively cooked foods. Another factor may be insufficient exercise, though one must be careful in making any positive assertion here, for, as Boles remarks, "letter carriers are said to be a constipated lot." The other types of constipation are due either to adhesions, pressure of other organs or of new growths upon the bowel, or to reflexes from eyestrain, chronic appendicitis, gallbladder disease, inflammation of the female adnexa, or of the stomach, liver or pancreas, etc. In infants one must also at times reckon with lack of ability or desire to use the expulsive forces necessary for defecation.

THERAPY

In an ancient recipe for rabbit stew one is enjoined to "first catch your rabbit." How sound that advice is when applied to the subject in hand; first be sure that the patient before you is suffering from simple constipation before you undertake to treat him. Gynecological, proctoscopical, sigmoidoscopical, roentgenological, internological (if I may coin the word) examinations may reveal many primary or secondary organic causes for the constipation; give the patient the benefit of these examinations, and only if they are convincingly negative consign him to the class of either spastic or atonic constipates, and treat him accordingly.

(a) **General Treatment.**—It has been loudly proclaimed in certain quarters that any case of simple constipation can be absolutely cured without the use of any drug, or, indeed, of any remedial agent or measure other than certain "mental cathartics"; that is to say, if we can get the patient to cease being constipation-minded, he will cease to be constipated. This is doubtless true in the main, but it is a fact worthy of careful note that those practitioners who have enjoyed most success with this method have been handling principally patients of sufficient means that they could sojourn for a period of several months in an agreeable sanatorium or resort, or travel at sea or abroad for a like period, without suffering the least disruption in their affairs. Such patients are the exceptions and do not concern us here. Of course much can be done, and must be done, in the attempt to overcome the neurological imbalance of most of our constipated patients, but I think that the present tendency to cry fie upon all practitioners who resort to the prescription of enemas, drugs, etc., for their work-a-day patients is not only stupid and silly but is actually subversive of the best interests of medical practice, the aim of which is, after all, to cure or to alleviate by some practicable means the ailments of those who toil and moil and are made ill thereby.

(*b*) **Diet.**—The atonic individual will nearly always be found to be taking too little "roughage" in his diet. Such patients will greatly profit from the addition to the menu of lettuce, celery, the endives, spinach, carrots, beets, string beans, figs, dates, raisins, and cooked fruits, especially prunes. It is in these cases, too, that bran serves its best purpose; it contains a considerable amount of indigestible cellulose which by its bulk adds to the distention of the intestine, and also gently titillates the mucous membrane by reason of the spicate shape of its particles. Cowgill and Anderson (1932) have shown that the washed and unwashed preparations are of equal value, thus disposing of the contention that the contained phytin is an important laxative. Bran must be taken in rather large amounts and indefinitely. It may be taken stirred up in water after meals, but most patients will soon tire of this dose; nor is it necessary to make a "medicine" of it for there are many pleasant bran recipes available—for cookies, muffins, breads, cakes, macaroons, biscuits, etc. Many patients take it enjoyably stirred up with other foods or else to replace in part or whole the morning cereal, in which case it is eaten with sugar and cream. Those persons, however, in whose intestinal tract excessive cellulose digestion takes place, will not do well upon bran which will only add to their distress from gas; in these cases agar is often useful. Agar passes through the intestinal tract without undergoing bacterial digestion and merely softens and adds bulk to the feces by virtue of its property of retaining water. It is best used in the form of shreds or a coarse powder, for when finely pulverized it may produce colic, according to Fantus. It may be necessary to employ agar in several tablespoonful doses; it may be incorporated with the foods just as described in the case of bran. Psyllium is a small brown seed that exudes a considerable amount of mucilaginous material when it is moistened. The dose is 2 to 4 teaspoonfuls stirred up with twice as much hot or cold water until a gelatinous mass is formed, which is then taken with cream or sugar, with stewed fruit, or in soup; a combination with agar has recently become commercially available. In the small amounts in which it is taken, psyllium does not usually increase gaseous distention.

The spastic individual is usually not one for whom it is advisable to prescribe "roughage," for two reasons: In the first place, he needs antispasmodic measures (bromides for awhile are sometimes very profitably used in these cases) rather than the introduction of substances calculated to stimulate peristalsis; and in the second place, he is often the victim of colitis (see p. 427) or of a fissure, the healing of which will in itself correct the constipation. Of course if he is a decidedly neurasthenic person he must be treated as such; the reader is advised to turn to Alvarez' discussion of the treatment of nervous indigestion on page 404. Drugs or enemas must nearly always be used for awhile in these cases.

Much water should be drunk by all constipated persons.

(*c*) **Exercise.**—General exercise of the body is of importance in atonic cases, but massage of the abdominal muscles, or its substitute, the rolling of a 6- to 8-pound ball over the abdomen for about ten minutes each morning, has been frowned upon of late because of the danger of causing injury to deep structures by abuse of these measures. In spastic cases, exercise is of course valuable for its general tonic effect, but it is doubtful if it directly affects the constipation.

(*d*) **Habit.**—The stool should be visited by every person every morning after breakfast. Too often housewives, who are very busy at this time, "put it off" until the desire is no longer felt. When the necessity of this regular daily visit is impressed upon constipated patients they often accept

28

the advice and carry it out with a grim determination, but this very grimness often defeats their purpose, for defecation is accomplished only by the maintenance of a very nice balance between contraction *and* relaxation. A few puffs of a cigarette, a few peeps at a newspaper or magazine, is a recipe well known to many men. Sometimes placing the feet upon the round of a chair so that the thighs are flexed on the abdomen is helpful; certainly the principle is anatomically and physiologically sound.

(*e*) **Enemas.**—It is very probable that the habitual use of enemas is much to be preferred to the habitual use of cathartic drugs, but it is well to bear in mind that the attempt should be made to gradually lessen the amount and the frequency of the enemas just as we do of the drugs. There are enemas *and* enemas. The daily injection of a quart of nice warm comfortable water is worse than useless; it soothes the bowel, lulls it to sleep as it were, and, though it may flush out a great deal of the fecal material, has never yet cured constipation. What is wanted is the injection of not more than a pint of water and that preferably cool: thus congestion is lessened in the hemorrhoidal area and the sluggish bowel is given some stimulus to act. McKenney says: "Should the pelvic colon and rectum be emptied in this way, after breakfast, daily for a week and every other day for another week, then, perhaps, once a week for awhile, it is not at all uncommon in a few weeks to have daily unaided natural bowel movement with restoration of sensation and tone to the lowered bowel. A large, hot enema, on the contrary, soothes the bowel, causing loss of sensation with no incentive to contraction and thus the bowel distends easily and loss of tone is the result."

The content of the enema also deserves the closest attention of the physician. Hirschman has recently emphasized, what others have long ago stated and proved, that the ordinary soapsuds enema is so irritating to even the normal bowel that for some time after its use the mucous membrane presents an angry red appearance; yet it is the enema nearly always ordered and used. Says Hanes: "Yet when an enema is ordered in a hospital, soapsuds will be given in 90 per cent of cases unless no soap can be found or a guard is by to prohibit its use." The routine enema should be of physiologic saline or of 1 per cent sodium bicarbonate (1 teaspoonful to the pint of water). Irritating substances must of course be added to the enema at times, but this should be done only when there is reason to believe that plain water, physiologic saline, or sodium bicarbonate solution will not serve the purpose.

Levy has reported a formula with which he claims to have gotten very good results in cases that have resisted milder measures. He makes a mixture of 5 cc. of rectified oil of turpentine, 25 cc. of cotton seed oil, 45 cc. of glycerin, and 45 cc. of soft soap. One to 2 teaspoonfuls of this mixture are added to 4 ounces of water which is injected into the rectum by means of a rubber bulb syringe holding exactly this amount. The action is quick and complete.

Graham pointed out some years ago that if rapid evacuation of the rectum and pelvic colon is desired, a 5-grain (0.3 Gm.) quinine dihydrochloride suppository will promptly produce a large but not a watery stool. Glycerin suppositories have of course been in use since time out of mind.

The Oil Enema.—This subject is considered under a separate heading here because I believe it worth while to thus draw especial attention to it. About twenty-five years ago (1909–10), Lipowski wrote somewhat extensively upon what he believed to be a common type of constipation, namely, that in which there is excessive absorption of fluid from the colon with the resultant abnormal drying out of the fecal masses; these hard fecal masses cause congestion of the colonic mucosa, and the congested mucosa resorbs excessive amounts of fluid. The oil enema breaks in on this vicious circle by keeping the feces soft and thus preventing the congestion which permits the exaggerated resorption—but it must be properly given, that is to say, the oil must make contact with the liquid contents of the ascending colon, which it will then keep in a semiliquid state in two ways: First because it is in itself nonabsorbable, and second, because it interferes with the diffusion of water into mucosa. Fantus (1930) describes the technic as follows:

"For self-administration, the patient should have everything prepared before going to bed, so that he does not have to get up after taking the injection. The bottle of oil is placed in a basin of hot water until it has acquired blood heat (100 F.). An ordinary fountain syringe might be used, provided the nozzle has a sufficiently large bore to permit the oil to pass readily. Though it is intended that the oil should be introduced slowly, the bag usually has to be hung from 2 to 3 feet high owing to the viscosity of the oil, which makes it run rather slowly. The clip should be placed within easy reach of the patient. Having poured the warmed oil into the bag, the patient lies on the left side with a folded towel and a firm pillow underneath the buttocks. The nozzle is inserted into the anus, and the oil permitted to flow. Should the patient experience distress or desire to move the bowel, the flow of the oil is checked and the patient remains quiet until the desire has passed. It might then be possible to introduce an additional quantity of oil. It is usually best, however, to be satisfied with the introduction of an amount that can easily be retained. A piece of absorbent cotton or a woman's sanitary towel or both may be applied to prevent accidental soiling of the bed, for the passage of flatus may be accompanied by a spurt of oil. The patient should understand that, unless the oil remains in the intestine for several hours at least, satisfactory results cannot be expected."

In the beginning, the patient may not be able to retain more than 70 cc., but is usually able in the course of time to build up to 250 or even 500 cc. In children, 50 to 100 cc. may be reached; in infants, 15 cc. Of course after awhile the attempt must be made to reduce the quantity of oil and increase the time interval between injections.

Olive oil, poppy seed oil, oil of sesame, cotton seed oil, and petrolatum are used for this purpose. The latter would seem to be preferable to all the others for the reason that it is nonsaponifiable; some of the fatty-acid products of saponification form soaps which are irritant.

The reader is here advised that water enemas are much more valuable than oil for the breaking up and removal of *impacted* feces.

(*f*) **Drugs.**—I believe that the few drugs discussed below constitute a quite sufficient list of cathartics for use in the treatment of constipation, bearing in mind that one should always have at least a hope of bringing about a return to that normal state of affairs in which all medication is unnecessary.

1. *Cascara Sagrada.*—This drug is a mild yet reliable cathartic, though one occasionally finds a patient in whom it fails to act. When there is complaint of griping, investigation usually discloses that it is being taken in overdose. It acts by stimulating colonic peristalsis and at the same time decreasing antiperistalsis; the "defecation reflex" is perhaps also stimulated. The ideal dose is one that will produce a single formed, but slightly soft, stool in the morning when it has been taken on retiring the previous night. The dose of the aromatic fluidextract necessary to accomplish this is from 1 to 3 drachms (4 to 12 cc.). The drug may be taken before meals and at bedtime, or all in one dose at bedtime. It is sometimes possible to gradually reduce the dosage. Fantus gives the following dosage of the aromatic fluidextract for children:

		Cc.
Child, 6 months old		1
Child, 18 months old		From 2 to 3
Child, 3 years old		4
Child, 5 years old		From 4 to 8

The adult dose of the plain fluidextract is 15 to 60 minims (1 to 4 cc.), but this preparation is so bitter that it seems needlessly cruel to prescribe it for adults, and children can hardly be made to take it at all. The use of cascara sagrada in patients with the spastic type of constipation is very doubtfully advisable.

2. *Senna.*—This drug is more powerful than cascara sagrada and also much more prone to cause griping and general abdominal soreness. It acts by stimulating peristalsis in the colon and is definitely contraindicated in spastic constipation and any type of intestinal inflammation. The dose of the fluidextract is ½ to 1 drachm (2 to 4 cc.), if taken at one time, or 8 to 16 minims (0.5 to 1 cc.), several times daily. Four to 8 minims (0.25 to 0.5 cc.) of the tincture of belladonna added to each dose will antagonize griping. The official syrup has a full dose of 1 drachm (4 cc.) and the aromatic syrup of the N.F., 2 drachms (8 cc.). Children prefer the latter; 15 drops for an infant of one year. Such nostrums as "castoria" and "syrup of figs," which owe their chief value to senna, should not be used. Senna may also be pleasantly taken as the compound glycyrrhiza powder, which is official; adult dose, 1 drachm (4 cc.) or more, stirred up in water.

Dosage of compound powder of glycyrrhiza for children (Fantus)

Age of child.	Gm.
6 months	0.60
1 year	0.90
2 years	1.20
3 years	2.00
5 years	3.00

3. *Aloe.*—Aloe increases the tone of the colon very greatly, sometimes almost to a spastic condition; its griping tendency is notorious. The official pill, which contains 2 grains (0.12 Gm.), is likely to be too large (I believe it will be omitted from U.S.P. XI). Fantus offers the following prescription:

			Gm.
℞.	Powdered aloe	gr. xxiij	1.5
	Powdered soap	gr. xxiij	1.5

Mix.   Make a mass and divide into 30 capsules.
Label: One three times a day after meals.

"If this daily dose is insufficient, the patient may be directed to use two or three of these pills, as required, and to return for another prescription when the quantity prescribed has been consumed. After regularity of bowel evacuation has been secured by means of such pills for a week or two, one dose a day is dropped weekly or monthly, as the case may permit, provided the desired effect continues; and, in this way, the cathartic habit may be avoided. When failure after faithful and repeated trial renders it apparent that the patient seems incurably constipated, then it is best to give him a prescription for pills of sufficient size to secure a thorough evacuation when one daily dose is taken. Such a pill is to be administered at bedtime on the day that the patient has been without a bowel movement. . . . "

The active principle, aloin, should be reserved for use only when excessive action is needed—it may be given in a pill containing from 2 to 5 grains (0.12 to 0.3 Gm.).

4. *Phenolphthalein.*—This is a yellowish-white, odorless and practically tasteless powder, which stimulates peristalsis in both the small and large

intestines when taken in even very small amount; the effect upon the large intestine predominates. An excellent drug this, which has but one great fault, namely, that a small dose sometimes acts excessively while a large dose may at times fail to act altogether. This variability of action very probably depends upon the amount of alkali in the intestine available for its solution. It is usually given at bedtime and in the morning produces a stool very like the normal bowel movement. The adult dose is from 1 to 3 grains (0.06 to 0.2 Gm.), though it is said that as much as 15 grains may be given with safety. Infants of eighteen months may be given as much as ½ grain (0.03 Gm.). The National Formulary contains a formula for a cocoa and sugar flavored tablet containing 1 grain (Tablets of Phenol- phthalein, N.F.). A great many nostrums rely upon phenolphthalein for their principal or sole active cathartic ingredient; they are for the most part pleasing little tablets, but there is no good reason why the physician should not prescribe the drug in its Formulary preparation. A sufficient number of skin eruptions have been shown to be due to the prolonged use of phenol- phthalein to warrant one in taking this possibility into account in urticarias and erythemas; the literature of such cases was reviewed by Netherton, in 1924. It is also said that colic, rapid pulse, palpitation, difficult breathing, general uneasiness, and even collapse may be caused by the drug in suscep- tible persons, but these cases are extremely rare.

The prolonged use of large doses of phenolphthalein will many times aggravate a preexisting colitis, and, according to some authorities, will even give rise to the condition in a previously normal bowel.

5. *Isacen.*—This is a synthetic substance, somewhat resembling phenol- phthalein, which was introduced by Guggenheim, in 1925. His studies, and those of Katzenelbogen and Güder, early established it as a valuable remedy in the treatment of chronic constipation. In the United States, Einhorn and Rafsky (1926) have reported on its successful use in the treatment of 47 chronically constipated elderly persons in an institution, all of whom were more or less chronic invalids. The drug is apparently a safe one, for it is not absorbed into the circulation even when taken in enormous quantities. However, Fuld has warned against giving it to individuals who have abnor- malities in the region of the cecum, in which cases it may cause severe ab- dominal pains or frequent insufficient evacuations with rectal tenesmus.

Isacen passes through the stomach unchanged, is slowly disintegrated in the alkaline intestine, and exerts its cathartic effect upon the lower colon. It is marketed in tablets containing 0.005 Gm. of the drug. Taken at bed- time, a soft stool may be expected in the morning. To begin with, only one tablet should be given on several successive nights, allowing this time to elapse for the full effect of the drug to become apparent; if, however, this amount is not sufficient to produce the desired result, two, or even three or four, tablets are permissible.

6. *Apocodeine.*—Alvarez (1916), and others, reported that this drug was an efficient cathartic when given either orally or hypodermically, but Schwartze (1931) failed to find any experimental pharmacological evidence of its alleged effects other than the fleeting increase in peristalsis which ac- companies the administration of other circulatory depressants. In Stockton and Hoffmann's (1932) use of the drug under clinical conditions in 22 patients, there was not only failure of cathartic action but some nausea and occasionally indications of narcosis occurred; severe local reactions fol- lowed intramuscular injection.

7. *Liquid Petrolatum.*—Liquid petrolatum is the most harmless of all the cathartic substances, for it is nonirritating, indigestible, nonabsorbable and incapable of undergoing bacterial decomposition. Even the main objection which has been urged against it, namely, that it coats the intestine with an

impervious material that hinders the egress of secretion and the ingress of digested food substances, is no longer tenable, for it is now known that the oil remains distributed throughout the feces in the form of globules, merely softening the mass by its incorporation therein. It would therefore seem to be the ideal drug to use in the treatment of chronic constipation, and indeed it is coming to be looked upon as such by many experienced practitioners. A limitation, however, and a very great one, should be borne in mind: In cases of atonic constipation we want something that will stimulate the sluggish intestine to some exertion on its own account, and this stimulation will not be supplied by liquid petrolatum. In spastic constipation it serves excellently; here there is usually some irritation of the mucous membrane also, which seems to be soothed by the oil. Fantus says of it further: "In intestinal stasis due to crippling of the intestine, whether from kinks or other forms of obstruction, or even malignant tumor, its effects are most likely to prove valuable; and it is most especially of use if the obstruction is located in that portion of the bowel that ordinarily has to deal with formed hard fecal masses. Hence its special value in intestinal disturbance located in the left side of the abdomen."

The dose of liquid petrolatum is from 4 drachms (16 cc.) upward, the proper dose for a given patient to be determined only by trial; that dose which produces a daily stool without leakage of the oil from the anus is the correct one. For my own part, I have yet to see a normally active, ambulatory patient who obtained satisfactory results with the oil without occasional slight staining of the clothing, though many practitioners have assured me that they have patients who are able to achieve so nice a balance in the matter of dosage that this accident never occurs. Most patients find that if taken during or just after a meal it causes some discomfort, which is doubtless due to interference with gastric digestion; it is therefore best given at bedtime, or it may be given in small doses an hour or more before meals.

The investigations of Bastedo have clearly shown that the liquid petrolatum of the U.S.P. is just as good as any that is put out under fancy trade names; there is therefore no good reason why these special brands should be prescribed by the physician, the more especially as the U.S.P. article is cheaper. The oil is bland, odorless, tasteless, and colorless, and can be taken from the spoon by most patients without any difficulty. It can be easily flavored, however. Hinton has found that in 500 cc. of the oil any one of the following flavoring oils is satisfactory: Anethol, 10 drops; oil of almond, 15 drops; oil of cloves, 10 drops; oil of cinnamon, 5 drops; oil of peppermint, 15 drops; oil of spearmint, 15 drops; and methyl salicylate, 25 drops. Fantus suggests that the oil combination used in the flavoring of aromatic elixir might be used to make liquid petrolatum aromatic; a combination of this sort would be: Oil of orange, 2 cc.; oil of lemon, 0.5 cc.; oil of coriander, 0.2 cc.; oil of anise, 0.05 cc.; and liquid petrolatum, 1000 cc.

Emulsification lessens the oiliness of the substance and is said to combat the tendency to leakage. A number of proprietary brands of emulsified liquid petrolatum are now on the market and are rapidly gaining in popularity. Of this class of preparations, Fantus writes: "The worst that can be said about them is that they are more expensive than the same quantity of liquid petrolatum, containing as they do from 25 to 60 per cent of the active agent. The dose of 1 tablespoonful is recommended for them with the suggestion that the activity of the emulsified oil is greater than that of the plain oil, a statement that remains to be proved. That the agar in some of these preparations is of any laxative value whatever cannot be asserted, as the largest amount of agar in any of the specimens examined was equivalent to about 1.5 per cent of agar [see Warren, L. E., in the Bibliography— H. B.], which is about 2 per cent of the average (U.S.P.) dose of agar. As agar acts exclusively by its bulk, it would be absurd to expect any action from so small a proportion of the usually required dose." The New and Nonofficial Remedies (1933) contains the following emulsions: Abbott's Mineral Oil Emulsion, Petrolagar, Petrolagar (Unsweetened), Petrolagar (with Milk of Magnesia), Petrolagar (with Phenolphthalein), Squibb's Liquid Petrolatum with Agar, Squibb's Liquid Petrolatum with Agar and Phenolphthalein, and Maltine with Mineral Oil and Cascara Sagrada. A much advertised emulsion, that is not accepted in the N.N.R., is Agarol, regarding which the following warning of Sagal (1927) should be earnestly heeded:

"It is surprising how few in the medical profession, as well as among the laity, know of the high phenolphthalein content of one of the emulsions of liquid petrolatum marketed under the name of 'Agarol.' The impression gained from the advertising matter and the circulars supplied by the manufacturers of the preparation is that it represents merely a mixture of mineral oil and agar. The label on the bottle exhibits the words 'mineral oil' and 'agar agar' in large type, and the word 'phenolphthalein' in minute letters. Little wonder that the latter ingredient is generally overlooked. Physicians advising its use, as well as patients using it, do not realize that they are being weaned away from the use of pills or tablets, containing phenolphthalein as their active ingredient, to the use of this liquid, which contains phenolphthalein in considerable dosage.

"The composition of the preparation was reported among several others by the Chemical Laboratory of the American Medical Association in the Journal, May 30, 1925; but unless specifically sought for, the information is easily overlooked. I have come across numerous cases of colitis, which were aggravated or perhaps produced by the prolonged use of this preparation, often on the advice of a physician who did not suspect the presence of such an active ingredient as phenolphthalein to the extent of 6 grains to each ounce, or 3 grains to the average dose.

"The use, or rather the misuse, of this compound is so general that the profession ought to be apprised in a forcible way of its true composition."

(*g*) **Yeast.**—I think that this much exploited remedy for all the ills to which the flesh is heir deserves no place in any serious treatise on therapeutics. From time to time a paper appears in which its virtues are extolled, but the findings always fail of confirmation. Let us leave yeast to the quacks—certainly it is much less harmful than many another substance with which they dabble to the detriment of mankind. For an exposé of the method employed by the manufacturers to obtain advertising material from eminent physicians, see Brit. Med. Jour., 1929, 1, 973.

(*h*) **Bacillus Acidophilus.**—Since the pioneer writings of Metchnikoff on the dietotherapeutic rôle of lactic acid-producing micro-organisms, so many hastily set up claims have had to be abandoned, that I think the present attitude of scepticism which most scientists maintain toward the whole subject is not at all to be wondered at. However, we know now beyond doubt that *Bacillus bulgaricus* cannot be implanted in the human intestinal tract and that *B. acidophilus* can. A number of very sincere workers have claimed that intractable cases of constipation, or diarrhea, or intestinal fermentation can be controlled or cured by the transformation of the intestinal flora from one that is predominently gram-negative to one that is predominantly gram-positive—a number of other workers deny this, or at least have failed to succeed with the method. Kopeloff, who has been the most indefatigable student of the subject, has found no correlation to exist between constipation and the absence of *B. acidophilus* in fecal specimens; about 50 per cent of individuals seem to harbor the organism. The aim of this type of therapy is, therefore, to implant the organism by feeding living cultures and at the same time to give large quantities of lactose to provide the preferred source of energy for the bacterium in the intestinal tract. The amount of the lactose necessary seems to be at least 1 to 3 ounces (30 to 90 Gm.), though much larger quantities are sometimes employed; the required amount of the culture is extremely variable. Weinstein *et al.* (1933) found that when successfully implanted the organism often persists for several weeks after the use of milk has been discontinued; they therefore favor long-continued treatment with periodic interruptions.

Preparations.—The questionnaire of the Council on Pharmacy and Chemistry of the American Medical Association (Jour. Amer. Med. Assoc., 87, 172, 1926) revealed the fact that most of the foremost students of this subject do not believe that intestinal implantation of *Bacillus acidophilus* can be brought about by the use of such preparations as broth cultures, concentrated cultures, blocks, candies, tablets, or oil suspensions. I shall therefore list here only the acidophilus *milk* preparations appearing in the N.N.R., for 1933, and such supplements to that publication as have reached me at the time of writing. These preparations are marketed in bottles, should be kept on ice and consumed within the period of time stated on the label, the daily dose being the amount required to accomplish the desired purpose; 500 to 1000 cc. is probably the average daily adult dosage; Acidophilus Milk—Towt, Acidophilus Milk—Fairchild, Acidophilus Milk—Lederle, Cheplin's Acidophilus Milk.

HEMORRHOIDS

Internal hemorrhoids are masses of redundant tissue caused by the dilatation of capillaries, arteries or venules just inside the anal sphincter. They cause trouble either by reason of the fact that they are ulcerated and thus give rise to considerable pain when scraped by the feces, or by their bleeding, or by their prolapsing which necessitates their frequent manual replacement up behind the sphincter, or by the fact that they become strangulated after having passed out through the sphincter. The so-called "external" hemorrhoids are really only tags of skin that are vascular and that become troublesome when inflamed. A great deal of anal itching is usually associated with hemorrhoids.

THERAPY

Palliative Measures.—Prolapsed hemorrhoids are best sprayed with cold water, or a cold compress may be applied, in order to reduce the congestion; they may then be gently returned through the sphincteric canal by manipulation with the oiled fingers. Other palliative measures than this I think are no longer justified in view of the excellent results now to be attained by employment of either of the two curative measures; however, of the following prescriptions, the first is for an astringent rectal suppository, the effect of which can be modified by changing the proportion of tannic acid:

℞.			
	Tannic acid	gr. xv	1.0
	Balsam of peru	ℳxxij	1.5
	Bismuth subcarbonate	℥iiss	10.0
	Oil of theobroma	℥iv	16.0
	Cerate	℥ss	2.0

Make ten suppositories.
Label: One three times daily.

And the second is for an analgesic suppository:

Ŗ. Powdered opium...................................... gr. vj   0.4
    Extract of belladonna.............................. gr. ij   0.12
    Ethyl aminobenzoate............................... gr. xviij   1.2
    Oil of theobroma.................................. ℥iij   12.0
    Make six suppositories.
    Label: One before bowel movement.

For a discussion of the treatment of anal pruritus, the reader is referred to page 679, in the section on Diseases of the Skin.

Curative Measures.—(*a*) *Surgical.*—It is now urged by surgeons that hemorrhoids that are causing discomfort be removed by operation, a plea that is heartily endorsed by most nonsurgical practitioners since the operation is practically always successful, is not dangerous, does not incapacitate the patient for a very long period, and oftentimes cures a stubborn constipation as well as the case of piles. However, the profession should not overlook the fact that the injection method of treatment has withstood the test of time; it is presented below.

(*b*) *Quinine and Urea Injection.*—In 1916, Terrell advocated the use of quinine and urea hydrochloride injections in the treatment of hemorrhoids. At that time the method was looked upon with considerable disfavor, but it has since won many advocates all over the world. Terrell has since (in 1927) reported his use of it in about 5000 cases and believes it to be suitable in about half of all cases of hemorrhoids. I quote his technic:

"Quinine and urea should not be used in inflamed, strangulated or external piles, but is a specific in that large class of chronic internal hemorrhoids, the chief symptoms of which are protrusion and bleeding. A hemorrhoid that is badly ulcerated and bleeds freely will seldom bleed again after the first treatment. To those who have a prejudice against all forms of treatment other than operative, and I know there are many such, I would suggest the use of quinine and urea solution to tide over the bad surgical risks, made so from excessive hemorrhoidal bleeding. You will be surprised how quickly the hemoglobin index will improve.

"About 50 per cent of those with protrusion are relieved of this symptom immediately after all the tumors have received one injection. With those situated lower in the anal canal, the prolapse will disappear gradually, although a marked reduction will be noticed from the beginning of treatment. Soon after a hemorrhoid is injected with quinine and urea solution, it loses some of its flexibility and becomes more or less fixed, when it can be felt very plainly with the finger introduced into the anus. This lessening of mobility accounts in many cases for the sudden relief of prolapse, for a noticeable diminution in the size of the tumors does not begin for several days after treatment. In a few days, a hemorrhoid that has been injected with a solution of quinine and urea has a glazed appearance, and is very much paler in color. A fibrosis with local anemia of the parts has been produced. On account of the fibrosis, the blood vessels are constricted, and, since the parts are denied the usual amount of nourishment, an atrophy is the result. Although the question is open to criticism, I believe this is the manner in which a cure is produced.

"I have experimented with various strengths of solution in some of my cases, and have finally come to the conclusion that 5 per cent is approximately the right strength for the average case. Sometimes if a hemorrhoid seems resistant to treatment, as occasionally it does, I use a 10 per cent solution with better results.

"It is my custom to inject one hemorrhoid each succeeding day until all are treated; but, if the sphincters are relaxed, there is no objection to treating two or more hemorrhoids at one time. After all the hemorrhoids have received a treatment, the patient is asked to return once a week until a cure is effected, which takes about six weeks for the average case. At these visits, treatments are alternated from one side to the other, that is, the piles on the right side are injected at one visit and those on the left at the next, so that each hemorrhoid is treated once every two weeks, which, I think, ordinarily is often enough. There is no attempt made to dilate the sphincters, nor do I draw the hemorrhoids down, as is advised by some operators. Personally, I think a Brinkerhoff anal speculum is the instrument of choice in bringing the tumors into view. It is small, conical in shape, and very easily introduced. The pile selected for treatment is cleansed with an antiseptic solution, preferably iodine and alcohol. Enough of the quinine and urea solution is then injected into the pile to slightly distend it. The needle must be very small, and should be inserted at a point as far away from the skin margin as possible, the slide in the speculum being used as an aid in doing this. The injection should be made through and not into the mucous membrane; otherwise a slough is likely to occur. During the course of treatment there are no restrictions whatever placed on the patient. He is allowed to proceed about his business as usual.

"Most of those who come to me for the treatment of hemorrhoids are more or less constipated, and since the latter condition most often precedes and is the cause of the former, I deem it necessary that the treatment of both be taken up at the same time. Eliminating appendicitis, bile tract infections and other like intra-abdominal conditions as causes, I have been greatly surprised to find how easily many cases of long-standing constipation are relieved. Most patients while under treatment for constipation need encouragement more than all else, and visiting the physician at regular intervals for six weeks or so, while under treatment for hemorrhoids, offers an excellent opportunity for this. At the same time, other measures deemed necessary are used. Relief from constipation, when possible, is a decided aid in the treatment of the hemorrhoids, and no doubt lessens greatly the likelihood of a recurrence.

"In properly selected cases of hemorrhoids, treated with quinine and urea, as outlined, rarely does a patient complain of pain during or following a treatment. If the work is done carefully, gently, and without haste, 90 per cent of the patients will not know when the injections are made. During the past year, in treating 185 patients, 3 have had pain due to complications, which I will describe. In one of these there occurred an edema of the skin below the point of injection, and it was apparently quite painful for two days. I think the injection was made too near the skin line, a danger I advised against in my last paper. In the second, there developed during the course of treatment a well-marked fissure, which necessitated excision. This may have been a coincidence, but I am inclined to believe it was the result of infection from treatment. In the third, there occurred a small marginal abscess a short time after the first visit. After incision and drainage it soon healed, when treatment of the hemorrhoids was continued without further trouble. A complication, such as one of the above occurring now and then, serves to remind the operator of the necessity of a more careful technic.

"During the year, every patient treated by the method described has been cured. It is fair to state, however, that among this number there were a few resistant to treatment, sometimes as along as twelve or fourteen weeks being required for a complete disappearance.

"In another group, five or six in number, a hard, fibrous hemorrhoid would persist after the others, softer and varicosed, had disappeared. Such a condition is usually anticipated at the first visit, if the examiner is experienced, and a careful inspection is made. The patient should be told at this time that it will be necessary to excise the hard growth, which may be done before or after the softer hemorrhoids are gotten rid of by quinine and urea. In most of the cases with this complication, unless very slight, I have advised an operation at the hospital, when a complete removal of all the hemorrhoids is done.

"The treatment of hemorrhoids by the injection of quinine and urea appears simple, and it is; but a thorough knowledge of rectal diseases is essential if one expects uniformly good results. Most important of all is a realization of the class of cases to which it is suited, and its limitations. I hope no physician will attempt to use the remedy until these ideas are thoroughly grasped."

(*c*) *Alcohol Injection.*—On the Continent alcohol is apparently preferred to anything else for injection. The objectionable features of transient fever, subsequent hemorrhages and occasional necroses, which have been cited as drawbacks to this method, have been reported to be practically eliminated by Boas (1931) by the reduction in the concentration of the alcohol from absolute, or 95 per cent, to 70 per cent.

(*d*) *Phenol Injection.*—In England, and to some extent in America also, phenol, 5 per cent in olive or cotton seed oil, is preferred. The mixture is self-sterilizing. Hiller (1932) has stated that he looks upon the injection of 1 to 2 cc. beneath the mucosa *well above* the hemorrhoid, and none into the hemorrhoid itself, as a marked improvement in technic.

CATARRHAL JAUNDICE

This condition is principally encountered in children and young adults and more often in males than in females, though middle-aged and even elderly patients are not rare. We know practically nothing of the pathology of the affection for it is never fatal and the autopsy material upon cases suffering an accidental death is too small and contradictory to be of any value. It is generally assumed, however, that there is a catarrhal condition of the mucosa of the upper gastro-intestinal tract and the bile ducts, and that the ampulla of Vater is plugged with mucus. The symptoms are malaise, sometimes mild headache and dizziness, occasionally pain in the liver region, nausea and perhaps vomiting—both these latter symptoms being especially marked if the patient refuses to go to bed—slight fever, a normal or subnormal temperature, slow pulse, jaundice, bile-stained urine and clay-colored stools, more or less general pruritus, and a mental depression which is sometimes quite profound and is not infrequently associated with an unwonted irritability. The gastric symptoms usually persist for only a few days, but many patients suffer a return of nausea and dizziness if they attempt to assume the upright position at any time throughout the course of the malady. The average duration of an attack is from three to six weeks, though some degree of jaundice often persists for a long time in a patient otherwise apparently quite recovered. Dietary indiscretions, the abuse of alcohol, and exposure to cold are usually mentioned in the etiology of catarrhal jaundice, but I do not think that the causative rôle of any of these factors has ever been convincingly shown. The disease is often epidemic and is almost certainly infectious in nature, though no specific organism has as yet been convicted; there is much presumptive evidence pointing toward "droplet" respiratory infection.

In making the diagnosis it should be remembered that almost all the types of liver and bile duct disease may produce jaundice with little or no pain; chronic pancreatitis, carcinoma, hemolytic, and Weil's infectious jaundice are to be ruled out. In lobar pneumonia, jaundice is probably always latent but may appear clinically; it may sometimes be seen in relapsing fever, sepsis and tuberculosis, is often present in malaria and always present in yellow fever. Many chemical poisons may cause jaundice: Arsenic, antimony, acetic acid, carbon tetrachloride, cinchophen, chloroform, phenylhydrazine, potassium chlorate, phosphorus, picric acid, snake venom, mushroom poison, trinitrobenzene, tetrachlorethane, trinitrotoluol. It may appear in eclampsia and following accidental or operative trauma; it may arise from any one of a number of mechanisms in chronic heart disease (its sudden appearance in myocardial insufficiency points toward pulmonary infarction), and is one of the symptoms following the transfusion of incompatible blood. The ordinary icterus neonatorum, in which the infant seems unaffected, is probably physiologic.

THERAPY

The treatment is entirely empirical and is based upon the assumption that there is a subacute inflammation of the stomach and duodenum. A light soft diet, devoid of fats, is usually prescribed. Toast, gruels, junket, custards, rice pudding, cereals, fruits, and vegetables are all permitted in small quantities, though most clinicians feel that milk should be withheld or that only skimmed milk should be given.

It is the general practice to start off with a dose of calomel and then to keep the bowels open with a daily saline purge, but I do not see why these patients should be so persistently dosed with the salines when other drugs of proved value in the treatment of chronic constipation may be used, the more especially as notoriously large doses of salines are required to move the bowels of a bedridden patient. That the patient *should* be bedridden all experienced practitioners are agreed. Hot applications over the liver region are also felt to be of value; perhaps fomentations (stupes) are to be preferred to the use of a hot-water bag, but it seems needlessly hectic therapy to force this sort of thing upon the family attendant when the patient is no more dangerously ill than is the catarrhal jaundice victim.

To provoke an alteration in mucous membrane secretions, ammonium chloride is used in 7½-grain (0.5 Gm.) doses; the following prescription is acceptable:

℞.	Ammonium chloride...............................	ℨiv	16.0
	Syrup of citric acid.................................	℥j	32.0
	Water to make....................................	℥iv	128.0

Label: Teaspoonful in water three times daily after meals.

Nonsurgical drainage of the gallbladder (Lyon duodenal tube method) is said to be of value in these cases; the subject is more fully discussed under the treatment of cholecystitis on page 446. Whether or not there is an actual disturbance of calcium metabolism in jaundice *per se*, remains a controversial point, but there is little doubt that the routine preoperative administration of calcium in the obstructive type of the malady has a beneficial effect upon the hemorrhagic diathesis. Some physicians use the drug also in catarrhal cases; for method of administering calcium salts, see page 714. Relief of the itching is discussed on page 450. The use of cinchophen in something less than antirheumatic doses, as favorably reported by Brugsch and Horsters (1924), would seem doubtfully advisable as a routine in view of what we have recently learned of this drug's ability to cause liver injury.

CHRONIC GALLBLADDER DISEASE

Although chronic cholecystitis and cholelithiasis are possibly separate entities, they are nevertheless so similar in their symptoms and in the therapeutic measures with which we attempt to control them, that it is legitimate and convenient to discuss the two conditions here under the common title of "chronic gallbladder disease." The victims of this disease are more often women than men and are usually near or past their fortieth year. "Female, fair, fat and forty" used to be a diagnostic alliteration of my student days—but not a very accurate one, I am convinced, for many persons who are described by none of these adjectives do have the disease. The symptoms are those of dyspepsia, such as acid eructations, nausea, flatulence, heart burn, and especially chilliness and a feeling of weight in the abdomen after eating. During acute exacerbations there is pain and tenderness in the gallbladder region, chilliness, malaise, more or less precordial oppression, and perhaps a slight bit of fever. There are usually frequent asymptomatic periods. A typical attack of gallstone colic—which is an acute condition not to be confused with the chronic state just described—occurs almost invariably in the middle of the night; the patient experiences excruciating pain in the upper right quadrant of the abdomen, which radiates all over the abdomen and into the back, the shoulders, and even down the arms; she sweats profusely, is usually much excited and assumes many different positions, both in and out of bed, in an attempt to put an end to the agonizing pain. Such an attack usually persists only a few hours, but it may last for several days with remissions. When palpation becomes possible, on the subsidence of pain, it will be found that the gallbladder region is exquisitely tender; usually some degree of jaundice appears also after the paroxysm is over, or at least the urine will be bile-tinged and the feces undercolored. Chronic obstructive jaundice is rare in gallbladder disease unless there is an accompanying chronic cholangitis of considerable degree. It is to be noted that "gallstone colic" may occur in cases of chronic gallbladder disease in which there are no gallstones present.

Gallstones are supposed to be formed as the result of infection of the gallbladder, stasis of bile, or alteration in the chemical composition of the bile; as yet we have very little exact information on the subject. In chronic gallbladder disease, either with or without gallstones, the pathology in and about the gallbladder varies greatly: There may be a simple catarrhal inflammation with moderate swelling of the mucous membrane; or the viscus may be distended with mucopurulent material; or there may be many adhesions binding it in a distorted shape to the liver, pylorus and duodenum; or it may be much thickened and contracted and show actual erosions of the mucous membrane. Gallstone colic is due to spasm of the inflamed muscular viscus, to its distention with bile, or to the temporary lodgment of a stone in the cystic, hepatic, or common duct; but the cause of the much more vague constitutional symptoms of chronic, nonparoxysmal gallbladder disease is no more definitely known than is indicated in the statement that "the gallbladder becomes a focus of infection." Lyon believes that not only does the gallbladder become a distributing center for what he calls "poisoned bile," through its lymphatic connections with the liver and pancreas, but that hepatitis and cholangitis also play a prominent part in the pathologic picture; his position is that the liver, the gallbladder and the ducts are guilty of initiating a vicious circle since they pour into the duodenum "poisoned bile" which, being taken up by the mesenteric veins and lacteals is conveyed throughout the body "to exert a harmful effect on all tissues." I do not believe that he has proved the "poisonous" nature of this bile; indeed, I think that all observers with any pretension to scientific acumen must agree with Carlson when he says: "Koch's postulates are still good science and good medicine. Has Lyon or Smithies reproduced the disease by putting the duodenal return into the duodenum of well persons or dogs?"

Gallstones were first recorded by Gentile da Foligno in the fourteenth century.

THERAPY

(a) **General Treatment.**—In chronic gallbladder disease, with or without stones, a regulation of the diet is very important for two reasons: First, because the dyspepsia must be treated, and second, because substances which contain much cholesterol are thought to favor the formation of stone. Egg yolk in any form, sweetbreads and brains, and in general any excessively fatty substances are to be avoided. Fruits and vegetables may be taken, cereals, milk, poultry, fish (except salmon, mackerel and herring), and lean red meats in moderation. Most patients do well to avoid acid salad dressings, cheeses except cottage cheese, pork, fried foods, spices in excess, alcohol, thick or thin gravies, and often coffee.

Olive oil has long had the reputation of stimulating the secretion of bile, but I do not know that any one has proved that gallbladder cases suffer from a lack of bile. If clinicians would carefully study the work of experimental physiologists they would know that bile is entering the intestinal tract practically all the time; nor is this flow apparently interrupted in patients with gallbladder disease, if one can judge from the color of the stools. Certainly, stasis sometimes takes place in these cases, but the thing then needed is not an increase in bile secretion but some measure which will overcome the mechanical (inflammatory) obstruction to its egress into the duodenum. It will be stupid to deny that olive oil is often helpful in these cases, but the relief which it gives probably rests solely upon its ability to overcome the hyperchlorhydria and reflex pylorospasm that many times accompany chronic gallbladder disease. It is usually prescribed in a dose of a teaspoonful a half hour before meals and on retiring; the addition of a little lemon juice makes it more palatable for many individuals. This use of olive oil may serve to keep the bowels open—but it may also make the patient fat, a thing certainly not to be desired in view of the operation which always hovers as a possibility.

Spa treatment is often of value in cases of chronic gallbladder disease, not so much because of the mineral content of the waters as for the fact that a large quantity of water *per se* is drunk, and also by reason of the really tremendous psychic readjustment which takes place in many people when they visit a pleasant health resort.

Methenamine (urotropin) is *not* a biliary antiseptic; Burnham long ago laid that ghost.

(b) **Nonsurgical Drainage (Lyon Duodenal Tube Method).**—In 1917, Meltzer suggested that if a strong solution of magnesium sulphate were placed in the duodenum by means of the duodenal tube, evacuation of the gallbladder might take place due to the relaxation of the sphincter of Oddi, and probably also with the aid of the contraction of the gallbladder itself, according to his "law of contrary innervation." Lyon (1919) tested the matter upon human beings, and upon his findings has based a method of nonsurgical "drainage" for which great claims are made by himself and others. The duodenal tube is introduced and, when its tip is ascertained to be in the correct position in the duodenum, 40 to 50 cc. of 33 per cent magnesium sulphate solution is introduced. In a little while, bile begins to flow out of the tube; at first it is light lemon colored (A bile); then it changes to a more viscid consistency and is golden brown or green (B bile); and then it changes again and becomes much lighter and thinner than either of the two previous specimens (C bile). The A bile is said to come from the common bile duct, B from the gallbladder, and C from the liver itself (*i. e.*, freshly secreted bile). There is very little proved fact to support these assumptions. To be sure, the sphincter is relaxed, as it will be made to relax also by the use of 5 per cent peptone, or 0.5 HCl, and the bile flows out of the tube—but it is not shown that bile eliminated from the body in this way is of any more benefit to the patient than if it were eliminated by passing down the intestinal tract. Indeed, Soper (1925) has found that he obtains just as good clinical results when he gives his patients a concentrated solution of magnesium sulphate without using the tube at all; ½ to 2 ounces (15 to 60 cc.) of a saturated magnesium sulphate solution, flavored with a small amount of the compound tincture of cardamom, mornings before breakfast. And Howard has shown that the concentration of the drug in the duodenum is the same whether taken first into the stomach or directly through the tube; magnesium sulphate is not chemically altered in the stomach to an extent that could possibly be of any importance. Lyon cites many cases in which improvement in symptoms has followed upon single or repeated drainages with the duodenal tube, but study of his book and his subsequent publications has left me very sceptical of the value of the method. The enthusiasm of himself and his followers is at times almost hilarious, but they claim results in almost all the ailments to which man is heir, and they certainly do not show that the mental attitude of their patients is not tremendously affected by the atmosphere of almost religious awe with which the institution of a duodenal "drain" has come to be surrounded. With Carlson, I must say that I do not understand how the results reported can be due to drainage of a patent bile system and the removal of some of this bile from the duodenum. "Pus in the bile may be significant," says Carlson, "but what symptom is induced by this pus acting in the intestine? We are swallowing bacteria every day. There are a few bacteria that are specifically toxic in the intestine. There are a few toxins poisonous by mouth, but, so far as I know, we could eat pus, ordinary pus, and not be influenced, excepting esthetically. It is not clear, therefore, that finding bacteria or pus in the duodenal content means injurious effects from the bacteria or bile lower down."

(*c*) **Gallstone Colic.**—In a very mild attack, a simple enema of warm physiologic saline, or of 1 per cent sodium bicarbonate, will often bring relief; a dose or two of a carminative (prescription on p. 412) nicely supplements this treatment. Hot fomentations, as described on page 131, should be applied to the gallbladder region. In a severe attack, none of these measures is of any avail; morphine will bring relief, however, but it must often be given in a dose of ¼ grain (0.015 Gm.) repeated at one-hour intervals for several doses, or it may be given in a ½-grain (0.03 Gm.) dose at the outset—these patients tolerate doses of opiates which would otherwise be quite dangerous. According to the work of Macht, who has shown that papaverine, narcotine, and narceine are more potent than morphine in causing inhibition of gallbladder contractions, pantopon would be indicated instead of morphine in gallstone colic, since this drug contains the isolated alkaloids of opium in their natural proportions. The average dose of pantopon is ⅓ to ½ grain (0.02 to 0.03 Gm.), by mouth or hypodermically. A dose of $\frac{1}{120}$ grain (0.005 Gm.) of atropine sulphate is usually combined with the first dose of morphine, but it would probably be better to give it in a larger dose in order to relax the pylorospasm with which we are often having to deal here. In a recent small series of cases, Bauer *et al.* (1931) caused prompt relief by slowly injecting intravenously 20 cc. of a sterile 5 per cent solution of calcium chloride. Beware, proceed calmly here, even though the patient is writhing in pain; see page 714 for the reasons. In rare cases, light or even relatively deep general anesthesia must be instituted in order to bring release from the agony. Return to full diet after the attacks must be very gradual.

Medical measures, though they will carry a patient through an attack of colic, will not cure gallstones, that is to say, we know of nothing that will effect the dissolution of the stones, and so long as they remain these attacks are liable to recur. However, it is perhaps not the part of wisdom to rush off to the operating room every patient who has had an attack of gallstone colic, for there is no evidence that delay occasions any serious threat to the welfare of the patient whose colic has been mild, and, on the other hand, there is always the chance that the attacks may be very infrequent. However, when a stone has become impacted in the common duct, or when the attacks are frequent and the general health failing, operation is certainly indicated. Common duct operations are the most dangerous—a fact upon which many surgeons base a plea for operation in any case in which gallstones have been diagnosed with certainty, since the removal of the stones from the bladder saves the patient the risk of a possible operation for stone impacted in the duct. Stones reform in about 10 per cent of cases and a second operation is considered indicated in somewhat less than this proportion of cases. Miller's (1932) recent study of the association of cardiac pain with disease of the gallbladder is of interest in that it has caused a number of surgeons to recall instances in which "heart trouble" disappeared after cholecystectomy.

CIRRHOSIS OF THE LIVER

The study of the cirrhoses of the liver has only recently been taken up again with vigor after having been neglected for a very long time. Anyone, therefore, who writes upon the subject today must do so with the certain knowledge that tomorrow all that he has to say may be shown to be quite wide of the truth, for much has been learned in the last few years. "The subject is ripe for investigation," says Rowntree; "it awaits the touch of a Richard Bright." But, pending the arrival of the new Bright, I must content myself with a more or less conventional presentation of the subject, merely directing the interested reader to the studies of the following investigators: Counsellor and McIndoe; Whipple; Davis and Whipple; Greene *et al.;* Mann *et al.;* Rous; Graham; Opie and Alford; and Rowntree *et al.*

The cirrhoses may be divided into (*a*) portal, (*b*) syphilitic, (*c*) Hanot's, and (*d*) obstructive biliary. Of these types, it may be said that Hanot's, if it really exists as a disease entity, is of so rare occurrence that it cannot be dealt with in this book (the same statement regarding rarity applies also to Banti's disease, Wilson's disease, and hemochromatosis, in all of which cirrhosis forms a part of the picture). The syphilitic affections of the liver were dealt with in the chapter on Infectious Diseases (see p. 178); it should be noted, however, that portal cirrhosis may occur in an individual who also has syphilis, *i. e.*, every case of cirrhosis in a syphilitic is not necessarily a case of syphilitic cirrhosis. Obstructive biliary cirrhosis occurs as a complication of chronic gallbladder disease, and is relieved or not accordingly as the measures directed toward the cure of the gallbladder condition succeed or fail. Portal cirrhosis, then, alone remains for consideration here.

The clinical entity which we recognize as portal cirrhosis results from prolonged inflammatory, degenerative or proliferative changes in the liver, which are believed to occur in the following sequence: (*a*) Degeneration of cells in the periphery or the lobules caused by poisons carried in the portal vessels, (*b*) proliferation and contraction of interstitial tissue about the remaining cells and the bile ducts, which attempt repair by means of a resort to hyperplasia, and (*c*) portal obstruction and the more or less successful attempt to overcome it by the establishment of a collateral circulation. The surface of the liver is usually "hob-nailed" and the organ diminished in size, but it may be enlarged and smooth due to the deposition of fat. The spleen is also frequently enlarged, whether merely by reason of venous congestion, or because the liver is not an isolated organ but exists as part of a "splenohepatic" system, is not known. Infections, toxins, overactivity of the liver, the excessive deposition of pigments—any one or all of these factors may be the causative agent in a given case. Excessive use of alcohol has long been blamed for the production of most of the cases, and I do not know of any studies that have ever seriously challenged this opinion; however, it should be noted that investigators are beginning to stir in the matter and that Mallory is already willing to risk the opinion that it is the copper in the distilled spirits, rather than the alcohol itself, that is the harmful agent; the studies of Hall and Mackey (1930) seem to confirm this opinion at least for the experimental animals employed. Certainly alcohol is not the only agent that causes cirrhosis, for the disease occurs in nondrinkers and also among Mohammedans and the Chinese, whose lower classes at least do not use much alcohol. Attempts to statistically correlate a rise or fall in cirrhosis incidence with the alcohol-prohibitive measures that have been tried out in various parts of the world are worthless, all countries having explicitly or tacitly admitted that such measures notoriously fail to control alcohol consumption. Friedrich Müller, according to Rowntree, says that cirrhosis is uncommon in Munich, where beer is used almost exclusively, while in Basel, where the people from the surrounding provinces of France use particularly a great deal of absinthe, it is quite common.

Portal cirrhosis occurs most frequently in the early forties and terminates fatally in the early fifties. Men are more frequently affected than women in about the proportion of 2 to 1. The early symptoms are dyspeptic and are rarely recognized, though the new tests of hepatic function should make diagnosis easier now than it was a few years ago. In a fully established case the patient has lost much weight and energy, has a muddy complexion, sunken eyes, and a sharp nose on which there are distended venules; he complains of dyspepsia and perhaps of hemorrhoids and of an itching skin. Engorgement of the veins in the abdominal wall and elsewhere is a striking evidence of the attempt that is being made to establish a collateral circulation. Ascites occurs in more than 50 per cent of cases, the abdomen sometimes containing as much as 15 liters of fluid. Both the spleen and the liver may be found to be enlarged. Jaundice is rare, but the urine is usually scant and highly colored. Purpura and a tendency to easy bleeding are very usual, and profuse hemorrhage from the stomach, due to the anastomoses formed about the lower end of the esophagus, is a frequent and serious occurrence. In far advanced cases such symptoms of hepatic insufficiency as malaise, nausea and vomiting, headache, depression, loss of memory, and delirium or coma may be seen. It should be noted that the majority of patients do not die from this hepatic insufficiency, however, but from complicating disorders, such as circulatory failure, hemorrhage, ascites, and intercurrent infectious disease, particularly pneumonia and a rapid tuberculosis.

John Brown described a case of cirrhosis in 1685, and John Andre, in 1788, and Matthew Baillie, in 1818, both wrote on the subject, but the first adequate account was that of Laënnec, who gave the disease its name in 1819.

29

THERAPY

1. **Diet.**—It is of course imperative that alcohol be denied the patient, but in the case of habitual heavy drinkers it may sometimes be advisable to withdraw the drink by rapid diminution in the quantities allowed rather than by the more radical procedure of cutting off all the supply at once. Milk should form the staple article of diet but this must be supplemented by other foods, of course; vegetables, cereals, bread, and cooked fruits are to be preferred to meats, which should always be allowed infrequently and in small quantities. Eggs, spices, and condiments, and fats of any kind are usually not to be allowed at all. The frequent drinking of small quantities of mild saline water has long been looked upon as of value in depleting the portal circulation, and many of the older generation of practitioners believed that it was the mineral waters that caused their patients to be temporarily improved while sojourning at a spa, but we now take the liberty of believing that the psychic effect of such a sojourn is its most valuable contribution to therapeutics. For a consideration of the low-salt, low-fluid factors in the diet, see under *diuretics*, page 451.

2. **Iodides.**—Iodides are often employed, as in the treatment of syphilis, in the hope that the overgrowth of connective tissue might thus be corrected, but I do not know that the survival of this practice rests upon any more secure footing than the rather vague clinical impression that it is of some value. It is of course an extremely difficult matter to put to the test of controlled clinical experimentation.

3. **Focal Infection.**—It is generally agreed that all demonstrable foci of infection should be eradicated if this can be accomplished consistently with the safety of the patient; that such treatment serves to arrest the process of the disease can rarely, if ever, be shown, for whatever contribution the infectious process may have made toward the establishment of the disease has become accomplished fact long before the diagnosis of cirrhosis is made.

4. **Dyspepsia.**—In the beginning of this chapter (see p. 403) are discussed measures for the treatment of dyspepsia; they nearly always fail when instituted for the control of the dyspepsia accompanying cirrhosis of the liver, the reason being that such dyspepsias are due to congestion throughout the gastro-intestinal tract and that they are relieved only when the congestion is made to decrease, *i. e.*, when the cirrhotic process is abated or arrested.

5. **Itching.**—Sponging with a hot solution of sodium bicarbonate followed by dusting with talcum powder, or the application of 1 per cent menthol in alcohol, or an ointment of 1 per cent phenol, may be tried. Sometimes sweating brings relief, either induced by applied heat or the use of pilocarpine nitrate: $\frac{1}{10}$ to $\frac{1}{5}$ grain (0.006 to 0.012 Gm.) by mouth or hypodermically, repeated so as to maintain mild diaphoresis. Lichtman (1931) obtained a very good relief in 2 cases with the oral administration of ergotamine tartrate (gynergen), $\frac{1}{60}$ grain (0.001 Gm.), three times daily; it may also be given subcutaneously or intramuscularly once a day in a dose of $\frac{1}{20}$ to $\frac{1}{60}$ grain (0.005 to 0.001 Gm.). Snell and Keyes (1933) were successful many times in their 7 cases, though occasionally a dose was completely without effect. In the experience of Rowntree and many others, calomel has proved the most effective agent; it is used in doses of $\frac{1}{4}$ to $\frac{1}{2}$ grain (0.015 to 0.03 Gm.) hourly for four doses a day (omitting the usual saline) for periods of three or four days. Sodium thiosulphate is also sometimes antipruritic when given intravenously in a dose of $7\frac{1}{2}$ to 15 grains (0.5 to 1 Gm.), to be repeated as necessary.

6. **Hematemesis.**—For the treatment of gross hemorrhage from the stomach, see page 425. Checking of bleeding from esophageal varices can only be approached by ligation of the coronary veins of the stomach or resort to the other surgical procedures (see p. 452).

7. **Ascites.**—(*a*) *Paracentesis.*—Soon or late all cases have to be tapped. This tapping is a procedure which it were idle to attempt to describe here since its technic can only be learned in the clinic. The indications, however, are another matter; they are well stated by Kern:

"Tapping should not be delayed so long that serious displacement of the diaphragm and excessive intra-abdominal tension have occurred. Something might perhaps be said in favor of the possible usefulness of moderate effusions as promoting the development of collateral circulation by giving external support to the splanchnic circulation; but there is no doubt that too long delay of tapping is inadvisable. Some external abdominal compression should be used after paracentesis to prevent as far as possible rapid distention of the portal tributaries and reaccumulation of effusion. The operation should be performed as frequently as the reappearance of ascites, in considerable amount, requires."

(*b*) *Diuretics.*—It is generally agreed among practitioners that all of the older diuretics nearly always fail to reduce ascites of hepatic origin. Novasurol (merbaphen) and salyrgan (mersalyl) have, however, acquired a considerable vogue since 1925, when novasurol was studied by Rowntree, Keith and Barrier in combination with their low-fluid, low-salt diet and ammonium chloride. The two drugs are 10 per cent aqueous solutions of organic mercury compounds containing about 33 per cent of mercury, and for all practical purposes may be considered as interchangeable. The more recent reports comprise a total of 84 cases of portal cirrhosis with ascites, treated as follows: (*a*) A low-fluid, low-salt diet containing 800 cc. of water and inorganic ions as follows: sodium, 0.49 Gm.; potassium, 1.76 Gm.; calcium, 0.23 Gm.; magnesium, 0.2 Gm., and chlorine, 0.74 Gm. An additional 800 cc. of water is allowed. Ammonium chloride (or ammonium nitrate, which is better tolerated by the digestive tract) is given in doses of 75 to 150 grains (5 to 10 Gm.) daily, and novasurol is given in doses up to 2 cc. intramuscularly or intravenously every third or fourth day, the tolerance of the patient for the drug being first determined by the intramuscular injection of 0.5 to 0.75 cc.

Duncan and Rudy (1926) write as follows of a diet which complies with the above requirements: "No salt or sodium bicarbonate is to be added to any foods either in the cooking or at table. Allen has pointed out the necessity of excluding all foods high in salt, such as bacon, ham, corned beef, tongue, salted or dried fish and smoked or preserved meats; baker's bread, cakes, canned fruits, vegetables and soups, as well as prepared cereals, such as corn flakes, are not permissible; milk and cheese have an incompatible chloride content. Fruit in the form of apples, oranges and grapefruit, cereals, as oatmeal, farina, shredded wheat, puffed rice with thick cream provide an available variety for breakfast. Eggs and salt-free meat, salt-free homemade bread with sweet butter and tea and coffee (in moderation) are permissible. Home-prepared, salt-free soups, fresh vegetables (canned vegetables must be brought to the boil three times and the water discarded each time to eliminate chlorides) may be added for lunch or supper. Horse-radish, vinegar, pepper and other flavoring materials if properly used make the diet palatable. Medications, nasal sprays and mouth washes may be used only when the salt content is known to be minimal. The same precautions are to be exercised in the choice of solutions for douches and colonic irrigations."

Chapman, Snell and Rowntree (1931) describe the results: "About 80 per cent of the 84 patients have shown some response to treatment: about 47 per cent excellent results, 32 per cent fairly satisfactory results, 21 per cent poor results. In spite of the time required for this type of treatment, it is preferred by many patients to paracentesis. It is also apparent that ascites recurs much more slowly after medical treatment than after paracentesis. Mild toxic reactions occurred in about 35 per cent of this group of cases and consisted chiefly of diarrhea, chills, fever and hematuria detectable only on microscopical examination of the urine. In only a few instances were these reactions particularly severe, and in most cases it was possible to carry the treatment through to a successful conclusion in spite of them."

8. Surgical Treatment.—A number of short-circuiting operations to divert blood from the collateral circulation, as well as measures to establish additional connections between the portal and the general circulations have been employed with variable results. The best known of these, the Talma-Morison omentopexy, is believed by Höpfner to be beneficial in only one third of the cases, which is in agreement with the opinion of Eliot and Culp; Snell (1931), in a recent review, is no more sanguine. The operation is accompanied by high immedate mortality. Splenectomy, though giving great relief in some cases by removing a substantial burden from the portal circulation, is also accompanied by high surgical risk and not generally productive of so excellent results as in Banti's disease.

9. Hepatic Insufficiency.—In advanced cases in which there is very definite depression of liver function, perhaps especially of glycogen storage, such symptoms appear as loss of memory, delirium, convulsions and coma. These manifestations of toxemia may usually be made to disappear, at least temporarily, under the administration of adequate amounts of water and carbohydrate. Althausen (1933) points out that extra sugar may be conveniently and easily given by employing a high carbohydrate diet with additional feedings of 50 to 100 Gm. of glucose in fruit juices three times daily; he deplores the routine giving of 500 cc. of 10 per cent glucose solution several times daily intravenously as though that were the only known method of forcing carbohydrate nutriment. However, he recognizes the advantages of continuous intravenous infusion (venoclysis) in selected cases. Hendon (1930) has given 500 Gm. of glucose daily in this way for five successive days in instances of severe hepatic damage. Available evidence (Ravdin, 1929) does not indicate that there is any advantage in employing insulin also unless there is proof of its deficiency.

DISEASES OF THE RESPIRATORY TRACT

LARYNGITIS

Acute laryngitis appears rather suddenly with a dryness and tickling in the throat and some pain on swallowing; oftentimes there is tenderness to pressure made upon the protruding portions of the voice box in the neck. The voice becomes husky and speaking is not only painful but is also provocative of extreme weariness. Cough may not be present in the beginning but it usually develops quite soon and serves to eliminate considerable amounts of mucus. Not infrequently the voice is completely lost during the few days' duration of the attack.

Laryngitis usually follows the exposure to sudden changes of temperature, sudden climatic changes, the inhalation of irritating materials, or the excessive or faulty use of the voice. Occasionally the condition becomes chronic; in these cases there is nearly always a discoverable source of chronic infection in the nasopharynx.

THERAPY

Rest of the body, and especially rest of the voice, are the most important elements of treatment. Complete silence for forty-eight hours works wonders in these cases, but is practically never possible of enforcement.

Confinement to a room in which the temperature is maintained at an even level and the air moist is helpful. Some patients like to apply cold compresses to the throat. The use of a steamy inhalation mixture, such as is described under the treatment of Catarrhal Fever (see p. 30), is soothing. Gleason says that the taking of 10 drops of dilute nitric acid, in a glass of water every two hours, is often helpful in the aphonia of singers and speakers, a statement which is fully corroborated by the experience of many of the older practitioners.

The use of drugs to control the cough is doubtfully advisable since it serves a benign purpose; when it becomes too severe, however, the preparations described under the treatment of Catarrhal Fever (see p. 26) should be considered.

Oftentimes reeducation in the use of the voice is necessary for those who are suddenly thrust into a public-speaking career.

BRONCHITIS AND EMPHYSEMA

Sydenstricker, of the United States Public Health Service, has recently pointed out that the use of death rates as an index of the prevalence of disease has become so universal that the problems and aims of public health are set forth almost entirely in lethal terms when statistics are used. Valuable statistics these, but their use unfortunately sometimes serves to obscure the fact that there is still a tremendous amount of "ill health" in the world, even though people so fortunate as to dwell in civilized lands do not die so young as they did a few decades ago. What doctor of any experience at all needs to be told that the ailments of most individuals are seldom dangerously severe, though they are nevertheless of very great importance both to the individual and the community? Among these important affections that make people simply "sick," acute and chronic bronchitis and emphy-

sema hold a prominent place; indeed, together with the common cold in
its various stages, they occupy the *most* important place, for it is certain
that an upper respiratory infection is the diagnosis most often made in home
visits in Great Britain and the United States—doubtless this is also the
case in the other north temperate countries as well. Look well, therefore,
to the upper respiratory tract, you who read these pages, and try before you
die to contribute something to the success with which we may hope to
approach its affections.

I shall not pretend that a therapeutic distinction can be made—at least
by myself—between acute bronchitis and the common cold, with its more
severe forms known as grippe and influenza. I refer the reader to page 25,
where the treatment of Catarrhal Fever is described. The winter cough,
often becoming a year-round cough, of late middle-aged and elderly people,
coupled with shortness of breath and cyanosis on exertion, *i. e.*, that which
we call chronic bronchitis and emphysema, *may* be just that, but the wise
practitioner makes a careful search for a possible underlying cardiovascular
disease, aortic aneurysm, gout, syphilis or some other debilitating disease.
The treatment of these twin afflictions has advanced hardly at all since the
days of our great-great-grandfathers. Moderation in all things, the quiet
and regular life with the shunning of all vigorous pursuits, a residence in the
South during the winter—all of these measures are quite helpful to the few
for whom they are possible. The treatment of cough is described under
Catarrhal Fever (see p. 26).

BRONCHIECTASIS

Chronic dilatation of the bronchial tubes, which is secondary to tuberculosis, pneumoconiosis, tumor of the lung, etc., is characterized by the
paroxysmal coughing up of large quantities of extremely foul-smelling sputum which settles out into three distinctive layers on standing. The fingers
are clubbed and there is a webbed appearance in the roentgenogram. Provided there is free drainage, *i. e.*, free expectoration, bronchiectasis *per se*
does not usually cause very marked constitutional symptoms.

It would seem, from the work of Klare and Reusse, that children can
have extensive bronchial pathology of this sort without exhibiting the characteristic symptoms above described.

THERAPY

The general hygienic treatment of tuberculosis, combined with postural
treatment designed to facilitate drainage of the cavities, is employed in
bronchiectasis. In advanced cases the prognosis is poor. Measures to
control expectoration are described in the treatment of Tuberculosis (see
p. 245). It is the consensus of opinion that thoracoplasty, lobectomy, cauterization, artificial pneumothorax and the other surgical procedures should
be used only as a last resort. Mainzer (1931) recommends bronchoscopical
aspiration in each case, following the removal of the pus from the bronchi
by the injection of a medicated oil that acts as an antiseptic in the dilated
air cells.

ABSCESS OF THE LUNG

Abscess of the lung may follow a severe bruise of the chest wall or a
penetrating wound of the lung, or it may occur during the course of chronic
pulmonary tuberculosis, or it may occur as a sequela of pneumonia, espe-

cially the influenzal type of pneumonia. Its occurrence following operations in the mouth and throat of adults is notorious, particularly when general anesthesia has been employed. Whatever the cause, the cardinal symptoms and signs are: Cough and explosive expectoration, foul breath and foul sputum, elastic tissue in the sputum, dulness on percussion over a circumscribed area, and positive x-ray findings. Sometimes the symptoms of sepsis, such as intermittent fever, sweats, high leukocytosis, etc., are present. However, diagnosis is by no means always easy and not infrequently is made only at the autopsy table.

THERAPY

The use of an inhalant, such as is described on page 30, is indicated, and also the creosote and guaiacol preparations (see p. 242). These measures have little more than placebo value, however. The best medical treatment is postural: Placing the patient with head lower than feet and the affected side uppermost; this favors drainage but also increases the patient's discomfort.

Considering the relative frequency with which abscess of the lung is seen, very little has been accomplished toward its satisfactory treatment. Of course the problem is a very difficult one. Most long-standing cases eventually come to operation, but the results of surgery are not too brilliant either. Miller, Lambert, and others state that operation during the acute phase of abscess carries with it a mortality of 65 to 70 per cent.

PLEURISY

Pleurisy, which is usually abrupt in onset, often follows exposure to cold, or it may be a sequela to some other respiratory affection; in a few cases neither antecedent condition appears in the history. There is a stabbing pain in the side, which is aggravated by breathing and changes in posture; usually a hacking cough, which also aggravates the pain; increased respiration, leukocytosis, several degrees of fever; and a number of typical physical signs, the chief of which is a leathery friction rub. In some cases the pain is referred to the abdominal region, which makes differential diagnosis somewhat difficult; also, in some instances, the patient never at any time experiences any pain. Sometimes the onset is marked by pronounced chill.

Pleurisy with effusion differs very little in its onset from the dry variety, but when the inflamed pleural surfaces begin to be separated by the fluid, the pain disappears and dyspnea develops; it is not in order in this book to describe the numerous other physical diagnostic signs of effusion. Occasionally a patient feels very little subjective distress whatever.

The immediate prognosis in both forms of pleurisy is good. A dry case usually clears up gradually in two to three weeks; a case with effusion is often protracted much beyond this period. However, the fact that an attack of pleurisy is looked upon as presumptive evidence that the individual who suffers it is tuberculous, makes the disease of much more serious import. Some physicians of vast experience maintain that *all* cases of pleurisy are tuberculous; others hold that all cases not accompanied by the signs of a known infection, such as typhoid, are tuberculous; others are doubtful regarding dry cases (only 4 of Fulton and Hahn's (1931) 40 cases developed pulmonary tuberculosis during an average period of observation of seven years) but believe all cases with effusion to be of tuberculous origin; while there are those who, lacking positive evidence of tuberculosis in a first attack, always make a diagnosis of tuberculosis in any patient who has pleurisy twice, whether with or without effusion.

Boerhaave (1668–1738) was the first to show that pleurisy is an affection of the pleura alone.

THERAPY

The patient with dry pleurisy should be kept at rest—indeed he will impose the most absolute immobility upon himself, usually lying on the affected side with the shoulder depressed and the arm stretched along the body. Compresses are hardly worth using for relief of the pain. The best measure is the application of adhesive plaster strips (2-inch width) with the chest in the expiratory position. They should pass from the vertebral column to the midline in front, at right angles to the column, not slanting with the ribs; begin below and let each strip slightly overlap its predecessor. The cough does not usually require special treatment if the affected side is immobilized in this way. In severe cases, 1 grain (0.065 Gm.) of codeine sulphate, or ¼ grain (0.015 Gm.) of morphine sulphate, should not be withheld in the beginning. A number of physicians believe that calcium and parathyroid extract are effective at times in preventing effusion or promoting its resorption; for methods of administering these drugs, see page 714.

When fluid appears in sufficient quantities to aggravate the condition of the patient it should be removed by paracentesis. The indications for, and the technic of, this procedure are to be learned in an apprenticeship upon the wards and not from the pages of a book. Attempt should not be made to remove the effusion by diuresis or catharsis, for the fluid cannot return with sufficient rapidity through the inflamed serous membrane to make up for the loss of water by way of the kidney or bowel; the patient will thus only be weakened to no purpose. Blisters are also of little or no value.

The necessity for looking upon an individual who has once had an attack of pleurisy as a tuberculosis suspect is of the utmost importance, since by accepting such an attack as a sign from the gods that a readjustment of the mode of life is in order, we may sometimes entirely prevent the appearance of a frank pulmonary tuberculosis.

GAS BURNS IN CHEMICAL WARFARE

In the next great World War, poisonous gases will undoubtedly play an even greater part than they did in the latter days of that terrible conflict which is just a few years behind us. Therefore, despite the existence of the League of Nations, the World Court, Disarmament Conferences and other such millennial agencies, I feel obliged to treat of the therapeutic aspects of the subject in this place.

Local Treatment of the Respiratory Tract.—The following is a quotation from Page's excellent paper, read before the section on Laryngology, Otology and Rhinology at the meeting of the American Medical Association, in 1922.

"When we entered the war, the enemy was using mixed gases, thrown over with shells from trench mortars and by heavy artillery. The attacks usually began with gases which produced excessive sneezing and lacrimation; this being followed by the more poisonous gases, mustard and phosgene. Mustard gas, so called because its odor resembles that of mustard oil, classified as a vesicant, causes inflammation, blistering, discoloration of skin, acute conjunctivitis and intense inflammation of the respiratory passages

Its action is caustic, the extent of damage or destruction of tissue depending on the degree of concentration and the time of exposure. Its action may be delayed over a few hours to two or three days.

"Phosgene is classified as a lung irritant of suffocant type, which, in the alveoli and lung tissues, causes exudation of large quantities of frothy mucus; acute pulmonary edema, and death, by flooding the air spaces.

"One of the most important and arduous duties of the throat and ear service throughout the war, after the introduction of poison gases, was the treatment of gas burns of the respiratory tract.

"Our first observations [at Base Hospital 32] were made on a convoy of patients received, March 23, 1918, gassed in the Lorraine Woods, American sector, March 21 and 22, 1918. The gas attack was made with shells thrown from mortars and heavy artillery and was concentrated around the dugouts of Companies K and M, One Hundred and Sixty-fifth Infantry. When the attack began, all had on their gas masks and kept them on for two or three hours, when they were informed by their officers that it would be safe to remove them. Many claimed that they felt a burning sensation in the lungs while they had on their masks, but, from reports made by others, it was evident that they removed their masks too soon and that the masks afforded perfect protection while they kept them on. The first severe effects of the gas were felt in the eyes, at varying intervals of from one to three hours. The respiratory effect developed from a few hours to several days after the attack. A number of these patients had no symptoms of gas poisoning until they had slept under blankets which had been exposed to the gas.

"We had rarely witnessed such suffering and distress as these patients manifested, with skin burned and discolored, eyes swollen shut, spasms of choking, vomiting and struggling for breath, with the lungs literally drowned by their own secretions, they writhed in pain until they became unconscious from want of oxygen.

"Nausea, retching and vomiting, with pain and oppression over the chest, were among the earliest and most persistent symptoms, followed later by coughing and spasms of the glottis, with excessive discharge of frothy mucus often mixed with blood. Hemorrhages from the nose and lungs were among the rare symptoms. A deeply cyanosed and lead-colored face, labored respiration, rapid pulse, restlessness, constant and spasmodic efforts to expel the profuse frothy expectoration was the usual clinical picture during the first few days. The pain and distress in the lungs and epigastric region was often very intense.

"The pathology of gas burns is similar to that of an escharotic chemical applied to the tissues. If gas sufficient to produce serious effects is inhaled, there results an extreme engorgement of all the vessels and capillaries of the lungs, followed by the outpouring of a serous exudate from the injured bronchial and alveolar linings. In this stage, the patient might be drowned by the edematous exudate which fills the lungs, to the exclusion of the air. As in other inflammations of a severe degree, the outpouring of the fluid exudate from the blood is followed by deposit of fibrin on the injured surfaces. Thus, the bronchial passages, already wholly or partially denuded of epithelium, became lined or even occluded by a fibrinous membrane similar to that seen in diphtheria. This greatly hindered respiration and adhered to the mucosa with such tenacity that coughing was ineffectual to dislodge it. Necrosis of the bronchial walls and lung tissue resulted in a varying degree from exposure to the gas. These areas were, of course, promptly invaded by whatever bacteria were present in the respiratory tract, resulting in ragged, foul ulceration of the larynx, trachea and bronchi, and in multiple abscesses of the lung.

"After the first few days, the burned areas became infected and began to suppurate. As the necrotic process advanced, large quantities of exudate consisting of broken down tissue, tube casts, greenish-gray masses of membrane and sometimes necrotic lung tissue, were thrown off from the air passages. During this stage, the breath was very foul from the gangrenous discharges, and the patient, utterly exhausted from absorption of poison and the constant spasmodic and ineffectual effort to expel the accumulated slough, very often would lapse into a semiconscious state.

"In the milder forms of mustard-phosgene poisoning, we found the nasal, laryngeal and bronchial mucosa red, dry or edematous, in the early stages. The general appearance was not unlike an ordinary laryngitis or bronchitis. After a short time, the membranes began to pour out large quantities of mucus. In many of these cases of mild gassing, the patients recovered in a few days, and, in those patients who had been exposed to a high degree of gas concentration, the mucosa showed an intense hyperemia and dryness at first, followed later by flooding of the air passages with the frothy mucus, often mixed with blood. After two or three days, the burned areas were covered with a fibrinous membrane. These patches were found in the vestibule of the nose, on the turbinates and, in some instances, extending into the accessory sinuses. The mouth and pharynx seemed to show resistance to the caustic action of the gases, owing, probably, to the character of the epithelial lining; while the larynx, especially the arytenoid region, seemed to be particularly vulnerable. Burns were often found to be deep, with infiltration and edema about the vocal bands, causing aphonia, which occasionally persisted for weeks and months. The tracheal lining was usually burned in irregular patches. In many cases, the entire lining of the trachea extending into the small bronchi was involved. Edema of the lungs was always present to a greater or less extent when there had been exposure to the mixture of mustard and phosgene in any high degree of concentration. Bronchopneumonia with multiple abscesses was not infrequently present.

"At this time (March 23, 1918), when we received our first convoy of patients at Base Hospital 32, the Allies had not developed any treatment which was satisfactory for the effects of poison gases in the respiratory tract and lungs. Alkaline washes and sprays apparently increased the suppuration and aggravated the condition. We felt at liberty to institute any form of treatment that promised relief; and as I had had several years' experience in the treatment of laryngeal and bronchial affections with intra-tracheal medication, it seemed to be applicable in the conditions arising from gas intoxication. The first object of the treatment was to relieve pain and the exhausting spasms and ineffectual cough without the use of opiates; and next, to obtain better drainage of the lungs and respiratory tract. For these purposes, it was found intratracheal medication was the most effective. Medication in oil solution was introduced with the tracheal syringe during inspiration. Skilled assistants soon learned the trick of introducing the syringe and administering the medicated oils in the trachea and bronchi. In some patients who were peculiarly sensitive to any kind of throat medication, it was at first necessary to spray the pharynx with a 2 to 4 per cent solution of cocaine, before introducing the syringe.

"The principal medicines used were solutions or emulsions, in liquid petrolatum or olive oil, of either bismuth, iodoform, antipyrine, guaiacol, or camphor menthol. The following formula was found to be the most generally effective in the majority of cases: Guaiacol, camphor menthol, 5 per cent of each in liquid petrolatum or olive oil. From 1 to 3 drachms of this mixture was introduced into the trachea two or three times a day in the severe cases.

"When the oil solution reached the deeper bronchi a few seconds after introduction, the first effect produced was a cough, which expelled the contents of the bronchial tubes, often consisting of tube casts and diphtheritic membrane, grayish green, with pus, and other products of suppuration which had accumulated in the trachea, and which previous efforts of coughing had not been sufficient to expel. The natural drainage of the lungs was facilitated by the action of the camphor menthol on the inflamed, swollen mucosa, while the guaiacol acted as an antiseptic and anesthetic. The necrotic membranous exudate became more easily detached under the action of the liquid petrolatum, and easier breathing and better oxygenation were at once noticeable, as well as a diminution of the coughs and spasms. Relief of pain, with a sense of comfort throughout the lungs, usually followed with rest and better oxygenation; the general toxic condition of the patient improved.

"Without exception, these patients expressed themselves as receiving great relief, and, when suffering, requested the treatment. Those who received the treatment usually made a quick recovery, and most of them were able to return to the lines in a surprisingly short time, considering their condition when they entered the hospital. Of the 6000 gas patients who passed through our hospital, only 2 died. These deaths occurred within the first twenty-four hours after admittance. The results were so encouraging at Base Hospital 32 that the treatment was recommended in the official bulletin of the Allied Gas Service, in April, 1918."

Pierce has recommended the substitution of oil of peppermint in the petrolatum, as being more efficient than the other volatile oils in breaking down the frothy mucous discharge.

Findings of the Chemical Warfare Service.—Throughout the period of the United States' participation in the war, this service conducted experimental studies on animals, and in so far as was possible upon man also, under the able leadership of Frank P. Underhill, whose untimely death in 1932 was a great loss to our profession. The recommendations for systemic treatment, with particular regard to phosgene as it was the gas almost exclusively used toward the end, may be summarized, as follows: There are three types of cases, (a) those lightly gassed, the principal symptom being slight dyspnea; (b) so-called *blue* cases, with very pronounced respiratory distress and evidence of edema; and (c) the *gray* cases, with pronounced edema and almost utter inability to breathe, and often a shocklike condition also. In the *blue* cases, by analogy to animal studies, venesection to the extent of 0.5 per cent of the body weight is felt to be indicated as soon as practicable after gassing. If the temperature rises rapidly and a fall in blood concentration occurs (the two changes are simultaneous), a second and even a third withdrawal of the same quantity of blood may be made. If the *gray* stage is entered, in which there is a considerable fall in the temperature and marked increase in blood concentration, large quantities of fluid are to be given—by mouth if possible, as well as by intravenous infusion or intraperitoneal injection of normal saline. Such increase in edema as may, but is not likely to, follow this introduction of fluid is looked upon as of little moment if it be accepted that the cause of death is the excessive concentration of the blood and not the edema *per se.* Regarding oxygen, it may be said that the increasing concentration of the blood causes it to circulate less rapidly, which reacts upon the heart efficiency, and the two conditions combined cause the tissues to suffer from lack of oxygen and the nervous mechanisms to approach a condition of narcosis. The administration of oxygen is therefore distinctly indicated, but oxygen alone will not remove or alleviate the cause of the trouble, namely, the blood concentration.

Treatment of the Skin Burns.—Phosgene does not cause skin burns, but so-called "mustard" and lewisite do. I quote from the paper of Commander E. W. Brown, U.S.N., written in 1928:

(a) *Mustard*.—"The first step in the protection of the skin against the effects of contact with mustard is prompt and complete removal. Mustard enters the skin very quickly and, unless its removal is accomplished without loss of time, a serious burn will surely result. The first essential is to prevent further exposure to mustard from contaminated clothing or equipment, which would be a source of danger both to the casualty and to those attending him. This should be removed at the earliest possible moment.

"A bathing procedure, if possible, using shower baths with hot water and soap, is organized for all personnel suspected of contamination with mustard vapor. The eyes are prophylactically treated with boric acid lotion. This is followed by the issue of fresh clothing. Mobile bathing units for this purpose were assigned to army divisions on the western front toward the end of the World War. If the patient has been exposed only to mustard vapor the bathing procedure and change of clothing will usually be effective if carried out within thirty minutes.

"Liquid mustard is removed from the skin by sponging with an organic solvent, such as kerosene or carbon tetrachloride, in which it is soluble. If the mustard has been in contact with the skin for more than one or two minutes, it will be absolutely essential that the area be treated with fresh portions of the organic solvent every two or three minutes and massaged with the hand continuously after each application, the entire operation continuing for thirty minutes. This technic will prevent blistering if commenced within twenty minutes after exposure to the mustard."

(b) *Lewisite*.—"The most suitable treatment for the vapor burns of lewisite is the use of a ferric hydroxide paste which consists of a suspension of fine colloidal nongranular ferric hydroxide in pure glycerin. This paste is applied profusely over the burn and covered with an impervious dressing.

"Promptness in removing liquid lewisite from the skin is even more imperative than in the case of mustard. Lewisite is completely destroyed by the application of a 5 per cent solution of sodium hydroxide, which must then be quickly removed by washing with soap and water. This method will undoubtedly save life by preventing the absorption of a lethal quantity of arsenic through the skin after extensive exposure. A more effective procedure, which has proved successful with animals, is excision of the skin of the burned area and adjacent region. This may be regarded as a life-saving procedure for a period as long as twenty-four hours after the burn has been received, provided the lewisite has been already neutralized with the sodium solution."

Tear Gas.—There is irritation of the eyes, lacrimation, and a tendency toward salivation and irritation of the throat, and slight rubefaction and mild burning of the more tender portions of the skin. Col. Vedder (1925) says that there is no effect upon the lungs in any concentration that will be met with in the field, a statement which doubtless applies as well to the conditions under which the gas is used against mob gatherings. However, upon exposure to somewhat more than the usual concentration it may require twenty-four hours before the eyes feel perfectly normal again, and it is conceivable that enough irritation of the eyes and throat may occur in such instances to pave the way for secondary bacterial invasion with ensuing conjunctivitis and pharyngitis.

When the contents of a tear-gas gun are directly discharged against the skin or into the eyes, McNally (1932) finds that prompt washing of the skin with 50 per cent alcoholic solution of sodium sulphite, and the eyes with 0.4 per cent sodium sulphite in 25 cc. water and 75 cc. glycerin, effectively relieves distress.

DISEASES OF THE KIDNEYS

NEPHRITIS AND NEPHROSIS

Introduction and Classification.—So far as is yet known, the first description of kidney disease was that of Aetius (500 A. D.), who is said to have found at autopsy that certain cases of dropsy were associated with hardening of the kidneys. Rhazes (860–932 A. D.), the great Arabian clinician, probably also recognized the entity but no further advance toward its understanding was made until Avicenna, that "convivial Omarian spirit" at the court of Bagdad, noted that in dropsy the urine was thin, watery and increased in density. Then Saliceto, in the middle of the thirteenth century, provided the classical description of edema associated with contracted kidney, and Malpighi (1628–94), aided by the great discoveries of Harvey (1578–1657), established the function of the capillaries. Thus were laid the foundations upon which Richard Bright (1789–1858) was able to erect his anatomico-pathologico-clinical classification. A hundred years have now passed since the last of these fundamental contributions was made, and it seems that we have about reached a position from which it has become possible to view the disturbances in normal physiology associated with nephritis with greater advantage to the patient than accrued to him from the exclusive study of renal pathology necessary in an earlier day. Many attempts are being made to clear the way completely for this new manner of considering the disease by simplifying the classification of types to a point where this phase of the subject will cease to be confusing. Indeed the necessity for any very rigid classification at all has come to be looked upon with considerable doubt, since the physician rarely deals at the bedside with any one of the forms pure and unmixed except in very acute cases.

Certainly it will suffice us to employ here for therapeutic purposes some such simple conception as that depicted in the accompanying figure. Here the toxic nephritides are regarded as including acute and chronic glomerular and tubular nephritis and nephrosis, and they are all looked upon as being the renal manifestations of the operations of some deleterious agent which causes inflammatory and retrogressive changes in these structures and which is also probably, in some particulars demonstrably, affecting the other active tissues of the body as well. The other type, arteriolosclerotic nephritis, is considered to be the late expression in the kidney—in the form of sclerotic changes in the glomeruli and tubules as a result of progressive constriction of their arterioles and capillaries—of a similar process in the finer arterial structures throughout the body, most probably as the result of the prolonged action of some toxic agent not derived from the kidney. The following simple descriptions of the above types must suffice.

Toxic Nephritis.—Acute diffuse glomerular nephritis usually makes its appearance rather insidiously, in children several days or weeks after apparent recovery from one of the acute streptococcic infections, such as tonsillitis, scarlet fever, rheumatic fever or erysipelas. Cases occurring during a subacute bacterial endocarditis are usually looked upon as "focal" rather than "diffuse," the differentiation being made on the smaller number of glomeruli found to have been involved in the rare specimens that come to autopsy, plus the absence of hypertension and edema. Gainsborough (1932) has very well remarked, however, that the absence or presence of edema cannot afford a very critical division since the beginnings of tissue edema

461

are invisible. In the common or diffuse form there are present both edema and hypertension, but the former is rarely of the marked pitting sort seen in chronic nephritis, and the latter is usually not inordinately high and very rarely may not be present at all. There is more or less albumin in the urine but the characteristic feature of these cases, in addition to the hypertension, is the presence of red blood cells and red cell casts, often enough to cause the urine, which is diminished in amount, to have a smoky brown color. The prognosis as regards life and recovery without permanent sequelae is quite good in these cases; indeed, better perhaps than is usually believed, as shown by the careful study of Tallerman (1932), in whose 27

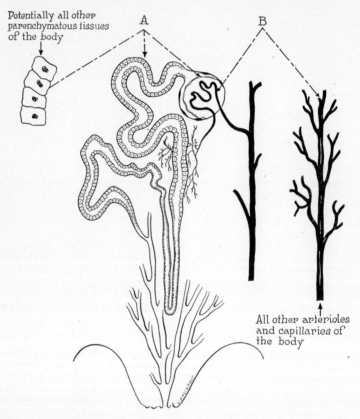

A. Site of disturbances in toxic nephritis.
B. Site of disturbances in arteriolosclerotic nephritis.

consecutive cases, followed up for periods of eighteen months to three and one-half years after discharge from hospital, only 2 died and only 4 showed any evidence of persisting renal damage. The future course seems to be independent of the initial severity of the symptoms, except that Van Slyke has observed that in cases in which the plasma protein has fallen to a low level the tendency to become chronic is marked. However, a most alarming picture may at times develop, the characteristics of which are vomiting, headache, visual disturbances, frequently a slowing of the heart and respiratory rates, coma, convulsions and ultimately death. This syndrome, which is variously termed "uremia," "pseudo-uremia," or "convulsive uremia," is apparently unrelated to the retention of nitrogenous products and has been shown by Blackfan to be caused most probably by cerebral edema. Cases advancing toward chronicity often develop subacute exacerbations during which there is some elevation of temperature and the urine is clouded with blood and casts, but as the glomeruli are gradually destroyed during months and years the urine contains less blood and fewer erythrocytic casts, and finally nitrogenous retention, manifested by rise in blood urea and creatinine, makes its appearance foretelling uremic termination—though it has been remarked that in all *fatal* cases of chronic nephritis characterized by severe nitrogen retention there is an acidosis severe enough in itself to be the actual cause of death. It has also come to be increasingly recognized in recent years that severe secondary anemia is an accompaniment of decreasing renal efficiency, though it may also appear early in the acute cases.

The striking characteristics of tubular nephritis, which distinguish it in its pure form from the glomerular type, are hyaline, waxy and fatty casts but no blood or blood casts in the urine, marked and persistent edema, and albuminuria without hypertension or nitrogen retention. This type may also appear acutely in children in the course of streptococcal infections, or as a mild form complicating Asiatic cholera, diphtheria, malaria, syphilis, typhus, yellow fever and possibly other infectious diseases. It is the nephritis sometimes caused by mercury, also the nephritis seen in pregnancy. If, in addition, there is observed an increased blood cholesterol, refractile globular bodies in the urine, a low metabolic rate, a marked disturbance in the ratio of serum albumin to serum globulin, and a tendency toward a protracted course with relatively frequent complete recoveries or death from intercurrent infection without the appearance of signs of severe inflammatory renal disturbance—in these cases the diagnosis of lipoid nephrosis is made, which is considered by some observers to be a rare entity not directly related to inflammatory nephritis.

Arteriolosclerotic Nephritis.—This type of kidney disease is only one element in the cardiovascular-renal syndrome, which begins with "essential" hypertension, progresses to arteriolar disease of the body as a whole and not solely of the kidneys, and ends often in cardiac or apoplectic death before kidney complications of a serious nature have appeared. The urine is much increased in amount and low in specific gravity and contains often only a small amount of albumin and a few hyaline casts. Edema is not a usual feature of the pure form, but ultimately uremia appears in association with the slowly increasing nitrogen retention. More rapidly progressive cases are designated "malignant."

The Essential Unity of Nephritis.—In the attempt to view disease as a natural response to disturbed physiology one is ever beset by visual temptations to see it only in a series of histopathologic pictures, and is thus traduced from achieving a complete vision of the full significance of conglomerate manifestations. To avoid this error in so far as is practicably possible in the present instance, and to enable us more easily to look upon nephritis as essentially a systemic affection, we must bear in mind that with diverse and often overlapping manifestations in the kidneys, the occurrences characteristic of the malady are only necessary adjustments in normal renal function, our knowledge of which function is comprised in the following fundamental observations: (*a*) That albumin and casts are normally passed by the kidneys; (*b*) that products of protein destruction are normally eliminated through the kidneys; (*c*) that the kidneys normally both secrete and reabsorb water and salts; (*d*) that they maintain the osmotic pressure of the blood at a constant level, and (*e*) that they share at all times in the maintenance of acid-base balance in the body.

(*A*) That the passage of albumin and casts may be regarded as a normal thing is evidenced by their presence in the urine after strenuous exercise, by the "functional" albuminuria of adolescence, and by the passage of albumin after the ingestion of excessive amounts of albumin (as egg albumin, for instance) at any age; furthermore, it is by no means unusual to find an occasional hyaline cast in the urine of a normal person, and Addis (1926) and his co-workers have shown that both casts and albumin can be found in almost every specimen of normal urine provided certain precautions are taken.

(*B*) The normal catabolism of protein consists chiefly in the deamination of amino-acids with the elimination of ammonia, which combines with carbon dioxide to form ammonium carbonate, is then dehydrated to the carbamate and ultimately to urea, which final waste product is excreted in the urine at a daily rate of 30 to 40 Gm. when the blood urea level is normal. The efficiency of this renal excretion is maintained long after the secreting units in the kidneys have been quantitatively much reduced by disease. Other nonprotein nitrogenous products normally appearing in small quantities in the urine are uric acid, creatinine, amino-acids and ammonia.

(*C*) The accepted explanation of the secretion of fluids and solids by the kidney is that of Cushny, according to which the glomeruli filter off enormous quantities of fluid containing all the noncolloidal constituents of the plasma, which fluid is then reduced to the quantity and concentration characteristic of urine by a process of reabsorption in the tubules, the urine ultimately being composed of the excess of fluid not needed by the body, normal constituents of the blood which have been present in it in excessive quantities, and all abnormal substances such as drugs, foreign proteins, etc.

(*D*) The filtration-reabsorption process also aids in maintaining the osmotic pressure of the blood unaltered.

(*E*) The extent of the kidneys' participation in the maintenance of acid-base balance is insignificant in comparison with the activities of the lungs, but it is very important nevertheless for it is by the renal route, together with the bowel, that the nonvolatile sulphuric and phosphoric acids resulting from protein catabolism are eliminated. The final economic advantage which the body derives from employing this excretory route lies in the fact that the ammonia used to accompany the passage of these acids is formed directly in the kidneys, thus conserving the fixed bases of the blood and maintaining the alkali reserve.

Obviously, in view of the above considerations, the matters requiring closest attention in nephritis, from the standpoint of their systemic or local origin and causation, are albuminuria, edema, hypertension, nitrogen retention, acidosis, anemia, lipemia, and hypothyroidism.

Albuminuria.—The oldest of the fixed conceptions regarding the origin of the albumin in the urine was that it was the direct result of the renal lesion; that is to say, that the albumin was a product of the degeneration of the functional units in the kidney. But this belief has almost entirely given way before the point, so trenchantly made by Christian, that in patients dying of infection relatively early in the course of a nephritis characterized principally by degenerative changes in the tubules (tubular or chronic parenchymatous nephritis, or nephrosis), the daily amount of albumin in the urine has been often far in excess of what could possibly come from degenerating renal epithelium. Therefore the opinion has come to be almost universally held that the explanation of the albuminuria is in the passage of albumin through the walls of blood vessels, most probably "glomerular capillaries, thus presupposing the occurrence of a functional change in a colloid membrane of which the microscope gives no evidence" —a surmise, to be sure, but entirely in consonance with the hypotheses by which we account for many other phenomena. Albumin may possibly normally pass through the capillary walls all over the body, with exception of the three sites of which Simonds (1932) recently reminds us: the alveolar walls of the lungs, the choroid plexus of the brain, and the glomeruli of the kidneys (to this latter there is, however, some qualification, as earlier pointed out). Now in each of these locations the capillary endothelium is covered on its outer surface by a layer of closely adherent flat epithelium and, at least in the glomeruli, as shown by McGregor (1929), these two layers are separated by a thin hyaline basement membrane. To Simonds it therefore appears probable that albuminuria is due to retrogressive changes in this epithelial layer of the glomeruli. However, entrenched as we may be in either of these two very rational conceptions that the cause of albuminuria lies solely in demonstrable or nondemonstrable changes in the kidney, there can be no longer any excuse for cursorily dismissing the accumulating evidence that the nature and source of the albumin, and the cause of its appearance in the urine, are to be found elsewhere. Volhard's (1914) explanation of the influence of a hypothetical poison arising in the tubules did not greatly challenge the old position since it merely assumed that this poison caused the increase in permeability; and Fahr also explained the occurrence on approximately the same basis. Aschoff (1917) had, however, in the meantime gone a step further and postulated the increase in glomerular permeability upon a toxic damage of the whole body. But the wide departure from accepted beliefs has been that of Epstein (1921), whose views on this point are essentially those of Munk (1925), namely, that there occurs in this malady a general metabolic disturbance of such nature that there is a shift in the plasma proteins toward the coarser globulin fraction, albuminuria then resulting when the kidneys excrete this foreign "denatured" protein in a quite physiologic way and without any increase in their permeability. Storm has of course raged round this view, and many observers have accepted as final the independent studies of Hewitt (1927) and Cavett (1930), who have been unable to find any differences in the protein of urine and plasma. However, Thomas and his associates, Schlegel, Andrews and Welker, in work which they have been reporting since 1928, are strongly supporting the foreign protein position. Thomas, recently, by departing entirely from the optical rotation and chemical methods of Hewitt and Cavett, and turning to the admittedly more delicately accurate immunological precipitin method of Hektoen, has been able to demonstrate some quite astonishing things. The protein excreted during the first hours of an artificially induced uremia in his dogs reacts strongly to an anti-liver precipitin, indicating the presence of liver tissue without serum proteins in the urine; central nervous system, muscle and spleen proteins have also been identified. Gradually this tissue reaction becomes weaker and is finally masked altogether by the serum reaction. In these later portions of urine, Welker has succeeded in identifying a toxic peptone radical attached to the protein molecules. Thomas' present belief is that, normal or damaged, the kidney is able to retain within its circulation those proteins which are normal to the body and will excrete proteins foreign to it. The excretion of serum proteins in nephritis indicates that these proteins have become so altered that they no longer conform to the requirements of the organism and are therefore excreted as such. As a result of general damage to parenchymatous tissue in nephritis, this conception postulates the releasing of tissue proteins into the intercellular spaces, from which they enter the circulation as relatively nontoxic tissue proteins and are excreted by the kidneys only because they are foreign to the blood. Shortly, however, as the process proceeds, the cells are further damaged, the protein is split so as to lose its identity, and as this splitting is carried to the proteose-peptone stage the split products become highly toxic. At this point, then,

30

they unite in the blood stream with a normal molecule of serum protein, the two combined form a foreign protein and are excreted, though the combination retains the precipitin identity of serum protein. The very rational comment of Leiter (1931) upon all such reasoning, namely, that in other diseases associated with pronounced tissue destruction—widespread tumor metastases, starvation, severe infectious diseases, acute yellow atrophy of the liver, etc.—there is usually no marked appeárance of albumin in the urine, is of undeniable force; nevertheless, I believe that this approach of Thomas *et al.* is the most promising that has so far been made in the attempt to understand albuminuria.

Edema.—I think that quite as certainly as we now generally admit that albuminuria may have its cause in some factor or factors which the eye cannot always detect in the autopsied kidney, so must we likewise grant that the histologic features of 2 cases may be the same on postmortem examination, though the one patient died with edema and the other did not. And so the physiologic approach must again be made, examining factors regulating fluid balance between the fixed tissues and the blood current, so far as our present knowledge has revealed them: (1) The water and salt excretory function of the kidneys, (2) variations in capillary permeability, (3) osmotic and hydrostatic pressure relations within the capillaries.

Water and Salt Excretion by the Kidneys.—It has long been the consensus of opinion that the increase of water and chlorides in renal edema is due to the inability of the damaged kidneys to excrete them, but it is certainly equally rational to maintain that these substances are not excreted simply because they are held by the tissues, and therefore never presented for elimination. All the more does this latter assumption seem to be the likely one in view of the repeatedly confirmed observation that in the normal kidney approximately 90 per cent of the functional units are always at rest; one feels that were the water and sodium chloride presented to the kidney during nephritis quite as they are at any normal time, this tremendous reserve of structure coming in part or whole into action would be able to more than counterbalance the crippling effect of the loss of a relatively few units damaged by disease. Now, just recently, two bits of information have come to light which seem to me to disprove quite convincingly the assumption that the lowered excretory function causes the edema. Loeb (1932) and his associates very carefully studied a patient with gross edema and a normal individual who was maintained on a "salt-poor" régime; when sodium chloride was given to these two individuals, both retained the salt and water, the retention being greatest in the edematous individual; however, after the base of the blood of the normal subject had been returned to its normal level by the ingestion of sufficient salt, continued ingestion of salt caused no further retention of either it or water. The implication of this is plain: So long as the tissues require salt to make up for a shortage they retain all that reaches them in the blood, water being likewise held in fulfillment of well-known physicochemical laws—a process with which the kidney has nothing whatever to do. The second piece of information is the beautifully clear-cut demonstration of Lashmet (1931) that not only is edema due to tissue thirst for chloride but also that it is actually thirst for chloride in a specific form; when he gave sodium chloride to edematous patients the edema increased regardless of the daily fluid intake, but when he gave an equivalent amount of chloride in the form of hydrochloric acid, the edema promptly decreased without any relationship to the intake of fluids, and the chloride content of the urine was multiplied several times. Barker (1932) accomplished the same remarkable result by substituting potassium chloride for sodium chloride. Here again we have a comedy of errors that plays itself out behind the scenes of the renal theater.

Variations in Capillary Permeability.—As the assumption is made that increased permeability of the glomerular capillaries accounts for albuminuria, so too can it be made to account for edema—the tissues become water-logged simply because the systemic capillaries become permeable to such a degree that flooding is inevitable. This may be the right and true explanation, but I know of no sound experimental or clinical studies that have served to substantiate it; indeed, the passage of water and its contained diffusible molecules is always so rapid in both directions through the capillary walls that it is impossible to conceive of any factor that could influence it only in one direction. Leiter has therefore well pointed out that those who employ the term "increased permeability" can only mean by it an increased passage of plasma proteins or other colloids out of the vessels —which is a contravention of actual experimental evidence.

Osmotic and Hydrostatic Pressure Relations Within the Capillaries.— The plasma proteins, consisting of albumin and globulin in a relationship to each other of 1.5–2.5 to 1, together with a very small amount of fibrinogen, do not serve as a source of nutrition for the tissues and hence do not pass freely out of the vessels. Their chief function was pointed out by Starling so long ago as 1895, namely, the maintenance of balance between colloid osmotic pressure and electrolyte hydrostatic pressure within the capillaries, the hydrostatic pressure being measured in terms of the force exerted by the diffusible crystalloids in attempting to escape from the capillaries in fulfillment of the laws of diffusion, the osmotic pressure being measured in terms of the force exerted by the relatively nondiffusible colloids in opposing this attempt through fulfillment of the laws of osmosis. Epstein (1917) first drew attention to the bearing of this struggle upon the problem of edema, but the first actual measurement of the relationship of the two combatant forces in edema was made by Krogh (1922), who showed in a single case that as a result of considerable loss of plasma colloid through albuminuria the balance of forces was markedly tipped in favor of the filtration of fluids from the blood into the tissue spaces, an observation that has been many times confirmed. Having established that the total colloidal osmotic pressure is greatly reduced through the loss of proteins, and that as a result fluids pass into the tissues in abnormal quantities, it remained necessary to answer the objection offered in the work of Linder, Lundsgaard and Van Slyke (1924), who found that the greatest decrease in plasma proteins does not always correspond to the greatest extent of edema, and that, indeed, a marked decrease in plasma proteins is even compatible with absence of edema. The partial answer had, however, apparently already been made in the studies of Govaerts (1925), who showed that albumin molecules have a much higher osmotic pressure than globulin molecules; therefore a serum with 5 per cent of protein may yield a much lower osmotic pressure than another serum with the same amount of protein if the first has less albumin and more globulin than the second. The following is now accepted as an explanation of what takes place: When the total protein of the plasma falls as a result of albuminuria, the ratio of albumin to globulin is reversed, the proportion of globulin to albumin becoming greater; however, the large globulin molecule exerting a lower osmotic pressure than did the small albumin molecule which it replaces, the attempt at compensation usually fails, and edema appears. That the globulin effort may succeed, however, has been shown by Salvesen (1926), whose patient showed a complete lack of edema in spite of months of gross albuminuria, which was an unintelligible state of affairs until it was found that in him the globulin had risen to such extent as to completely make up the albumin loss. On the other hand, a relatively small increase of albumin, even though accompanied by a corresponding fall in globulin so that total protein does not rise, may be sufficient to alter the degree of edema very noticeably. Moore and Van Slyke (1930) have observed an almost perfect correlation between reduction in plasma protein content and presence of edema in 75 cases, though Krogh's (1929) placing of normal plasma protein osmotic pressure at about three times that of capillary filtration pressure would allow a considerable fall in the proteins without the appearance of edema.

A complete explanation of the edematous process is not offered by this protein-disturbance conception, as the earlier discussion of the specific ionic factor indicated, but it certainly brings us a great step toward complete understanding. The unanimity of opinion regarding the low protein content of edema fluid, together with the evidence adduced by plasma protein reduction in animals by the process of plasmaphoresis, as employed by Leiter (1928) and more recently by Barker and Kirk (1930), strongly support the thesis.

Hypertension.—In the arteriolosclerotic (cardiovasculorenal) type of chronic Bright's disease an assumed preliminary period of spasm of the finer arteries and arterioles is succeeded by a process of fibrosis throughout the entire circumference of the intima without the nodular distribution and fatty degeneration with deposit of lipoids that characterize the ordinary type of arteriosclerosis. The lumen of the vessel is gradually narrowed and finally obliterated entirely and replaced by a core of connective tissue. In the kidney, the afferent vessels to the glomeruli, and the extensions of same to the tubules (see figure, p. 462), are affected; but these changes are not limited to the renal arterioles, for they have been seen by Simonds (1932) in the spleen, pancreas, liver, suprarenals and surrounding fat, and by Kernohan, Anderson and Keith (1929) in the skeletal muscles. Obviously, the increase in quantity of the urine is rationally explained upon the basis of increased blood pressure and decreased resorptive capacity of the tubules. The causes of hypertension in this type of the disease are not to be sought primarily in the kidneys; they are the causes of "essential" hypertension, whatever they may be, and indeed many patients die of cardiac failure or vascular accident without ever showing any signs of renal involvement, though, of course, death in uremia is by no means uncommon in the group. The belief that the rise in the blood pressure is a compensatory process to overcome the narrowing of some of the glomerular arterioles dies hard, however, despite the fact that it has several times been shown that plugging of the glomerular arteries, bilateral ligation of the ureters, or even removal of the kidneys produces no elevation in blood pressure. In their excellent brief review of nephrosclerosis as it occurs in children, in whom they feel that exogenous and endogenous poisons and toxins can usually be ruled out as etiologic agents, Mitchell and Guest (1931) describe such an array of effects upon growth, development and nutrition as make it difficult to ascribe all the symptomatology of this disease in children to occlusive lesions exclusively. They feel that further metabolic studies are urgently necessary. Do not many things point to an underlying allergic or metabolic dyscrasia in adults also? Essential hypertension, and with it cardiovasculorenal disease, is still almost a complete mystery; it is not a kidney disease *per se.*

In those types of toxic nephritis in which hypertension also appears, I see no reason for avoiding the assumption of a general systemic action of the offending agent to produce a generalized spasm of arterioles and capillaries. Indeed, something of the sort must take place, for in some cases of acute glomerular nephritis the rise in blood pressure actually precedes any abnormal urinary findings. Major (1930) has stated that in some cases, studied very early, a constriction of the skin capillaries can also be demonstrated before the appearance of typical symptoms. The reason for hypertension in all types of nephritis may therefore be looked upon as lying outside any potential causes that may be histologically demonstrated in the kidneys.

Nitrogen Retention.—It is probably the almost universally held belief that studies of the relative ability of the kidneys to excrete dyes and concentrate solids in the urine, and the determination by chemical methods of the fluctuations of nonprotein nitrogen (uric acid, creatinine and particularly urea) in the blood, provide together a reliable index of the impairment of renal function in nephritis and, further, that the well-known symptoms of clinical uremia are a direct result of "poisoning" by the retained products after they pass a certain point of concentration in the blood. The strongest arguments in support of this faith are: (*a*) The sudden imposition of an extra burden upon an already diminished renal functional capacity, such as excessive vomiting or diarrhea or an intercurrent acute infection, is reflected in added evidences of functional impairment. (*b*) So long as the patient is able to clear the blood of potential retention products by increasing the quantity of urine to counterbalance the lowered ability to concentrate it, uremia does not occur. (*c*) Retention occurs during other destructive kidney diseases, such as tuberculosis, pyelonephritis, polycystic kidney, malignancy, etc., and when there is an obstructive process, such as bilateral ureteral calculus; when this latter is relieved, the retention ceases. (*d*) It is difficult to see how diminished ability to concentrate the urine could be the result of anything but renal functional impairment. (*e*) Uremia is nearly always accompanied by marked retention.

However, there is also a host of facts of at least speculative interest which may be arrayed against a too blind acceptance of this faith. (*a*) Unless we admit the possibility of other extrarenal factors conditioning retention we must accept its appearance as evidence of destruction of two thirds of the renal tissue, for it has been shown that in conditions other than nephritis adequate elimination occurs if only two thirds of one kidney remain. (*b*) Use of the new standard clearance tests have shown that it is the persistence of impaired renal function rather than the height of the rise of the retained products that determines the prognosis in acute nephritis. (*c*) To account for intervals of relatively good renal functioning in the presence of a far-advanced lesion we employ the phrase "stage of compensation," though how this can be justified if it is assumed that all of the trouble is in the kidney I am sure I do not know. (*d*) An individual with such slight renal symptoms that we refer to him as only *potentially* nephritic, may suddenly go into a type of uremia, following an accident, anesthetic or the like, with very bizarre manifestations in the blood chemistry: A fall in retention products while the condition is becoming rapidly worse, or a tremendous rise in the same during a period of distinct clinical improvement. Looking upon such occurrences as an indication of what is going on solely in the kidneys makes them very difficult to understand, but if they are accepted as at least partially due to some generalized, or perhaps even specialized, but at any rate extrarenal metabolic upset, then the task is lighter. (*e*) Renal function may be markedly impaired in such a nonrenal condition as pernicious anemia, and of course inability of the urine to concentrate solids is an outstanding symptom in diabetes insipidus. (*f*) Experimental animals live from five to ten days with a large part or all of the kidney tissue removed and die without having shown any of the characteristic uremic symptoms. In man also, obstruction and complete anuria with a consequent high rise in retention products does not cause uremia, nor does it appear during the anuria of bichloride of mercury poisoning. (*g*) There is a pronounced hereditary tendency to develop nephritis. (*h*) Other profound changes in the physical chemistry of the body, such as those already discussed in connection with edema and albuminuria, argue in favor of nitrogen retention being of the same nature, rather than comprising merely the damming back in the blood of products which the kidney is unable to excrete.

It certainly seems to me that we cannot rest content with our present understanding of retention. If nephritis is really a general or special metabolic disturbance, with other manifestations as well as those in the kidneys, then it is quite rational to look elsewhere than the kidneys for at least a part of the cause of retention. Of course the possibilities are very great. Thomas (1931) believes that in nephritis the level of the nonprotein nitrogenous products in the blood is simply the level at which osmotic and chemical equilibrium with the tissues must be maintained under the peculiar conditions obtaining in the disease; when the equilibrium is satisfied the kidneys excrete the excess over the demand, regardless of the level. He offers the timely reminder that the body will remain in nitrogen equilibrium, the kidneys doing their share of the work, whether the total nonprotein nitrogen of the blood is 25 or 100 mg. per cent. The production of some substance foreign to normal catabolism, probably with a special affinity for the nerve cells, must at least be postulated to account for uremia, the more particularly as the peculiar diazo reaction remains unexplained. "Undetermined" or "rest" nitrogen rises disproportionately in nephritis; perhaps some poisonous fraction of this is converted into one of the known waste products normally (Foster suggests the analogy of guanidine's conversion into creatine), but fails to undergo the change in nephritis. Retention remains one of the great challenges of medicine.

Acidosis.—In the terminal stages of nephritis acidosis is usually present to a marked degree, in most instances roughly paralleling nitrogen retention. Phosphates and sulphates are retained in the blood, there is decreased formation of ammonia by the kidneys, and as a result direct depletion of the alkali reserve takes place. This depletion is sometimes even augmented by an increased excretion of alkali by the kidneys and the loss of additional base through vomiting, for in advanced nephritis the free hydrochloric acid in the stomach is often very small in amount. All of this may come about merely as a result of diminished renal functional ability, but I feel that we will be wise to reserve final judgment in this instance, for these things too may be but a part of the general metabolic disturbance in nephritis. Elucidation of the point in a speculative fashion would require us to go deeply into the subject of acid-base balance, for which space is not here available.

Anemia.—Just how or why destruction of a certain portion of kidney tissue causes anemia is not known. Certainly there must be other factors than just the local disturbances concerned, for in some cases of nephritis the hemoglobin poverty appears surprisingly early, and sometimes it does not appear at all. The reduction of protein in the blood through albuminuria is probably etiologically important. McLester (1932) feels that in chronic arteriolosclerotic cases, in which blood protein level is maintained, much of the anemia is directly chargeable against unnecessary dietary restrictions.

Lipemia.—In some cases of nephritis the blood serum becomes cloudy or almost milky in appearance due to an abnormal content of fatty acids, cholesterol esters and phosphatides. The phenomenon apparently bears a direct relation to reduction of blood protein, particularly the albumin fraction, but the reasons for its appearance are still entirely speculative; it may be an attempt to maintain osmotic pressure, or it may be looked upon with equal legitimacy as just another evidence of the general metabolic nature of the disease, marking an excessive production or mobilization of lipoids, or an inability to utilize or remove them from the blood stream.

Hypothyroidism.—Low basal metabolic rates have been recorded a number of times in nephritis, but a reclassification of the disease which would ascribe fundamental significance to these observations is not warranted upon the basis of any evidence yet accumulated. In his recent exhaustive review, Leiter (1931) expresses his doubt that the incidence of such rates is any greater than might be expected to occur secondary to undernutrition, therapeutic diets, inactivity and possibly other factors not directly related to the intimate nature of the malady.

It seems to me that even in this brief review of the physiologic factors associated with or underlying the nephritic state it must be apparent that the conception of the malady, nephritis, as a fundamental unit whose primary cause lies outside the kidneys is at once most rational and most profitable; rational because it offends none of the accepted canons of scientific approach; profitable because it greatly simplifies the problems of therapy. The objection that the only visible evidences of pathology are to be found in the kidneys is of small weight; do we not recognize the diseases of allergy, deficiency diseases, and the diseases of metabolism, in whose victims we can find no definitely causative lesions when we place their dead bodies upon the slab? The picture of a separate entity, "lipoid nephrosis," which belongs outside the frame, was first drawn by Müller, in Germany. The work has apparently made no lasting impression in France and has only recently occupied British observers to any great extent, but here in America, Epstein's interest in the subject has caused it to receive much attention. However, I think that most astute observers are now of the opinion that in these cases we are most likely dealing only with tubular (chronic parenchymatous) nephritis dignified by a new title. Murphy and Warfield, in 1926, were apparently of the opinion that "pure" cases of nephrosis, though rare, do occur; but four years later Warfield finds great difficulty in differentiating between nephritis and nephrosis; "One can have pure tubular degeneration and on top of that one can have inflammation, or one can have inflammatory lesions, the so-called 'acute glomerular nephritis,' and on top of that have degenerative processes leading to large amounts of albumin in the urine and to the presence of the doubly refracting lipoids which are so characteristic of pure cases of so-called 'degenerative' nephritis or nephrosis." Leiter (1931) admits that the nephrotic type of glomerulonephritis can symptomatically mimic nephrosis down to the last detail, but believes that the pathologic differentiation can be made if there is skill and interest enough on the part of the pathologist. However, Bell (1929), even when employing the fine technic of McGregor, was unable to make this distinction, though Leiter feels that the cases were "probably not pure lipoid nephrosis." Many "pure" cases of nephrosis, just as some "pure" cases of nephritis, undoubtedly recover, but most of the former die from intercurrent pneumococcic or streptococcic infections. It is not known what would happen if infection did not occur, but Gainsborough stresses the importance of noting that the cases of glomerular nephritis which present at some time the nephrotic syndrome in purest form are those which have the longest course and greatest chronicity. Leiter says that true uremia never occurs; it *couldn't*, says Gainsborough, and still be a case of "pure" nephrosis by definition! I shall not go on with this—the nephrosis protagonists are bravely championing their views and may be able some day to offer more than academic proofs of their validity.

The Importance of Full Nutrition.—However much it may shock our preconceived ideas, the time has now certainly come for full recognition of the fact that protein restriction, Karell and other semistarvation diets, are completely outmoded procedures. The reasons for this are so clear that they lend themselves to terse statement: (*a*) Nephritis, either acute or chronic, is a wasting disease; Harrop has well pointed out that, disregarding edema, the patients are almost invariably underweight. Full feeding is certainly the best weapon against wasting and cachexia. (*b*) Anemia, which has come to the fore as a matter of considerable importance in nephritis, always calls for food, particularly proteins. (*c*) The belief that the kidneys can be spared by restricting protein intake is quite incorrect because if the requisite amount of protein is not supplied in the food it will be derived from the tissues, and in the end the kidneys will have nitrogenous waste products to eliminate just the same. The patient is thus in effect eating himself in order to keep alive, a rather unpleasant if not dangerous extremity in adults, absolutely inimical to growth and development in the young. In McCann's (1931) edematous patients, the nitrogen of the high-protein diets was most probably stored as deposit protein, since the non-protein nitrogen of the blood did not increase. Peters and Bulger conclude from their extensive investigations that presumably the blood proteins lost through albuminuria may be also replaced; the clinical impressions of many physicians support these observations, so that, other things being equal (see acidosis, p. 478), it is doubtful if there is any harm whatever in prescribing liberal protein feeding even in the presence of considerable retention. The hemorrhagic state in acute nephritis is also no contraindication. Indeed, the contention that a meat diet is harmful has never been substantiated. The affirmative animal experiments of Newburgh and his associates have been equally confirmed and denied by other investigators. It would seem to be Newburgh's present belief that the harmful effects observed in his rats may have been due to substances associated with the proteins which he fed in enormous quantities. His normal human subject lived for six months on 4177 calories, 327 Gm. of animal protein daily (truly, says Moulton, a gargantuan diet!), while engaging in nonstrenuous activities; as a result he developed both albuminuria and cylindruria, but both disappeared completely ten days after cessation of the diet. Nephritis, therefore, was not caused, and it is certainly open to legitimate doubt whether the lesions produced in animals are directly comparable to those of chronic toxic nephritis in man; they bear no relationship to those of the arteriolosclerotic type. Thomas writes that the Greenland Esquimo on a carnivorous diet exhibits no increased tendency to vascular or renal disease, and Lieb finds no evidence of kidney disease in Arctic explorers who have lived on an almost exclusive meat and fish diet for years. McClellan and Du Bois (1930) have studied Stefansson and Anderson during one year while they lived on an Arctic meat-fat type of diet and found no demonstrable injury of any sort. McCay reports that the incidence of nephritis is no greater among the meat-eating Europeans in India than among the Bengali who get very little good protein, while Gunewardine writes me that in Ceylon essential hypertension is very common. Summarizing, then, we lack proof and even strongly suggestive evidence that meat eating is harmful. (*d*) If the assumption is correct that toxic destruction of proteins is taking place, an additional reason is provided for high-protein feeding, since under these conditions more is needed to maintain nitrogen balance. The necessity is freely granted in typhoid fever, streptococcic infections, etc., where a considerable degree of such destruction is known to occur; McCann has found that even in tuberculosis, in which there is only slight toxic destruction, the minimum level of nitrogen balance can be reached only by taking from two to two and one-half times the caloric requirements of a patient in bed. The actual computation of diets can be based entirely upon the needs of a normal healthy individual of the patient's age, height and weight, though certain advantages in making definite alterations in the protein, water, salt, acid and base allowances will be considered in the immediately following paragraphs. McLester (1932) feels that for economy in nutrition, carbohydrate should provide 50 per cent, preferably more, of the caloric value of the ration in order to assure that the protein will be used for repair rather than burned for the production of energy. "The type of food chosen, provided these specifications are met, is of little importance, with one exception: The protein should in large part be of high biological value such as is found in meat, milk and eggs. In general it can be said that if the adult with nephritis takes a quart of milk daily, two eggs and one large serving of meat, his need for protein will be covered and no harm will be done his kidneys." In so-called "lipoid nephrosis," Epstein favored marked fat restriction, but Schiff (1932) is reporting good results by looking upon the high lipoid content of the blood as an evidence of lipoid-want and meeting the indication with a diet rich in fat, especially egg yolks, beginning with two or three and increasing quickly to five daily, given with sugar and orange juice; meat, vegetables, etc., are of course also employed. Matters to be discussed in the succeeding pages will suggest the advisability of other alterations in individual cases.

The Importance of Protein in Controlling Edema.—The absolute advisability of supplying at least the full normal daily amount of protein, which is 1 Gm. for adult males, 0.75 Gm. for females, per kilo body weight, is directly corollary to the discussions of albuminuria and edema in the preceding pages. Even higher than normal quantities of protein are being used, 150 to 200 Gm. or more, but it is probable that enthusiasts will tend eventually toward figures around 100, which is above normal for an average individual but still not usually unpalatable. However, McCann's fifteen-year-old patient's condition was stationary at 75 Gm., but showed immediate and marked increase in serum protein, carbon dioxide combining power of the blood and urea clearance, and decrease in red cell and cast content of the urine, when this quantity was doubled. McLester's (1932) experience has been similar. Experimentally, Kerr, Hurwitz and Whipple have found that regeneration of serum proteins is quickest on a meat diet, slower on bread and milk, and slowest during fasting. The deposit of protein in the tissues may increase the edema for awhile until the slowly rising serum proteins draw it out again and diuresis begins.

Water, Salt, Acid and Base Allowances.—Study of the preceding pages will have prepared the reader for the statement that also in these particulars therapy has been considerably rationalized. It is not electrolytes and water so much as the way in which they are given that matters. The tissues are holding water and chlorides and are eager for more chlorides, as I have said before, but it is not *sodium* chloride that they want. Loss of sodium is a characteristic phenomenon associated with diuresis and the reduction of edema; sodium chloride administered is retained and edema increases if the nephritic state is at all severe or advanced. An absolutely salt-free diet (see p. 451) is certainly not advisable for the following reasons: (*a*) Such a diet is woefully unpalatable and causes nausea and vomiting, headache and legache, and a host of other symptoms; (*b*) moderate reduction is easier and in the end more effective because it can be continued for a long period; and (*c*) the substitution of other chlorides has become quite practicable in the light of recent studies.

The average daily salt ration in America is about 10 Gm., water intake probably 2000 cc. The salt can be considerably reduced without difficulty since most of it derives from its addition to foods during preparation, most raw foods being salt-poor. The principal exceptions that are likely to be included in the average dietary are milk, butter, cheese, preserved meats, fish and breads. Simpson (1931) writes: "In a normal diet of an average person which includes these latter articles the salt intake, exclusive of salt as a condiment, will not exceed 3 Gm. daily. The unpalatability of a salt-poor diet can be overcome, partly, by using such highly flavored substances as pepper, mustard, vinegar, lemon juice, spices, garlic, onion, etc. The rather commonly held opinion that such condiments and foods are harmful to kidney structure is not supported by experimental work." Briefly, allowing any foods desired but forbidding the use of salt either in kitchen or dining-rooms, means permitting 3 Gm. daily; this may be raised by actual additions of salt, lowered by omitting milk, butter or any other of the worst offending articles.

Simpson feels that if the output of urine keeps within 300 cc. of the intake of water the patient, though he may be somewhat edematous, is in little danger of becoming water-logged. The keeping of a graphic chart of intake and output, as he advocates, will be found very helpful, for on it the physician can watch this relation from day to day and month to month; the contents of the twenty-four-hour urine container should be measured at a stated hour each morning before bowel movement, and the measurement at the same time of the amount of water remaining in a measured quantity supplied at the beginning of the twenty-four-hour period will avoid the bothersome measuring of each drink. However, the newer practice of substituting other chlorides for sodium promises to very much lighten the difficulties of water and salt restriction. Calcium chloride having been shown to be an effective diuretic but very disturbing to the gastro-intestinal tract, Keith, Barrier and Whelan, in 1924, substituted ammonium chloride for it, in daily doses of 5 to 16 Gm. (75 to 240 grains) in connection with a low-salt, low-fluid regimen. The drug is often quite effective; one of their patients lost 11 pounds (5 Kg.) in eight days, and in a single day the urine amounted to 2350 cc. Lashmet (1931) has taken a step in advance of this by showing that it is the reaction of the total ash of the diet that is the important thing. He uses a diet that is neutral in reaction and then assures the acid reaction of the total ash (the incombustible inorganic residue) by the administration of ammonium chloride, as above, or the use of from 100 to 200 cc. of N/10 hydrochloric acid daily. Under such a regimen, diuresis often occurs independently of the fluid intake. But the most important of the newer contributions seems to me to be that described below.

The Importance in Diuresis of Sodium Replacement by Potassium.— Barker (1932) noted in the study of edema in dogs that when potassium chloride was substituted for sodium chloride in equal amount at any period during fluid storage, a prompt and marked diuresis occurred. After repeatedly confirming this observation, he has made excellent clinical application of the fact in edemas of both nephritic and cardiac causation, employing all the factors concerned in the physiologic approach to the subject. Table 46 contains all the details. Briefly, the patients are given a liberal diet which is adequate in every respect except that a small amount of viosterol had best be used now and then to overcome the deficiency in vitamin D. The total amounts of specific mineral agree closely with Sherman's (1930) average of 150 American dietaries except in the inverted ratio of potassium to sodium. The diet is properly high in protein and has an acid ash. No sodium chloride is used in either kitchen or dining-room, but the patient is given 5 Gm., occasionally more, of potassium chloride crystals in a salt shaker each morning; with this he salts his food and at the end of the day places the remainder in water and drinks it. Twelve of 16 patients, both nephritic and cardiac cases, have lost their edema under this regimen. No significant changes in blood sodium or potassium were noted, despite the poisonous nature of the potassium ion, no ill effects have followed after as long as a year and a half, one individual with pronounced nephrotic syndrome requiring 10 Gm. potassium chloride daily to remain edema-free. In contrast to the use of acid or acid-forming salts, as described above, this treatment has not caused a shift in the acid-base balance. This work of Barker seems to me to be of very bright promise. It is particularly gratifying to find in it the explanation of Osman's (1930) disturbing report of diuresis following the administration of alkalis, *i. e.*, Osman gives alkali in the form of large quantities of potassium salts.

Diuretic Drugs.—*Acid Salts and Calcium.*—The use of the acid salt, ammonium chloride, has been discussed above; ammonium nitrate is often substituted. Calcium chloride acts also as an acid-forming salt and has been used successfully at times in per orum daily doses of 10 to 20 Gm. (150 to 300 grains), but is quite disturbing to the gastro-intestinal tract. It may be given intravenously, however, in doses of 5 to 10 cc. of a 10 per cent solution. It would seem that the sodium antagonizing effect of calcium is also a factor here, for calcium lactate, in daily amounts of 10 to 20 Gm. by mouth, is occasionally effective. O'Donnell and Levin (1931) have also had success with calcium gluconate given subcutaneously in doses of 15 to 30 grains (1 to 2 Gm.) in 10 to 20 cc. of water, at intervals of two days or more; the drug may also be given intramuscularly or intravenously. Parathyroid extract, in doses of 20 to 50 units at intervals of one or more days, has given very divergent results. Peters and Eiserson (1929) have confirmed the earlier finding that serum calcium rises and falls directly with the excursions of plasma protein. See page 714 for precautions when injecting calcium salts.

Novasurol (Merbaphen) and Mersalyl (Salyrgan).—Most physicians believe that these two very similar mercury compounds are contraindicated in nephritis. In Sprunt's (1930) study of kidneys at autopsy, renal damage was found to have occurred in 1 of 6 cases in which novasurol had been given in the absence of any known contraindication. However, in Keith, Barrier and Whelan's series novasurol produced beneficial effects in 3 cases after the patients had taken sufficient ammonium chloride to render the urine decidedly acid. After a preliminary intramuscular injection of 0.5 cc. to observe the effect, the drug was given intramuscularly or intravenously in doses of 0.5 to 2.5 cc.; no deleterious effects were noted. Barker and O'Hare (1928) have had a similar experience. From the historical point of view, Leiter cites the interesting fact that Richard Bright gave mercury to his edematous nephritics until they salivated, but was not convinced of the wisdom of the procedure.

Caffeine, Theobromine and Theophylline.—These members of the xanthine group practically always fail to promote diuresis in nephritis.

Urea.—In daily doses of 30 to 90 Gm. (1 to 3 ounces), stirred up in water, urea is sometimes slowly effective in inducing diuresis, but is usually discontinued after a little while because the effect is rarely commensurate with the rigor of the ordeal.

Sweating.—In accordance with the belief that it is the high nonprotein nitrogen content of the blood *per se* which induces the fatal termination in nephritis, sweating would be theoretically indicated because the perspiration contains 30 per cent more of these retention products than does the blood. However, even though induced only by the use of hot-water bags and plenty of blankets, sweating is a very debilitating activity. A hypodermic of $\frac{1}{12}$ grain (0.005 Gm.) of pilocarpine nitrate is very effective in bringing out the perspiration, but it also not infrequently causes vomiting and hiccup, and may bring about collapse with a very slow pulse. If there are pulmonary complications the danger of precipitating pulmonary edema is very great.

Catharsis.—Some physicians favor the daily dose of a saline cathartic, but the practice certainly makes it impossible to maintain any exact knowledge of the patient's ability to eliminate through the kidneys. Proprietary

TABLE 46.—LOW SODIUM-HIGH POTASSIUM DIET WITH ACID ASH FOR USE IN EDEMA
(AFTER BARKER)

Ingredients

Fruits:
    3 servings daily, fresh or stewed, but should include either prunes, .plums, cranberries
    or currants once daily.
Vegetables:
    2 large servings daily, especially beets, carrots, Brussels sprouts, yellow corn, kohl-
    rabi, lettuce, mushrooms, peas, spinach, kidney beans, parsnips.
Meat:
    2 servings daily.
Eggs:
    2.
Milk:
    1 glass.
Cream:
    ½ glass.
Butter:
    Salt-free, 6 squares.
Cereal:
    Oatmeal or wheatena; farina, puffed wheat or rice occasionally.
Bread:
    Graham bread, 3 large slices or 6 small slices daily.
Rice, macaroni or spaghetti:
    1 serving daily
Potato:
    1 serving.
Jelly, preserves or honey:
    2 level tablespoonfuls.
Sugar:
    Ad libitum—at least 1 tablespoonful.

Sample Menus

1	2	3
Breakfast	*Breakfast*	*Breakfast*
Stewed currants	Plums	Stewed prunes
Oatmeal	Wheatena	Farina
Two poached eggs	Scrambled eggs	Soft cooked eggs
Graham toast	Graham toast	Graham toast
Sweet butter	Sweet butter	Sweet butter
Honey	Jelly	Honey
Cream	Cream	Cream
Sugar	Sugar	Sugar
Dinner	*Dinner*	*Dinner*
Roast beef	Broiled steak	Broiled lamb chop
Mashed potatoes	Buttered macaroni	Buttered spaghetti
Buttered beets	Stewed tomatoes	Buttered spinach
Sliced peaches	Banana salad	Grapefruit cup
Graham bread	Graham bread	Graham bread
Sweet butter	Sweet butter	Sweet butter
½ glass milk	½ glass milk	½ glass milk
Supper	*Supper*	*Supper*
Broiled chicken	Broiled liver or sweet-	Broiled whitefish
Buttered rice	breads	Mashed potatoes
Jelly	Baked potato	Buttered Brussels sprouts
Lettuce salad	Celery salad	Pineapple and nut salad
Orange cup	Cherries	Graham bread
Graham bread	Graham bread	Sweet butter
Sweet butter	Butter	Jelly
½ glass milk	Jelly	½ glass milk
	½ glass milk	

Menu	Pro-tein	Fat	Carbo-hydrate	Cal.	Vitamin				
					A	B	C	D	E
1	89.3	140.4	235.9	2565	+++	+++	+++	+	++
2	77.2	131.4	215.7	2355	+++	+++	+++	+	++
3	84.2	130.1	227.6	2417	++++	+++	+++	+	++

Mineral Content

Ca	Mg	K	Na	P	Cl	S	Fe	Acid	Base
0.660	0.278	3.362	1.126	1.514	1.485	1.139	0.0177	46.4	34.0
0.627	0.268	3.263	1.038	1.332	1.556	0.975	0.0156	42.6	34.6
0.638	0.299	3.483	1.061	1.471	1.47	1.177	0.0168	45.4	40.5

Notes

All foods are to be prepared without salt and no salt is to be served with meals. Potassium chloride (from 2 to 5 Gm. in shaker) may be given as salt substitute. Spices—cinnamon, sage, paprika, pepper, cloves, nutmeg, allspice—may be used. Small servings of citrus fruits may be added after fluid volume is established. Additional vitamin D to be supplied.

Coffee or tea, 1 cup daily.

This diet is designed preferably for the treatment of convalescent and ambulatory patients. Very ill patients will have difficulty in eating all the diet, in which event, the diet may be reduced, the same food substances to be given, but in smaller amounts.

---

saline mixtures should not be used unless it is positively known that they contain no other salts than the nonabsorbable ones desired to produce the cathartic effect. The following salines are effective:

1. Magnesium sulphate (Epsom salt): ½ to 1 ounce (16 to 32 Gm.).

2. Magnesium citrate: Principally used as the solution of magnesium citrate, an effervescing preparation in 12-ounce bottles; dose 1 bottle or less. Milk of magnesia can be converted in part into magnesium citrate by the addition of a fruit acid, such as lemon or orange juice.

3. Sodium sulphate (Glauber's salt): Dose ½ ounce (16 Gm.).

4. Potassium and sodium tartrate (Rochelle salt): Dose 2½ drachms (10 Gm.).

5. Sodium phosphate: Dose 1 drachm (4 Gm.); there is also a pleasing effervescent preparation with a dose of 2½ drachms (10 Gm.).

6. Compound effervescing powder (Seidlitz powder): Dose, the contents of one blue paper (sodium bicarbonate and Rochelle salt) and of one white paper (tartaric acid), dissolved separately in water, and then mixed.

Mechanical Measures for Reduction of Edema.—Extensive hydrothorax or abdominal ascites, if causing respiratory embarrassment, is usually relieved by paracentesis. Recently, Bland and White (1930) have read a paper on the use of the Southey tubes, which has provoked considerable discussion and revealed that the profession retains a quite justified faith in the efficacy of mechanical drainage of fluid from the edematous legs following the opening of the skin. Acupuncture, which is the making of six or more punctures in either extremity with an 18-gauge needle, and the making of long deep incisions are the older methods and have their very great efficacy marred considerably by the many obvious disadvantages associated with causing the person and bed of the patient to be soaked in fluid; for the patient able to sit up with the feet in a small tub they are excellent. When the Southey technic is employed the fluid is led off through tubes.

In Pemberton's (1932) opinion, the value of gentle massage in promoting redistribution of fluid is too much overlooked in this country.

Anuria.—There are equally cogent arguments in favor of forcing or restricting fluids, though Murphy (1933), summarizing an abundant experience, says: "After using both methods in many cases, it is concluded here that the administration of fluids gives the best results in quantities varying from 2000 to 3000 cc. daily. Fruit juices and water given by mouth, glucose solution (500 cc. of 10 per cent solution) by vein, or water administered by rectum accomplished satisfactory results. To promote diuresis is the main object of treatment. Objections have been made to the use of large quantities of fluids on the ground that it favors the formation of edema and especially edema of the brain. Anuria, if unchecked, leads to an early uremia and it involves more danger to the patient than edema. Hot wet packs, applied twice or three times a day, in conjunction with adequate fluid consumption, frequently bring relief. Packs do not benefit the patient by extracting fluid or poisonous substances through the skin but they aid in promoting diuresis." In acute cases, or acute exacerbations of chronic cases, decapsulation, or simply incision into the kidney, have upon rare occasions increased the amount of urine. The first theoretical explanation of the result is that these operations relieve the tension of the kidney induced by the compensatory effort to overcome the diminished circulation in the glomeruli, and I don't believe it; the second, that the circulation of the organ is improved through the entrance of new blood vessels through the new capsule, seems equally unsatisfactory, for experimental studies have shown that after decapsulation an efficient collateral circulation is rarely, if ever, established. Diathermy has been recommended in the German clinics.

Anemia.—The high protein diet is the best safeguard and cure; indeed, in arteriolosclerotic nephritis, the poverty of the blood is the principal reason for the full protein diet, since here we do not have to combat great protein loss. The usual hematinics fail in nephritis; at times blood transfusions are imperatively required.

Acidosis.—Undernutrition is well known to promote acidosis, which is another argument for full feeding in nephritis. Mitchell and Guest remind us of the faulty synthesis of glycogen in acidotic states as an important factor in the poor development and growth of young nephritics. Even in the severe acidosis of advanced cases, the necessity for reduction of protein will not arise if we heed the report of Lyon *et al.* (1931), whose careful work showed that the readjustment of the diet to give an alkaline ash will often result in a decrease in the acidity and considerable amelioration in symptoms; measures by which this may be accomplished are: Reduction in meat, rice, macaroni, bread, cereals; increase in fruit and vegetables; addition to the diet of figs, molasses and raisins. If the patient remained on an acid diet, Lyon was able to overcome its acidifying effect, while retaining all the advantages of feeding meat, etc., by supplementing it with sufficient alkali by mouth to keep the urine alkaline; in some instances he had to do this even though a basic diet was being employed.

It is possible of course to induce a state of acidosis with the acid-forming salts used in combating edema, though this rarely happens. Barker's method of using potassium chloride is a superior diuretic measure upon this head also.

Hypothyroidism.—A number of observers—Campanacci, Eppinger, Epstein, Liu, Molnar and others—have reported the favorable production of diuresis by the employment of enormous doses of thyroid substance in nephrotic cases. The results are by no means always obtained, but the fact seems to be established that individuals exhibiting the low basal metabolic phase of the malady can sometimes tolerate astonishing amounts of this ordinarily very toxic agent. Epstein gave as much as 4 Gm. (60 grains) of desiccated thyroid daily. One patient received 1.5 Gm. (22 grains) daily for five months, followed by a total of 137 mg. of thyroxin in eleven weeks, with no striking effect on the basal rate and no symptoms of toxicity. Leiter believes that this is not true hypothyroidism in spite of the rate, that a tolerance above normal may be found in other edematous states, and that the matters of absorption, destruction, excretion need to be studied in view of the differences between this sort of reduced metabolism and that encountered in true myxedema. Platt (1929) failed to demonstate thyroxin in the urine of one of the nephrotic patients while being dosed in the above extravagant manner.

Hypertension.—The treatment of essential hypertension must remain entirely unsatisfactory until the causes of the rise in pressure are elucidated. The several measures designed to relieve this condition are discussed on page 559.

Uremia.—The treatment of uremia is the treatment of acute and chronic nephritis, *i. e.*, the attempt should be made to prevent the occurrence of a severe uremic state. When convulsions and coma have developed, death is almost certain to take place in a short time, nor do I know of any remedial measures that have been shown to have any appreciable efficacy in staying the end. Resort is often had to the withdrawal of 500 to 1000 cc. of blood, with the simultaneous administration of an equal quantity of physiologic saline. I wonder in how many cases this procedure has really been of value?

Nonuremic Convulsions in Children.—In the presence of this syndrome, which Blackfan regards as caused by edema of the brain, magnesium sulphate is given in large doses—1 to 2 ounces (30 to 60 cc.) of a 50 per cent solution by mouth or rectum every four hours. Strangely enough, profuse catharsis is seldom induced. If this method of administration does not check the cerebral symptoms and reduce the blood pressure, Blackfan now injects intramuscularly, since he has found this route just as satisfactory as the intravenous, formerly advocated. Usually 0.2, occasionally 0.4 cc., of a 25 per cent solution per kilogram (2.2 pounds) is the dose; the effects are usually seen in fifteen to thirty minutes, but failing, the injection can be relatively safely repeated after two or three hours. He has had no alarming toxic symptoms follow the use of the drug parenterally, but it is well to be prepared to combat respiratory depression by the slow intravenous injection of a few cubic centimeters of 25 per cent calcium chloride solution. The fact that the mechanism of this action of magnesium sulphate is not entirely understood should not militate against its careful employment in these emergencies.

DISEASES OF THE BLOOD-FORMING ORGANS

CHRONIC SECONDARY ANEMIA

Under the above title may be conveniently grouped the anemias seen in the following conditions: (*a*) Chronic blood loss, as in the case of patients with peptic ulcer, bleeding hemorrhoids, uterine lesions (especially fibroids), and sometimes in cirrhosis of the liver. (*b*) Chronic nephritis, jaundice, tuberculosis, cancer. It has become habitual to refer to the anemia in these cases as a matter of course, but the actual fact is that we do not know why it occurs. (*c*) Intestinal parasites, especially hookworm and the broad tapeworm. (*d*) Chemical poisons, such as lead and the coal-tar derivatives. (*e*) Pregnancy and the puerperium. (*f*) Infectious diseases and septic states. Such conditions as the following, in addition to a number of the acute infectious diseases: Chronic arthritis, pyelitis, dental and nasal infection, endocarditis, cholecystitis, salpingitis, osteomyelitis, etc. (*g*) Idiopathic. A large group of cases; in Leake and Evans' careful study of 63 cases of secondary anemia, 15 were described as "cause unknown."

In chronic secondary anemia there is usually a reduction in both the number of red cells and the amount of hemoglobin, but the hemoglobin is reduced to the greater extent. Sometimes there are a few reticulocytes (young red cells) in the circulation. The symptoms are usually predominantly those of the underlying disturbance, but in the idiopathic cases the symptoms are pallor, weakness on exertion, shortness of breath, slight puffiness about the ankles, and perhaps a soft heart murmur. Medical students, and frequently practitioners as well, often have the idea that pallor means anemia. That this is not true is demonstrated by that class of industrial workers who rarely see the sun and are of a nearly deathlike pallor, and yet are no more often anemic than are persons from any of the other walks of life. Pallor is one of the symptoms of marked secondary anemia but all pallid persons are not necessarily anemic.

THERAPY

The attempt to increase the number of red cells and the amount of hemoglobin in secondary anemia is a worthy one, but it must always be looked upon as secondary in importance to the search for the causative factor and the eradication of the same where that is possible. Such measures as are described below, therefore, are to be looked upon as constituting merely symptomatic treatment, though as such they have a very considerable importance.

1. **Iron.**—Every clinician of any experience knows that a patient who has secondary anemia will have the hemoglobin content of his blood raised by the prolonged use of iron unless he is moribund and unable to respond to any therapy; to be sure, it may not be very greatly raised in all cases, but the height of the hemoglobin increase is sufficient in most cases to indicate the value of iron therapy in secondary anemia. There has been entirely too much broadcasting of the results of animal experimentation performed under conditions not at all comparable to those obtaining in practice. Who will believe that the failure of animals to respond to iron therapy after they had been rendered anemic for a very short period by a few severe bleedings has anything to do with the subject? Whipple and his co-workers (1925) have

shown that when these animals are bled in only small amounts and over a long period of time, *i. e.*, when conditions are rendered comparable to those obtaining in the human, then iron therapy is effective. And, as I have said before, iron therapy is effective in practice even though it is not known why a patient, who is apparently taking sufficient iron for the needs of the body in his daily food, should nevertheless profit by the use of additional iron in the form of a drug. It is very easy for interested parties to exploit much of the experimental work of the last few years in favor of the expensive (and to them profitable) *organic* iron preparations. I shall not review in this place the controversy which raged for many years between the champions of organic *versus* inorganic iron, for it is all settled now: *Inorganic preparations are fully as effective and in some cases more effective than the organic preparations;* the latter are therefore not superior as a class, and only one or two having special merit will be described in this book.

The following are satisfactory preparations of iron.

Blaud's Pill (Pill of Ferrous Carbonate, U.S.P.).—The conventional dose is 2 pills after meals three times daily, but much larger doses are often needed to obtain full effect; Sargant (1932) has effectively employed 150 grains (10 Gm.) daily in powdered form in capsules when smaller dosage has failed. The U.S.P. pills are quite stable and are superior to proprietary substitutes which are urged upon the profession because "Blaud's pills don't keep." They *do* keep! Practically all patients can take Blaud's in moderate doses without any gastro-intestinal disturbance.

Mass of Ferrous Carbonate, U.S.P. (Vallet's Mass).—This may be prescribed in pills or capsules in the same dosage range as Blaud's pills; thus when giving the large doses of ferrous carbonate it is sometimes convenient to use this mass for the reason that considerable may be packed into a single capsule.

Saccharated Ferrous Carbonate, U.S.P.—Prone to slowly deteriorate; ferrous carbonate had better be given in the form of the above mass or as Blaud's pills.

Reduced Iron, U.S.P.—A grayish-black, tasteless, nonastringent, insoluble powder. Must be given in capsules. A dose of 1 grain (0.06 Gm.) three times daily is conventional, but for full effect from 45 to 90 grains (3 to 6 Gm.) must be given daily. This preparation is best given just before meals to allow the HCl of the gastric secretion to have full effect upon it; it does not cause gastro-intestinal disturbances.

Ferrous Lactate, N.N.R.—A mild iron preparation, which, because of its feeble taste, may be taken without difficulty. The dose range is from 1 to 20 grains (0.06 to 1.3 Gm.) depending upon the age and size of the individual. Because of its liability to oxidation, it is best prescribed in solutions containing much sugar. Syrup dissolves 4 grains to the ounce (0.25 Gm. to 30 cc.).

Iron and Ammonium Citrate, U.S.P.—This is a freely soluble preparation with a slightly iron-saline taste. The conventional dose is 4 grains (0.25 Gm.) three times daily after meals but it is often necessary to give from 60 to 120 grains (4 to 8 Gm.) daily to obtain full effect. On the higher doses gastro-intestinal disturbance is not unusual. *Iron Citrate Green— P.D. and Co.* is an N.N.R. preparation that contains proportionately more ammonium citrate and is therefore said to be less painful and less likely to produce coagulation of proteins when used subcutaneously or intramuscularly than the U.S.P. preparation. The daily dose is ¼ to 1½ grains (0.015 to 0.1 Gm.); ampules of ¼, ¾ and 1½ grains are available. However, it has never been certainly proved that the injection of iron is the least whit more satisfactory than its use by mouth—*though* it brings the patient back to the office oftener.

31

Cacodylate of Iron.—This is another preparation for injection, embodying the virtues of both iron and arsenic. I do not think it a necessary preparation since the injections must be given daily, are quite painful, *and exactly similar results can be obtained when the iron and arsenic are given by mouth.*

Tincture of Ferric Chloride, U.S.P.—This preparation is both acid and highly astringent, yet, to judge from its popularity in the treatment of anemia in the northern United States, one would believe it to be the only iron preparation available; in the malarial belt down South they know better. The dose is 10 minims (0.65 cc.), well diluted, three times daily after meals; it is usually considered necessary that it be taken through a glass tube to protect the teeth. The *Tincture of Ferric Citrochloride* has fewer incompatibilities.

Measures must oftentimes be instituted to overcome constipation in those taking iron over a long period, for even the less astringent preparations are prone to induce costiveness after a time. Aloe is much favored in these cases as it has its activity increased by the presence of iron salts. The reader is referred to the discussion of constipation (p. 431).

2. **Arsenic.**—There is a firmly entrenched clinical impression that arsenic is of value in the treatment of secondary anemia especially if combined with iron. Iron and arsenic combinations cannot be made in solution unless the arsenic is used in the form of *Solution of Arsenous Acid, U.S.P.*, dose, 3 minims (0.2 cc.), for the salts of iron are incompatible with all other forms of arsenic in solution. Arsenic trioxide, in an average dose of $\frac{1}{60}$ to $\frac{1}{30}$ grain (0.001 to 0.002 Gm.), may be combined with any of the irons in capsule or pill; or a 3-minim (0.2 cc.) average dose of the solution of potassium arsenite (Fowler's solution) may be administered in water before meals and the iron preparation be taken after meals.

I know of no valid reasons why the more expensive sodium cacodylate should be preferred to the older inorganic preparations of arsenic, except the magic of the needle which holds so many uncritical physicians in mystic thralldom. The injections are painful, they many times cause the patient to have a very offensive garlic breath, and they force his attendance at the office of his physician every day for a long period. Decidedly, the treatment of secondary anemia by the injection of iron and arsenic, when the same results can be obtained by the simpler per orum medication, is opposed to the best interests of modern practice.

3. **Spleen Marrow.**—There is nothing new in the idea of using either spleen or bone marrow in the treatment of anemia, but Leake (1923) has given new life to this type of therapy by undertaking a careful study of the combined effects of the two substances. The following line of reasoning serves him for a working hypothesis: "(*a*) The production of red blood cells is not constant and maximum for existing red bone marrow, but, more in accordance with the general economy of nature, is regulated by the rate or extent of erythrocyte destruction, and a margin of reserve remains for the functioning of existing red bone marrow, with extension of the erythrogenic centers occurring only when this margin of reserve is exhausted under conditions of extraordinary stress. (*b*) The spleen, usually accepted as the organ chiefly concerned with the removal of the older erythrocytes from the circulation, elaborates, in proportion to the number of red blood cells removed, and possibly from them, a hormone capable of stimulating erythrocyte production. (*c*) This splenic hormone, being carried by the blood, lodges in the erythrogenic centers of the red bone marrow, either by means of an affinity of its own for them, or through the agency of a receptive substance in them capable of binding it. (*d*) Under the influence of this combination, and possibly with the destruction of the hormone or hormones

concerned in the process, the activity of the adult erythropoietic system is regulated."

Preliminary experimentation on dogs and rabbits, with adequate controls, showed that spleen substance and red bone marrow were powerful erythropoietic agents, and that they were indeed more powerful when used together than separately. The findings were confirmed on normal humans, and it was found that desiccated preparations were effective when given in capsules. Not only was a marked rise noted in the number of circulating red blood cells (amounting to over 15 per cent in the case of the combined materials), but the hemoglobin content was also found to be considerably increased. In addition, it was noted that, although the hemoglobin did not rise as rapidly as did the red blood cells, the hemoglobin increase was better maintained than was that of the red blood cells when the administration of the materials was stopped.

Applying these findings in the clinic, Leake and Evans have treated 63 cases of secondary anemia with a mixture in equal proportions by weight of desiccated spleen and red bone marrow, a 5-grain (0.32 Gm.) capsule of this mixture being given three times daily, before meals, with plenty of water. With improvement of the blood picture, this dosage was diminished at first to 2 capsules and then to 1 capsule daily, the administration being withdrawn as soon as the erythrocyte and hemoglobin content of the blood remained constant. Seventy-five per cent of the individuals in the series showed moderate or marked improvement on the basis of objective and subjective clinical findings plus definite evidences in the blood. Giffin and Watkins (1930), using bone marrow alone in 98 cases, were unable to obtain satisfactory results. However, a number of confirmatory reports have appeared in which the spleen-marrow dosage of Leake and Evans was employed. Thalhimer, for instance, has shown that in a group of 46 patients with secondary anemia, a definite increase in hemoglobin and circulating erythrocytes occurred in 89 per cent, employing the same dosage as that of Leake and Evans. In many cases the erythrocyte increase occurred in from one to three days, but the hemoglobin rise was more tardy and gradual. It seemed to require six to eight weeks of treatment for the improvement to become permanent. The withdrawal of treatment in 3 cases that had responded quickly was followed by a moderate fall in the blood count; when treatment was resumed, a rise again took place in hemoglobin and erythrocytes, which would seem to point to more than coincidence in these cases.

4. **Liver.**—In standard anemia dogs, which perhaps represent to some extent the counterpart of certain types of secondary anemia in the human, Whipple and Robscheit-Robbins have found that liver is the most efficacious agent in promoting blood regeneration. In the human, however, liver feeding has not been so uniformly productive of good results in secondary anemia as in pernicious anemia. The more recent literature has been quite contradictory and confusing, but the facts that seem principally to have emerged (Murphy, 1933, and others) are that whole liver diet (or injections of the extract in solution) plus iron is sometimes more effective than either agent alone, and that liver extract, as ordinarily used in pernicious anemia, is of little value in secondary anemia. Whipple *et al.* (1930) have, however, described a fraction present in extract which they have designated "secondary anemia liver extract"; with this some successes have been reported. Cheney and Niemand (1932) have used the Lilly Secondary Anemia Liver Extract No. 55 with Iron, in 50 cases, giving an average of 12 Gm. (3 drachms) daily, in single or divided doses in whatever vehicle was preferred, for three weeks. They felt some doubt about the superiority of their results as a whole to what might have been attained with large doses of iron alone, but in anemias due to hemorrhage they thought the

combination could be recommended. Richter *et al.* (1932) used an extract containing the active secondary anemia fraction combined with glycerated ferric chloride in defibrinated blood serum—theoretically including all the factors concerned in blood regeneration. Though their studies convinced them of the great difficulty of ascribing proper values in this type of therapy, they felt that the improvement in a certain proportion of their 112 patients was definitely ascribable to the use of the preparation.

5. **The Dietary Factor.**—The studies of Sherman have shown that the body requirement of iron is just barely covered in the ordinary dietary; therefore, individuals who do not eat sufficient animal protein and fruit and green vegtables, but partake instead of excessive quantities of cereals, potatoes, fish, etc., are liable to develop secondary anemia. This factor of dietary deficiency bears looking into in every case.

6. **Hydrochloric Acid.**—More will be said on this head when discussing pernicious anemia, but it is worth while mentioning here that Mettier and Minot (1931) have found that even in secondary anemia it is advisable to investigate the acid strength of the gastric juice, since in their studies iron was more potent in stimulating blood regeneration when absorbed from an acid than from an alkaline medium within the intestinal tract. If gastric analysis is not considered to be justified in the average case, the simple administration of hydrochloric acid (see p. 410) will certainly do no harm; especially in pregnancy anemia would this seem to be an advisable measure.

7. **Copper.**—As a result principally of the experimental studies of Hart, Steenbock, Waddell, Elvehjem and Sherman (1928–32), we have come to recognize that in the presence of copper the salts of iron are more effective in hemoglobin synthesis. Apparently the copper does not affect the assimilation of iron, since iron given alone is stored, but it does seem to function in the conversion of such stored iron into hemoglobin. Current investigations indicate that other elements, particularly manganese and germanium, may also be associated with the process. The findings in regard to copper are quite clear-cut, but the reader is reminded that they apply to rats in whom anemia has been produced by iron starvation. Comparable studies of the rôle of copper in human hemoglobin economy have not been made, and therefore the copper therapy methods that are being so extravagantly advocated really have no scientific foundation as yet; however, no harm is probably being done. The following prescription will enable one to give the three hematinics in a capsule:

℞.   Arsenic trioxide.................................... gr. j   0.06
     Copper sulphate.................................... gr. v   0.30
     Mass of ferrous carbonate .... ℥iiss   10.00
     Make 30 capsules.
     Label: One three times daily after meals.

For prescribing the iron and copper in a bottle, the following is palatable and pharmaceutically compatible; it contains 8 grains (0.5 Gm.) of the iron salt and ⅙ grain (0.01 Gm.) of the copper sulphate per dose—for an infant the copper salt should be cut in half and the iron reduced to 2 grains (0.12 Gm.) in order to avoid gastric irritation.

℞.   Copper sulphate.................................... gr. v   0.3
     Iron and ammonium citrate......................... ℥iv   15.0
     Syrup of orange................................... ℥ij   60.0
     Water to make..................................... ℥iv   120.0
     Label: Teaspoonful three times daily after meals.

8. **Blood Transfusion.**—Not all the anemias of pregnancy respond well to the usual measures employed in the treatment of secondary anemia.

Sometimes blood transfusion, even repeated transfusions, are necessary to save life in these cases. Some students of the subject are beginning to believe that this difference perhaps sets off a separate type of malady from the milder "physiologic" secondary anemia of pregnancy and the puerperium. Despite the many reclassifications of the anemias, the right one has obviously not yet been made.

CHLOROSIS

Chlorosis is a type of anemia that has two peculiar characteristics: First, that it occurs practically exclusively in girls between puberty and twenty-five years of age; and second, that, though quite common in the latter part of the nineteenth century, it has died out so rapidly that a case is now one of the greatest rarities. In the United States by far the majority of the patients were Irish immigrant girls of the working classes. The points which differentiate this disease from chronic secondary anemia are the greenish pallor, most marked about the eyes, and the fact that the red blood cells, themselves reduced somewhat in number, are so devoid of hemoglobin that in a stained preparation they appear definitely achromic, often being mere rings. Constipation and dyspeptic disturbances, a low-grade fever, and perverted appetite, are other frequent symptoms.

Practically nothing is known of the etiology and pathology of this strange affection.

THERAPY

The treatment is that of secondary anemia. To be sure, the disease is self-limited, but iron may be said to possess specific properties in that it will cut the duration of the attack in half or even more. For a description of iron preparations, see page 481. To change the general hygienic surroundings of these girls, to treat their constipation (see p. 431), and to improve their diet was always found to be additionally helpful.

SIMPLE ACHLORHYDRIC ANEMIA

This apparently new clinical entity has been described under a variety of names: Achylic chloranemia, idiopathic hypochromemia, hypochromic anemia with achlorhydria, primary hypochromic anemia, chronic chlorosis, etc. Most of the patients are women between the ages of thirty and fifty years, though the disease is not unknown in men. There is a host of symptoms, which probably prevented the earlier recognition of the syndrome as a unit; however, the principal ones are achylia, anorexia, tongue appearance like that in pernicious anemia, paresthesias and other nervous changes, fingernails and toenails with spoonlike depressions, discomfort and flatulence following meat so that carbohydrates are mostly eaten, possibly diarrhea, menstrual disturbances, pallor, the general lackadaisical symptoms of secondary anemia, a blood picture practically indistinguishable from that of chlorosis, and a history of long standing. A number of observers feel that this is really chlorosis of a chronic sort in women, and occasionally men, older than those who had the disease when it used to be described as "green sickness" of young girls.

THERAPY

Most observers have been in agreement that one of the outstanding characteristics of the disease is its favorable response to iron if given in especially large doses and for a long enough period. Fresh air, good food and rest—the elements of the old treatment of chlorosis—are also of value here. Hydrochloric acid is used as in any other achlorhydria, but the consensus of opinion is that it is usually of little value except perhaps to check a postprandial diarrhea or flatulence. Liver therapy is not effective. Both Mills (1931) and Waugh (1931) have had better success with iron when reinforcing it with copper. Apparently the disease always recurs unless the iron is taken continuously; Haden (1932) has found that after the blood returns to normal, 10 grains (0.6 Gm.) of ferrous carbonate three times daily is a good maintenance dose in most cases; Dameshek (1933) uses a total daily amount of 15 grains (1 Gm.) iron and ammonium citrate or 8 grains (0.5 Gm.) of reduced iron.

THE ANEMIAS OF INFANCY

Premature infants almost uniformly develop anemia as the result, it is assumed, of the curtailment of the period allotted for the deposition of iron. The anemia of twins, which is almost as common as that of premature infants, is somewhat similarly explained. A third form of infantile anemia, which occurs in infants fed too long on an exclusively milk diet or on a diet predominantly of milk with an inadequate supply of green vegetables or other iron-containing food, also may be explained on the "iron depot" theory of Bunge, though Czerny and his school trace the origin of this alimentary anemia to the toxic or hemolytic effect of the fat of milk (in the United States, Bass, Denzer and Herman failed to confirm Czerny's contention). There is also undoubtedly a correlation between iron deficiency in the pregnant woman and nutritional anemia in the infant which bears much further investigation.

THERAPY

A few years ago, as a result of gross clinical misinterpretation of animal experimentation, many pediatricians were led into the condemnation of iron in the treatment of the anemias of infancy. That this was hasty action seems now to be quite generally admitted, for as a matter of fact iron is of great worth here, though it is certainly true that recovery takes place without it. Upon this head Bass and Denzer have written:

"Why are there not more dire results when iron is not administered? In other words, what happens to anemic children who do not receive iron? In the group of children with mild anemia there is a strong tendency to spontaneous improvement and sometimes to cure with advancing age. Thus, many of these babies develop into children somewhat pale and generally inferior, and the infantile anemia responsible for their condition may be forgotten entirely. Another group of infants succumb to intercurrent infection, and the anemia plays an important but often unsuspected part in the fatal outcome. One of us [Bass, see Bibliography] has called attention to the relation between pneumonia and anemia and the beneficial effects of transfusion. A third group of infants develop anemia of such severity that transfusion becomes an emergency measure. . . . When seen at this late stage of anemia, one is apt to forget that iron therapy earlier in the disease might have prevented a catastrophe, or at least rendered drastic measures unnecessary."

Infants and children may be quite as freely dosed with iron salts as adults; indeed, it would seem to be necessary to use uniformly larger doses in them. A satisfactory preparation for use in youngsters is the saccharated ferrous carbonate, U.S.P., which has a sweetish taste that only later turns ferruginous. The drug is only partially soluble in water. Its official dose is 4 grains (0.25 Gm.) but it is often used in very much larger dose than this; Bass and Denzer habitually employ from 30 to 60 grains (2 to 4 Gm.) daily in infants. Grulee and Sanford (1931) have found the intraperitoneal injection of iron satisfactory; irrespective of the weight of the child, they gave 5 cc. of colloidal iron as ferric hydroxide, the solution containing 8 mg. of colloidal iron. The injections were given twice a week for eight injections, but the rise in hemoglobin did not begin until after the last of them had been given. Ultraviolet irradiations were also employed "to assist the body in its assimilation of iron."

In a series of 34 children, Lewis (1931) has obtained better response from iron and copper than from iron alone; he used from 15 to 60 grains (1 to 4 Gm.) of saccharated ferrous carbonate daily, and 0.5 per cent copper sulphate solution, from 1 to 2 teaspoonfuls three times daily. Lewis, Mackay (1931) and Parsons (1931) have recently remarked upon the interfering effect of intercurrent infection upon the rate of blood regeneration. Maurer *et al.* (1932) have found that infants failing to improve on an iron and copper mixture, made good gains when liver extract was given in addition— 2 cc. of concentrated liver extract in 20 per cent alcohol, three times daily. Other forms of liver therapy have also been used successfully: Liver juice, cooked liver, scraped liver (1 to 2 ounces daily), powdered liver (2½ to 6 drachms); they have likewise all failed as in the other secondary anemias.

Of course in what has been written here in regard to the treatment of the anemias of infancy I do not mean to imply that *all* such anemias are best treated with iron, copper, liver, etc. Obviously, the anemias secondary to the avitaminoses, rickets and scurvy, are to be attacked by eliminating or alleviating the cause, and in the anemia of syphilis, tuberculosis and prolonged pyogenic infections, iron administration is not of primary importance.

MISCELLANEOUS ANEMIAS

Idiopathic aplastic anemia, myelophthisic anemia, and Gaucher's disease are rare entities that will not be described in this book. The first two are surely fatal despite all treatment, but it would seem that splenectomy is possibly life saving in an occasional case of Gaucher's disease.

Banti's disease, which partakes of the nature of both anemia and cirrhosis, is sometimes completely arrested by early splenectomy. In hemolytic jaundice, which is a familial disease characterized by chronic anemia, jaundice and splenomegaly, the success of splenectomy is so great that the majority of all reported cases are said to have been cured by this surgical measure. Von Jaksch's disease, an entity frequently associated with rickets in children, tends to recover spontaneously; splenectomy often does not change the blood picture.

Since its first description by Herrick, in 1910, in all about 200 cases of sickle cell anemia have been mentioned in the literature, and a great many of these have been described in detail. It is a familial, hereditary disease limited almost exclusively to the negro race; at the present writing (late

1933) only 2 cases have been reported in white persons in whom there could have been no possible admixture of negro blood. The peculiar paroxysmal abdominal crises of the disease are as yet unexplained. It is stated that about 7 per cent of Negroes have the sickle cell trait, though only a relatively few develop the active phase; those who do so usually die before the age of thirty years.

PERNICIOUS ANEMIA

Pernicious anemia is a chronic deficiency disease which progresses, usually with remissions, to a fatal issue, unless the patient ingests or receives by injection an adequate amount of a specific substance which is apparently absent from the stomach, in which case the chief manifestations of the disease can be held in abeyance apparently for an indefinite period of time.

The outstanding feature of the disease is the peculiar anemia. There is diminution in the number of red cells, white cells, and blood platelets; the red cell diminution is greatest, counts of 500,000 or less not being unusual. The hemoglobin is somewhat reduced but not in proportion to the reduction in the number of red cells; consequently, there is always a color index higher than one. In addition, there is marked anisocytosis with macrocytes predominating, marked poikilocytosis, and diffuse and punctate polychromatophilia. A variety of nucleated red cells, and occasionally mitosis, is seen. In the beginning of a remission there is an increased number of reticulated red cells.

Symptomatically the onset is insidious, the patient usually appearing for the first examination with most of the characteristic symptoms present in some degree. There is complaint of languor, muscular weakness, and shortness of breath on exertion. As a rule there is little or no weight loss in the beginning, but if the gastro-intestinal symptoms are marked the patient not infrequently becomes thin. A simple pallor is sometimes seen but a lemon-yellow tint to the skin is more usual. A heart murmur of the "hemic" type is almost the rule. Slight puffiness of the ankles is a frequent finding; in rare cases the edema is much greater. And then there are, in addition, the gastro-intestinal and central nervous system symptoms. The former may at one time or another include all the dyspepsias, with periods of diarrhea being especially prone to occur; tongue and stomach findings are the most constant. The tongue is off and on sore and raw, particularly around the edges, and may at times be slightly ulcerated; it is nearly always smooth, red, and glazed, and without any furring. The chief finding of moment in the stomach is a great diminution in HCl; in fully established cases of the disease there is a constant achylia. Careful examination will reveal the involvement of the central nervous system in about 80 per cent of cases. Paresthesias are most frequent, but a diminution in the objective senses, such as to vibration and posture, are not infrequent; sometimes the clinical picture is that of a posterolateral sclerosis. The patients are generally irritable and extremely difficult to handle; definite psychoses are occasionally encountered. The spleen is palpable in about 40 per cent of the cases; marked enlargement of the liver is not so frequently noted in the living patient, but at autopsy both the organs are found to be somewhat enlarged. Other constant findings at autopsy are the extension of hyperplastic red bone marrow into portions of the medullary cavity of the long bones ordinarily occupied by fat only; the "tiger lily" appearance of the heart; the presence of hemosiderin granules in a number of the organs; and, in many cases, the presence of foci of sclerosis in the cord and sometimes in the brain also. Marked atrophy of the gastric mucosa is oftentimes noted, but I do not think this observation is of very great importance in view of the well-known rapidity of the postmortem changes in the stomach.

The disease occurs among rich and poor alike, among urban and rural dwellers regardless of type of occupation. Only a few cases have been reported in childhood and adolescence, and the malady is very rare between twenty and thirty, but after this latter age the incidence increases rapidly up to the age of seventy; in extreme old age it is again very rare. There has come to be more than a suspicion of familial and hereditary tendencies. In the United States, England and France, more men are affected than women, but in Germany, Finland and Scandinavia the reverse seems to be true. Classical addisonian pernicious anemia is very rare in the tropics.

THERAPY

. There was little significant advancement in the treatment of pernicious anemia from the time that Addison described the disease in 1855 until Minot and Murphy, in 1926, announced that liver contained a principle which stimulated blood regeneration. These Harvard investigators, whose work was based directly upon the painstaking investigations of Whipple and his associates, who worked with dogs, found that a diet rich in liver was regularly followed by a remission of the disease, without the employment of the time-honored therapeutic agents, arsenic and transfusion. They first reported 45 cases, but later brought the number up to 105 cases. Since that time the mortality rate for pernicious anemia has declined at every age-group; so uniformly successful has been the treatment, indeed, that the few failures reported are looked upon with suspicion—either, it is felt, the liver was not properly taken or else the diagnosis was faulty. Full explanation for this magic is not yet at hand, but the classical studies of Castle and his associates, in the period 1928–33, have demonstrated almost beyond doubt that pernicious anemia is a deficiency disease conditioned by the lack of a specific intrinsic factor which is present in normal gastric juice but not in that of an individual with this disease. It is considered that the function of the intrinsic factor is to interact with an extrinsic factor supplied in the food to produce a hemopoietic substance active in preventing pernicious anemia in normal individuals and in checking its progress in ill individuals when given to them in some form derived from liver, kidney or brain tissue, in which it is apparently stored. The investigations of Morris and his co-workers (1932) suggest that the substance may exist preformed in gastric juice, but their findings are as yet unconfirmed. Strauss and Castle (1932) now believe the extrinsic factor to be closely related to vitamin B_2, if not vitamin B_2 itself.

The results of the specific therapy as employed throughout the world today are as follows:

(*a*) *Blood Changes.*—Beginning four to seven days after therapy is begun, the reticulocytes rise to a peak (often preceded by a minor peak) on about the ninth day, the height of which is inversely proportional to the level of the red cells, other things being equal; by the twenty-first day return to normal has usually taken place. After this the red cells begin reaching the circulation in a more mature form; in two to four months the count is within normal limits, by which time the hemoglobin increase, which began more slowly, has also usually reached normal.

(*b*) *Objective Changes.*—Usually the skin begins to acquire color in the first week and later becomes healthy and moist in appearance. The mucous membranes share in this improvement and the tongue returns to normal in most instances; persistent tongue lesions are felt by some observers to be associated with marked cord involvement. Isaacs, Sturgis and Smith advise painting the lesions with 1 to 2 per cent silver nitrate. Hemic murmurs, edema and spleen palpability disappear.

(*c*) *Subjective Changes.*—The improvement in state of mind is usually rapid and marked. Appetite, physical strength and sexual power return. The gastro-intestinal symptoms disappear, though if there has been normal bowel activity looseness may supervene for a short time. Dizziness, blurred vision, headache, dyspnea disappear.

(*d*) *Effect on the Neurological Findings.*—Improvement in the blood and in the subjective and objective findings is not always correlative with improvement in the nervous symptoms. Marked improvement is often seen, particularly in the more recently acquired disturbances, and patients with flaccid paralysis may completely regain their ability to walk, bedsores are quite likely to heal and incontinence to disappear; nevertheless, a return of the deep reflexes is seldom demonstrated, and, says Connery (1931) of his series, "a return of vibratory sense has never been completely effected in any instance where this has been completely lost." Subacute combined degeneration of the cord may develop during vigorous treatment with liver, although certainly in the vast majority of instances the progress of this neurological disturbance is arrested by the therapy.

(*e*) *Effect on Childbearing.*—Pregnancy used to be looked upon as a calamity in the life of a woman with pernicious anemia, but reports are beginning to appear (Eyding, 1933) of women carried through safely to term and giving birth to healthy babies.

(*f*) *Effect on the Gastric Acidity.*—Connery and Jolliffe (1931), and Heere (1928), have each reported a patient who showed a return of free hydrochloric acid following liver therapy.

(*g*) *Resistance to Therapy.*—In their original paper, Minot and Murphy indicated that infection could inhibit the effectiveness of the therapy, an observation which has been substantiated in many subsequent reports. However, McCrie (1932) has recently reported 1 and Carey (1931) 3 cases which progressed to a typical pernicious anemia fatal termination in the absence of infection and under adequate therapy. We cannot yet be certain that liver resistance is not occasionally encountered.

Liver and Liver Extract Routinely by Mouth.—The calf's liver may be taken either raw or lightly cooked, provided the water employed in cooking is added to the completed dish, for the active principle is soluble. Many recipes have been made available but of them all most patients tire in time. Falconer (1931) has described his own experience in taking raw liver in large cachets—an easy method which does away with the trouble of "lightly" cooking and also makes it possible to use the tough, fibrous, and hence cheaper cow's liver. The cachets must be filled just before using else they become soggy and liable to come apart in the mouth. Kidneys are about one half, sweetbreads about one third as valuable in treatment as the liver. The liver may be eaten at one or be divided between all the meals of the day. Farquharson and Graham (1930) have found a broth made from beef or pork liver to be inexpensive, palatable and effective in treatment. It is made as follows: Five hundred grams of liver are finely ground in a meat chopper, care being taken to save all the juice. Two glasses of water are added, and it is transferred to a fruit jar, shaken for a moment and allowed to stand for eight to twenty-four hours, if possible in an ice chest. Finally it is heated to the boiling point, and after cooling sufficiently it is strained through cheesecloth. By twisting round and round, as much fluid is expressed as possible and the total amount of fluid obtained is given to the patient every day. It may be taken cold or hot, and various flavoring agents—onions, soup powders, tomatoes—may be added if desired. In addition, the diet must be fully adequate in meats, fresh vegetables, fruits and dairy products. Liver extract may be taken in solution in any pleasing beverage or mixed with other foods. The preliminary studies of Herron and McEllroy (1933) indicate the possibility of greatly reducing whole liver dosage by autolyzing the liver; Squibb's autolyzed concentrate is recommended in dosage of 4 to 6 or more teaspoonfuls for ten days and thereafter 1 teaspoonful daily. Fouts and Zerfas (1933) are studying the substance made by interaction of liver or liver fractions and hog gastric tissue.

It is now generally agreed, as the result of the experience of recent years, that the dosage required to induce remissions and maintain health in the usual uncomplicated case of pernicious anemia in an individual under fifty years of age, is daily, by mouth, 250 Gm. of liver, or the amount of extract (N.N.R.) derived from 400 Gm. of liver. Conner (1932) has been using marine liver extract (N.N.R.) in daily doses of 3 to 6 ounces (90 to 180 cc.). The rate at which complete remission is reached varies quite directly with dosage, *i. e.*, when the number of red cells is less than 2,000,000 per cubic millimeter, usually about 150 Gm. of liver, or liver extract (N.N.R.) derived from 250 Gm. of liver, daily, will cause the red cells to increase by about 1,300,000 per cubic millimeter in a month. If the ingested quantities are doubled, the cellular increase will proceed at about 2,500,000 in a month, which is about the maximum possible speed. Great heed, however, should be given the recent plea of Minot (1932) against standardized therapy, as it is undoubtedly true that the specific agent here is too often being used upon the basis of one criterion only—an increase in the number of red cells—without thought for the other demands of the body for this potent agent, or of the necessity of building up a store of the substance against times of special need. A patient omitting his dose on one day should make up for it on the next. As Davidson (1932) has recently stated, there is a considerable body of opinion to the effect that subacute combined degeneration occurs less frequently, and when present responds better, when whole liver is given instead of extracts, but I think it quite likely that mere matters of dosage are at fault here, for a number of observers have opined that to overcome neurological manifestations requires heroic administration. Witness one of Farquharson and Graham's (1930) cases: *J. W., aged thirty-nine, nervous manifestations increase greatly while on extract equivalent to 150 Gm. liver daily, a maintenance dosage. When ordered to take daily broth made from 1000 Gm. liver, nervous manifestations almost completely disappear.* This was a change from extract to whole liver surely, but it was also a tremendous quantitative change.

Single Massive Doses of Liver Extract by Mouth.—Encouraged by scattered favorable reports in the literature, Connery (1931) has made a thoroughgoing study of massive dosage in 6 patients under complete control. Administration in each instance was as follows: Case 1, drank 30 vials in buttermilk, Cases 2 and 6, each 50 vials in water through Rehfuss tube into stomach, Cases 3 and 5, respectively, 48 and 30 vials by the same method. Case 4 received 50 vials through gastric lavage tube. Patients 2 and 6 vomited a mixture of extract, gastric juice and saliva about one hour after receiving the extract; Patient 1 vomited in fifteen minutes. In these cases progress was in all respects comparable with that of other patients receiving daily liver therapy. Connery feels that the method has value in carrying moribund patients through a period of emergency and so gaining their confidence that day by day therapy will be continued when the peak of advantage from the single massive dose has been reached.

Liver Extact by Rectum.—The results are so variable and the disagreeableness of the procedure so great that the method must be considered hardly practicable.

Injection of Liver Extract.—The original extract prepared by Cohn, Minot, and others, in 1927, was unsuitable for parenteral injection, but by 1930, Cohn, McMeekin and Minot, and West and Howe, had sufficiently purified the active principle as to make this method of introduction practicable. Perhaps the purest preparation so far produced has been made by Dakin, West and Howe (1931), who suggested that the active principle is probably a dipeptide of β-hydroxyglutanic acid and γ-hydroxyproline; in their more recent investigations this view does not seem to have been substantiated. Wilkinson (1931), in England, has also been using a highly potent preparation. However, the first to demonstrate the real effectiveness of parenterally administered active principle was Gänsslen, in Germany, whose extract is being extensively employed on the Continent under the name of "Compolon." If I translate him correctly, Gänsslen's present view is the following: "We see from these examples, which make no pretense to completeness, that there has appeared in the new and fruitful realm of liver therapy a great field for investigation with important practical and theoretical successes. Several questions are already ripe for discussion, many still await solution; to work toward their elucidation is a task for the widest circles, so that by a critical trial on a broad basis the right preparation will find its use in the right place." Now this does not seem to me to warrant the wave of almost hectic enthusiasm which is sweeping our own country at this time. There can be no doubt that there are circumstances in which it is of distinct value to have available an actively potent substance which may be given parenterally, such as in a moribund patient, or a "resistant" case when the resistance may be due to poor alimentary absorption, or in an individual who is absolutely unable to take the whole liver or extract by mouth, but to advocate the sweeping replacement of oral by parenteral administration, merely because the latter is at the moment cheaper, appears to me not to be in keeping with the tenets of sound therapeutics. This is of course merely the viewpoint of one who is primarily a pharmacologist, but I have been delighted to find Musser (1932) expressing the same feeling from the practical standpoint of a research clinician. Let us delay as long as possible before we foist upon pernicious anemia patients that slavery to the needle which is the bane of the diabetic's existence. Strauss and Castle; Meyer, Richter and Ivy; Connery and Goldwater; Conner; Middleton; Murphy; Isaacs; Sturgis, and others are thoroughly investigating the subject in this country. The question of dosage has by no means been thoroughly worked out. To date, late 1933, only preparations advocated for intramuscular or subcutaneous injection have been accepted for N.N.R. The Chappel extract for subcutaneous or intramuscular use is said to have an initial dose of 2 cc., a maintenance dose of 2 cc. at intervals of ten to twenty days; the new refined and concentrated Lederle extract for intramuscular use, 3 cc. for three or four successive days, thereafter 3 cc. at weekly intervals, but in complicated cases, etc., the dosage "must be determined for each patient"; the Parke-Davis extract for intramuscular use, 2 cc. daily "until the red blood cells and hemoglobin have reached normal," thereafter 2 cc. every two or three days; the Lilly extract No. 343 for intramuscular use, "determined by the condition of the patient—daily intramuscular injection of 2 cc. has been followed by maximal reticulocyte count—the maintenance dose varies with the individual patient."

Hog Stomach Preparations by Mouth.—A great advance in therapy has been initiated by the practical discovery of Sturgis and Isaacs, in 1929, that hog's stomach, desiccated and defatted, and taken by mouth can replace liver with at least equal effectiveness from all standpoints. Their findings have been corroborated by Conner; Snapper and du Preez; Wilkinson, Gänsslen; Brower and Simpson; Davidson; Henning and Brugsch, and many others all over the world. It is believed that the "intrinsic" substance postulated by Castle exists in an enzyme-like form in the stomach tissue and that it acts on the muscular coat while the stomach is being ground up in the fresh state, the stomach tissue here taking the place of Castle's "extrinsic" or food factor; the active principle thus formed is retained in the stomach preparation and, when swallowed, is rapidly absorbed and becomes at once available for use by the patient. Just which part of the stomach contains most of the substance has not been determined: Conner has found all parts satisfactory, Henning and Brugsch have obtained best results when using pyloric mucous membrane, Sturgis and Isaacs obtained no result from the muscular coat, only a poor one from the mucous membrane, and complete effects from the use of all parts together. The N.N.R. preparation, ventriculin, is made from the whole stomach. The relative cheapness of this article seems destined to cause it to practically supersede liver preparations; it is, however, insoluble and cannot be brought to a boil without destroying the active principle. Apparently it is much less distasteful to patients than is liver; none of Brower and Simpson's 15 patients expressed an aversion to its continuous use. Stomach and liver preparations can be used interchangeably, each in suitable dosage of course, when such alternation seems advisable for the sake of varying the diet.

Sturgis and Isaacs, in their careful studies, have worked out the beginning dosage of ventriculin on the basis of 10 Gm. daily for each million deficit in the red blood cells. For example, with a red count of 1,000,000 there is a deficit of 4,000,000; the dose is then 4 x 10 or 40 Gm. daily. When the red cell level reaches 2,000,000, the deficit is 3,000,000 and the dose is 30 Gm. The maintenance dosage to be used indefinitely to prevent relapse after the blood has become normal probably varies somewhat with different patients, but the experience of the authors just referred to, and borne out widely by others, is that 10 Gm. daily for five or six days a week is satisfactory in most cases.

The hog stomach preparation may be taken in water, milk, orange or tomato juice, or as a thick purée (heated to taste but not boiled) or emulsion, and may be eaten with or between meals. An extract has not yet been obtained in usable form, but the recent investigations of Wilkinson and Klein (1932) indicate that it may soon be made available. The very interesting studies of Morris, Schiff and their associates hint that perhaps we may be very near to the time when one injection of a substance ("addisin") obtained from hog stomach will suffice to control the anemia and other symptoms for a period of several months—let us be hopeful but hard to convince!

Brain Diet.—Ungley (1931–32) has shown that a diet of 240 to 480 Gm. of beef or sheep's brains, uncooked, is only about one third as potent as comparable dosage with liver; there is therefore no reason, other things being equal, for employing this tissue in therapy. But he has found also that the effect of the brain diet upon the neurological symptoms is much greater than upon the other symptoms, and therefore feels that its combination with adequate amounts of liver or stomach preparations is worthy of further trial.

Vitamin Therapy.—The reports of Wills (1931–33), in India, have enlivened the search for the possible vitamin factor in the active substances specific in pernicious anemia. She successfully used yeast ("marmite") rich in Vitamin B in the treatment of cases of tropical macrocytic anemia, a condition with the blood picture of true pernicious anemia but differing from the latter in its other symptomatology. Gilroy (1931) showed in feeding experiments in rats that if liver extract is added to a diet deficient in vitamin B, satisfactory growth results, while the control animals fail to show a similar improvement. Davidson (1931) has failed in two cases of true addisonian pernicious anemia and succeeded in one, and feels that any benefit following the use of vitamin B is due merely to improving the efficiency of the gastro-intestinal tract. However, Godall (1932) has maintained 19 patients very satisfactorily without relapses for periods of six to twelve months by the use of marmite alone (*i. e.*, six to twelve months at the time of his report); the maintenance dose never exceeded 1 drachm (4 Gm.) three times daily. Most of his patients found the marmite palatable when stirred in water or milk or spread on bread and butter and welcomed it as a change from or as a pleasant solution to the difficulty of obtaining liver in remote districts. Ungley (1933) has also tried marmite and found that doses of 4 ounces (120 Gm.) daily usually produce a variable and submaximal response as compared with liver therapy and that the remission is more slowly obtained than with liver extract in large doses. In view of Strauss and Castle's belief that the active substance will ultimately be found to be, or to be closely related to, vitamin B, this new investigational trend must be watched with the greatest interest.

Transfusion.—Prior to the institution of liver treatment, undoubtedly blood transfusion produced better and more permanent results than any other therapeutic measure. It is by no means a cure but it has certainly brought many a moribund patient back to life, and in some cases it has probably been responsible for the occurrence of a remission. Such cases as do respond with a remission may require anywhere from five to fifteen transfusions before a normal blood count is approached. The utmost extension of active life attainable by the use of this measure probably follows upon transfusion of 350 to 450 cc. at intervals of three to five days, as advocated by Jones (1926), instead of giving larger transfusions at longer intervals. A number of observers still feel that the transfusion of about 500 cc. of blood is the most valuable of all emergency measures, placing the intravenous injection of liver extract as second best. Others feel that the danger of serious reactions following transfusion should always weigh against it if liver suitable for injection is available. Davidson stated, in 1932, that he had seen three fatal terminations to the reaction following transfusion in the preceding two or three years, though he still feels that the measure is extremely valuable in selected cases for the relief it gives to the anoxemia from which every organ in the body is suffering.

Iron, Arsenic and Hydrochloric Acid.—It is believed that in pernicious anemia the breakdown products of the red cells are stored in the body and are available at once for the manufacture of hemoglobin should normal blood formation occur as the result of a natural remission or of treatment with one of the new specifics. However, in a few cases the amount stored may not be sufficiently great, as has occurred in the experience of both Beebe and Lewis (1931) and Davidson (1932). In one of the patients of the latter, the blood count remained at 3,500,000 and the hemoglobin at 70 per cent despite large doses of ventriculin, liver and liver extract, but upon the addition of 90 grains (6 Gm.) of iron and ammonium citrate daily the blood level rapidly rose to 5,500,000 and 100 per cent. Sargant (1932) also felt that the use of enormous doses of iron—150 grains (10 Gm.) of Blaud's pill in powder form in capsules daily—was productive of strikingly beneficial results in several cases of subacute combined degeneration in which liver therapy alone was apparently failing.

It is generally agreed today that arsenic no longer has any place in the treatment of pernicious anemia.

Since the overthrow of the intestinal contamination theory of the etiology of pernicious anemia by the newer studies which have shown the disease to belong among the disorders of deficiency, there seems little rationale for the continued employment of hydrochloric acid. However, a number of physicians continue to prescribe it in doses of ½ to 2 drachms (2 to 8 cc.), well diluted and taken as a routine with meals, finding that flatulence and diarrhea that are not alleviated by the use of liver or stomach are kept well in check by the addition of this measure. Wilkinson and Brockbank (1930) have obtained better results by the use of pepsin also, employing a mixture of three parts of the glycerite of pepsin (B.P.) and one part of dilute hydrochloric acid, and ordering 2 drachms (8 cc.) to be placed in 6 to 8 ounces (180 to 240 cc.) of water, which may be flavored with orange or lemon juice, and sipped throughout the meal.

ERYTHREMIA
(Polycythemia Vera (Rubra))

Erythremia is a rare disease occurring in all races, in either sex, and usually after the age of fifty. The cause is unknown but the disease has a distinct familial tendency. The studies of Moehlig and Bates (1933) point toward the possible causative rôle of pituitary disturbances. The patient complains of lassitude, weakness, loss of weight, dizziness, tinnitus, congestive sensations especially in the hands, dyspnea, gastro-intestinal disturbances, and often severe headache, muscular spasms and neuralgias of the extremities. Examination reveals red cyanosis of the face and hands (though it is said that an occasional patient may be actually pale, but I much doubt that any victim of this disease is at *all* times pale), a greatly enlarged spleen, congested conjunctivae, and a typical blood picture. The red cells are increased to from 8,000,000 to 14,000,000; there are a great many immature cells present and differences in staining are marked; the number of white cells is usually two or three times the normal; hemoglobin is more than 100 per cent. Although the total blood volume is much increased, the increase in plasma is not in direct proportion to that in cells, with the result that viscosity is much increased. Despite the diffuse capillary dilatation that is known to occur in this disease, I think it is quite surprising that the heart rate is not greatly increased and the organ itself hypertrophied more often than is actually the case. Kidney function is usually impaired and both blood pressure and basal metabolism sometimes increased.

Erythremia is a fatal disease but there are remissions in most cases. Death seldom occurs under five years and may be deferred as long as twenty years, though this is unusual; if directly attributable to the erythremia, it is consequent upon the increased sluggishness of the circulation or is due to a vascular catastrophe, such as hemorrhage or thrombosis.

THERAPY

Phenylhydrazine Hydrochloride.—This is the most promising remedial agent as yet suggested for the treatment of erythremia. In 1924, Owen reported a case in which he had successfully used it, and in 1925 he brought the number of cases up to five. These patients were all benefited by the drug, as was evidenced by a uniform decrease of the hemoglobin and red cells, a great improvement in all the symptoms, and a reduction in blood pressure of the three individuals who had hypertension. Since that time a large number of case reports has appeared in the literature, in most of which the drug had been used very successfully. The dosage plan advocated by Owen is the one usually followed: (*a*) Treatment may be safely begun in most instances with 3 grains (0.2 Gm.) daily for three or four days, then 1½ grains (0.1 Gm.) daily until the leukocytes increase in number or the hemoglobin falls below 100 per cent; (*b*) with the advent of either of these two occurrences, usually after several weeks, the 1½-grain dose may be given every second or third day, or the drug may be stopped altogether, resuming medication when the hemoglobin and red cells rise or the leukocytes begin to fall; (*c*) gradually the interval between doses can be lengthened with the hope of ultimately maintaining the blood count within normal limits on 1½ grains once a week. However, the experimental studies of Giffin and Allen (1928) indicate that the leukocytosis cannot always be taken as a reliable index for therapy since the increase in the white cell count may be at times predominantly due to the breaking down of red cells and at other times to stimulation of the hematopoietic system; it very doubtfully indicates damage to liver cells. In Stealy's (1932) valuable experience of seven and one-half years' medication of one patient he several times felt justified in continuing with the drug through a period of extreme leukocytosis unaccompanied by much decrease in the red cell count. His dosage was a total of 2.1 Gm. of the drug divided into daily doses of 0.1 Gm. each; after each such dosing period there was an interval of one and one-half months without drug treatment. Instances of acquired tolerance to the drug, requiring increase in dosage, have been reported, but in Stealy's experience such periods of tolerance were always temporary.

It has been suspected that injury to the liver or kidneys might result either from the drug itself or from excess hemolysis, but clear-cut proof of this has not been forthcoming. Certainly its use should be carefully checked by studies of the blood and not be allowed to depend upon its effect upon other symptoms such as the pain in an extremity; rapid hemolysis may be fatal of course. Giffin and Conner feel, from a review of the literature and their own experience, that (*a*) patients should be kept ambulatory as much as possible; (*b*) advanced cases confined to bed should not receive the drug; (*c*) and it should be given with greatest possible caution to those above sixty years of age, to patients with marked arteriosclerosis, and to those who manifest evidence of thrombosis or advanced visceral injury.

Acetylphenylhydrazine.—Stone *et al.* (1933) have used this drug satisfactorily in 2 cases over periods of seven and four and a half years and believe it to be superior to the above preparation because it is probably less toxic and the dosage is easier to regulate. They give 1½ grains (0.1 Gm.) by mouth in capsules for seven to ten days, carefully observing the red cell count meanwhile; the drug is then discontinued for two weeks, regardless of the result that has been achieved, because of its cumulative effects. Thereafter, in their cases, 1½ grains at intervals of five to seven days sufficed to maintain the blood normal and the patients symptom-free.

Potassium Arsenite.—Forkner, Scott and Wu (1933) have obtained distinct improvement in all of their 6 patients by saturating with Fowler's solution in the conventional way except that they have liked to reach 20 minims (1.2 cc.) three times daily instead of stopping at 10 minims as is usual in other conditions.

"Addisin."—Morris (1933) suggests the trial of this preparation in erythremia as well as in pernicious anemia (see p. 493).

Benzene (Benzol).—The good results following the use of benzene in a number of single case reports from the German clinics prompted McLester to try it in a single case in the United States (1914). He also obtained good results, but I do not know of any report of its extensive trial since that time, probably for the reason that it was found to cause a reduction in the leuko-cytes out of all proportion to the erythrocyte reduction.

Other Measures.—Irradiation of the spleen is contraindicated since there are a number of cases on record in which the procedure has increased the severity of the disease; irradiation of the long bones, however, seems to be of some value, improvement taking place in most cases. The usual practice is to apply a rather large dose to the long bones, the scapula, the sternum, the pelvis, and eventually the vertebral column, or the ribs. The effect is temporary, and Minot says that as time goes on the therapy often becomes ineffective. A considerable, or even a sudden inconsiderable, decrease in the leukocytes of the circulating blood indicates that the leuko-cyte-forming tissue of the bone marrow is being injured and calls for immediate cessation of the treatment. The following references to this type of therapy will be found in the Bibliography: Hollaender, Stolkind, and Kingsbury; Pack and Craver. Sgalitzer (1932) has reported the occurrence of long remissions in a number of instances following general irradiation.

In one case, Jacobi (1931) found that considerable relief from the pain in extremities was afforded by daily intravenous injection of 250 cc. of physiologic saline for a period of three weeks.

Splenectomy has apparently upon rare occasions been of value, but so also has exactly the opposite measure, namely, the administration of large amounts—as much as 250 Gm. daily—of fresh spleen tissue (Haberfeld, 1931).

Frequent extensive bloodletting brings temporary relief but not permanent benefit.

LEUKEMIA

Leukemia is a relatively rare and always fatal disease of unknown etiology, characterized chiefly by the presence in the blood stream of large numbers of abnormal white cells. It is a disease of fowls and the lower mammals as well as of man. It occurs more frequently in males than in females; a familial tendency has not been proved. Chesterman (1925) has noted the great rarity of leukemia in the Congo, where enlargement of the spleen due to malaria, trypanosomiasis, and other tropical diseases is common.

Acute leukemia occurs usually in individuals under twenty-five years of age. It is rapidly fatal, death occurring within a few days to a few weeks at most. The attack is usually superimposed upon an acute infection, such as tonsillitis or a furuncle. There is malaise, headache, high fever, extreme prostration, and a rapidly increasing pallor. Ulcerative lesions appear in the mouth and throat, and marked enlargement of the regional lymph nodes of the neck occurs very rapidly; lymph nodes elsewhere in the body, and also the spleen, are slightly enlarged. Bleeding occurs both externally and internally from the mucous membranes and sometimes also in the fundus of the eye; hemorrhages of the skin are almost the rule. There is very severe anemia due to a rapid decrease in the number of red cells and the amount of hemoglobin; at the same time the number of white cells is mounting, though it rarely attains the great height seen in the chronic form of the disease. Lymphocytes usually constitute more than 90 per cent of the white cells but sometimes myeloblasts predominate. Immature red cells are also present in large numbers.

Chronic leukemia is insidious in its onset, but usually causes death from

32

anemic exhaustion, hemorrhage, or intercurrent infectious disease, for which the resistance is much lowered, in about three years; a few cases last as long as ten years, but true spontaneous remission never occurs. The most prominent symptoms are marked enlargement of the spleen, which causes great discomfort, pallor, dyspnea, dizziness, gastro-intestinal disturbances, loss of weight, and progressive weakness. Hemorrhage and fever are much later in their appearance than in the acute form of the disease. In lymphatic leukemia the spleen is not usually much enlarged but there is marked general enlargement of the lymphatic glands, a finding which is quite unusual in the myelogenous type; even the tonsils and the Peyer's patches in the intestine show proliferative changes. The glands are at no time inflammatory. The blood is pale in color, with a low red count and much reduced hemoglobin; immature and abnormal red cells are present. In the myelogenous type of the disease there is an increase in white cells to from 100,000 to 1,000,000 or more; polymorphonuclear, eosinophilic and basophilic leukocytes are relatively and absolutely increased, the lymphocytes are relatively reduced but absolutely increased, and immature cells from the bone marrow are present. In lymphatic leukemia the white count is rarely increased more than to 200,000, and consists almost exclusively of pathologic lymphocytes. Chronic myelogenous leukemia occurs most often in individuals between twenty-five and forty-five years of age; chronic lymphatic leukemia in those between forty-five and sixty.

THERAPY

1. **Acute Leukemia.**—There is nothing to describe.
2. **Chronic Leukemia.**—*Irradiation.*—There are two schools of opinion with regard to the value of irradiation. The minority group feels, with Isaacs (1930), that all x-ray radiation is stimulating and not killing, the majority holds the opposite view and maintains that in *skilled hands* irradiation is of distinct value. Both the spleen and long bones are usually treated, but dosage, etc., do not seem to be matters upon which there is perfect accord. In the series of 130 cases of Minot, Buckman and Isaacs (1924), 78 patients were irradiated, 52 were not; the average duration of life in the treated group was only 0.46 year longer than in the untreated group, from which they concluded that irradiation had little effect in prolonging life. The statistical studies of Hoffman and Craver (1931) show that slightly more than one third of the patients die within two years, more than one half within three years, and two thirds within four years of onset. Using the nonirradiated group of Minot *et al.* as controls, they found that the radiation treatment of their 82 cases caused an average increase of about ten months in the duration of efficient life—"a period of efficiency and usefulness that the patient otherwise could not hope to enjoy"; in a recent clinic on the subject, Elliott and Jenkinson (1933) expressed themselves similarly.

Benzene (Benzol).—In 1910, Selling reported on the toxic effects of benzene as witnessed in 2 fatal and a number of mild cases, in which there was a profound reduction in both red and white cells. He later confirmed these findings in rabbit experiments. Koranyi, in Germany, was the first to use the drug in the treatment of leukemia, since which time (1912) a large number of cases has been reported from Germany and Austria and a few from the United States and other countries. The present status of the drug may be described as follows:

(a) EFFECTIVENESS.—In most cases it seems to be nearly or quite as effective as irradiation; however, in an occasional case it provokes no desirable response whatever.

(*b*) DOSAGE.—The usual method of administration is to give the benzene in gelatin capsules prepared just before using, each capsule to contain 0.5 Gm. of benzene with an equal amount of olive oil, these capsules to be swallowed during the meal. On the first day four capsules (2 Gm.), on the second day six capsules (3 Gm.), on the third day eight capsules (4 Gm.), and on the fourth day and to continue at this dose—see *dangers* below— ten capsules (5 Gm.). If in spite of the administration of the drug in a capsule with olive oil the stomach is disturbed, the capsules may be coated with phenyl salicylate, which will generally prevent their solution until they reach the intestines, where the alkalis will dissolve and break up the salicylate.

(*c*) DANGERS.—The most frequent unpleasant symptoms from the use of benzene are gastric disturbances, which range in all degrees from simple irritation to loss of appetite, vomiting, hiccup, etc. More or less persistent headache and dizziness and kidney and bladder irritability should be danger signals, to be heeded by withdrawal of the drug. It should also be noted that the action of benzene persists for some time after the patient ceases to take it; therefore too great care cannot be taken in watching the results of its administration. Not only must unpleasant symptoms be noted and good judgment be used as to whether or not the drug should be continued, but the blood must be repeatedly counted, and when the white cells are reduced to 20,000 the advisability of immediately discontinuing treatment should be seriously considered. The occurrence of anemia should also cause the treatments to be stopped. Smith, who has reported a number of cases in the United States, writes as follows:

"There is nothing more certain in benzene therapy than this: the practitioner who prescribes the drug without making frequent blood counts is courting disaster. We have only to point to the blood picture of the table [*i. e.*, of a case responding favorably to treatment] to justify the statement that there is no possible way of guessing what the count will be on the basis of the last; and, therefore, of judging whether the dose should be held stationary, increased, decreased or stopped altogether. I am firmly convinced that such judgment must be constantly exercised, under the threat of having the disease jump out of bounds on the one hand, or of producing disaster on the other.

"One can guess that the rise of the count after a fall will be slower and more gradual than a drop. This is illustrated several times in the table. Nothing in it is more striking than the abrupt way in which the count drops from a point around 30,000 to 6000 or 7000. If the blood curve were ruled graphically, the chart would resemble a fever chart of a disease full of crises: it *is* a series of blood crises. In other words, the leukocytes have all along *stepped up* and *fallen down*. Just how gradual will be the step upward cannot be calculated: one time in two weeks, another, in eight weeks, perhaps. The drop comes abruptly, but what is more important, 'when we least expect it,' if such an expression can be allowed.

"Nowhere can the last sentence be better illustrated, nor can the potential dangers of the drug be better emphasized, than in the happenings recorded as of between June 1 and July 20, 1914. The patient had been getting the largest doses of benzene he had ever had, and to the end of a course extending over four months, it seemed to be making no impression on the leukocytic curve. So it was stopped, for the double reason that the treatment seemed at last ineffectual, and because I was afraid to continue such large doses. My surprise and interest was keen, then, to note a drop from 24,000 to below 7000. The cells remained at or near this point on no benzene at all for six weeks. There seems but one explanation available, and that just now suggested: After an indefinite time and after an uncertain degree of saturation has been reached, the leukopoietic tissues seem not only to become immune to benzene, but are actually stimulated by it.

"The effect of this experience is to cause doubt as to how to handle the drug when the count stays high when we are pushing it. Shall we stop, or shall we continue? I feel that if the patient has already been taking benzene for several weeks and the curve is still ascending, or even at a standstill, the safest plan is to stop it for awhile. The drop may come then. At any rate, one cannot get away from the reported cases in which, under benzene, the leukemia assumed a fulminant form, and the patient rapidly succumbed. Whether or not these flare-ups are due to the benzene is not clear; but there is a type of benzene poisoning which is certain; a practical loss of leukocytes with aplastic anemia superadded."

Other Remedies.—Forkner and Scott (1931) have recently reawakened interest in the use of Fowler's solution by their report of good results; the former has (1932) laid down the "rules" for the use of the drug, which are, in summary: (a) Begin with 5 minims three times daily in orange juice with or immediately after meals, increasing on the third and fourth day to 6 minims per dose, and continuing in this manner to about 10 minims per dose, thereafter increasing 1 minim per day until advent of pronounced toxic symptoms or until leukocyte count approaches normal. Then omit medication for two to five days, and thereafter decrease by 1 minim per day down to a maintenance dose of 5 to 8 minims thrice daily. Continue this dosage indefinitely. (b) Disregard mild toxic symptoms. (c) Patients who become nauseated and who vomit, or who believe they cannot take Fowler's solution, will be able to take it if it is well masked in orange juice or other vehicle.

When employed as arsphenamine, arsenic is dangerous; a number of acute deaths have been reported.

Transfusion has often been effectively employed to offset the tendency toward hemorrhage and to temporarily relieve the anemia until it has been possible to irradiate the patient sufficiently to produce results. Splenectomy is nearly always fatal.

For many years it has been known that intercurrent infections during the course of leukemia are accompanied by a fall in the number of leukocytes. Gamble (1927) has treated 2 cases by the therapeutic production of malaria (for methods, see p. 187 in the article on Syphilis). In each of these cases, there was a prompt fall in leukocytes to half the previous number. Following the termination of the paroxysms, however, the leukocytes rose, in three and six days respectively, to approximately their previous level. Lucherini had better results in his case: The leukocytes fell from 250,000 to 4400 after twelve paroxysms, and at the end of the reported observation of the case, six weeks after paroxysms were stopped with quinine, the blood count was, leukocytes, 5800, erythrocytes, 4,400,000, hemoglobin, 52 per cent; the differential count was said to be normal.

In 1931, Hueper and Russell produced an inhibitory serum in rabbits which they used with apparently remarkable effects in one human case, but I have heard nothing further of this.

HODGKIN'S DISEASE

(Lymphadenoma; Lymphogranulomatosis)

Hodgkin's disease is an affection of the lymph nodes of unknown etiology and invariably fatal termination. It is fairly widespread throughout continental Europe, England and the United States, but I do not know of any statistics regarding its incidence in other parts of the world. Males are more frequently affected than females, the majority of cases in either sex occurring between the ages of fifteen and thirty-five. Negroes and whites are equally affected.

In the usual form of the disease the patient notices a gradual, nonpainful, discreet enlargement of glands in the cervical region; in the beginning the enlargement may be unilateral but both sides are almost invariably involved ultimately. In most cases the axillary and then the inguinal glands, and finally both superficial and deep glands all over the body, become involved. Moderate enlargement of the spleen, and often an increase in the size of the liver, take place. The patient loses weight and becomes cachectic. General pruritus of a very severe and persistent type is a not infrequent early symptom. A peculiar feature of the disease is the frequent alternating febrile and afebrile periods. The enlargement of cervical, mediastinal, retroperitoneal or mesenteric groups of nodes may cause symptoms which make the picture a very complex one. Initial involvement of the retroperitoneal nodes without subsequent mediastinal or peripheral manifestations is infrequent. The disease usually terminates in death within two to three years, though many patients have lived a few years longer than this; cachexia and profound anemia, mechanical obstruction of one sort or another, or intercurrent infection is usually the immediate cause.

Malpighi (1628–94) gave the first vague account of this disease, which was fully described by Thomas Hodgkin in 1832. The recent report of Gordon (1933) indicates that he and his associates at St. Bartholomew's Hospital may have found a virus that is intimately associated with the disease.

I have presented briefly here only the most usual type, of which there are numerous variations. Histologic examination of an excised node shows very definite alterations in structure which cannot be described here for obvious reasons; likewise, the blood picture in the various types of Hodgkin's disease is a topic that is still in a state of too great confusion to warrant its discussion in a book of this sort.

THERAPY

Irradiation.—The application of radium or x-rays to the enlarged nodes causes a great reduction in their size and consequently leads to considerable amelioration of symptoms. The effect is always temporary, however, and the response to subsequent courses of treatment is less satisfactory. Finally a point is reached at which there is no response at all. It is quite doubtful whether these agents really extend the length of the patient's life, though there is no denying that they make his existence much more comfortable; it is possible to match every case of exceptionally long survival under irradiation with a case given no treatment at all.

Arsenic.—This is the only drug of any value, the dosage scheme of Forkner (see p. 500) sufficing here also. The nodes recede temporarily under this treatment, but, as in the case of irradiation, the ultimate course of the disease is not affected. Perhaps the best type of therapy is the use of x-rays or radium with arsenic between the courses.

Surgery.—It is now generally conceded that the removal of glands by operation is inadvisable in the vast majority of instances. Even the removal of a single gland for purposes of diagnosis should be postponed until it is certain that the procedure is absolutely necessary.

Serum.—On the basis of l'Espérance's evidence in favor of the view that Hodgkin's disease is an atypical type of tuberculosis due to the avian type of organism, Utz and Keatinge (1932), in Australia, have produced a protective serum in hens, with which they have produced surprisingly good results in human cases; further details are awaited.

PURPURA

The two principal purpuric diseases are purpura hemorrhagica and idiopathic purpura, the cause of neither of which is known. Both are preeminently diseases of the young though no age is exempt. Purpura hemorrhagica more often affects females than males. In this type of purpura, which was first described by Werlhof in 1735, there is marked diminution in the number of circulating blood platelets and the bleeding time is much prolonged. Spontaneous capillary hemorrhages may occur into any of the tissues, bleeding from the uterus, nose and mouth, and into the retina being the most common. The cutaneous hemorrhages vary from a few petechiae to extensive ecchymoses, though the latter are rare. There is usually some fever. The bleeding often begins without any warning and persists intermittently for days or weeks, when the patient dies from exsanguination; or the course may be much more abruptly fatal. Some cases recover. A chronic form of the disease is recognized; it does not develop from the acute form but is chronic throughout. These patients give a history of having bruised and bled easily for many years before the onset of the attack in which the diagnosis is made from finding the platelets below normal. They bleed intermittently during a number of years, some dying and others apparently recovering completely. In idiopathic purpura there is no abnormality in the blood but the permeability of the small vessels appears to be altered. In the simple type of this disease the purpuric lesions appear in crops which recur at intervals of weeks to years, usually without any other symptoms. Another type (Schönlein's disease) begins with malaise, fever, sore throat, and polyarticular pains, all of which usually precede by some time the eruption, which often partakes of the nature of purpura, urticaria and erythema in combination. In the third form (Henoch's purpura) abdominal or renal crises occur due to the extravasation of blood into the intestines or kidneys; there may or may not be concomitant crops of purpuric lesions in the skin, without which, of course, the diagnosis is extremely difficult. Idiopathic purpura is not fatal; with advancing years the attacks tend to become milder or to disappear altogether.

THERAPY

Transfusion.—No satisfactory treatment has been evolved for idiopathic purpura, though calcium, by reason of its presumed ability to alter capillary permeability, has had its advocates from time to time. Except to overcome the anemia consequent upon severe hemorrhage, transfusion is not indicated since there is not a shortage of platelets in this disease. In the treatment of purpura hemorrhagica, however, transfusion has an important place. Larrabee (1923) has well discussed the subject as follows:

"The objects of transfusion are, as in all hemorrhagic diatheses, twofold: First, to mitigate the anemia. This is not very important in the disease under consideration, except in severe and advanced cases. In straight purpura hemorrhagica there is no trouble with the red cell forming function of the marrow, and once the bleeding has ceased, recovery from anemia is usually prompt and satisfactory. The second and more important object of transfusion is to control the bleeding. This implies supplying enough platelets to permit natural hemostasis to occur.

"The primary object of transfusion being to increase the number of platelets in the patient's blood, the question arises as to how largely the count is affected by this procedure. In our experience, a single transfusion seldom increases the patient's platelet count by more than 20,000. Obviously, it is desirable to give large transfusions. The patients are mostly young persons, with normal hearts, and there is little danger from over-transfusion. They can safely and advantageously receive as much blood as the donors can safely supply. We do not, therefore, advise small transfusions. [Some observers do, however; Jones and Tocantins (1933) favor 100 to 300 cc.; Potts (1932) got better results by giving 8 to 10 cc. whole blood intramuscularly, and suggests that some activating agent, not platelets, is formed from the disintegration of the clot at the point of injection.]

"For the same reason we feel strongly that citrated blood is greatly inferior, in this disease at least, to whole, unmodified blood. In citrate transfusions, large numbers of platelets stick to the gauze filter and to the glassware, as can easily be proved by staining scrapings from the latter. To show how considerable the loss is, 0.1 per cent of sodium citrate was added to the blood of a patient whose platelet count was 102,000. After a half hour the citrated blood contained only 18,000 platelets. The loss is very much less if paraffined tubes are used. For example, a donor's platelets were 280,000 immediately before a transfusion by Kimpton's method. A count of the platelets in a small quantity of blood left in the tube at the end of operation gave 220,000. I am aware of the paradoxical fact that, while citrate is used to prevent coagulation of blood outside the body, its action when injected is to shorten coagulation time, and that it has been used clinically for this purpose; but this has little to do with purpura hemorrhagica, in which coagulation time is not impaired. Indeed, there is reason to believe that citrate injections act by destroying platelets, thereby releasing substances that assist coagulation [see Neuhof and Hirshfeld in the Bibliography]. I would not go so far as to say that citrate transfusions should never be used in the disease under consideration—some good observers have had success with them. But both theory and experience seem to point unmistakably to the superiority of other methods when they are available. Perhaps direct, arm-to-arm transfusion by the original Crile technic has theoretical advantages, but for practical uses paraffined tubes are, of course, preferable. All of our transfusions have been done by the Kimpton-Brown method.

"Another point is that usually more than one transfusion will be needed. Indeed, the first one may have no visible effect. A brief consideration of the facts already noted readily explains this. Hemorrhages generally begin when the platelets have fallen to some fifty or seventy-five thousand. By the time the patient comes to the table for this first transfusion, they may have fallen so far below this number that a single transfusion, however large and however efficiently performed, will not put them back to the point at which bleeding will be controlled. Several may be needed and, in view of the short life of the platelet, the intervals must be brief—not more than forty-eight hours. Even when the hemorrhages have been controlled, there is no certainty that they will not recur. If they do, transfusion should be repeated at once without reference to the presence or absence of anemia. Nothing is gained by delay, especially if the platelet count shows steady diminution; control will be more difficult each day one waits. Only boldness and persistence in transfusing will save life in severe cases. One cannot begin to feel safe until the patient has gone on without bleeding for a period considerably beyond the life of a platelet—say, ten days.

"Let me add that the platelet count is not a very good criterion. Platelet counting is at best inaccurate. After cases have gone on for a month or so, they are apt not to run true to type, and we have been much perplexed by a discrepancy between our counts and our stained smears. The former may show more than 100,000 platelets, and yet they may be almost absent from the smears. The presence or absence of bleeding from the nose and gums is a more reliable guide."

Splenectomy.—This operation has assumed a position of great importance in the treatment of purpura hemorrhagica in the last few years due to the accumulated data which show that there is an increase in the number of platelets following splenectomy in experimental animals and also in the human when the operation has been performed for the relief of other conditions. The operative mortality is very slight, and symptomatic cure, plus a considerable increase in the number of platelets, has resulted in the majority of cases. Washburn (1930) collected the reports of 48 cases; 70.7 per cent showed good results, 16.8 per cent were definitely improved, 4.2 per cent were slightly improved, and 8.3 per cent died. Pemberton (1931) reports the results of 41 operations at the Mayo Clinic, 1923–31: of the 39 patients living, 36 were well. Eliason and Ferguson (1932) have studied the results in 213 reported cases and feel that splenectomy is the most effective method of controlling the disease though they by no means believe it proved that the spleen is the organ at fault. It will be extremely interesting to have subsequent reports on as many "cured" cases as possible after the lapse of a few more years, for some of the functions of the spleen are known to be eventually taken over in large part by other members of the reticulo-endothelial system. Giffin and Halloway write: "The recurrence of petechiae in some of the cases, the slowness with which the bleeding time becomes reduced, and the variability in connection with the recovery of the retractility of the clot, indicate that although a change has been brought about by splenectomy sufficient to arrest gross hemorrhage, the finer mechanism of coagulation requires a complex readjustment on the part of the organism, which may or may not become complete and permanent. A few of the patients have remained somewhat anemic. However, the uniformly good results indicate at least a temporary cure."

Some observers have felt that the operation is definitely contraindicated in acute cases, but Washburn believes that "acute" here should be defined as "acutely bleeding."

Irradiation.—Irradiation of the spleen with small doses of x-rays occasionally benefits a patient somewhat. Minot and Buckman report that increases in the blood platelet count and a distinct decrease in bleeding have occurred in some of their patients simultaneously with tanning of their skin by sunlight. The experimental work of Laurens and Sooy has demonstrated a definite increase of the blood platelets after irradiation of white rats with the mercury vapor quartz lamp, and offers a rational basis for the application of this method of treatment to cases of purpura hemorrhagica. Sooy and Moise, and a number of others, have reported good results with heavy ultraviolet irradiation, some going so far as to produce painful hyperemia. Mason's (1932) long experience with the treatment has led him to favor the use of smaller doses.

Liver.—Liver or liver extract has been used as in pernicious anemia, but the reports so far are not convincing of its value.

HEMOPHILIA

Hemophilia is a hereditary disease of unknown etiology in which the coagulation time of the blood is markedly prolonged. It is transmitted by the female but occurs only in the male; about two thirds of the male offspring of a female conductor are hemophiliacs, while about one third of the female offspring do not become conductors. The disease usually makes itself apparent at an early age. External or internal hemorrhage of an oozing type occurs following the most trivial injuries; spontaneous bleeding is rare. Obstinate epistaxis is common, so also are hemorrhages into and about the joints, the latter causing deformities much resembling those of tuberculosis. Hemophiliacs nearly always succumb before adulthood is reached, either during the course of a profuse hemorrhage or from the cachexia and anemia resulting from frequently repeated sublethal bleedings.

In the Babylonian Talmud (second century, A. D.) it is stated that circumcision is to be discontinued in a family in which it has caused two successive fatalities; this is looked upon as the earliest reference to hemophilia. The first clear account in modern literature was that of Otto, in 1803. The disease was named by Schönlein in the middle of the nineteenth century.

THERAPY

The use of anticoagulants and other remedies and measures employed in the control of hemorrhage are described on page 425. Blood transfusion. usually hastens coagulation for a period which is long enough for clotting to take place; the effect of a transfusion lasts at most only about three days, however, from which it will be seen that as a measure to keep the patient alive for an indefinite period it is of very limited value. Hemophiliacs, especially those who are only mildly afflicted, can be carried safely through a surgical operation if transfused just before incision and repeatedly during the healing stage of the wound. On the other hand, since severe hemorrhage results in decreased clotting time, Lawson *et al.* (1932) have deliberately bled a patient, 500 to 600 cc., every five to six weeks, apparently with good symptomatic results.

Minot and Buckman write that the use of protein sensitization in the treatment of hemophilia is worthy of note. The nonsensitive patient is given 3 to 4 cc. of sheep or horse serum subcutaneously, and after ten days, having become sensitive, about 0.2 cc. of the same serum intradermally. The reaction may be repeated at will by subsequent intradermal injections, as the skin reaction does not desensitize the patient. Eley and Clifford (1931) have reported that in their 8 cases the method was of convincing benefit in the prevention or control of bleeding from superficial injuries but of no value in controlling hemorrhage from the larger vessels or in preventing effusions into the joints or the occurrence of subcutaneous hematomas or intestinal bleeding. In the capillary, but not in the venous blood, there was a definite reduction in coagulation time.

When theelin, lutein and several preparations of whole ovary are added to hemophilic blood in the test tube, decreased clotting time results; normal blood is not so affected. Clinical application of this fact, based upon the sex-linked transmission of the disease, has recently been made, though suggested so long ago as 1904, by Grant, in England. Birch (1933) has obtained best results with 40 to 120 grains (2.4 to 7.2 Gm.) daily by mouth of preparations of whole ovary or 50 to 200 rat units when given subcutaneously or intramuscularly. Successful ovarian graft into the abdominal wall in one case gave normal results for five months. In a single case, carefully studied, Kimm and Van Allen (1932) brought the laboratory findings to normal by two 4-grain (0.25 Gm.) intramuscular injections spaced from twelve to twenty-four hours apart; three doses in twenty-four hours were necessary for permanent control of spontaneous bleeding. White (1932) has observed marked improvement in 3 cases through the intramuscular injection of 1 to 3 ampules of theelin every four days.

The administration of mixtures of all the known vitamins, as also liver feeding, have been variously reported upon, but I am not convinced that the results merit present description of the methods.

HEMORRHAGIC DISEASE OF THE NEWBORN

Spontaneous bleeding into any of the tissues of the body occurs between the fourth and tenth days in about 1 per cent of all newborn infants. The cause is unknown; practically the only abnormal finding is an increased coagulation time of the blood. The state is self-limited, but if untreated is fatal in about half the cases.

THERAPY

Several subcutaneous or intramuscular injections of 10 to 30 cc. of human blood, repeated at four- to eight-hour intervals, are usually sufficient to stop the bleeding. In the more serious cases intravenous or intraperitoneal transfusion of from 30 to 80 cc. is perhaps to be preferred. Vincent writes "the iso-agglutinins and their receptors are not entirely developed at birth and probably isohemolysins are not present in infants' blood." This means that the selection of a donor in accordance with the blood groups to ensure compatibility, though desirable, is not strictly necessary in transfusing these very young infants. The blood is usually given by the father without any preliminary tests being made.

AGRANULOCYTOSIS

It has been interestingly pointed out by Pepper that so long ago as 1857 the entity which we now designate "agranulocytosis" was clearly recognized as to its terminal clinical features, but it was not until 1922 that Schultz reported the first series of cases in which all the laboratory and bedside findings were included to form the characteristic picture that bears the title today. Since Schultz's report a prodigious literature has sprung into being and the nosological possibilities have been shown to be truly appalling, but it is necessary for us here to keep the presentation as simple as possible, else we are lost. Agranulocytosis, then, is an apparently widespread disease whose outstanding characteristics are the following: (*a*) It is a disease chiefly of middle-aged women of the middle and upper classes, rarely if ever seen in Negroes, and occurring only occasionally in infants and very old people. (*b*) There is an orderly sequence of events. First, a complete or nearly complete disappearance of the myelocytes, and about four days after this event the granular leukocytes are either absent or nearly absent from the blood stream. Second, about two days after complete or all but complete disappearance of leukocytes from the blood stream the clinical onset begins, often with dramatic suddenness, with collapse, chill, fever, red throat or ulcerative stomatitis, perhaps jaundice, stupor and death—unless the manufacture and maturation of myelocytes is resumed. Third, sepsis develops in many cases before the end, the organisms concerned being the normal inhabitants of the oral cavity or lower intestine. Fourth, practically all of the recurrent cases conform during their actively ill periods to the above specifications, so that in recurrent agranulocytosis we have a state of affairs much like that in pernicious anemia, *i. e.*, periods of symptomatic activity alternating with periods of asymptomatic remission.

One of the diagnostic criteria of Schultz was that there be no reduction in blood platelets, but cases are now being seen in which there is both a hemorrhagic tendency and a reduction in the number of red cells, so that there are complicating features of purpura hemorrhagica and even of aplastic anemia. The importance of recognizing these facts is that splenectomy, which is of such great value in simon-pure purpura, might be very harmful in agranulocytosis with purpuric features. All work to date indicates that the granulopenia (reduction in leukocytes) is due to bone-marrow aplasia, or, in the sense of Fitz-Hugh and Krumbhaar's observations, to maturation arrest in the myeloid series, rather than to a destruction of cells in the blood stream. It would seem that complete absence of granular cells for seven days, more or less, is incompatible with life; many patients die before ulceration, necrosis and sepsis have had time to develop, the only finding, in addition to the overwhelming collapse, being a mild redness of the throat utterly unable in itself to cause or hasten death. Invasion of the defenseless tissues by whatever bacteria are at hand is therefore probably a beneficent thing, since infection and sepsis may stimulate the bone marrow to renew the maturation of myelocytes.

The etiology of the disease is as yet unknown and the difficulties lying in the path of further investigation are prodigious, for Roberts and Kracke's (1931) careful study of 8000 blood counts has shown that 1 out of every 4 patients, in Atlanta, Ga., may be expected to have a mild granulopenia; the proportion is even 1 out of 2 in females between the ages of forty and sixty. Pepper (1931) believes that the granulopenic reaction may be on an allergic basis; Corey and Britton (1932) suspect an association with adrenal insufficiency; no attempt to show a specific micro-organism in a definite etiologic rôle has as yet been entirely successful. Perhaps some exogenous factor may produce granulopenia in susceptible persons; benzene and the benzene nucleus present in the arsphenamines have already been convicted in a few instances as is well known. Kracke (1932) has produced granulopenia unassociated with anemia in rabbits by the use of benzene; the recent bedside observations of Madison and Squier (recorded below) indicate that some related drugs now in common use might profitably be looked upon with suspicion. The following is but a partial list of drugs in whose composition the benzene nucleus occurs once or by linkage several times:

Acetanilid
Actephenatidin (phenacetin)
Acid and basic fuchsins
Arsphenamines
Atoxyl
Balsam of Peru
Balsam of tolu (1)
Benzoic acid and sodium benzoate
Benzoin (2)
Benzaldehyde (3)
Benzyl alcohol
Benzyl benzoate
Bismarsen
Brilliant green
Bromsulphalein
Compound cresol solution (lysol)
Creosote
Dimason
Fluorescein
Gentian violet
Guaiacol
Hexylresorcinol
Iodoxybenzoic acid
Mercurochrome
Nitrobenzene (4)
Phenol
Phenolphthalein
Phenolsulphonphthalein
Phenoltetrachlorphthalein
Phenylhydrazine hydrochloride
Phentetiothalein sodium
Picric acid
Proprietary "headache remedies"
Pyrogallol
Resorcinol
Saccharin
Salicylates
Scarlet red
Scarlet red sulphonate
Stovarsol (acetarsone)
Tannic acid, tannates and synthetic tannin compounds (5)
Tar
Tetrabromphenolphthalein sodium
Thymol
Thymol iodide
Tryparsamide
Uva ursi
Vanillin (6)
Zincphenolsulphonate (sulphocarbolate)

Bayer-205 and Fourneau-309 and 270 probably also belong in the list.

(1) present in syrup of tolu.
(2) present in tincture and compound tincture of benzoin.
(3) present in bitter almond water, the spirit of bitter almond and in perfumes.
(4) included because a constituent of some perfumes and perfumed soaps.
(5) also present in tea and the tincture of krameria.
(6) present in vanilla.

In order to include the condensed polynuclear compounds the following must be added:

Aloe	Naphthalene
Betanaphthol	Rhubarb
Bismuth betanaphthol	Santonin
Cascara	Senna (1)

(1) present also in compound glycyrrhiza powder and in many laxative nostrums.

Other related substances are the quinoline derivatives and the acridine dyes:

Quinolines	Acridine dyes
Cinchophen Neocinchophen	Acriflavine Proflavine

When we realize that the opiates are condensed polynuclear compounds and that the other alkaloids are now generally conceded to be compounds in which at least one nitrogen atom forms part of a cyclic system it is seen that the whole affair has appalling possibilities. However, it will be noted that antipyrine, antipyrine salicylate (salipyrin), melubrin and amidopyrine (pyramidon), and allonal and amytal compound (both containing amidopyrine together with a barbiturate) are not included in any of the above lists, and this I think is the saving feature. They are not truly benzene but rather pyrazolon derivatives. Here, with these drugs and compounds, would seem to be the point of departure for the new investigations.

THERAPY

It seems to me altogether impossible to truly evaluate the different forms of treatment at the present time, for several reasons: (a) The tendency toward spontaneous recovery naturally invites a claim of cure for the last agent used; (b) it is not yet known how many of the recoveries are really only remissions; (c) there are records of response to a given agent in one attack and failure to respond to the same agent in a subsequent attack; (d) the mortality statistics range between 25 and almost 100 per cent, but until the remission-recurrence factor can be fully taken into account in a large series studied through several years, such figures must remain of little value; (e) such statistical analysis as is already in existence is quite contradictory, Taussig (1931) showing the superiority of x-ray treatment, Jackson et al. (1932) of nucleotide. What follows, therefore, is merely a statement of methods. General supportive measures are of course necessary, particularly cardiac stimulation and the supplying of adequate nourishment in easily assimilable form. Griffith (1932) records a case in which he felt that the forcing of fluids through a Jutte tube passed through the nose into the stomach and left in place for seven days, by means of which 120 to 130 ounces (3600 to 3900 cc.) of a high carbohydrate liquid diet (not specified, but I should think that 10 to 15 per cent glucose solution would be satisfactory) were given, resulted in overcoming the dehydration, and causing good kidney function, without disturbing the hematopoietic system or overloading the heart by fluids introduced intravenously. Isolation, in the attempt to prevent infection, would certainly seem to be a rational procedure.

The Withholding of Drugs Containing Pyrazolon Derivatives.—Just before going to press I have had the privilege of discussing with Drs. Madison and Squier, of Milwaukee, their rather astonishing findings, which are as yet unpublished. In their series of 14 consecutive cases there was a history in each instance of amidopyrine (pyramidon) having been taken immediately prior to the clinical discovery of granulocytopenia: in 7 cases combined with a barbiturate and in 7 cases alone or in combination with drugs other than barbiturates. Five of these patients were being treated in the hospital for other conditions, in the handling of which amidopyrine was being employed, when the agranulocytosis appeared. In the nine instances in which the drug was withheld there were only two deaths (the mortality was 100 per cent in the remainder of the group), both patients having been moribund when the diagnosis was made; all who recovered from the acute attack are living and well after an interval varying from two years to three months at the time of this writing. One patient, who had had his initial attack eighteen months previously and who had been in a state of complete remission for ten months, took 5 grains (0.3 Gm.) amidopyrine in the evening—within three hours he had a chill, in the morning symptoms had returned and he was found to be almost agranulocytic. Another patient whose first attack had developed during the administration of a compound containing amytal and amidopyrine had recovered from the attack and had had a normal granulocyte count for three weeks when she was given two capsules of the compound; before administration the count was 6850, two hours later it was 3200 and twelve hours later it was 1200. The count then gradually returned to normal. Two weeks later she was given amytal without the pyramidon and showed no alteration in the granulocyte count.

Nucleotides.—On purely empiric grounds, nuclein therapy was suggested in the days of Metchnikoff to increase the germicidal power of the blood in diseases of microbic origin, but Doan (1932) has shown that the increase in leukocytes reported to have been stimulated by the use of these products of cell breakdown was well within the limits of normal fluctuation in the light of modern hematological studies. However, stimulated by the observations of Sabin, he has undertaken a restudy of the hypothesis of leukocyte disintegration products as the stimulus of leukocyte production. The result has been the introduction into the therapy of agranulocytosis of the product known at first as nucleotide K-96, but now designated pentnucleotide, N.N.R. Jackson and his associates of the Harvard group describe the use of the product as follows (1932):

"As the series has become larger it has become increasingly obvious that medication, to be effective, must be intensive and continuous. Of the nucleotide K-96 preparation 10 cc. (equivalent to 0.7 Gm. of the solid), should be injected intramuscularly twice a day until the white blood cell count has very definitely risen: 10 cc. should then be given intramuscularly once a day until the white blood cell count has been essentially normal on at least three consecutive days. Thereafter the patient should be watched for a possible relapse. In certain resistant cases an increase over the usual dose brought a marked increase of white blood cells, after smaller doses had produced little or no effect. In desperately ill cases the contents of one vial should be diluted to 100 cc. with warm sterile saline and injected slowly intravenously each morning for four days. On the evening of each of the same days, 10 cc. (undiluted) should be injected intramuscularly. At the end of four days the intravenous injections may be discontinued but the bidaily intramuscular injections should be kept up until the white blood cell count has definitely risen, after which daily single intramuscular injections are to be continued until the white blood cell count has been at a normal figure for at least three consecutive days.

"To the intramuscular injections there are, as a rule, few if any unfavorable reactions attributable to the material. An occasional patient may have nausea, precordial distress and dyspnea, immediately following an injection. Rarely there may be chills and fever several hours later, but we believe that an improved method of preparing the material has largely eliminated these features. To the intravenous injections there is usually an immediate reaction of dyspnea and palpitation and in an occasional case there may be chills and fever several hours after the injection. The intravenous injection should, therefore, not be used in the presence of myocardial damage.

"No improvement is to be expected during the first few days of treatment. In fact the patient may appear to become worse. This is no indication that eventual recovery will not take place and is no reason for discontinuing treatment. The white blood cell count may even fall during the early days of treatment but this fall can be attributed to progress of the disease occurring before the nucleotide can sufficiently effect the production of white blood cells."

Madison believes it wise to continue minimal stimulation of the granulopoietic centers after recovery by the administration of nucleotide at two- to four-week intervals or bone marrow extract (see below) in daily doses of 1 to 3 Gm.

Bone Marrow Extract.—Watkins and Giffin, of the Mayo Clinic, have been using the extract of yellow bone marrow with reputedly good results; Madison is also well impressed by the effects obtained through the oral administration of 20 to 30 Gm. daily throughout the acute stage.

Adenine Sulphate.—Reznikoff (1933) has reported the use of this drug in 15 uncomplicated cases with recovery in 11 of the patients; in severely complicated cases it was not effective. The suggested dosage is 15 grains (1 Gm.) of adenine sulphate boiled in 35 to 40 cc. of physiologic saline solution, given warm, intravenously three times a day for at least three days.

Blood Transfusion.—Since no technically satisfactory method of transfusing leukocytes alone is at present available, whole blood transfusions are resorted to, but it must be admitted that the rationale of the method is open to legitimate doubt since the transfusion of 500 cc. of blood can theoretically only raise the leukocyte content of recipient's body by 6 per cent. Hemorrhage might be expected to be more productive of bone-marrow stimulation. However, Doan feels that transfusion is a rational procedure on the basis of its nucleic acid content. Kracke states that the blood of an individual who has recovered from the disease should be used if possible. One or more transfusions of 250 to 500 cc. are usually given; sometimes a transfusion is given daily or on alternate days until the leukocytic rise is well advanced.

x-Ray.—Roentgen therapy in this disease is certainly a two-edged sword, as pointed out by a number of observers, and there is no escaping the fact that the difference between the dose which will stimulate the hematopoietic tissues and that which will destroy them cannot be accurately known to the roentgenologists since it most probably varies widely from individual to individual; therefore the assumption upon which therapy is based, namely, that there is a fixed stimulatory threshold below which primary destruction of cells does not precede regeneration, is—well, assumption. Doan, indeed, believes that such good results as may be obtained are directly chargeable to destruction of myeloid foci with a liberation of autogenous nucleotide and resultant initiation of maturation.

Matters of dosage and technic of course cannot be discussed here; those interested should study the paper of Waters and Firor (1932).

Arsphenamines.—The use of the drugs of this group was apparently begun in the attempt to check proliferation of organisms of the Vincent type, but since the recognition of the entirely secondary rôle of the oral process it is doubtful if the practice will survive; furthermore, the possibility of bone-marrow damage seems to me absolutely to condemn it.

Fetal Tissues.—There are several reports of the feeding of raw, ground fetal calf spleen, or a mixture of fetal spleen, marrow, thymus, hypophysis, and blood serum; as much is given in orange juice as the patient can be gotten to take.

Liver Extract.—Kracke advocates the per orum administration of liver extract as in pernicious anemia. Paine *et al.* (1933) obtained remissions in all of their 5 cases.

Nonspecific Proteins.—Nonspecific protein therapy (see p. 327), especially by the intravenous route (see p. 191), has been advocated tentatively by Brooks (1932).

Local Therapy.—The usual treatment for severe stomatitis is considered to be indicated by most observers (see methods on p. 400), who feel that the danger of blood-stream invasion is thus lessened, but others feel that the continuous swabbing of the lesions with various antiseptic solutions serves only to disturb the patient and really accomplishes nothing else since in severe cases organisms will multiply and enter the system from even the cleanest mouth. Griffith made daily applications of an erythematous dose of ultraviolet light to lesions in which streptococci predominated, hoping for the same good result which is sometimes obtained in erysipelas.

DISEASES OF THE CIRCULATORY SYSTEM

FUNCTIONAL DISTURBANCES OF THE HEART

Psychogenic and emotional cardiac neuroses are usually seen in persons of a definite neurotic type and often with a history suggestive of a neurotic ancestry. There is complaint of transitory palpitation, rushing of blood in various parts of the body, throbbing, and many other symptoms which are described with the particularity so habitual to the neurotic. When there is pain it is usually felt over the left chest where the heart is supposed to be rather than under the sternum where the organ is actually located. Not all of these patients are neurotics, however, for in an occasional individual of quite robust mental and physical habit the fear of heart disease, and the consequent development of a functional heart disturbance, follows upon the shock of a sudden cardiac death in a near associate. In the condition known as effort syndrome, soldier's heart, irritable heart, or neurocirculatory asthenia, the symptoms—giddiness, faintness, palpitation, precordial pain and breathlessness—are the symptoms of effort and mark the patient as one who is physically inadequate to the ordinary stresses and strains of an active life.

THERAPY

These patients comprise a very considerable portion of the "heart" cases seen in an average general practice, and the fact that the elements of their treatment can be set down in a relatively few lines of print by no means justifies a contemptuous attitude toward this group of sufferers—for sufferers they are, as any physician knows who will honestly recall the agonies of his student days when he diagnosed upon himself nearly all the known maladies. The more robust of these individuals will be cured by the complete examination and the reassuring statements of a doctor in whom they have confidence, but what is needed by the majority of the patients is just exactly the hardest thing in the world to supply, namely, an entire readjustment to life. If there is some one thing which is causing the basic unhappiness upon which the cardiac neurosis is engrafted, the bringing of that thing out into the open and the attempt to reconstruct a life in which that particular fact is accorded no more than its proper share of importance, will oftentimes greatly relieve the patient, though if he is basically neurotic the relief will usually be only temporary. Freudian "psychoanalysis," with its ridiculous symbolism, its unsound premises, and its unscientific deductions, is absolutely worthless. In no case must a cardiac neurotic be permitted to continue in the belief that he has the least thing the matter with his circulatory apparatus, but there are ways and ways of assuring him of this fact. Perhaps the best method is to demonstrate his freedom from symptoms while enjoying some diversion in which he is for a time freed from his inordinate load of cares; to ridicule or to scold is almost certainly to toss him to the quacks.

The avoidance of physical and mental fatigue is important and can usually be accomplished in some degree if the patient is at all tractable. A long night of sound sleep is worth much. Hirschboeck (1928), among others, has emphasized the value of sedative drugs in those who are not able to put themselves to sleep by the time-honored counting of sheep and similar devices, though there is a popular medical and lay opinion that these drugs should not be used. "Bromides, barbital (veronal) and its innumerable offspring may be used with success, their administration being supplemented with a word of warning as to the evasion of any advice from the community grandmothers contrary to its use. The danger of forming a habit is to my mind nil, except in the few instances in which patients have felt that if a little is good more is better. The necessity for not advising the patient of the nature of the remedy, except that it is not a 'dope,' is obvious. An alternation of remedies is advisable in long-standing cases, and its practice never reveals any tendency to habit formation."

In effort syndrome cases the definite attempt to build up the patient's tolerance for that amount of physical exertion which is necessary in his occupation should be made, but it is seldom possible to bring him up to the normal of physical endurance. Carefully graded exercise, with special stress upon the necessity of obtaining not only a long night's sleep but a midday rest as well, is desirable.

PERICARDITIS

Pericarditis rarely if ever occurs except as a complication of one of the infectious diseases, particularly tonsillitis, sinusitis, tuberculosis, scarlet fever, acute rheumatic fever, pneumonia, and general sepsis (septicemia), though as a terminal condition it is sometimes recognized in chronic nephritis. In fibrinous pericarditis without effusion the symptoms are those of the primary disease plus pain in the precordium, or referred to other parts of the body, and a characteristic friction rub heard upon auscultation. When effusion occurs the patient usually becomes anxious, more or less cyanotic and dyspneic, and often very restless. Pressure on nerves and other structures may cause cough, aphonia, difficulty in swallowing, hiccup, vomiting, etc. The pulse rate usually rises very high and becomes irregular. The area of dulness at the base of the heart is increased and there may be actual bulging of the precordium; the apex impulse usually disappears. As the fluid increases the friction rub diminishes and, with a large effusion, the heart sounds are no longer audible.

Despite the glibness with which it is usually described, pericardial effusion is by no means always easy to diagnose. The prognosis in fibrinous pericarditis is always good; in the effusion cases, if the fluid is tuberculous or becomes purulent, death is the usual outcome, but in rheumatic cases the fluid is usually absorbed.

Pericarditis was probably first described by Avenzoar, of Cordova, in the twelfth century.

THERAPY

The treatment of pericarditis is the treatment of the primary disease. An ice-bag placed upon the precordium in the robust, or hot applications in the puny, asthenic individual, are usually successful analgesic measures. Codeine, 1 grain (0.065 Gm.), or morphine, ¼ grain (0.015 Gm.), should not be withheld if the pain is sapping the patient's strength, though it is well to restrict the opiates as much as possible because of their effect in locking the bowel. Salines, or enemas, are definitely indicated to prevent abdominal distention or straining at stool, both of which increase the load upon the heart. Aspiration of fluid brings such great relief in the effusion cases that it is held to be advisable to employ the procedure early and frequently, except perhaps in the rheumatic cases, in which remarkably quick subsidence of the effusion sometimes takes place. When the fluid becomes purulent, the attempt to establish surgical drainage must be made at once.

33

ENDOCARDITIS

There are four types of acute endocarditis. The rheumatic type develops during the course of an attack of rheumatic fever and is usually heralded by an increase in severity of this disease, *i. e.*, more discomfort and a rise in fever. Precordial pain, increase in pulse rate, murmur, and often a considerable dilatation of the heart appear later. Acute bacterial endocarditis is also usually a secondary affair complicating one of the acute infectious diseases. Its diagnosis is usually based upon the appearance or increase in the signs of sepsis (septicemia) and the finding of a positive blood culture, though cardiac symptoms are sometimes prominent also. Some of these cases are so rapidly fatal as to have earned the appellation "malignant endocarditis." Then there are the cases of subacute bacterial endocarditis in which the patient with a preexisting valvular lesion experiences a reinfection of the endocardium from an infectious process in the teeth, tonsils, middle ear, or other focus. The disease runs an obscure febrile course until a murmur of growing intensity is detected, or petechiae on the extremities and visible mucous membranes and signs of splenic or kidney infarction make their appearance. Positive blood cultures, nearly always of nonhemolytic streptococci, are usually easy to obtain and assist in making an early diagnosis. Death is usually caused by cerebral embolism. And finally there is the type of nonbacterial endocarditis which is apparently an independent disease. The patient becomes suddenly and acutely ill with fever, marked prostration, vomiting and pain in the epigastrium, and after twenty-four hours the appearance of palpitation, dyspnea, precordial pain, etc., indicate the cardiac involvement. Recovery from the acute attack usually takes place in a week or ten days but convalescence is very slow.

I believe that Matthew Baillie (1761–1823) was the first to describe endocarditis.

THERAPY

In all forms of endocarditis the patient must be kept absolutely quiet, to which end the use of the ice-bag, or in the asthenic individual hot applications over the precordium is indicated; opiates should be used if pain and restlessness are severe. In the rheumatic type of the disease the salicylates have no effect upon the endocardial process. Acute bacterial (malignant) endocarditis is best treated as a case of sepsis (see p. 159), the symptoms of which, indeed, usually dominate the picture. No treatment so far devised seems to be successful in subacute bacterial endocarditis; according to Kinsella, nonspecific protein therapy and attempts to immunize the patient with vaccines and serums tend only to shorten his life. In nonbacterial endocarditis the use of the ice-bag and opiates to induce rest are efficacious measures during the acute attack. During convalescence from any of the types of endocarditis the attempt should be made to strictly enforce a prolonged period of rest.

ACUTE MYOCARDITIS

Acute myocarditis is always secondary to one of the acute infectious diseases, being particularly prone to occur during or after an attack of influenza, scarlet fever, typhoid fever, diphtheria (especially if antitoxin is too long delayed or given in too small doses), rheumatic fever, or sepsis. There is usually a decrease in blood pressure with an increase in heart rate and the appearance of some sort of irregularity, though in diphtheria bradycardia occasionally occurs and is almost invariably fatal. When acute heart failure makes its appearance the symptoms—cyanosis, dyspnea, dependent edema, signs of accumulation of fluid in various portions of the body, etc.—

are the same as those of heart failure from any other cause. Because of the similarity of the symptoms in endocarditis, vasomotor circulatory failure, and myocarditis, the diagnosis of the latter condition is a doubtful one at best; this is well shown at the autopsy table where myocarditis is often demonstrated though it had not been suspected during life, and where, on the other hand, a diagnosis of the condition is sometimes discovered to have been unfounded.

THERAPY

The factor of greatest importance in the treatment of acute myocarditis is absolute rest. Not only should rest be enforced in all known cases, but in suspected cases as well, *i. e.*, in all attacks of the acute infectious diseases, particularly those listed above, the patient should not only be kept in bed but must lie quietly in the bed and must remain therein until long after the subsidence of the acute symptoms of the disease. Sudden rising up out of bed and resumption of the ordinary round of duties, without a preliminary period of strength testing by daily increases in the amount of pillow propping, is especially dangerous.

During the course of an acute myocarditis drugs are usually of little value. Most physicians look upon digitalis as a dangerous drug here because of its tendency to accelerate an already established heart block. Certainly it should not be used in a larger dose than 15 to 30 minims (1 to 2 cc.) three, or at most four, times daily, and only then if the physician is able to visit the patient at frequent intervals. In diphtheria it is usually considered to be contraindicated. Caffeine citrate by mouth is usually stated to be of value, but there are few recorded clinical studies of its action. The average dose of the drug is 5 grains (0.32 Gm.), but Taylor (1914) found it necessary to give twice this amount four times daily; his results were on the whole only moderately good and the drug caused unpleasant nervous symptoms in all cases. Caffeine sodium benzoate, the best of the hypodermic preparations, has an official dose of 3 grains but is also sometimes given in doses as high as 10 grains (0.65 Gm.); it is perhaps the best preparation to use when only an occasional dose of caffeine is to be given, but when the drug is to be given frequently during the day and for several days in succession, the oral route is preferable. The fact should not be overlooked that the persistent use of caffeine in large doses invariably causes a fall in blood pressure which often persists for some time after medication ceases. In severe acute heart failure epinephrine (adrenalin) is often useful as an emergency stimulant. Eggleston states that when used intramuscularly in doses of from 5 to 10 minims (0.32 to 0.65 cc.) of the 1: 1000 solution every ten or fifteen minutes for six doses the maximum stimulation of the heart is obtained with the minimum of vasomotor constriction.

AURICULAR FIBRILLATION

This, the commonest of the persistent arrhythmias, is now believed to be due to a self-perpetuating ring of excitation—the so-called "circus movement"—originating about the mouth of the superior vena cava in the right auricle. The result of this circus movement is to maintain a series of small rapid fibrillary contractions of the auricle, only a relatively small number of which are responded to by the ventricle. The result is a pulse which is usually rapid and extremely irregular both as to time and force, but may be quite slow and almost regular in some cases. Due to the failure of some of the weak ventricular contractions to open the semilunar valves or to initiate a pulse wave in the aorta, the pulse rate at the wrist is often less than at the apex. Exercise increases both the rate and irregularity of the contractions. Auricular fibrillation is a frequent occurrence in heart failure due to the usual causes, but it also occurs in individuals who have no valvular or myocardial disease. When it occurs in heart failure the arrhythmia merely alters to some extent the other preexisting symptoms, but in the paroxysmal auricular fibrillation of unknown origin the patient is often suddenly attacked with precordial pain, dyspnea, vertigo, nausea, pallor, and perhaps even collapse. These attacks may be recurrent, or a single attack may persist for months or years; individuals at or past middle age are the most frequent victims of this type of arrhythmia.

Sir James Mackenzie (1853–1925) was the pioneer in the scientific investigation of all the arrhythmias.

THERAPY

Digitalis.—In the entire range of medicine there is nothing more spectacular than the response of a decompensated heart with auricular fibrillation to digitalis properly administered. For the details of the use of the drug see page 529. The pulse rate is decreased, while at the same time the strength of the individual ventricular contraction increases, diuresis is established and edema disappears, dyspnea, cyanosis, etc., diminish—in short, compensation is reestablished and the patient's life is saved. But the auricular fibrillation is not cured. By the employment of proper doses during the acute stage, and the continued use during months or years of a maintenance dose of 5 to 10 minims (0.32 to 0.65 cc.) of a standardized tincture three times daily, compensation may be maintained, but the heart will continue to beat irregularly—perhaps not quite so irregularly as before treatment was instituted, but no amount of digitalis, over no period of time, will restore the normal rhythm. In the days before quinidine appeared upon the scene this was considered a very satisfactory result and is still so considered by many astute practitioners of long experience. And, indeed, if we can restore a patient to fair activity by the use of digitalis alone, an activity which may continue for fifteen years or more despite the persistence of the fibrillation, and can do this without incurring any of the risks which appertain to quinidine therapy, and can have our patient feeling subjectively quite as well as under quinidine therapy, who shall say that the digitalis treatment of auricular fibrillation is obsolete? Quinidine therapy will be described below with no attempt to minimize its value, but the reader is counselled to ponder long and well the satisfactory results which are regularly obtained with digitalis in the treatment of this condition.

Quinidine.—(a) *History.*—Quinine, the drug used in the specific treatment of malaria, has been used by physicians for its supposed sedative action on the heart for more than half a century. It was not until 1914, however, that Wenckebach, of Vienna, recorded its deliberate use in the treatment of auricular fibrillation. He has described his experience as follows:

"In 1912, a patient presented himself in my office wishing to get rid of his attacks of auricular fibrillation. He knew that this was the so-called perpetual or complete arrhythmia and that his attacks ceased for the most part spontaneously after from two to fourteen days. He was a stout man, aged about fifty, able to do a good deal of bodily exercise and even during the attack to walk for four or five hours. From this fact it was clear that the efficiency of his heart and circulation was only slightly diminished by the attack. He did not feel great discomfort during the attack but, as he said, being a Dutch merchant, used to good order in his affairs, he would like to have good order in his heart business also and asked why there were heart specialists if they could not abolish this very disagreeable phenomenon.

On my telling him that I could promise him nothing, he told me that he knew himself how to get rid of his attacks, and as I did not believe him he promised to come back the next morning with a regular pulse, and he did. It happens that quinine in many countries, especially in countries where there is a good deal of malaria, is a sort of drug for everything, just as one takes acetylsalicylic acid today if one does not feel well or is afraid of having taken cold. Occasionally, taking the drug during an attack of fibrillation, the patient found that the attack was stopped within from twenty to twenty-five minutes, and later he found that a gram of quinine regularly abolished his irregularity.

"I was greatly struck by this fact, and afterward tried this sort of treatment in many cases of auricular fibrillation. My success was disappointing, in that quinine abolished auricular fibrillation in only a few cases and in those cases only when the onset of this form was quite recent, never when it was of several years' duration. At the same time, I found that even in those cases in which auricular fibrillation was not abolished, the drug had a marked soothing action on the often terrific rate of the ventricle."

Stimulated by these observations, Frey, in 1918, undertook to study the clinical pharmacology of various cinchona derivatives (quinine, quinidine and cinchonine) in patients with auricular fibrillation. Finding the most effective therapeutic agent to be quinidine, he chose its more soluble sulphate for extensive trial. (In this present article wherever the word quinidine is encountered quinidine sulphate is to be understood.) In his first publication Frey reported 10 cases, in 6 of which he was able to convert the fibrillatory mechanism into the normal sinus rhythm, results which have since been amply confirmed, at first in Germany and later all over the world.

(b) *Action.*—So far as the drug's actions are at present understood, they are assumed to be the following: (a) It mildly paralyzes the vagus, (b) it lowers the rate of sinus impulse discharge, (c) it causes a slight decrease in auriculoventricular conduction, (d) it lengthens the refractory period of cardiac muscle and slows conduction in the muscle, (e) it lessens the excitability of cardiac muscle. The useful therapeutic action depends upon its effect on circus movement. By lengthening the refractory period it slows and abolishes circus movement, but also, by reducing conduction in the muscle, it tends at the same time to fix circus movement. Therefore, whether quinidine is to abolish or to fix circus movement would seem to depend upon whether its preponderant effect is upon the refractory period or upon conduction, a more or less selective type of action which is not at present definitely predictable.

(c) *Effectiveness.*—Wolff and White (1929) have reported the successful restoration of sinus rhythm in 65 per cent of their large series of 177 cases; this seems to be about the average of what is accomplished nowadays. However, Stroud *et al.* (1932), who have obtained about the same initial success, have now become less sanguine after studying some of their cases for as long as seven years, since the duration of life in these cases was only slightly over a year longer than that of patients who were considered unsatisfactory for quinidine therapy and exactly the same as that of patients who had received quinidine but without the restoration of normal sinus rhythm. Wolff and White also feel that there is no definite evidence that quinidine prolongs life or reduces mortality. The following is offered as a statement of the more important elements which probably condition success with the drug:

1. The predilection of quinidine for the abolition or fixation of circus movement, an unpredictable element in every case.

2. The idiosyncrasy of the patient for cinchona derivatives, which may be so great as to effectively eliminate the possibility of success with the drug.

3. Dosage and management of the patient (discussed in detail below).

4. Selection of cases. Barrier (1927) writes: "Not all patients with chronic fibrillation should receive quinidine; a competent myocardium is the criterion in selecting cases. I eliminate the aged, and those with marked hypertorphy, chronic heart failure, active endocarditis, or significant changes in the T waves or Q-R-S complexes of the electrocardiogram." This writer also says that the duration of fibrillation is not a trustworthy criterion on which to prognosticate the restoration of normal rhythm, in which, however, he is not in accord with the opinion of the majority of observers, who feel that short duration much improves the prognosis under the drug. Levy (1927) employs the following criteria for the elimination of unsuitable cases, which coincide with those of the members of the Cardiac Club of London, as reported by Hay: (a) Badly injured hearts, especially with marked enlargement and long-standing valvular disease; (b) hearts which, after rest and digitalis, evince but little evidence of reserve strength; (c) a history of embolism; (d) patients with an idiosyncrasy for cinchona derivatives; and (e) occasionally, patients giving a history of cardiac pain which ceased after the onset of fibrillation. It is evident that if these criteria are followed the number of patients eligible for quinidine therapy is limited. I think it worthy of note that in Maynard's series in which there was 71 per cent success in 53 cases, complete restoration of sinus rhythm was actually accomplished in 90 per cent of the cases in which the degree of compensation was classed as good.

5. Spiro and Newman write that there would seem to be an element of luck in the use of quinidine. "In a certain case we were about to give up the use of quinidine in despair, and the patient begged for another dose. Another dose was given; the pulse became regular and has remained so. In another case, after days of rather heavy doses of quinidine without success, the quinidine was discontinued and the pulse became regular. It seemed that discontinuing the quinidine caused the pulse to become regular. This uncertainty of action makes it difficult to judge how much to give the patient and when to stop."

There is little to be said in regard to the duration of the relief except that it is very variable; sometimes lasting for only a few days, perhaps most often for several months, and occasionally for more than a year. Maynard (1928) has presented evidence to show that there is a definite tendency for auricular fibrillation to become permanent. Sinus rhythm may be established five, six or even seven times over a period of years, but the time finally comes in the majority of cases when further attempts are unsuccessful.

.(d) *Dangers.*—The greatest danger in the use of quinidine is that one may establish with it ventricular tachycardia or an actual ventricular fibrillation, which is a very serious matter. It is generally advised that quinidine be stopped after the onset of a persistently high ventricular rate, and this is certainly a safe policy, but, as a matter of fact, this increased ventricular rate may be due to the slowed auricular rate, or to the conversion of auricular fibrillation into auricular flutter, in both of which cases it might be advisable to increase the dosage of the drug—from which it will be seen that the administration of quinidine is by no means a simple matter.

Embolism is another potential danger, but not nearly so great a one as was believed in the early days of the drug's use. In the dilated, noncontracted appendages of the auricle of auricular fibrillation mural clots are formed. So long as fibrillation is present and the auricle does not contract as a whole these clots are relatively harmless, but with the disappearance of fibrillation and the reestablishment of total auricular contraction, they are dislodged and forced out into the peripheral circulation, where embolic catastrophe takes place. So much for the theory, but I do not feel that we have reliable evidence of the occurrence of this phenomenon any more often after quinidine therapy than during the course of a nontreated fibrillation or uncomplicated heart failure *per se;* Viko, Marvin and White (1926), Parkinson and Campbell (1929), Lewis (1932), Weisman (1932), and Stroud *et al.* (1932) concur in such opinion.

Sudden syncope and collapse occurs with relative frequency. It is nowadays usually ascribed to idiosyncrasy for the drug, but the fact should not be overlooked that a few deaths of this sort have been reported.

Spiro and Newman describe the following danger signs during the administration of quinidine:

"1. Showers of petechiae. The patient should be examined daily, the conjunctivae, the mouth, and the body in general, to see if there are any petechiae. If there are, the quinidine should be at once discontinued. Frequently the heart becomes regular for a few seconds only, and the showers of petechiae are then caused.

"2. Signs of respiratory distress, a sort of air-hunger, with slight cyanosis, dizziness, anxious expression and a cold sweat. In such cases the quinidine should be discontinued and caffeine given. Caffeine is an absolute antidote.

"3. An increase in pulse rate, the pulse running 125 or over. The quinidine should be stopped. As a rule, if the quinidine is discontinued the tachycardia will stop. There is danger of producing ventricular fibrillation if quinidine is carried beyond this point.

"4. Of course, an embolus naturally will stop one from the use of quinidine."

(*e*) *Methods of Use.*—In Auricular Fibrillation Associated with Heart Failure.—I quote Spiro and Newman's excellent summary of their method (1928):

"A patient who is troubled with auricular fibrillation should have his food and fluid intake, his rest and his exercise regulated. He should be given digitalis. When the pulse is slow, from 72 to 80, and the pulse rate at the wrist equals the rate at the apex of the heart, the output of urine balances the fluid intake and there are no signs or symptoms suggesting decompensation, he probably is ready for quinidine. One should now try to determine whether the heart chambers are contracting vigorously enough to make it unlikely that the chambers could contain an unorganized clot. The patient should be taken, not sent to the roentgenologist, and the amplitude of the heart's pulsatory waves studied.

"1. If there is great difficulty in seeing any motion, the patient is not ready for quinidine.

"2. If the motion seen is so slight as to make a mere flicker, the patient is not ready for quinidine.

"3. If the patient is rotated until the left shoulder touches the fluoroscopic screen, and he takes a short breath, in this position the apex of the heart becomes visible and the motion should be easily and distinctly seen. If motion is distinctly seen, the patient is probably ready for quinidine.

"4. If the patient is rotated until the posterior part of the right shoulder touches the fluoroscopic screen, one is now looking through the patient's back; the margin of the left ventricle should contract and relax in a quite decided manner, and there will be no difficulty in seeing this fairly vigorous motion. If numbers 3 and 4 are satisfactory, the patient should be sent to the hospital and treatment begun with quinidine, the patient being kept at absolute rest in bed.

"The quinidine is given, 4 grains (0.26 Gm.) the first day, 8 grains (0.5 Gm.) the second day. This is supposed to determine whether there is any idiosyncrasy to the drug. If there is none, the quinidine is increased 8 grains (0.5 Gm.) every twenty-four hours for ten days, or until the patient is taking 72 grains (4.7 Gm.) in twenty-four hours, a reasonable interval intervening between the doses. Quinidine is given day and night. If after the end of ten days the heart is not regular, the drug can be discontinued and the digitalis started again in fairly large doses for from one to three days and then the quinidine started again. It is now known that there is no idiosyncrasy, so a dosage of from 32 to 40 grains (2 to 2.6 Gm.) is given in twenty-four hours, and this dosage is pushed until the previous dose is reached. We have given as high as 96 grains (6 Gm.) in twenty-four hours. There are published records of 200 grains (13 Gm.) in twenty-four hours.

"If not successful in six days more we discontinue the effort, get the patient up and about, and advise another attempt in from thirty to sixty days, using the interim for improving the patient's general muscle by regulated exercises. If we are successful in either the first or second attempt the patient receives quinidine for an indefinite period (ration dose, 4 grains [0.26 Gm.] three times a day).

"Recently we have been trying the method of not discontinuing the use of digitalis at once on starting quinidine, and are satisfied with the results. We now continue the digitalis at the same dosage as on the day we believed the patient ready for quinidine, as, for example:

"First day: Tincture of digitalis (or equivalent in powder), 20 minims (1.25 cc.) at 7 A. M., 12 noon, 7 P. M.; quinidine, 4 grains (0.26 Gm.) at 10 A. M.

"Second day: Digitalis, 10 minims (0.6 cc.) at 7 A. M. and 7 P. M.; quinidine, 4 grains (0.26 Gm.) at 10 A. M. and 3 P. M.

"Third day: Digitalis, 10 minims (0.6 cc.) at 7 A. M.; quinidine, 10 A. M., 4 P. M., and 8 P. M.

"Fourth day and after: Digitalis discontinued; quinidine given according to the dosage in the first part of this paper."

IN PAROXYSMAL AURICULAR FIBRILLATION OR IN CHRONIC AURICULAR FIBRILLATION NOT ASSOCIATED WITH HEART FAILURE.—It is the belief of Riecker (1925) that the ventricular tachycardia and even the ventricular fibrillation which sometimes occurs under quinidine can often be prevented by using concomitantly the auriculoventricular blocking effect of digitalis. After bringing the heart in condition with digitalis (see above), he discontinues the digitalis and begins quinidine within twenty-four hours; then, upon the accomplishment of a return to normal rhythm, the quinidine is stopped and the condition is maintained by the use of maintenance doses of digitalis—usually about 30 minims (2 Gm.) of a standardized tincture per day. The majority of observers, however, do not attempt to forestall ventricular tachycardia in this way with digitalis, but when the excessive acceleration of the ventricular rate makes its appearance they stop the quinidine simply. Barrier (1927) expresses the opinion of many when he says that digitalis definitely retards the restoration of normal mechanism and that it should not be given previous to the administration of quinidine unless there is heart failure, and that in cases in which digitalis is constantly needed to maintain cardiac competence quinidine is not indicated.

AURICULAR FLUTTER

This is a condition in which the auricles develop a rate of 200 to 300 per minute, only a few of these impulses passing over and initiating a ventricular contraction. The ratio is usually 2 to 1, with a ventricular rate of 120 to

170. The symptoms are those of auricular fibrillation plus heart failure, but there is a predominant rhythm even though the pulse is irregular. Flutter is more rarely encountered than fibrillation; it is also more often transient than permanent.

THERAPY

Quinidine.—The review of the literature made by Colgate and Mc-Culloch (1926) definitely points to circus movement as underlying all the arrhythmias whether of the auricle or ventricle, which would make of fibrillation, flutter, premature systole and paroxysmal tachycardia only different degrees of the same process. Theoretically, then, quinidine is indicated in all of these arrhythmias, but actually the drug has not succeeded very well in flutter. Parkinson and Bedford's (1927) experience is quite typical; they succeeded in restoring the normal rhythm in only 3 out of the 15 cases of flutter in which they used the drug. Gager (1931) has reported an interesting case of auricular flutter coexistant with complete heart block which he restored to sinus rhythm and A-V conduction by the use of quinidine; he cites two similar instances of restoration in the literature.

Digitalis.—Digitalis is used in flutter to slow the ventricular rate by increasing the auriculoventricular block. After the pulse is slowed the continued use of smaller doses of digitalis converts the flutter into fibrillation; it is said that cessation of digitalis medication then causes the reappearance of normal sinus rhythm. In Parkinson and Bedford's series of 52 cases, digitalis restored normal rhythm in one third, established auricular fibrillation in a third, and failed altogether in the other third. Hamburger has not had very great success with the method. He finds fibrillation easy enough to produce, but states that in his experience there has usually been reversion to flutter upon the discontinuance of the digitalis.

Vagus or ocular pressure oftentimes temporarily reduces the ventricular rate.

PAROXYSMAL TACHYCARDIA

In this condition the patient becomes aware of a sudden great increase in the heart rate, usually to from 120 to 180 beats per minute. The rhythm is regular and the rate is not decreased during rest. Such a paroxysm may persist for hours or even for many days, and the attacks may recur frequently for weeks, months, or years. Individuals without demonstrable cardiac pathology are just as liable to these paroxysms as are the victims of heart disease; the young are more often affected than the old. The attacks terminate just as suddenly as they arise, and in most instances without having caused any disturbance other than distress and palpitation; in cases of long duration, however, mild symptoms of heart failure supervene, and there are even a few recorded deaths.

THERAPY

Mechanical Measures.—Pressure on the vagi in the neck, especially the right vagus, often terminates an attack by stimulation of the inhibitory function of this nerve. Pressure should not be made upon both nerves at the same time; Hume (1930), strangely, finds that if he does not succeed with pressure on the *left* vagus, right vagus pressure is a waste of time. Pressure upon the orbit is sometimes effective also. There are individuals who can stop an attack by indirect stimulation of the inhibitory mechanism, such as by deep breathing or holding the breath, vomiting, swallowing a hard bolus of food, or by assuming various postures.

Quinidine.—This drug is sometimes effective in controlling the paroxysms. Barrier (1927) writes: "I have found quinidine fairly reliable in auricular paroxysmal tachycardia. Most patients who take the drug consistently are relieved of attacks; in others who take it only when attacks become numerous it is difficult to gain an idea as to its efficiency." The doses used by most observers are much smaller than those employed to obtain the full effect of the drug in fibrillation: A daily dose of 1.2 Gm. (0.4 Gm. three times a day) is considered a safe dose to be taken over a long period. Levine and Fulton succeeded in 8 cases out of 10; Parkinson and Nicholl, Lean, Ottol, Wolferth, Sprague and White and others have also been successful, though failures are reported with perhaps as great frequency. One need not fear embolism in this use of the drug. Singer and Winterberg have given it intravenously in 9 cases; the doses were 0.4, 0.5, 0.75 Gm., average 0.5 Gm. In 6 of the cases the attack was stopped in from a few seconds to ten minutes.

Digitalis.—Failure usually results from the use of this drug here. However, Levine and Blotner (1926) have presented 4 cases in which keeping the patient digitalized (beginning with full doses and finally employing maintenance doses of approximately 2 grains of leaves, 0.13 Gm., per day) has been effective in preventing recurrence in those prone to have many attacks during a year. This is a small number of cases, but it is suggestive that the failure of most workers to get satisfactory results may be due to their small dosage of the drug.

Acetyl Cholin.—Stepp and Schliephake (1925) reported full and almost instantaneous control of recurring tachycardia by intramuscular injection of 0.5 to 1 cc. of a 20 per cent cholin derivative solution; the heart rate fell from 240 to 84 in five minutes, but there was extreme substernal discomfort. Starr (1933) has caused immediate termination of 24 attacks in 9 patients by the subcutaneous injection of acetyl-β-methylcholin. In a few instances the drug plus carotid pressure was successful where carotid pressure alone had failed; failure, which was infrequent, was ascribed to inadequate dosage. Average effective dosage has seemed to be between 30 and 50 mg. The injection is followed by a sudden sensation of warmth in the face, hyperpnea, sweating and salivation; the patient should be prone when injected. Starr has found that atropine sulphate, $\frac{1}{50}$ grain (0.0012 Gm.), intravenously terminates the reaction almost at once. An asthmatic attack seems to be precipitated in susceptible individuals and momentary heart block has also been noted in a few instances. Both dyspnea and substernal pain followed one injection, but these symptoms were overcome by the use of atropine.

Other Drugs.—Wolffe and Bellett (1931) succeeded in 3 of 5 cases in which one or more commercial ampules of afenil (calcium gluconate) were administered intravenously; the patients complained for a few minutes of a burning in throat or rectum, intense heat and sometimes nausea—after publication, they observed a death in a few moments after the injection by the same route of 10 cc. of 10 per cent calcium chloride, but analysis shows the patient to have been undoubtedly a very poor risk for any radical therapy. Atropine, physostigmine, epinephrine, strophanthus, parathyroid extract, all have successes and failures to their account. Healy (1931) maintaining a highly acid urine with high-fat diet, supplemented with acids and in 1 case whisky, has lessened the incidence of attacks in 3 cases treated. Sampson and Anderson (1932) have used potassium acetate in 25 per cent solution effectively in about 50 per cent of 58 cases of paroxysmal tachycardia or premature systole. Two to 4 Gm. (30 to 60 grains) every six to eight hours was the most usual dosage but individual variations were between 1 and 6 Gm. (15 to 90 grains).

PREMATURE SYSTOLES

Premature systoles occur at some time in the life of most individuals and they are therefore the most common of the arrhythmias. The phlegmatic often do not notice them at all, but in the nervous individual the abnormality is quite annoying. The heart usually "thumps" or "turns over" and then there is a long pause before the next beat occurs; this compensatory pause, due to the occurrence of an extrasystole during the period of diastole, may be felt at the wrist and is usually equal in length to the time of two normal beats. These premature contractions, when they occur over a long period of time, may become a serious matter in that the patient often loses appetite and the ability to sleep, and may even suffer a considerable impairment in general health, because of nervous worry. If unassociated with any demonstrable cardiac pathology, as is usually the case, premature systole is quite without direct significance, but since this phenomenon sometimes heralds the beginning of serious heart maladies it is always incumbent upon the practitioner to make a thorough examination of his patient before pronouncing the matter of no moment.

THERAPY

These cases are oftentimes very difficult to treat for the reason that it is one thing to tell a patient that his heart is quite alright and another to get him to believe it in face of the heavings of which he is aware in his chest. Many individuals are quite capable of believing that what the physician tells them is true during the busy daylight hours, but when night comes and they lie bedfellows with their misbehaving hearts apprehension grips them hard. The wise physician will not overlook the advantage of reestablishing the habit of sleep by the use for a while—several weeks if necessary—of $7\frac{1}{2}$ to 10 grains (0.5 to 0.7 Gm.) of veronal upon retiring.

Quinine and Strychnine.—Wenckebach, the Austrian authority on arrhythmias, has written as follows (1923): "I have found strychnine in small doses helpful in cases of extrasystole in otherwise normal as well as in diseased hearts, but very often it did not act strongly enough, or it lost its action very soon. In these last cases I tried the combination of quinine and strychnine and found that this form of treatment had complete success in the great majority of my cases. I have given from 0.3 to 0.4 Gm. (5 to 6 grains) of quinine daily, plus 2 or 3 mg. ($\frac{1}{30}$ to $\frac{1}{20}$ grain) of strychnine through periods of ten days. My experience with this treatment since the years 1915 has been so favorable that I am convinced that whoever will try it will come to the same conclusion."

Quinidine.—Barrier's experience (1927) agrees with that of most observers. "I have been able to abolish this arrhythmia in more than 90 per cent. Premature contractions arising in either the auricle or the ventricle yield equally well to the treatment, which, as a rule, need not exceed three doses of 5 grains (0.32 Gm.) a day. After a short time, from 5 to 10 grains (0.32 to 0.65 Gm.) suffices. The disadvantage is that the pulse is usually higher, owing to the action of quinidine on the vagus. The advantages are that it tides the patient over a nervous period of cardiac consciousness, and impresses him with the fact that something can be done for him. He usually stops treatment because it is more troublesome than the disability, but he feels that this is his weakness rather than the physician's."

Potassium Acetate.—(See p. 522.)

Rest and Exercise.—In Otto and Gold's (1926) careful study of hospitalized cases, rest in bed and atropine had no effect on the number of premature contractions. Exercise and epinephrine increased the number; quinine, quinidine and digitalis decreased the number.

HEART BLOCK

(Stokes-Adams Disease)

Varying, but usually lesser grades, of heart block occur not infrequently during the course of the acute infectious diseases, especially those of the respiratory tract, and also as a result of vagus pressure or of massive digitalis therapy. But chronic heart block known as Stokes-Adams disease is a definite symptomatic entity, the block being due to arteriosclerotic, syphilitic, tuberculous, rheumatic, or adipose changes in the conduction tract; it should be noted, however, that at autopsy some cases have been found to exhibit no lesions of the bundle. The victims of this disease usually have a pulse rate of between 25 and 40 and suffer fainting spells which often occur at such frequent intervals that the patient is in almost constant anguish. The disease usually makes its appearance in individuals past middle age, and in its milder grades is not incompatible with a normal duration of life, especially in those who are fortunate enough to live in partial retirement, but from one of the syncopal attacks the patient finally does not recover.

This disease was first described by Robert Adams, in 1826, and shortly thereafter by William Stokes—both leading members of the great Dublin school of the first half of the nineteenth century.

THERAPY

It is a great pity that medical science and art has as yet evolved no entirely satisfactory agent for the relief of these sufferers. The drugs to be described below are only occasionally effective.

Atropine.—Atropine paralyzes the vagus endings and should therefore release the heart from vagal inhibition, but as a matter of fact we do not as yet definitely know to what extent the ventricles are under this control. It is known, however, that vagus tone as a whole in man is greatest under thirty years and markedly decreases after fifty—which fact in itself would be quite sufficient to explain the usual failure to quicken the heart in Stokes-Adams disease, most of whose victims are elderly. The drug is used in large doses, $\frac{1}{20}$ to $\frac{1}{12}$ grain (0.003 to 0.005 Gm.), subcutaneously.

Epinephrine.—Epinephrine is used because of its well-known ability to stimulate the sympathetic innervation of the heart and thus to cause an increase in rate.

Feil summarizes experience with the drug as follows: "There is clinical evidence that the subcutaneous injection of epinephrine in cases of partial heart block may overcome the delay in conduction, restoring it to normal; in 2:1 block, the mechanism may be restored to normal or dissociation may follow. In complete block, normal sequence may result or no change occur. In the latter event acceleration of the auricles and the ventricles usually results. In cases of frequently recurring attacks of Stokes-Adams' syndrome, the syncopal attacks may be abolished. From the clinical report of the English observers and from my report, the effect of the subcutaneous injection may be said to last about twelve hours. The dose administered to adults of average weight is from 0.3 to 0.6 cc. of a 1:1000 solution, injected subcutaneously. The danger in administration of epinephrine to patients with a considerable degree of arteriosclerosis or with hypertension (and in many cases of complete heart block there is an elevated systolic maximum pressure) must be weighed against the dangers and the discomfort of the syncopal attacks. Doubtless, epinephrine therapy is justified in the treatment of patients with frequently recurring syncopal attacks, in view of the usual urgency of the patient's condition and because of the satisfactory results obtained in the reported cases. In no event should epinephrine be administered intravenously. The use of epinephrine subcutaneously offers relief from Stokes-Adams' attacks and doubtless stimulates the new center of impulse formation in complete heart block, by way of the sympathetic endings. There appears to be little or no danger in the use of epinephrine in this type of case when it is properly administered. Intravenous injection results in greater concentration of epinephrine in the blood stream, and it is this factor that is probably responsible for the grave reactions reported in the literature." Schwartz and Jezer (1932) consider that the use of the drug may be a life-saving measure in patients whose syncopal seizures are due to a slowing of the ventricular rate, but that it is contraindicated when the attacks are the result of ventricular fibrillation, and that its use in such patients may result in death.

Ephedrine.—Miller (1925) recorded an increase in ventricular rate from 38 to 55 per minute following subcutaneous injection of 1½ grains (100 mg.) of ephedrine. Hollingsworth (1927) relieved rapidly occurring seizures in thirty minutes with 50 mg., orally. Continued use of the drug prevented the attacks, while its omission was followed by a recurrence forty hours later. Stecher (1928) recorded similar success. Parade and Voit (1929–31) described a case in which oral use of the drug gave almost continuous relief for over two years; when discontinued, the attacks returned and the patient died in a seizure before aid could be given. In a single very severe case, Wood (1932) has prevented attacks for eighteen months by the daily or twice daily oral use of 24 mg.; at one time when the patient was unable to procure the drug for four days, minor attacks began within thirty-six hours and continued until relieved by ephedrine.

Barium Chloride.—Cohn and Levine (1925) have described their use of this drug as follows: "The periods of standstill are presumably due to the fact that the ventricles, for the moment, contain no mechanism for initiating stimuli. On account of the existence of complete heart block, they can, of course, receive none from the auricles. It occurred to us, therefore, in complete heart block, to make use of the knowledge gained in animal experiments that calcium or barium tended to increase the irritability of the ventricles as indicated by the development of numerous ectopic ventricular beats or ventricular tachycardia. The same effect has been obtained in the experimental animal as a result of barium chloride, even when complete heart block is produced by clamping the bundle of His. If this were so, the ventricles, because of the increased irritability, either through some new ectopic focus or by the action of barium on the idioventricular pacemaker, would not permit a long pause of inactivity to occur. In 3 patients suffering from Adams-Stokes disease, whose histories are here reported, the attempt was made to observe whether an effect comparable to the one observed in experiments might be obtained. Accordingly, we decided to administer barium chloride, in doses of 30 mg. (½ grain), three or four times a day by mouth. . . . The effect of its action was striking in all three cases. The attacks, which had persisted until barium chloride was given [atropine, digitalis and epinephrine having failed—H. B.], ceased entirely on the day on which it was started. The effect in Case 1 was extraordinary. Previous to the administration of barium chloride, the patient's condition had constantly become worse until, on the day on which it was started, he resembled patients in the status epilepticus. He was passing in and out of attacks of syncope constantly, being conscious only about one half the time. The day following the giving of barium chloride, there were no more attacks or long pauses, although complete heart block persisted. Although barium chloride was given by mouth in doses of 30 mg. (½ grain) three times a day for only two days, he remained free from attacks for some weeks. There was a similar direct relationship between the cessation of attacks and the administration of barium chloride in the other two cases. All 3 patients left the hospital free from attacks."

Herrmann and Ashman (1926) report a case in which ⅓ grain (0.02 Gm.) of barium chloride every four hours failed to be effective, but when larger doses were used excellent results followed. They gave ⅔ grain (0.04 Gm.) every four hours, then later ⅚ grain (0.05 Gm.) every four hours for a week, then the latter dose three times a day for eight weeks, and finally once a day. The pulse rate rose steadily to 46, 54, 64, and 72, and at the time of report the patient had been back at work as a salesman for ten weeks without further attacks. So far as I am aware no subsequent report on this most interesting case has been made.

Heard, Marshall and Adams have reported a case (1927) in which barium chloride was no more effective in relieving the attacks than were atropine and epinephrine, and it must be admitted that the reports upon the use of some of the other drugs discussed above often contain a statement to the effect "after barium chloride had produced no satisfactory results." Parsonnet and Hyman (1930) record failures in eight consecutive cases.

Thyroid.—Upon the whole, the use of thyroid substance, or thyroxin, which causes tachycardia in the normal individual, has been very disappointing in this malady. Blackford and Willius (1917) did, however, record good results in 4 cases.

CHRONIC NONVALVULAR HEART DISEASE

A very large proportion of the patients in whom symptoms of cardiac derangement have developed after the age of forty may be classified as having chronic nonvalvular heart disease. They have neither endocardial, pericardial or valvular lesions and their disability seems to depend entirely on inefficiency of the muscle. The cases may be placed more or less satisfactorily in Christian's three groups. (a) Patients who at any age complain of great exhaustion or of palpitation following slight exertion. They do not have true dyspnea, but experience uncomfortable sensations in connection with respiration, are often sensitive to pressure in the region of the apex, and their heart rate is easily accelerated. Examination reveals a normal heart, but with perhaps a few extrasystoles and a rather tapping pulse; there are no evidences of past or present edema or passive congestion. Usually an adequate cause for the condition can be found in antecedent infections, in debilitating diseases with a too short convalescent period, or in occupational overfatigue together with worry and loss of sleep. (b) Patients, usually past forty, in whom the chief departure from normal is in the size of the heart, hypertrophy often being very marked. Just what causes this hypertrophy, and why the hypertrophy should result in dysfunction, has never been satisfactorily explained. There may or may not be a soft to loud systolic murmur best heard at the apex, but it is important to bear in mind that the mitral insufficiency is the result, and not the cause, of the myocardial insufficiency. This cardiac enlargement would seem to mark the beginning of a train of events which practically always ends in cardiac decompensation. (c) Relatively uncommon are the patients with true chronic myocarditis. At autopsy there may be found small foci of perivascular infiltration with lymphocytes and plasma cells, or, far less frequently, a focal or a widespread fibrosis with definite evidence of injury to the muscle fibers. These chronic myocarditis cases are indistinguishable clinically from those, above described, who have hypertrophy and no other change.

THERAPY

Myocardial Fatigue.—The practitioner who will assure patients with simple myocardial "fatigue," those described in group (*a*), that they have no heart disease and are sure to get well renders a real service to mankind, for these patients form a large class of chronic invalids who burden their friends with their "weak" hearts; and all because an incorrect diagnosis was made in the beginning. Rest and reassurance, with a gradual return to full physical activity, is all that is needed in these cases; indeed, their easy curability is the chief mark by which they may be distinguished from effort syndrome (see p. 512). Regarding the use of digitalis in these patients, Christian writes:

"The type of heart in which digitalis invariably does not cause any striking change in function is the heart that is normal in size, sounds and function. This to my mind is the striking example of when digitalis should not be used, not that it is harmful but because it is not beneficial. Patients that I have grouped as having myocardial fatigue are in this class, and yet one often sees them in their own opinion entirely dependent on a daily or twice daily dose of 5 drops of tincture of digitalis, which, by the way, would be about 2 to 4 minims (0.12 to 0.24 cc.) daily or possibly as little as 1¼ minims (0.075 cc.). Others of these patients may take small doses of digitalis at intervals when their heart is 'bad,' getting an immediate relief, all of which goes to show that for such patients digitalis in such doses is not a cardiac medicine but one that works directly on the mind."

Hypertrophy and Chronic Myocarditis.—These cases, those described in (*b*) and (*c*) above, often present very considerable diagnostic difficulties by reason of the fact that a regular rhythm is frequently maintained, but there can be no doubt about the proper treatment; decompensation here, as in other types of heart failure, indicates digitalis. Therefore, for the details of therapy the discussion of heart failure (p. 529) must be referred to. Regarding the rationale of the employment of digitalis here, witness Christian (1928):

"Therapy in the group of patients just described is, as a rule, very satisfactory. Since many of these patients who respond so well to digitalis therapy do not have auricular fibrillation, it has always been a mystery to me why it is so generally thought and taught that digitalis is strikingly effective only in the presence of auricular fibrillation. I have evolved the following explanation of this belief and teaching. Digitalis is so generally thought to be measured in its effect by slowing the pulse that when the pulse is not strikingly slowed it is considered that digitalis is not effective, and its other effects are not recognized. These patients at rest often have only a slightly accelerated pulse rate, and it is true that digitalis changes it very little. However, for digitalis to stop dyspnea and cough or to cause a loss of edema and a great diuresis is certainly just as great a therapeutic triumph as to have it slow the cardiac rate. Another explanation may be that, since this type of case is not recognized as being primarily cardiac, the patient does not receive digitalis and consequently the physician has no opportunity to see the striking effect that would have been in evidence had the patient been given digitalis. Or possibly the physician does not weigh his patients, and so fails to appreciate the great loss in weight from the removal of edema that has occurred as a result of digitalis. If by giving a patient digitalis I can cause in ten days a loss of weight of from 60 to 70 pounds (27 to 32 Kg.) from the disappearance of edema, and such often occurs, or can stop the dyspnea and cough, to me these things are as striking effects as slowing the pulse from 140 and higher to 75 or 80. In these patients with myocardial disease, in my experience, the therapeutic results with digitalis are no better when auricular fibrillation is present than when the rhythm is regular. I feel that the time has come when the teaching that digitalis therapy is effective only in the presence of auricular fibrillation should be given up by every one. Its continuance does positive harm, for the physician often says, 'The pulse is regular, digitalis will not be effective, so I will not give it.' Of course, the man who reasons thus will never see a strikingly satisfactory result from digitalis in a patient with regular rhythm, simply because to that type of patient he never gives digitalis.

"Another popular idea about patients with myocarditis is that they should not receive digitalis, since digitalis increases the work of the cardiac muscle and the diseased muscle will be injured by digitalis. After having given digitalis, sometimes in large doses or over long periods of time, to patients with myocarditis, I am convinced that there is no basis whatever for this idea. The heart may be too diseased to respond satisfactorily to digitalis, and all cardiac patients sooner or later reach this stage, but that digitalis in therapeutic doses is dangerous to them I feel sure is not the case."

In cases of cardiac enlargement, even though there be no signs or symptoms of decompensation, Christian (1933) also uses digitalis continuously in amounts just short of toxicity and feels certain that there is no reason to fear deleterious effects from such therapy.

HEART FAILURE

By heart failure is meant the state of broken compensation in which the heart is no longer able to perform the amount of work necessary if the body as a whole is to maintain a condition of normal activity. When first seen, the patient is in bed, usually propped up on several pillows, has a depressed though anxious expression, is breathing with difficulty, may or may not be cyanotic (in mitral disease the cheeks are often flushed, whereas pallor is characteristic of aortic lesions), and has a rapid and usually arrhythmic heart. Edema of the lower extremities is usually present and perhaps even anasarca with fluid in the serous cavities. The urine is usually scant and contains albumin and casts; often also there is congestive cough and sometimes, especially in aortic disease, complaint of cardiac pain. This state of affairs may result from a recently acquired or a long-standing valvular lesion, or it may be a part of the picture in chronic nonvalvular heart disease previously described (see p. 526). Obviously, a description of the differences in the physical findings in the various types of heart failure has no place in this book, nor is it in order to describe the various premonitory symptoms by which the onset of complete decompensation of this sort may be recognized. The important thing, from the therapeutic standpoint, is that it is the state of the myocardium that gives cause for concern, heart failure being solely and simply muscle failure. Therefore, the treatment of the extreme degree of this failure, to be described below, will be in modified form the treatment of the lesser degrees as well.

THERAPY

1. **Rest, Diet, Sedatives and Analgesics.**—Rest in bed is usually self-imposed in cases of severe failure, though it is astonishing how long individuals of indomitable will are sometimes able to keep on their feet; it is of

course imperative if cure is to take place that the patient *does* go to bed, even though he is able to repose there only in a sitting posture, for the heart muscle, like all other muscle, requires physiologic rest if it is to recuperate. In the normal heart the length of diastole (the resting period) is approximately one third longer than systole and the total amount of time during which the heart is at comparative rest depends directly upon the amount of muscular exercise being performed by the body, since exercise regulates heart rate; therefore, if we are to obtain the maximum of rest for the heart (remembering that heart failure is merely myocardial exhaustion) we must enforce the maximum of rest for the body. This is by no means the same thing as saying that every case of decompensation will show direct profit by being sent to bed, for the factors of arrhythmia, edema and congestion, etc., are grave perpetuators of the broken down state, but it does mean that, other things being equal, the patient who takes to his bed early and rests while he is in it, has the best chance of recovery, be his decompensation slight or great. To the end of providing complete rest it is often advisable to employ sedatives. Fifteen grains (1 Gm.) of sodium bromide three times a day will lessen apprehension in the beginning and make for greater quiet, or, if the patient is sleepless, 10 grains (0.65 Gm.) of the bromide may be combined with an equal quantity of chloral hydrate for a sleeping potion. Chloral hydrate is known to be a circulatory depressant but it is so only in *large* doses, much larger than the one indicated here. Paraldehyde is preferred by some physicians because it is not at all depressant to the heart; it is, however, very nasty and difficult to take, the dose being from 1 to 4 drachms (4 to 16 cc.), administered either on crushed ice or in one of the higher alcoholic vehicles (see p. 785). Veronal, in a dose of $7\frac{1}{2}$ to 10 grains (0.5 to 0.65 Gm.), is also useful, but it must be borne in mind that this drug is relatively slow in action.

For the treatment of cardiac pain, it is sometimes advisable to give $\frac{1}{8}$ to $\frac{1}{4}$ grain of morphine, or the nitrites may be employed as in the treatment of angina pectoris (see p. 542).

With the details of diet this book is not primarily concerned; it must therefore suffice to say that the patient should receive small but frequent feedings of such substances as vegetable purées, lightly cooked red meats, chicken, fish, well-baked breads and well-cooked potatoes and green vegetables, rice, tapioca, custards and ice-cream. That is to say: Feed the patient a light and well-cooked diet, and feed him small amounts and often. In the presence of marked edema, the matters discussed in the chapter on Nephritis, particularly with regard to the salt and fluid intake, apply here also. Some physicians prefer the radical Karell diet for a few days to a week, then gradually adding other foodstuffs as the symptoms abate under treatment. This diet consists in 800 cc. of milk distributed during the twenty-four hours, and certainly combines a restriction in fluids with a small amount of food; the fact should not be overlooked, however, that the amount of food supplied by this diet is very inadequate and that the patient thus fed is considerably undernourished while on the diet; it seems to me to be completely out-moded in cardiac as well as in nephritic edema.

2. **Digitalis.**—Elsewhere (p. 516) I have said: "In the entire range of medicine there is nothing more spectacular than the response of a decompensated heart with auricular fibrillation to digitalis properly administered. The pulse rate is decreased, while at the same time the strength of individual ventricular contractions increases, diuresis is established and edema disappears, dyspnea, cyanosis, etc., diminish—in short, compensation is reestablished and the patient's life is saved." Just as satisfactory results are obtained in nonfibrillating decompensation also, a fact which has been attested by many competent observers (see Luten and Marvin in the Bibliography,

34

and Christian's testimony as quoted on p. 527). Of course, in these non-fibrillating cases the reduction in rate is oftentimes not spectacular because the increase in rate may not have been as great as in the fibrillating cases—but all the other manifestations of powerful action, such as reduction of edema, dyspnea, etc., are shown. Especially is this true, according to Marvin, if the decompensation occurs during the course of what has been described in this book as "chronic nonvalvular heart disease." Only in the occasional syphilitic case is the drug effective, and in rheumatic decompensation without fibrillation it would seem to be almost valueless; but these latter cases are relatively rare in occurrence.

(a) *Choice of Preparations.*—The disadvantages of all of the drugs of the digitalis group have served as a constant stimulus in the search for pure principles suitable for subcutaneous and intravenous administration, but, despite these investigations, the chemistry of digitalis and the other members of the group is still very imperfectly understood. Of the isolated principles, digitoxin and digitalin together probably represent very nearly the crude drug digitalis. The digitalin on the market, however, is not the true digitalin, but the different brands consist of mixtures of two or more principles. Several digitalis preparations have been introduced into therapeutic use with the claim that they are composed either of pure principles or of purified extracts of digitalis, and that they are devoid of certain disadvantages possessed by the U.S.P. preparations. I have been repeating almost verbatim the opinion of the American Medical Association Council on Pharmacy and Chemistry, the arbiter in these matters, which further says (N.N.R., 1933, p. 154): "It may be said at once that there is no proof that any of these proprietary preparations can be used to greater advantage than digitalis and its galenicals in the majority of cases of cardiac disease." This being the case—and the truth of the statement is attested by the experience of great numbers of competent observers—I shall not concern myself with these preparations in this book, save for the few whose intravenous or rectal use is described elsewhere. That is to say, for the routine treatment of heart failure with digitalis by mouth, only the U.S.P. preparations will be considered, and the following N.N.R. preparations will not be discussed: Digalen-Roche (Cloetta); Digifoline-Ciba, Digitalin, Crude; Digitalin, True; Digitalin, "French"; Digitalin, "German"; Digitos; Digitoxin; Digipoten; Digitan (Digipuratum). Digitol is a fat-free biologically standardized tincture of digitalis, and is now sold merely as such, though it was formerly held that its freedom from fat lessened gastric irritation, a claim which is no longer tenable since Hatcher and Weiss have convincingly shown that the vomiting caused by digitalis is a reflex from the heart and is not due to irritation of the gastro-intestinal tract. The fact that this fat-free tincture does not become turbid when mixed with water, as does the U.S.P. tincture, in nowise increases its therapeutic worth.

Coming now to the U.S.P. preparations there are the leaves, the tincture, and the infusion (the fluidextract having been omitted from the tenth revision). And, since the work of Weiss and Hatcher and the careful observations of very many practitioners have shown that the official infusion does not represent the drug completely, it, too, will be omitted from discussion in this book. Therefore, the description of digitalis therapy, to follow, will be a description of the use of the official leaves and tincture only, except when rectal and intravenous uses are discussed.

(b) *Rapid Digitalization by Mouth.*—EGGLESTON METHOD.—In 1915, Eggleston revolutionized digitalis administration by the demonstration that, using biologically standardized leaves or tincture, the body weight of the patient may be utilized for the estimation of the approximate total amount of the drug which will be required to obtain its therapeutic effects.

Of good standardized preparations this approximate amount will be 15 minims (1 cc.) of the tincture, or 1½ grains (0.1 Gm.) of the leaf, for each 10 pounds of body weight. Thus, in a patient weighing 156 pounds, the approximate dose at which full effect may be expected would be 234 minims (15.6 cc.) of the tincture and 23½ grains (1.56 Gm.) of the dried leaf— figures which are arrived at by the simple procedure of inserting, in the figure representing the patient's weight in pounds, one decimal from the right for the tincture and two decimals from the right for the leaf.

Eggleston has described the use of his method for rapid digitalization as follows:

"1. When the patient has received no digitalis within the preceding ten days.

"(a) *In Urgent Cases.*—From one third to one half of the total calculated amount is administered at the first dose. After an interval of six hours, from one fifth to one fourth of the total is administered. After a second six hours, from one eighth to one sixth is administered. Thereafter, if more digitalis is needed, about one tenth of the total may be repeated every six hours until maximal digitalization is secured.

"(b) *Rapid, for Nonurgent Cases.*—About one fourth of the calculated total is to be given at each of the first two doses, six hours apart. Thereafter about one tenth to one eighth of the total is given every six hours.

"2. When the patient has been taking digitalis within the preceding ten days.

"Before further digitalis is prescribed, the patient is to be subjected to the most careful examination, including the use of polygraphic or electrocardiographic records if available, to determine whether or not there are any evidences of digitalis action.

"(a) *When Evidences of Digitalis Action are Absent.*—The procedure is the same as outlined above, except that the total amount of digitalis required is to be reduced to 75 per cent of the total calculated.

"(b) *When Evidences of Partial Digitalization are Present.*—It is best not to attempt to administer more than one half of the total calculated amount of digitalis, divided equally between the first three doses. In urgent cases in this group, however, one may administer 75 per cent of the calculated amount, preferably in three equal doses, and then if digitalization is not quite complete, one tenth of the total amount may be prescribed every six hours."

Regarding the effectiveness of this method of digitalization, and the safeguards to be employed in its utilization, Eggleston writes as follows:

"The observance of a six-hour interval between doses allows time for complete absorption of the preceding dose and the development of its full action on the heart, so that if the patient is examined just before the administration of each dose, dangerous intoxication can be absolutely prevented. In practice it is perfectly safe to give the first three doses without personally examining the patient before the second and third doses if the one nursing the patient is properly instructed to look for nausea, vomiting, or slowing of the pulse to 60 or less a minute before giving the succeeding dose, and to stop administration if any of these phenomena appear. . . .

"By its employment [*i. e.*, the Eggleston method] it is usually possible to produce maximal digitalis action in from twelve to eighteen hours, and marked therapeutic effects frequently appear within six hours after the initial dose. By its use it is possible to dispense with the intravenous or intramuscular administration of ouabain, amorphous strophanthin, or other digitalis body in the great majority of cases of heart failure."

OTHER METHODS.—While yielding full credit to Eggleston for leading the profession into bolder digitalis therapy, many physicians have come to doubt the value of utilizing the body weight for the determination of the dose. Levy and Mackie (1927) write: "It affords a false sense of security on the basis of a formula which yields only an approximate figure. The range of variation, both above and below, may be considerable in individual patients, because of differences in absorption and susceptibility. This range is sufficiently wide to include the limits of therapeutic dosage as determined by clinical experience. Successful digitalis therapy requires careful study of idiosyncrasy and individual requirements." The following pertinent questions, which are not easy to answer, are often asked by the general practitioner: How many patients, as seen in the home, have an accurate knowledge of their normal weight before the onset of edema? How are we to weigh them in the home? And if we succeed in doing so, how much allowance must be made for retained fluid which is not to be included in the individual's weight?

The alternative to employing the weight method of determining dosage is to accept a certain total dose as that which clinical experience has shown to be effective in accomplishing digitalization in the majority of cases, and then employing portions of that dose according to some arbitrary scheme. Examples follow.

1. In the report of Robinson, White, Eggleston and Hatcher, made to the Council on Pharmacy and Chemistry of the American Medical Association, in 1924, the following dosage is advocated: "The total average dose of fairly active standardized digitalis by the mouth for inducing full therapeutic effects within from thirty-six to forty-eight hours in an adult who has not received digitalis within ten days is about 22 grains (1.5 Gm.) of the leaf or 225 minims (15 cc.) of the tincture. The total dose may be divided into several equal parts given every four or six hours, or one half or one third of the total calculated dose may be given at once, and the remainder in two portions after intervals of four or six hours. If there is doubt about recent medication, smaller doses of from 1½ to 4½ grains (0.1 to 0.3 Gm.) of the leaf, or from 15 to 45 minims (1 to 3 cc.) of the tincture, should be given three or four times a day, with observation for toxic symptoms or signs on each occasion before the next dose is administered."

2. The following dosage scheme, which is very satisfactorily employed in practice by many physicians, is here given in the form in which I have been presenting it to my students for several years (a slight modification of Clendenning's method):

Rapid digitalization (one to two days for full effect).
First day—
Leaf: 6 grains (0.4 Gm.) every six hours for four doses
     or
Tincture: 1 drachm (4 cc.) every six hours for four doses.
Second day—
Leaf: One half the dosage every four hours for four doses
     or
Tincture: One half the dosage every four hours for four doses.
Thereafter: Such dosage as is shown to be necessary after a period of observation in which the drug is withheld entirely.

(c) *Slower Digitalization by Mouth for Ambulatory Patients.*—In mildly decompensated bed-ridden patients who are not seen by the physician at frequent intervals, it is neither necessary nor wise to employ the large dosage just described above. Also, in ambulatory patients, who are seen only at relatively long intervals, it is very dangerous to use large doses. In the report of Robinson *et al.*, cited above, the following dosage is suggested for such cases.

"Ambulatory adult patients who are seen only at intervals of a week or more may be given 1½ grains (0.1 Gm.) of the leaf or 15 minims (1 cc.) of the tincture three times a day by the mouth for a week or two, with the warning to reduce this to one dose daily if toxic symptoms appear."

Pellini, writing of his experience with 250 ambulatory cases at Bellevue Hospital (New York), states: "We set our upper limit of digitalis at 45 minims per day for the ambulatory patient with cardiac disease, and if no beginning improvement followed the dosage after one week's trial we felt that he was a hospital case. We realize that this is conservative, but we feel that we must be conservative as our patients are not under constant observation and are not able to see us except at clinic nights. We have never attempted any of the rapid digitalization methods at the clinic as we feel that patients requiring such medication should be in the hospital. . . . One not infrequently meets a physician who believes that the giving of digitalis in more than very small doses to the ambulatory cardiac patient is attended with the danger of sudden death. We doubt whether any well-informed physician would agree with this. Of our patients who died while under digitalis medication, we know the cause of death in each instance and in none of them could the death be attributed to digitalis. In fact, our hospital experience shows that many patients are forced to enter the hospital in a dangerous condition because of insufficient digitalis medication."

The careful studies of Gold and DeGraff (1930) have shown that daily doses of leaf ranging from 2 to 6 grains (0.12 to 0.4 Gm.), and occasionally as high as 9 grains (0.6 Gm.) suffice to maintain compensation in ambulatory patients.

For several years I have been teaching the following dosage:

Slow digitalization (four to seven days for full effect).

Leaf: 2 grains (0.13 Gm.) every four hours for four doses each day

or

Tincture: 20 minims (1.3 cc.) every four hours for four doses each day.

Administration to stop after full effect is obtained, maintenance dose to be determined thereafter.

(*d*) *Maintenance Dosage.*—Pardee's investigations have shown that digitalis disappears from the body at the rate of 22 minims (1.5 cc.) of the tincture, or 2½ grains (0.15 Gm.) of the leaves, per twenty-four hours, findings which have been confirmed by the electrocardiographic studies of Bromer and Blumgart (1929). Theoretically, then, the daily administration of this amount, either as tincture or leaf, would suffice to maintain a state of saturation once such a state had been established by one of the systems of administration previously described. As a matter of practical experience, however, this is not always found to be true, for in some patients these amounts will be larger than necessary and in others much too small; in Pardee's own investigations, individuals were found who varied from one half to four times this average rate of elimination. And the decreasing need of the heart for the drug as general circulatory improvement takes place must also be taken into account. On this head, Gold and DeGraff write: "For instance, after digitalization, patients may often go for months without the drug and without symptoms of failure. This obviously signifies that the effect of digitalis on the heart is partly direct and partly indirect as the result of the general improvement in the circulation which, though initiated by the drug, tends to sustain itself after the drug has been eliminated or destroyed. Nevertheless, it is often assumed that in order to retain the effects produced by the initial doses of digitalis, it is necessary to keep up the 'saturation' by giving daily doses equal to the amount of the drug eliminated a day. This view does not take into consideration the tendency for the circulation to remain improved without the drug. We believe that the theory has been simplified at the expense of the facts. From our studies we feel fairly certain that the degree of 'saturation' with digit-alis necessary to produce the best results in the initial digitalization is fre-quently in excess of that necessary to maintain the effects so induced over long periods of time."

A safe procedure is to use 22 minims (1.5 cc.) of the tincture, or 2⅕ grains (0.15 Gm.) of the leaves, as the daily *test* dose for maintenance, vary-ing the amount as is shown to be advisable by a careful study of each indi-vidual case.

(e) *Rectal Administration.*—Levy's studies (1924) have shown this method of administration to be quite feasible. He employed it in 31 cases, a desirable therapeutic effect being obtained in each instance. Initial effect was seen in two and one-half to nine and one-half hours, usually in two and one-half hours. The technic is described as follows:

"The preparation employed was an aqueous solution of purified extract of digitalis leaves called 'digitan.' One cubic centimeter of the liquid con-tained the equivalent of 1½ grains (0.1 Gm.) of powdered leaf. . . . Early in the course of the work a tincture of digitalis was used. The alcohol was occasionally found to be irritating to the rectal mucosa unless the dose to be given was diluted to such volume that the enema, because of its bulk, was often expelled. No such difficulties were encountered with the use of the aqueous preparation. The digitalis tincture, properly diluted, may be em-ployed for rectal use.

"With one exception, the entire dose of digitalis was given at one time. The patient received a preliminary cleansing enema. After evacuation, from 8 to 20 cc. of digitan was given by rectal tube and washed through with 25 cc. of tap-water. A rectal tube of small caliber was inserted to a depth of about 6 inches (15 cm.) from the anal orifice. The funnel into which the digitalis was poured was held about 15 inches (37.5 cm.) above the level of the anus. After the tap-water had been allowed to flow in, the tube was clamped, left *in situ* for fifteen minutes and then slowly withdrawn. The patients were carefully instructed to resist any desire for a bowel movement for at least six hours."

The method is of value in those cases of decompensation in which con-gestive nausea and vomiting (not to be confused with the same symptoms caused by the drug itself) are present before digitalis therapy is begun. When the rectally administered digitalis has begun to exert its effect the vomiting usually ceases, after which the usual type of administration by mouth should be started.

(f) *Intravenous Digitalis and Strophanthin* (Ouabain).—The need for intravenous methods of digitalization rarely arises now that large doses are being used by mouth, for, though the full effect is usually not apparent under twenty-four to forty-eight hours, the beginning effect of these full doses may be seen in two to four or five hours, as shown in the independent studies of Robinson and Pardee; thus a life-saving degree of digitalization may be accomplished quite rapidly enough by oral administration in the vast majority of cases. Even those patients who are vomiting because of congestion need not be treated intravenously nowadays since Levy has demonstrated the simplicity and practicability of rectal administration (see above). However, a patient is occasionally seen in whom it is apparent that digitalization must be accomplished in minutes rather than hours or days if life is to be saved; for such, the following intravenous methods are available. Intramuscular or hypodermic methods are not described in this book because of their utter unreliability.

1. INTRAVENOUS DIGITALIS.—I quote at some length from the thorough

studies of Pardee (1928), who used three preparations—digalen, digifoline solution, and digitan hypodermic solution.

Rate of Action.—"There is usually a definite slowing by five minutes after administration, a marked slowing by fifteen minutes and a still greater decrease by thirty minutes. From then until two or three hours after the administration, the rate becomes slightly slower and remains about at this level for the next twelve or twenty-four hours, perhaps increasing slightly toward the end of the period. Different patients show some variation from this average curve, but on the whole it seems that this is a fair representation of the rate of onset of the effect of the intravenous dose, and it is probable that this rate of onset is similar in all patients whether or not they have auricular fibrillation."

Dosage.—"The dosage should be regulated by the patient's normal weight and by the amount of digitalis which he has taken during the previous two weeks. For a patient who has not had digitalis within this time, the dose of these intravenous digitalis preparations (*i. e.*, any one of the three) should be 1 minim per pound of the patient's weight, if a prompt and definite effect is desired. This is one half of the estimated full therapeutic dose and is as much as should be given for fear of producing marked signs of poisoning in occasional very susceptible persons.

"Should the first dose not produce clinical improvement in two hours, I would give another dose one fourth the size of the first (¼ minim per pound of body weight), and would repeat this at two-hourly intervals if no clinical improvement or no signs of toxic digitalis action were observed. Only four of these subsequent doses should be given, however, for it is not safe to exceed the average full therapeutic dose when dealing with very sick patients. In such patients, severe toxic effects may set in before clinical improvement and the toxic effects may not be recognized in the moribund patient. . . .

"Should the first dose produce clinical improvement and the patient still be urgently ill after four hours, a dose one fourth the size of the first may be given and if clinical improvement progresses, six hours or more may be allowed to elapse before the third dose. With continued improvement oral administration may now be used and the dosage regulated according to the apparent need for digitalization. . . .

"When a patient who has recently been receiving digitalis is found to be in a condition demanding intravenous therapy, the problem of dosage is extremely difficult. There is no way of telling how much of the full therapeutic dose of digitalis is active within the patient. We must proceed slowly in order to keep short of a strongly toxic dose. It is plain from the charts [which I have omitted—H. B.] that the strong initial effect of these digitalis preparations will have appeared by thirty minutes after administration, so it seems proper to give the small dose recommended, ¼ minim per pound body weight, and to repeat this at thirty- to forty-five-minute intervals until a therapeutic or toxic effect is produced or until four doses have been given. This will represent the initial dose of 1 minim per pound and the patient will have received it in from one and one-half to two and one-half hours. One should proceed after this as has been described, repeating the dose according to indications at from two- to four- or six-hour intervals, or changing to oral administration if clinical improvement has set in. . . .

"Some will, of course, hesitate to use doses of the size recommended intravenously. [The American Medical Association Council on Pharmacy and Chemistry is of opinion (N.N.R., 1933) that the first dose should be ⅛ minim per pound body weight and that this may be repeated at two-hour intervals until improvement occurs, poisoning becomes apparent or a total of 1 minim per pound has been reached, which under no circumstances should be exceeded in seriously ill patients.—H. B.] However, it should be remembered that some years ago there was just as much hesitation about using doses of this size by mouth. There has been enough experience with this intravenous dose of 1 minim per pound to make it plain that in previously untreated patients it is quite safe, and I do not hesitate to recommend it for producing a prompt effect in any emergency in which digitalis is indicated. If it seems preferable to approach this seemingly radical dosage by a gradual process, a dose of $\frac{1}{4}$ minim per pound may be used, to be repeated at forty-five-minute intervals for four doses and then, if digitalis is still needed, every two or three hours, the physician observing the patient for toxic effects before each dose but never giving more than a total of eight of these doses."

Precautions.—"The only precaution observed was for one to inject the solution slowly, taking thirty or forty-five seconds to complete the injection so that it will mix well with the blood and not arrive at the heart in great concentration. If a hypodermic needle is used for the intravenous injection, it is not possible to inject too rapidly. . . . Great caution is necessary in giving full doses of digitalis to patients who are critically ill. It should never be given as here recommended unless the physician is present before each dose to determine that there are no toxic effects from the previous doses."

2. INTRAVENOUS STROPHANTHIN OR OUABAIN.—Amorphous strophanthin is the official preparation, but crystallized ouabain, a glucoside obtained from *Strophanthus gratus,* is the drug most often used because of its greater activity. Ouabain deteriorates rapidly in ordinary glass containers but may be kept in hard glass ampules or in buffered solution for several months without appreciable change. The commercially available ampules contain a dose in buffered sterile physiologic saline solution and bear an expiration date. Wyckoff and Goldring made a study of intravenous ouabain therapy, in 1927, at the Bellevue Hospital in New York. Of their two hundred and forty-eight injections, one hundred and sixty-three were followed by definite cardiac effect. The initial effect was noted in from five to twenty minutes, which is no earlier than was obtained by Pardee (see p. 535) with intravenous digitalis preparations, but it seems that the maximum effect was obtained in about one hour, as contrasted with two hours in the case of the digitalis preparations. In patients who had been given no digitalis during the preceding two weeks, an initial dose of $\frac{1}{120}$ grain (0.0005 Gm.) was given, this dose being followed by smaller doses, usually $\frac{1}{600}$ grain (0.0001 Gm.), every half hour until a lasting effect was obtained. The average total dose per patient, regardless of body weight, was $\frac{1}{68}$ grain (0.00095 Gm.); in terms of milligrams of ouabain per pound of body weight the average was 0.0067 mg. In patients with auricular fibrillation, where therapeutic effect can be readily and easily noted, these observers felt that ouabain as administered by them was safe, but in patients with a regular rhythm they enjoined caution, as follows: "When ouabain is given to patients with regular sinus rhythm, greater care must be used. In these patients clinical improvement seems to be the only criterion for full therapeutic effect; and since moribund patients may not show clinical improvement, there is greater danger of overdosage."

(*g*) *Strophanthus by Mouth.*—Strophanthus preparations are absorbed from the stomach and intestinal tract so inadequately as well as so irregularly that their oral administration is both unsafe and therapeutically unsatisfactory. The sublingual route of administration has been championed by Cornwall, who has gone so far as to assert that "the method is a convenient one which does away with the necessity for hypodermic technic"—which, if it were true, would be most welcome news. Unfortunately his work fails to reveal any convincing evidence in support of the belief. Eggleston and White (1927) have shown in careful clinical investigations that both the sublingual and perlingual (dorsum of tongue) methods of administration are unsuitable for therapeutic use of strophanthin, since neither of them results in the absorption of the drug and the development of its action on the heart.

(*h*) *Clinical Toxicology of Digitalis.*—There is an unfortunate confusion in the literature of the terms "digitalization" and "toxic effects"; indeed, it would seem that in the minds of many writers they are synonymous. . But Reid (1927) has called attention to the fact that this is not true, and I fully agree with him in his condemnation of the statement (Editorial in the Jour. Amer. Med. Assoc., September 10, 1927), "Complete digitalization will cause nausea, vomiting, complete loss of appetite for days, disturbance of vision, and generally a diminished secretion of the urine, although in the early stages of the large doses of digitalis the excretion of urine is increased." The toxic effects of digitalis are well known to be the following: Nausea, loss of appetite, vomiting, diarrhea, headache, drowsiness, mental confusion, visual disturbances, coupled rhythm, partial or complete heart block, simulation of any of the other spontaneous arrhythmias, diminution in secretion if urine, and urticarial and scarlatiniform rashes. To be sure, the administration of digitalis to the point of obtaining its full effects—*i. e.*, the achievement of "digitalization"—is usually marked by evidences of mild toxicity, but to single out certain of these symptoms as invariably marking complete digitalization, is erroneous and dangerously misleading. Gastric symptoms do not occur in all cases even if the patient is seriously poisoned, and the studies of Gold *et al.* (1931) have shown that an initial stimulation of the vomiting reflex may be succeeded by depression of the same, so that to rely greatly upon nausea and vomiting as measures of the degree of cardiac poisoning may be a very dangerous policy. Nor is the typical slowing of the heart always seen. Witness Reid: "In some instances, the order is written to repeat the dose unless there is vomiting or the pulse rate reaches 60. There is no objection to these directions provided too great reliance is not placed on their protective influence. It must be emphasized that there are some patients who may be seriously or even fatally poisoned by digitalis, and yet emesis does not occur. Also it frequently happens that the onset of ventricular extrasystoles, if the latter are felt at the wrist, may prevent the pulse rate from dropping to 60 a minute." On the same point, Pardee states, "Slowing of the heart is of course a well-recognized toxic effect of digitalis, but it is not so well realized that acceleration of the heart or the onset of irregular heart action may also be a toxic digitalis effect. If the heart of a sick patient becomes more rapid or becomes irregular, the physician might possibly attribute this to the cardiac condition becoming worse. This may indeed be so; but if considerable amounts of a digitalis preparation have been given to the patient, it may be a sign of toxic action and indicate cessation of digitalis rather than its continuation." To list disturbances of vision as among the invariable signs of full digitalization is also misleading, for flickering disturbances are perhaps more often absent than present when digitalization is reached.

In short, then, by full digitalization is meant the administration of digitalis until its full therapeutic effects are obtained, at which time there usually also appear mild symptoms of toxicity. The physician should familiarize himself with *all* the signs of toxic action and not be content to recognize merely the most familiar ones, such as nausea, drowsiness and excessive slowing of the rate.

The use of either epinephrine or ephedrine in a patient taking digitalis is dangerous.

(*i*) *Digitalis Dosage for Children.*—It is usually considered that children require proportionately larger doses of digitalis than do adults, but the matter has never been exhaustively studied for the reason that complete heart failure is very rare in children. In children with normal hearts, the studies of McCulloch and Rupe (1921) indicate that between 8 and 20 kilos (17.6 and 44 pounds), or up to the approximate age of four years, children respond more readily to digitalis than do children above this weight and age, and that older children require a larger amount per unit of body weight than is required by adults with heart failure. However, there is some reason to doubt the exactitude with which the appearance of toxic symptoms, which determined the end-point in these normal heart observations, can be compared with the appearance of full therapeutic effects in adults with diseased hearts.

3. The Use of Diuretics.—Christian (1924) has written, "For the great majority of cardiacs with edema, digitalis is a wonderful diuretic and all that is needed. Occasionally it needs to be helped." There are very few reports, however, indicating either the proportion of cases in which resort is had to the diuretic drugs or the percentage of successful results which follows upon their use. The present discussion of their merits cannot therefore be as complete as one might wish.

(*a*) *Theobromine and Theophylline.*—The most valuable clinical study of the xanthine diuretics that has been performed to date is that of Marvin (1926). Prior to the appearance of his report, though the literature abounded in studies of the effects of diuretics on normal animals, one sought in vain for a satisfactory study of a considerable group of patients on which might be based a critical appraisal of the *clinical* value of theobromine and theophylline. Marvin studied 77 patients with advanced congestive heart failure and no evidences of nephritis; all had gross subcutaneous edema and many, in addition, hydrothorax or ascites or both. After thorough digitalization had been accomplished and maintenance dosage established and after the amount of diuresis thus accomplished with the patients in bed and restricted to a fluid intake of 1200 cc. daily had been determined, the use of the xanthines was begun.

Three drugs were employed, theobromine sodium salicylate, theobromine and theophylline, singly if successful, in succession if unsuccessful. Theobromine sodium salicylate dosage: 40 to 80 grains (2.6 to 5.3 Gm.) daily for five or six days; theobromine in gelatin capsules, 10 grains (0.6 Gm.) three times daily for two days; theophylline (theocin), 5 grains (0.3 Gm.) three times daily for two days. The results in the 77 cases are as shown in the table (Table 47). The arteriosclerotic hypertensive group was overwhelmingly in the majority among those who experienced loss or reduction in edema under this treatment.

"With regard to the relative potency of the three drugs studied . . . the superiority of theophylline is too apparent to require extended comment. The distressing nausea and vomiting that so often attend its use lessen the enthusiasm one might otherwise feel for this excellent preparation. In favor of theobromine sodiosalicylate there is apparently little to be said, except that it is tolerated in huge doses. . . . A statement frequently made in behalf of theobromine sodiosalicylate is that it is freely soluble in water, while theobromine is relatively insoluble: a statement quite without significance in view of the fact that the increased solubility decreases its diuretic potency.

"Theobromine appears to be used but seldom, although our results indicate that it is far more valuable than its more soluble relative theobromine

TABLE 47.—EFFECTIVENESS OF XANTHINE DIURETICS AFTER DIGITALIS IN HEART DISEASE

Total number of cases.	Edema.					
	Removed by digitalis alone.	Cases remaining.	Removed by diuretics.	Much reduced by diuretics.	Partially reduced by diuretics.	Unaffected.
77	36 (47 per cent)	41	13 (31 per cent)	5 (12 per cent)	5 (12 per cent)	18 (44 per cent)

sodiosalicylate. It not infrequently causes diuresis when the latter preparation has completely failed, and it is equally free from undesirable side-actions. That absence of water solubility is of no importance whatever is indicated by the fact that theophylline, the most potent of the xanthine diuretics, is equally insoluble."

REPETITION OF DIURETICS.—"There were many opportunities for repeating diuretics that had been given once without result. The repetition was found valueless; in no instance was there a response to subsequent courses of a drug that had proved useless at its first exhibition. Not infrequently, however, patients who had shown no diuresis after theobromine sodiosalicylate reacted most satisfactorily to theophylline. If the customary doses of these drugs were found ineffective, they were often repeated in larger amounts: 5.3 Gm. of theobromine sodiosalicylate daily, 3 Gm. of theobromine daily, and 2 Gm. of theophylline daily being the usual maximal doses. In no patient of the present series did increased dosage cause diuresis after the customary doses had failed, and the larger amounts of theophylline invariably provoked severe vomiting, which sometimes persisted for several days. It was sometimes necessary to administer an effective diuretic five or six times to cause the complete disappearance of edema; with a single exception, the diuretic response to the first course of the drug was the greatest. This was probably due, in part at least, to the fact that there was a larger amount of edema fluid available for removal at the beginning of treatment."

(b) *Novasurol (Merbaphen) and Salyrgan (Mersalyl).*—Novasurol is the double salt of sodium mercurichlorphenyl oxyacetate with diethylbarbituric acid (barbital). It was introduced a number of years ago in Germany for the intravenous treatment of syphilis, but its pronounced diuretic properties were early noticed and first reported by Saxl and Heilig (1920). Salyrgan, which is prepared by the action of mercury acetate and methyl alcohol on salicylallylamido-o-acetic acid and subsequent conversion to the sodium salt, is a more recent product. In the last few years numerous reports have appeared on the diuretic effects of these drugs, most of them favorable—to the effect, indeed, that these mercurials are superior to all other diuretics in congestive heart failure. The actions may be summarized as follows: (a) The excretion of water and chlorides is greatly increased, the increase in chloride excretion exceeding that of the water; (b) diuresis, when it occurs at all, begins within two or three hours after the injection, reaches its maximum in from eight to twelve hours, and thereafter steadily declines; (c) diuresis has usually ceased within twenty-four hours, but occasionally extends into the next day; (d) there is little or no effect upon inflammatory exudates; (e) a certain number of individuals exhibit unpleasant, and even alarming, reactions. There is difference of opinion as to the site of action, whether upon the kidneys themselves or upon extrarenal tissues; most probably it is a combination of both types of action.

The N.N.R. preparations consist of ampules of 1 cc. of 10 per cent solution; dose 1 to 2, or at most 4 cc., at intervals of four to seven days. Either the intramuscular or intravenous route may be employed, the latter preferably. As evidence of the relief often afforded by these drugs, a typical case report is here given (Crawford and McIntosh, 1925):

"Case 2.—S. M. Hosp. No. 4851. The patient was a man thirty-one years of age. On admission he was dyspneic and cyanotic. The heart was enlarged and there were systolic and diastolic murmurs to be heard at the apex. The pulse was rapid and irregular. There were moist râles all over the chest but no fluid in the pleural cavities. The liver was enlarged and there was well-marked ascites. There was edema of the legs. Digitalis slowed the heart but failed to alter the edema. Diuretin also failed to produce any action. Theocin produced a slight diuresis but caused symptoms of gastric irritation. Novasurol injection produced a marked improvement. Dyspnea and cyanosis disappeared. The edema of the legs and the ascites disappeared and the liver was reduced in size. Improvement continued without further injections. The diagnosis was mitral stenosis; auricular fibrillation; acute cardiac decompensation."

Hyman and Fenichel (1932) have given salyrgan in 69 cases, producing satisfactory diuresis in 64. Keith *et al.* have shown that these drugs are oftentimes more effective if combined with a low salt, low fluid diet, and ammonium chloride in large amounts. The reader is referred to the discussion of these matters in the chapter on Nephritis (p. 461).

Marvin (1926), it should be noted, doubts the superiority of this new diuretic. He points out that many of the enthusiastic statements in the literature are not supported by case records or details of the medication other than the employment of novasurol, and that certainly in some instances digitalis and the xanthine diuretics were discarded as ineffective when inadequate doses had been given. In Marvin's comparative study of the effects of novasurol and theophylline he used cases of advanced congestive heart failure characterized by large amounts of edema and no evidences of renal disease. They were kept in bed on a restricted daily fluid intake and thoroughly digitalized. As soon as the diuresis from the digitalis had ceased, or was it apparent that diuresis would not occur, an adequate dose of novasurol was given, to be followed, when its diuretic effect had ceased, by an adequate dose of theophylline (or the practice was reversed, the theophylline being given first to be followed by novarsol). The results were determined by measurement of the urinary volume, reduction of edema and changes in body weight.

It would seem from Marvin's work that, if digitalis has been given full chance, and that if either the novasurol or the theophylline is given in sufficient dose, there is little to assist one in choosing between these two diuretics, for each drug failed to cause diuresis in the same number of cases and was partially or entirely successful in the same number. It is important to note, however, that novasurol caused diuresis after theophylline had failed much more often than theophylline succeeded after a novasurol failure. In the studies of Herrmann *et al.* (1933) there was shown to be a distinct advantage gained from alternating the older xanthine diuretics with these newer mercurial drugs.

NOVASUROL TOXICITY.—Marvin observed undesirable side-effects in the majority of instances, but in only 2 of the 26 patients were these serious enough to prevent further administration. He felt that abscesses could be avoided by giving the drug intravenously but that colitis and collapse could not be adequately safeguarded against. Wiseman (1932), too, has preferred the intravenous route, but in a remarkable case in which he maintained satisfactory diuresis during a period of five years with the practically uninterrupted injection of 2 to 4 cc. of salyrgan at intervals of five to seven days, toxic effects were not seen, though they did appear when he changed to novasurol. The only occasions on which diuresis did not follow the injections were when the abdomen was greatly distended with fluid, "which presumably caused pressure on important veins"; after paracentesis the diuretic response was at once obtained.

Hyman and Fenechel (1932) saw no evidence of renal damage in their series.

(c) *Urea.*—Urea as a diuretic has been alternately praised and condemned for some years, perhaps due to a paucity of reliable clinical data upon which to base the rationale of its use. In a rather limited study, Crawford and McIntosh (1925) have used it satisfactorily in cases of advanced heart failure where the other usual methods did not suffice to remove the edema. In these cases, urea in doses of 1 to 2 ounces (30 to 60 Gm.) per day increased the amount of the urine and reduced the edema. The response after administration was rapid, but the effect passed off in a short time, unless the dose was repeated. They gave the drug in a little water after meals; it is objectionable in taste.

Others have given up to 90 or 100 Gm. daily.

(d) *Acid Salts* (*Ammonium Chloride, etc.*).—It is becoming a rather firm clinical impression that the best use of these drugs is to prepare the way, as it were, for the mercurial diuretics. Read the subject of edema in the chapter on Nephritis, particularly the portions pertaining to water and salt excretion and acid-base balance.

(e) *Mechanical Measures for Reduction of Edema.*—See page 477 in the chapter on Nephritis.

4. Catharsis.—Saline cathartics are not so much used nowadays since we have learned more about the proper employment of digitalis; however, they have an important and proper use, for in some cases in which digitalis and the diuretics have failed to completely reduce the edema, and especially to entirely "wring out" the liver, catharsis will accomplish this desirable end. The acceptable saline cathartics are listed on page 477.

5. Quinidine.—Quinidine has come to have an important place in the treatment of heart failure. The use of the drug is described in the discussion of auricular fibrillation, on page 516.

6. Oxygen.—Used as in the treatment of pneumonia (see p. 132), oxygen is beginning to have a vogue, but because of the difficulties in the way of accurately judging the real value of such measures, it seems to me too soon to be certain of its worth. Hamburger, Katz, Colin (1932) and their associates, after a study of the literature and several cases of their own, felt that the rôle of oxygen will probably prove to be to add to the comfort of patients who have definite pulmonary complications—congestion, consolidation, infarction, edema, etc. "Miracles are not to be expected, and in the presence of prolonged, advanced, progressive cardiac disease, as is true also of other available therapeutic measures, oxygen cannot achieve the impossible."

7. Thyroidectomy.—In a small series of patients with congestive heart failure who had practically no cardiac reserve after prolonged periods of adequate medical treatment with complete rest in bed, Blumgart *et al.* (1933) have performed total ablation of the normal thyroid gland. They are convinced that the return of the ability to be up and about without symptoms or signs of congestive failure warrants resort to the measure in instances in which the operative risk would be fair.

ANGINA PECTORIS

Angina pectoris is a serious malady that is widespread throughout the world, affecting everywhere men much more often than women. It has probably been recognized since classical times, but the first complete descrip-

tion of the disease was made by Heberden before the Royal College of
Physicians in London, in 1768. Angina pectoris is preeminently a disease
of the intellectual classes, those upon whom rest the political, professional
and business worries of the world, but it is by no means unknown among
purely physical laborers; indeed, Boas and Donner (1932) are pursuing
investigations which already point to an astonishingly high incidence among
the industrial working classes. The age of onset is usually in the late fifties,
fewer cases occurring in the forties, and cases below thirty being extremely
rare. The actual cause of the malady is unknown. One explanation for the
pain is that it arises directly out of spasm of the coronary arteries, but the
view that is rapidly gaining the most adherents is that it is the result of
anoxemia of the myocardium and is therefore muscular in origin. The coincidence of angina and anemia, functional nervous and mental disturbances,
gallbladder disease, and particularly diabetes mellitus is beginning to be
statistically studied. The symptoms are very typical and it is upon them
and the history that diagnosis must be based for the physical signs and
laboratory findings are not characteristic. The anginal attack is a sudden
vicelike gripping of the thorax, usually centering behind the sternum, with
pain that is more often crushing than knifelike, and accompanied by an
agonal sense of impending death. When the pain radiates it is nearly always
into the left shoulder and down the left arm. Such an attack may be precipitated by unusual exercise or, in the more severe cases, by the most ordinary movements of the body; in some cases emotional stresses or crises are
the more potent causes. The paroxysm is characterized also by one other
conspicuous feature, the immobility of the patient; he may elect to stand
or to sit bolt upright (he rarely reclines), but whatever his posture he retains it fixedly, rarely even emitting a groan despite his pain, until the attack
has passed. The paroxysm may last only a few seconds or it may persist
for several minutes; if it lasts more than a quarter hour, the observer does
well to suspect coronary occlusion (see p. 549). The disease does not run
a typical course, but the average individual dies within five or six years
after the initial seizure; some die in the first attack and others there are
who live fifteen or twenty years with the affection, though these latter are
perhaps rare. Some individuals have several seizures during each day,
others have them less frequently, and in rare instances there may be a
period of a year or more entirely without attacks. Death is either sudden in
an attack or it may occur as a result of coronary occlusion; or of course the
patient may succumb to heart failure or other complications, but it is astonishing how often angina recedes before intercurrent diseases.

THERAPY

(a) **For Immediate Relief.**—*Nitrites.*—Lauder Brunton introduced
amyl nitrite in 1867 and William Murrel nitroglycerin in 1879. These two
drugs are now more often used than any others to promote rapid coronary
dilatation and relief from the anginal spasm. Amyl nitrite by inhalation
often brings relief in thirty seconds to one minute and may be conveniently
carried on the person in the form of a box of the 5-minim (0.32 cc.) "pearls,"
one of which is easily crushed in the handkerchief for inhalation. There are
several objections to this preparation, however. The relief is not so certain
as with nitroglycerin, especially in the severe cases; the odor is often objectionable to patients and also to others who may be nearby when the necessity to use it arises; and the effect persists for only fifteen minutes to half
an hour at most. Nitroglycerin is usually preferred for the following reasons:
It may be conveniently prescribed in the form of hypodermic tablets of

$\frac{1}{100}$ grain (0.00065 Gm.) which are not volatile, do not quickly deteriorate, and are less expensive than the amyl nitrite pearls; several tablets may be taken at one time with as great convenience as a single tablet; and the effect lasts for half an hour to an hour. It is slower in action, however, than the amyl nitrite, two or three minutes being required for full effect. The average dose of this drug is one tablet ($\frac{1}{100}$ grain) to be dissolved under the tongue, but it must often be used in much larger doses, as in the following severe cases reported by Ingals and Meeker:

"Nitrites are among the most valuable remedies, but they are commonly given in insufficient doses. X found the most satisfactory preparation a hypodermic tablet of nitroglycerin of $\frac{1}{100}$ grain, which was found to act more promptly and effectively than otherwise, when allowed to dissolve on or beneath the tongue. In this way its full effects were experienced in from one to three minutes, whereas, if it had been taken into the stomach, only about half the efficiency was experienced, and it did not appear for about ten minutes. Frequently two or more of these tablets were taken at once, and they were repeated every few minutes until the desired effect was obtained. Often as many as ten or a dozen were taken in two or three hours. As much as 15 to 20 hundredths of a grain three times a day has been recommended in severe cases. A physician told me of one patient who took 100 of the $\frac{1}{100}$-grain nitroglycerin tablets in one day with the effect of relieving a severe angina, and at that time he said the pain had not returned for three years. X usually took four or five of the tablets daily, and when the pain was worse or more persistent, ten or twelve. Frequently after these larger doses he would be entirely free from pain all the next day. From my personal observation, I think these large doses are often needed; and if the physician feels his way with gradually increasing doses, no harm will come from them unless they cause too much headache. Osler thinks nitroglycerin is too timidly used and is then abandoned as ineffective. . . . The patient should be warned of the possible dizziness, the flushing of the face and the headache resulting from its use, and should be assured that these disorders will do no harm. I have found it a good plan to give the patient $\frac{1}{100}$ grain or more at once, so as to learn its effects before he leaves my office. After the susceptibility has been determined, it is best to give a full dose when attacks come on. It may be repeated as often as necessary to accomplish the result, except when it causes too much headache. The headache is sometimes relieved by repeating the dose. The remedy does no harm even from prolonged use."

Prodger and Ayman (1932) have pointed out that the earlier physicians were more fearful of possible harmful effects from nitroglycerin than are we of today. In their own series of 110 cases they observed 4 alarming reactions, but Sprague and White (1933) have observed such reactions in only 3 of their 900 cases in private practice. This certainly does not seem to me a very alarming proportion; however, the latter authors point out that it is an easy routine procedure in the office to try $\frac{1}{400}$ to $\frac{1}{200}$ grain (0.00015 to 0.0003 Gm.) sublingually in each new case.

Sodium nitrite, erythrol tetranitrate and mannitol hexanitrate are not suitable for use in an acute seizure, but are described in conjunction with the other remedies (see p. 544) employed in the attempt to lessen the frequency of attacks.

Alcohol.—Heberden advised the use of this drug in his original description of the disease in the following words: "Quiet, and warmth, and spiritous liquors, help to restore patients who are nearly exhausted and to dispel the effects of a fit when it does not soon go off." We should not allow the present pother over alcohol as a "poison" to blind us to the virtues of this drug, for it will sometimes bring about prompt relief from the attack, occasionally being effective when the nitrites fail. The dose should be large, 1 to 3 ounces (30 to 90 cc.) of a good whisky or brandy.

Oxygen.—Boothby (1932) has pointed out the advantages that might accrue from a brief administration of oxygen to the patient whose attacks usually come when he is at rest and who could probably manipulate the apparatus himself. However, the dangers of keeping oxygen under pressure in the home for long periods are certainly great.

Morphine.—For the relief of a prolonged attack morphine may be necessary, but when the attack persists for more than five minutes and requires a large dose of morphine to bring it under control, coronary occlusion should be strongly suspected (see p. 549).

Harmful Drugs.—The experience of Cottrell and Wood (1931) indicates that both epinephrine and ephedrine should not be used in angina.

(b) **To Lessen Frequency and Severity.**—*Rest and Relaxation.*—If the overworked, overworried, overwrought individual with angina pectoris can be brought to relinquish in whole or in large part his professional or business affairs, and can be brought to adopt the mode of life of a person of indolent habit and independent means, and can be induced to journey south in a leisurely fashion during the inclement months, going preferably to a spa, and can be reeducated to eat slowly of light foods in small amounts—that is to say, if all that is practically impossible for the average competing individual in a work-a-day world can be accomplished, then the patient may be said to have the best chance of prolonging his life beyond the four or five years allotted to most of his fellow sufferers. Even under these ideal circumstances, however, resort is practically always had to the following measures in an attempt to lessen the severity of the disease.

Nitrites.—Erythrol tetranitrate and mannitol hexanitrate are not suitable for the control of an acute paroxysm for the reason that their effect does not usually come on until twelve or fifteen minutes have elapsed but it then lasts in some degree for three to five hours, which causes these preparations to be preferred in attempting to forestall the attacks. In an individual who is having many attacks during the twenty-four hours it is sometimes possible to lessen both their number and severity for a time at least by the faithful use of either of these preparations; the result is especially gratifying in the cases characterized by nocturnal attacks which make the nights very miserable. Erythrol tetranitrate is obtainable in $\frac{1}{4}$ and $\frac{1}{2}$ grain (0.015 and 0.03 Gm.) tablets; the effective dose is $\frac{1}{2}$ to 1 grain (0.03 to 0.06 Gm.) every four to six hours. The mannitol salt is not always easily obtainable in America, but in England it appears on the market in $\frac{1}{4}$, $\frac{1}{2}$ and 1 grain (0.015, 0.03 and 0.06 Gm.) tablets; it has the same dosage as the erythrol. Both these preparations are quite expensive.

Sodium nitrite produces its effect in about five minutes, but this effect usually persists no longer than an hour or two hours at most. It also causes gastric disturbances in most individuals. The drug is given in capsule in a dose of 2 to 3 grains (0.13 to 0.2 Gm.). Many practitioners feel that this salt is more effective in patients having more or less continuous pain if it is combined with an equal amount of sodium or potassium iodide.

Theobromine and Theophylline.—The first report of an attempt to utilize the vasodilator effect of the xanthine diuretics in the treatment of angina pectoris was made by Askanazy, in 1895, and was followed, in 1902, by the following enthusiastic statement by Breuer: "In regard to the effect of theobromine I can, on the basis of now more than five years' experience, only confirm the results of Askanazy throughout, and I cannot refrain from saying that I consider his recommendation of theobromine in the treatment of cardiac asthma and of angina pectoris to be one of the most praiseworthy therapeutic attainments of the last ten years." The drugs have been slow, however, in becoming popular with the profession, probably for the reason that they nearly always cause unpleasant symptoms after a while if taken in effective doses. A thorough study of a number of these xanthines has been reported by Gilbert and Kerr (1929), a summary of which I shall present here:

CONDITIONS OF THE STUDY.—There were 86 patients, all ambulatory but none engaged in hard manual labor. The bowels were kept open with liquid petrolatum or several glasses of warm water on rising, occasionally a cathartic; no other drugs were used. Rest before and after meals was enjoined but the daily life was not otherwise altered.

DOSAGE AND ADMINISTRATION.—The customary doses were as follows: Theobromine, 5 grains (0.3 Gm.); theobromine sodium acetate, 10 grains (0.7 Gm.); theobromine sodiosalicylate, 10 grains (0.7 Gm.); theobromine calcium salicylate, from 7½ or 10 grains (0.5 or 0.7 Gm.); theophylline, 2 grains (0.1 Gm.); theophylline sodio-acetate, 4 grains (0.3 Gm.); theophylline-ethylenediamine, from 1½ to 3 grains (0.1 to 0.2 Gm.). These drugs were usually given in capsules, except theobromine calcium salicylate (theocalcin), and theophylline-ethylenediamine (euphylline), which were given in the tablet form. Four doses a day were usually given, but this, as well as the dosage, was shifted about when made necessary by unpleasant after-effects. In the same way the time of administration was varied and shifted about to the time when it was found to cause the least untoward effect. In some cases it was given before meals, and in some cases after meals. "A physician patient discovered that, while he had nausea when the drug was taken either on an empty stomach or after meals, he had no ill effects when he took part of his meal, then the drug, and then the rest of his meal. This we found to apply in a great many cases. Another patient discovered that she had unpleasant symptoms only when she took the theobromine and had tea with her meal."

The drug was usually given for the first four days of each week and omitted the last three because in this way it was felt that nausea and other unpleasant symptoms were best avoided (though it should be noted that Musser, 1928, has reported a series in which theophylline-ethylenediamine was taken for many weeks without any unpleasant symptoms; at least he reported none), and because a tolerance is prone to appear in many patients. Because of this latter tendency, the drugs were in the beginning alternated, using one one week and another the next, or shifting them about from time to time. Later in the study each of the preparations was tried in succession, and then the two were alternated that gave the best results with the least discomfort, adhering still to the four-day dosage and three-day rest periods.

RESULTS.—I have summarized the results in Table 48. If there was any difference between the theobromine preparations it was in favor of the acetate salt, probably because of its 60 per cent theobromine content against 46 per cent in the salicylate. Theophylline-ethylenediamine seems to have come out best in the trial, because though at times it seemed not to be quite as effective as the theobromine preparations, there were some cases which responded to it which did not respond to theobromine. In some instances in which there was inadequate response with 1½ grains (0.1 Gm.) four times a day, very satisfactory results followed doubling the dose.

UNPLEASANT EFFECTS.—The untoward effects consisted of nausea most frequently, emesis, a burning pain in the epigastrium or under the sternum, palpitation, dizziness, headache, "nervousness" and a few other scattering complaints. These symptoms are grouped under untoward effects and classified again as none, slight, moderate or marked, as shown in Table 49.

Only two patients who experienced marked nausea had even moderate

35

relief, but each of these obtained a moderate degree of relief with slight or moderate untoward effects when shifted to another one of the drugs. On the basis of a minimum of untoward effects, theobromine calcium salicylate more than challenged theophylline-ethylenediamine, but the beneficial effects of the theophylline were perhaps slightly greater and, as previously

TABLE 48.—EFFECTIVENESS OF XANTHINE DIURETICS IN ANGINA PECTORIS

	No. cases.*	Effect on pain.			
		Marked.	Moder-ate.	Slight.	None.
Theobromine..................	14	3	6	1	4
Theobromine sodium acetate.......	69	37	11	1	20
Theobromine sodium salicylate.....	69	38	10	1	20
Theobromine calcium salicylate....	39	27	3	2	7
Theophylline sodium acetate.......	14	2	5	1	6
Theophylline-ethylenediamine......	43	28	3	3	9
Totals......................	248	135 (54 per cent)	38 (15 per cent)	9 (3 per cent)	66 (28 per cent)

* The total number of patients was only 86, but a trial of several of the drugs was made on each.

mentioned, it replaced the theobromine salt rather well when the latter had failed.

Benzyl Benzoate.—In 1921, Spach reported 6 cases of angina pectoris in which more or less complete relief followed the use of benzyl benzoate, and, in 1924, Babcock reported 20 cases similarly treated. Of Babcock's cases, 6 were so distinctly relieved as to justify daily employment of the

TABLE 49.—UNPLEASANT EFFECTS OF XANTHINE DIURETICS IN ANGINA PECTORIS

	No. cases.*	Marked.	Moder-ate.	Slight.	None.
Theobromine..................	14	4	3	1	6
Theobromine sodium acetate.......	69	8	9	16	36
Theobromine sodium salicylate.....	69	8	7	13	41
Theobromine calcium salicylate....	39	0	0	7	32
Theophylline sodium acetate.......	14	6	3	3	2
Theophylline-ethylenediamine......	43	2	1	7	33
Totals......................	248	28 (11 per cent)	23 (10 per cent)	47 (19 per cent)	150 (60 per cent)

* The total number of patients was only 86, but a trial of several of the drugs was made on each.

drug for many months, a few were slightly relieved, and the remainder were not helped at all. The drug is probably effective in Babcock's opinion only in those cases in which vascular tension or spasm produces such a degree of intra-aortic pressure as to pinch the sensory nerve endings richly supplied to the aortic coats, in accordance with Sir Clifford Allbutt's explanation of angina pectoris.

Regarding dosage, Babcock says: "As a general rule, 30 drops, poured directly from the bottle, are ordered four times daily. In no instance have harmful effects been detected. Administered in milk or cream, it does not appear to disturb the stomach."

Sedatives.—In a few cases, 10 to 20 grains (0.65 to 1.3 Gm.) of sodium or potassium bromide three times daily will serve to lessen the number of paroxysms, while there are other individuals who will be able to get through the night by taking a full dose of veronal (barbital) upon retiring—10 grains (0.65 Gm.). Codeine sulphate, ½ to 1 grain (0.03 to 0.06 Gm.), is much more likely to prevent the night attacks. However, the number of patients with true angina who are relieved by the use of sedatives is extremely small.

Digitalis and Quinidine.—There is no indication for the use of digitalis in the treatment of angina pectoris except when congestive heart failure supervenes. Fenn and Gilbert (1932) believe that the possibility of the drug actually causing cardiac pain has not received the attention it deserves, a thesis which is likely to prove difficult to defend. Quinidine is definitely contraindicated.

Magnesium Chloride.—In cases responding to none of the other remedial agents, Bandman (1933) has tried intravenous injections of sterile 10 per cent solution of magnesium chloride thrice weekly, beginning with 5 cc. and gradually increasing to 10 cc. Immediate reaction of heat, much as occurs in connection with injections of calcium salts (see p. 714), was noted in each instance. Twenty-nine of his 50 patients showed considerable diminution in frequency and severity of attacks, the greater number being among those who also had hypertension. During the course all other medication was discontinued; twelve injections were given in the majority of instances.

Surgical Procedures.—At the present time two surgical measures are before the profession, cervical sympathectomy and paravertebral alcohol block. Both are major procedures and should therefore be resorted to only in the most severe cases. However, since they do give a considerable degree of relief from pain in the majority of cases, and as the early objection to their use—namely, that the absence of pain as a warning signal would lead to overindulgence and earlier death in most cases—has not been statistically supported, I see no reason why these surgical measures should not become increasingly popular for the relief of those cases *in which there are no signs of grave cardiac pathology*.

(*a*) CERVICAL SYMPATHECTOMY.—Jonnesco, in France, reported the first operations of this kind in 1916, but the work was not considerably studied until interest was revived in it by Coffey and Brown, in 1923, in the United States. Yater and Trewhella (1931), following a very poor result, were led to scrutinize the type of treatment very closely. From their study of the literature and their own experience, the following case, for and against the procedure, was made out:

For: (1) Complete relief of the original pain in 40.5 per cent of cases and partial relief in 27 per cent; (2) low immediate operative mortality when cases associated with syphilitic aortitis are eliminated.

Against: (1) No relief or only partial relief in 53 per cent of cases; (2) postoperative appearance of annoying paresthesias, new pains or other evil complications in 31 per cent of cases; (3) effectiveness of nitrites for individual attacks of pain is certainly much more than 40.5 per cent of cases; (4) apparent absence of influence upon the course of the disease.

According to Telford (1932), the operation has never found favor with British physicians, and I am sure that in America it will be decreasingly performed except in exceptionally severe, but uncomplicated, cases.

(*b*) PARAVERTEBRAL ALCOHOL BLOCK.—The most recent review of this method, introduced by Swetlow in 1926, which I can find is that of Levy and

Moore (1931). There were available records of 68 cases, including their own 9, but only 49 with adequate data. Results: (a) 51 per cent of the patients obtained complete or almost complete relief, improvement was noted in 34 per cent, and in 15 per cent the operation was a failure. Benefit varied from slight and temporary to striking and long lasting (1 case, sixteen months); (b) a majority of the patients after injection suffered from hyperesthesia of the chest wall and painful, sometimes terribly painful, intercostal neuritis; these distressing symptoms sometimes lasted for six weeks; (c) many patients had fever for a few days to a week after operation; in 2 cases, effusion into the left pleural cavity followed the injection. Molitch and Wilson (1931) have reported an instance of Brown-Séquard paralysis which lasted for many weeks.

Glucose and Insulin.—Smith (1933) has reported his careful study of 6 severe cases in which he used glucose and insulin for periods varying from two to seventeen weeks; 5 units of insulin before breakfast and before the evening meal, each dose being followed by 30 Gm. of glucose taken with the meal. All conditions as to work, rest and other medication were maintained during the study just as before it began. In all instances the relief obtained after being on the treatment for awhile was almost complete and when the pain returned after the conclusion of the study it was again overcome by return to the glucose-insulin therapy. Smith feels that anginal pain is related to faulty carbohydrate metabolism in the heart and that insulin acts immediately through its stimulating effect upon glycogen metabolism in the organ and progressively by promotion of the combustion of fat, thus leading to the early resolution of atheromatous changes in the coronary arteries. The new trend in thinking with regard to angina, which approaches the manifestations in the disease as evidences of "altered physiology" (I find this term mightily pleasing for it is one more weapon with which to batter at the wall of dead-house pathology which the last generation erected around us), is most interesting.

Muscle Extracts ("Circulatory Hormones").—Following the preparation by Schwarzmann (1928), of Odessa, of an extract from skeletal muscle with which he was able to demonstrate depressant circulatory effects, there has appeared on the Continental market a considerable number of such substances, the principal ones being myoston, myotrat, angioxyl, entonon, lacarnol and padutin (formerly kallikrein). This last, the preparation of Frey-Kraut, is obtained from the urine but formed in the pancreas, and to it has been applied the title "hormone." Indeed, it seems probable that its true hormonal action upon vessel caliber will eventually be shown; it is furthermore likely that the active ingredient in all the extracts from muscles and other organs depend for their activity upon the content of this substance.

So far as I am able to determine (it is a difficult literature because of the multiplicity of preparations), the effect in hypertensive cases is very variable and probably upon the whole of little value, but in angina pectoris excellent results seem often to be obtained—severity and frequency of attacks both being favorably influenced. The majority of writers upon the subject, as well as most of those experienced with the extracts who answered von den Velden's (1931) questionnaire, are in agreement upon the point. The most recent publication to come to my attention is that of Fleishmann (1932) who, having reported favorably to von den Velden on 25 cases of angina pectoris, now substantiates that opinion upon a much larger experience. The controversy over superiority among the preparations, and the details of administration, need not concern us here for the new substances are not yet so far as I am aware generally available in this country.

CORONARY OCCLUSION

The correlation of bedside and pathologic findings in coronary occlusion, with the resultant recognition of it as a definite clinical syndrome, has taken place only in this present century. Thrombus formation is the commonest cause of the interference with the coronary circulation. As in angina pectoris, the victims are usually men past fifty years of age. Except when death is sudden, the salient features of acute occlusion are the following: (*a*) Sudden severe anginoid pain, which is substernal or upper abdominal; (*b*) pinched, ashen gray or very pale facies often associated with a feeling of impending death; (*c*) acute emphysematous distention of the lungs with dyspnea or orthopnea and moist crackling râles at the lung bases, together with the onset of acute heart failure; (*d*) an early thready pulse with almost any form of arrhythmia; (*e*) sudden drop in systolic pressure; (*f*) a diffuse, scarcely palpable cardiac impulse; (*g*) distant heart sounds and often a gallop rhythm; (*h*) a localized, evanescent pericardial friction rub; (*i*) short, mild fever with leukocytosis; and (*j*) inversion or iso-electric position of the T wave and sometimes evidence of intraventricular block in the electro-cardiogram. Coronary occlusion is often associated with or is the cause of abdominal signs and symptoms, and occasionally it will closely simulate an acute surgical condition of the abdomen. Frequently the underlying coronary pathology is entirely overlooked, and these cases are diagnosed as "acute indigestion." One should listen carefully to the history of the attack as given; the prior history, especially, will often give an inkling of the nature of the attack from the mild angina and shortness of breath described by the patient. Fixation in a definite position is not the rule as it is in a severe attack of angina pectoris.

Many of these patients die after lingering for a few days to weeks, but a certain number recover to a surprising extent. Conner and Holt (1930) have studied the records of 287 cases and find (*a*) immediate mortality in first attacks, 16.2 per cent; (*b*) 75 per cent of the survivors were in good health at end of one year, 56 at two, 21 at five, and 3.4 per cent at end of ten years; (*c*) a single attack only was recorded in 67 per cent of all the patients, two attacks in 24 per cent, three attacks in 4 and four to seven attacks in 5 per cent.

THERAPY

Morphine.—Large doses are required to relieve this pain, perhaps as much as $1\frac{1}{2}$ grains in the first twenty-four hours.

Nitrites.—This group, so valuable in the treatment of angina pectoris, is of little value here.

Sedatives.—Even with the large doses of morphine the patient is not infrequently in a state of continuous mental anguish. Scopolamine hydrobromine (hyoscine hydrobromide) may be safely used in addition to the morphine in hypodermic doses of $\frac{1}{300}$ to $\frac{1}{200}$ grain (0.0002 to 0.0003 Gm.). Later, the milder sedatives may be effective, such as sodium bromide and chloral hydrate, 10 grains (0.65 Gm.) each, or $7\frac{1}{2}$ to 10 grains (0.5 to 0.65 Gm.) of veronal (barbital).

Digitalis.—Full digitalization is indicated in the presence of rapid heart failure. For methods, see page 529.

Theobromine and Theophylline.—As in angina pectoris, the xanthine diuretics are sometimes of value for their ability to dilate the coronary vessels. Musser (1928) has reported a number of cases in which theophylline-ethylenediamine, especially, was of some value in patients with a mild degree of occlusion. For the methods of using these drugs, see page 544.

Oxygen.—Barach (1932) has reported favorably upon the effects of oxygen, administered as in pneumonia, in 4 cases; Gilbert (1933) also believes it to be of value.

Complications.—Ventricular tachycardia seems to call for quinidine; Levine (1932) has found epinephrine of great value in the opposite condition, heart block. There is increasing impression that insulin should be withheld if possible in diabetics; Levine feels that death was caused by its use in one case against his wishes.

Rest.—Patients who survive the acute stage are in constant danger of sudden death, and should not only be kept at absolute rest in bed for at least a month, but should be permitted finally to return to only very restricted activity.

AORTITIS AND ANEURYSM

(See under the Treatment of Syphilis, p. 177)

THROMBO-ANGIITIS OBLITERANS

(Buerger's Disease)

This peculiar disease is an inflammatory infection of the deep-seated arteries and veins and the superficial veins of the lower extremities, occasionally of the upper extremities. It occurs principally in middle-aged male Jews, though women, in whom it seems to be a milder affection, and Gentiles are occasionally afflicted. The etiology of the disease is entirely unknown, but it is generally conceded that excessive smoking plays some part. The independent studies of Sulzberger and Harkavy and their associates indicate that there may be such a thing as allergic sensitiveness to tobacco underlying many of the cases. The character of the lesion suggests either a toxic or bacterial exciting factor; there is acute inflammation with occlusive thrombosis, organization or healing, canalization of the clot, disappearance of the inflammatory products, and the development of fibrotic tissue that binds together the artery, vein and nerves. The cardinal signs and symptoms of the disease, which usually develops insidiously, are pain in the calves or feet, which is severe and cramplike, and is aggravated by walking but not usually by standing; pallor of the limb when it is raised above the horizontal position and great redness (rubor) when it it dependent; coldness of the extremity; and lack of pulsation in the arteries affected. Migrating phlebitis of the superficial veins is of frequent occurrence. Ultimately, ulceration and gangrene occur in the great majority of cases. Taube (1931) has reviewed 26 cases in the literature and added 2 of his own in which vessels other than those of the extremities were affected.

The disease was first described by Leo Buerger, in 1908. Kaunitz (1931) has been developing the thesis, in a very interesting fashion, that this and related vasomotor and trophic disturbances are the present-day expression of ergotism.

THERAPY

This disease being of unknown etiology, of serious import, and as yet without a specific remedy, it is to be expected that a large number of remedial agents and measures shall have been tried. I shall discuss here only those that seem to be holding their own as therapeutic procedures, but in attempting to evaluate them the reader cannot give too much consideration to the following statements of Perla (1925): "Thrombo-angiitis obliterans is an extremely chronic disease, often lasting as long as fifteen or twenty years. More than 80 per cent of all cases give a history of remissions during which the patient is free from all symptoms. These remissions occur spontaneously at almost any stage of the disease and last from a few months to several years, frequently as long as five, ten and even fifteen years. . . . Temporary arrests have been reported as cures following almost every new therapeutic innovation. In this disease, particularly, a temporary arrest of one year is not evidence of more than a remission." In Silbert's recent (1930) valuable study of a large number of patients, he has shown that of a group of 460 patients with untreated thrombo-angiitis obliterans, 64 per cent had an amputation of one extremity during the first five years of illness and 46 per cent an amputation of the second extremity during the first ten years. Therefore, it would seem that the successful treatment would be one that not only relieved the suffering of the patients in a large series but also presented the majority of them with intact extremities after a period of five years from onset.

General Routine.—The pain, which is probably largely due to diminution in blood supply to the muscles since it is increased by exercise, should certainly be primarily treated by rest. Rest in bed for a month or more is imperatively necessary in every case no matter in what stage it is first seen, and when improvement takes place the return to partial activity should be extremely gradual. Another indication, upon which practically all observers are agreed, is the necessity to promote collateral circulation. For this purpose heat is employed, either by means of the electric pad or the electric bulb cradle, or by any other means by which heat may be applied to the affected extremity continuously for a long period of time; after the patient becomes ambulatory, diathermy may be suitable—I write "may be" advisedly, for I am still sceptical of the superior merits of this method of applying heat. During a period of migrating phlebitis heat is not well borne. Five to 15 grains (0.3 to 1 Gm.) of potassium iodide is given twice or thrice a day during the whole period of treatment by many physicians, but it is doubtful whether structural changes in the vessel walls, reduction of the viscidity of the blood, or hastened absorption of these nonspecific cellular exudates actually do follow upon its use.

Patients who refuse to stop smoking rarely improve under treatment.

Passive Exercise.—Buerger employs the following method of improving the circulation: "The affected limb is elevated, with the patient lying in bed, to from 60 to 90 degrees above the horizontal, being allowed to rest upon a support for from thirty seconds to three minutes, the period of time being the minimum amount of time necessary to produce blanching or ischemia. As soon as blanching is established, the patient allows the foot to hang down over the edge of the bed for from two to five minutes, until reactionary hyperemia or rubor sets in, the total period of time being about one minute longer than that necessary to establish a good red color. The limb is then placed in the horizontal position for about three to five minutes, during which time an electric heating pad or a hot-water bag is applied, care being taken to prevent the occurrence of a burn. The placing of the limb in these three successive positions constitutes a cycle, the duration of which is usually from six to ten minutes. These cycles are repeated over a period of about one hour, some 6 to 7 cycles constituting a séance." The number of séances per day varies for individual patients.

Intravenous Sodium Chloride.—Hypertonic solution of sodium chloride has gradually and practically completely replaced all other substances for intravenous injection. Silbert describes the method as follows: "The solution is prepared in freshly distilled water, filtered, and immediately sterilized. At the present time, 5 per cent sodium chloride is used, 150 cc. for the first injection and 300 cc. for all subsequent injections. The injections are at first given three times a week, later, twice a week, and the length of intervals further increased as the patient improves. The injection is given into a superficial vein in the usual manner by the gravity method; the fluid is allowed to run into the vein slowly during ten minutes, and the patient is kept flat on his back during this period. If care is taken, the superficial veins will not be injured or become thrombosed, so that the same vein can be punctured again and again. If the solution has been properly made, chills or fever should rarely, if ever, follow the injection. . . .

"No other means of treatment has been regularly employed in the cases that we have treated. . . . During the injection, the blood volume is increased and the patients often state that they feel warm; the face becomes flushed and the superficial veins engorged. They often complain of thirst. The excretion of the 15 Gm. of sodium chloride injected takes place through the urine within forty-eight hours—approximately two thirds of the salt being excreted the first day, and one third the second day. The administration of hypertonic salt solution produces a certain amount of blood destruction. A slight amount of urobilin may appear in the urine, and a reduction in hemoglobin and red blood cell count will occur. As the majority of patients with thrombo-angiitis obliterans have a high hemoglobin and red cell count, a slight blood destruction is of no serious consequence. No symptoms of anemia have ever been produced even in patients who have been treated for a very long time; but if a mild anemia should occur, the injections should be stopped for a time, or diminished. No injury to the heart or to the kidneys has ever been seen, in spite of prolonged treatment in many cases. It is advisable to examine the urine and to repeat the blood count once a month to follow any changes that may occur. On theoretical grounds, it would seem that the repeated increase in the blood volume, necessarily stretching the vascular system, is responsible for the improved circulation and the development of the collateral blood supply that results. Another possible factor is the dilution of the blood with resulting decrease of viscosity.

"Improvement may be noted immediately, but more frequently not until at least a few weeks have elapsed. In many cases treatment must be continued for several months before definite evidence of improvement appears. The first subjective evidences of benefit are usually the increase of warmth in the extremities, with a diminution of pain. Objectively, the increase in the temperature of the extremity and the growth of new nails are first seen, then healing of an ulcer, if one is present, and finally the development of pulsation in previously occluded or collateral vessels. In addition, a gain of weight and improvement in the patient's general health was also noted. The healing of ulcers has been the usual rule in nearly all of the cases listed as 'improved,' although in a few cases from eight to ten months of treatment were necessary. In about one third of the patients who have been treated for over a year, a return of pulsation in the previously obliterated or in a collateral vessel has been found. When a patient has been restored to good health, the intervals between treatments have been lengthened to once a month and less. No patient has been discharged as cured, as it was felt that this would be unsafe; but no patients who have been kept under observation in this way have had a recurrence of symptoms. The best general evidence of the value of the treatment will be seen from the statement that the majority of the patients, many of whom have been unable to work from periods of from six months to three years, were able to return to work and were restored to economic usefulness. The treatment must sometimes be continued for months.

"In some instances the treatment is without results, and some of the failures have been in advanced cases in which gangrene had already set in. Even in these patients, however, the treatment has sometimes proved of value. In the last four of these patients, treatment for at least two months had been given before amputation became imperative. In all of these, amputation at the middle of the leg was performed and a successful result was obtained. It scarcely needs to be stated that when amputation becomes inevitable it is important to give the patient a stump below the knee if at all possible. While amputations below the knee have occasionally been successful in cases of thrombo-angiitis obliterans in which treatment has not been given, this is certainly the exception rather than the rule, as will be apparent to any one who sees a large number of these crippled men. Four consecutive successful amputations at the middle of the leg are not many, and it is far from my desire to claim that all such amputations will meet with equal success. The fact is recorded as possible evidence of the value of the saline treatment administered to these patients, but only further experience can demonstrate whether this was not merely a coincidence." Burke and Meyerding's (1931) study of 102 amputations at the Mayo Clinic failed to establish any criteria for determining a site for amputation.

In 1931, Silbert reported that among the 225 typical cases and 64 borderline cases treated by this method during the preceding eight years, amputations had been necessary in only 8.3 per cent; 84 per cent of the patients showed symptomatic improvement and 67 per cent had been able to return to work.

Foreign Protein Fever Therapy.—Any of the fever-producing methods (see p. 187 in chapter on Syphilis) are employed. Barker (1931) has analyzed the results after treatment of 150 cases at the Mayo Clinic: Marked improvement, 49 per cent; slight to moderate improvement, 27 per cent. In a follow-up study upon 113 of these patients for from one to five years, it was seen that no recurrence had occurred in 24 per cent, that 14 per cent were again relieved by the same treatment, that 3 per cent were relieved without treatment, that 18 per cent submitted to ganglionectomy, and that 13 per cent responded to no treatment save amputation. It was not particularly stressed in the report, however, that upon 28 per cent of these 113 patients there were no data at all.

Sympathetic Ganglionectomy.—In a recent report Adson and Brown (1932) have stated that quite considerable improvement resulted from operation in 83 per cent of their 104 patients (100 patients plus 4 who had both upper and lower extremity involvements). My impression is that most surgeons of experience in the disease do not believe that such results are obtainable in the ordinary run of cases, that is to say, that perhaps a preponderance of relatively early cases is seen at the Mayo Clinic.

VARICOSE VEINS

Varicose veins of the legs are seen principally in early and middle adult life and more often in men than in women. The cause is not yet elucidated but lies presumably in the atony of tissues which permits stretching of venous walls and the consequent insufficiency of the valves. The superficial varicosities are usually seen on the inner aspect of the calf and thigh and the inner and posterior aspect of the knee, but when the tributaries of the external saphenous vein are principally involved they appear on the posterior and outer aspects of the limb. The veins appear as tortuous bluish cords beneath the atrophic shiny pigmented skin; often the ankles present a doughy induration. Erythema and eczema are common, but the most serious complication is the sluggish chronic varicose ulcer. This ulcer appears on the lower third and usually inner aspect of the leg, tends to attain very great size, and is extremely resistant to treatment. The subjective symptoms of varicose veins are a feeling of weight in the legs and dull aching pain, which is much relieved when the patient lies down or elevates the legs on a chair. Spontaneous disappearance of the varicosities does not take place.

THERAPY

Walking exercise favors venous return but standing is very bad for these patients. Great care should be taken to avoid even the slightest injuries to the legs as trauma favors the development of ulcer, but unfortunately just the class most often affected with varicosities, *i. e.*, the laboring class, can least afford to seriously heed this admonition. The wearing of elastic stockings, or the employment of the woven elastic bandage, brings considerable relief to many individuals. The legs should be elevated during every moment that it is not absolutely necessary for the patient to be standing.

Surgical Measures.—The two procedures most employed are ligation of the long saphenous vein at its point of emergence from the fossa ovalis (Trendelenburg operation), and the stripping out of a section of the vein between two small skin incisions (Babcock operation). Varying success accompanies these surgical measures, but Berntsen has shown (1927) that there is a 0.7 per cent incidence of embolic deaths.

Injection Treatment.—The substances used for injection of the veins provoke a coagulation thrombosis or, when injected in hypertonic solution, provoke irritation, injury, and even destruction of the intima, thus producing adhesion of the vessel walls. The injection treatment dates from 1851, when Pravaz introduced the use of ferric chloride, but, because of the danger of embolism following the introduction of substances which merely cause coagulation thrombosis, it did not become popular until 1911, when Linser, in Germany, became interested in the obliteration of veins by mercuric chloride during antisyphilitic therapy; he continued to use this substance until 1923, when he changed to sodium chloride solution. Meanwhile, and quite independently, Sicard of Paris, and his associates, Paraf and Forestier, were working with sodium salicylate. Recently, many substances have been tried but those now most used are the following: Sodium salicylate, sodium chloride, invert sugar (popularized through the studies of Nobl, in Vienna), quinine dihydrochloride and urethane (introduced by Genevrier), glycerin, sodium morrhuate, and a mixture of sugar and sodium chloride.

(*a*) *Solutions.*—Forestier describes his use of salicylate solutions as follows: "Twenty per cent solution: Sodium salicylate, 1 Gm.; distilled water, 5 cc. (sterilized for one ampule). Thirty per cent solution: Sodium salicylate, 1.5 Gm.; distilled water, 5 cc. (sterilized for one ampule). Forty per cent solution: Sodium salicylate, 2 Gm.; distilled water, 5 cc. (sterilized for one ampule). Two, three and even four of these ampules may be injected at the same time at different points. . . . As a rule we do not exceed a total of 5 Gm. of sodium salicylate at a time. . . . Generally we begin the treatment by injecting 3 or 5 cc. of the 20 per cent sodium salicylate solution. During the next sitting the same concentration is used if a proper reaction has been obtained; if not, the 30 per cent is injected. In cases responding feebly to the treatment, the 40 per cent solution should be injected."

Sodium chloride is usually employed in 20 per cent solution, from 2 to 12 cc. being injected at the various points. It has recently been stated that the 20 per cent sodium chloride solution need not be boiled "as it is self-sterilizing." Apropos of this, Schussler has cryptically remarked, "I tried this once, got an infected thrombus, and have boiled my solution ever since."

Nobl's sugar formula is 75 per cent glucose and 5 per cent sucrose, but latterly a 75 per cent solution of glucose alone has been much used. From 2 to 12 cc. are injected at the various points.

Genevrier's quinine formula is: Quinine dihydrochloride, 0.4 Gm.; urethane, 0.2 Gm.; distilled water, 3 cc. Forestier writes: "The content of one ampule is as a rule sufficient to make injections at two or three points. No more than 6 cc. of solution should be injected in one day."

Wolf (1931) employs glycerin and water in the proportions of 126 Gm. of glycerin and 200 cc. of water.

Wright, in England, introduced the use of sodium morrhuate; the usual dosage is 2 to 10 cc. of 5 per cent solution, in very obstinate cases, 2 to 8 cc. of a 10 per cent solution; 3 per cent is used in stellate or "spider-burst" veins.

Kern (1931) uses a mixture of equal parts of 50 per cent dextrose and 30 per cent sodium chloride solutions; in other words, 100 cc. of his mixture contains 25 Gm. glucose and 15 Gm. sodium chloride.

(b) *Technic.*—Schussler (1928) described the technic as quoted below, and informs me, in 1933, that he has made no substantial changes:

"The technic is important, and hence will be given in detail. It can be acquired only after long practice, and should not be attempted by those who find arsphenamine injections difficult, as the technical skill required to inject a tortuous, thin-walled, freely movable varicosity is often considerable. The patient sits upright on the table, with the legs horizontal. Two soft rubber tourniquets are applied, one about the ankle and one just above the knee, or higher if necessary. A 10-cc. eccentric tip Luer syringe and a 26-gauge half-inch needle are used. From two to four prominent points are selected and marked with ink, and the area is cleansed with 95 per cent alcohol rather than with iodine. The injections are made slowly, to allow time for distribution of the solution and for contraction of the veins. This forces out the contained blood and allows the solution to act in full concentration, thus completely destroying the intima of the vessel. A gauze sponge is pressed on each puncture site as the needle is withdrawn from it, and held long enough to prevent leakage. When all the injections have been completed, and before the contracted veins have had time to dilate again, a thick pad of cotton is placed over them, and a 4-inch Ace elastic bandage is firmly wound on, extending from one tourniquet to the other, the ends being fastened to the skin with adhesive tape. Ten minutes later the tourniquets are removed and the patient may go home. He is advised, however, to keep off his feet as much as possible until the next morning, and to apply a hot water bottle or electric pad during the night. This procedure is repeated every other day, the bandage being readjusted each time, until no more varicose veins can be found. A few days later the bandage is permanently removed, and after a final inspection the patient is dismissed with instructions to return in six months, and again at the end of a year, so that any recurrences may be dealt with before they become large."

However, Forestier writes as follows on these matters (1928): "There are three different postures available for the injection: Standing on a table, sitting or lying down. We state at once that we discard the use of compressive bandages to cause the veins of the patient to project. We have used the standing and sitting postures for a long time because these postures facilitate the puncture of the vein, but it is necessary for the same posture to be continued throughout the duration of the injection, and, as it is desirable for the muscles to be released, the sitting position is generally more suitable than the standing posture. For the last three years we have been giving the preference, as Sicard and Gaugier do, to the recumbent position, because, as one may well anticipate, it tends to give better results; the vein not being filled with blood, the injected liquid in contact with the endothelium is in a greater concentration."

It should be noted also that some workers do not inject as often as every two or three days but preferably at one-week intervals.

(c) *Choice of Solution.*—Both the salicylate and salt solutions cause pain upon injection, and both cause slough if injected outside the veins; Tunick and Schmier (1929) say that sodium chloride causes the less severe cramp but the more severe slough of the two. Salicylate solution may rarely cause the typical systemic salicylate poisoning. Quinine and sugar solutions may also cause slough, particularly, it seems, if the solution goes half in and half out of the vein, but they are certainly less apt to do so than the previously mentioned salts. Quinine does not cause cramp when injected but cinchonism is of course on record. The sugar solution may cause cramps and will always do so in mixture with sodium chloride. Sodium morrhuate causes no systemic reaction if absorbed, unless it be the very rare generalized eczema which Wright thinks may be an evidence of idiosyncrasy, no cramps but perhaps slight burning on injection; Smith (1932) says that in more than 4000 injections he had only three sloughs of moderate degree, though he believes that he was out of the vein more often than that. Tunick and Nach (1932) and Schussler (1933) also prefer this to all other solutions.

If the escape of solution is suspected, a diluent should be injected subcutaneously—physiologic saline or plain sterile water; Kilbourne (1930) prefers 1 per cent procaine hydrochloride solution to the amount of 5 to 10 cc. The injection of 5 cc. of the patient's own blood from a neighboring varix has also been recommended not only as diluent but also to aid in absorption of the damaged tissue through the marked hyperemia it causes. Dry heat may also hasten absorption. If slough occurs it is best to excise it at once—*in the operating room, not in the dispensary or office.*

(d) *Effectiveness of the Injection Method of Treatment.*—Forestier (1928), one of the pioneers in this work, reported successful obliteration without recurrence in 85 per cent of the cases; more recent experience is confirmatory: de Takát's (1931), recurrences in 10 per cent of 800 cases; Weeks and Miller (1932), recurrences in 7.5 per cent of 200 cases; Lewis (1932), recurrences in 7 per cent of 848 cases. A plea for return to surgical measures, or at least a combination of surgery and injection, is nevertheless made by Howard, Jackson and Mahon (1931) on the basis of recurrence in 79 per cent of 66 cases. However, this latter report surely cannot be representative of the results obtained by most practitioners, for the method seems to be increasing in popularity.

(e) *Dangers and Contraindications.*—It would seem that the incidence of embolism after this type of treatment should be very great, but as a matter of fact it is negligible. McPheeters and Rice (1928) found reports of approximately 53,000 cases, with only 7 deaths from all causes. Compare this mortality of 0.0024 per cent with the 0.7 per cent mortality from embolism alone following the surgical type of treatment. More recently, Silverman (1931) has reviewed the literature and found that among the many hundreds of thousands of patients that have now been injected, there are at least on record only 20 in whom embolism developed; of these, 15 died. Definite contraindications to the injection method include cardiac and renal disease accompanied by venous stasis and dilatation of veins, hypertonus, lack of patency in the deep veins and a thrombophlebitic edema, hyperthyroidism, active tuberculosis or any other acute infectious disease, advanced pregnancy, and present or recently subsided phlebitis. Old persons with enfeebled health should not be given injections. The presence of varicose ulcers does not contraindicate the injection method; indeed, it constitutes one of the best means of hastening the disappearance of these ulcers. It is unanimously agreed that injections should be limited in most cases to the veins below the knee, and that under no circumstances should they be made above the middle of the thigh. The reason for this is that the suction action of the deep veins of the pelvis predominates in the upper course of the saphenous vein where the positive pressure is low; the danger of embolism is thus increased.

Varicose Ulcer.—When I was in residence at the New York Skin and Cancer Hospital a certain number of years ago, we used to treat ambulatory cases in the clinic with salves and no hope, or an occasional Unna paste boot, but when we could get a bed in the house and a patient who could occupy it for the requisite number of weeks or months, we did cure them. The patient was put to bed, the ulcer cleaned, and a gridiron of narrow adhesive straps criss-crossed over it. Various wet antiseptic dressings were then applied continuously in the beginning, and later the exuberant granulations were cut down with the silver nitrate stick, which was also used upon occasion to touch up the sluggish edges here and there. They got well at last (shall I ever forget the old Irish woman who knitted sweaters for the entire staff, twice round!), but I do not think the dressings had anything to do with the result. The more blithely they went out, the more disgruntled they returned, however, for we were not doing enough with the recumbent position, and in those days we hadn't begun injecting the veins to attack the matter at its roots. Now all that is changed, for the majority of ulcers gradually heal after successful obliteration of the veins, and those which do not are apparently surely healed by one of the two new methods described below.

The Occlusive Compression Bandage.—The advantages of this method, which was developed by Wright (1930–32), in England, and is being used with astonishing success all over the world, are the following: (*a*) The varicose circulation is abolished, forcing the blood through the capillaries and thus reestablishing aeration of the tissues; (*b*) the edema is reduced, thus bringing the edges of the ulcer closer together and pressing the raised margins of an indurated ulcer down flat; (*c*) the delicate granulations and new epithelium are not only protected from dressing trauma, but the wound is actually dressed in its own secretions—the "pansement spécifique" of Besredka; (*d*) pain is abolished in the majority of cases; (*e*) work and exercise aid rather than hinder the cure; (*f*) the cure is rapid—"frequently an ulcer of the size of the palm of the hand, if of short duration, will heal within seven days"; (*g*) the ulcer is cleaned more quickly than by antiseptic methods and fetor rapidly disappears; (*h*) varicose veins that had been deeply buried in edema are brought to the surface and rendered injectible; (*i*) the scar is supple without adherence to the bones; (*j*) expense is saved; (*k*) and no special training or skill are required to apply the treatment.

DETAILS.—(1) The uppermost veins are injected (Wright uses 5 per cent sodium morrhuate) from above downward. (2) The leg is then wound with an elastic-adhesive bandage very firmly and evenly over a longitudinal strip on both sides, the tightness of the winding being proportional to the swelling and induration, sometimes using practically all of one's strength —"the almost invariable cause of failure is the looseness of the bandage." (3) No treatment of any kind is applied to the ulcer, neither eczema, phlebitis or periphlebitis being considered a contraindication; indeed, Wright considers associated arterial disease and diabetes to be practically the only contraindications to the entire treatment. (4) If the ulcer is of the painful type, aspirin powder is blown in with an insufflator and the patient is given a hypnotic for a few nights, the latter not so much for the pain but because "she has fed the ulcer with salves, antiseptics, lint and gauze for so long that she thinks terrible things are happening under the bandage." The pressure under the ulcer if it is a particularly painful one is sometimes increased by applying a small firm absorbent pad stuck onto the bandage with adhesive and then pressed into the ulcer bed with another turn of the bandage; especially useful is this procedure in treating ulcers in the sulcus under the malleoli where the bandage does not grip very tightly. (5) The patient is instructed to wash off the discharge if it seeps through with a nail-brush and soap, and to protect the clothing with a dressing over the weeping area, and also to wear a long stocking over the whole. Work and as much walking exercise as possible are mandatory. (6) The subsequent visits are dependent upon the size and location of the ulcer (over the malleoli, movements will loosen the bandage; copious discharge will necessitate frequent changing; disappearance of edema will also require reapplication). (7) Upon each removal of the bandage the veins are injected again in the previous order and also any others that have become accessible, and if the ulcer is large and a good sheet of granulations has developed, grafts are inserted under them on the fibrous bed—insinuation of small implants, darning in threads of skin, or injecting a suspension of skin in saline. "Grafting may be repeated and it is always well to have a graft waiting in the center of the last patch of ulcer to receive the edges as they close in, otherwise there is often an annoying delay at the last." (8) Finally, when the ulcer is healed and all veins obliterated, the former often being accomplished first, a Unna paste boot, or preferably one of the new Klebro bandages is applied for three months to consolidate the cure. Thereafter, either of the above—the Klebro being changed four times a year, or an elastic stocking—may be required.

Wright finds that eczema may develop under the bandage, or if previously present may get worse during treatment; however, so far as the patient will permit, he ignores it and is often rewarded by disappearance of eczema, ulcer and edema all together. Failing, he employs interchangeably bandages impregnated with rivanol 1:1000, ichthyol 5 per cent and aluminum acetate 5 per cent. Blisters developing under the bandage do not cause him to alter the treatment, overlapping each turn of the bandage with two thirds of its width, plus the greatest care in application, has usually avoided cutting with resultant linear ulceration in very edematous legs.

Rubber Sponge Supportive Bandage.—This method of therapy developed by McPheeters (1931) has been called by him the "venous heart" treatment and rests on the belief that the patient's heart will pump fresh arterial blood filled with oxygen and tissue food to the ulcerated area but that the circulatory apparatus must be artificially aided to carry off the products of combustion and ketosis which cause the local acidosis and tissue death. To this end he applies a rubber sponge tightly to the ulcerated area and then causes the patient to walk a great deal, so that with each step the elastic sponge performs a "systole and diastole" by which serum, lymph and venous blood are actively pumped away from, and arterial blood into, the affected tissues at the same time that all the advantages of constantly applied firm pressure are obtained. Unless the patient exercises he will suffer intolerable pain; with exercise he will find that the normal soreness and the edema rapidly disappear and "ideal conditions are maintained for the ulcer-healing, the end-results are reached in a comparatively short period, and the patient continues on at work during the entire period." The treatment is of course absolutely contraindicated in the bedridden.

DETAILS.—(1) Cleanse the skin and ulcer area with gauze and benzine and apply 10 per cent silver nitrate to the ulcer, which will stimulate but is of no value at the first dressing of a badly infected and necrotic ulcer. (2) Apply some ointment that will *remain soft* to the ulcer, cover it with fluffed gauze and four layers of sheet wadding or cellucotton. (3) Bandage in place directly on the ulcer a good grade rubber bath sponge (firmest possible) that is 1 inch larger than the ulcerating area, using a plain 3-inch gauze bandage and being careful that the whole does not slip to one side. (4) Apply a 4-inch Ace bandage from just below the knee to the toes, over the sponge and dressing, applying it as a double figure-of-8 about the foot and ankle. (5) Convince the patient of the absolute necessity of walking as much as possible. (6) The dressings are to be changed as often as necessary to prevent saturation. "Every two days is preferred. The rubber sponge can be boiled up and used again when soiled, but should be discarded as soon as it has lost its 'kick' and has become firmly pressed together." After healing, the subsequent treatment is practically the same as in the method of Wright (see above).

The Unna Paste Boot.—This dressing, several times referred to above, is made and applied as follows: (*a*) Mix 100 Gm. of gelatin into 400 cc. of water and allow to stand overnight; then bring to boil and add 100 Gm. of zinc oxide and 400 cc. of glycerin which have been previously rubbed together to smoothness; boil while stirring for fifteen minutes. (*b*) Cool to a bearable temperature, or heat to same if the paste has already hardened, and paint with a wide camel's hair brush over the ulcerated area, which, together with the leg, should have been thoroughly cleaned first, the latter shaved also. Now apply a spiral bandage and a second coat of paste and repeat until the desired rigidity is attained. The entire space from ankle to knee is usually covered. In the older type of treatment, when the secretion began to seep through, a window was cut over the ulcer and antiseptic and cleansing applications made directly to the raw surface, the leg being held fairly stiffly encased in the paste boot; now, as described above, the Unna dressing is more often applied on the dry surface after healing of the ulcer. When wet dressings are being applied, the boot is usually changed every two weeks, every three weeks at least.

ESSENTIAL HYPERTENSION

(Hyperpiesis; Hypertensive Cardiovascular-renal Disease)

Permanent elevation of the blood pressure without known cause is a disease of high incidence and great seriousness. Recent studies of a number of independent investigators have shown that it is present in about 1.6 per cent of the population in the United States and Canada, a figure which is probably too high to hold for England and the Continent, since the reflection of the thought of European physicians in the literature does not show them preoccupied with the disease; the incidence in other parts of the world is not accurately known to me, but the assumption of rarity in China, India and tropical lands everywhere is probably gratuitous, since a number of physicians have taken kindly exception to a statement to that effect in the first edition of this book, informing me that they see numerous cases in these countries. The matter is ripe for investigation, all the more in that the result of statistical studies might help to disabuse us of the notion, whose validity is far from proved, that it is the kind of life we lead in America that causes the disease. Here with us hypertension ranks with tuberculosis and cancer as causes of death, the actual exitus being due to apoplexy, heart failure and nephritis, probably in that order.

The symptoms which bring the patient—usually between forty and fifty, as likely, perhaps, to be a man as a woman, often obese—to the physician, and thus lead to discovery of the high blood pressure, are usually disturbances in kidney function, cardiac and respiratory complaints, vertigo, dyspepsia, bleeding from the mucous membranes, loss of weight, retinal hemorrhage, persistent morning headaches, unusual drowsiness, and transient palsies and aphasia. The height of the systolic pressure varies greatly; it may be only 160 or it may rise above 300. Of course the height of the diastolic rise depends upon the state of the heart and vessels, hypertrophy and arteriosclerosis being usually early complications of the malady, but the impression that a constant diastolic pressure of 120 is not compatible with more than two years of life is contradicted by many records. Indeed, it seems high time to reinvestigate the disease in the light of the new and promising assumption that the changes in the finer vessels are caused by, and are not themselves the cause of, the hypertension. Let us begin just a little to twitch about under the mantel of *exclusive* cellular pathology thrown over us by Virchow. May this not be essentially a disorder of general metabolism, or an endocrine disturbance—we do not yet know *all* there is to be learned of these humoral affairs. Ayman's investigations of the earlier phases of the disease cannot be too warmly supported; already he is willing to speak tentatively of psychic disturbances before the onset of circulatory symptoms. And is not the hereditary tendency already granted? Murphy, Grill *et al.* have shown that the histologic quite like the clinical manifestations in "malignant" cases differ from those of ordinary cases in degree only.

THERAPY

The best opinion at present, since the etiologic position of chronic interstitial nephritis has been overthrown, is that hypertension is merely a symptom without a known uniform causation. Therefore treatment of this serious malady must remain entirely unsatisfactory until the various causes of the rise in pressure are elucidated. The measures to be described below are designed to lower pressure solely in an attempt to prevent the deadly sequelae of a maintained hypertension—heart failure, apoplectic stroke, kidney dysfunction. Ayman's (1931) studies are showing the ease with which successful therapeutic reduction of blood pressure may be simulated by many factors operating on the extreme lability of blood pressure and the excessive reactivity which characterizes the hypertensive personality. He requires persistent systolic drops of at least 30 mm. as a criterion for therapeutic effect even in studies in which all the controllable factors are well in hand. Perhaps it is well to point out also that no treatment is often the best treatment, at least for awhile, *i. e.*, some patients will only be made unnecessarily miserable instead of being helped if it is hinted to them at all that their blood pressure is high.

Rest.—I quote Mosenthal:

"The best available means at the present moment to reduce the blood pressure in essential hypertension is to obtain nervous relaxation in the patient. This is glibly said but hard to accomplish, for it means untold effort on the physician's part and limitless cooperation by the patient. Occupation, home life, social obligations and many other factors must be studied and their rough corners rounded off. . . . The regulation of occupation, family relations and other personal affairs must remain an individual matter. It is a good plan to have the patient visit the office once a week and talk over such topics for a few minutes. Eventually a way out may suggest itself.

"A good routine of relaxation is one or two hours' rest after lunch and at least eight hours in bed at night. In severe cases, one day a week in bed may be recommended. At times, more or less prolonged rest in bed may be of value.

"It is gradually becoming appreciated that exercise within the limits of cardiac power is beneficial. Apparently sedentary individuals are more subject to hypertension than physically active persons. The late Theodore C. Janeway found that even strenuous physical exertion, such as tennis, was helpful in younger persons. Moderate exercise as walking, golfing or restricted setting-up calisthenics serve to keep the voluntary and cardiac muscles in better condition and promote more satisfactory well-being than if a more sheltered regimen is pursued."

All else is of quite secondary importance compared with the necessity to accomplish nervous relaxation in the patient. If this cannot be accomplished without drugs, there should be no hesitation in employing the sedatives. Sodium or potassium bromide, 10 to 20 grains (0.65 to 1.3 Gm.), or barbital (veronal), 1 to 2 grains (0.13 to 0.26 Gm.) may be given two or three times daily for their general quieting effect; phenobarbital (luminal), ½ to 1½ grains (0.03 to 0.1 Gm.), may also be used two or three times daily, but disagreeable symptoms are more liable to appear than in the use of the other two drugs. Or if the patient requires no sedatives during the day but cannot sleep soundly for eight hours at night, full doses of barbital, 7½ to 10 grains (0.5 to 0.65 Gm.), or chloral hydrate, 20 to 30 grains (1.3 to 2 Gm.) if given alone, or 10 to 20 grains (0.65 to 1.3 Gm.) if combined with 10 grains (0.65 Gm.) of sodium bromide, may be employed upon retiring. Experience teaches that the best effects are obtained by the alternation of sedative drugs.

Diet.—All the dietary restriction that the hypertensive patient needs is in quantity if he is obese or if there is a gobbling fulsome tendency in his family; for every bit of evidence in favor of any particular *qualitative* change in diet it is possible to find a sufficient amount of recorded contrary evidence to invalidate the whole contention. The entire subject of food, fluid and salt intake has been discussed in the chapter on Nephritis and cannot be repeated here.

Cathartics.—Alvarez, McCalla and Zimmerman (1926) have demonstrated conclusively that constipation has no effect on blood pressure in men, and that in women it is associated with lowered pressure; findings which should dispose once and for all of the "intestinal auto-intoxication" myth. This statement is not to be taken to mean that routine use of cathartics is to be deplored in the treatment of hypertension; by no means, for constipation, with its attendant straining at stool, is one of the arch enemies of these individuals. See the treatment of this condition, page 432.

Bleeding.—On this point I quote from Elliot's (1927) excellent review: "Bleeding is an ancient therapeutic measure in this condition now generally discredited. Perhaps the condemnation of the practice has been unwarrantably severe. Purely as a matter of personal experience, I would regret to abandon it entirely in high blood pressure. In the plethoric individual with threatened heart failure of the type known as 'high blood pressure stasis,' a good bleeding will sometimes postpone the breakdown. In the presence of apoplexy prodromes, venesection may serve to tide over the crisis. The reduction of pressure, especially diastolic pressure, resulting from a free abstraction of blood may last for several days. In addition to its emergency use, there is something to be said for the employment of

36

venesection repeatedly carried out to a moderate depletion at appropriate intervals in plethoric cases. This applies particularly to individuals with blood counts above normal. These cases have been designated 'polycythemia hypertonica' by Giesböck and may be identified by their ruddy apoplectic appearance and blood count over 5,000,000."

Iodides.—Sodium or potassium iodide, 5 to 15 grains (0.32 to 1 Gm.) three times daily, are employed by many physicians in all cases even though there is no evidence of a syphilitic involvement. I think we have very little scientific warrant for this sort of routine "alterative" medication, though the statement, "it can't do any harm," is probably a true one. And in many cases it seems to accomplish much good! Intravenous administration is unjustified.

Digitalis.—When heart failure threatens or occurs it should be treated just as at any other time. The additional practice has arisen in the last few years of attempting to forestall the cardiac catastrophe by placing the patient on digitalis before the heart shows signs of failing; full digitalization is not attempted usually, the patient being placed on maintenance doses after a short period of somewhat higher dosage in the beginning. The reader is referred to the discussion of heart failure which begins on page 528.

Vasodilators.—The number of careful students of this disease who are beginning to oppose the use of all vasodilator measures in treatment seems to be slowly growing. However, like it or not, the practically universal employment of drugs of this class is a fact which must be faced; it is a rare case, indeed, of this malady in which they are not at some time administered. And, as a matter of fact, I believe their use to be quite justified: not as a routine, to be sure, for such use will often cause a nitrite to be administered when digitalis is really the drug indicated, and not in advanced cases certainly, when they do very little good anyway; but if the periodic use of these remedies can bring about a temporary amelioration of symptoms in early cases, especially a lessening of headache, nervousness, tingling and dizziness, which often outlast the lowering of the blood pressure, and if these effects can be obtained without danger to the patient—as they can—why, then, should the use of drugs of this class be discountenanced? No one any longer believes them to be of the least curative value, but while results can be obtained with them, which is not for very long in any case, they are nearly always quite powerful as palliatives.

(a) *Nitrites.*—Erythrol tetranitrate and mannitol hexanitrate are the longest lasting in their effect upon the blood pressure and are therefore to be preferred. The former salt is obtainable in ¼- and ½-grain (0.015 and 0.03 Gm.) tablets; the effective dose is ½ to 1 grain (0.03 to 0.06 Gm.) every four to six hours or as indicated. The mannitol salt is not always easily obtainable in America, but in England it appears on the market in ¼-, ½- and 1-grain (0.015, 0.03 and 0.06 Gm.) tablets; it has the same dosage as the erythrol. Both these preparations are quite expensive.

Sodium nitrite is second in point of duration of effect to the above two salts, but it has the disadvantage of causing gastric disturbances in most individuals. It is given in capsule in a dose of 2 to 3 grains (0.13 to 0.2 Gm.), often combined with an equal amount of sodium or potassium iodide, at intervals to be determined in each case.

Nitroglycerin is the least durable in its effect upon the blood pressure, but it is the preparation often preferred for the following reasons: It does not usually disturb digestion; it may be conveniently prescribed in the form of hypodermic tablets of ¹⁄₁₀₀ grain (0.00065 Gm.), which are not volatile, do not quickly deteriorate, and may be easily dissolved under the tongue. The dose is one or more tablets as required. The drug is much cheaper than the erythrol or mannitol salts.

Amyl nitrite is very little used in the treatment of hypertension because of the brief duration of its effect.

Stieglitz (1930), believing that the nitrate radical of bismuth subnitrate is liberated as the nitrite radical by bacterial action in the intestine, and that the latter is then slowly and evenly absorbed to produce hypotensive action, has suggested the administration of bismuth subnitrate as in the treatment of diarrhea. During the five years preceding his report he had used the drug, in doses of 10 grains (0.6 Gm.) three times daily in capsules, in 200 cases with highly satisfactory results. Wilson's (1932) experimental studies have to some extent established the probability of the allegedly even absorption taking place and Bruen (1932) has shown that effective blood pressure reduction takes place in normal persons, but Ayman (1932), in a group of 15 carefully studied and controlled patients, has been unable to repeat the success of Stieglitz in even a single case though he continued treatment for from three to nine months. However, Stieglitz (1932) has pointed out that the drug is useless in the presence of extensive arteriolar sclerosis, which he believes accounts for Ayman's failure. The latter observer also reported some type of upset apparently due to the drug in three of his patients, but in Stieglitz's series (400 cases at the time of the last report) no toxic manifestations have been observed.

(b) *Sulphocyanates* (*Thiocyanates*).—The use of sulphocyanate to reduce blood pressure was described by Pauli in the early years of the present century, but the disagreeable symptoms attending the employment of his large doses caused the drug to be neglected until revived by Westphal, in 1924. The chemical and pharmacological properties of sulphocyanate are distinct from the hydrocyanic acid group with which its name would seem to connect it. Its effect upon the blood pressure is generally found to be slower but more lasting than that of the nitrites. Among those who have found the drug useful upon the basis of resultant hypotension and relief of symptoms are Smith and Rudolf (1928), Gager (1928), Palmer, Silver and White (1929), Fineberg (1930), Goldring and Chasis (1931), and Palmer (1932). The drug may be given in a dose of 1½ grains (0.1 Gm.) three times daily, though both Fineberg, and Goldring and Chasis, were successful only with 5-grain (0.3 Gm.) doses; the former gave the drug continuously for three months. Any vehicle is acceptable; the incompatibilities are quinine bisulphate, tincture ferric chloride, syrup ferrous iodide, spirits of ethyl nitrite. However, only 2 of the 25 patients of Egloff *et al.* (1931) reacted favorably—"and even in these two the reaction was not particularly striking." The dosage was 15 grains daily the first week, 10 grains daily the second and 5 grains daily the third week. Ayman's (1931) conclusion from an exhaustive review is that there is no clear evidence in the literature to show that the sulphocyanates have any value except in the early functional stages of the disease. Occasional toxic results, such as uncomfortable weakness, anginal symptoms, exfoliative dermatitis and coryza, have been reported following the small doses; the larger doses are extremely likely to produce all of these symptoms in an aggravated form and in addition a toxic psychosis. This latter seems to be quite regularly preceded by a stage of weakness, so that this may perhaps be looked upon with relative safety as a warning sign to reduce or omit the drug for awhile. Severe kidney damage is thought to increase the liability to intolerance but other contraindications have not been definitely worked out. It would certainly be the part of wisdom to omit using the drug in a patient who has anginal symptoms.

Cucurbocitrin.—Following Barksdale's (1926) experimental study of watermelon seed extract (cucurbocitrin), Althausen and Kerr (1929) reported a series of 40 patients that responded favorably to treatment with the drug. Seward (1932) and a few others have also reported successes in a goodly proportion of their cases. Of Seward's patients, 11 took 300 to 400 mg. daily (in capsules of 50 mg. "Citrin") and 12 took 600 to 800 mg. A reduction of $\frac{30}{10}$ mg. mercury was obtained, plus symptomatic relief, in 9 patients after a period of twelve days to two months—certainly a doubtful result in so variable a disease. Response to second and third courses was quicker. Basing the evaluation of their data on Ayman's criteria for therapeutic effect in this disease, Gargill and Rudy (1931) were not convinced that the drug had any value in their series of 29 patients.

Muscle Extracts ("Circulatory Hormone").—See page 548, in the section on Angina Pectoris.

Hyperventilation.—Starling was the first to demonstrate and clearly recognize the tremendous "depot" or blood-storage capacity of the capillary bed in the lungs, but he really underestimated the full capacity, which Blumgart and Weiss (1928) showed to be about 21 per cent of the total circulating blood volume. Hyperventilation—pulmonary distention—will of course increase the size of this storage bed, and as it also apparently retards the return of blood to the left side of the heart and therefore lessens the quantity of blood passing into the aorta with each systole, it is theoretically correct to assume that, other things being equal, hyperventilation could reduce systemic blood pressure. As a matter of fact such reduction is easily demonstrable in the laboratory using animals and has also been shown by Vincent and Thompson (1928) to occur to the extent of a 25 per cent drop in normal human beings. Rappaport (1929) has made clinical application of these facts in hypertension, employing deep-breathing exercises with good effects in a small number of cases. The patient is taught very slowly and gradually to fully expand his lungs and is then requested to do so four to six times daily for a period varying in individual cases— in the beginning not to exceed five to seven minutes, however, Rappaport particularly warned against having these exercises performed in anything but the quietest manner—"breathing exercises that make the patient work are doomed to failure." Recently, in Kief, Berljand and Weinstein (1931) administered oxygen daily, for fifteen to twenty minutes as in pneumonia, for ten to fourteen days, to a group of 25 patients and obtained quite considerable reductions in blood pressure by the end of the period in 23 of the individuals. These observations are perhaps not yet of practical value but are recorded here as a rational attempt at physiologic therapeutics which certainly is worthy of further trial, especially the simple method of Rappaport. Of course bearing in mind the hyperreactive personality of the hypertensive, he will probably vitiate the chance of good effects by his manner of approach to these exercises if he is allowed to know that they are directly designed to lower his blood pressure.

Treatment of the Apoplectic Stroke.—During the period of bleeding, the application of an ice-bag to the head and the placing of the feet in a warm mustard bath are time-honored remedies. It is the usual practice to raise the head and lower the feet. The attempt to reduce blood pressure and decrease the hemorrhage by venesection is now discountenanced.

After recovery from the acute attack, potassium iodide in large doses (beginning with 5 grains (0.32 Gm.) three times daily and increasing to as much as the patient can tolerate) is employed in the attempt to promote resolution of the clot; but this medication must not be begun until several weeks after the hemorrhage.

Stimulants of whatever sort are contraindicated during the acute stage, but later the use of $\frac{1}{40}$ grain (0.0015 Gm.) of strychnine sulphate several times daily is thought to aid in maintaining the muscle tone; massage, passive exercises and electrical applications are, of course, also indicated.

ARTERIOSCLEROSIS

Arteriosclerosis is a disease characterized by hyperplastic, hypertrophic, fibrotic, calcareous, and necrotic changes in the vessel walls, resulting ultimately in diminution of the normal elasticity plus weakening and deformity. The etiology of the condition has been well stated by Mosenthal: "A summary of the many causes that have been detailed thus far (advancing years, dietary excesses, nervous strain, muscular exertion, tobacco, alcohol, various poisons, chronic and infectious diseases) reveals a long list of habits and events of which every living human being is to some extent at least a victim. These are the external influences that assail us. Men being more exposed to them than women, it is only natural that arteriosclerosis is much more prevalent in the former than in the latter." That a definite hereditary factor is responsible for the development of this condition in some individuals much earlier than in others living under the same stress and strain is beginning to be tentatively stated.

The statement that "a man is as old as his arteries" may serve for lay opinion but it is not a strict expression of medical truth, for we not infrequently encounter a young, middle-aged or elderly individual with tortuous and quite "hard" arteries who is in excellent general condition. This is not to deny, of course, that in many cases there is a gradual loss in mental and physical vigor. In most cases the blood pressure is not raised, but when it is, that is to say, when essential hypertension and arteriosclerosis are coexistent, then the prognosis is much more grave. The following is the order of frequency with which most investigators have found the organs to be affected, those organs most frequently affected being also most markedly affected: spleen, brain, kidneys, adrenals, pancreas, heart, gastro-intestinal tract, lungs, liver and diaphragm. Localized arteriosclerosis is of course usually a much more serious affair than the general form.

The great anatomist Scarpa (1747–1832) was the first to record the opinion that arteriosclerosis is a disease of the inner coats of the arteries.

THERAPY

The treatment of localized arteriosclerosis is really the treatment of chronic nephritis, or of cardiac failure, or of essential hypertension. For the victims of generalized arteriosclerosis who suffer gradual mental and physical deterioration there is nothing to do save to direct their lives in as pleasant channels as possible; nor can one write much of an edifying nature about the prevention of the condition. To avoid the competitive hurly-burly of life as much as possible, to avoid too quick returns to full activity after attacks of the acute diseases, to submit to the fullest treatment for the chronic affections, and to select one's parents as carefully as may be, are all measures of presumptive value.

DISTURBANCES OF THE THYROID GLAND

CRETINISM

Cretinism is an affection originating during fetal life or in infancy, characterized by retarded mental and physical development, and due to the absence or more or less complete atrophy of the thyroid gland. Practically nothing is known of the cause of this abnormality. It occurs all over the world but is most prevalent in goitrous regions, though, curiously enough, it is relatively rare in North America; however, with regard to this last point, Stoddard's (1933) recent study indicates that in Wisconsin, and by inference in other Great Lakes regions and in the Pacific Northwest, the condition of endemic cretinism is probably quite imminent. Among preserved records the first reference to cretinism is that of Paracelsus, in the sixteenth century, though it was doubtless very prevalent long before that.

Most patients do not come under observation until they are six to eight months old because failure to develop normally is not often noticed before that age. In typical cases the general appearance is characteristic, regardless of the child's age. The hair is dry, coarse and usually scanty; the face is broad, with a wide flat nose, thick lips, protruding tongue and heavy jaw; the fontanels remain open, the forehead is low, the abdomen is large, and there is often an umbilical hernia; bony growth is delayed, but the hands and feet are large and the toes and fingers short and thick; dentition is delayed, the temperature is subnormal, the skin is dry, and the tissues have a doughy feeling but do not pit upon pressure. Constipation is the rule. Cretinous individuals are undersized physically and very much stunted mentally. Their characteristic response to questioning is a wrinkling grin, and their ultimate mental development is usually into a clownish sort of childishness in which they seem very happy; any type of idiocy, however, may be seen. The state of untreated cretinism is not incompatible with the attainment of full years, but most victims of the affection succumb fairly early to one of the infectious diseases.

THERAPY

The response of cretins to the administration of desiccated thyroid substance (*nota bene:* this substance is *not* an extract, therefore the term "thyroid extract" is not permissible; see also the note regarding differences in brands on p. 569) is well known to everyone. Osler has written: "Not the magic wand of Prospero or the brave kiss of the daughter of Hippocrates ever effected such a change." And truly written, for the change is as rapid as it is remarkable. One needs but to start with a small dose, build it up as tolerance and necessity dictate, and then watch during the brief space required for the conversion of an imbecile into a rational being. Regarding dosage, Kerley writes from his wide experience: "The required thyroid dosage is very readily learned; the child adjusts itself to the amount it requires. We usually begin with about ¼ grain twice a day, and then increase as necessary until we get results; overdosage is followed by perspiration, irritability, and bed-wetting. However, having thus sung the praises of one of our most prized specifics, the plague of meticulousness that is upon me compels the admission that most of the contributions on cretinism in the literature relate solely to the spectacular change wrought by the drug in infancy. Few cases are followed through for the rest of their lives, and such as are, present few evidences of a complete recreation of the mentality. Therefore, in presenting three of Kerley's case reports below, I have several objects in view: First, to demonstrate the progress which may be expected in these cases; second, to indicate the dosage required, and, third, to show the end-results which may be hoped for.

"Case 1.—I. H., female, age twenty-four years, height 62 inches, weight 130 pounds. Absence of thyroid gland. Physically robust, is good at housework, can write her name but cannot compose a letter, can sew well, has no appreciation of mathematics, cannot add a column of figures, multiply or divide, enjoys moving pictures. Not interested in boys, never reads newspaper, is interested only in the comic section. Apparent mental age about ten years. Taking 10 grains of desiccated thyroid daily. Came under observation at the age of three years and was still nursed by the mother, weight 15 pounds But two lower incisor teeth had been cut, very stupid, played with a rattle, showed no interest in surroundings, unable to sit unsupported, could support the head after the second year. General physical appearance typically cretin. Given 1 grain of desiccated thyroid daily. After ten months of treatment attempted to talk. When four years old she required 2½ grains daily. At ten years of age the height was 47½ inches, weight 44½ pounds. At this time she was taking 6½ grains of desiccated thyroid daily.

"Case 2.—E. L., female, age twenty-five years, weight 139 pounds, height 62⅜ inches. Absence of thyroid gland. She is competent at housework and handwork, no appreciation of mathematics, never reads newspaper, inclined to be antisocial. Has no girl friends. Interested in opposite sex. For past eight years she has worked in a leather factory, salary $15.00 a week. Unable to take a promotion. Reads and writes well, but cannot compose a letter. Spelling is good but when writing a letter inserts words which have no bearing upon the subject. Interested in moving pictures and comic section of newspapers. Always enjoyed good health. Menstruated at fourteen years of age, periods regular. Taking 7½ grains of desiccated thyroid daily. First seen at the age of two months, typical text-book type. Mother refused to have child photographed because of 'awful appearance.' Given 1½ grains of desiccated thyroid daily; usual improvement. First walked at fourteen months; began to talk at the eighteenth month."

A report, in 1931, reviews the dosage in this case: Five years of age, 2½ grains; ten years, 5 grains; fifteen years, 7 grains; twenty years, 9 grains; twenty-four years, 12 grains. After a few months on 12 grains, extreme nervousness caused reduction to 9 grains, which was diminished, still because of nervousness, during next three years to 3 grains at twenty-seven years; thyrotoxicosis symptoms here caused the drug to be withheld for forty-one days, but 2-grain dosage was resumed on reappearance of myxedematous symptoms; at thirty-one years, 2½ grains.

"Case 3.—H. F., female, age twenty-two years, weight 104 pounds, height 63 inches. Absence of thyroid gland. Attended school until seventeenth year; at this time she was in the seventh grade, usually attained by girls in the twelfth year. Is particularly clever at playing the piano from memory. Musical instruction by professional teacher a failure. Has social tendencies but appreciates her defects and is resentful. Is particularly good at housework, takes entire charge of two rooms in the family apartment, cannot compose a letter without assistance. Penmanship very poor, is moody, cries readily, particularly deficient in mathematics, takes telephone messages correctly, if not too long. First menstruated at fourteen and a half years. Is fond of opposite sex. No interest in newspapers. Memory is excellent. Taking 2½ grains of desiccated thyroid daily. Came under observation at the fifth month, weight 9 pounds, text-book case. Prompt response to desiccated thyroid, 1 grain daily. Smiled at six months, walked at fourth year. Formed sentences at the fifth year."

MYXEDEMA AND HYPOTHYROIDISM

Spontaneous myxedema is a chronic affection associated with a gradual fibrosis and atrophy of the acini of the thyroid gland, and characterized by impaired mentality, overgrowth of fat and connective tissue, and pronounced change in appearance. The disease occurs all over the world, but is most frequent in goitrous regions. It is usually a disease of women at about the time of the menopause, but approximately one eighth of the cases occur in men and a very small number in children. Of the cause of the thyroid shrinkage practically nothing is known; it is said that the disease has a familial tendency.

In the usual case of myxedema the first symptom is a gradually increasing mental sluggishness combined with a feeling of bodily weariness which is not appeased by any amount of resting. The face assumes a coarsened, masklike expression, with often a transverse furrow across the forehead and an area of brownish pigmentation over the cheeks. The skin is dry and scaly and the hair falls out. The false edematous deposits, which do not pit upon pressure, occur in all the subcutaneous tissues, making it appear as though the patient has stored up much fat; the extremities are chiefly affected, however. The temperature is below normal, there is a secondary anemia and a reduction in pulse rate and basal metabolism, and the patient complains of constipation, unusual sensitiveness to cold, and pains in the muscles and joints. The occurrence of "myxedema heart" as a typical entity is not agreed to by all observers: Marked enlargement, slow feeble beat, insufficiency absent or present—all resisting digitalis but clearing up promptly under thyroid therapy. In recent years evidence has been accumulating to show that these patients are unusually prone to arteriosclerosis, chronic nephritis, and arthritis, fibrous myocarditis and coronary sclerosis, but since the age of onset of all of these conditions coincides closely with that of myxedema, it is going to require very careful work to establish the interrelationship. Cardiac enlargement, associated with hypothyroidism and disappearing under thyroid therapy, has been reported a number of times and has given rise to the phrase "myxedema heart."

In recent years a number of observers have been calling attention to the probable frequency with which individuals are relegated to the scrapheap of "neurasthenia" when they are suffering from a mild hypothyroidism in which the full myxedematous picture never develops. Such patients may show one or more or none of the classical symptoms of real myxedema, but it is astonishing how many other symptoms not usually associated in a diagnostic connection with thyroid dysfunction will clear up on specific treatment. For instance they may be underweight, not sensitive to cold or suffering from a marked dryness of skin; indeed they may not even feel mentally sluggish, though they nearly always grow inordinately tired by the end of the day. Menstrual disturbances, rheumatic or abdominal pains may bring them under observation. Warfield (1930) considers that a basal metabolic rate which is consistently no lower than minus 10 per cent is justification for the tentative diagnosis and therapeutic test in these cases. However, it is worthy of note that in the carefully studied series of Thurman and Thompson (1930), 11 of 196 patients with basal rates of 11 to 45 per cent below average normal (in only 8 was it lower than minus 25 per cent) were found to be clinically normal, 172 were suffering from various pathologic conditions not helped by thyroid therapy, and only 13 appeared to be really in a state of "hypothyroidism without myxedema" as evidenced by marked improvement under thyroid-substance therapy. They concluded that if the depression in basal rate is less than 21 per cent below the average normal, underfunction of the thyroid is usually not present.

THERAPY

In the summer of 1891, Murray described before the British Medical Association the first case of myxedema ever treated by the administration of the thyroid gland of the sheep. His patient, a woman of forty-six, regained good health and lived to be seventy-four, dying in 1919 of heart disease. Since the reporting of this classic case, many thousands of patients have been thus treated and cured, and it has now become apparent that such failures to restore the patient to complete health as do occur are due to one or more of the following factors: (*a*) The use of a nonpotent specimen of the drug. The U.S.P. desiccated thyroid substance is described as the thyroid glands of animals which are used for food by man, freed of connective tissue and fat, dried and powdered and containing no less than 0.17 per cent nor more than 0.22 per cent of iodine in thyroid combination. However, Hunt (recently corroborated by Means, 1933) has shown that there may be a great variation in the strength of the drug as prepared by different manufacturers, a fact which certainly places the practitioner with his occasional case of this disease in a quandary. The only solution of this difficulty so far suggested is to determine the dosage with a particular preparation solely upon the basis of therapeutic results. The isolated thyroxin has not sufficient advantages over the desiccated substance to justify its greater expensiveness. (*b*) The beginning of treatment too late in the disease. It is the exceptional case of far-advanced myxedema that completely recovers under even the most careful treatment. (*c*) Lack of cooperation upon the part of the patient. After a considerable degree of recovery has taken place very many individuals refuse to continue with the proper dosage required to complete and maintain their cure. (*d*) The careless taking of overdoses by patients, who, having once experienced the resultant thyrotoxic symptoms, are evermore reluctant to take sufficient doses to maintain them in a normal condition.

It is the universal practice to administer the thyroid substance in two stages: (1) The initial dosage, designed to restore the patient to a normal level of metabolism, and (2) the maintenance dosage, which is the smallest amount necessary to keep the metabolism within normal limits.

Initial Thyroid Dosage.—The patient is best put to bed, or at least required to spend much of the time in bed during the initial stage of treatment. In Sturgis and Whiting's (1925) study the patient was weighed at the beginning, given 2 grains (0.12 Gm.) of thyroid substance three times daily for five days, and the pulse counted each morning by herself or some member of the family at rising time. In this way a check on the basal pulse rate is obtained with the elimination of such factors as the influence of food and muscular activity. At the end of five days the patient is to be weighed again and if only 2 or 3 pounds (0.9 or 1.4 Kg.) have been lost, and the pulse rate is not above 80 and there are no signs of overaction, such as palpitation, dyspnea, excessive warmth, dizziness or nausea, administration may continue until a normal pulse rate is obtained or such toxic symptoms appear.

Maintenance Thyroid Dosage.—The object in this stage of the treatment is to determine, by reducing the dosage, just how much will be required to keep the patient normal, trying at first to maintain this state on 2 grains (0.12 Gm.) daily. Once the correct dosage is determined it is likely that the patient will have to continue employing it with slight variations through the remainder of her life; few recoveries have been recorded. In the experience of Sturgis and Whiting with 25 patients, it was found that 14 required 2 grains daily; 6, 3 grains; 2, 1 grain; and 3, 1½ grains. "Occasionally a patient has taken as much as 6 grains as a maintenance dose for a short period, but this amount has invariably produced symptoms of overdosage if continued for any length of time." These observers strongly advise hospitalization in the beginning so that therapy may be frequently checked by basal metabolic determinations. In their experience these patients are about in a condition normal for them when their rate is minus 5 or 10 per cent. They find also that the initial weight loss as a consequence of the disappearance of the nonpitting edema is usually made, with 5 to 10 pounds additional, as a result of the improvement in general nutrition.

Thyroid Dosage in Hypothyroidism without Myxedema.—The dosage here is about the same as in true myxedema. Warfield's patients are taking 3 to 5 grains daily; he usually begins with 2 to 4 grains and checks the metabolic rate after ten to fourteen days, being satisfied also with a minus 10 reading. "It is not the figure of the basal metabolic rate but the well-being of the patient which is the criterion for dosage."

Auxiliary Therapy.—The eruptions or other reactions which sometimes accompany thyroid therapy in the beginning can at times be avoided by the simultaneous administration of small doses of the solution of potassium arsenite (Fowler's solution). Where there is an extreme degree of idiosyncrasy, desensitization must be attempted with minute doses—$\frac{1}{1000}$ grain daily to begin with and gradually increasing after a few days. Where this is not practicable, the thyroid substance will have to be given intermittently in as large doses as can be tolerated. Koehler (1927) has pointed out the occasional paradoxical necessity for the use of sedatives in the initial stage; particularly in the nervously unstable type of individual; barbiturates serve well here. Christian (1925) warns of the especial need of digitalis in cases complicated by cardiac insufficiency, for as the myxedematous condition improves more work is demanded of the heart; anemia too should be corrected.

SIMPLE GOITER

Simple goiter is a diffuse, symmetrical, noninflammatory enlargement of the thyroid gland which is caused by the distention of its alveoli by an excessive deposit of colloid. Since the earliest times the view has probably been held that the incidence of this affection is in some way associated with the water supply. The Chinese of fifteen centuries B. C., as well as the Greeks and Romans of the western Classical Age, have left attestations of this belief, and relatively recently "discovered" races, such as the natives of interior Africa and the American Indians, were also convinced of the relationship. However, it remained for the Swiss, Grange, to first propose the hypothesis that it is an insufficiency of iodine in food and water that is the causative factor. His observations were made in 1840, at which time, due to his efforts and especially those of Chatin in France, iodine prophylaxis was attempted in Switzerland, France and Italy. The present theory of the association of iodine starvation and colloid goiter is due to the painstaking researches of Marine and his associates and really constitutes a "new" discovery, for the work done during the middle of the last century had long since been forgotten. That goiter is most prevalent in regions where the water, soil or indigenous vegetables, cereals, fruits and milk are poorest in iodine, is now generally recognized. In Asia and Continental Europe these regions correspond to the Himalayan and Alpine mountain ranges, in England to the valley of the Thames and Derbyshire, in South America to the Andes plateau, and in North America to the region about the Great Lakes and the St. Lawrence River, and the Cascade mountain region of Oregon, Washington and British Columbia, with less important foci in the Rocky Mountain states and those of the upper Mississippi valley. That residence near the sea is in itself a safeguard against the development of the disease, as would seem to be indicated by the relative infrequency of its occurrence along the Atlantic seaboard of the United States, is disproved by the fact of its great prevalence on the northern Pacific coast and also in New Zealand, in which latter country most of the habitations are coastal and none more than 100 miles inland. In accepting this relationship of iodine starvation to goiter it is necessary, however, to go a step further and postulate that the disease develops only in those in whom some other as yet unknown factor or factors are operating, for it would otherwise be impossible to account for the escape of many individuals in goitrous regions and the appearance of sporadic cases in nongoitrous regions. The work of McCarrison with goitrogenic diets, and particularly his demonstration of certain positive goiter-producing substances present in cabbage, ground-nut, bran and maize, and possibly in certain other cereals, marks a great advance in knowledge. Webster has shown that the iodine content is of no importance here and that the active agent in cabbage is thermostabile and water-insoluble. According to Marine (1932) it is probably of cyanide nature. Suk (1932) has apparently shown rather definitely the importance of cabbage as an etiologic agent in the diet of certain Carpathian highlanders in Ruthenia. Further developments along this new investigative line are awaited with great interest.

Simple goiter develops most frequently at the age of puberty and is more frequent in girls than boys; it also not uncommonly appears in women during pregnancy and lactation. The symptoms it causes are usually few or none, save the psychic disturbances consequent upon the disfigurement. A small proportion of goiters disappear spontaneously but most of them persist to some extent throughout life. When serious symptoms arise they are usually due to the displacement of the larynx and trachea, with disturbance of respiration, or to circulatory disturbances due to pressure upon contiguous nerves.

PROPHYLAXIS

Methods.—At the present time the prophylactic measures employed are the following:

1. The administration of a tablet containing ⅙ grain (0.01 Gm.) of an organic iodine compound once a week throughout the school year (or throughout the duration of pregnancy). Such preparations contained in the 1933 N.N.R. are: Iodocasein, Iodostarine, Stearodine and Oridine.

2. The addition during a period of two or three weeks twice a year of sufficient sodium iodide to the municipal water supply to bring the iodine content up to fifty parts per billion during that time.

3. The use of iodized table salt. The Swiss Goiter Commission advises the addition of 5 mg. of iodide per kilogram of salt; in the United States, the iodized table salts generally contain forty times this much, *i. e.*, about 200 mg. of potassium iodide per kilogram of salt. It is recommended that this salt be used in cooking and at table by all persons throughout the year.

Efficacy of the Methods.—Iodine was first used on a large scale in the prevention of human goiter by Marine and Kimball in the school population of Akron, Ohio, in 1917. Of 2190 school girls who took 30 grains (2 Gm.) of sodium iodide twice a year for three years, only 5 developed goiter, while of 2305 also observed for three years but who did not take iodine, 495 developed goiter. Since the publication of these studies numerous communities in America and Europe have employed the prophylactic use of the element with very satisfactory results. In the table below (Table 50) I have summarized the 1928 report of Kimball on the experiments conducted in the state of Michigan during the period 1924–28.

These figures do not constitute an absolute comparison between the state of affairs in 1924, before any iodine had been taken, and in 1928, after

TABLE 50.—IODINE PROPHYLAXIS OF SIMPLE GOITER IN MICHIGAN (1924–28)

Locality.	Children examined— 1924.	Goiter percentage.	Children examined— 1928.	Goiter percentage.
Midland County...............	3,645	41.6	984*	8.8
Wexford County...............	3,984	55.5	1,553†	17.3
City of Grand Rapids (1923)....	26,215	30.0	39,435	9.0
City of Muskegon..............	7,710	33.3	8,250	10.7
	Total number 41,554	Average percentage 40.1	Total number 50,222	Average percentage 11.4

* City of Midland only.
† City of Cadillac only.

iodine had been taken for four years, for the simple reason that, as pointed out by Kimball, all the children included in the survey were not taking iodine throughout this period—some were not taking it at all and others doubtless in an ineffectual fashion. However, the table does indicate the very great success to be met with in even these large-scale prophylactic experiments with all their shortcomings from the scientific standpoint. It is the belief of those who have watched these surveys that under ideal conditions the incidence of goiter could be reduced to practically nothing.

In a more recent report Kimball (1931) has shown very strikingly the difference in goiter incidence in Detroit, where prophylaxis is officially and routinely practiced, and Cleveland, where these conditions do not obtain (Table 51). In the lower portion of the table is shown the decrease in goiter incidence through the years in Detroit.

TABLE 51.—GOITER INCIDENCE IN CITIES USING AND NOT USING PROPHYLACTIC IODINE

Comparison of Incidence of Goiter in School-children of Detroit and of Cleveland

	Total incidence of goiter in regular schools, 1924 (per cent).	Total incidence of goiter in special schools, 1930–31 (per cent).	Hyperplastic or iodine deficiency goiter in special schools, 1930–31 (per cent).	Number of examinations.
Detroit........	36	12	0.3	5075
Cleveland.....	34	30	18.0	3175

Yearly Report of Incidence of Goiter in Detroit*

	1924.	1926.	1927.	1928.	1929.	1930.	1931.
Incidence of goiter.......	36%	9.7%	7.7%	7.2%	5.2%	3.1%	2.1%
Number of examinations..	3,000†	69,805	78,085	115,535	107,853	141,366	114,969

* From Detroit City Health: School Health Service, Annual Reports, vol. 13–14.
† Approximately.

Regarding the prevention of goiters that develop before birth, Kimball writes as follows: "We are privileged to report here the observations of the physicians of Houghton County doing obstetrics and pediatrics. The report was given by Dr. W. A. Manthei of Lake Linden, who states that before prophylaxis became general it was not at all uncommon to see babies with definite goiters at birth. He and his associates discussed this fact and looked forward with eagerness to see whether the general use of iodized salt, or iodine prescribed throughout pregnancy, would change this condition. To date they have not seen a single case of congenital goiter when the mother has used iodine. From their observations so far the continued use of iodized salt has been found sufficient; yet many prescribe additional iodine during this period, such as 1 grain (0.065 Gm.) of sodium iodide or one or two organic iodine tablets a week." The studies of Hudson (1931) have shown that iodides given to the mother pass through the placenta and are absorbed by the thyroid of the fetus, so that if a child is born of a mother who has received iodides throughout her pregnancy, it is not because of a deficiency of iodine in the fetal thyroid.

Comparison of the Methods.—Perhaps the best plan of them all is the use of the organic iodine tablet once each week throughout the school year, but this plan should be employed only under the supervision of the school physician who will exclude from treatment all children having adenomata of the thyroid. The principal advantage of this tablet over sodium iodide as originally used by Marine and Kimball is that it is easier to get it regularly taken, particularly if chocolate coated.

When iodine is added periodically to the water supply of a city, those who drink this water obtain no more iodine than is habitually taken throughout the year by the inhabitants of regions whose soil and water are relatively rich in iodine. It is not thought that this can be harmful, but, on the other hand, it is very doubtful whether the measure has any very real value in the prophylaxis of goiter.

When the iodized salt method of prophylaxis is used iodine is in effect administered to an entire community in the attempt to prevent the development of simple goiter in children and pregnant women. Objections to this type of campaign are by no means new. Kimball has pointed out that Rilliet of Geneva was the first to stress the possibility of harm from the use of iodized salt, in 1858. He read a paper on this subject before the Academy of Medicine in Paris, in which he described 4 cases typical of what is today commonly called toxic adenoma. These patients had been using potassium iodide in their cooking salt in the proportions of 1 part to 10,000 parts of salt. The relation between the use of iodized salt and the duration of the symptoms was not clearly established by Rilliet. He also described two patients who had left the mountainous region of Geneva and had gone to the seashore, and, breathing the sea air which is heavily laden with iodine (according to the theories of that time), had become as toxic as the two patients who had used the iodized salt. The same year, M. de Boinet wrote a letter to the commissioners of the Academy, Messrs. Chatin and Trousseau, in which he pointed out the fallacies and dangers of Rilliet's deductions from such a small number of cases. He doubted the statement that iodine in the sea air would be sufficient to cause such immediate toxicity, preferring to believe that the condition was already present and brought out by some other factor. Furthermore, he made the point that, in view of the large number of goiters under treatment by Rilliet and his many friends, and in a country where goiter was so prevalent, there should have been more than 2 cases affected by this treatment. However, Rilliet's warning note as to the possible dangers of the use of even small amounts of iodine in the treatment of goiter carried more weight than the deductions of de Boinet, the result being that the entire profession immediately stopped the use of iodized salt.

And now again, since the revival of this method of prophylaxis, papers are appearing emphasizing its dangers. For my own part, I may say that

I am by no means convinced that the advocacy of the general use of iodized salt is entirely wise, since I think that anyone who has had intensive dermatological training will always carry the notion that skin eruptions may be caused in this way. The criticisms based upon the preparation's alleged ability to cause thyrotoxicosis (see Hartsock and Jackson in Bibliography) would seem to be of the same general nature, *i. e.*, they are based largely upon clinical impressions, which, though of very great value, cannot be accepted in lieu of statistical proof in a matter so important as this. Kimball's (1928) studies of large groups of individuals in the state of Michigan certainly unearthed no evidence to the effect that this prophylactic method is dangerous.

"Every adult who had goiter was urged to come in and receive a careful study of his goiter with diagnosis and suggestion for treatment. Also, each physician called up his goiter patients and advised them to come to this study and to bring any friend or neighbor who had a goiter problem. . . . We found it necessary to make four distinct classes and to classify each patient before dismissal.

"Class 1 comprises patients who have used iodized salt alone for a period of from one to four years. Of those in class 1, 88 per cent have used iodized salt continuously for four years and 12 per cent have used it at least one year.

"Class 2 includes those who have used no iodine, or at least none before the development of hyperthyroidism.

"Class 3 consists of those who have used iodized salt continuously but have also used other forms of iodine, such as external applications or compound solution of iodine.

"Class 4 comprises those who took iodine on prescription or otherwise but had never used iodized salt.

"The fact that approximately three fourths of the people of Michigan are using iodized salt forms the basis of an excellent experiment. While studying a group that has used iodized salt for a period of years, we also have a group which purposely or otherwise has not used iodine in any form. All are adults with goiter, many of which are large adenomatous goiters of long standing. . . . A concise summary of the 1229 cases studied is found in the accompanying tabulation (Table 52).

TABLE 52.—IODINE PROPHYLAXIS AND HYPERTHYROIDISM

	Class 1— iodized salt.	Class 2— no iodine in any form.	Class 3— iodized salt plus iodine.	Class 4— iodine but no iodized salt.
Number of cases..............	655	419	114	41
Hyperthyroidism cases..........	27	233	20	8
Hyperthyroidism percentage.....	4.1	55.5	17.5	20.0

"From my observations of all adults with goiter who came for study in three different communities, I feel sure that there is no basis for the statements that iodized salt might induce hyperthyroidism in long-standing goiters. By study and comparison of the 27 cases of hyperthyroidism, or 4.1 per cent of those who had used iodized salt and later developed the disease, with the larger number, 233, or 55.5 per cent of those who had not used iodine yet had developed the same condition, I feel that the etiology of hyperthyroidism lies within the individual. I also feel that these etiologic factors are increased or aggravated by endemic goiter, and by preventing endemic goiter we are thereby preventing, in the future, many cases of hyperthyroidism."

Hartsock, previously referred to as a severe critic of the use of iodized table salt, has stated, in 1932: "No one at the present time sees cases which are very suspicious of this [thyrotoxicosis caused by table salt]. The explanation I do not know, and I am very much confused in my own mind about the whole thing." McClure (1932) has shown that there has been a marked decrease in the number of goiter operations in the Detroit and Ann Arbor areas since the use of the salt began, though the number of operations of all sorts has increased. This same author states that no single case of hyperthyroidism has developed as the result of massive iodide therapy over long periods in the Johns Hopkins Hospital syphilitic clinic, in a series of 6000 patients, and only 1 or 2 cases have come under suspicion among the 3000 patients in the similar clinic at the Henry Ford Hospital.

THERAPY

The treatment of simple goiter by the same methods as are employed in prophylaxis sometimes accomplishes an astonishing diminution or even total disappearance of the enlargement. However, the cases of long-standing goiter that are favorably affected are very few. Up to sixteen or seventeen years of age the response is better; in Marine and Kimball's studies in Akron, Ohio, of 1182 children with goiter at the first examination who took iodine, 773 thyroids decreased in size, while, of 1048 children with goiter at the first examination who did not take iodine, only 145 decreased in size.

ADENOMA

A certain number of goiters are nodular and are therefore, but perhaps erroneously, considered adenomatous. A few of these nodules have the structure of fetal thyroid and are assumed to arise from embryonal cell nests, but the great majority of them seem to be encapsulated masses of adult thyroid tissue. Many observers believe these nodules to represent areas of disorderly growth in response to some unknown stimulus, and that a state of hyperthyroidism can be initiated from such a nodule without diffuse involvement of the gland. However, the studies of Rienhoff, confirmed by both Dunhill and Hertzler, are beginning to influence opinion; studies in which it was shown that the involutional changes occurring in the thyroid glands of patients with exophthalmic goiter who were undergoing remission revealed striking similarities to the histologic picture seen in nodular goiter; Cole and Womack have made the same observation in their experimental production of nodular goiter in dogs. This would make of these nodules neoplasms in no sense of the word, but involutional bodies whose number and size depend upon the number of remissions and exacerbations in the gland. The fact that cases of so-called "toxic adenoma" develop in long-standing cases of so-called "adenomatous goiter" may simply mean that the diagnosis of toxic adenoma is made during a particularly fulminating exacerbation in a gland that has undergone many milder exacerbations and remissions. The fact that exophthalmos is unusual in these cases need not set them apart as a separate type of thyrotoxicosis, for most of the cases develop after the middle thirties, at which time this symptom is also unusual in the nonnodular cases.

THERAPY

Most surgeons believe that all nodular goiters should be removed because of the occasional development of malignancy on a nodular base, or because of the fact that thyrotoxicosis may appear later in life. Foster's comment on this attitude seems to me most excellent: "This appears a radical view in the face of the fact that discrete adenomata are not rarely palpable in the thyroids of elderly persons who had recognized an abnormal 'gland' in their necks years before. Considering the adequate supply of hazards in modern life it seems both conservative and judicious for the family physician to make an occasional examination of a young person with an adenoma of the thyroid, and reserve decision on developments."

The treatment of "toxic adenoma" is identical with that of thyrotoxicosis (see below).

THYROTOXICOSIS

(Exophthalmic Goiter; Graves' Disease; Basedow's Disease)

Thyrotoxicosis is the name given to a peculiar complex of symptoms of which the chief are enlargement of the thyroid gland, an increase in the basal metabolic rate and a decrease in weight and strength, a characteristic nervous syndrome, exophthalmos usually, and a tendency to gastro-intestinal crises of nausea and vomiting. Shirer (1933) has shown that there is a state of hypermotility of the gastro-intestinal tract, the degree of which, however, is no index of the severity of the disease. The classic description of the disease is that of Caleb Parry, in 1786, though the paper of Graves, in 1835, was the first to attract wide attention; Basedow described it again in 1840. Thyrotoxicosis occurs far more often in women than in men and principally between the ages of fifteen and thirty-five. No race is entirely exempt; even in the Negro we have recently been shown (Herrmann, 1932) that the state is not rare. It is believed to be a relatively rare disease throughout the world, but doubtless many mild cases are constantly being mistaken for neurasthenia, psychoneurosis, and cardiac disorders unrelated to thyrotoxicosis. The accepted belief that the disease is more frequent in large cities than in rural districts is not supported by the fact that of 2700 fatal cases in the United States in 1925, 1700 were recorded as rural. Likewise, the opinion that the incidence is highest in goitrous areas is beginning to be shaken.

The patients are usually restless, nervous and irritable long before any other disturbances are noted. The appetite increases during this period and there is not infrequently a gain in weight. When the patient finally visits the physician, however, she usually presents the following signs and symptoms: Loss of weight despite a normal or even increased appetite; rapid pulse rate, usually accompanied by palpitation; a great emotionalism, either of the depressed or exhilarated type, perhaps even with the development of a pronounced psychosis; muscular tremor, especially noticeable in the extended fingers, combined with easy muscular fatigue; complaint of insomnia; excessive sweating and discomfort in warm weather; a basal metabolic rate much above the normal, and not uncommonly glycosuria and hyperglycemia; usually some degree of exophthlamos; and the history of a number of attacks of nausea, vomiting and diarrhea, during which all the symptoms are much aggravated. Considerable thyroid enlargement is the rule and some enlargement is detectable in practically all cases. Hyperplasia of the thyroidal tissue is the most frequent finding at autopsy, but it does not seem that this bears a constant relationship to the clinical symp-tomatology, for this hyperplastic state is compatible with a normal or even myxedematous condition. A gradual increase in lymphoid tissues all over the body and hyperplasia of the thymus gland is found in most thyro-toxicosis autopsies. There are surprisingly many variations from the typical in this disease; Wohl (1932) has particularly directed attention toward cases that successfully masquerade as other entities with little to call attention to the underlying thyrotoxic disturbance, and Lahey (1931) writes of an "apathetic" type which is probably too seldom recognized. Clute (1930) draws the following conclusions regarding this disease and pregnancy from his study of the large material at the Lahey Clinic: (a) With proper treatment pregnancy is not unnaturally terminated in most cases; (b) pregnancy is distinctly an added burden which should be avoided if possible; (c) babies born of thyrotoxic mothers, or of mothers who have had thyroidectomy, are normal; (d) pregnancy does not cause the disease nor does pregnancy after thyroidectomy cause recurrence; (e) thyroidec-tomy can be undertaken during pregnancy with safety to both mother and child.

The etiology of this disease is still unknown, one school of observers holding that the occurrences in the thyroid gland are the primary cause of the abnormal state, the other that thyrotoxicosis is a general constitu-tional disease, perhaps originating in an upset of the autonomic nervous system, of which the thyroid symptoms are only a part. The secondary etiologic rôle of acute or chronic infectious processes, fear, trauma, oper-ative procedures, nervous strain, or acute nervous shock are affirmed and denied with equal fervor and authority. A type of autonomic imbalance, differing from thyrotoxicosis by absence of asthenia, heightened metabolic rate and loss of weight, is usually looked upon as a separate entity.

THERAPY

The nature of this disease is such that most of its victims have their malady diagnosed when it is at its height, the experience of practically all physicians consisting merely in watching its defervescence. Not that active therapeutic procedures are not instituted whenever consent for their employ-ment can be gained, but the effect of any of these measures upon the dura-tion of the disease in the "long run" is certainly open to doubt. "The average duration of hyperthyroidism," says Barker (1924), "associated with diffuse hyperplasia of the whole thyroid gland is probably two or three years, no matter how you treat it (medically, surgically or radiologically). You may, it is true, compel a subsidence of the symptoms by treatment, but rarely a cure until this time has elapsed; moreover, after recovery from an attack, these patients are prone to recurrence later in life." Read (1924) has studied the course of 189 patients, 35 of his own and the remainder from eight other published reports. Eighty-six of these individuals received x-ray treatment, 48 were treated surgically, and 55 were given no specific therapy; but it cannot be assumed of this latter group that, because they were relatively untreated, they were intrinsically mild cases, for, as a matter of fact, most of them were taken from Kessel and Hyman's well-known group containing some very sick individuals. Now the results in all these cases, at least so far as the basal metabolic rate is concerned, were prac-tically the same, regardless of the method of treatment: A marked fall oc-curred from the original high point to a low point which was reached in from four to five months; thereafter, there was again a slight rise for sev-eral months, but not to the original height, another fall, and then again another slight rise at about the sixteenth month; at twenty-four months,

37

the average basal metabolic rate of all patients remaining in the series was plus 10 per cent, practically a normal figure.

I am quite aware that I would seem to be preaching a therapeutic nihilism here, but actually nothing is further from my desire. What I do wish to impress upon the reader is this: No one type of treatment is the ideal for all cases, neither surgery, medicine, nor x-ray; all claim 75 to 80 (occasionally 90) per cent of "cures," thus tacitly admitting a rather large percentage of failures; and no one has as yet compiled a satisfactory review of a series of cases followed for as long as fifteen years. This latter point is very important, for, as Foster says, "a woman may be 'cured' at thirty, still well at forty, and suffer a recrudescence during menopause at forty-five." Hyman and Kessel (1931) state that in persons under thirty-five years of age the spontaneous course is toward recovery in from 60 to 70 per cent of instances, but that in patients above this age it is rarely so. In what follows I shall merely attempt to set down my own conception of the relative value of the three types of treatment. That my position is open to attack is a matter of course since every position must be until we have a specific therapy in this disease.

(a) **The Importance of Rest and Diet.**—There are three types of treatment available in thyrotoxicosis: medical, surgical and roentgenological. Differing as they do in aim and method they are nevertheless in agreement on one point, namely, that rest and a full diet are essential to success with any type of treatment. I think it can therefore be said with surety that rest and full diet are the most important elements in the treatment of the disease. Surgeons do not like to operate unless the patient has gone through a preparatory period of rest and full diet; the roentgenologists do undertake the handling of cases without such a preliminary period, but only because their results are slowly obtained, and they insist upon the institution of a regimen of rest and full diet concomitantly with their course of treatments; and, as regards the medical type of treatment, rest and full diet are practically the whole of the therapy.

(b) **Medical Treatment.**—This is the type of treatment most frequently employed, yet it is the one about whose results we know least. It consists in instituting primarily a period of complete rest and full feeding, to be followed by a gradual return to as near full activities as can be accomplished, the sole object and aim of the method being to promote an earlier economic and social rehabilitation than occurs in the entirely untreated case. It is of course based upon the assumption that thyrotoxicosis is a constitutional disease with a marked tendency to be self-limited. The patient is put at complete rest in bed and the attempt is made to accomplish complete mental rest as well. Both these objects are often best attained in a hospital, but as a matter of fact most of these cases are treated in the home. In any case, success will hardly crown the attempt unless the economic and other stresses under which the patient is laboring are materially reduced. Often such a reduction can be accomplished by merely denying the access of certain persons to the patient, but usually the difficulty is not so easily overcome. The employment of sedatives is nearly always necessary at least in the beginning. Sodium or potassium bromide, 10 to 20 grains (0.65 to 1.3 Gm.), or barbital (veronal), 1 to 2 grains (0.13 to 0.26 Gm.), or amytal, $\frac{3}{4}$ grain (0.045 Gm.), may be given two or three times daily for their general quieting effect; phenobarbital (luminal) $\frac{1}{2}$ to $1\frac{1}{2}$ grains (0.03 to 0.1 Gm.), may also be used two or three times daily, but disagreeable symptoms are perhaps more liable to appear than in the use of the other two drugs. Small doses of scopolamine hydrobromide (hyoscine), $\frac{1}{300}$ to $\frac{1}{200}$ grain (0.0002 to 0.0003 Gm.) at six-hour intervals, are not contraindicated, though one should always bear in mind the uncertainty and .

irregularity in action of this drug. If sedatives are not being employed during the day and it is desired to ensure full eight hours sleep at night, full doses of barbital, 10 grains (0.65 Gm.), or amytal, 1½ to 5 grains (0.1 to 0.3 Gm.), or chloral hydrate, 20 to 30 grains (1.3 to 2 Gm.) if given alone, or 10 to 20 grains (0.65 to 1.3 Gm.) if combined with 10 grains (0.65 Gm.) of sodium bromide, may be employed at retiring time. Paraldehyde is preferred by some physicians because it is not at all depressant to the heart; it is, however, very nasty and difficult to take, the dose being from 1 to 4 drachms (4 to 16 cc.), administered either on crushed ice or in a vehicle with high alcohol content (see p. 785). Experience teaches that the best effects are obtained by the alternation of sedative drugs.

Full feeding in these cases means simply giving the patient all she will eat. Usually the appetite is quite ravenous in the beginning and is best satisfied by numerous small feedings between the three full meals. The theoretical value of holding down the protein content of the diet because of its specific dynamic effect has not been borne out in practice; indeed, at least in America, the preference seems to be for a predominantly carbohydrate diet, which obviates the necessity of limiting fats as advocated by McCarrison.

Under this treatment the basal metabolic rate and the pulse rate gradually fall and the patient's subjective symptoms markedly recede; then, after a variable number of weeks, *i. e.*, when it is no longer felt that anything is being accomplished by further insistence upon absolute rest, the attempt is made to slowly return the individual to her, or occasionally his, former economic status. It is freely admitted by those who champion this type of treatment that a full rehabilitation is not always accomplished, perhaps is not accomplished even in the majority of cases, but it is maintained that surgery and roentgenology do no more. I can only repeat that we have practically no statistical evidence of the value of this "medical" treatment. The reasons for this are obvious: It is principally employed by general practitioners who have not the follow-up facilities of the large clinics; it is not often persisted in until the program is fully executed for the reason that many individuals feel forced to resume their full activities as soon as moderate subsidence of symptoms makes this possible; and, finally, for the reason that many patients who begin such a course of treatment weary of the time consumed and yield to the promise of quicker relief held out by the surgeon.

Two statistical studies of the value of such treatment are available. Bram's (1929) report may be simply presented in Tables 53 and 54, which follow. These 2000 cases comprise the patients studied during nineteen years with the exception of all cases suspected to be toxic adenoma, which were referred for surgical treatment at once. Division was into (*a*) early cases: metabolic rate not above 20, heart rate not above 100, weight loss not above 20 pounds, duration of subjective symptoms one to six months; (*b*) cases of average severity: rate 20 to 60, pulse rate 100 to 150, weight loss many times exceeded 40 pounds, duration of symptoms six months to ten years with average of about fifteen months; (*c*) advanced cases: all symptoms very severe and "quite a few" presented cardiac decompensation with edema and ascites, duration of symptoms one to ten years or longer with average of about three years; 20 per cent of this series had been previously operated with temporary or no relief, myxedema being superimposed in a few, acromegaly in one. Unfortunately the division of the total cases among these three groups is not given in the report.

The results of treatment in terms of economic and social restitution are shown in Table 55. Summarizing this report of the results of rest and diet treatment of 2000 cases, it may be said that after periods of observation

TABLE 53.—FOLLOW-UP RECORD OF 2000 GRAVES' DISEASE PATIENTS TREATED BY MEDICAL MEANS

Follow-up.	Number of patients.	Per cent.
At least 3 years	387	19.35
At least 4 years	433	21.65
At least 5 years	558	27.9
At least 6 years	222	11.1
At least 7 years	165	8.25
At least 8 years	95	·4.75
At least 9 years	82	4.1
At least 10 years	58	2.9
Totals	2000	100

TABLE 54.—END-RESULTS IN 2000 CASES OF GRAVES' DISEASE TREATED MEDICALLY

	Number of patients.	Per cent.
Perfectly well	1819	90.95
Persistent exophthalmos (slight or moderate) otherwise perfectly well	53	2.65
Heart enlargement (chiefly objective)	41	2.05
Myxedema (in previously thyroidectomized patients)	27	1.35
Persistent exophthalmos and heart enlargement	22	1.1
Persistent exophthalmos, heart enlargement and post-operative myxedema	12	0.6
Persistent exophthalmos and postoperative myxedema	7	0.35
Postoperative myxedema and heart enlargement	19	0.95
Totals	2000	100

of three to ten years, 90.95 per cent regained complete health; 5.8 per cent are in good subjective health and restored to social and economic usefulness, though still presenting exophthalmos, heart enlargement, or both; 3.25 per cent present some myxedema with or without some exophthalmos and cardiac enlargement—cases in which thyroidectomy had occurred months or years prior to the institution of medical treatment.

TABLE 55.—DURATION OF ABSTINENCE FROM PERFORMANCE OF CUSTOMARY DUTIES DURING MEDICAL TREATMENT OF GRAVES' DISEASE

	Number of patients.	Per cent.
Performing usual duties while under treatment	344	17.2
Abstaining from customary work—		
1 month	176	8.8
2 months	235	11.75
3 months	405	20.25
4 months	212	10.6
5 months	128	6.4
6 months	120	6
7 months	96	4.8
8 months	104	5.2
9 months	54	2.7
10 months	47	2.35
11 months	43	2.15
12 months	36	1.8
Totals	2000	100

The second statistical study is that of Kessel and Hyman, which, though comprising only a small number of cases, is nevertheless of great value for the complete analyses of results which were made. In 1921, these observers instituted a study of 50 unselected cases of fully developed thyrotoxicosis in order to determine the natural history of the disease and to establish an index for the evaluation of therapeutic measures. From the group were excluded (a) patients who had thyroid enlargement without other manifestations of thyrotoxicosis, and (b) those who, with or without thyroid enlargement, presented sympathomimetic symptoms without sufficient elevation of the basal metabolism to warrant the diagnosis of thyrotoxicosis. Included in the group were (1) patients with a significant elevation of metabolism on repeated readings, (2) patients whose illness was sufficiently severe to warrant residence in a hospital where beds were at a great premium (two exceptions), and (3) patients from the poorest sections of the city, who were subjected to constant economic strain (one exception). The treatment of these patients in the hospital consisted in the attempt to provide for them complete physical and mental relaxation and a high caloric diet. Foci of infection were extirpated or drained, phenobarbital (luminal) was used as a sedative, and, after four to six weeks, the syrup of ferrous iodide, from 5 to 30 minims (0.3 to 2 cc.) three times daily, was used to "hasten the involution of the thyroid." After an average hospital stay of six weeks the patients were sent to the country and were given small tasks. In another two to six weeks they were returned home and permitted a gradual resumption of responsibilities, being instructed as to their disease and warned that the condition was arrested rather than cured and that recurrence was a distinct possibility. The families of these patients were warned that they should be protected but not coddled.

In 1927, the status of this group of patients was again reported upon. Of the 50 patients, 8 had died: 1 of carcinoma of the stomach, 2 of cardiac failure, 1 of infection, 1 of status lymphaticus, 2 of thyrotoxicosis, and 1 of thyroidectomy. Ten patients considered their progress unsatisfactory, sought some form of specific therapy, and were therefore considered failures from the standpoint of this study. One of these went to an endocrinologist and was lost from the study; another received radium treatments and obtained excellent results—"the only noteworthy result of radium therapy that we have observed." Eight were operated; 1 died immediately, 1 made good progress, the results in 3 cases were good but not particularly brilliant, and in 3 the operative results were indeterminate. Three patients were lost from observation. Thirty-one patients were successfully followed, 25 for more than four and one-half years and 14 for over five years. The recorded progress of these patients I shall attempt to summarize below.

Subjective Symptoms.—The subjective sypmtoms did not entirely disappear in any of the patients. "Economic restitution is by no means analogous to freedom from subjective complaints. As a general rule, however, it is fair to say that the subjective symptoms in these patients have strikingly and markedly diminished."

Exophthalmos.—Thirteen of the 24 completed records did not show appreciable change; 7 had decreased slightly and 4 had increased.

Tremor.—Many of the patients retained a fine tremor, but in no instance was it complained of nor did it interfere with the patient's occupation.

Goiter.—"In no instance did the goiter completely disappear, though in 4 patients it was noticeable only to the examiner."

Basal Metabolic Rate.—The average basal metabolic rate on admission was plus 43 per cent. At the end of six months it had fallen to plus 22 per cent, at the twelfth month to plus 17 per cent, at two years to plus 14 per cent, and at three years to plus 10 per cent. In the fourth year there occurred a slight rise to plus 15 per cent, in the fifth year to plus 17 per cent, and in the sixth year to plus 19 per cent. The small total number of cases in the series has caused individual rises in these years to disproportionately raise the average level of the metabolism. For instance, in the fourth year the rise to plus 15 per cent is due entirely to four high readings, the average of the remaining readings being plus 8 per cent; and in the fifth and sixth years the omission of four high readings would have brought the average readings down to plus 13 and plus 17 per cent respectively. "It should be understood that all readings were taken while the patients were ambulatory, so that they are, if anything, slightly higher than would be obtained in patients who were in bed. Many of our patients who were progressing satisfactorily could not leave their work to come to the hospital for metabolic readings. An example of this is patient 10, who had a rate of minus 2 per cent in her thirty-sixth month and who, owing to her work, was unable to report for a basal metabolic reading thereafter [since reported as plus 4 per cent in the fifty-ninth month—H. B.]. A reading has not been made for patient 16 since her third month. This patient lives out of town and we hear from her only by letter. Patient 19, who had a basal metabolic rate of plus 7 per cent at one year, has not been able to come for a reading since, though we are still in communication with her at the sixty-second month. She has just had another baby, and cannot leave it to come to the hospital. Patient 23, whose last reading was plus 16 per cent in the sixth month, lives out of town, and writes to us that he does not have any symptoms referable to exophthalmic goiter. Had these patients been able to call on us, the average basal metabolic rate would have been materially lowered. Nineteen readings of zero or an actual minus will be seen, contrary to the usual statement that these patients do not reach normal or subnormal readings unless they are the subjects of specific therapy. The basal metabolic rate that reached normal in the twelfth month has remained well within normal limits throughout the following five years."

Weight.—The average weight gain in the first and second years was 18 pounds (8.2 Kg.), and an average gain of 11, 12 and 13 pounds (5, 5.4, and 5.9 Kg.) was maintained in the third, fourth and fifth years, respectively. "At the end of six years, 6 patients show a loss in weight, and 25 have gained weight, the average difference in weight between the first and last weight being 14 pounds (6.4 Kg.)."

Social and Economic Restitution.—"Social and economic restitution is the most important desideratum from the standpoint of the patient, and may be independent of any of the subjective and objective manifestations. In this group, there is an average period of hospitalization of six weeks and an average period of rest in the country of five weeks, which is followed by variable periods of rest at home. By the third month 15 were restored; by the six month all but 3 patients were economically restored. Of the 3 patients who had a prolonged convalescence, one was a malingerer and another was an old woman with essentially abdominal symptoms, due to a cholecystitis. The third was a young girl who, despite the period of prolonged convalescence, has made favorable progress since. During the remainder of the period of observation, little or no economic or social incapacitation has occurred. . . .

"Worthy of comment, too, is the number of pregnancies that have occurred. Eight of the patients have borne twelve normal children, without exacerbation of symptoms, and the pregnancy, labor and children have all been normal. The test of labor was adequately met in all instances.

"Economic restitution occurred for an average of fifty-two months in the fifty-seven months' average span of observation in this group. The average time for social and economic restitution was four and a half months, and during the remaining fifty-two and a half months these people were able to assume their burden as wage-earners or housewives in the trying circumstances of metropolitan life. They all had residual symptoms, usually negligible, sometimes annoying, but never sufficient to cause them to go to bed, partially due to the fact that a day or even a few hours in bed among this class of patients is far too great a luxury. Doubtless the same symptoms in the more leisurely walks of life would have resulted in variable periods of incapacitation."

I wonder what the average practitioner, who does not report his cases, is accomplishing with the medical plan of treatment. We all know that many women have thyrotoxicosis who do not become surgical or roentgenological cases; and yet they are practically all under the care of a physician at some time, for the malady is of such nature that few individuals afflicted with it would fail to present themselves at least for a diagnosis. And they do not die, for the thyrotoxicosis mortality in the registration area of the United States is about on the level of that of erysipelas and leukemia, though it is undoubtedly true that some cases are incorrectly recorded as cardiac deaths. Must it not be evident that these individuals are being treated by some such plan of "skilful neglect" as that which has been discussed above? Since I expressed this query in the first edition of the book a number of general practitioners have kindly written me to say that they feel their results to be quite satisfactory, but that so much propaganda has been built up for surgery that patients' friends often make the régime an impossible one to observe to the end. The situation with regard to the use of iodine seems to be about the same. Surgeons are complaining that many patients are made worse by its use and that they thus lose the opportunity to operate at the optimum time. Doubtless this is so in some instances, but what the surgeons are prone to forget is that not all the cases of thyrotoxicosis come into their hands, and that not all physicians are using iodine unskilfully. Hyman and Kessel (1931) now begin, at once the patient is put to bed, with the administration of 0.2 to 0.5 cc. of the saturated solution of sodium iodide three times daily. They have seen patients continue to present symptoms or even grow worse while in the uphill phase of the disease, but do not feel in the least that the iodide is responsible for the persistence or exacerbation of the symptoms. Thompson *et al.* (1930) have treated 24 patients with iodine alone, either continuously or intermittently for periods of from one and a half months to three years—a year or more in 13 instances—but their data are by no means comparable with those presented above because with three exceptions all the patients remained at work and thus eliminated the effect of rest, one of the most important weapons with which to fight the disease. Even so, they found that in the mild cases the patients often responded satisfactorily and in some instances apparently recovered entirely. In moderately severe and severe cases there was rarely more than temporary improvement and some of the patients of course grew worse. Langmead (1929) has shown that iodine treatment apparently improves the circulatory system, as shown by Read's formula, more definitely and more permanently than it improves the basal metabolic rate, which indeed often resists reduction for quite a long time. I wonder if most practitioners know of this useful formula of Read? It is as follows:

$$\tfrac{3}{4} \ (\text{P.R.} + \tfrac{3}{4} \ \text{P.P.}) - 72 = \text{the metabolic rate,}$$

where P.R. is the pulse rate and P.P. the pulse pressure (*i. e.*, difference between systolic and diastolic blood pressures). Taking a normal patient with, say, a pulse rate of 72 and the pulse pressure of 40, the formula would give:

$$\tfrac{3}{4} \ (72 + 30) - 72, \text{ which is equal to } + 3.$$

The formula should be applied under basal conditions; it has been found by a number of observers to serve as a sufficiently accurate index of progress in all but the severest cases, in which the true rate is higher than that given by the formula. In 1931, Gale and Gale revised the formula, as follows:

$$P.R. + P.P. - 111 = \text{the metabolic rate.}$$

They find this very serviceable at the bedside.

It is undoubtedly the consensus of opinion among English and German as well as American observers that prolonged treatment with iodine is not successful, but the French school does not at all agree with this stand. Bondreau (1927), Labbe (1928), and Dautrebande (1928) maintain that the drug must be administered for a very long time and gradually be brought up to quite enormous doses, equivalent, in fact, to four or five times our usual doses and administered five or six times daily. I wish that such heroic dosage would be given a trial on this continent. (Iodine matters are discussed further on p. 585.)

(*c*) **Surgical Treatment.**—1. *Indications.*—The chief indication for the removal of the thyroid gland in the opinion of most surgeons is simply the presence of thyrotoxicosis; that is to say, it would seem to be the consensus of surgical opinion that surgical treatment is indicated whenever the diagnosis is made. However, there is a considerable body of opinion in opposition to this position, and by many internists it is considered highly desirable that this opposition should grow. As already mentioned above (see p. 577), Read has shown that in a large group of patients the ultimate, and for the most part even the immediate, effects upon the metabolism are no more marked under surgical than under roentgenological or medical treatment. Occasionally, to be sure, rapid subsidence of most of the symptoms follows immediately upon the operation, but these cases are the exception and not the rule; and do we not sometimes also see unaccountably rapid improvement in a patient who is being "skilfully neglected"? Few leaders in surgery deny that practically all the patients become medical cases again after they leave their hands, but what is not so often stressed by them is that surgery usually claims credit for the primary improvement which follows upon any vigorous type of treatment, whether enforced bed rest (medical treatment), surgical removal or *x*-ray ablation of the gland. I doubt very much the value of any statistical studies of postoperative results that do not show the condition of the patients five years or more after the operations have been performed. This the surgical reports cannot do for the reason that at once after the operation the patient becomes in effect if not in actual fact a medical case. Witness the report of Frazier and Mosser (1928) upon the end-result after surgical treatment of a large number of cases: "In this clinic it is our practice to follow all patients who have been operated on for at least five years. As far as possible this is done by personal examination, although patients who live at a considerable distance are seen less often than those near at hand, letters or examination by the family physicians being substituted." This fact does not deter these authors, however, from describing as end-results the status of patients whose ratings are "based on an average postoperative interval of ten months." This sort of evidence is not convincing. And I wonder how many practitioners will subscribe to their statement, typical of the attitude taken by many surgeons, that "The treatment for recurrence is, of course, reoperation." Crile is now advocating denervation of the suprarenals; it might be good fun if we began sending in all recurrent cases to have this neat little operation performed. Furthermore, I think it not impertinent to enquire how those who advocate surgery in all cases explain away the fact that their present high praise of preoperative iodine therapy as enabling them to perform more single-stage operations and to greatly reduce their operative mortality constitutes a tacit acknowledgment of the fact that, before iodine days, they were clamoring for the right to operate *repeatedly* and *dangerously* upon patients whom they have not yet proved their ability to cure more reliably than by any other method.

Those who oppose indiscriminate surgery nevertheless admit that the surgical method has its legitimate indications. (*a*) It is generally felt that adenomata do not spontaneously disappear, and that when thyrotoxicosis develops in an individual having an adenomatous goiter surgery is the method of choice if ultimate cure is to be achieved. (*b*) In a fulminating case of thyrotoxicosis complicated by preexisting myocardial degeneration, surgery is the method of choice because of the quick relief from the worst symptoms which may follow its employment. (*c*) In a case of thyrotoxicosis without preexisting myocardial complication but of such severity that the patient is forced to bed, is highly excited, is rapidly losing strength, and is liable to develop heart failure at any moment, it used to be agreed by even the most implacable foes of surgical treatment that here the knife was called for; but nowadays all observers are not so sure. The surgeons delay in these cases until iodine has brought the patient into a satisfactory condition, *i. e.*, a condition in which he will not disturb the operative mortality statistics in the upward direction; there are those who are wondering whether this is not also a good starting point from which to continue with their medical treatment—omitting the operation!

2. *The Preoperative Iodine Treatment.*—It was the great Kocher's unfortunate diatribes against the use of iodine in thyrotoxicosis that for many years deprived the profession of the aid of this valuable remedy in preparing cases for surgery. However, release from this thralldom finally came in 1922, when the epoch-making tests of Plummer, at the Mayo Clinic, following close upon the preliminary and independent studies of Neisser, and Loewy and Zondek, in Germany, fully established the efficacy of the drug. Iodine is now almost universally used to prepare patients for operation. The studies of Gutman *et al.* (1933) failed to substantiate the recent claims in the German literature that diiodotyrosine is superior to the other forms of iodine, though they found it just as good.

METHOD OF EMPLOYMENT.—The following description of method, that of Clute (1926) and his associates at the Lahey Clinic in Boston, is typical.

"As nearly as possible, the patients have been treated throughout their illness along the same general plan. They have been kept in bed after admission to the hospital, with the exception of a few severely toxic cases, who have been given lavatory privileges. Fluids have been given as freely as possible, and every patient has been urged to eat as much food as possible. Extra meals have been given whenever the patient could eat them. During this period, the total calories consumed have averaged from 2600 to 2900 in twenty-four hours. On the morning after admission, a basal metabolic test has been done, and this test repeated either daily or every other day while waiting for operation.

"In patients not dangerously ill, we have waited until after the first metabolic test before giving compound solution of iodine. The treatment of the severely toxic cases has consisted of the immediate administration of the solution without waiting for the preliminary metabolism tests. In treating the latter type of case, we have endeavored to give from 50 to 100 minims (3 to 6 cc.) of the drug within the first twenty-four hours after admission. It has been given in divided doses of 5 or 10 minims (0.3 or 0.6 cc.) each, by mouth and rectum. It may be given subpectorally, if necessary, well diluted in salt solution.

"The drug should be well diluted whether given by mouth or by rectum, and 5-minim doses given repeatedly are preferable to single large doses.

We have found that compound solution of iodine diluted with cool water is not unpleasant to most patients. Occasionally it is preferably diluted with milk. It may be given by dropping the requisite amount on a piece of dry bread [or giving it in grape juice].

"To the patients not dangerously ill on admission, we have given 10 minims of the solution three times a day. This is continued during the pre-operative period and for several days after operation. In cases in which we have anticipated a serious postoperative reaction, we have doubled this dose on the day preceding and the day of the operation. It is essential that the drug be continued through the operative period if reactions are to be avoided.

"When we have performed a subtotal thyroidectomy in multiple stages, we have continued the use of compound solution of iodine during the entire interval between the operations. It has been our custom to give but 10 drops a day, however, during these intervals. In general, the use of the solution has been omitted four or five days after the operation is completed."

In some clinics it has now become the custom to continue doses of 10 minims (0.6 cc.) once a day or in divided doses, for six weeks to two months after operation. If potassium iodide is substituted for Lugol's solution, which is advisable on the ground of being as effective and less offensive, the saturated solution of potassium iodide should be used in only one sixth to one fifth the quantity of the Lugol's solution; i. e., Lerman and Means (1931) used 6 minims of potassium iodide solution, or 30 minims of Lugol's solution, with equal effect. The advisability of using smaller doses both pre- and postoperatively has been investigated rather thoroughly; the studies of Thompson et al. (1930–32) are the most exhaustive. They believe it to be doubtful if more than 5 drops of Lugol's solution daily is ever needed, even taking into account the varying responses in the same patient from time to time.

The mode of action of the iodine is not understood, though the work of Rienhoff indicates that there is fostered an accumulation of colloid which may by pressure prevent the absorption of thyroxin into the circulation. However, it should be noted that quantitative or qualitative abnormalities in thyroxin have never been proved. The claim of Holst, Lunde and their associate workers that there is a certain insoluble blood iodine fraction which is increased in all cases of toxic goiter and may be reduced by oral treatment with iodine, has been confirmed by the studies of Dodds et al. (1932), but substantiation has not as yet been found for the further belief that this fraction may be made to serve as a measure of the toxic secretion by the thyroid; indeed, Dodds' findings were quite to the contrary. Curtis et al. (1933) believe that the significance of the total blood iodine in thyroid disease is similar to that of the blood sugar in diabetes mellitus and blood calcium in parathyroid disease, for they found it lowered in thyroid hypo-function and elevated in hyperfunction; it was always elevated by any form of iodine medication.

IMMEDIATE EFFECTS.—Under iodine, nervous tension soon relaxes, basal metabolism falls on the average between 2 and 4 points daily, the pulse rate is markedly lowered, sleep and appetite improve, and a gain is made in both weight and strength. The ideal improvement for surgical purposes is usually considered to be reached in from ten to twenty days. Why a small number of individuals should resist the salutary effects of the drug, and a few even be made worse by it, is not understood. In the beginning of this new iodine preparation for operation it was urged that adenomatous cases should not be so treated for fear of aggravating the severity of their condition. We now believe that this fear was ungrounded. That patients may become refractory to iodine and show an increase in metabolism, perhaps with an increase in severity of other symptoms also, is well recognized. There is difference of opinion regarding correct procedure here. Most observers believe that iodine administration should be undisturbed, but Thompson has found that if it is omitted (usually for one month), the refractoriness disappears. Both Graham and Coller have observed similar responses. Surgeons often wish to operate at once upon the appearance of refractoriness, but the above observations would point to the advisability of delay, economic factors permitting.

EFFECT UPON SURGICAL PROCEDURE.—In recent years the improvement in surgical procedure made possible by preliminary iodine and rest is very great; several clinics now operate more than 80 per cent of their cases as single-stage subtotal thyroidectomies. In a few specialized clinics, by reason of skilful surgery plus organized teamwork between surgeon, internist, anesthetist and nursing staff, the operative mortality has been reduced below 3 per cent, in some instances even to 1 per cent and less; but the reader will do well to note Foster's recent statement that in general hospitals, where this perfected coordination is not possible, the mortality is still about 15 per cent; Hyman and Kessel (1931) say "Well over 10 per cent."

3. *Acute Postoperative Crisis.*—This reaction consists in a severe exacerbation of all the symptoms of thyrotoxicosis. The metabolism, fever and pulse rate rise very high, nausea, vomiting and often diarrhea are present, and the excitement and restlessness not infrequently reach maniacal proportions. At present, with the persistence of the iodine therapy through the postoperative period, these crises are not so frequent or usually so severe as formerly, but they still occur.

The iodine must be continued, though it will often have to be given by rectum. Goodrich (1931) has reported excellent results in very severe reactions from the intravenous injection of 15 grains (1 Gm.) of sodium iodide, repeated at twelve, eighteen, and twenty-four hours, and thereafter twice a day for one day and once a day for two days. In one instance he gave the second dose after three hours. Others have had similar experiences. Fahrni (1932) has given larger doses: 15 to 30 grains (1 to 2 Gm.) once or twice during the first twenty-four hours. Dehydration should be counteracted by hypodermoclysis of 2 to 4 liters of fluid during the twenty-four hours. During this attack, glycogen stores are exhausted very quickly, fats are only partially burned, and acidosis follows—an important fact that has been fully recognized only since it was reemphasized by Major, in 1923. Glucose must be given intravenously to counteract this condition. Foster writes: "Not less than 100 Gm. of glucose is required during twenty-four hours to prevent acidosis under the conditions of a thyrotoxic crisis. This amount is conveniently given by using a 50 per cent glucose solution, 20 Gm. being administered intravenously every four hours for five or six doses during twenty-four hours." The venoclysis method of Hendon (see p. 164) is also being very satisfactorily used.

The control of the excitement and restlessness is in most cases very difficult. One-quarter- to ½-grain (0.015 to 0.03 Gm.) doses of morphine are usually employed, often with the addition of another sedative drug: chloral hydrate, 10 to 20 grains (0.65 to 1.3 Gm.), barbital (veronal), 5 to 10 grains (0.03 to 0.06 Gm.), phenobarbital (luminal), ½ to 1½ grains (0.03 to 0.1 Gm.), amytal, 1½ to 5 grains (0.1 to 0.3 Gm.). Small doses of scopolamine hydrobromide (hyoscine), $\frac{1}{300}$ to $\frac{1}{200}$ grain (0.0002 to 0.0003 Gm.), may be safely used together with morphine, though one should always bear in mind the uncertainty and irregularity of this drug's action.

4. *Postoperative Tetany.*—This condition is rare, but even in the best clinics an occasional case is seen, perhaps about once in every thousand thyroid operations. For methods of treatment, see the article on tetany.

(d) **x-Ray Treatment.**—The latest statistical studies of x-ray therapy in thyrotoxicosis cases followed for a period of several years, such as those of Means and Holmes; Sanger; Krause; Barclay; Jenkinson; Loucks; Holzknecht; Groover *et al.*; Pfahler; Stevens; and Sielmann show that so-called "cures" result just as frequently following this type of therapy as any other; herewith the results of Groover *et al.* (which are typical of many reports) in Table 56.

TABLE 56.—RESULTS OF x-RAY TREATMENT IN THYROTOXICOSIS
Classification of Cases

	Number.	Per cent.
Mild	37	12
Moderate	157	51
Severe	111	37
Total	305	100

Results of Treatment

	Number.	Per cent.
Cured of hyperthyroidism	271	88.85
Improved	26	8.52
Unimproved	8	2.63
Total	305	100.00

This being true, it would certainly seem that x-ray ablation of the gland should be the method of choice of those who consider removal or destruction *in situ* of this structure necessary for the accomplishment of a cure. It has the following advantages over surgery: (a) The procedure is simple and will usually be accepted by all classes of patients; (b) mild reactions, characterized by nausea, vomiting and malaise, and lasting only twenty-four to forty-eight hours, are rare; (c) ambulatory patients, who cannot or will not give up their usual activities, can be treated just as well as the bedfast; (d) patients are not subjected to the psychic trauma of the preparation for operation; (e) in the event of failure it may still be followed by surgery (Stevens, 1931, has quoted both Crile and Rogers to the effect that the alleged production of dense adhesions does not increase operative difficulties to a degree that is of any moment at all); (f) there is no appreciable mortality chargeable against the method. Of course a large tumor with pressure symptoms is an indication for surgical removal, but if there is evidence of great toxicity in these cases, preoperative roentgen treatment will reduce the operative mortality.

(e) **Cardiac Complications.**—The treatment of heart failure and auricular fibrillation occurring in a thyrotoxicosis patient is no different from that in any other patient. To be sure, the symptoms will oftentimes be discouraging in their persistence, but that is a fact for comment, not consternation.

In the treatment of the tachycardia that is a distinguishing feature of the disease, and for the relief of palpitation that so often distresses the patient, many physicians find quinine most satisfactory. The hydrobromide is most often used, but any other salt would probably act as well. The average dose is 2 grains (0.13 Gm.) in a capsule three or four times daily but many patients require larger doses and show considerable tolerance for the drug; Bram (1932) has found that the tolerance recedes as the patient improves. Read prefers quinidine (methods applicable here, on p. 522).

(f) **Miscellaneous Drugs.**—Physostigmine, quinine in very large doses, ergotamine, sodium fluoride and a number of other drugs have been reported to have a more or less specific type of action, but the accounts are too conflicting as yet to warrant analysis here.

GENITO-URINARY INFECTIONS AND STONE

GONORRHEA

Gonorrhea would seem to be as old as man, for very many of the ancient writings that have come down to us, both religious and secular, contain references to this "flow of semen" disease. However, so far as we now know, the true nature of the discharge and the recognition of the infectious and venereal nature of the malady were not recorded until quite late in the Middle Ages. Fernel, in the sixteenth century, seems to have differentiated gonorrhea and syphilis; apparently the disease was very common at that time, but in John Hunter's day (1728–93) we find the two diseases again confused; Ricord, in 1838, finally established the separate entities. In 1879, Neisser discovered the causative gonococcus. Regarding the present incidence of the disease, it can only be said that it is very prevalent all over the world, but whether it is on the increase or decrease cannot be stated with any positiveness; the available statistics are so incomplete and contradictory as to be of compartively little value.

The subject will be considered here under the following heads: (*a*) Gonorrhea in the male, (*b*) prophylaxis, (*c*) gonorrhea in the female, (*d*) vulvovaginitis of infants.

(A) GONORRHEA IN THE MALE

Gonorrhea is contracted during the act of sexual intercourse and appears primarily as an infection of the anterior portion of the urethra, the early involvement of the urethral glands, however, playing an important part in maintaining the infection. The average incubation period is three to five days. Profuse purulent discharge is the rule and is usually accompanied by painful micturition. Edema of the parts is not often sufficient to prevent free voiding, but infiltration of the corpus spongiosum is sometimes sufficient in degree to destroy the elasticity of the urethra so that on erection the penis curves downward, giving rise to the very painful symptom known as chordee. When the infection spreads behind the sphincter, which occurs in the majority of cases between the second and fourth weeks, the so-called "posterior" urethritis is established; in its train often come prostatitis, epididymitis, and seminal vesiculitis. Gonorrheal arthritis, first clearly described by Brande, in 1854, and endocarditis are serious complications which occur, of course, only after the organism has entered the blood stream in considerable numbers, which is thought by many observers to occur in the majority of cases. If the gonococcus is conveyed to the conjunctiva by the hands or other contaminated object an acute infection often resulting in blindness follows; that this catastrophe does not occur with greater frequency than is the case is solely due to the fortunate fact that the organism perishes very quickly outside the body, though cases of its survival on damp towels for ten or eleven hours are on record (Engering). In most cases of gonorrhea there are few systemic symptoms beyond malaise and a slight headache, though the leukocytosis is indicative of a general reaction. Psychic disturbances are often quite pronounced, but they are probably for the most part engendered by the patient's fear that what he looks upon as his moral dereliction will be discovered.

In Vecki's (1925) delightfully caustic review of the status of therapy in gonorrhea, he draws attention to the fact that from the time of Lallemand in the seventeenth century down to Desormeaux, who devised the first urethroscope in the middle of the nineteenth, preeminence in the genito-urinary field was held by France. This was a period of internal medication, local attack upon the disease being made hardly at all. Then leadership was transferred to Vienna, where Sigmund introduced the urethral syringe; thence to Berlin, though Neisser's discovery of the causative organism was made in Breslau; back again to Paris, where Janet devised his syringe in 1893; and finally to North America, with Valentine's introduction of his glass-tipped irrigator. At the present time the disease is being attacked locally by the use of antiseptic solutions in injections and irrigations, and systemically by the ingestion of drugs that are antiseptic when excreted by the kidneys, and also by the intravenous introduction of the new dye combinations. But the one treatment which, in the opinion of many observers, would be the best of all, has never been given a thorough trial on a large scale. That treatment is to put the patient to bed, just as though he had pneumonia or any of the other febrile infectious diseases, maintain the diet light but ample, give large quantities of water and keep the bowels open to prevent pelvic congestion, and leave the urethra severely alone. Obviously, there are many economic and social factors which will probably always militate against a thorough trial of this scheme of treatment; however, all of us who have had much experience in the treatment of gonorrhea have occasionally had the opportunity of trying this "skilful neglect" in a modified way, usually with gratifying results.

A few months after the entry of the United States into the World War, in 1917, there appeared in the Journal of the American Medical Association a series of articles on the treatment of venereal diseases prepared under the direction of the Surgeon-General of the U. S. Army by the following advisory committee: Lieut. Col. F. F. Russell; Dr. W. A. Pusey, Chicago; Dr. F. R. Hagner, Washington; Dr. G. W. Wende, Buffalo; Dr. S. Pollitzer, New York; and Dr. H. H. Morton, Brooklyn. For much of the text and arrangement of what follows in this book concerning the treatment of gonorrhea in the male, I am deeply indebted to this series of articles; indeed, my aim was originally, and still is, merely to weave into the excellent treatise of these gentlemen those things that have seemed to me of most value in the literature since 1917.

ACUTE ANTERIOR URETHRITIS

General Management.—The patient should be urged to refrain from exercise as much as possible and to rest in the prone position whenever he can do so. Insofar as it is possible, the diet should be bland and light with absolute abstention in the particulars of highly seasoned foods and alcohol. Much water should be taken (ginger ales, etc., are spiced and should not be used), but it is probably a mistake to render the urine alkaline in order to lessen its irritation; the normal acidity, which will already be somewhat lessened by the increase in fluid intake, is a valuable defense against ascending infection. Coitus and all sexual excitement should of course be interdicted. The correction of constipation (see p. 431) is indicated in order to lessen pelvic congestion as much as possible. The scrotum should be carried in a suspensory and the penis in a loose bag into which the discharge can drip unimpeded; constricting bandages are to be avoided so that there may be no interference with the return circulation.

The drug that has the most valuable soothing effect upon the inflamed mucous membrane is the oil of sandalwood. It is given in capsules in a dose of 8 to 15 minims (0.5 to 1 cc.) three times daily after meals. This drug often disturbs digestion and causes loss of appetite; severe pain in the back and an increase in urethral discomfort are sometimes complained of. The proprietary preparations (N.N.R. 1933), Arheol and Santyl, are said to be fully as effective and less liable to give rise to objectionable symptoms. The former occurs in capsules containing 3 grains (0.2 Gm.), 9 to 12 of which are to be taken daily; the latter in capsules containing 6 minims (0.4 Gm.), 4 of which are usually given three times daily. These preparations, as indeed the oil of sandalwood itself, are best prescribed alone.

Methenamine (urotropine), methylene blue and hexylresorcinol are sometimes given by mouth in the attempt to sterilize the genito-urinary tract from above, but the practice is not general. For the methods of using these drugs see page 616.

In very severe anterior urethritis with intense reaction, profuse discharge, and great swelling and edema, it is good judgment to wait for some sub-sidence of the symptoms before beginning treatment by injections. In the meantime the parts should be kept clean, the penis held in hot water for fifteen minutes at a time every few hours, and hot sitz baths given every three or four hours to relieve distress. If pain on urination is very great it may be relieved by an injection into the urethra, five minutes before urina-tion of 1 cc. of 1 per cent cocaine hydrochloride. The oil of sandalwood will in most cases sufficiently relieve the pain to make this rather dangerous medication with cocaine unnecessary.

The two-glass test should be made at each examination for the purpose of determining: (a) If the posterior urethra has been affected; (b) the amount of pus secreted. The urine passed during gonorrhea appears turbid from admixture with pus, and in it are little clumps or masses of desquamated epithelium. After standing, the pus settles to the bottom of the glass and a cloud of mucus appears floating above it. As the patient proceeds toward recovery, the pus disappears, but the hypersecretion of mucus continues and occasions a cloudiness of the urine, giving it a mucilaginous appearance. After the mucus disappears, the "clap shreds" persist for months, because isolated portions of mucous membrane are not covered with epithelium and are still secreting pus.

In the two-glass test, if the anterior urethra alone is affected the first glass of urine will be cloudy and the second glass clear; but if the posterior urethra is involved both glasses will be turbid from the presence of pus. This is accounted for by the action of the "cut-off" muscle which forms a barrier between the anterior and posterior urethra. It prevents pus in the anterior urethra from flowing back into the bladder; so that in anterior urethritis alone the pus in front of the cut-off muscle is washed out in the first flow of urine, while the last of the urine will flow over a clean surface and remain clear, i. e., the first glass will be turbid, the second clear. On the other hand, in posterior urethritis, the cut-off muscle holds back the pus, as it does the urine in the bladder, and the pus flows back into the bladder and renders all the urine turbid. When the urine in posterior urethritis is passed into two glasses, the second glass is turbid as well as the first. If it is desired to determine the condition of the anterior urethra in posterior urethritis, it can readily be done by irrigating the anterior urethra with physiologic saline solution and collecting the washings in a glass for in-spection.

Local Treatment.—The local application of antiseptic and cleansing solutions to the urethra is made in the form of injections and irrigations. These treatments are usually begun as soon as the case is diagnosed unless it is of the extremely severe type already mentioned above. Some physi-cians prefer and use injections exclusively, others employ only irrigations;

but perhaps the most usual practice is to irrigate the patient in the office and to have the injections employed by him at home. *Injection technic:* Before injections, the patient should wash out the urethra by urinating. For these injections an acorn-tipped syringe should be used, the tip being firmly pressed into the meatus, and the penis held under moderate tension. The injections should always be given with the utmost gentleness, and if they produce distress their strength should be reduced. In order to be effective a sufficient quantity of fluid must be injected to distend the anterior urethra; a syringe of at least 15-cc. capacity is needed. The solution should be held in the urethra for at least five minutes. *Irrigation technic:* A glass irrigator is filled with the fluid and suspended at a height of 2 to 4 feet (0.6 to 1.2 meters) above the penis. The irrigations should be given as hot as can be comfortably borne—110 to 115 F. (43 to 46 C.). Most irrigations are given with the patient standing at a sink, but it is perhaps preferable to have him sitting well forward on the edge of a chair with his shoulders against the chair back. The glass irrigator tip is pressed against the meatus and the anterior urethra distended with fluid; then by a short release of pressure of the tip a return flow is allowed. This is repeated until thorough irrigation of the anterior urethra is obtained. If it is desired to irrigate the posterior urethra (*i. e.,* in the presence of posterior urethritis), the anterior urethra should first be washed out; then the tip should be firmly pressed against the meatus and the anterior urethra dilated with fluid. The patient is then instructed to take a long breath and to try to urinate; this releases the cut-off muscle, and the fluid flows into the bladder. The bladder is filled with fluid but should not be distended beyond the point of comfort. After the bladder is filled the patient empties it by urination.

Injections are usually given three or four times daily at intervals of four to eight hours, usually combined with one or more irrigations. When irrigations alone are employed, it is customary to give four if possible in the twenty-four hours.

I shall not attempt here a direct comparison of the antigonorrheal properties of the various solutions used locally for the reason that most physicians of unbiased experience hold that, while an occasional case may respond excellently to the use of one drug from start to finish of the treatment, in the vast majority of cases it is necessary to alternate drugs before permanent results are obtained. What follows is therefore mainly a statement of the dosage of the various drugs used in injections and irrigations.

1. *Silver.*—Collargol is used for injection in the strength of 0.5 to 1 per cent; protargol in the strength of 0.25 to 1 (rarely 2) per cent; and argyrol in the strength of 2 to 5 per cent. For irrigations any of these organic silver preparations may be used in the strength of 1: 1000.

Of these three preparations, the two most used are protargol and argyrol. It is popularly believed that they both deteriorate rapidly. That this is not true was shown by Pilcher and Sollmann (1924) who found that: (*a*) Protargol solutions become poorer in ionic silver and therefore less efficient, but not sufficiently to be of much clinical importance even in one year. (*b*) Argyrol, on the contrary, becomes richer in silver ions, and therefore more antiseptic but also more irritant. The changes in argyrol solutions start rapidly, so that a week might modify the clinical response.

Another contention often made with regard to the action of the protein silver compounds is that, while their immediate antiseptic activity depends entirely upon the silver ions present, there is in these compounds some reserve "colloidal silver" which becomes slowly available during a long contact with the tissues. This ghost has also been laid by Pilcher and Sollmann, who write that "the entire antiseptic efficiency resides in the silver ions that are present or become immediately available. The colloids doubtless, however, diminish the irritative effects of these silver ions by reason of their demulcent action."

The presence of blood greatly diminishes the antiseptic action of the protein silver compounds (Pilcher and Sollmann).

2. *Mercurochrome-220-Soluble.*—There is considerable misunderstanding in regard to the strength in which this drug is best employed in the urethra, due, I believe, to the unfortunate fact that in the original report in which Young, White and Swartz (1919) introduced the drug there was a footnote stating that trials of a 2.5 per cent solution were being undertaken; the report was based, however, on experience with a 1 per cent solution. At the present time, at the Brady Urological Institute in Baltimore, where Young and his associates have been studying the drug, it is employed in the anterior urethra in a strength of 0.5 to 1 per cent, only very rarely in a solution stronger than 2 per cent (Jour. Amer. Med. Assoc., 101, 467, 1933). This is the example followed by most practitioners. Such a report as the recent one of Rupel, in which there is described the use of a 5 per cent solution in 104 cases without evidences of harmful action, is impressive but wants considerable confirmation before it can be generally recommended, the reason being the tendency among nonspecialized practitioners to jump to the conclusion that what can be used with safety in the anterior urethra is also acceptable in the posterior urethra and bladder. Mercurochrome contains about 26 per cent of mercury, and, if it is used in strong solutions in regions from which it is not promptly drained away, it is quite easy to get sufficient absorption to produce mild mercurialism, as evidenced by transient albuminuria. A 5 per cent solution in the anterior urethra would appear, according to Rupel, to be free from this danger; but daily injection of such a solution into the posterior urethra and bladder is distinctly contraindicated in the present state of our knowledge.

Mercurochrome precipitates with silver nitrate and zinc sulphate; it may be used alternately with the silver preparations but should not be used concurrently with them. In general, salts of heavy metals will precipitate mercurochrome. It precipitates with acid substances (not, however, with the saturated solution of boric acid), and with alkaloidal salts, such as cocaine hydrochloride, procaine hydrochloride (novocain), and quinine and urea hydrochloride. It seems that the fresher the mercurochrome solution, the less likely are these precipitations to take place. White (1923) suggested that when it is desired to use a local anesthetic with mercurochrome, a 2 per cent solution of benzyl alcohol be employed; this has been found to be compatible with the dye.

3. *Acriflavine.*—This dye is used for irrigation in aqueous solution in the strength of 1: 4000 to 1: 8000; Young says (1926), "preferably the latter." The usual concentration for injection is 1: 1000, but this strength is often irritating, the base being less so than the hydrochloride. Herrold and Culver (1927) have reported that acriflavine does not produce any subjective or objective symptoms of irritation in a dilution as low as 1: 400 in water containing 10 or 15 per cent of gelatin. "The drug is first added to distilled water for the desired strength and then heated to about 60 C.; then the gelatin leaves are placed into the mixture and stirred until dissolved. . . . The gelatin acriflavine mixture solidifies at room temperature, so it was necessary to use 8-ounce wide vacuum jars which kept the gelatin in a semifluid state for from ten to twelve hours. This is practicable for office use since it is necessary only to heat the mixture each morning and place it in the vacuum jars."

Boyd (1928) reports exceptional success with the following technic, using a 1: 1000 solution of the English preparation (Boots) of acriflavine.

38

After voiding, the patient lies down and from 1 to 2 drachms (4 to 8 cc.) of the solution is injected into the urethra, being held in with finger pressure back of the glans. A piece of absorbent cotton, about 1 by 3 inches, is then laid over the meatus with its ends carried back above and below the penis, and another similar piece is wrapped around the penis. The patient then releases pressure on the urethra and is kept lying for ten to fifteen minutes with the penis held upright. By the end of that time nearly all of the acriflavine has oozed out of the urethra into the cotton. Two such treatments are given daily for one week before beginning with the irrigations and injections with other drugs.

4. *Mercurophen.*—Shivers describes his method of using this drug as follows: "In acute gonorrheal urethritis the injection of mercurophen is preceded by an irrigation of the anterior urethra with a warm 1: 8000 potassium permanganate solution. This cleanses the parts and dissolves the plugs of mucus in the mouths of glands. One or 2 drachms (4 to 8 cc.) of a 1: 4000 solution of mercurophen is then carefully injected and held in the anterior urethra for five minutes. The patient is then given a 1: 9000 or 1: 10,000 solution of mercurophen for home use. He is instructed to use a blunt nose glass syringe, with a bulb tip, holding about 2 drachms (8 cc.). These injections are to be taken following every other urination and retained in the urethra for at least five minutes. If the irritation from these injections lasts more than a few minutes the number taken should be reduced to two or three times a day, following urination."

5. *Metaphen.*—This drug is used for irrigating in the strength of 1: 10,000 to 1: 5000.

6. *Pyridium.*—This azo dye is used in the form of the commercially prepared 1 per cent solution, which is diluted to a 0.5 or 0.3 per cent solution for irrigation or injection.

7. *Potassium Permanganate.*—This drug is used for irrigating in the strength of 1: 8000 to 1:3000, the usual range being between 1: 5000 and 1: 3000.

8. *Astringents.*—In acute anterior urethritis the astringents are absolutely contraindicated. It is true that they relieve the patient of his greatest annoyance—the urethral discharge—but on the cessation of the treatments for a few days, the urethral strippings or the morning discharge often shows an abundance of gonococci. The appearance of a cure and the sense of security this affords the patient are thus entirely false. Writing of the use of astringents in this stage of the disease, Pelouze, who has won wide recognition as an authority on his subject, says: "It does reduce the patient's respect for a serious disease that is one of society's greatest menaces, and is sure to be the cause of many innocent infections."

Intravenous Mercurochrome-220.—The intravenous use of mercurochrome in the treatment of sepsis is discussed at some length elsewhere in this book (see p. 160). Regarding its use in the treatment of gonorrhea, Young (1932) and his associates are apparently still enthusiastic, as are also a number of independent investigators; however, the literature has become rather voluminous and is not of a nature that permits of evaluating the actual part played by mercurochrome in accomplishing the cure, since the intravenous injections (technic and other details, p. 163) are nowadays always given in conjunction with the usual type of local treatment. Redewill, Potter and Garrison (1929) continue to recommend that the drug be given in 50 per cent glucose solution, and believe that the routine use of mercurochrome in glucose solution, plus intramuscular injections of foreign protein (see below) has been of considerable value as used by them throughout the Asiatic Fleet.

Acriflavine Parenterally.—Use of this drug intravenously in gonorrhea has not been shown to be consistently worth while. Hughes and Birch (1933) have recently found in a small series of cases that its deep subcutaneous injection causes urethral discharge to disappear quickly, but relapses were common and the pain at the site of injection was quite considerable; furthermore, other immediate and delayed reactions caused them to abandon the trial.

Diathermy.—Attempts have been made in recent years to apply a high degree of heat directly to the urethra by means of the diathermy apparatus, but the objection to the methods has been that in all of them it is necessary to introduce a metal instrument into the highly inflamed anterior urethra, a procedure certainly contraindicated in the treatment of acute anterior urethritis. Redewill's (1927) method is a distinct advance in this type of therapy. He fills the urethra with a mercurochrome solution in gelatin, which is held *in situ* by the simple expedient of placing a rolled-up condom over the glans and securing the same by a rubber band that encircles the corona; the electric terminals of the diathermy apparatus are then applied to the outside of the penis. His observations have shown that as much heat as can be borne by the patient can be easily established in the urethral canal in this way. However, as only 112 F. (44.4 C.) can be attained in the surrounding tissues, and the gonococcus can survive 1 or 2 degrees more than this for at least half an hour in culture, it is easy to see that direct sterilization is perhaps too much to hope for, but of course there is always the possibility of stimulating the local defensive mechanism in this way. Diathermy has been disappointing in the experience of most observers.

Miscellaneous Measures.—There are few, if any, signs of immunity in gonorrhea, which indicates that it would certainly be difficult to produce gonorrheal antibodies artificially. All the older vaccines have failed to make a place for themselves and I doubt if any of the newer methods of the French, or the "intradermal immunization" recently described by Corbus (1932), in America, will have any happier fate. More direct methods of foreign protein therapy aiming at the stimulation of leukocytosis (and inferring that this means phagocytosis as well), seem more rational; the orthodox procedures are described on page 327. Fever therapy (methods, p. 187) is also being tried.

DECLINING ANTERIOR URETHRITIS

Under the treatment of acute anterior urethritis, as described above, the acute symptoms of the disease usually disappear very promptly, but if treatment is discontinued at this point, even though the discharge has ceased and only a few shreds remain in the urine, a relapse is certain to occur in from two to three weeks, since a few gonococci have been left in the tissues and extensive reinfection thus invited. In cases that have run a favorable course under treatment, the discharge has become watery and scant in about three weeks' time. Microscopical examination shows few or no gonococci, but many newly formed desquamated epithelial cells. The urine in the first glass is clear or slightly turbid, but contains many long mucous filaments. When the case has reached this stage, the task remains of curing the residual gonorrheal lesions. These consist of catarrhal inflammation of the mucous membrane, erosions, periglandular infiltrations, and infiltrations of the submucous tissues.

1. **Use of Astringents.**—Since the use of the antiseptics hitherto has been solely for the purpose of destroying the gonococci, it is well to supplement them now by the use of astringents whose purpose is to overcome the catarrhal condition of the mucous membrane. The following are acceptable preparations:

Zinc sulphate	gr. xij	0.75	
Resorcin	gr. xxiv	1.5	
Water	℥iv	120.0	

or

Zinc sulphate	gr. iv to xij	0.25 to 0.75	
Phenol	gr. iv	0.25	
Water	℥iv	120.0	

or

Zinc sulphate	gr. x	0.65	
Lead acetate	gr. xx	1.3	
Water	℥iv	120.0	

or

Zinc permanganate	gr. i to ij	0.06 to 0.12	
Water	℥iv	120.0	

It is well to alternate one of the astringent preparations with one of the antiseptics, giving each twice daily. Again it should be said that these astringents are indicated only in the terminal stages of gonorrhea, and that they should be given neither in acute gonorrhea nor in the presence of acute complications in the posterior urethra.

2. **Provocative Irrigation.**—Under astringent plus antiseptic treatment, as above outlined, the discharge soon stops and the urine becomes clear and free from pus; but numerous small clap shreds persist. When this stage is reached, a provocative irrigation of 1: 4000 solution of silver nitrate should be given. If gonococci are still present, this causes the return of a profuse discharge in which the organisms will be found. The occurrence of such a discharge after provocative injection necessitates a return to treatment for acute urethritis.

3. **Use of Sounds.**—When no relapse follows the provocative silver nitrate irrigation, and the urine is clear but contains many shreds, dilatation of the urethra about every five days is necessary to get rid of the remaining lesions and bring the urethra back to normal. The dilatations are made with a sound large enough to distend the urethra, and if the meatus is too small to admit a 28 or 30 French sound, a meatotomy should be done. Gentle finger massage of the urethra is then practiced over the sound while it is lying in place.

Each dilatation should be followed by a copious irrigation with a 1: 10,000 silver nitrate solution; an irrigation with the same solution should also be made on days when the sound is not introduced. Hand injection of one of the astringents may also be used in conjunction with the irrigations.

It is in this stage of the disease that copaiba is used to stimulate the mucous membrane toward repair. The drug is practically insoluble, but can be gotten into solution by incorporating with it an equal amount of the U.S.P. solution of potassium hydroxide. The following prescription, containing 15 minims (1 cc.) of copaiba to the dose, is acceptable:

℞. Copaiba	℥j	30.0	
Solution potassium hydroxide	℥j	30.0	
Peppermint water to make	℥iv	120.0	
Label: 1 teaspoonful after meals.			

Copaiba lends its peculiar odor to urine and breath and sometimes causes an urticarial or measles-like rash. The urine gives a false nitric acid test for albumin.

Treatment by dilatation and irrigation should be continued until the shreds disappear from the urine. In most cases this is eventually accomplished, but occasionally persons will be observed who do not respond to this treatment; these are likely to improve rapidly under a daily irrigation of potassium permanganate. It is possible to treat gonorrhea too long and to cause the discharge to persist by the simple irritation of injections. In such cases there will be a secretion free from gonococci, which on squeezing will appear at the meatus as a small transparent glycerin-like drop, and which will cause sticking together of the meatus in the morning. If treatment is stopped at this point the mucous discharge will often disappear spontaneously.

After five or six weeks of treatment, if the discharge has stopped and the urine is free from filaments, and the prostate and vesicles are not involved, treatment may be suspended, though the patient should be kept under observation for several weeks more. A culture and an examination with the urethroscope are also advisable.

POSTERIOR URETHRITIS

Posterior urethritis develops in most cases between the second and fourth weeks, due to spontaneous spread of the infection or to injudicious instrumentation. In severe cases there should be complete bed rest and cessation of local treatment of the urethra. Fluids should be urged upon the patient, but not more active diuretics because the frequent evacuation they engender may overtax the bladder. For relief of pain, saline cathartics to relieve pelvic congestion, sitz baths, and the oil of sandalwood (see p. 590) are indicated; it is sometimes necessary to give an opiate. Some physicians hold that when all other measures fail to relieve tenesmus and pain, the instillation of a few drops of 1: 500 to 1: 100 solution of silver nitrate through a soft rubber catheter or a deep urethral syringe, is indicated. But most practitioners are against the practice for the reason that the introduction of any instrument at this time is almost certain to set up one of the dreaded complications; also, the silver nitrate may itself cause more or less tenesmus.

After the posterior urethritis has become subacute, which it usually does quite promptly, resort is had to injection or, more usually, to irrigation with any of the following: protargol or argyrol, 1: 1000 to 1: 500; silver nitrate, 1: 10,000; potassium permanganate, 1: 8000 to 1: 3000; acriflavine, 1: 8000; mercurochrome, 1: 1000.

Success in treatment depends very much on the treatment of the complications.

EPIDIDYMITIS

Immediately on the development of epididymitis all treatment and instrumentation of the urethra should be stopped, the patient put to bed on a light diet and plenty of water, the scrotum immobilized by a bandage going under it and over the thighs, and hot or cold applications made. Foreign protein therapy, diathermy, the intravenous use of sodium iodide, the application of scrotal irritants such as 50 per cent guaiacol in glycerin, and most of the other special types of therapy have not been shown to have great value; perhaps intravenous calcium gluconate injections may prove to be of a little more worth—Herrold (1930) injects 10 cc. daily for three or four days and then three and finally two injections weekly for about a month. According to Campbell (1927), who has described the treatment of 3000 cases in Bellevue Hospital, New York City, a modified constriction hyperemia produced by tight rubber band compression about the scrotal contents has apparently given good results in some cases. The fever usually quickly subsides with the patient in bed, but epididymotomy is sometimes necessary to relieve the pain; it was indicated in 1 of every 15 of Campbell's cases. He writes: "The question of when one should operate presents the most difficult problem. Persistence of pain is the chief criterion at Bellevue. If pain does not disappear within forty-eight hours after confinement to bed

and application of the suspensory and ice-cap, we operate. If pain is sufficient to keep the patient awake the second night after admission, the case
is surgical. Some time ago a nonsubsiding temperature was our criterion.
Pain has proved a better guide, since we have found patients suffering
sufficiently to be kept awake at night who were afebrile. When the epididymitis has been exposed in these cases, gross evidence of abscess formation has been seen. In all cases disclosing gross evidence of suppuration,
operation has been performed without delay." The average period of
hospitalization in Campbell's series was between three and four days for the
nonsurgical cases, and between seven and eight days for the surgical cases.

PROSTATITIS

In acute prostatitis the patient should be put to bed, be given a light
diet and plenty of fluids, and hot or cold applications, the oil of sandalwood
(see p. 590) or opiates to relieve the pain. Hot sitz baths are helpful, or
continuous irrigation of the rectum with hot physiologic saline solution.
Catheterization should be resorted to only if absolutely necessary; the injection into the urethra of 1 cc. of a 2 per cent cocaine hydrochloride solution may precede the introduction of the catheter. When abscess forms, surgical
evacuation of the pus is necessary if the symptoms persist for more than a
few days.

In chronic prostatitis, which occurs in most cases of long-standing posterior urethritis, massage of the prostate through the rectum is the only
measure of great value. It should be performed several times weekly,
according to indications in the individual case, but some patients do not
bear this treatment well at all and are probably harmed by it. In nearly
every case the verumontanum is diseased and requires particular attention.
The usual method of treatment is to apply 20 per cent solution of silver
nitrate directly on it through the urethroscope. A severe reaction, with
discharge and bleeding, follows, but the treatment may be safely repeated in
eight to ten days. Tincture of iodine is sometimes substituted as it is less
painful. Usually a half-dozen treatments suffice, but if the condition has
existed for a long time, the submucous infiltration will have to be treated by
posterior dilatation.

SEMINAL VESICULITIS

Acute seminal vesiculitis usually occurs during the course of acute prostatitis and its treatment is the same; anterior urethral injections, massaging
and stripping of the vesicles are contraindicated.

Chronic vesiculitis as a rule develops by the extension of a chronic
inflammatory process through the ejaculatory duct; the duct, however,
remains patulous and sterility is not caused. The treatment consists in
stripping the contents of the vesicles once in five to seven days. This empties them of their inspissated contents, relieves distention, and thus allows
the muscles to rest and recover their tone. The inflammatory thickening
around the vesicle is also absorbed as the result of the massage. Usually
this treatment must be protracted for many months, and difficult it is, for
these patients are often neurasthenic and most aggravating. The danger
of setting up an epididymitis causes stripping to be contraindicated under
the following conditions: (a) The existence of acute vesiculitis, (b) blood in
the expressed material, (c) excessive tenderness. It seems that the operation of seminal vesiculectomy has been practically abandoned and vasotomy
is not in very good favor. The studies of McCarthy and Ritter (1932)
point toward the possibility of seminal vesicular lavage becoming a practicable procedure for those specially trained.

GLANDULAR URETHRITIS

Many intractable cases of gonorrhea lasting for years are caused by a chronic inflammation of Morgagni's crypts. These cases are usually characterized by a persistent morning drop of moisture at the meatus and a tendency toward exacerbation of the discharge upon the slightest provocation. Urethroscopic examination shows the mouths of the crypts either open and pouting or occluded by a growth of epithelium. These cases should be treated by dilatations with a full-sized sound followed by irrigations; the few glands that resist this treatment may be destroyed by the galvanocaustic needle introduced through the urethroscope—an operation to be performed very skilfully if stricture formation is to be avoided.

FOLLICULITIS AND COWPERITIS

Suppuration of one of the urethral follicles with abscess formation occasionally occurs in gonorrhea. If it does not open into the urethra by the time fluctuation occurs, it should be incised—from within the urethra if the abscess is connected with the urethra, otherwise a urinary fistula may result. Cowperitis is treated by incision from without.

CHORDEE

Before going to bed the penis should be given a prolonged immersion in hot water and the bladder emptied. A cool sleeping room, light covers, and a towel around the waist and knotted in the back to force sleeping upon the side, tend to prevent attacks. When the attack comes, the patient should again immerse the penis and testicles in cold or hot water and should empty the bladder before returning to bed. Attempts to "break" the chordee should be strictly forbidden. When the patient is subject to recurrent attacks of this very distressing symptom, sedatives are certainly indicated (for a list of sedatives, see p. 578). In some cases ⅛ grain of morphine in suppository upon retiring may be necessary.

GONORRHEAL ARTHRITIS AND ENDOCARDITIS

The treatment of gonorrheal sepsis with joint or endocardial localization is the treatment of the acute gonorrhea plus the treatment of sepsis. Sepsis is discussed on page 158, nongonorrheal endocarditis on page 514. Of course in the arthritic complication, immobilization and the application of heat are indicated; sometimes joint aspiration, and occasionally incision and open drainage, are required. Porter and Rucker have reported prompt and lasting relief from both local and constitutional symptoms following aspiration and subsequent air insufflation in knee-joint involvement.

(B) PROPHYLAXIS OF GONORRHEA

We know very little of the value of venereal prophylactic measures in civilian life, such knowledge as we have being derived entirely from army statistics. It is certainly the feeling among most of those who had to do with these matters during the recent World War that prophylaxis was successful in bringing about a marked reduction in the incidence of all three of the diseases, syphilis, chancroid and gonorrhea. What follows here is a description of the measures employed in the prophylactic stations of the American Army in Paris during 1918–19. Dr. Joseph Earle Moore, of Johns Hopkins Hospital, who was the inspector of these stations and had twenty-five of the seventy-two under his immediate control, has made a statistical study of the results and believes that the man who failed to take the treatment was more than seven times as likely to contract disease as the man who did take it. Of course the earlier the treatment is applied, the more effective it is against all three diseases, syphilis, gonorrhea and chancroid; the difference in its value when applied six or seven rather than one hour after exposure is very great. Moore says that it is still of some value, especially against syphilis, as late as eight hours after exposure and is worth while giving even as late as twelve hours.

Methods.—Three methods of prophylaxis were available (*a*) the use of a packet or tube to be carried at all times or issued upon demand, (*b*) the use of prophylactic stations, where materials were supplied but were applied by the soldier himself, and (*c*) the use of prophylactic stations where materials were both supplied and applied by a trained staff held to some extent responsible for the success of the prophylactic treatment. The use of the packet had been tried and pronounced a failure in the American Navy before the World War, and it was also said to have failed in the New Zealand Expeditionary Force in France. In the American Army in France, packets or tubes were issued only sporadically and we have no knowledge as to their value, though many medical officers gained the impression that, as used by the men, they were practically worthless. The use of prophylactic measures by the soldier himself in a station provided for the purpose was also shown to be only partially satisfactory because of the indifference with which instructions were carried out. The method finally adopted, therefore, and the only one from which we have derived any statistical studies of worth, was the presumably expert application of the prophylactic measures by trained soldier attendants in the prophylactic stations which it was compulsory for soldiers to attend who had exposed themselves to infection.

As a first step the patient was instructed to urinate. Then he was provided with a pint of warm water in a basin and a gauze wipe, with which he washed thoroughly, while the attendant dropped liquid soap on the penis. The next step was the injection of a drachm (4 cc.) of a 2 per cent protargol solution (recently, 10 per cent argyrol is perhaps more often used) into the urethra by the attendent. The patient then held the meatus firmly between the thumb and forefinger for five minutes, from time to time allowing a drop to escape from the meatus so that all parts of the urethra were kept in contact with the solution. At the end of five minutes, the protargol was allowed to escape without pressure so that a few drops remained. One-half drachm (2 Gm.) of 33⅓ per cent calomel ointment was next rubbed thoroughly by the patient, under the observation of the attendant, into all parts of the penis for five minutes, special attention being paid to the retracted prepuce, the frenum and the glans. Finally the penis was wrapped in toilet paper to protect the clothes, and the patient instructed not to urinate for four or five hours.

Technic of Prophylaxis for the Female.—I quote Moore (1929), of Johns Hopkins Hospital:

"Have the patient urinate. Place the patient in the lithotomy position. Wash the genitals and adjacent parts with soap and water. Give a douche of 2 quarts of sterile water, temperature 100 F., followed by 2 quarts of ½₀₀₀ mercuric chloride solution, and wash external parts with the latter. Dry the vagina and vulva by sponging. Swab the entire vagina, through a speculum, with a 2 per cent protargol solution, or 10 per cent argyrol solution, freshly made; reach every fold and especially the posterior vault and external os. Swab the entire vulva in the same way, reaching every recess and endeavoring to facilitate the entrance of the solution into the openings of Skene's ducts and Bartholin's glands. Inject enough of the same solution into the urethra to distend it moderately and let the patient hold her finger (in a rubber glove) against the meatus to retain the solution for from three to five minutes.

"Douche the vagina and vulva with a small amount of sterile water, and sponge dry with gauze. Apply calomel ointment to the cervix, vagina, vulva, and adjacent parts, rubbing thoroughly into the recesses and folds of the mucous membranes and skin, and taking at least ten minutes for the operation. Do not use more than 4 Gm. (1 drachm) of calomel ointment in the vagina. Cover the external parts with oiled silk or waxed paper securely and instruct the patient to allow ointment to remain for several hours before washing the parts."

(C) GONORRHEA IN THE FEMALE

Gonorrhea in women is usually indicated subjectively in the beginning by a feeling of unusual dryness and discomfort about the genitalia; this is soon followed by a burning sensation and the appearance of a discharge, which is accompanied by smarting on urination and increase in frequency. The infection is limited in its distribution, for it is only in the very young and the very old when the cornified layer of epithelium has not yet formed or has disappeared that the vagina itself is involved early. The primary points of localization are in the urethra, the urethral (Skene's) glands, the vulvovaginal (Bartholin's) glands, and the endocervix. The vaginal walls and the structures around the vaginal orifice become hot and rough and tender but they are not in themselves infected by the gonococcus in the beginning. The discomfort of acute gonorrhea in women usually passes away very quickly, but the process nearly always becomes chronic, just as in the male. The natural barriers against the upward extension of the infection into the uterus and the adnexa are very great, but once this extension takes place the resultant endometritis, salpingitis, etc., are serious affairs indeed.

Noeggarath, in 1872, was probably the first to lay stress upon the importance of latent gonorrhea in the female.

THERAPY

General Management.—The patient should be urged to refrain from exercise as much as possible and to rest in the prone position whenever she can do so. A bland light diet is helpful, and absolute abstention in the particulars of overseasoned foods and alcohol highly desirable. Much water should be taken (ginger ales, etc., are spiced and should not be used), but it is probably a mistake to render the urine alkaline in order to lessen its irritation; the normal acidity, which will already be somewhat lessened by the increase in fluid intake, is a valuable defense against extension of the infection above the meatus of the urethra. The drug that has the most valuable soothing effect upon the inflamed urethral orifice is the oil of sandalwood; for particulars of its use, see page 590. Antiseptics are sometimes given by mouth in the attempt to sterilize the genito-urinary tract from above, but the practice is not general. For the methods of using these drugs, see page 616.

The correction of constipation is indicated (see p. 432) in order to lessen pelvic congestion as much as possible, but it should be accomplished by the use of drugs, not enemas; the spread of gonorrhea into the rectum is by no means unusual. Coitus and all sexual excitement should of course be interdicted. Sedatives are used if indicated (for a list of sedatives, see p. 578). A pad of cotton should be worn over the external genitalia and frequently changed in order to avoid irritation from the discharge. Treatment of gonorrhea during pregnancy involves no danger to either mother or child.

Local Treatment in the Acute Stage.—If inspection and gentle manipulation show that the infection is confined to the meatus and the vulvovaginal (Bartholin's) glands, the local treatment should be of the simplest, for experience teaches that the acute stage of gonorrhea quickly passes in women. Instrumentation should certainly be avoided for two reasons: (a) It is painful, and (b) it is extremely likely to cause a spreading of the infection. Using a dressing forceps and a small ball of cotton, paint the affected parts with 20 to 30 per cent argyrol solution, or 2 to 4 per cent protargol solution, neither of which will cause much irritation. Silver nitrate, in 1 to 5 per cent solution, is sometimes used but it is nearly always excessively painful. After the treatment, the use of an antiseptic and drying dusting powder is very comforting to some patients but seems to increase the discomfort in others. Crossen, who employs 1 part of xeroform and 3 parts of boric acid, advocates the use of the powder after each treatment unless it increases the smarting and burning; the parts should of course be thoroughly dried before the powder is dusted in.

A profuse discharge may usually be taken to indicate that the infection has spread up into the vagina. Do not attempt instrumentation while there is still much tenderness; this stage will soon pass and then the speculum can be introduced and the cervix and the vaginal vault inspected. Therapy here consists in the painting of the cervix and the vaginal walls with the same strength silver preparation as was used in the earlier treatment of the vulva. The dusting powder should also be tried in the vagina. Mayes (1926) reported a series of cases in which he used 4 per cent mercurochrome in the vagina without any evidence of mercurialism, the vaginal mucosa being much less absorbent than that of the urethra.

It is usually considered that no attempt should be made to enter the urethral (Skene's) glands or the vulvovaginal (Bartholin's) glands with direct medication during the first several weeks. The above-described local applications, given at first every two to four days and gradually at longer intervals, should suffice for office treatment. When the discharge is profuse, the patient may be instructed to take a mild antiseptic vaginal douche twice a day, using one of the following preparations: (a) Prescribe the U.S.P. compound solution of cresol (writing for "Lysol" is to be discountenanced since this product is advertised under exaggerated and dangerous claims, such as that it is nonpoisonous), of which 1 teaspoonful is to be added to 2 quarts of water; (b) prescribe 4 ounces of a 10 per cent solution of potassium permanganate, 1 teaspoonful of which to 2 quarts will make approximately a 1: 5000 solution; (c) prescribe 2 ounces of the U.S.P. solution of formaldehyde (formalin), 6 drops of which to 2 quarts of water will make approximately a 1: 5000 solution. As usually used in the home, i. e., with the patient upright on the stool, the value of these douches is certainly questionable; in some instances they undoubtedly increase the irritation by being used too frequently. Astringent douches are entirely contraindicated. Bichloride of mercury is much too dangerous to be employed in the douche and is being rapidly dropped by the profession. Either the cresol, potassium permanganate or formalin preparations, in the proportions used for the douche, will also serve to cleanse the external parts when changing the pad.

Treatment in the Chronic Stage.—Chronic gonorrheal discharge that persists more than three or four weeks is due to the localization of the infection in the urethral (Skene's) glands, the vulvovaginal (Bartholin's) glands, or in the cervix.

(a) *Urethral Glands.*—Stevens and Heppner write (1920): "In the treatment of chronic urethritis, installation of from 1 to 3 per cent solutions of silver nitrate, and local application of stronger solutions of the same drug through a short female endoscope are useful in the absence of glandular involvement or strictures. . . . Infected ducts and glands should be destroyed, best by the actual cautery or fulguration electrode introduced through a skenoscope. Strictures should be dilated or incised." Crossen prefers a preliminary attempt to sterilize the glands with argyrol. He describes his method as follows (1926): "To treat these conditions apply a pledget of cotton soaked in a 20 per cent solution of cocaine, pushing a part of it a short distance into the urethra. Leave this in place five minutes and then proceed as follows: If the duct is open, inject a 25 per cent solution of argyrol into it with a hypodermic syringe. Use a needle the point of which has been filed round and smooth, so it will easily pass into the duct without penetrating the wall. Fill the duct with the solution so that it comes in contact with all the recesses. This injection is repeated every few days, at the same time that other infected structures are treated."

(*b*) *Vulvovaginal Glands.*—Here again, Crossen advises the preliminary attempt to sterilize the glands with once or twice weekly injections of 25 per cent argyrol or 5 to 10 per cent protargol. In most cases, however, this treatment fails and the glands must ultimately be incised and drained, or excised if the process has become chronic. Stevens and Heppner write: "Although it is usually impossible to palpate a normal Bartholin gland, an infected gland can be detected in the majority of instances. A palpable gland is usually infected; consequently its removal is advisable, notwithstanding failure to find the gonococcus on examination. Occlusion of the duct may be but temporary and is not a contraindication to this procedure. An important factor in this connection is our observation that, following operation for removal of one series of fifty-two palpable glands, the ducts of which were occluded or in the secretion from which no gonococci could be demonstrated, these organisms were found in 29 cases in the secretion from the wound. It therefore seems probable that the infection may be dormant in this location for a long period of time, and reinfection of the urethra, Skene's glands or cervix with subsequent extension to the pelvic organs eventually occurs."

(*c*) *Acute Endocervicitis.*—It is important to bear in mind that the primary object of treatment in acute endocervicitis is to so hold the disease in check that it will not spread upward into the body of the uterus and out into the fallopian tubes. Sometimes the acute cervical condition is apparently cured, but perhaps more often it becomes chronic, and in a certain proportion of these chronic cases the endometritis and salpingitis, which were escaped during the acute stage, finally develop. Acute endocervicitis is treated by (1) measures directed toward the destruction of the organisms, and (2) measures designed to lessen the pelvic congestion.

1. DESTRUCTION OF THE ORGANISMS.—Since there is a certain amount of inflammation of the vaginal vault in most cases in addition to the endocervicitis, the usual practice is to remove as much of the discharge from the cervix and vault as possible (using cotton applicators), and then to paint the vault and cervix with 4 to 10 per cent silver nitrate solution, or 4 to 10 per cent protargol, or 20 to 30 per cent argyrol. A thin strip of gauze, saturated with either of the solutions, is then placed in the cervix, where it is allowed to remain for twenty-four hours. Many other antiseptics are used, but most practitioners prefer the silver preparations. Skene, according to Crossen, usually used a mixture of tincture of iodine 2 parts and phenol 1 part. Usually the vault is dried after such a treatment, and then packed with cotton tampons with the liberal use of the antiseptic dusting powder. This pack may remain in place for twenty-four hours to two days, depending upon the amount of discharge, and should then be renewed. It is the usual practice to apply the silver preparations only at four- to seven-day intervals. Brady (1925), at the Johns Hopkins Hospital, has reported very favorably on the use of mercurochrome; twice a week the cervix and vault are painted with a 20 per cent solution of the drug, and a small amount of

cotton on a thin wire applicator is well soaked in the solution and carried through the cervical canal to the internal os. There have been no instances of mercurialism following these treatments.

2. REDUCTION OF PELVIC CONGESTION.—The attempt is often made to relieve pelvic congestion, and perhaps also to draw some of the deeper-seated organisms to the surface, by utilizing the hygroscopic action of glycerin. In this treatment the dusting powder is omitted when packing the vagina, and the inner surface of the first tampon is saturated with 10 per cent ichthyol-glycerin or protargol-glycerin. Such packs are not allowed to remain longer than twelve to twenty-four hours.

Perhaps more uniform success attends the use of the hydrotherapeutic douche. From 8 to 16 quarts of tap-water, as hot as can be tolerated, should be used as a vaginal douche during twenty to thirty minutes. The patient must be on her back with the hips elevated. Meaker (1926) writes: "The effect of prolonged wet heat is at first vasoconstriction, both arterial and venous, which allows passive venous congestion to disappear. Then follows a period of normal healthy circulation, often lasting for several hours before the hydrotherapeutic benefit is lost. ... As palliation, the depleting douche relieves pain, limits the spread of inflammation, and helps in the absorption of exudate. In many cases, notably those of endocervicitis and of mild salpingitis, a course of depletion may result in a permanent cure, the improved circulatory conditions allowing the tissues to regain enough of their natural resistive powers so that they are able to overcome infection."

Diathermy has been employed with rather limited success: Williams (1932), who obtained satisfactory results in about one fourth of his cases, feels that the response is due to the increased vascularity induced rather than to actual thermal destruction of the gonococci (see also p. 595). The use of the Elliott distensible vaginal bag, through which water is run continuously for an hour, beginning at 115 F. and increasing ¾ of a degree per minute up to 130 F., induces the same sort of circulatory changes most likely; Holden and Gurnee (1931) have reported upon its quite satisfactory use.

Chronic endocervicitis, as also endometritis and salpingitis, are potentially surgical conditions and are therefore not discussed in this book. For the same reason I have not included a discussion of the entity known as "leukorrhea," which, if looked upon as a malady to be treated by purely medical measures, irrespective of its varied etiology, will often cause surgical help to be withheld at the only time when it might save function or even life.

(D) VULVOVAGINITIS OF INFANTS

Gonorrhea outranks in incidence a large number of the infectious diseases in children, running perhaps second to measles and outnumbering smallpox and scarlet fever. Its greatest frequency is in girls up to the age of five years, but it may occur at any age up to puberty. The disease is contracted indirectly from infected adults, through such media as clothing, bed-clothing, towels, diapers, baths, sponges, and innumerable other household materials. Perhaps the chief disseminator is the common toilet seat. Rape and precocious sexual contacts are infrequent causes. In hospitals and asylums vulvovaginitis is often epidemic and is extremely difficult to eradicate. The symptoms are painful urination and pain on walking, pronounced redness and edema of the external genitalia, coapted labia majora, and a thin watery secretion which soon develops into a thick, yellow, offensive discharge. The gonococcus can be demonstrated in about 50 per cent of cases. Sometimes all the symptoms are very mild and the condition soon clears up, but most cases cause considerable discomfort and last from three to six months, during all of which time there is at least potential danger of infection of the eyes; other complications are fortunately rare. Stein's (1923) criteria for cure are (*a*) disappearance of clinical evidence of the infection, (*b*) three negative smears at intervals of one week after suspending treatment, and (*c*) a period of observation equal in time to the duration of the treatment.

THERAPY

Cleanliness.—Unquestionably the most important single element in treatment is the promotion of cleanliness. Daily tub baths and the use of clean undergarments should constitute a part of the routine treatment. For the protection of others, the child should be made to wear a vulvar pad at all times, to stay away from school and from playmates, to wash the hands thoroughly after each use of the toilet, and to protect the toilet with a towel, followed by washing with 1 per cent compound solution of cresol. She should sleep alone, and all her clothing and bed-clothing should be washed separately, after preliminary steeping in 1:50,000 bichloride of mercury solution.

Injections of Silver.—The daily injection of argyrol is perhaps the most frequently employed treatment. After a review of many other methods, Yesko (1927) recommends the following procedure: With the child in the sacrodorsal position, the genitalia are washed either with soap and water or with boric acid solution. Then by means of a soft rubber catheter, 1 ounce (30 cc.) of a 25 per cent solution of argyrol is introduced into the vagina and kept there approximately four or five minutes. The vulva is then freely painted, either with the argyrol solution or with 1 to 2 per cent mercurochrome solution. For use between treatments, this author prescribes a suppository containing 20 per cent argyrol, one to be introduced by the mother in the morning and one at night.

Douches.—A few physicians favor the use of douches in addition to the injections. Bichloride of mercury, 1:10,000, or potassium permanganate, 1:2000, or saline solution, are usually employed.

Dakin's Solution Plus Mercurochrome.—Norris and Mickelberg (1922) use the surgical solution of chlorinated soda (Dakin's solution), 1 per cent in olive oil. Three ounces (90 cc.) of this are placed in the vagina morning and evening; the external parts are also washed with it. In refractory cases they dry the vaginal mucosa thoroughly with hot air, after which 1 or 2 per cent mercurochrome solution is applied. This drying treatment is carried out three times a week, the object being to develop a more resistant vaginal mucosa. They report cure in an average time of twelve weeks in 63 cases.

Saline Douches Plus Mercurochrome.—Williams (1928) employs twice daily hot vaginal douches with saline solution. Immediately after the morning douche, the cervix is exposed through a urethroscope and mercurochrome is applied to the cervical canal by means of a nasal applicator. Coming out, all parts are painted thoroughly; a few drops of the solution are instilled into the urethra. Williams' experience has convinced him of the superiority of 5 per cent mercurochrome solution over 2 per cent of the same, 2 per cent ointment of mercurochrome, or 40 per cent argyrol.

Silver Nitrate in Ointment.—In 1920, Gellhorn, at Washington University, introduced a method of treatment that has since been much employed, the advantage claimed for it being that the antiseptic remains for a long time in contact with the diseased structures. One per cent of silver nitrate in equal parts of lanolin and white petrolatum is injected into the vagina through an ordinary glass syringe to which is attached about 3 inches of soft rubber catheter tubing. The tubing is slowly pushed inward the entire length of the vagina, and the latter is then very slowly filled to capacity with the silver salve. The excess of salve oozing back through the hymenal opening is not wiped off, as it serves to cover and protect the irritated vulva and its surroundings. One such treatment is given every day without any additional douching. Every seventh or eighth day, after a day of rest without any treatment, a smear is examined and the injections are continued if gonococci are present.

"The 1 per cent silver nitrate salve has been used in my service at the City Hospital on children ranging in age from nine months to twelve years. Under the older forms of treatment, these children had been confined in the wards for several months; the older ones were kept out of school and exposed to all the harmful influences that emanate from the adult inmates of venereal wards in public hospitals. Moreover, the very chronicity of the affection caused the interest of interns and nurses to wane, and this still further prolonged the stay of the little patients. Happily, this condition no longer prevails. Results are obtained promptly, and the number of weeks in which the children are evacuated is less than the number of months that was formerly required."

Mercurochrome in Ointment.—Stein (1923) has substituted 1 per cent mercurochrome for the silver nitrate in the ointment injection method just described above; his results were equally gratifying. More recent observers have increased the strength to 2 per cent.

Vaccines.—Very little success has been had with biologicals, as is to be expected (see p. 595).

CHANCROID

Chancroid is, next to gonorrhea, probably the commonest of the venereal diseases in the male. It would seem that the organism is able to maintain a saprophytic existence in the female, for the ulcerations are comparatively rare in women, even in those who are known to have been the direct infecting source of men. The bacillus of Ducrey is the causative agent but is very difficult to find. Diagnosis is therefore usually made upon clinical findings, having always uppermost in mind the necessity to make thorough dark-field examination to eliminate the possibility of the lesion being syphilitic in origin. The incubation period is one to several days, at the end of which time there develop one or more small ulcers with a dirty base; these usually spread rapidly, by contiguity and continuity, discharging more or less pus, bleeding freely, and causing destruction of tissues. The most frequent site of the initial lesion is the coronary sulcus, but the process may begin at any point on the penis. As the ulcerations spread, there is much subjective pain and objective inflammation and swelling of the affected parts. In the individual with a long foreskin there often occur varying stages of phimosis and paraphimosis. In about 50 per cent of the cases, especially those remaining ambulatory, the draining lymph glands are affected, giving rise to the condition known as bubo.

John Hunter (1728–93) clearly distinguished between true syphilitic chancre and this false, "soft" chancre. Ducrey discovered the causative organism in 1889.

TREATMENT OF THE ULCERS

1. **Cleanliness and Soothing Measures.**—Chancroid occurs almost exclusively in those who are negligent and unclean in their habits. Simple

use of plenty of soap and water after coitus will nearly always prevent this infection. Also, if the patient can be made to rest, to partake of simple but nourishing food, and to keep himself clean, many early cases will heal without much spread or the development of bubo. Hot boric acid (saturated solution) soaks or compresses are usually used several times daily, or the lesions are irrigated with hot potassium permanganate 1:15,000 to 1:10,000. After these treatments it is well to apply a dusting powder, such as thymol iodide (iodoform is preferable if the patient does not have to go about among people from whom his illness must be concealed), best covered with a little gauze spread with petrolatum. Dry powders alone form a crust under which the pus accumulates. When possible, it is perhaps best to substitute moist dressings, using the same solutions employed for irrigation. A much used dressing in very acute cases is one wet with one part of the N.F. solution of aluminum acetate (Burow's solution) to 10 or 15 parts of water. Black wash, the lotio hydrargyri nigra of the B.P., which is a suspension of mercurous oxide, obtained by mixing 0.685 Gm. of calomel with 5 cc. of glycerin and 95 cc. of lime water, is also much used.

Rosenwald Method.—In 1923, Rosenwald introduced his well-known treatment in which the following modification of black wash is used:

Calomel	℥j
Zinc sulphate	℥ij
Fluid opium camphorated	℥ij
Lime water	℥viij

The calomel and lime water are mixed and allowed to stand two days, with frequent shaking; the other ingredients are then added and the preparation is ready for use. Young (1926) has stated that at his clinic at the Johns Hopkins Hospital this lotion has replaced all others, but he points out that the treatment is sometimes so painful as to require the previous use of novocaine; I wonder if this is not because in Young's modification of the formula he has substituted paregoric for the fluid camphorated opium, which is the stronger preparation used by druggists in making their paregoric. Further, Rosenwald directs that the ingredients be measured by volume and not by weight, which makes a tremendous difference in the case of calomel.

Rosenwald describes his technic as follows: "A thin film of cotton about 1 inch by 3 inches is laid on the palm of the hand. The mouth of the bottle is now placed on the cotton, and a few shaking movements saturates the cotton, leaving a slight deposit. The entire length of the film is treated in this manner. The 'buttered' side of the cotton is now placed around the penis covering the ulcerations, and the foreskin drawn over the cotton. The pain produced by this application is variable, but not intense enough to require any anodynes. The patient is instructed not to remove the cotton but to return the next day for further treatment. The cotton is now removed and every chancroid is plainly outlined and limited. Chancroids from the size of a pin-point to the extent of a silver dollar are shown plainly. The uninfected skin has not been damaged in the least. What moisture is present is wiped off with a little cotton and some of the following ointment applied.

"Formula by weight:

"Zinc oxide	ℨj
Starch	ℨj
Boric acid	ℨj
Gum camphor	ℨj
Carbolated vaseline, 3 per cent	℥xij

"After the second day the chancroids begin to drop out, leaving a clean, granulating surface which heals with remarkable rapidity. The ointment is applied daily till healing is completed."

Circumcision.—In some instances it is necessary to make a dorsal slit of the prepuce, but this should be postponed until it is certain that progress in treatment cannot be made without it. Circumcision is usually considered contraindicated in all cases, however at the Cleveland City Hospital a few years ago it was decided to try the effect of surgical procedures. The result of circumcision in 171 cases was that the stay in hospital was reduced from twenty-three and four-tenths days to eighteen days and not one bubo developed. This was considered to definitely establish the value of operation, according to Rauschkolb (1930), because: (1) There are no complications, such as buboes, balanitis, phagedena and phlebitis of the dorsal vein; (2) the likelihood of early diagnosis of syphilis, by dark-field examination of ulcers rendered accessible, is increased; (3) the care of the lesions is made easier through their greater accessibility.

2. **Abortive Treatment.**—This type of treatment is described by Pusey, Hagner *et al.*, as follows: "In a certain proportion of cases of chancroid, abortive treatment is successful. The principal of all methods of abortive treatment is to convert the infected ulcer into a sterile one by the use of some destructive agent. This may be either the actual cautery, or one of several strong chemical caustics.

"The thermocautery is perhaps the best agent for this treatment. The ulcer is thoroughly cleaned and well dried. Then the entire area of it is seared with a cherry-red cautery. Every particle of diseased tissue must be destroyed. It should be done under a general anesthetic, preferably gas.

"Chemical cauterization is done as follows: The ulcer is well cleaned, being first irrigated and then dried. Then a pledget of cotton wet with 5 to 10 per cent solution of cocaine hydrochloride or novocain is applied to it. After anesthesia is produced the ulcer is dried as thoroughly as possible, preferably with blotting paper, in order to prevent the running of the chemicals subsequently to be applied. After it has been thoroughly dried, the entire surface of the ulcer, both edges and base, is touched with pure liquid phenol (carbolic acid) applied on a small cotton swab, care being taken to let no infected point escape. Then the excess of phenol on the surface is taken up, and nitric acid is applied lightly in the same way. The ulcer should be flushed immediately with sterile water to stop the action of the acid. Instead of nitric acid a saturated solution of zinc chloride can be used. This is as active a caustic as nitric acid, and its action should be stopped as quickly after application by flushing with water.

"After cauterization in any of these ways, the wound should be dressed with cold compresses of boric acid solution or similar bland solution. There results an acute inflammatory reaction, the slough is thrown off, and in successful cases, a healthy granulating surface is left."

In successful cases, healing follows quickly upon this abortive treatment, and the danger of bubo is almost eliminated. However, if the destruction of the infected area has not been thorough, more harm than good is done, for the larger ulcer produced by the treatment only becomes infected from the focus that has been left. The procedure is definitely contraindicated in the following instances: (*a*) When the diseased area is so extensive, or so situated, that its destruction would result in considerable deformity; (*b*) when there is intense inflammation with much edema; (*c*) when there is inguinal adenitis.

3. **Strong Antiseptics and Escharotics.**—It is in the cases of sores that have not been successfully aborted, or that do not respond to simple cleansing and mild antiseptic measures, that resort must be had to the use of

strong antiseptics and escharotics. Measures coming under this head are legion; only a few of the most typical will be described below. A direct comparison of the efficacy of these measures is not attempted for two reasons: First, there is no way of predicting which of them will succeed in a given case, and, second, in some cases they all fail, the disease running a course of many months, during which time much destruction of tissue takes place, until the infection finally wears itself out.

Argyrol Crystals.—Argyrol crystals are applied directly to the sores once daily for three to four minutes, followed by a moist dressing of 10 per cent argyrol or 1 per cent protargol. This treatment is sometimes so painful that preliminary local anesthesia is necessary (see below).

Copper Sulphate.—The ulcer is first anesthetized with a 10 per cent cocaine solution, and then either with or without preliminary curettement with an applicator wound firmly with cotton, a 25 per cent copper sulphate solution is applied. This is left in contact for three or four minutes and then sponged off, to be followed either by a dusting powder such as thymol iodide and covered with gauze spread with petrolatum, or wet compresses, such as are described under the head of cleanliness and soothing measures (see p. 606), are employed. The copper sulphate is generally reduced to 10 per cent for the subsequent treatment administered at two- or three-day intervals.

Copper Sulphate Plus High-frequency Current.—I quote the description of the method as given by Robbins and Seabury (1917):

"A small pledget of cotton is wet with 10 to 20 per cent solution of cocaine and applied to each lesion. After four or five minutes the field is carefully cleansed with soap and water and dried. Each lesion is then thoroughly wiped out with a cotton wound applicator until bleeding ensues. This is arrested by sponging, and when only serum exudes from the wound, this is collected for examination by dark field or stain, as may be the choice of the operator.

"A 25 per cent solution of copper sulphate in distilled water is now applied to the sore, and the short high-frequency spark from a rather fine-pointed vacuum electrode is applied directly to the sore for one to three minutes, depending on the extent of the ulceration. Especial care is exercised in carrying the point of the electrode well down into any fissure or undermined edge, and the area of application should extend over the edge of the sore about $\frac{1}{16}$ inch into the doubtfully healthy area.

"The current is not turned off until every crack and crevice has been thoroughly treated and the surface of the sore is changed to a dark greenish gray. It is then wiped dry and some antiseptic powder is lightly applied to the entire mucous surface of the preputial cavity. If the sore is exposed, it should be covered with a thick moist dressing, for which any very dilute antiseptic solution may be used, as a 1:10,000 or 1:20,000 mercuric chloride solution; or even tap-water answers nicely in most cases. This should be changed once or twice daily, and must not be allowed to stick.

"The patient is instructed to return in two days, and, if the work has been carefully done, the wound will present a perfectly healthy granulation that will go on to complete healing in a few days. If the sore does not look clean, the application is repeated at the second visit. The patient returns each second day. If the original sore was large, or if a small sore does not seem to be closing rapidly, we have made it a practice to apply, at each visit, either a 10 per cent copper sulphate or a 5 per cent silver nitrate solution. We do not hesitate to repeat the original cauterization at any time we have reason to think the chancroidal infection is not completely eliminated.

"The complete success of this, as of any other method, is dependent on careful, thorough work. There is more danger of too little cauterization than of too much, and thorough cleansing at the time the sore is destroyed must not be forgotten. Again, the after-care, especially with ulcus molle outside the preputial cavity, and with ulcus molle miliare, is of the utmost importance. If one fails to carry the electrode to the bottom of the cavernous ulcer, then one is lost. It heals over the surface, and in two or three days breaks out anew, larger and deeper than before.

"If the dressing on an exposed surface is not changed once daily, and moistened at least three or four times, in many cases one will not succeed."

Tartar Emetic.—The first to employ antimony and potassium tartrate intravenously in the treatment of chancroid were McDonagh, of London, and Potter, of Melbourne, in the second decade of this century. On the American continent there is no record of its use prior to 1925, but since that date there have appeared the reports of Goodman, Kingsbury and Peck, and Jones. It would seem that the pain, discomfort, discharge and edema, are all markedly reduced under this treatment and that rapid repair of the ulcer takes place. Jones (1927) reports 27 cases, 23 of which "showed excellent results." In his series, an initial dose of 3 cc. of a 1 per cent solution of tartar emetic, increasing 1 cc. with each dose up to 10 cc., with the administration at four-day intervals, seemed to be amply sufficient. No authors report serious reactions, though coughing, salivation and vomiting, all of which clear up in a few hours, are to be expected from these large doses of tartar emetic. The method certainly merits further study.

Rupel (1926) has also reported a small series of cases in which daily local applications of a 0.5 per cent solution of the drug were made. His results were better in his opinion than those obtained on the average with other local treatment. The applications are well tolerated at the strength used, but he found 1 per cent solution to cause considerable burning pain.

TREATMENT OF BUBO

I quote here from the excellent discussion of this subject by Cole (1929):

"Occasionally in a chancroidal bubo, if it be detected early and if the patient be placed in bed, the inflammation will subside and disappear by simple rest alone. At other times, by the use of hot applications or by ice applications, the same can be achieved. Nevertheless, it has been our general experience that if the bubo has reached any size it is almost bound to go on to suppuration or to a stage in which it will be necessary to have some type of intervention.

"In the past the treatment of chancroidal buboes has been almost entirely surgical. At one time even dissection out of the entire mass was recommended, but since this resulted in bad cases of elephantiasis this procedure has been discarded. Another type of therapy which has been quite popular and is still widely used is to wait until the mass has begun to soften and until fluctuation is present. Then the abscess is incised, drained, and the cavity packed with iodoform gauze or with gauze saturated in boracic acid solution. Still another procedure that is widely employed is to inject into the cavity a 10 per cent iodoform emulsion in sterile olive oil, along with this using iodoform gauze drains. This type of therapy undoubtedly has its place and it may be that there are isolated cases where it is to be recommended in preference to any other form of treatment.

"However, in the last few years the injection treatment of buboes has become quite popular, and in our experience is preferable to any other method of treating the average case coming under observation. It gives a large percentage of cures (as high as 92 per cent in some of our statistics), and this in a very short time, three to four days in many cases; seldom over two weeks.

"For this type of treatment rest in bed is absolutely essential, and preferably in a hospital bed. One observes the bubo from day to day, watching it closely until such a time as fluctuation is noted, with softening over the glands. A slight nick with a sharp knife, 1 cm. in length, is then made near the base of the surface, slanting down toward the thigh. Under gentle expression the pus is allowed to run out as much as it will. Following this a compression bandage is applied, using plenty of gauze immediately over the gland in order to get heavy compression for a period of twenty-four hours. During this time the patient is supposed to lie flat in bed with his legs unflexed, in order to get as much pressure locally as is possible. The bandage is then removed, the pus in the cavity is completely evacuated by pressure with the fingers, and under aseptic precautions 1 or 2 cc. of Mencière's solution (iodoform, guaiacol, eucalyptol, and alcohol (95 per cent), each 10; balsam of Peru, 30; ether, 100) is injected into the cavity of the gland. A Record syringe is used for this purpose, the nozzle of the syringe, without a needle, being simply forced into the small aperture that has been made twenty-four hours before, the elbow of the syringe being pressed up firmly against the skin in order to prevent the fluid from escaping. This fluid, which causes severe burning for a few seconds, is allowed to remain in the cavity of the gland for one minute. It balloons out the cavity in such a way that all the interstices and pockets receive a certain amount of the preparation which is antiseptic, astringent, and reducing in its properties. The hope is that the cavity will be entirely sterilized from this contact with the fluid. The fluid is then allowed to run out from the opening and is gently expressed to get out all of the remaining Mencière's solution. After this another heavy compression bandage is applied and allowed to remain in place for forty-eight hours. The patient is again advised that he must not flex his legs, but should keep them extended in order to have heavy compression over the area. At the time that the bandage is removed one may note that some clear serum runs from the opening of the gland cavity. This simply indicates an irritation type of fluid and is of no moment. The fluid is pressed out, another compression bandage is reapplied and allowed to stay on for another twenty-four hours. At the end of this time, if the cavity still continues to discharge pus, another injection of Mencière's solution will have to be made according to the technic described above.

"In a large proportion of the cases, if the technic is properly carried out, one treatment will suffice in curing the bubo. In certain of them, if pus is noted instead of serum, one or two more injections may be necessary. The injection should not be repeated in less than three days. It has been our experience that with this injection technic hospital bed days have been enormously lessened and likewise sick days for the patient."

Mencière's solution was first used in the treatment of chancroidal bubo by Lassère, a French army surgeon, in 1920.

BALANITIS

Balanitis, of which erosive and gangrenous types are recognized, is a fairly uncommon affection, even in large venereal clinics, but its grave character when unrecognized entitles it to very serious consideration. It is an infectious venereal disease due to the symbiosis of a fusiform bacillus and a spirochete, both of which are anaerobic and structurally resemble those found in Vincent's angina. The lesions, which develop quickly on the glans or foreskin, usually are single, in contradistinction to chancroid, and do not give rise to bubo, though there is sometimes an inguinal adenitis. The pus is of a characteristic foul odor. The local and constitutional symptoms vary with the severity of the infection. Owing to the fulminating nature of the inflammatory process, phimosis is an early and annoying complication. Extension of the disease is commonly very rapid, the glans and the prepuce, and in some instances even the entire shaft of the penis, being destroyed by gangrene in a surprisingly short time.

THERAPY

The key to the treatment of this disease lies in the fact that the organism does not flourish when exposed to oxygen. The usual practice is to open the prepuce by a dorsal slit, so that the glans is completely uncovered, then keeping the parts clean either by wet dressings or by continuous irrigation with 2 per cent solution of hydrogen dioxide. Most cases heal rapidly under this treatment, especially if the parts are kept exposed to air at all times when the oxidizing agent is not being used.

The use of arsphenamine intravenously, as in the treatment of syphilis, is said to hasten recovery.

Sutton has described the use of subcutaneous injections of oxygen in a resistant case as follows:

"When I first saw the patient, five days after the onset of the disease, almost the entire dorsum of the penis was involved, the skin and subcutaneous tissues being soft and gangrenous. During the following thirty-six hours the infection continued to spread, despite the frequent and liberal use of hydrogen peroxide, by irrigation and by moist packs.

"At this time subcutaneous injections of oxygen were begun, by means of an ordinary hypodermic needle connected to an oxygen tank through a small rubber tube, and repeated every four hours. The normal tissue surrounding the affected area was first treated, the flow of gas being regulated by means of a small screw clamp encircling the outlet tube. Afterward the involved structures also were thoroughly impregnated with the gas. Within six hours the progress of the disease was checked, and within twelve hours it was completely under control. Shortly afterward the slough began to separate, and recovery, aside from the deformity resulting from loss of tissue, was prompt and uneventful."

GRANULOMA INGUINALE

Granuloma inguinale is a chronic infectious, ulcerative process, usually involving the genitalia or neighboring parts, and showing no tendency toward spontaneous healing. Most of the cases are seen in young adult negroes, with perhaps an even distribution between the sexes. The disease is probably not venereal since wives or husbands often are not affected though continuing to cohabit with an infected mate. The process begins as a small moist papule which rapidly ulcerates; thereafter, invasion of the surrounding tissues by the elevated, reddish, often shiny, delicately skinned granulomatous proliferations is gradual and eccentric. Where moist, the lesions are superficially ulcerated, but where dry they are cracked. Adenopathy is characteristically absent, though the occurrence of elephantiasis of the genitalia, or of a leg, signifies involvement of the lymph channels. Except for the presence of the lesions and a slight itching or burning sensation, the patients experience little discomfort. The discharge from the ulcerating areas is held by some observers to have a quite characteristic odor, but having once seen the entire staff of a reputable hospital led temporarily away from their correct clinical diagnosis of epithelioma by the asseveration of an expert on this disease that he "smelled granuloma in the ward," I am extremely doubtful of the value of this diagnostic sign. Wilson's (1930) study of a small series indicated rapid progression and a tendency toward stillbirth in cases complicating pregnancy.

Granuloma inguinale was first recognized by MacLeod, in India, in 1882, but it was first accurately described by Conyers and Daniels, in British Guiana, in 1896. In 1905, Donovan, in India, first described the organism now believed to be causative, but, strange to say, it is not definitely known as yet whether this organism is a protozoan or a true bacterium. It is found in all parts of the lesions, but especially in the deeper areas, where all other organisms are absent. Campbell (1927) has written, "Numerous descriptions to the contrary notwithstanding, we believe there is nothing peculiarly characteristic or diagnostic in the histologic picture." The geographic distribution of the disease is very wide, including India, southern China, Australia, West Africa, the East and West Indies, and parts of North, Central and South America. Its widespread presence in the United States is now generally recognized, though undoubtedly it is more prevalent in the South than elsewhere.

THERAPY

Tartar Emetic.—Antimony and potassium tartrate was first used in the treatment of this disease by Aragao and Vianna of Brazil; it is now looked upon as a specific remedy. The lesions are caused to progressively involute and the Donovan bodies to disappear. It is usual to use a 1 per cent solution beginning with 2 cc. intravenously and increasing 1 to 2 cc. at a time until 10 to 12 cc. are being given at a dose. The injections are given at intervals of two to three days. Ten or twelve injections often clear the lesions sufficiently that it is difficult to hold the patient for further treatment, but Gage has stated that, to avoid relapse, weekly injections should be given for two or three months after entire healing, followed by two injections monthly for four months.

The solution is usually sterilized in the autoclave, though it has been pointed out that serious symptoms may arise from the formation of decomposition products of the drug when submitted to high temperatures. It may also be sterilized by passage through the Chamberland filter. Extreme care must be exercised in giving the injection, for even a very small amount placed outside the vein is very painful and causes a brawny induration that ruins the site for subsequent injections. If given too rapidly, excruciating pain will be felt in the arm and shoulder. The occurrence of dizziness, coughing, vomiting, marked diarrhea, and pains in the extremities are signs that the limits of tolerance have been reached; thereafter the drug must either be reduced or suspended altogether for a time.

In the series of 150 American cases, collected by Fox (1926), in which results of treatment by tartar emetic were mentioned, complete or almost complete healing took place in 78 (52 per cent), and various degrees of improvement in 31 cases (20 per cent). This does not impress one as the sort of results usually accomplished by "specifics"; indeed, there are other evidences in the literature that all is not yet as well as it might be in the treatment of this disease with tartar emetic. Crutchfield (Galveston, Texas, 1926) says, "We speak of antimony and potassium tartrate as a specific, and perhaps it is; but in a certain number of cases improvement occurs for a time, and then a point is reached at which improvement no longer obtains." Michael (Houston, Texas, 1926) says, "In my experience, response to treatment has not been as satisfactory as one is led to believe." And then there is Fraser, in South Africa (1925), in whose hands the drug was by no means specific: Of 16 cases, 6 healed completely, but 10 derived no benefit whatever. Perhaps we shall some day gain some understanding of these failures which at the present time are quite baffling. Hazen *et al.* (1932) have obtained indifferent results and turned to radiation with *x*-rays, which they describe as "reasonably effective"; however, when they prepared their own solution of tartar emetic instead of relying upon the commercial preparation, both subjective and objective improvement was observed in all patients in their small series. One thing has been universally observed, namely, that in the presence of syphilis as a complication, response to the tartar emetic is much less complete.

Antimony Sodium Thioglycollate.—Randall (1924) has presented evidence that this drug (now described in New and Nonofficial Remedies) may prove to be preferable to tartar emetic in that it is less toxic and apparently considerably more effective. Several of Randall's patients who were intolerant to tartar emetic took the new drug without reactions. The dose is 0.05 to 0.1 Gm. dissolved in 10 to 20 cc. of sterile water every third to fourth day until fifteen to twenty-five injections have been given. The number of cases thus treated is as yet not very large. Hazen *et al.* (1932) have used antimony thioglycollamide with "striking therapeutic response" in 3 cases; Senear and Cornbleet (1932) and Patch and Blew (1930) have also used the drug successfully, though I believe the thioglycollate is usually considered to be less toxic.

Fuadin.—Williamson (1933) and his associates have recently reported enthusiastically upon their success with this new trivalent compound of antimony and sodium in 14 cases. Their treatment consisted of twelve intramuscular injections on alternate days of a 7 per cent solution; the first injection was of 1.5 cc., the second of 3.5 cc. and the subsequent injections each of 5 cc. No reactions considered dangerous were observed though 3 patients experienced generalized subacute joint pains after certain of the injections, persisting at times long enough to cause postponement of the subsequent injection one day.

LYMPHOGRANULOMA INGUINALE
(Climatic Bubo)

This is a specific venereal disease which always follows sexual exposure and therefore is seen with extreme rarity in children. Men predominate among the victims of the inguinal form, but the anorectal localization is seen often enough in women (occasionally in men also) to probably equalize the sex distribution. The initial small lesion on the external genitalia is not often seen, but it is known that the incubation period after exposure is between ten and thirty days. Usually the glands of only one side are involved but bilateral cases are on record; there is gradual progression until a fist-size mass bound together by periadenitis is formed, and then breakdown and fistula formation takes place; a thin seropurulent fluid drains for weeks and months. Occasionally, however, no break-down occurs. French observers have regarded involvement of the iliac gland as pathognomonic. The rectal cases usually lead to serious stricture interfering with defecation. The systemic symptomatology is mild. Frei (1925) has developed an antigen reaction which is positive in all cases. The causative organism is known to be a filtrable virus; mice, the guinea-pig and monkey are serving as experimental animals with which it is hoped to learn more of the nature of the malady.

It is now thought that John Hunter treated cases of lymphogranuloma inguinale because of some descriptions in his "Treatise on Venereal Diseases," published in 1786; Chassaignac, in 1859, also described similar clinical pictures, but the individuality of the disease and its probable venereal nature was only truly pointed out by Durand, Nicholas and Favre, in 1913. Originally considered to be only tropical in its distribution, it is now recognized as occurring practically everywhere, though until quite recently most of the reports have come from European countries. DeWolf and Van Cleve (1932) have made the diagnosis in 58 cases in the Cleveland City Hospital, between August, 1930, and March 15, 1932, which indicates a considerable prevalence in the United States. According to Findlay (1932), the entity is still extremely rare in England.

THERAPY

As in the therapeutic approach to all relatively "new" diseases, a host of drugs has been tried here, but the only one which apparently gives fairly consistent results is tartar emetic, used as in granuloma inguinale (see p. 613). Nonspecific protein therapy (methods on p. 327), hot air, ultraviolet rays and x-rays have also been employed. DeWolf and Van Cleve state that their results have been rather unsatisfactory with all the measures, though the use of tartar emetic intravenously has been begun too recently to permit of any opinion of its efficacy. Five cases have been treated by excision of the involved inguinal glands, as recommended by some of the European observers; the results were good in the first 4 so treated, in the fifth a sufficient time had not elapsed to warrant the inclusion of a progress report at the time of publication. Sulzberger and Wise (1932) write, "At present roentgen therapy of the glands or surgical extirpation of the deeper lymph structures and repeated puncture of the more superficial ones seem to offer the best results." I find no record of American employment of the vaccines which have been used with some success (Hermans, 1929; Hellerström, 1931) abroad.

NONTUBERCULOUS URINARY TRACT INFECTIONS
(Cystitis, Pyelitis, and Pyelonephritis)

Urinary infection should probably be considered no more a clinical entity than hematuria or pyuria. Whenever the diagnosis is made, it should be looked upon merely as a warning that a thorough urological investigation is indicated in order to determine if possible the underlying pathologic condition responsible for the infection. The following signs and symptoms are indicative of nontuberculous infection of the tract. Kidney: Fever, chills, prostration, kidney pain or tenderness; bacteria, pus and perhaps blood in the urine; in addition there may be the symptoms of cystitis. Bladder: Frequency, burning, bacteria and pus in the urine, and pain which may be referred to the penis, meatus, urethra, scrotum, perineum, rectum, or the inner surface of the thighs. The organisms most often present in the causative rôle are the bacilli of the colon group, with the staphylococci next and the streptococci third; all other organisms are found only rarely.

THERAPY

General Considerations.—In fulminating cases of urinary tract infection, absolute rest in bed, with hot fomentations to the kidney region or the perineum, the pushing of fluids, and the employment of sedative measures are imperative. The following prescription, containing ½ grain of luminal, ⅚ grain of extract of hyoscyamus, and 5 grains of pyramidon to the dose, is useful.

℞.	Phenobarbital (luminal)............................	gr. vi	0.4
	Extract of hyoscyamus.............................	gr. x	0.65
	Amidopyrine (pyramidon).........................	℥j	4.0

Make twelve capsules.
Label: One capsule every four hours.

The luminal is sedative, the hyoscyamus has a belladonna-like action in relaxing smooth muscle, and the pyramidon is analgesic. Of course in the thoroughly septic patient the treatment is that of sepsis (see p. 159). In these latter cases, the temptation to operate is strong, but, as Barney has well said, "the recollection of the pathology, the knowledge that in more than 50 per cent of the cases the infection is bilateral, and the experience which has seen patients in other equally bad states recover, will perhaps stay the hand that is eager to grasp the knife." Drainage of the kidney pelvis through a catheter is sometimes considered to be indicated. There is a firmly entrenched clinical impression that the use of methenamine (urotropin) before drainage is established will serve only to increase the edema and thus tend to increase the blockage of the canal. Certain it is that defective drainage at any point in the urinary canal must be corrected, for to leave a patient with urinary stasis is to invite reinfection. The difficulty lies in the recognition of the presence of stone, tumor or diverticula. Injury to any part of the tract is also an inciting cause of infection; injury from exposure, from the use of irritating drugs, or following instrumentation. Also in all cases, mild or severe, foci of infection, which may be a constant source of reinfection of the tract, must be searched out and dealt with.

Young, Scott and Hill (1924) have advised the use of mercurochrome-220 by mouth to combat the primary source of infection, which is often in the intestine. The drug is given in capsules, each containing 1½ grains (0.1 Gm.), three times daily. "Treatment may be continued ten to fourteen days without much discomfort, but should then be discontinued for several days. The effect of this internal medication is to reduce the bactericidal count in the feces. The bile becomes strongly antiseptic." The treatment has not been used much as yet. Redewill *et al.* (1930) believe that it is often worth while to change the intestinal flora by implantation of *Bacillus acidophilus;* for methods see page 439.

In the majority of cases of urinary tract infection, at least in adults, it becomes necessary to resort to the use of internal antiseptics (those given by the mouth) or external antiseptics (those applied directly to the mucous membrane by injection or irrigation). In ulcerative cystitis, topical applications of silver nitrate or electrical fulguration may be necessary.

Internal Antiseptics.—I would wish the reader to take whatever dogmatic statements appear in this section on internal "antiseptics" with one or more grains of salt, for the longer I study the literature of this subject the more firmly do I become convinced that direct comparison of the clinical efficiency of the several drugs is hardly possible. Sometimes, indeed, it would seem that Gordon (1932) was right when he said in a discussion in ew Orleans: "I have used all types of urinary antiseptics, from pyridium down the list. I have never seen any effect on the bacteriological content e urine. I think the best urinary antiseptic is water, and plenty of it."

kalis.—At present it would seem that pyelitis in infants and children treated by alkalizing the patient. How this alkaline treatment cures puzzling, especially in view of the work of Helmholz (1922), who showed that the degree of alkalinity of the urine obtained by any regimen is probably not sufficient to inhibit bacterial growth. Many of the cases, however, are quickly cured. Sodium bicarbonate, 15 to 30 grains (1 to 2 Gm.) four times daily, is usually used, but Freeman (1924) recommends the following dosage plan: 5 to 20 grains (0.32 to 1.4 Gm.) every hour day and night, or every hour during the day and a double dose at bedtime, at 10.00 P. M., and possibly again at 2.00 A. M.

In adults, the use of alkalis rarely lessens the infection, but it does often-times reduce the symptoms of irritation.

Methenamine (Urotropin).—Urotropin depends for its value as a urinary tract antiseptic upon the fact that in acid medium part of it is con-verted into formaldehyde, which is a valuable antiseptic substance. In the absence of bacteria the reaction of the urine is usually acid, and even when neutral or alkaline from disease or diet, regulation of the latter and adminis-tering acid-producing drugs, such as sodium biphosphate, will quickly render it acid. In the presence of certain infections, however, it is not always pos-sible to produce an acid urine. *Bacillus proteus vulgaris* readily decom-poses urea into ammonia, thus producing a strongly alkaline urine; both staphylococci and streptococci are prone to decompose urea, and even the typhoid bacillus sometimes breaks it up; colon and paratyphoid bacilli probably never do so, however.

The usual method of giving the drug is to alternate it every two hours with doses of sodium biphosphate; that is to say, the patient gets a dose of sodium biphosphate at 8.00 A. M., urotropin at 10.00 A. M., sodium biphos-phate at 12.00 noon, etc. In adults it is customary to distribute from 45 to 90 grains (3 to 6 Gm.) of the urotropin through the twenty-four hours. In children the following dosage may be employed three times daily: Under one year, ½ to 1 grain (0.03 to 0.06 Gm.), one to three years, 1 grain (0.06 Gm.), three to five years, 2 grains (0.13 Gm.); these doses may be cau-tiously increased very considerably—indeed, Campbell (1932) has written: "While there are children with an idiosyncrasy for methenamine, as a rule it may be given in doses whose basis of computation is 12½ grains (0.8 Gm.) daily *per annum*. For example, a two-year-old child receives 25 grains (1.6 Gm.) a day. Seventy-five grains (5 Gm.) a day is the average maxi-mum that my associates and I employ in children, although we have ad-ministered still larger doses without untoward effects."

The sodium biphosphate may well be given in lemonade or in some such prescription as the following, which contains about 15 grains (1 Gm.) of the drug to the dose:

℞. Sodium biphosphate...............................	℥j	30.0
Syrup of citric acid	℥j	30.0
Water to make....................................	℥iv	120.0
Label: One teaspoonful every four hours.		

Recently, the invariable ability of sodium biphosphate to render the urine markedly acid has been questioned, and ammonium chloride and acid ammonium phosphate have been used instead, with perhaps better results; either one may be substituted in the above prescription in the amount of 1½ ounces (45 Gm.), which will give a dose of 24 grains (1.5 Gm.).

Moderate doses of urotropin will cause hematuria in a small number of individuals, the bleeding being due to the production of a hemorrhagic cysti-tis. Bloedorn and Houghton (1922) were not able to produce it at will, and they believe that it occurs only in those individuals who have an idiosyncrasy for the drug. It has been claimed (Abt, 1917) that the drug causes severe and fatal nephritis; if this is so, the cases must be extremely rare. Skin rashes, catarrhs of various mucosae, and digestive disturbances, though rare, have also been reported.

The intravenous use of urotropin does not seem to be necessary or even justified in view of the rapid absorption obtained upon oral administration; however, it has been successfully used by Braasch and Bumpus (1925), of the Mayo Clinic, in 76 cases of acute and subacute infection. They used 5 cc. of a 10 per cent solution daily. "Even though no attempt is made to acidify the urine it is remarkable how frequently the fever is controlled and symptoms alleviated. None of the gastric upsets associated with its oral administration was noted, and this much smaller dosage seems to produce effects equivalent to those formerly obtained by a much larger dose by mouth."

Although urotropin was introduced as a urinary antiseptic in 1895 and has been very much used since that time almost as a routine in urinary tract infections, the actual existing body of evidence does not very strongly support the claims made for its efficacy; especially does it seem to be ineffective if diuresis is practiced at the same time. In 1912, Burnham showed that on the customary doses not more than one patient out of five gives a positive test for formaldehyde in the urine, and Hinman (1913–15) found that only 5 per cent of 318 bladder urines studied by him were bactericidal and only 17 per cent were completely bacteriostatic. He further showed that at the kidney level the drug was of no value for the reason that the urine does not remain in the renal pelvis long enough to permit the conversion of urotropin into formaldehyde, and that the same conditions prevail in the bladder if urination is frequent. His conclusions were that the drug is of no value above the bladder and only in the bladder if fluids are restricted. Even the custom of alternating with doses of drugs which will increase the acidity of the urine will not offset the reduction in antiseptic efficiency consequent upon dilution of the formaldehyde. These findings have been amply confirmed both in Europe and America, despite which the practice of giving large quantities of water or diuretic drugs during urotropin treatment is still popular. The matter must not be misunderstood: Many times the forcing of water or the giving of diuretics is of more value than to attempt disinfection—but in these cases urotropin should not be used, for under the circumstances it will be of no avail and its employment will only needlessly subject the patient to the chance of an induced kidney irritation.

The earlier claim that urotropin is itself a diuretic was entirely disproved by the work of Ruh and Hanzlik (1922).

Methylene Blue (Methylthionine Chloride).—When methylene blue is given by the mouth only about 50 per cent of it is excreted by the kidneys, the remaining half being eliminated mostly in the stools, which often become as highly colored as the urine. The drug undergoes much decomposition in its passage through the blood, some of it appearing in the urine in the form of leukoderivatives which are, for the most part, nonbacteriostatic. Considerable amounts of the dye may also be decomposed by bacterial activity, as is often observed in patients with pyuria, whose urine may acquire only a dirty green hue even when large doses of the drug are ingested.

From 3 to 6 grains (0.2 to 0.4 Gm.) of the drug four times a day is a ⟩od average dose, but 10 grains (0.6 Gm.) have been given without causing ᵗative or toxic symptoms; the 1-grain (0.06 Gm.) dose, so often em-ᵉd, is too small. Methylene blue should not be given continuously over ᵧ long time, and it is contraindicated in cases of severe nephritis, for been shown that the excretion of a small fraction of a grain in these ᵃy be prolonged for several weeks.

ᵃn writes: "Personal studies show that methylene blue is a very weak and slow germicide. It will not kill the staphylococcus, streptococcus or *Bacillus coli communis* under twenty-five minutes even in a 1:10 dilution, and even after forty-eight hours' exposure it shows little selective power as a germicide. As a bacteriostatic, however, it is very selective and powerful in its action. It completely inhibits the staphylococcus in a 1: 150,000 dilution, the streptococcus in 1: 80,000, and the colon bacillus, however, in only a 1: 1000 dilution."

Acriflavine.—This drug is used in the form either of the hydochloride or the base, the latter being considered less irritating. For full effect with these drugs the urine must be kept alkaline by doses of sodium bicarbonate which have to be determined in each individual case but are usually between 2 and 3 drachms (8 and 12 Gm.) daily. Average dosage is from 2 to 4 grains (0.12 to 0.25 Gm.) twice daily, best administered in capsules. Davis (1932), who has long been studying urinary antisepsis, favors this drug, though in his experience as in that of many others, nausea, vomiting and diarrhea are not infrequent accompaniments of the administration. Perhaps in some instances the sodium bicarbonate is responsible in part for these symptoms.

Quinine.—Quinine is occasionally used by practitioners as a urinary antiseptic by mouth, but there is practically nothing in the literature regarding its efficacy. Any of the salts may be employed in doses just short of those causing cinchonism; that is to say, the daily dose must be separately determined in every case. It is known that the bactericidal action of quinine is not hindered by the coincident presence of pus. The subject would seem to beg for investigation.

Phenyl Salicylate (Salol).—This drug is still sometimes used by mouth as a urinary antiseptic, but I know of no investigations showing that it has any value other than its very doubtful function as an intestinal antiseptic.

Hexylresorcinol (Caprokol of the N.N.R.).—This drug, which is an alkalized resorcinol, was introduced as a urinary tract disinfectant following the investigations of Leonard, at the Johns Hopkins Hospital, during the years 1914–24. It is claimed to have the following advantages: Administrable by mouth, chemically stable, nontoxic in therapeutic doses, nonirritating to the urinary tract, bactericidal (not merely bacteriostatic) in high dilution in urine of any reaction, secreted by the kidney unchanged in sufficient percentage to impart active bactericidal properties to the urine. An outstanding feature of the drug's action is the symptomatic relief, particularly of vesical irritability, that is said to be an early occurrence in practically every instance in which it is properly used. Sterilization of the tract is said to be accomplished in most cases but requires a considerable time: staphylococcus, streptococcus, and *Bacillus pyocyaneus* yield the more readily, *B. coli* is more resistant.

The drug appears on the market as Caprokol in two forms. The capsules each contain 2⅕ grains (0.15 Gm.) dissolved in olive oil, and are intended for adult use. The solution contains 2½ per cent of the drug dissolved in olive oil, and is intended for use in infants and children; 1 drachm (4 cc.) of this solution contains 1⅓ grains (0.1 Gm.) of the drug. During the first few days on hexylresorcinol the patient often has diarrhea and perhaps some griping; in occasional cases there is also nausea and vomiting. All of these symptoms disappear if the use of the drug is persisted in. Hexylresorcinol must be given on a full stomach, *i. e.*, just after meals three times daily.

The first wave of enthusiasm past, there has been much difference of opinion regarding the efficacy of the new drug; its cost, which seems to me quite excessive, certainly does not increase its attractiveness. Leonard has stated four factors which he believes control the drug's effectiveness:

"1. The dosage must be adequate. On less than from 0.45 to 0.6 Gm. three times a day (from 3 to 4 capsules immediately after each meal), the surface tension of the urine will not be lowered sufficiently to obtain the maximum disinfectant action.

"2. Fluids must not be forced. This procedure raises the surface tension of the urine, and thereby robs it of its bactericidal action. In many instances, quantities of water may be a prime necessity. Under these circumstances it is just as well to postpone active antiseptic therapy until the amount of fluid ingested can be safely reduced.

"3. Sodium bicarbonate is contraindicated for the reason that it raises the surface tension of the urine, and, like large quantities of water, thereby robs the urine of its bactericidal properties. Hexylresorcinol is equally efficacious in alkaline and in acid urine.

"4. The course of treatment with hexylresorcinol must be sufficiently prolonged. Among the organisms commonly found in urinary tract infections, those which are most resistant to surface tension changes in the test tube (colon group) are most resistant to the action of hexylresorcinol in vivo. Urinary infections by *Bacillus coli* and related types ordinarily require from sixty to ninety days' continuous treatment with the drug. If combined with the usual local measures, the course of treatment will be shortened and the percentage of ultimate cures increased."

Recent studies in the bacteriology laboratory indicate that organisms grown in the presence of hexylresorcinol may acquire an increased sensitiveness to the germicidal properties of formaldehyde; the reverse of this proposition is not true. Leonard (1927) has suggested that cases which have for some time resisted the action of hexylresorcinol might well be placed on urotropin, with a reasonable chance that the latter drug might be found under these circumstances to possess a quite unusual degree of germicidal activity.

Pyridium.—This intensely red azo dye of the pyridine series is now having some vogue. It is usually given orally in the form of 2 tablets three times daily, each tablet containing 1½ grains (0.1 Gm.). The manufacturers suggest the following dosage for children: one half to one year, ¼ tablet twice daily; two to five years, ½ tablet twice daily; six to eight years, 1 tablet twice daily. Or it may be given as a 0.5 per cent aqueous solution, as follows: one half to one year, 1 drachm (4 cc.) thrice daily; two to five years, 2 drachms thrice daily; six to eight years, 4 drachms thrice daily. Pyridium is incompatible with mercury and silver and all mineral acids, and is contraindicated in uremia and in severe disorders of the kidneys of a noninfectious type.

Chemotherapy.—Young (1932) and his associates have recently reaffirmed their confidence in the advisability of supplementing the other methods of therapy by the intravenous injection of mercurochrome in selected cases.

External Antiseptics for Lavage of the Renal Pelvis.—1. *Silver Nitrate.*—The experimental work of O'Conor, in 1921, though probably misunderstood since it was interpreted as derogatory to silver nitrate as an external antiseptic, served the very valuable purpose of bringing out a defensive expression of urological opinion, which was overwhelmingly to the effect that silver nitrate is our most valuable agent for renal lavage. Injections into the pelvis are made by the use of a small syringe attached to a ʰthral catheter, never using more than 3 to 5 cc. The number of injections ᵗo be regulated by the patient's reaction. Some patients are very little ʳed, and in them the treatments may be given two or three times a this may have to be kept up for months. Other patients, however, ᵒnsiderably and may even go into shock after one of these treatments. It is believed that the silver nitrate is effective not only by reason of its superficial destruction of organisms, but also because it destroys to some extent the mucosa of the passages, and that in the reparative reaction thus called forth, with its accompanying increase in vascularity, many of the deeper organisms are also destroyed.

As to strength of solution, I believe Braasch's statement, made in 1915, still represents the opinion of the majority of urologists:

"Silver nitrate is unquestionably a very valuable aid in the treatment of renal infection. Recently Geraghty called our attention to the use of a denser solution of silver nitrate, advising as high as 5 per cent. It has been my experience, however, that it is not necessary to use such dense solutions. It is best to commence with a solution, say 1: 500 or 1: 1000 and gradually work up to 1 per cent. I think 1 per cent is just as efficacious as 2 or 3 or 5 per cent. Five per cent can cause considerable reaction; I have seen a number of cases that have given evidence of renal insufficiency as the result of a 5 per cent injection of silver nitrate. It is difficult to understand why silver nitrate should be of so much more value in some cases of renal infection than in others. It has been my experience that silver nitrate is of value in the great majority of cases. We have recently reviewed several hundreds of cases and there were very few that were not benefited by its use, and many of them were evidently cured."

Pyelitis in Infancy and Childhood.—These cases clear up in the course of time under routine treatment, or even without any treatment, in the great majority of instances. However, a review of the pediatric literature leaves the impression that there is a certain definite group that do not get well. In cases of this sort, the use of pelvic lavage has become more popular since the work of Kretschmer and Helmholz, in 1920. Of course, special instruments and special training are required, and a general anesthetic is necessary, particularly in boys; but the lavage seems to be feasible and curative in many cases. Poulsen (1923), in Denmark, has reported considerable success by ignoring the pyelitis and merely washing out the bladder twice weekly with 2 per cent silver nitrate (1 per cent in boys), until the urine is sterile on two successive examinations. The only new therapeutic measure of promise is the employment of the ketogenic diet to render the urine sufficiently acid to be bacteriostatic (for methods, see p. 641). Helmholz (1932) has employed this measure quite successfully in a number of instances at the Mayo Clinic.

2. *Other Drugs.*—Argyrol is sometimes used in a 1 per cent solution, mercurochrome-220 or gentian violet in 1 to 5 per cent solution, acriflavine in 1: 1000 strength. None of these solutions are as much favored as silver nitrate. Young, White, Hill and Davis (1923) also report good results with meroxyl, but very little experience has been had with this substance.

External Antiseptics for Bladder Irrigation.—The following is a list of the solutions most often used:

Silver nitrate, 1: 10,000 to 1: 5000 (follow by saline irrigation).

Argyrol, 1: 100.

Potassium permanganate, 1: 8000 to 1: 5000.

Mercurochrome-220, 1: 200.

Mercurophen, 1: 10,000.

Gentian violet, 1: 500.

Acriflavine, 1: 8000 to 1: 6000.

The dyes should be retained for two or three hours if possible in order to secure full penetration.

McDonald (1915) has repeatedly urged the use of quinine bisulphate, which, in the strength of 1: 2000, causes very little irritation. She has found it especially useful in the treatment of cystitis in women. I do not know whether the drug has been given a trial by many other practitioners.

Bacteriophage.—A number of reports have appeared in recent years extolling the value of bacteriophage therapy in the ailments under discussion, but none of them present entirely satisfactory evidence that the bacteriophage was actually the agent responsible for the improvement noted. Most of the series have been small and practically all of them are uncontrolled. *Bacillus coli* infections, particularly in the acute and subacute stages, are the ones which are most often promptly terminated, but, to repeat, until we have a very large series of cases in which alternate patients just as they come are untreated as controls, it will not be possible to feel certain that the claims of cure as now presented have any value. It is believed that the patient should be given sufficient alkalis, perhaps be placed on a basic diet also, to render the urine distinctly alkaline if best results are to be obtained. If the bacteriophage is to be injected subcutaneously, the usual dosage is between 2 and 3 cc. on alternate days for three times. Usually no very great discomfort is caused, but both local and general reactions of very great severity have often been observed; it should be noted that, no matter what the protagonists of bacteriophage therapy say, this constitutes foreign protein shock therapy, whatever else it may be. When instilled locally, Schultz (1932) says that approximately 5 cc. of the undiluted 'phage should be placed in the kidney pelves and at least 30 cc. in the bladder, all in one dose. The patient should lie down and retain this (*i. e.*, should not urinate) for as many hours as possible. It is usually considered of advantage to give the treatment at night, together with a dose of a hypnotic by mouth. The instillations are sometimes repeated once or twice at intervals of two days. Cowie and Hicks (1932) do not place more than 10 cc. in the bladder; these authors have given a good description of their methods of developing the bacteriophage, which are of course too long and technical to include here.

Ketogenic Diet.—Helmholz and Clark introduced this type of treatment (for methods, see p. 641) in 1931 and in their experience as well as that of many others treating these conditions in children it has been highly satisfactory. Rennie (1933), however, feels that it will succeed only if there are no abnormalities of the urinary tract. Equally good results are beginning to be tentatively reported in adults. Wilson sterilized the urine of 20 patients whose colon bacillus infections had endured from seven months to eighteen years. In long-standing cases this required from one to three weeks though ketone bodies may be made to appear in the urine on the second or third day of treatment. We do not know as yet how long it is necessary to persevere with the diet after sterilization has been accomplished nor what proportion of relapses is to be expected.

Fuller (1933) has concluded from his careful studies that the effective factor in this treatment is l-β-oxybutyric acid.

ESSENTIAL HEMATURIA

This is a condition of renal bleeding, the etiology of which has not been [deter]mined; it is usually symptomless, though the patient may actually [bleed] to death therefrom. There are of course many theories as to its [etiolo]gy, but the findings in the kidneys have not been sufficiently con[firmed to] establish the cause. Hunner (1932) has been intensively investi[gating th]e subject for many years and feels that in most instances ureteral stricture may have the important etiologic rôle. Stewart, of Edinburgh, first described the malady, in 1794.

THERAPY

The whole operative gamut has been run in these cases. Recently, with the perfection of the technic of ureteral catheterization, nonoperative procedures have come to be preferred. The usual measures employed, singly or together, are intrapelvic injections, intramuscular or subcutaneous injections of horse serum, oral administration of calcium lactate. As pointed out by Braasch (1913), it is probable that best results follow not the mere filling but the actual overdistention of the renal pelvis until the patient complains of lumbar pain; this distention can best be accomplished—and maintained for several minutes—by plugging the distal end of the ureteral catheter. Levy (1922) reports that in a series of 30 cases in the Johns Hopkins Hospital, nonoperative and operative measures have been about equally successful in stopping the bleeding. Some of his cases apparently cleared up without any treatment, but a careful review of the charts showed that many of them had had a pyelogram done in their routine examination. He looks upon a pyelogram with gravity flow as really constituting a distention of the renal pelvis, so that these patients actually were treated while being given the x-ray examination. Dilatation of the ureter is of course indicated on the basis of Hunner's theory.

In essential hematuria there are usually spontaneously alternating periods of bleeding and no bleeding, which it is well to bear in mind in weighing the value of any new form of therapy with its claims as to number of remissions after treatment. The mere passage of a ureteral catheter has often stopped the bleeding.

STONE IN THE URINARY TRACT

Urinary stones, or calculi, consist of amorphous collections of granules of urinary salts gummed together and embedded in a structureless albuminous substance. The great majority of these stones form originally in the calices or pelvis of the kidney. If there is no obstruction anywhere in the urinary tract, the stones pass down into the bladder and out through the urethra without giving rise to symptoms, but if they are arrested at any point, there they lodge and continue to grow. It must also be assumed in some instances that the stone is capable of affixing itself to the mucous membrane, for cases are seen in which a large stone is present without any obstructive abnormality to account for its retention. Stones in the bladder may either be halted there by some obstruction to their passage out from the kidney, or they originate there as deposits on some foreign substance introduced by the patient, or as encrustations on inflammatory lesions. With the various hypotheses put forward to explain this phenomenon of stone formation I cannot deal here: suffice it to say that there seems to be a hereditary factor concerned; that vitamin A deficiency possibly plays a contributory rôle; that hematogenous infection often precedes and almost invariably succeeds the lodgment of a stone, but that stones do not form in the vast majority of persons who have hematogenous urinary tract infections; and, finally, that the disease is unilateral in most cases, but that there is at present no way of foretelling the patient's tendency to the development of stone on the other side. The male victims of this malady greatly preponderate.

In kidney stone there may be just a constant but fluctuating aching pain

in the loin of the affected side, or radiating into the lower back, the abdomen
or leg. Constant or intermittent hematuria is oftentimes remarked, and
sometimes there is the passage of "sand." Bladder symptoms, such as frequency, urgency and burning, are not unusual even when the bladder is free
from lesions. The most characteristic manifestation of the presence of stone
is an attack of renal colic. The pain strikes quickly in the kidney region,
but soon radiates down into the abdomen, the thigh and leg, the scrotum (or
vulva), and sometimes into the opposite kidney region (the so-called
"renorenal reflex"). There is nausea, vomiting and gaseous distention during such an attack, which may last for a few minutes to several days, but
probably endures for four to twelve hours in most cases. If complete obstruction occurs there will be hydronephrosis on the affected side and perhaps anuria, even though the opposite side is not obstructed (the so-called
"reflex anuria").

In general the symptoms of stone in the bladder are not very characteristic. The most usual complaints are of frequency, hematuria, the passage
of sand, difficult urination, sudden stoppage in the flow of urine, and pain
running down to the head of the penis. Tuberculosis, prostatic enlargement, and vesical neoplasm must be carefully ruled out.

In urinary stone, infection of the tract, with all its usual signs and
symptoms, is an almost certain complication soon or late.

Apparently, Domenico Marchetti, in 1633, performed the first operation
for renal calculus. The treatment of vesical stone was made a specialty
early in the Middle Ages by quacks who "cut" only for stone, and these
operative procedures were not effectively gotten out of their hands until the
sixteenth century.

THERAPY

Dietary restrictions are usually of two sorts: If the calculi are of uric
acid the amount of meat is much reduced and no glandular organs (sweetbreads, etc.) permitted at all in order to keep the diet "purine-free;" if of
oxalates, the patient is not permitted to eat potatoes, beans, spinach,
tomatoes, endive, strawberries and plums, or to drink cocoa or chocolate.
Actually, however, there is no proof that such restrictions are in the least
helpful. It seems also to be the consensus of opinion that alcohol should
not be allowed. The most valuable preventive measure is undoubtedly the
drinking of large amounts of water. The use of sodium biphosphate, in
some such prescription as that on page 617, for short periods is also thought
to be of some use. Certain mineral springs in Europe and America have a
high and apparently deserved reputation for bringing about the fracture of
small stones; the fragments are ultimately passed. The use of turpentine
(the rectified oil of turpentine of the U.S.P.) in 10-minim (0.65 cc.) capsules, three times daily for a week at a time, has also been recommended
since ancient times. Urotropin, in such dosage as recommended on page
617, is of very doubtful value as a solvent of urate stones in the bladder;
sodium or potassium acetate, in a dose of 15 grains (1 Gm.) three or four
times daily, will probably accomplish just as much. When dealing with
phosphatic stones, nitrohydrochloric acid, in some such prescription as that
ı page 678, has been much used, but any measures that will render the
ne acid are probably of equal value.

ın the presence of severe colic, morphine and atropine are of course
freely, a ¼-grain (0.015 Gm.) dose of the former and $\frac{1}{100}$-grain
ı6 Gm.) of the latter; the morphine will probably have to be re-
Bauer *et al.* (1931) recently slowly injected 20 cc. of a sterile 5
solution of calcium chloride in a small series of cases; in practically
there was prompt relief of sufficient degree that sleep was possible

and the use of morphine was avoided. In one case the injection gave almost instantaneous relief though morphine had not been effective. But the reader is cautioned to be careful here, for reasons stated on page 714.

Most individuals with stone must ultimately submit to instrumental or operative interference, measures which of course are not dealt with in this book. Also the treatment of urinary tract infection is an important part of the therapy.

40

DISEASES OF THE NERVOUS SYSTEM

SYDENHAM'S CHOREA
(St. Vitus' Dance)

Chorea is one of the common diseases of childhood. It may occur at any age but most cases are seen between the fifth and fifteenth years. The disease is more frequent in occurrence in girls than boys and in the poorer than in the richer classes. Negroes and full-blooded American Indians are rarely affected. When the child is brought to the physician for the first time, the parent usually states that for a week or more it has been fidgety, emotional and excessively clumsy. Upon observation the patient will be seen to be in almost constant jerky motion; grimacing and purposeless movements of the face and head are the most usual phenomena, but any part of the body may share in the wriggling or writhing motion. There is also much muscular incoordination, as shown frequently by the overpassing of objects with the hand or in difficulties in locomotion. Except in the most severe cases, these movements cease during sleep and are to some extent under voluntary control; at least firm, kindly commands will often cause them to be restrained for a brief space. The speech is often choppy in character, sometimes being entirely unintelligible; in a relatively few cases the child is entirely unable to speak. The usual mental involvement is in the direction of dulness, carelessness and loss of memory, though not infrequently this state is broken into by intense emotional storms. Appetite and the general condition usually remain good despite some loss of weight and the development of more or less anemia. Headache and muscular weakness are always complained of. The most frequent complication is endocarditis. The duration varies from several weeks to many months, sometimes to more than a year. Death is very rare, and when it occurs is due to general wasting plus intercurrent sepsis and heart failure. Relapses and recurrences are not uncommon in this disease.

Since the middle of the last century the effort has been made, both in Europe and America, to link together rheumatic fever, acute endocarditis and chorea. Undoubtedly the presumptive evidence in favor of such an association has a certain weight, but to date all efforts to statistically prove the contention have failed. First we must make certain of the causative organism in either rheumatic fever or chorea; the streptococcus is *not* as yet thoroughly convicted. Chorea has also many times been seen to follow upon an attack of one of the other infectious diseases, particularly scarlet fever, but again this has not been shown to be more than coincidence. Bits of evidence pointing toward calcium deficiency are appearing now and then.

Sydenham provided the classical description in 1686. During the early part of the fifteenth century, one of the waves of crazy fanaticism which characterized the period took the form of a dancing mania among certain groups of physically degenerated people; one such group, "dancing" toward the chapel of St. Vitus in Zabern, gave the disease its other title—though the etiology of this affair of perverted crowd psychology bears probably no relation to that of the disease we have here under consideration.

THERAPY

Rest.—Absolute bed rest is the single most important element in the treatment of chorea. Whether this rest should be secured within or without the family circle must be decided in each individual case. The sedative drugs (for a list, see p. 578) are by no means contraindicated and can perhaps be used with profit in most severe cases; of course their dosage must be reduced according to the child's size and age. Poynton would add chloretone to the list of useful sedatives in this disease; he states that 5 grains (0.32 Gm.) three times daily is of value if given under proper supervision—which of course must mark the use of sedatives *always* in children. Tepid sponge baths are nearly always soothing, and in some cases an excellent reaction follows upon the use of the ice pack (*i. e.*, wrap the patient in blankets with a sheet wrung out of very cold water next his skin).

Salicylates.—Those who look upon chorea as a rheumatic meningo-encephalitis consider the salicylates to be indicated. For a description of their employment in rheumatic fever, see page 149. I know of no studies that show these drugs to be of the least value in chorea.

Arsenic.—This drug has been employed here empirically for many years. Usually it is given in the form of Fowler's solution (the solution of potassium arsenite of the U.S.P.) in ascending doses. The method most often employed is to begin with 3 minims (0.2 cc.) three times daily and increase this dose by 1 minim (0.065 cc.) each day or each second day, until 10 minims (0.65 cc.) are taken at each dose; this dose is then continued for a week unless toxic symptoms appear earlier. The symptoms most often sought for are puffiness under the eyes or about the ankles, or gastro-intestinal disturbances. The possibility of arsenical neuritis should always be borne in mind, however, for this rather serious consequence of prolonged arsenical therapy has been seen, without any premonitory edematous or gastro-intestinal symptoms, more often than is commonly believed. I know of no statistical studies of the efficacy of arsenic treatment; the presumptive clinical evidence is far from being unanimous in its favor. Of course the disease is almost too variable in its severity and course to make careful studies of nonspecific remedies possible; however, Abt's statement, made in 1916, would probably find more endorsers today even than it did when it was made: "I want to say a word about arsenical treatment and rest in bed. For years I have had children brought to me with chorea. One of my colleagues might have a case in an opposite bed. I would say, 'You treat with arsenic and I will treat without.' The baby without arsenic, but with rest in bed, would recover just as rapidly as the other child treated with arsenic. The child's term in the hospital would be no longer than with the arsenical treatment. . . . It seems to me the treatment of these cases of chorea, especially in neuropathic children without heart lesions and no evidence of infection, is to take them away from their family, feed them, keep them absolutely quiet in bed, give them hot baths, and they generally recover in a short time."

Nirvanol.—This drug, which is phenylethylhydantoin, was introduced as a hypnotic but soon ceased to be used for that simple purpose because of the rash it caused. Now, for a number of years, it has been employed in the German clinics to produce "nirvanol sickness," a complex consisting of fever, rash and eosinophilia which appears usually in from six to twelve days after the first dose of the drug; in a certain number of patients the course of the malady is much shortened. Latterly, nirvanol has begun to be used in all countries, but the results are rather difficult to appraise, since most of the series have been rather small, and in some success has been marked while in others considerable doubt of the drug's action has been expressed. However, most observers feel that nirvanol is often effective in rather sharply checking chorea, particularly the severe cases, but that it is highly doubtful if it is advisable to use an agent as toxic as this in such a self-limited disease as chorea. In addition to the symptoms mentioned above, there may appear swelling of the face, stupor, and agranulocytic blood changes. The few deaths charged against the drug have not been proved but it seems certain that the reaction may be very frightening. Dosage: 5 grains (0.3 Gm.) distributed throughout the day, usually 1½ grains (0.1 Gm.) three times daily; larger doses have been used—10 grains per day, in one report 15 grains. Administration is usually stopped when the rash or fever appears or in any case after ten or twelve days of medication. It is still a moot point whether the reaction is of a specific idiosyncratic nature or is due to a simple cumulative toxic effect; I think it worthy of note how often sudden improvement has occurred in those cases in which there occurred a high fever. Examining the blood frequently to attempt early detection of deleterious cellular changes, certainly seems the part of wisdom. Use of this drug, which is very "strong" to say the least, might be better justified if someone were able to show that the subsequent incidence of cardiac disease is materially lowered. (Bibliography: Schmal, 1925; DeRudder, 1926; East and Cullinan, 1930; Pilcher and Gerstenberger, 1930; Ray and Cunningham, 1930; Dennett and Wetchler, 1932; Weinfeld and Cohen, 1932; Schick *et al.*, 1933.)

Fever Therapy.—In 1931, Sutton tried out at Bellevue Hospital the fever method of treatment which has been steadily in use with excellent results in several Continental clinics since its introduction, by Kern, in 1923. Twenty-four cases were treated, the average duration of symptoms after treatment was started being only eight or nine days—results which were much more satisfactory than those obtained with other types of treatment. Fever therapy methods are described on page 187; Sutton found that most of her patients required a febrile period of about a week, some of them rather longer.

Other Measures.—Lumbar puncture, the intravenous injection of phenol or arsphenamine, the use of serums, autoserums, or vaccines as specific agents—none of these measures have proved their worth.

HICCUP

Hiccup is produced by a sudden clonic spasm of the diaphragm accompanied by a spasmodic closure of the glottis. It occurs not infrequently in the fetus, detectable as regular, short, quick jerks at the rate of 15 to 30 a minute; they are visible and palpable, and the muscle sound of the diaphragm as well as of the body striking the uterine wall can be heard. If occurring during labor it is sometimes not interrupted by the birth of the child and continues for a short time afterward; DeLee has seen a baby born hiccupping so loudly that it could be heard in the next room. The greatest incidence of hiccup in infancy occurs during the first three months, principally among breast-fed babies, probably due to overdistention of the stomach with food and swallowed air. In adults it may be caused by inflammatory or pressure irritation of the phrenic nerve or reflexly through the vagus. It may be a symptom of almost any disease but the entities with which it is most often associated are neurosis, epilepsy, encephalitis, brain tumor, Addison's disease, and functional, organic, traumatic and acute infectious processes anywhere in the gastro-intestinal tract. Apparently it also occurs reflexly in diseases of the pleura and pericardium as well as in some of the chronic constitutional diseases. And some surgeons of experience, as pointed out by Wade (1932), look upon the occurrence of postoperative hiccup as a warning of impaired renal function. In addition to which there are the idiopathic and epidemic cases!

THERAPY

Most cases in infants are transitory and of no serious importance. The infant should not be permitted to suck the breast when it is empty or the bottle in such way as to take in large quantities of air, and after feeding it should be held upright to aid regurgitation. Sometimes it is necessary to give a spoonful or so of hot water or weak sodium bicarbonate solution or diluted lemon juice. Of course the more serious cases may also be seen in infants. In adults the most important thing, of course, is to make every effort to locate and treat the underlying cause of the trouble, which is very much easier to say than to do. The actual measures directed against the spasms are of course legion, as is the case in all maladies of vague and variable etiology; the following seem most often to have been of assistance.

Sedatives.—The whole gamut is run—bromides, chloral, barbiturates, paraldehyde, belladonna, compound spirits of ether (Hoffmann's anodyne), hyoscine, opiates and even apomorphine. Mention of benzyl benzoate is rather frequent in recent years; Cadham (1925) says that it found greatest favor with physicians during the well-known Winnipeg epidemics, but he felt that evaluation of any remedy was very difficult. It may be suspended with mucilage of acacia or prescribed in one of the higher alcoholic vehicles (see p. 785); Ruhräh prefers to give the drug in sweetened milk. See also the sedative measures employed in whooping cough; these are sometimes successful here.

Cocainization.—In persistent cases, Lichtenstein (1928) has obtained good results with a dilute cocaine-epinephrine solution containing a very small amount of phenol, applied to both nostrils on pledgets of cotton.

Carbon Dioxide.—Carbon dioxide in various proportions with oxygen, delivered from the usual apparatus, has been very favorably reported upon a number of times. Golden (1931) describes a simple, inexpensive method of inducing the inhalation of carbon dioxide, which has been effectively used by him. An ordinary paper bag of medium size and strength is placed over the patient's face and so held that it tightly encloses the mouth and nose, thus inducing rebreathing of an atmosphere whose carbon dioxide content steadily rises. Five of his 6 patients were relieved in from three to six minutes; one of them had been hiccupping for two days.

Fluids.—In postoperative cases in which impaired renal function is suspected, the "pushing" of fluids not infrequently brings relief.

Lavage.—Soper's method of keeping the stomach continuously cleaned out by siphonage (see p. 426) has been successfully employed a number of times.

Phrenic Nerve Operations.—Weeks (1931) believes that in intractable cases, when everything else has failed, the patient should be examined fluoroscopically to determine which side of the diaphragm is involved; the phrenic nerve on that side should then be exposed under local anesthesia, a stout silk ligature passed about it, and the nerve anesthetized—which seems to bring relief of about eight hours. Following this, traction is to be tried, this failing the nerve can be crushed; both failing points toward anastomosis below the site of section or blocking and indicates avulsion. In cases of bilateral involvement, it is said that the operative procedures can be bilaterally performed. Dollert (1933) states: "When contemplating phrenic nerve avulsion it is well to check up on the lung ventilation because insufficient ventilation following operation may cause death due to anoxemia."

Household Remedies.—The remedies most frequently employed with success in mild attacks are pressure on the back of the neck, holding the breath, swallowing a bolus of food, tickling the nose to induce sneezing, gentle compression of the upper part of the thyroid cartilage, sipping cold drinks, and swallowing finely cracked ice.

TRIGEMINAL NEURALGIA

(Tic Douloureux)

Trigeminal neuralgia is a disease of the gasserian ganglion, affecting one or all of the branches of the trigeminal nerve; the infra-orbital division is the most frequently affected, then the mandibular, and then the ophthalmic. The pain comes "out of a clear sky," and is described as shooting, stabbing, lightning-like, cutting, etc. It lasts but a few seconds to a few minutes, but during the time of its presence is perhaps as severe as any that man is ever called upon to experience. The patient remains motionless with a fixed grimace and oftentimes with some defensive posture of the body as a whole. The relief is usually complete upon the termination of the spasm. Such an attack may be precipitated by any minor essential movement, such as opening the mouth, swallowing, winking the eyes, talking, washing the face, brushing the teeth, etc. In the beginning there is often a considerable interval between seizures, and there may even be an asymptomatic period of several months to years, but finally in practically all cases the pain becomes continuous and affects all three divisions of the nerve. It is my belief that spontaneous recovery has never been recorded. In untreated cases, death may result from inanition consequent upon inability to eat or sleep.

Trigeminal neuralgia, which is a disease of those in or past the middle years of life, is of unknown etiology, though its association with carious teeth has often been remarked. It was first described by Avicenna (Ibn Sina), he who was called "the Prince of Physicians" at the court of more than one caliph at Bagdad, about the year 1000 of our present era; the first accurate description satisfying the present-day criteria was that of Fothergill, in 1773.

THERAPY

Nonsurgical Treatment.—None of the sedatives or analgesics are consistently of value save only opium, and even it must be given in rapidly increasing doses in order to control the pain; it is therefore used only when surgical relief cannot be obtained or is refused. It is also stated in the older literature that doses of the U.S.P. tincture of aconite sufficient to cause considerable lethargy and a slowing of the pulse to 50 or less, *i. e.*, beginning with 15 minims (1 cc.) three times daily and increasing, will sometimes afford temporary and partial relief.

Trichlorethylene.—This is a strong, sweet-smelling white liquid which was used for industrial purposes in Germany during the World War and was accidentally discovered to be of value in relieving trigeminal pain when Plessner presented before the Berlin Medical Society, in 1915, several workers suffering from chronic poisoning by the substance. Joachimoglu (1921) has apparently shown that, as a drug in the dosage in which it has now come to be employed, trichlorethylene is not toxic. The present method of administration is to place 20 to 25 drops on a piece of gauze and inhale (lying down because slight dizziness and drowsiness are occasionally caused) until there is no more odor; this three or four times daily for a period of four to six weeks. In those obtaining relief or cure, it is the practice to continue the treatment by inhaling on three consecutive days every two or three months. The mode of action of the drug remains a mystery. None of the patients develop anesthesia, which is now taken to indicate that in Plessner's original toxic cases, in which anesthesia was present, the poison was really some agent other than trichlorethylene (which makes this great discovery doubly accidental!). It is this lack of anesthesia which gives the drug its advantage over surgery, so that every sufferer from tic douloureux should be placed on a full course before being subjected to the operative relief measures. Glaser (1931), in reporting 15 of his own cases, has summarized the results obtained in the 177 reported cases as follows: (*a*) Complete relief, about 15 per cent; (*b*) partial relief from 13.3 to 74 per cent. The largest single series of cases in the literature is that of Kramer (1921), in whose 58 cases there is recorded complete relief in 11.9 per cent, partial relief in 66.3 per cent.

Surgical Treatment.—The surgical measures available at the present time are (*a*) the alcohol injection of the nerves near the foramina of exit from the skull; (*b*) the alcohol injection of the gasserian ganglion; (*c*) the operation of peripheral avulsion of the sensory root; and (*d*) the radical division of the sensory root. Nerve injection and avulsion would seem to afford relief for an average period of nine months; radical division affords permanent relief; relief from the ganglion injection seems to be permanent in most cases also. All of these measures have their advantages and disadvantages, their advocates and detractors. I believe the selection of the type of treatment to be employed in a given case is so serious a matter that it should not be treated of merely in passing in this book. However, I permit myself to council the reader to entrust his patient only to a surgeon who has had much cadaver and actual operative experience in these matters.

SCIATIC NEURALGIA

The majority of the victims of sciatica are males between the ages of thirty and sixty years. In most cases the pain begins in the sciatic notch or in the lower lumbar region and gradually extends down the course of the sciatic nerve. In the beginning this pain is often merely a dull ache that bothers the patient very little, but it finally becomes burning, sticking or lancinating in character, and radiates downward from the sciatic notch along the posterior aspect of the thigh into the calf muscles and foot. In many chronic cases the pain is ultimately confined to the outer aspect of the calf and foot, where it becomes persistent and causes as much discomfort as the pain in the thigh and buttock during the early stages. Tender spots and areas of paresthesia are frequently noted. Some individuals find the prone position on the unaffected side, with thigh and leg slightly flexed, absolutely essential for partial comfort, while others, particularly in the later stages, find walking gives greater relief. An attack of sciatic neuralgia may be relatively mild and persist for only a few days, but severe cases are protracted for weeks to months, during which time the patient is entirely incapacitated and suffers severely. Recurrence is the rule.

THERAPY

Removal of Foci of Infection.—Whatever may be the true cause of sciatica, *i. e.*, whether it be a ganglionitis, a periganglionitis, a neuritis, or an "idiopathic" neuralgia, it seems that the removal of all ascertainable foci of chronic infection brings about a more satisfactory result in this disease than in any other. The immediate response is often an increase in the severity of the symptoms, but the end-result is many times most gratifying. Therefore, the first duty in the treatment of a case of sciatica is to make a careful search for these foci and eliminate them if practicable.

Rest, Warmth and the Analgesic Drugs.—In the early stage of an attack, complete rest in bed and the application of some form of moist heat, or of diathermy, along the course of the nerve, especially in the gluteal region, are efficacious measures. If combined with the salicylates or cinchophens, as used in the treatment of acute rheumatic fever (see p. 148), the case is often controlled, though it is doubtful if these procedures lessen the total duration of the attack. Codeine sulphate, 1 grain (0.06 Gm.), or even full doses of morphine, must sometimes be used in the beginning of very severe cases. Counterirritants are not beneficial, and massage only aggravates the symptoms.

Injection Treatment.—Many severe attacks of sciatica, attacks that would normally last for many weeks or months if treated only by the above-described measures, have been reduced in duration to only a few days by perineural or epidural injection of physiologic sodium chloride solution. I give the technic of these injections as described by Strauss:

(*a*) *Perineural Injection.*—"In making perineural injections, the patient lies on the abdomen with a pillow underneath its lower part, and the feet projecting beyond the edge of the table or couch. A line is then drawn from the sacrococcygeal articulation to the lowest point of the postero-external border of the great trochanter. The point of puncture is 1 inch to the outer side of the junction of the inner one third and outer two thirds of the foregoing lines. A trocar and cannula about 20 cm. in length and 2 mm. in caliber is used in the injection. The point of the trocar ought not to project very far beyond the cannula. The needle is inserted directly downward through the gluteal muscles until the nerve is reached. When the nerve is touched, the patient feels a sharp, shooting pain down the leg, and there is very often involuntary contraction of the gastrocnemius muscles. When the nerve is struck, the trocar is immediately withdrawn, and a syringe attached to the cannula. Physiologic sodium chloride solution is then injected in amounts varying from 100 to 150 cc. Considerable pressure is sometimes necessary in order to force the fluid into the tissues, and in such cases, care must be taken that the needle is not forced into the nerve. Considerable pain may follow the injection, which, as a rule, subsides after an hour.

"It may be necessary to repeat the injection every other day until at least five are given, but as a rule three injections suffice. Alcohol should never be used for these injections."

(*b*) *Epidural Injection.*—"The epidural space in an adult begins at the lower edge of the first sacral vertebra, where the dura ends. It extends down to the sacrococcygeal articulation. At this level the injections are made. There are certain landmarks by which this opening, the foramen sacrale superius, may be identified. It lies at the end of the crest made by the spines of the sacrum. It has the shape of an inverted V or U, and is about 1 cm. wide and from 1.5 to 2 cm. in length. It is bordered laterally by two prominences, the cristae sacrales laterales, which are usually easily felt by the finger. The opening is covered by a dense fibrous ligament, the ligamentum sacrococcygeum. The opening lies generally 2 cm. above the end of the gluteal fold.

"The needle used for the injection should be about 8 cm. in length, and 1 mm. in caliber. I have used an ordinary steel needle previously tested as to its flexibility. If greater flexibility is desired, a needle made of platinum iridium may be used; but a broken needle need cause no alarm: it will do no harm if allowed to remain in the epidural space. The needle is to be inserted to a depth of 6 cm. to reach the second sacral vertebra. There is no danger of entering the subarachnoid space, because the dura ends at about the level of the first sacral vertebra; however, to be certain that this space has not been entered, it is well to wait for a few minutes before injecting to see whether there is an escape of cerebrospinal fluid. If possible, when inserting the needle, one should place the patient in the knee-chest position in order more easily to locate the landmarks. If the injection is made with the patient lying on the side with the knees and thighs flexed, the landmarks are not so easily discerned, and the gluteal fold usually lies above the foramen. It may be difficult, if not impossible, to enter the epidural space of very stout persons, especially of stout women. In such cases, recourse must be had to the nerve injection.

"It has been my custom to anesthetize the skin and tissue overlying the foramen and the ligament with novocain. In doing this, one must be careful not to cause much swelling, which might obliterate the landmarks. After the needle has been pushed through the skin, considerable resistance is met at the ligament. Once this resistance is overcome, the needle glides into the epidural space. If the patient is in the knee-chest posture, the needle is inserted into the body at an angle of 45 degrees. After it has passed through the ligament the needle is held so that it is horizontal to the body. During the injection, the patient lies on the affected side.

"The injection consists of warm sterile physiologic sodium chloride solution. To the first 10 or 20 cc. of solution is added 0.125 Gm. of novocain with epinephrine, and a few minutes are allowed to elapse after their injection to obtain the full benefit of their anesthetic effect. In all, from 60 to 80 cc. of solution are injected at a time.

"The injections are given at forty-eight-hour intervals. They may be given in the office, and the patient will have no difficulty in going home. It is preferable, however, for the patient to remain in bed during the intervals. The average number of injections required is three. Occasionally it may be necessary to give five, but sometimes two or even one suffice to relieve the condition. The most difficult cases to cure are the chronic ones in which the pain is along the outer aspect of the thigh. In some instances this pain persists even after several injections, and then treating the limb with superheated air in the Tyrnauer apparatus is efficacious. The heat treatment alone in the subacute and chronic cases is of no avail. Massage ought never to be used—it appears to do more harm than good. A patient may improve after several epidural injections but not be entirely cured. The injections of sodium chloride solution along the course of the nerve in the gluteal region may cause the disappearance of the pain. There have been no untoward results from the epidural injections. The knee jerk on the affected side has disappeared for a short time, and sometimes the patient complains of delayed micturition; but these symptoms soon disappear."

(c) *Alcohol-Novocain Nerve Block.*—Labat and Greene (1931) recommend injecting the individual lumbar or sacral nerves which are shown to be involved by the careful use of their electric percussion hammer. The solution used is 95 per cent alcohol and 1 or 2 per cent novocain, in proportions usually of 1 to 2, using 3 to 8 cc. for the injection. Paresthesias follow block of this nature and are occasionally severe and of long duration.

Fever (Foreign Protein) Therapy.—The recent vogue of sulphur injections, particularly in Germany, has included cases of sciatica, sometimes with good results (see Schlesinger, 1931), but I fail to appreciate the points made by those who ascribe to sulphur some virtues other than its ability to provoke the foreign protein type of reaction. For methods, see page 193.

Other Measures.—Of course, pain due to sacro-iliac strain, arthritis of the lumbar spine and of the lumbosacral and sacro-iliac or hip joint, anatomical anomalies, and pelvic and cord tumors must be ruled out in every case.

The old operation in which the nerve was stretched has been discarded, the results having been of little or no value.

CAUSALGIA

This syndrome, first observed by Weir Mitchell during the American Civil War, is a most distressing complication of gunshot injury to peripheral nerves. It has been observed quite frequently in veterans of the World War. The median nerve is involved most frequently in causalgia of the upper extremity, and the internal popliteal in that of the lower extremity. The hand or foot is hyperesthetic, hyperemic, glossy and dry, and extremely painful. The pain is first described as burning or throbbing, or like that produced by pin pricks, a red-hot iron or an injury of the flesh; it never ceases, day or night, and finally becomes paroxysmal. Another symptom frequently noted is an excessive sense of dryness, which causes the patient to keep the part soaked in water even though maceration and ulceration are thereby produced. The most pitiful feature of these cases is that the severe paroxysms are often induced by the performance of any ordinary and necessary act. The pain as a rule reaches its maximum intensity at five or six months after the injury, and then very, very slowly recedes, though the paralysis induced by the fixations in the effort to prevent paroxysms often persists after the disappearance of the pain.

THERAPY

Neurolysis, alone, does not control the pain in these cases. Sicard's suggestion of alcohol injection was first employed in the United States by Lewis and Gatewood, in 1920. The nerves affected are exposed under general anesthesia, and from 1 to 2 cc. of 60 per cent alcohol directly injected *above* the site of the original wound; as the injection is made the nerve swells and becomes white. Relief from the pain is almost immediate. Motor palsies, when caused by the alcohol, are rapidly recovered from.

MIGRAINE

Migraine is the name applied to a certain type of periodic headache that is associated with visual, gastro-intestinal and, to some extent, psychic disturbances. The individual who suffers from this disease is usually made aware of the approach of an attack by several days of malaise, perhaps accompanied by vague or definite gastro-intestinal symptoms; or the attack may come on more suddenly following a period of one or more hours of exceptional well-being; or—and this is not infrequently the case—the patient may recognize a night of more than usually sound and refreshing sleep as a warning signal. In most cases the headache is ushered in by visual disturbances; these may be of the nature of flashes of light, or of wriggling threads of light that pass across the field of vision, or of definite loss of visual acuity, and they may disappear before the onset of the headache or persist for some time after the pain begins. If the pain is confined to one side of the head, these visual phenomena are usually observed on the affected side only. The pain itself is most intense, and usually, though by no means always, confined to one side of the head. During the attack, which lasts from a few hours to several days, the patient is sometimes more depressed or confused than can be easily accounted for by the distraught state induced by the pain. In about 50 per cent of cases, nausea and vomiting occur at the height of the attack. The only sign of an inflammatory nature is the transient eosinophilia that is said to occur in a large proportion of cases.

Migraine usually appears in the early decades of life and tends to diminish in frequency and severity, and often to disappear entirely, as senescence approaches. It often is absent during gestation, and may disappear for a long period after one of the acute infectious diseases. Nothing is known definitely regarding the cause of this strange malady, though the tendency is known to be almost certainly hereditary. The similarity between migraine and the recognized allergic group—hay fever, asthma, urticaria, angioneurotic edema, etc.—has caused the suggestion to be made that it is truly a sensitization disease. Some observers have also placed it among the endocrine disturbances merely as a point of departure in their studies. That migraine and epilepsy are transmitted from generation to generation as an expression of the same underlying factor in the germ plasm, and that an individual with migraine is more likely to produce epileptic offspring than is an epileptic, is strongly suggested by Buchanan's studies. The coexistence of migraine and epilepsy is not significantly high, but momentary seizures much resembling *petit mal* sometimes alternate with, and may even replace the migraine attacks as age advances.

Women are the victims of this disease somewhat more often than men, or at least they more often have a severe form of the malady, and the upper social strata are more frequently afflicted than the lower. The variations in racial incidence are not known to me.

THERAPY

1. **Hygienic Measures.**—Most patients believe that the smoother and more even the tenor of their life, especially in the particulars of regularity in sleep and the eating of meals, the freer they remain from attacks; some, indeed, are even able to state with positiveness that a certain type of emotional or even physical indulgence will invariably induce the headache. Something of truth there must be in this, but I think its importance is exaggerated by many individuals, for the greatest success in regulating these matters often results in little or no decrease in either the frequency or the severity of the seizures. The correction of eyestrain, too, will sometimes bring about great improvement in a patient's condition, but these cases are rare. The elimination of foci of chronic infection is sometimes rewarded by a remission of many months; but almost invariably the attacks return after awhile, though they are oftentimes permanently lessened in severity. The intestinal auto-intoxication hypothesis still has its champions; as recently as 1921, Bastedo said, "I do not agree that headaches from decomposition products formed in the intestine are rare. I believe they are very common. I am one of those who believe that intestinal bacteria may produce toxic substances which cause headache." Certain it is that nearly every migraine patient is addicted to the habit of taking "a brisk saline purge" at the first hint of the prodromata, but I do not think it is apparent that he is much helped thereby. Chronic constipation, if proved to exist, of course demands correction; but that is a different matter.

2. **Symptomatic Measures.**—Rest in bed is nearly always self-imposed by sufferers from this disease, since it markedly lessens the throbbing of the head and of course decreases the bodily movements that so often give rise to added quirks of pain. Darkening of the room and the use of cold compresses are also helpful measures. In mild cases, any of the sedative drugs (for a list and dosage, see p. 578) may be employed, phenobarbital (luminal) being latterly preferred. In severe attacks, prohibitive doses would have to be employed in order to bring about any reduction in the suffering. Better results follow the use of the analgesics in mild cases, though their effectiveness seems to be much greater when the attack is beginning to wear off than when it is at its height. Sodium salicylate, or aspirin

(acetylsalicylic acid), either one in a dose of 5 to 15 grains (0.32 to 1 Gm.) at intervals of three hours for four or five doses, are often used; they sometimes serve only to make the patient more uncomfortable by reason of the perspiring induced. The advantage that the more expensive cinchophen and neocinchophen may have over the salicylates in acute rheumatic fever, namely, their lesser tendency to produce toxic symptoms (but see p. 151!) and gastric disturbances, does not justify their employment here where these toxic effects are not to be feared. A capsule of pyramidon (amidopyrine) and caffeine citrate, 5 grains (0.32 Gm.) of the former and 2 grains (0.13 Gm.) of the latter, three or four times during the twenty-four hours, is effective in some cases. Five grains (0.32 Gm.) of phenacetin (acetphenetidin), or 3 grains (0.2 Gm.) of acetanilid, may also prove effective if used several times at three-hour intervals; larger doses are seldom more effective and are more likely to cause the undesirable side-effects of this group: Sweating and chills, gastric disturbances, skin eruptions, renal irritation, methemoglobin cyanosis and collapse. The U.S.P. extract of cannabis (better known as Cannabis indica) formerly enjoyed the reputation of being almost specific when used in a pill containing ⅙ to ¼ grain (0.01 to 0.015 Gm.), not to be too often repeated, but has latterly fallen into a probably deserved disrepute. In some cases, codeine sulphate in a single daily dose of ½ to 1 grain (0.032 to 0.065 Gm.) is very effectively employed, but is open to the charges applicable to all the opium series: The locking of the bowel and the production of nausea and a general depression in the metabolic activities; habit formation, in the sense in which the term is understood in connection with the opiates, need not be feared from the use of codeine. Morphine is, of course, absolutely contraindicated. Trautmann (1928), in Germany, and Tzanck (1929), in France, have each reported good results with ergotamine tartrate (Gynergen, N.N.R.) in about 30 cases; dosage by mouth, ¹⁄₃₀ to ¹⁄₁₀ grain (0.002 to 0.006 Gm.) daily. In the United States, Ignelzi (1932) has successfully treated 6 patients, sometimes giving the drug intramuscularly when it failed to be effective by mouth. He also found that interval treatment with viosterol was helpful. It would seem to me that the nature of ergotamine is such that long-continued administration would not be advisable.

3. **Specific Measures.**—Those who are approaching the migraine problem from the allergy standpoint are reporting a certain degree of success in treating their patients by the various methods of specific desensitization and especially through the use of nonspecific protein therapy and the employment of measures for the diagnosis and treatment of food allergy, as developed by Rowe. It is suggested that the reader study the chapter on allergy, page 317.

EPILEPSY

Idiopathic or essential epilepsy is a disease characterized by a peculiar type of convulsive seizure and a tendency to mental deterioration. It occurs in individuals with a constitutional inferiority but with no demonstrable pathologic lesion, though physical stigmata, too numerous to list here, are often noted. In the majority of instances the onset of the attacks occurs before the twentieth year, in more than half before the fifteenth; but the time of appearance of the ultimate terminal dementia is very variable. In many cases the imminence of a convulsion is heralded by a warning visual, auditory, or other type of fleeting aura, which is followed, in about 50 per cent of cases, by the sinister epileptic outcry; then follow the sudden loss of consciousness, the defenseless fall, and the moment of pallor, cessation of respiration, and general muscular rigidity of the decerebrate type. Transition into the clonic stage, in which the body jerks rhythmically and violently, may be made suddenly and generally or in a disorderly manner, so that one side remains rigid while the other is already jerking. During this stage, which lasts from three to five minutes and subsides slowly, the skin is cyanosed, the pulse is rapid and feeble, the deep reflexes are greatly diminished, the blood pressure is low, the pupils are first constricted and then dilated and usually immobile to light, foam appears on the lips, bestial sounds are made, and the urine or feces may be violently ejected. Following the subsidence of this stage, the patient passes into a deep stupor of several hours, though in some instances he partially regains consciousness for a few moments and then falls into a more natural type of deep sleep. For a considerable time after awaking from this stupor, the state is either one of dreaminess, irritability, delirium, or mania during which acts of great violence may be committed. This is the classic *grand mal* seizure; the *petit mal* attack consists in only a momentary loss of consciousness, or some other sort of flashing sensory disturbance, without the occurrence of a convulsion and its sequelae. The *status epilepticus* is a state of affairs in which one convulsion succeeds another so rapidly that the patient practically never recovers consciousness; he presents all the signs of profound intoxication and usually dies from heart failure or pulmonary edema.

Between attacks the epileptic is a disagreeable antisocial psychopath, who is gloomy, irritable, suspicious, defensive, boastful and deceitful to cover his emotional poverty, violent, self-centered and uncomprehending. At all times the person with a severe case of this disease is a dangerous individual; those more mildly afflicted as to number and severity of fits, particularly if the symptoms do not appear until well on toward or into adulthood, suffer very much less mental deterioration.

Epilepsy was recognized as an entity in very ancient times. Sudhoff interprets the concept *bennu,* in the tablets of King Assurbanipal of Assyria (668–626 B. C.), as epilepsy, and the description of the disease written by Hippocrates (460–370 B. C.) would almost suffice for any present-day textbook. In the Middle Ages, it was customary to include epilepsy with the other diseases then recognized to be contagious—bubonic plague, tuberculosis, anthrax, scabies, erysipelas, trachoma and leprosy—and to ban the afflicted from the cities, or at least not to permit them to sell food and drink. At the present time, we are convinced that the disease is not infectious, and reasonably certain that heredity plays a part in its causation; but otherwise the etiology remains unknown and a satisfactory classification of the various types is still to be proposed. The claims of those who argue for the inclusion of epilepsy among the diseases of allergy become increasingly interesting, and Harris (1933) has shown that some cases are associated with a state of hypoglycemia, but still today, as a thousand or two thousand years ago, we must make the diagnosis by exclusion. There are four or five epileptics per thousand of population in the United States at the present time; in Continental Europe, perhaps no more than two or three. The disease is certainly increasing in incidence, but whether more rapidly than the general increase in population is not known.

THERAPY

(*a*) **Hygienic Measures.**—If essential epilepsy is incurable, and it probably is in the present stage of our knowledge, nevertheless very much can be done for these sufferers. But the physician who merely writes a prescription for a bromide or luminal, makes a few vague remarks as to dietary restrictions, suggests that the family make life easy for the patient, and then takes no vigorous and persistent subsequent steps to see that these measures are instituted to the fullest advantage of the patient, is shirking his bounden duty, for no individual is more prone to suit a treatment to his own convenience or whims, and finally to stop it altogether, than the epileptic.

It is probably true that the rehabilitation of the patient's hygiene, by which I mean his readjustment to his environment, is the single most important element in the treatment. These individuals are defectively equipped to cope with a social existence, and therefore must be especially protected. Fatigue is their greatest enemy, fatigue of mind, body or emotions; therefore they must be placed in such surroundings that they may perform light work (preferably remunerative so long as their mentality is alert to the significant facts of their plight), be much out of doors, bathe often and keep the skin in good condition, eat nourishing food but not much at a time, have alcohol, tobacco, and to a large extent tea and coffee, withheld from them, and be encouraged not by maudlin sympathy but by a rational optimism to enjoy the many advantages of life that may be theirs despite their handicap. For most epileptics, of whatever station in life, these desiderata can perhaps be best approximated in either a public or private institution, provided it is well conducted; but in many cases the readjustment is better accomplished without a too radical change in environment. Certain it is that to stop at once the education of a child or youth as soon as the diagnosis is made, is not justified unless the case be hopelessly severe from the beginning, for many of these children are precocious and will absorb much in their early years that will help to sustain them at a later time; furthermore, no one can predict with certainty that a mild case may not continue to be so always under proper care.

(b) **The Use of Sedatives.**—1. *The Bromides.*—The bromide salts were introduced into the treatment of epilepsy in 1853 and have since enjoyed an undisturbed and deserved preference over all other remedies until their position was recently challenged by luminal. In proper doses, and continued for a sufficient length of time, about 90 per cent of cases yield in some degree to these drugs; Binz, cited by Sollmann, gives the following compilation: Total abolition as long as drug is continued, 12 per cent; diminished number and violence of attacks, 83 per cent; no influence $2\frac{1}{2}$ per cent; number of attacks increased, $2\frac{1}{2}$ per cent. Long-continued use of the bromides in large doses leads to serious mental depression and nutritional disturbances, but the following signs enable the careful observer to avoid these dire consequences in most cases: foul breath and coated·tongue, rather sudden and extensive acne or any one of several other characteristic skin lesions, lethargy and mental dulness, slurring of speech, slow pulse, and a staggering gait. Either sodium, potassium or ammonium bromide alone will produce these "specific" effects in epilepsy, but there is a firmly entrenched clinical impression that a mixture of the three salts is more efficacious; they are used either in equal parts or in the proportions of 1 part each of potassium and ammonium bromide and 2 parts of sodium bromide, the "Erlenmeyer mixture." A much used preparation is the elixir of three bromides of the National Formulary, which is a colored and flavored preparation containing in one fluidrachm $4\frac{1}{2}$ grains (0.3 Gm.) each of sodium, potassium and ammonium bromide, *i. e.*, there is approximately 1 grain (0.065 Gm.) of bromide in 4 minims (not drops) of this elixir. The bromides are irritating to the gastric mucosa and should therefore be given well diluted; strontium bromide, being relatively free from this objectionable side action, is preferred by some physicians, but it is slightly more expensive than the other salts. It is generally believed that the N.N.R. synthetic compounds containing bromine—brometone, bromipin, bromural, carbromal and sabromin—are not as effective in epilepsy as the official preparations.

Bromide therapy is more effective in epilepsy if the diet is kept relatively salt-free, but resort to this measure is necessary only in those patients who are resistant to the action of the drug in safe doses. The concomitant use of strychnine, arsenic, atropine, digitalis, or sparteine is felt many times to increase the effectiveness of the bromide even though no definite indication for the use of these drugs is recognized. In the matter of dosage, I can do no better than set down Pershing's clear statement:

"In giving bromide the aim, of course, is to find such a dose, so combined with other remedies, that attacks will be prevented and yet the patient not seriously suffer from its prolonged administration. My average beginning dose for an adult is 20 grains three times a day in a liquid mixture. If that prevents attacks, but bromism appears, the medicine is not interrupted at all, but reduced 10 or 15 per cent at a time, until a dose that can be tolerated is found. Toleration may be increased by adding about 10 minims of tincture of nux vomica to each dose and also by adding arsenic, preferably as sodium cacodylate, from 0.002 to 0.005 Gm. ($\frac{1}{30}$ to $\frac{1}{12}$ grain). A laxative is often necessary, and the aromatic fluidextract of cascara can be added to serve this purpose. If the amount of bromide is inadequate to restrain attacks, it is to be increased cautiously. When a dose is found which is sufficient and is well tolerated, it is to be continued for a long time and then cautiously reduced. Dropping from three doses a day to two of the same strength is too great a change to make at one time, but one might change from three doses of 20 grains to two of 25 grains.

"But here is a matter of detail which . . . is so vital and so commonly neglected that it is necessary to emphasize it. The physician must not only know how much bromide by weight he wishes to give the patient but he must know just how much the patient actually gets. Eighteen grains may be too little and 22 grains too much. It not infrequently happens that a ready-made mixture of bromide is prescribed, without memory of its exact strength, with the direction to take a teaspoonful (which may mean anything from half a drachm to 2 drachms) and so the patient gets a dose somewhere between 5 and 40 grains without any certainty as to the exact amount. Now suppose this dose is not just right and an increase or decrease of 10 per cent is desirable, how is it to be accomplished? Is it any wonder that bromide gets the reputation of being ineffective, or of being so poisonous that its effects are worse than those of the disease?

"The remedy, of course, is simple, that is, for the physician to write the prescription giving the exact amount of each ingredient and then to have the patient measure the dose, which is usually a fluidrachm, in a small graduate glass, which will measure from 10 to 60 minims exactly. But vigilance is necessary. It is wonderful how much perversity patient and druggist can show in defeating the plan to have the dose accurately measured.

"In case the major attacks are held in check, but the minor ones remain as frequent as before, it will do little or no good to advance to large doses of bromide. Instead, from 5 to 10 minims of tincture of digitalis or half a grain of sparteine added to each dose may be of distinct service. Or, if there is much nervous irritability, from 2 to 4 minims of the deodorized tincture of opium with a corresponding increase in the laxative may be better."

The bromides are more effective in controlling *grand mal* than *petit mal*; also, success crowns their use more often in private than in sanatorium practice, principally for the reason that the more severe cases are encountered in institutions.

2. *Luminal (Phenobarbital).*—In recent years this drug has largely replaced the bromides. In *petit mal* it would seem to be no more effective than the classical drug, but in *grand mal* there is little doubt of its superiority. Not only are the attacks more often and more completely controlled,

but, and this is most important, the relief is usually unaccompanied by the mental and physical sluggishness that is so often the price of bromide relief. Luminal is insoluble and is therefore given in tablets or in powdered form in capsules. The following statement of Grinker is typical of the average experience with the drug in *grand mal* cases:

"There being very few cases of *grand mal* without an admixture of some *petit mal* attacks, I class under this caption the cases in which the attacks are principally of the major type, though occasional minor seizures are also recorded. There were under my observation 60 cases—40 for a period of three years, 10 during a period of five years, and 10 from a few months to seven years. Eight of the patients belonging in this group had no attacks in four years, and 20 none in two years, while the rest enjoyed immunity from seizures during periods varying from a few months to nearly two years. Three of my patients were uninfluenced by treatment; even maximum doses failed to produce the slightest effect on the attacks.

"The average dose was 2 grains (0.13 Gm.) of phenobarbital daily, given at night before retiring in nocturnal epilepsy, and during the day in the diurnal form. The benefits obtained from average doses of phenobarbital within a few days from the beginning of treatment were such that for some time at least I gave myself up to the belief that failure to obtain results in a given case of epilepsy meant that the dose of phenobarbital was inadequate. Like others I soon discovered that even in this, the most responsive group to the phenobarbital treatment, there are individuals who are refractory to the largest doses of phenobarbital; fortunately, these are exceptions. In a general way the statement still holds good that the convulsive variety of epilepsy almost always yields to phenobarbital in correct dosage, and that it is mostly the wrong dose which is responsible for unsatisfactory results and toxic symptoms."

In resistant cases, the dosage may be cautiously increased much above the average of 2 grains (0.13 Gm.) daily; perhaps 2½ grains (0.2 Gm.), three times daily for only a limited period, should not be exceeded. In mild, and indeed in some severe cases, the drug need be given during only five days of the week, the effect persisting during the subsequent two days, thus escaping the dangers of accumulation. Luminal sodium, the soluble form of the drug, is used when the tablets or capsules are refused and only a liquid medicament will be taken, or when it is necessary to administer the drug hypodermically. It is customary to prepare a 20 per cent solution in boiled and cooled distilled water; 15 minims (1 cc.) of this solution contain 3 grains (0.2 Gm.) of the drug. The dose of luminal sodium is 10 per cent greater than that of luminal.

Many physicians have noted that the bromides seem to lose their effect after the unsuccessful administration of luminal. This is a serious fact, for if the individual has been doing fairly well on the bromides and becomes worse on the luminal, we have then severely crippled our therapy. Grinker writes that in cases not responding well to luminal, he combines bromide with the luminal, and by gradually lessening the amount of luminal and increasing the amount of bromide, he believes that he obtains better success upon his full return to the latter drug. Another serious feature of luminal medication is the fact that, whether the administration is successful or not, stopping the drug is almost always followed by an increase in the incidence and severity of the attacks above that reached before the luminal had been started. However, Fox, in England, has recorded his observation that a second luminal attempt sometimes succeeds after an initial failure.

The following by-effects of luminal administration are infrequent but should always be borne in mind as possibilities, since they probably occur as often following small as large doses: (*a*) A dermatitis resembling that of measles or scarlet fever, though it is usually very itchy; Peterman (1931) has also reported an eruption exactly simulating bromoderma which followed a healed true bromoderma on the same sites; (*b*) a peculiar eruption upon the tongue; (*c*) states of apathy, mental sluggishness and slow speech much resembling those seen as a result of bromide therapy; (*d*) great muscular weakness; (*e*) extreme irritability, sometimes leading to violence; (*f*) a state of intoxication that may be mistaken for acute alcoholism; (*g*) and occasionally subacute and chronic epigastric pains.

Neither amytal nor any of the other barbiturates have been nearly as effective as luminal in most cases.

(*c*) **Dietetic Treatment.**—Fasting as a dietary measure in the treatment of epilepsy was first suggested by Guelpa and Marie, in 1910, but it was not until 1921 that Geyelin applied the suggestion in practice. Most of his children were freed from seizures during the period of fasting which produced ketosis, but the attacks returned sooner or later after the resumption of a normal diet. Repeated periods of fasting were thus shown to be impracticable in the maintenance of ketosis. However, in the same year, Wilder, while working with high-fat diets in the treatment of diabetes mellitus, suggested their use in the treatment of epilepsy as a means of producing ketosis and still supplying adequate food. This marked the beginning of the ketogenic diet, so called because the ketogenic factors outbalance the antiketogenic factors; but evidence has been accumulating to the effect that it is not the disturbance in the acid-base balance *per se* (*i. e.*, not any sort of sedative, anticonvulsant effect of the ketone bodies) but rather the dehydrating effect of starvation, or of a ketogenic diet, which is important in bringing symptomatic relief—an idea originally suggested by Fay (1929) and in the same year by McQuarrie. The hypothesis is that in epilepsy there is an increased production of cerebrospinal fluid in the nonextensible cerebrospinal space, that this increased pressure is associated with the convulsions in some causative or provocative relation, and that the effect of the treatment is the result of the removal of this surplus of extracellular fluid. Clinical attempts to test the hypothesis by simple reduction of the allowed fluids to a very low point have not been productive of satisfactory results in the hands of Fetterman and Kumin (1933), and Wilson and Limberger (1933); Fay (1933), however, believes that the method has considerable value.

The new method of attack of this ancient enemy was seized upon with avidity by the pediatricians, so that the earliest reports were of its results in the treatment of children; only relatively recently have comparable adult studies become available. Because of the differences in childhood and adult dietaries, it will be necessary to discuss the subject under separate heads below.

1. *Treatment of Children.*—Peterman, Helmholz, and Talbot, Metcalf and Moriarty have been the principal contributors to the literature of this subject. Peterman (1927) describes the method as follows (caloric food value tables will be found on p. 356):

"The diet is a low-carbohydrate, low-protein, high-fat ration adjusted for the individual patient. It is preceded by at least one week of starvation, or a longer period if necessary, until the attacks cease. During the starvation the patient is kept in bed and may be given water, clear broth, and bran wafers (no food value) freely. From 6 to 8 ounces of orange juice is allowed daily. At the end of the starvation period the prescribed diet is started abruptly.

"The basal metabolic requirement is calculated according to the Du Bois tables. From 25 to 30 per cent additional calories are allowed for energy exchange. The requirements may be simply calculated at 30 calories per pound. The total allowance should not exceed 1800 or 2000 calories.

Further adjustment is made to keep the weight at or slightly below normal for the patient's age and height. Overweight patients are not commonly seen. They are allowed to reduce the weight to normal. Children under five years of age are given a daily allowance of 20 Gm. of carbohydrate and 1 Gm. of protein per kilogram of body weight, with the remaining calories supplied in fat. Children over five years of age are given from 15 to 20 Gm. of carbohydrate, $2/3$ Gm. of protein, and the remaining requirement in fat. The vitamins and mineral salts must be supplied. Water is allowed freely. Salt is used to season. . . .

"The diet may be made palatable and attractive. The cooperation of the child must be enlisted and he must be carefully protected against all temptation. Any tendency to nausea or emesis can be quickly controlled with orange juice. Concomitant with the ketosis, when diacetic acid appears in the urine, the attacks usually cease or are greatly diminished in number. If the convulsions continue, the carbohydrate may be reduced to 10 Gm. and the fat pushed to the limit of tolerance. When the attacks are under control, the diet is continued for three months even through all ordinary illnesses. If there have not been further attacks, the carbohydrate is increased 10 Gm. After another month of freedom, the carbohydrate may again be increased. This procedure is continued until the carbohydrate reaches 50 Gm. At this time the fat may be reduced 15 or 20 Gm. During the next six months the carbohydrate may be increased 10 Gm. on alternate months, and the protein 5 Gm. alternating with the carbohydrate. The fat may be decreased every three or six months in proportion. No definite rule can be given. The changes are made according to the reaction of the individual. . . . Patients make much better progress if the protein is restricted carefully for the first year. It has been demonstrated that children over 5 years of age will make normal growth and development and will maintain a positive nitrogen balance on $2/3$ Gm. of protein per kilogram of body weight. This observation is substantiated by the recent report of Bartlett."

Peterman states, in 1933, that brewers' yeast concentrate is now added to the diet in 1-grain daily doses to insure adequate vitamin B content, and that calcium lactate is given in 1-grain amounts each day.

"The success of the ketogenic diet in the treatment of epilepsy is entirely a question of the ability to carry out the prescribed diet in careful detail. There must be a selection of cases—better perhaps, a selection of parents who are willing to cooperate and able mentally and financially to carry out the diet at home. The selection of cases also must exclude all patients with any evidence of organic lesions, and those patients who late in the disease have reached the stage of mental degeneration. If the diet is properly carried out, the proportions of carbohydrate, protein and fat may be gradually reversed to normal while the attacks are kept under control."

In 1932, a series of 85 cases was reported, 42.5 per cent of whom had been free of convulsions for from six months to three and a half years. The results reported by Helmholz and Keith (1933) of the Mayo Clinic are not quite so good: Of a total of 160 patients only 36 per cent were freed from their convulsions and 21 per cent improved; the fault is felt to lie in a much shorter contact with patients than is enjoyed by most physicians. In the series of both Peterman and Helmholz, as in the experience of all other observers, a considerable number of patients was much helped but not completely relieved of attacks. Dr. Peterman informs me he has found that fluid restriction adds greatly to the effectiveness of the regimen. He now (1933) allows only 300 to 800 cc. of fluids daily and never to exceed 1000 cc. at any time during at least the first three months after cessation of attacks has occurred.

Practical treatment (Peterman) of an epileptic child that cannot be hospitalized for fasting and ketogenic diet: (*a*) A definite daily regimen to include a long nap and a long sleep, meals at regular hours and a daily bowel movement; (*b*) restricted carbohydrate and protein and a high-fat diet; (*c*) fluid restriction to a minimum, at least to 600 or 800 cc. daily and less if convulsions continue; (*d*) phenobarbital in large enough doses to control any seizures which may occur after or until the above procedures are established.

2. *Treatment of Adults.*—The total number of calories to be given is estimated by multiplying the body weight by 16 if in pounds, by 35 if in kilograms, and then proceeding as shown in Table 57.

TABLE 57.—METHOD OF CALCULATION FOR KETOGENIC DIET IN ADULT EPILEPTICS
(BARBORKA)

Diet.	Carbohydrate, Gm.	Protein, Gm.	Fat, Gm.	Procedure.
1	Estimated calories $\times$ 0.035	Weight in pounds $\times$ ⅓	Estimated calories $\times$ 0.09	Continue for from six to seven days; test diet to determine whether or not total estimated calories are sufficient for maintenance of body weight.
2	Estimated calories $\times$ 0.02	Weight in pounds $\times$ ⅓	Estimated calories $\times$ 0.09	Continue for from one to two days; use as intermediate diet prior to production of ketosis, or have patient fast for two days and begin with diet 3.
3	Estimated calories $\times$ 0.015	Weight in pounds $\times$ ⅓	Estimated calories $\times$ 0.10	Continue for from three to five days; ketosis may develop at this stage.
4	Estimated calories $\times$ 0.01	Weight in pounds $\times$ ⅓	Estimated calories $\times$ 0.10	
5	Estimated calories $\times$ 0.008	Weight in pounds $\times$ ⅓	Estimated calories $\times$ 0.10	Continue indefinitely; diets 4, 5 and 6 to be used in order to develop or intensify ketosis if necessary.
6	Estimated calories $\times$ 0.006	Weight in pounds $\times$ ⅓	Estimated calories $\times$ 0.10	

Nausea or vomiting during the transition to the high-fat diet is usually controlled by small amounts of orange juice. When convulsive seizures persist in spite of the ketosis, a period of complete starvation save for the juice of two oranges a day (and the drinking of 1 to 2 quarts (1 to 2 liters) of water daily) is instituted for seven to ten days, after which the ketogenic diet is gradually resumed. It seems to be usually possible to determine whether benefit is to accrue at the end of six months but in some instances it is felt to be worth while persisting despite failure for as long as eight months to a year. The extent to which ketosis must be maintained in cases that are helped is a matter of individual determination.

In 1930, Barborka reported that of 100 adult patients thus treated, the attacks had been completely controlled in 12 and definite improvement had been shown in 44; thus 56 per cent of the patients were benefited. This observer has noted no deleterious effects from the relatively small amount of protein he allows (⅓ Gm. per pound body weight), but Regan (1931) has reported pellagra-like symptoms appearing in a patient whose protein intake had been reduced to considerably less than this (the Barborka allowance would have been 57 Gm.; the patient actually took only 36 Gm.) through refusal to eat certain foods; improvement immediately followed the resumption of higher protein feeding. Greer has reported a similar pellagra-like syndrome in a patient on low-protein allowance, which cleared up, however, when brewers' yeast was added to the diet. I think that most observers are now favoring diets of at least 1 Gm. protein per kilogram body weight; indeed, McQuarrie feels that even this is too low and that 1.75 to 2 Gm. would be preferable. I believe that this a quite rational contention in view of the part protein has been shown to play in the regulation of body fluids (see p. 467 in the chapter on Nephritis).

In the ketogenic treatment of pyuria (see p. 622) the necessity of rapidly achieving ketosis has been recognized. Wilson (1932), in England, describes the method by which he attempts to lessen the offensiveness of the regimen:

"The diet used has been varied with the patient, but the proportions of protein, fat, and carbohydrate have remained fairly constant: 60 Gm. of protein, 240 Gm. of fat, and 20 Gm. of carbohydrate. It would be idle to pretend that patients like the diet, but with care and a little imagination it can be robbed of most of its disagreeable features. We have to reconcile them to 240 Gm. of fat in the day, and to the almost total deprivation of carbohydrates. Protein is given in the normal amount.

"If fat is disliked in one form, it can be given in another. Let us suppose the 240 Gm. of fat are given as:

```
10 ounces of cream, 40 per cent, containing 100 ⎫
3½ ounces of butter              containing  90 ⎬ Gm. of fat
2 ounces of fat bacon            containing  36 ⎭
```

"The remainder of the fat is taken in meat and eggs. It is the butter and cream to which most patients object. If a jug of cream and a slab of butter with some diabetic biscuits are presented to the patient he will soon quarrel with the diet. As much as possible of both butter and cream should be used in cooking. A vegetable cream soup and a fruit food will not leave much cream to be taken with tea or coffee. In my experience of the diet I found the butter a stumbling-block. As we shall see presently, we have no carbohydrate to spare for breadstuffs or biscuits. There are two alternatives: To eat the butter with diabetic biscuits, or to use it in cooking in a vegetable purée, in buttered eggs, or in an omelette. If it is desired to reduce the butter or cream, half an ounce of olive oil night and morning will supply 30 Gm. of fat and provide a substitute.

"Only 20 Gm. of carbohydrate are allowed, and of this 10 Gm. have been used in the cream. The remaining 10 Gm. can be taken as fruit, a good vehicle for cream; or 5 Gm. may be given as fruit and 5 Gm. as milk in a custard, junket, or milk-jelly. In the American literature the patient is gradually broken into the diet by substituting fat for carbohydrates over some days, but this of course prolongs the agony, and in my experience embarking straightway on the full diet seldom leads to nausea."

Fuller (1933) states that at Queen Charlotte's Maternity Hospital they allow 14 ounces of 40 per cent cream daily, which contains 11 Gm. of lactose. If, however, a synthetic cream is made from butter and 3 per cent casein solution, with the aid of a mixer, all this lactose is eliminated with the exception of a trace in the butter. With this saving of 10 Gm. (plus) carbohydrate, it is possible to supply a diet of 250 Gm. fat and only 10 Gm. carbohydrate, or if the 20 Gm. carbohydrate is adhered to, the sugar saved by elimination of cream can be supplied in more satisfactory fashion in the form of extra fruit and vegetables.

(*d*) **Treatment of Hyperinsulinism.**—Harris (1933) has drawn attention to the state of hypoglycemia underlying some cases diagnosed epilepsy and successfully treated by the methods employed in the condition known as hyperinsulinism (see p. 383).

(*e*) **Treatment of the Attack.**—In a few individuals with a long aura, the use of amyl nitrite, by inhalation from a pearl crushed in the handkerchief, will sometimes abort an attack. During the course of a seizure about the only thing that can be done is to prevent injury insofar as is possible. A spoon or other hard object should be introduced between the teeth to prevent biting of the tongue, the clothing should be loosened, the mucus removed from the mouth, and the site of such gross injuries as may have been received in the fall protected as much as possible during the clonic period. Nocturnal epileptic attacks often precipitate the patient out of bed unless special safeguards are provided. The promotion of a quick return to consciousness by the use of cerebral stimulants is contraindicated, for such forced recovery from stupor is often obtained at the price of a terrific headache and very prolonged exhaustion.

(*f*) **Treatment of Status Epilepticus.**—The most usual methods of treating this state are by the use of strong purges, colonic irrigations with cold water, applications of ice to the spine, large doses of bromides, chloral hydrate, morphine, paraldehyde, luminal sodium, and chloroform. Bromides must be used in a large dose of 60 to 80 grains (4 to 5.3 Gm.), or chloral hydrate may be given in the same amount by rectum; morphine in a full dose is sometimes combined with either of these drugs. Grinker (1929) gives 3 to 5 grains (0.2 to 0.3 Gm.) of phenobarbital sodium intraspinally in 5 to 10 cc. of physiologic saline after drainage; intravenous injections of 3 grains (0.2 Gm.) every four hours may be made. Collier (1928) prefers paraldehyde to any other remedy; he gives it in a dose up to 8 drachms (32 cc.) in an equal quantity of olive oil by rectum. When a general anesthetic is necessary, chloroform is preferred to ether because of its quicker action. Robinson's careful studies at the New Jersey State Village for Epileptics convinced him that chloroform, pushed only to the point of producing complete relaxation, is the best remedy of all. Venesection should probably never be practiced unless injection of physiologic saline is made at the same time.

During the postconvulsive stupor, it may be necessary to continue the use of the anticonvulsants, for these patients are often in a state of motor unrest even after the convulsions have ceased. Supportive treatment is most important; atropine, alcohol, digitalis, caffeine, as indicated. The use of nutritive enemata and fluids by hypodermoclysis or intravenously may be necessary, bearing in mind the great metabolic upheaval that has been experienced by the body. Delirium is perhaps best controlled by scopolamine hydrobromide, $\frac{1}{200}$ to $\frac{1}{100}$ grain (0.0003 to 0.0006 Gm.).

Storchheim (1933), feeling that pulmonary edema with consequent or accompanying heart failure was largely responsible for the fatal termination in his 5 patients treated with sedatives or anesthetics, has turned to the intravenous injection of magnesium sulphate. He gives 10 cc. of a 25 per cent solution, repeating once or twice if necessary (dosage is further discussed on p. 479). Eight patients have so far been treated, all successfully; three have been brought safely through two attacks and one through four.

(*g*) **Miscellaneous Remedies in Epilepsy.**—The following remedies have had their advocates but have never been employed with anything approaching consistent success: Crotalin, acetanilid, acetylcholine, sodium borate (borax), protein desensitization, organotherapy (pituitary and thyroid substance), *Bacillus acidophilus* therapy, cervical sympathectomy, and removal of the colon. In connection with the claims that have been made for these agents, it is to be remembered that the epileptic often responds favorably to anything done to or for him, but it is only upon those measures that will produce results under any circumstances and time after time that our hopeful therapy can be based. In a certain proportion of cases, Swift is having success with an operation designed to relieve the disturbed mechanism of fluid storage in the reservoirs of the brain and subarachnoid spaces.

ENCEPHALITIS LETHARGICA
(Epidemic Encephalitis)

Encephalitis lethargica is an apparently new disease that first appeared in France in 1916 and has been occurring both sporadically and epidemically all over the world since that time. That the disease is of infectious nature is surmised from its acute course, the epidemic form in which it first appeared, and the nature of its pathologic foundation. A number of organisms and viruses have been brought forward in the allegedly causative rôle, but the true etiologic agent still remains unknown; that it is not identical with the herpes virus, and that it belongs to the neurotropic, invisible and filtrable virus forms is the opinion of most authorities—see J. B. Neal, Simon Flexner, and Stern in the Bibliography. During the recent St. Louis epidemic it was shown that the mosquito probably does not act as vector. It is believed by some investigators that the disease is not a new one but is identical with the "nona" of the 1890's and the outbreak of "sleeping sickness" of 1712. The theory of Watson that the disease has long been endemic in the Far East and was spread to other parts of the world as a result of the contacts of Asiatic and Occidental troops on the various fronts during the World War, is very interesting but unfortunately can hardly be put to the proof at this late day. I believe that most investigators no longer feel that there is any sort of connection between influenza and this disease.

The pathologic evidences of the disease are rather simple, consisting principally of cellular infiltrations in and about blood vessels, degeneration of ganglion and supporting cells, and the proliferation of glia; but the clinical manifestations are very complex. Indeed, I can permit myself only a brief description of the most usual characteristics, cautioning the reader that the greatest nicety is often required in differentiating between this disease and other psychiatric and neurological complexes. The onset may be sudden or gradual; usually there is an increasing drowsiness, often following a period of enforced activity (a number of observers have reported that all their cases have occurred in individuals who had been for a time under unusual mental or physical strain), slight fever, and diplopia or other eye-muscle disturbances. Salivation and "head cold" are perhaps as often absent as present. After the patient takes to bed, he usually lies with one or both lids ptosed, relaxed and absolutely quiet, apparently but not actually asleep; indeed, insomnia is of frequent occurrence despite the appearances of deep stupor. Other patients, however, manifest evidences of motor irritation from the beginning: The movements may be of the pillrolling, Parkinson type, or choreatic, or clonic-spasmodic. The mentality is usually impaired, especially as to memory, attention and orientation. Emotional disturbances are common, and in some cases marked alterations of character and oddities of behavior are outstanding features of the attack. Delirium sometimes alternates with periods of stupor. The cerebrospinal fluid may be normal, but in many cases there is an increase in globulin and sugar and a slight increase in the cell count.

During the four to eight weeks of the acute stage the mortality is quite high—in several counties in Missouri, in the period July-mid-October, 1933, there were over 1000 cases and 194 deaths; at this same time Japan was dealing with an epidemic in which there were 220 deaths in 427 cases. Convalescence is very slow, and in about 10 per cent of cases there is left some progressive disease of the central nervous system. These sequelae, which are the features of the malady that make it so much dreaded, may be of the form of persistent insomnias, Parkinson-like syndromes (paralysis agitans); autonomic pupillary, respiratory, cardiac, sphincter, etc., disturbances; mental impairment; psychoneurotic disturbances, etc. From these symptoms perhaps the majority of the patients recover completely in from six months to two years, but the others are left permanently disabled.

THERAPY

The description of therapy in this disease will require little space, since there is no specific remedial agent and only symptomatic treatment is available. During the acute stage, light but ample feeding, the forcing of fluids, the keeping of the body clean, and the protection of the patient from all annoying sensory stimuli are indicated. In the treatment of the insomnia or the excited states, of course resort must be had to full doses of sedatives (for list of these drugs, see p. 578). To control the parkinsonism and the upward rolling of the eyes that is so frequent and annoying, scopolamine hydrobromide (hyoscine), in a dose of $\frac{1}{200}$ to $\frac{1}{100}$ grain (0.0003 to 0.0006 Gm.) several times daily, is used. The careful studies of Cooper and Gunn (1931) show that harmalol hydrochloride, for which high hopes had been entertained, is at best only of adjuvant value to scopolamine, in doses of $\frac{4}{5}$ grain (0.05 Gm.) hypodermically or 8 to 12 grains (0.5 to 0.75 Gm.) by mouth. Juster's claims for stramonium in this condition have been confirmed by Shapiro (1928), Moren (1929), Jacobson and Epplen (1930), Worster-Drought and Hill (1930), Menard and Hurxthal (1931), and others. The powdered leaves are given at intervals of one or two hours until the good effect is obtained, after which a maintenance dose is used. In the beginning 15 to 30 grains (1 to 2 Gm.) may be distributed during the twenty-four hours, and Shapiro has found that a maintenance dose of 8 grains (0.5 Gm.) is well tolerated for many months; of the tincture, 60 to 90 minims three times daily has generally been found effective.

The treatment of the psychoneurotic sequelae, being largely systematic attempts at rehabilitation, cannot be described here. Arsenic, iodides, and indeed practically all the other specifics and near-specifics have been tried as aids to this process, and found wanting. Atropine has been given lately in Germany with apparently considerable success, as reported by Lewenstein (1931), Schenk (1931) and others. The dose is started at $\frac{1}{80}$ grain ($\frac{3}{4}$ mg.) thrice daily and increased by $\frac{1}{120}$ grain ($\frac{1}{2}$ mg.) twice daily until maximal therapeutic effects, or toxic disturbances, are obtained. In some instances, doses of $\frac{1}{6}$ to $\frac{1}{3}$ grain (10 to 20 mg.) daily are given for many months. However, mention should perhaps be made of the studies of acriflavine in Germany. Marx (1927) has reviewed the situation and ardently advocated the use of the dye. Of 40 cases, 14 were markedly improved, 22 were improved and only 4 were unaffected. These 4 were cases of extremely severe parkinsonism; however, among the 22 improved cases was also one of the same severity. Every other day he injects 1 in 200 (0.1 in 20) aqueous solution of the dye intravenously for six injections; then a 2 in 200 (0.2 in 20) solution every other day for six injections. The improvement was often shown by great change in the physical condition, especially the ability to walk for long distances without tiring. The facial expression and mental condition were also often improved. The only untoward effects of the dye were slight and brief nausea, and, in one case only, chills and fever of twenty-four hours' duration. Patients exposed to direct sunlight immediately after treatment complained of a short period of itching of the skin. Similar results have been reported in France by Laignel-Lavastine and Sterne (1932), using trypan blue in 1 per cent aqueous solution, 1 cc. injections intravenously at two-day intervals, followed by four injections of 2 cc. each at similar intervals; a month is allowed between courses. There is usually a slight nitritoid type of reaction but no serious toxic effects. A bluish tinge to conjunctiva and skin indicates the stopping point of the whole treatment.

Neal and Bentley (1932), reviewing the work of the Matheson Commission, have been unable to draw any definite conclusions regarding the results obtained with Rosenow's vaccine and Gay's hyperimmune rabbit brain vaccine.

DISEASES OF THE SKIN

IMPETIGO CONTAGIOSA

Impetigo is an acute contagious disease of the skin with a predilection for the face. It is sometimes spread among adult males by barber-shop infection, and an occasional case is seen in an adult female, but the great majority of patients are children within the school years. There are a number of varieties of this malady, but the most common one is characterized by a sudden crop of localized erythematous areas, upon which rapidly appear thin-walled vesicles and bullae; these lesions soon become pustular and then dry up quite rapidly, leaving thin, honey-colored, loosely attached crusts that drop off without scar formation, though the hyperemia fades out of the affected areas rather slowly. There is usually no itching. Both staphylococci and streptococci have been obtained from the lesions.

THERAPY

Ammoniated Mercury.—The most usual treatment of this condition is to thoroughly cleanse the parts with soap and water, breaking all bullae with gauze or a sterile tooth-pick, and then apply an ointment of 1 to 2 per cent ammoniated mercury, sometimes increasing to as much as 10 per cent. This suffices to cure most cases in one to three weeks, but of course to keep a grease applied to the face during working hours is objectionable to adults. In children, this objection does not apply for they should be kept out of school in any case.

Silver Nitrate.—Morrow has advocated the use of silver nitrate applied with a swab in 20 per cent solution after cleansing the lesions and opening the bullae. He and others have found this treatment very efficacious, but open to two objections: First, that there is some pain on application of the solution, and, second, that a black unsightly crust appears quickly and remains for three or four days. Sutton uses only a 10 per cent solution. The organic silver preparations (argyrol, etc.) have been found ineffective. After the application of the silver nitrate solution, Highman applies an ointment of ammoniated mercury or 10 per cent balsam of Peru.

Dusting Powder.—Morrow writes: "It is advisable to apply a dusting powder, preferably one containing ammoniated mercury in the strength of from 6 to 10 per cent, and a boric acid powder up to from 15 to 20 per cent. When impetigo is on the uncovered part, even without the silver, the powder form of treatment should be selected in preference to a grease. Customarily I have applied such a powder after swabbing with silver solution, and order its use by the patient several times daily."

℞.	Ammoniated mercury...............................	ʒiss	6.0
	Zinc oxide..	ʒv	20.0
	Talcum to make...................................	ʒij	60.0
	Make a dusting powder.		
	Label: Apply as directed.		

℞.	Boric acid..	ʒiij	12.0
	Zinc oxide..	ʒv	20.0
	Talcum to make...................................	ʒij	60.0
	Make a dusting powder.		
	Label: Apply as directed		

649

Salicylic Acid.—Lain states that after the secretions and scabs are removed by cleansing methods, he applies a 50 per cent alcoholic solution of salicylic acid in cases in which it is deemed that the patient can stand the treatment. This does not stain unless repeated and, in his hands, has been of especial value in preventing spreading.

Glycerin.—Kellert (1929), and more recently, Abramowitz (1931), have observed very rapid response in cases of impetigo neonatorum to the daily daubing all the body of a sterile 50 per cent solution of glycerin in water, after the bath.

Iodine.—One per cent iodine in alcohol is sometimes used to paint the lesions; the stain does not persist as long as that of the silver nitrate.

Copper and Zinc Sulphate.—Brownson writes: "In my opinion there is little need for treating the ordinary cases of impetigo so actively. I have used a modified form of *l'eau d'Alibour*, the favorite treatment of Saboraud. A modification of his remedy, which does very well, is made up of 1½ grains (0.1 Gm.) of copper sulphate and 3 grains (0.2 Gm.) zinc sulphate to the ounce (30 cc.) of camphor water. I often start by removing the crusts by a boric acid-starch poultice, and when removed, sop on the solution named several times a day, and its results are usually prompt. It is cleanly, and I can hardly see how it could be improved on. I think the results are fully as good as when stronger applications are used." In conjunction with this treatment he sometimes uses 1 per cent ammoniated mercury ointment at night and washes it off in the morning with soap and water, then applying the lotion during the day.

TINEA VERSICOLOR

This malady is characterized by the presence, usually only on the chest and shoulders, of a yellow or brown macular eruption that sheds very fine scales. There are usually one or more large plaques with numerous small lesions round about them. Itching is slight or entirely absent. The disease, which is caused by *Microsporon furfur*, is rather common among men, but is entirely harmless.

THERAPY

The disease yields readily to frequent applications of a saturated solution of sodium thiosulphate (sodium hyposulphite), but only if the affected areas are first vigorously scrubbed with soap and water and then dried before making the application. Crocker, cited by Sutton, has found the use of a 5 per cent solution of the thiosulphate, followed by a 3 per cent solution of tartaric acid, to be even more efficacious.

ERYTHEMA MULTIFORME

This disease is characterized by the rather sudden appearance of red to violaceous inflammatory lesions that, as the name implies, are multiform: they may be macular, papular, vesicular or bullous. The sites of predilection are the face, neck, arms, hands, legs and feet. Subjective symptoms are few or none, but the attack usually lasts from two to three weeks, and the same individual may be afflicted time and time again. The etiology is unknown, though many observers are inclining to the belief that this malady will eventually be placed among the allergic diseases; others feel that it is often due to a toxemia of intestinal origin.

THERAPY

There is no evidence that any of the internal remedies that have been recommended are of any use save the cathartics. Dieting and the taking of copious amounts of water are sometimes of value; perhaps the newer approach to food allergy which Rowe is making (see p. 332) might well be tried in recurring cases. At the New York Skin and Cancer Hospital we used always to give an initial dose of castor oil and then keep the patient on the Bulkley diet of rice (without sugar or cream), bread, butter, and water as long as he would cooperate—treatment that, plus the forcing of fluids, was thought to considerably lessen the duration of an attack. For local application, calamine lotion may be used (see pp. 668 and 168).

EPIDERMOPHYTOSIS

(Ringworm of the Hands, Feet, Groin, Axillae, Breasts and the Hairless Skin Generally)

This is a skin disease that, in one form or another, most people seem to have. The name is objected to because the causative fungus, *Epidermophyton inguinale,* is found in perhaps only a third of the cases, such names as trichophytosis and dermatophytosis being offered as substitutes. However, French, German, Italian, and, I believe, most of the British dermatologists have adopted the name epidermophytosis; also the majority of Americans. The principal forms of the disease are the following: (1) Vesicular, and (2) scaling, both of which predominate on fingers, toes, palms and soles; (3) macular, which is of two sorts, one (also called eczema marginatum or "jockey strap itch"), the well-known red, definitely marginated lesion occurring principally in the groin region, the axillae and beneath the breasts, and the other (tinea circinata), the slightly elevated, ringlike patches that occur principally on the face, neck and hands, and are spoken of as common ringworm of the body; and (4) macerated, the familiar lesion between the fingers or toes and beneath the breasts, presenting as an area of clean, white, sodden tissue of a varying degree of thickness. There are several other forms, less frequently encountered.

The disease is certainly contagious, but the problem of protecting against it, seeing its ubiquity and protean character, is a very difficult one indeed.

THERAPY

Treatment of epidermophytosis has never been entirely satisfactory, some cases resisting any and all sorts of measures, while others clear up very quickly under the simplest treatment (I distinctly remember cases, seen while working in Williams' clinic at the New York Skin and Cancer Hospital, that rapidly disappeared under the boric acid ointment being used at the time as a placebo!). To attempt to list all the preparations in use against this disease would be hopeless; I shall therefore content myself with mentioning some of the remedies in use by White, the well-known dermatologist of Boston, and appending a few other measures especially employed against the infections of the feet.

1. **Vesicular.**—After opening the deep vesicles antiseptically, apply any of the following: Ether, tincture of iodine; hot soaks of 1 per cent potassium permanganate solution; saturated solution of boric acid; 10 per cent alco-

holic solution of trinitrophenol (picric acid); 0.4 per cent copper sulphate; or paint with:

℞.	Oil of cinnamon	gr. xx	1.2
	Thymol	gr. xlv	3.0
	Alcohol to make	℥iv	120.0

or

℞.	Ether	ʒss	2.0
	Balsam of Peru	ʒj	4.0
	Collodion flexible	℥j	30.0

In the paper of Myers and Thienes (1925), in which the cinnamon-thymol mixture was first proposed, the original proportions were 2 per cent of oil of cinnamon and 5 per cent of thymol. The cinnamon oil is sometimes irritating, when it should be omitted from the formula.

2. Moist or Macerated.—Crude coal tar may be used in from 6 to 100 per cent strength, as:

℞.	Crude coal tar	gr. xlv	3.0
	Zinc oxide	gr. xlv	3.0
	Petrolatum to make	℥j	30.0

Or the Lotio Nigra ("black wash") of the National Formulary may be freely used; this is a preparation containing 8.75 Gm. of calomel, 15 cc. of water, and lime water to make 1000 cc.

3. Macular and Scaling.—Whitfield ointments 1 or 2:

Whitfield 1	Whitfield 2
Salicylic acid, 3 per cent	Salicylic acid, 6 per cent
Benzoic acid, 6 per cent	Benzoic acid, 12 per cent
Petrolatum to make	Petrolatum to make

or any of the following:

℞.	Salicylic acid	ʒss	2.0
	Precipitated sulphur	ʒss	2.0
	Lard to make	℥j	30.0

| ℞. | Mercurous chloride (calomel) | ʒiiss | 10.0 |
| | Lard to make | ℥j | 30.0 |

℞.	Red mercuric sulphide	gr. iss	0.1
	Salicylic acid	gr. xx	1.2
	Benzoic acid	gr. xxx	2.0
	Precipitated sulphur	gr. xlv	3.0
	Lanolin	℥j	30.0
	Petrolatum to make	℥ij	60.0

| ℞. | Yellow mercuric oxide | gr. ij | 0.12 |
| | Petrolatum to make | ℥j | 30.0 |

This long and varied list signifies, says White, but one thing—a confession of therapeutic weakness. But he then adds that he has of late been using a 2 per cent aqueous solution of mercurochrome-220 with most promising results. He swabs it on once a day and subsequently twice a day, permitting no bandages. At the appearance of small fissures, the applications become painful and must be stopped until healing has taken place.

Treatment of Lesions on the Feet.—The preparations in use by White for the treatment of the macular and scaling varieties are the ones most often used, though it is usual to have to shift about among them before accomplishing cure in a severe case. The following may be added to the list as they are often effective: A fresh 3 to 5 per cent iodine solution; or a 1 per cent potassium permanganate solution. Either of these last-mentioned solutions may also be applied to vesicular lesions if not very severe, but if the condition is bullous, the bullae should be aseptically opened and wet dressings of 1 part of solution of aluminum acetate and 15 parts of saturated solution of boric acid applied. Some cases, whether wet or dry, will stand no very irritating applications; for these, the coal-tar preparation of White seems best suited.

Taylor (1929) has reported excellent results in a small series of cases in which he froze the lesions with the ethyl chloride spray, a treatment attractive because of its simplicity and cleanliness. "To be effective, freezing should produce blanching of the skin (including the lesion itself) for a distance of at least 0.5 cm. beyond the periphery of the affected area; the blanching should be sustained for from one half to one minute. In most cases, one complete daily freezing of all lesions will suffice. Where the epidermis is thick, as in the plantar region, it may be advisable to apply the treatment twice daily; and from two to six or more applications of the spray may be required to secure subsidence of the infection." Plantar lesions are protected by a slight dressing between treatments but digital and interdigital lesions are not. Loose skin edges and overhanging margins of epidermis are trimmed away to give more effective access to the spray.

Prophylaxis.—Gould (1931) has reported good results with a powder of 20 per cent sodium thiosulphate in boric acid, applied to the feet and inside the footwear after a bath, or night and morning. Goodman (1931) recommends the following powder, his laboratory studies having shown the advisability of previously sterilizing the infusorial earth:

Ŗ. Phenyl salicylate (salol).............................. gr. xl   2.5
    Chloral hydrate...................................... gr. xl   2.5
    Purified infusorial earth (sterilized).................. ℥iv   120.0

Actual fumigation of the shoes may be accomplished by inserting in them a piece of blotting paper containing a teaspoonful of formalin; wrap tightly for twenty-four hours and air thoroughly before wearing again. There is no need of destroying clothing, as materials of all sorts may be sterilized safely by first washing, then soaking in 1:1000 bichloride of mercury for a day, and afterward thoroughly rinsing in water before drying.

Unfortunately, lack of space does not permit me to describe here the relatively simple and apparently successful method of large-scale prophylaxis in public baths employed by Osborne and Hitchcock (1931).

RINGWORM OF THE SCALP

Ringworm attacks the scalp only in children. The patches are round and scaly, but not centrally involuted as in similar affections of the glabrous skin; they are not completely bald, but contain numerous brittle or broken hairs and dilated or "débris-stuffed" follicular orifices. In the older patches there are usually many young hairs with fine shafts. In severe cases the whole scalp may be involved and the itching become quite intense.

THERAPY

(a) **Manual Epilation and Application of Antiseptics.**—This, the old treatment of ringworm of the scalp, requires anywhere from six months to three years to bring about a cure. The hair must be clipped short and maintained so, and the hairs in the affected areas plus those around the margins must be pulled out with the forceps. The scalp must be frequently and thoroughly washed with soap and water, and an antiseptic ointment, such as 10 per cent ammoniated mercury ointment, frequently applied over the surface. For application to the affected areas *per se*, the following are a few of the remedies used; they are all powerful irritants and are therefore to be employed with very great caution, especially as regards keeping them out of the eyes:

℞.	Chrysarobin	℥ij	8.0
	Chloroform to make	℥iv	120.0
	Careful!		

℞.	Chrysarobin	℥ss	2.0
	Petrolatum to make	℥j	30.0
	Careful!		

℞. Tincture of iodine.

℞.	Crude coal tar	gr. xlv	3.0
	Zinc oxide	gr. xlv	3.0
	Petrolatum to make	℥j	30.0

℞.	Resorcinol	℥iij	12.0
	Petrolatum		
	or		
	Glycerin to make	℥iv	120.0

℞. Whitfield 1 or 2 (p. 652).

℞.	Salicylic acid	℥ij	8.0
	Precipitated sulphur	℥ij	8.0
	Petrolatum to make	℥iv	120.0

℞.	Betanaphthol	℥j	4.0
	Precipitated sulphur	℥ss	2.0
	Petrolatum to make	℥j	30.0

(*b*) *x*-**Ray Epilation.**—There is no longer any doubt that preliminary epilation of the entire scalp by the use of *x*-ray, to be followed by the application of the antiseptics as above, is the best available treatment; Wise says that in his extensive experience at the Vanderbilt Clinic, the hair has come out in from seventeen to twenty-one days and regrowth has occurred within three months. However, I cannot refrain from cautioning the reader against placing his patient in the hands of just *any* upstart operator of an *x*-ray apparatus; this is a special technic, and, like all special technics, requires study and practice in order to obtain mastery. It is not easy to forget the unfortunate sequelae of unskilled roentgen ray or radium therapy.

(*c*) **Thallium Acetate.**—The occurrences of recent years have shown this drug to be entirely too toxic for employment in a benign condition such as ringworm. I shall therefore no longer describe it unless a restudy in the future proves the practicability of its use under conditions of wide marginal safety.

RINGWORM OF THE BEARD

The treatment of ringworm of the bearded region differs in none of its essentials from the treatment of ringworm of the scalp.

SEBORRHEIC DERMATITIS

This is probably the commonest of all skin diseases. In the scalp it is known as dandruff, which may be of the dry scaly or the moist greasy variety. In many cases lesions are also seen along the fringe of hair on the forehead, in the eyebrows, on the outer aspects of the nostrils, and behind the ears. The most frequent site of predilection other than the points mentioned is the sternal region; here the lesions are rounded, irregular or circinate, and are covered with greasy yellowish scales. The differentiation between seborrheic dermatitis, ringworm of the glabrous skin and psoriasis is not always easy to make. There may be much itching.

THERAPY

The remedies for this condition are of course legion, which is simply an indication of the relative ineffectiveness of them all. However, any one of the following plans of treatment will lessen the severity of most cases; some will be "cured," though return of the lesions is almost certain. Many dermatologists feel that a fatty diet predisposes to this condition, and therefore rigorously restrict the intake of certain foods; I used to feel in a rather superior fashion that dieting for dandruff was too amusing to be taken with entire seriousness, but now, with the allergists almost daily enlarging their field, I am no longer certain about many things. Other observers believe that a diet high in carbohydrate predisposes to this affection.

(*a*) **Ammoniated Mercury and Salicylic Acid.**—These drugs, as in the following prescription, may be thoroughly rubbed into the scalp one or two nights a week; it should be washed out with soap and water the next morning.

℞.	Ammoniated mercury	gr. xlv	3.0
	Salicylic acid	gr. x	0.6
	White wax	℥j	4.0
	Hydrous wool fat	℥v	20.0
	Petrolatum to make	℥ij	60.0

This contains 5 per cent of ammoniated mercury and 1 per cent of the salicylic acid; the quantities may be doubled, giving 10 and 2 per cent, respectively, but higher than this it is perhaps not advisable to go in the average case. On the nights when this ointment is not being used, Sutton advises the employment of the following lotion, which he accredits to Johnston:

℞.	Mercuric chloride	gr. ⅙	0.01
	Chloral hydrate	℥ij	8.0
	Spirit of formic acid (N.F.)	℥iv	15.0
	Castor oil	♏viij	0.5
	Oil of bergamot to give odor		
	Alcohol (80 per cent) to make	℥vi	180.0

(*b*) **Sulphur.**—This drug may be used in the form of a simple sulphur ointment, as the following:

℞.	Precipitated sulphur	℥j	4.0
	White wax	℥j	4.0
	Hydrous wool fat	℥v	20.0
	Petrolatum to make	℥ij	60.0

or it may be somewhat reduced in amount and combined with salicylic acid, as in the following prescription, in which the salicylic acid may be doubled in amount if considered desirable:

℞.	Precipitated sulphur	℥ss	2.0
	Salicylic acid	gr. x	0.6
	White wax	℥j	4.0
	Hydrous wool fat	℥v	20.0
	Petrolatum to make	℥ij	60.0

(c) **Resorcinol.**—This drug is used either as ointment or lotion in the strength of 1 to 6 per cent; the following prescriptions, much used in my day at the New York Skin and Cancer Hospital, contain 4 and 6 per cent. respectively:

℞.	Resorcin..	gr. xx	1.2
	Petrolatum to make.................................	℥j	30.0
℞.	Resorcin..	ℨiv	15.0
	Glycerin..	℥j	30.0
	Alcohol...	℥vj	24.0
	Water to make......................................	℥viij	250.0

Dark hair is not appreciably affected by resorcin, but the fact should always be borne in mind that this drug will stain light or white hair, especially if the patient exposes the head to the sunlight after an application of the ointment or lotion. Resorcin monoacetate is said to be less apt to do so; it may be substituted for resorcin in equal amounts. A satisfactory prescription would be written by replacing the chloral hydrate in the fifth prescription above by ℨiiss (10.0) of resorcin monoacetate.

SYCOSIS VULGARIS

This is a chronic, discrete, pustular folliculitis of the bearded region, caused by several strains of staphylococci. The essential lesions are either superficial or deep-seated papules or pustules pierced by hairs that are easily pulled out. The infection may persist for many months or years, and the resultant alopecia and scarring are sometimes quite considerable.

THERAPY

Here, as in the ringworm infections, the area must be epilated either by x-ray or forceps, and the antiseptic and stimulating drugs applied in ointment or lotion for a long period of time. The reader is referred to page 653, where ringworm of the scalp and beard is discussed, for I fail to follow the dermatologists in the fine distinctions they would have made in the treatment of the tineal and staphylococcic infections. x-Ray is said to cure about 40 per cent of cases. At the New York Skin and Cancer Hospital, Throne and Myers have obtained better results from nonspecific protein therapy (methods on p. 327). Others have had occasional success with bacteriophage.

LICHEN PLANUS

This is an inflammatory disease of the skin that is usually subacute in its onset, though it tends to run a chronic course and to recur many times after spontaneous recovery or "cure." It is characterized by the appearance, principally on the flexor surfaces of the wrists and forearms and the inner aspects of the knees and thighs, of intensely itching, glistening, red to violaceous, round, angular or star-shaped, plane-topped, pinhead-sized papules; at first these tiny papules, many in number, remain discrete, but they tend ultimately to coalesce into rough scaly patches. The disease not infrequently attacks the visible mucous membranes; other rare forms there are with which we cannot be concerned in this book. Lichen planus is a dry disease throughout its course, though pigmented areas or slightly atrophic spots are sometimes left behind after departure of the lesions.

THERAPY

Despite the frequency with which this disease is seen in practice, very little advance in its treatment has been made in many years. White believes that the cure depends mainly on natural evolution and that treatment is therefore principally palliative, an opinion in which many observers concur. However, it is usual to give preparations of arsenic and mercury by mouth (the arsphenamines usually fail when injected) and to treat the pruritus locally. Mercury administration is described in the section on Syphilis, arsenic in the section on Anemia—indeed its combination with iron in large quantities is thought to be of value in the treatment of lichen planus. Antipruritic measures are discussed on page 450.

Grossman (1932) has reported excellent results in a small series of cases in which he injected 1½ grains (0.1 Gm.) bismuth salicylate in oil intramuscularly once each week for ten injections; further studies will be awaited with interest. In the most stubborn cases, x-ray therapy is sometimes resorted to but with variable results.

PSORIASIS

Psoriasis is a common, nonitching, nonpainful, inflammatory skin disease characterized by a typical course, a typical appearance, and a typical distribution. Course: the disease usually develops between the ages of ten and thirty, runs a variable course, disappears spontaneously, and recurs and disappears again many times throughout the patient's life. Appearance: The lesions are papular, multiform, dry, reddish, and covered with white, gray or silvery imbricated scales. The scraping away of every one of the scales from a single papule reveals a very red, easily bleeding elevation; in long-standing cases many of the papular lesions coalesce to form thickened patches covering surprisingly large portions of the body. In the intervals between attacks the skin usually clears entirely. Distribution: The eruption is symmetrical, and, from a beginning usually on the elbows and knees, may spread all over the body; the scalp is often involved, but the face and the backs of the hands are frequently spared even when the involvement elsewhere is very extensive.

Psoriasis is rare in the Orient and in the tropics, and is much less frequent in the warmer than the colder parts of the temperate zones. Most patients are better in the summer and worse in the winter. The disease is extremely rare in full-blooded negroes and American Indians. Nothing is known of its etiology or of what part, if any, heredity plays in its causation.

THERAPY

While there are many cases of psoriasis that remain completely intractable, the duration of the average moderately severe attack can usually be much lessened by proper treatment. From my own observation of a relatively large number of cases, and a careful perusal of the literature, I am of the opinion that it is the local treatment alone that brings about this amelioration of symptoms. x-Ray therapy sometimes causes temporary improvement, but the occasional good result would seem to be bought at an excessively high price; to wit: prolonged treatment, such as is necessary in this disease, practically always lowers the white blood count more than can be entirely safe; if the treatment is unskilfully applied, the patient may be seriously burned (I have seen such a burn from one of the foremost clinics in the United States!); and the treatment may superimpose upon the lesions an itching, burning dermatitis. The use of autoserum, intravenous foreign protein, venipuncture, low-protein diet, x-ray stimulation of the thymus gland—all these measures have had their occasional successes, but I think that such results are utterly without significance in a disease so variable as this. The internal remedies recommended are legion, but the only one to which dermatologists return after their dallyings with other drugs—if they return at all—is arsenic. It is usually begun at 1 to 3 drops of Fowler's solution (U.S.P. solution of potassium arsenite) three times daily, and increased 1 drop per dose every other day until 10 drops are being taken after each meal; this dose is maintained for a week or ten days unless signs of slight poisoning supervene earlier, *i. e.*, puffiness under the eyes or about the ankles, or gastro-intestinal disturbances. It is not commonly realized that arsenical neuritis can also be produced with this method of administration. The best practice is perhaps to rest the patient for awhile after he has been held the week or ten days on the full dose, but some practitioners gradually reduce the dose and thus bring him back again by gradations to a nonarsenical basis. There is nothing to indicate that arsphenamine, or any of the other organic arsenicals, have any value here. Gold preparations are being used in this country by Throne, and in Germany manganese is having a trial, but I do not feel that the results warrant description as yet.

In the local treatment of psoriasis it is very essential that all the scales be removed before applying the remedial agent. This is usually accomplished by vigorous scrubbing with soap and water in a warm alkaline bath (see p. 668), but there are a few individuals who are made worse by the contact with water; for these, recourse must be had to the "grease bath," *i. e.*, the scrubbing of the body with some such preparation as the following, which is then to be thoroughly wiped off before applying the curative preparations:

℞.	Lanolin	℥v	20.0
	Glycerite of boroglycerin	℥ij	60.0
	Petrolatum to make	℥iv	120.0

The following preparations are perhaps those most used in treatment; the majority of cases will respond to any one of these, but in some cases the whole gamut will have to be run. All of these ointments should be worked into the lesions with a stiff tooth-brush, but they are not to be applied to other than diseased areas.

1. **Ammoniated Mercury and Salicylic Acid.**—For treatment of the scalp and face a combination of these drugs is employed, as chrysarobin and the other irritants will ultimately get into the eyes when used as long as is necessary in psoriasis. The prescription contains 2 per cent of salicylic acid and 10 per cent of ammoniated mercury; the former may be increased gradually to 5 per cent and the latter very cautiously to 20 per cent; in rare instances both are carried much higher than this:

℞.	Salicylic acid	gr. xl	2.4
	Ammoniated mercury	℥iij	12.0
	White wax	℥ij	8.0
	Hydrous wool fat	℥j℥ij	40.0
	Petrolatum	℥iv	120.0

2. **Chrysarobin in Ointment.**—This drug is undoubtedly effective in more cases than is any other, but it is extremely disagreeable to use as it stains everything brown with which it comes in contact. The stains are only partially removed from linen by the use of a chlorinated lime solution. Also the drug may at any time, especially on the upper ranges of its effective concentration, produce a dermatitis that is sometimes very aggravating. It is usually begun at 5 per cent strength and cautiously increased to 25

or even 35 per cent, though few cases will stand this latter concentration.
The prescription contains 5 per cent:

℞. Chrysarobin.. ʒiss   6.0
    Petrolatum....................................... ℥ij   60.0
    Lanolin to make.................................. ℥iv   120.0

A substance, cignolin, which is said to be chrysarobin minus a methyl
group in the formula has lately been introduced as a Bayer product on the
Continent; it is reputed to be three to five times as strong as chrysarobin
and without its propensity for causing kidney irritation upon being absorbed. Cowen (1932) has used it in the proportions of 5 to 10 grains to
the ounce in a simple ointment base with quite good results. Further studies
will be awaited.

3. **Chrysarobin in Collodion, Gutta Percha or Gelatin Film.**—The drug
may be prescribed in any one of these media to be painted on, a method
more acceptable to the fastidious patient but less effective than the use in
ointment; the gutta percha formula is to be preferred, as chrysarobin is
not soluble in collodion. The prescriptions contain 6 per cent, to be increased just as in the ointment:

℞. Chrysarobin.. ʒss   2.0
    Collodion (not the flexible) to make.................. ℥j   30.0

℞. Chrysarobin.. ʒss   2.0
    Solution of gutta percha (N.F. IV) to make........... ℥j   30.0

or the following may be written:

℞. Chrysarobin.. ʒij   8.0
    Soft glycerogelatin (N.F.) to make................... ℥iv   120.0

Such a gel is melted and applied with a brush and covered with a bandage.
Some physicians prefer the zinc oxide paste for vehicle:

℞. Chrysarobin.. ʒiss   6.0
    Zinc oxide... ℥j   30.0
    Starch... ℥j   30.0
    Liquid petrolatum to make.......................... ℥iv   120.0

4. **Tar.**—The following are forms in which this substance is frequently
applied:

℞. Tar ointment (U.S.P.)............................. ℥j   30.0
    Petrolatum to make................................ ℥iv   120.0

℞. Oil of cade (U.S.P.).............................. ℥j   30.0
    White wax... ʒij   8.0
    Hydrous wool fat.................................. ℥j ʒij   40.0
    Petrolatum to make................................ ℥iv   120.0

5. **Chrysarobin, Tar and Salicylic Acid.**—A compound sometimes successfully used during my time at the New York Skin and Cancer Hospital
had the following formula:

℞. Rectified oil of birch tar*........................ ʒiij   12.0
    Salicylic acid...................................... ʒvj   24.0
    Chrysarobin....................................... ʒvj   24.0
    Anhydrous lanolin................................. ℥j   30.0
    Soft soap to make................................. ℥iv   120.0

* In the interest of simplification of our armamentarium, I see no reason why this
preparation, the beloved Oleum Rusci of the dermatologists, could not in all instances
be substituted by the oil of cade, a U.S.P. preparation from which it surely can differ
slightly, if at all, therapeutically.

6. Coal Tar.—Coal tar is often better borne than the wood tars; it may be substituted in any of the above prescriptions. Goeckerman (1931) has seen some indications of hastened recovery if ultraviolet radiation to the point of tanning is carried on in conjunction with the coal-tar treatments. The lesions are wiped practically clean of the ointment and the light then directed onto the skin through a thin film of remaining ointment, the belief being that some new chemical substance, powerfully antipsoriatic, may be formed in the coal tar thus treated. Lesions are not retreated with ointment until several hours after the daily light treatment.

7. Unna's Chrysarobin-ichthyol Compound.—This much-used preparation is variously written, but I believe the following formula to be the one most often employed:

℞.	Chrysarobin.............................	ℨiss	6.0
	Salicylic acid............................	gr. xlv	3.0
	Ichthyol................................	ℨiss	6.0
	Petrolatum to make.......................	℥iv	120.0

8. Resorcinol.—This drug is used in ointment in the strength of 5 to 10 per cent; the prescription contains 5 per cent:

℞.	Resorcinol...............................	ℨiss	6.0
	Petrolatum...............................	℥ij	60.0
	Lanolin to make..........................	℥iv	120.0

9. Pyrogallol (Pyrogallic Acid).—This drug is used in ointment in the strength of 5 to 10 per cent; the prescription contains 5 per cent:

℞.	Pyrogallol...............................	ℨiss	6.0
	Petrolatum...............................	℥ij	60.0
	Lanolin to make..........................	℥iv	120.0

Pyrogallol stains tissues and clothing black and is too irritating to employ about the eyes or genitalia. A greater objection to its use, however, is the fact that it may suddenly be absorbed in sufficient quantities to cause serious systemic poisoning; in rapid cases there are cyanosis, dyspnea, convulsions and collapse, but in the slower cases chills, diarrhea and vomiting, acute nephritis with dark scant urine, and sometimes jaundice and glycosuria, are the outstanding symptoms. The indications are to empty the gastro-intestinal tract with emetics and purgatives, apply heat to the body, and stimulate; there is no specific antidote.

10. Betanaphthol.—This drug is probably less effective than pyrogallol, but it is also less dangerous; systemic poisoning of the phenol type may occur, however, from absorption through the skin, though the recorded cases are few. It is used in ointment in the strength of 5 to 10 per cent; the prescription contains 10 per cent:

℞.	Betanaphthol.............................	ℨiij	12.0
	White wax...............................	℥ij	8.0
	Hydrous wool fat.........................	℥j℥ij	40.0
	Petrolatum to make.......................	℥iv	120.0

or the following "peeling paste" of the N.F. may be applied for a short time twice a day:

℞.	Betanaphthol.............................	ℨiss	6.0
	Precipitated sulphur......................	℥j	30.0
	Petrolatum...............................	ℨiij	12.0
	Soft soap to make........................	℥ij	60.0

LUPUS ERYTHEMATOSUS

Lupus erythematosus is a chronic inflammatory skin disease characterized by the insidious development of small, pink, dry, macular patches with grayish adherent scales; which patches, both by extension and coalescence, form well-defined, thickened areas, varying in size from a small coin to the palm of the hand or more, and having in their center one large or several small thin, colorless or whitish, atrophic scars with gaping follicular orifices. The sites of predilection of this disease are the scalp, the regions about the ears, the cheeks, and the bridge of the nose; perhaps the next most frequent site is the backs of the hands. The mucous membranes are involved in about one fourth of the cases. When the lesions occur on both cheeks with a connecting bridge across the nose, the most typical distribution of all, the "butterfly appearance" is often glibly referred to—an unfortunate designation, for certainly in the vast majority of cases these patches resemble no butterfly ever seen or heard of.

The etiology of this malady is entirely unknown. The cases usually begin between the fifteenth and thirtieth years and run an erratic course throughout the rest of the patient's life, though spontaneous disappearance sometimes occurs. There are no constitutional symptoms, and the patient's welfare is disturbed only insofar as the unsightliness of the affliction alters his or her environmental reactions. The acute disseminate variety of the disease, with its severe general symptoms and grave prognosis as to life, is too rare to concern us in this book.

THERAPY

Local Treatment.—*x*-Ray, radium, carbon dioxide snow, ultraviolet light, high-frequency current—all these agents have more failures than successes to their credit, though instances of brilliant results with any of them may be cited. So, too, it is with the local application of drugs. I list below the remedies most frequently employed, but can only say that in my own experience in a large dermatological clinic, and from personal communications with dermatologists and a perusal of their literature, these agents have been found one and all to be sadly lacking in their ability to consistently produce the kind of results that are occasionally reported following their use.

1. **Sulphur.**—This drug is usually applied once or twice daily in ointment; the prescription contains 4 per cent, but it may be increased in strength:

℞.	Precipitated sulphur	gr. xx	1.2
	Petrolatum to make	℥j	30.0

2. **Sulphur and Salicylic Acid.**—These drugs are used in combination to be applied in ointment once or twice daily, or alternated with the sulphur alone; the prescription contains 4 per cent sulphur and 10 per cent salicylic acid, both of which may be gradually increased:

℞.	Precipitated sulphur	gr. xl	6.0
	Salicylic acid	℥iij	12.0
	White wax	℥ij	8.0
	Hydrous wool fat	℥j℥ij	40.0
	Petrolatum to make	℥iv	120.0

3. **Lotio Alba.**—This is a mixture of sulphurated potassa (U.S.P.) and zinc sulphate, usually applied once or twice daily. The following prescrip-

tion is for the mild form of the lotion, with which the treatment is usually begun; for a full description of the use of this *lotio alba*, see page 675.

℞. Zinc sulphate...................................	ℨij	8.0
Sulphurated potassa.............................	ℨij	8.0
Water to make..................................	℥iv	120.0

4. Ichthyol.—This drug is applied once or twice daily in ointment or collodion in 10 per cent strength.

℞. Ichthyol...	ℳxlv	3.0
Petrolatum to make..............................	℥j	30.0

or

℞. Ichthyol...	ℳxlv	3.0
Collodion (not the flexible) to make..............	℥j	30.0

5. Phenol.—Pure liquid phenol is washed over the lesions once a week with a cotton applicator.

6. Phenol-Lactic Acid.—The following mixture is applied with a glass rod over the surface of the lesions once every ten days to two weeks: Phenol, 1 part; lactic acid, 4 parts. The parts should first be cleansed with ether.

7. Trichloracetic Acid.—This substance is painted on the lesions with a cotton applicator once a week, the parts having first been cleansed with benzine to facilitate penetration.

8. Arsenic.—Equal parts of arsenic trioxide and acacia are made into a paste with a saturated solution of cocaine hydrochloride and spread over the diseased area, though no more than a square inch at a time should be treated. The paste is allowed to remain in place for twenty-four to forty-eight hours, when the slough is removed by poulticing.

9. Pyrogallol (Pyrogallic Acid).—This substance is applied in ointment twice a day to small areas for two or three weeks, the sloughs being removed from time to time by poulticing; the prescription contains 20 per cent, but this strength is sometimes doubled:

℞. Pyrogallol.......................................	ℨiss	6.0
Rosin cerate.....................................	ℨiv	15.0
Petrolatum to make..............................	℥j	30.0

10. Quinine and Iodine.—The patient is given 7½ grains (0.5 Gm.) of quinine sulphate three times daily for five to seven days, during which time the lesions are painted with the tincture of iodine once each day; after a week, during which the crusts are removed either spontaneously or by poulticing, another course of treatment is given.

Gold Salts Intravenously.—Gold salts of the type of Møllgaard's "sano-crysin," which have failed to win much support for themselves in the treatment of tuberculosis, seem to have found a place in the treatment of lupus erythematosus. At present in the United States, gold and sodium thio-sulphate, introduced by Schamberg and Wright in 1927, is the most extensively used preparation, though all those employed in Europe (triphal and krysolgan, principally) have their advocates here also. In matters of dosage, reactions and results there are probably no differences of note now that all the more toxic salts are no longer used.

Results.—As with all new therapy, enthusiasm ran high in the beginning but is now abating somewhat. There is no doubt that a large proportion of cases is favorably influenced and some apparently cured; probably 50 per cent altogether are helped considerably, but recurrences are beginning to be seen, so that it is not yet possible to know the duration of the effect with certainty.

Dosage.—The high dosage formerly used has been very considerably reduced and observers are able to report just as good results with the much smaller doses. I cannot review here all that has been written upon this subject, but believe that the present dosage and treatment plan of Driver and Weller (1931) represents average conservative practice: (a) An initial dose of 10 mg., followed one week later by 20 or 25 mg. and increased 10 mg. per week up to 50 mg., (b) in resistant cases the maximum dose is cautiously increased to 75 mg. and occasionally to 100 mg., (c) ten weekly injections with a rest period of four weeks between courses, continued until success or failure is apparent; the giving of as many as 100 to 150 injections to a patient has been several times reported, (d) if treatment is continued after untoward symptoms have developed, drop to 5 mg. or less and carefully determine patient's tolerance.

Monash and Traub (1931) have made preliminary report on successful local injections. They are not giving the drug intravenously in this series, but instead injecting into the diseased area, either intradermally, subcutaneously or under the mucosa, 10 to 25 mg. in 1 per cent concentration, with the addition of 0.25 per cent novocain. The slight swelling is controlled by cold applications.

Reactions.—The immediate reactions consist in (a) the anaphylactic type, much like the nitritoid reaction to the arsphenamines, (b) mild febrile reactions with malaise and headache, which may last a few hours to several weeks, (c) metallic taste in mouth. The delayed reactions usually occur after the second or subsequent injection and may last for only a few hours to several weeks: Digestive disturbances, stomatitis and gingivitis, albuminuria, hepatitis and jaundice. Skin reactions, resembling those of arsenic or mercury and usually characterized by pruritus, may be very serious, such as fatal exfoliative dermatitis. Focal reactions of the Herxheimer type also occur in the lesions; there are numerous unusual types of skin reaction which cannot be described here.

Würtzen (1926) has placed the number of deaths ascribable to gold injections at 18 per cent of cases treated, but this figure is by no means representative of what occurs today with the use of much smaller dosage. However, the various compounds should be employed only with the greatest care. It would seem that the definite contraindications to their use are disorders of kidneys, liver or spleen; active tuberculosis anywhere in the body; evidences of a lowered resistance; pregnancy; acute lupus erythematosus disseminatus; severe gold reactions. Throne *et al.* (1932) feel that an increase in blood sugar and decrease in chlorides and urea nitrogen are early signs of impending reaction, and that certainly at the first subjective signs—dryness of mouth and pruritus—treatment should be stopped and the use of sodium thiosulphate as antidote begun. Barber (1929) has recommended glucose injection. Throne also counsels the removal of any discoverable foci of infection before instituting treatment with gold.

Bismuth.—Recently, attention has been given to the possibility of using bismuth intramuscularly as in syphilis, but no definite conclusions can be drawn from the work as yet except that the toxicity is much lower and the risk of aggravating a tuberculous lesion is eliminated. MacKenna (1931) is obtaining good results with the local application of a 10 per cent ointment of bismuth oxychloride.

ECZEMA-DERMATITIS

That the identical process of spongiosis characterizes both eczema and dermatitis venenata histopathologically is now agreed. The occurrences are erythema, intercellular epidermal edema, microscopical and later macroscopical vesiculation, with or without the appearance of small isolated sub-vesicular papules. The lesions weep when the vesicles rupture and encrust when the high-fibrin exudate coagulates; scaling occurs if the keratinization process is much interfered with, and continued inflammation causes the skin to thicken with exaggeration of the normal lines (lichenification), and to lose its elasticity. However, there is one school of investigators which holds that when this state of affairs is set up by endogenous and undis-cernible causes we must call it eczema, all cases arising from demonstrable and exogenous sources (such as ivy, primrose, cosmetic, pollen, etc., poison-ing) then carrying the remaining designation, dermatitis. The other group of observers recognizes no such distinction and considers the terms "eczema" and "dermatitis" to be quite synonymous—the position which is taken by Jadassohn in Breslau, Bloch in Zürich, Urbach in Vienna, indeed, by nearly all the Continental dermatologists except Sabouraud and his school in Paris; in England, Norman Walker, in the United States, Highman, Pusey, Cole, Becker, Stokes and others champion the view. I shall present the therapy of the condition from this standpoint, but can only express the hope in passing that the gods who preside over these matters will soon see fit to send us a good serviceable name for the entity, so that one who goes about much in the clinics may have that at least to cling to.

THERAPY

1. GENERAL CONSIDERATIONS

Matters, etiologic and otherwise, bearing directly upon therapy have been the subjects of very intensive investigation throughout the world in recent years, and in America alone, since the appearance of the first edi-tion of this book, have given rise to at least four reviews of importance—those of Highman (1931), Becker (1931), Cole (1932), and Stokes (1932). From these, and a few other reports to be mentioned, I shall endeavor to devise a brief, practical statement of the larger phases of the subject as seen today. Attention to local therapy will then follow.

The Metabolic and Endocrine Factors.—It is now apparent after a good many years of exhaustive and expensive research that there are no meta-bolic and endocrine disturbances underlying eczema-dermatitis with any sig-nificant regularity. Therefore routine blood chemistry and basal metabolic studies are probably not justified, nor is the routine administration of glandular products, or of calcium or any of the alteratives. Urbach, Folin, Pillsbury and their several associates are finding evidences of local dis-turbances of metabolism in the skin but not such as can be determined by study of the general functions.

Splenic Extract.—I think that there is good reason to be extremely skeptical of the value of splenic extract about which there have recently been a number of enthusiastic trumpetings; Wien and Perlstein's (1933) review indicates little more than that it has limited usefulness in lessening pruritus and shortening the acute phase in eczema, though they believe it to be of more value in urticaria, dermatitis herpetiformis and secondary toxic exfoliative dermatitis. Purified extract of hog spleen is used: a daily subcutaneous injection of 2 cc. for seven days; injections on alternate days for the second week and twice or thrice weekly during the third and fourth weeks, depending of course upon the clinical response. There is frequently a local painful reaction and sometimes a general reaction with chill, fever and general malaise.

The Neurogenic Factor.—These dermatoses rarely heal in persons whose emotional apparatus is being often battered, for, as Sack (1927) has pointed out, the skin occupies perhaps the largest single place in consciousness and has the widest and most varied sensory appeal and the richest vasomotor and other nerve supply in the body. Well does Stokes say, "A mycosis may even be influenced by the stock market, and eczema by a course in French."

The Allergic Factor.—The importance of allergy in the causation has come to be generally recognized; indeed, Bloch and his school are maintaining that all cases are allergic in origin, but I think that not many observers are as yet willing to go that far. It is nevertheless certain that a most thorough search for the possible allergic factor should be made in every instance. Poison ivy, primrose, hair and fur dyes, inks (the Sunday rotogravure section), face powders, and a host of other domestic and industrial substances are already convicted, as are also a number of foods. Sensitization studies are often very difficult and the manifestations quite fickle in these cases, sometimes being present and at another time being absent, or sometimes being present but apparently without significant relationship to the symptoms. Doubtless the allergic response goes up and down with the responsiveness of the sympathetic nervous system to fatigue and irritation, as Stokes asserts, so that a patient who cannot wear a certain fur jacket this season but can do so the next may not be putting us to shame at all, but rather showing conclusively how much the allergic state is bound up with other affairs; perhaps our perky Miss by flaunting her coat flouts those stubborn fellows only who will see merely the immunological phases of the subject. I have suggested a connection of some sort with the fluctuations of the acid-base balance, but certainly have offered no proofs that this is so.

The reader must turn back to page 317 and study the subject of allergy, its detection and methods of treatment. The usual injection methods of desensitization have upon the whole been disappointing in the skin cases; the withholding of convicted foods is much more often rewarded by instant improvement. It seems to me that the methods devised by Rowe for the detection and treatment of food allergy are going some day to serve us excellently in eczema-dermatitis. Urbach, in Vienna, is apparently really obtaining good results with the peroral administration of peptones, but I wonder if his method of administering colonic irrigations to the patient while in a bath-tub or water-bed will eventually prove worth while.

In the approach to the very difficult problem of infantile eczema-dermatitis, all the food constituents have had their day of shame, but all save only the proteins have been able to raise their heads again. The theory of Towle and Talbot (1912) that fat intolerance underlay many cases was never really borne out by any subsequent investigations, and it seems that now it has been given the *coup de grace* by the failure of eczema-dermatitis incidence to drop coincident with the fat deprivation of the present period of economic distress. A few babies with mushy odorous ("pig-pen") stools and a pronounced blue reaction to the iodine test will improve when the starches are greatly restricted, and the ones with acid, green, loose stools will be helped by sugar restriction, but it is quite likely that such digestive disturbances only serve to make easier the wrong kind, or rate, or whatnot of protein absorption from the intestine. However, that there is oftentimes an intimate relationship between infantile eczema-dermatitis and protein sensitization has been several times reaffirmed since Blackfan first pointed it out, in 1916. I think the table of Smyth *et al.* (1931), whose findings practically paralleled those of O'Keefe and Rackemann (1929), is of considerable interest in showing the frequency with which the various food proteins give positive reactions. (Table 58 on the next page).

Unfortunately, however, these findings do not necessarily mean that withdrawal of the offending substance cures the disease. Smyth *et al.* obtained spectacular relief from dietotherapy alone in only about 30 per cent

TABLE 58.—ALLERGEN FREQUENCY IN POSITIVE REACTORS HAVING INFANTILE ECZEMA-DERMATITIS

Allergen Tests			
Positive.................. 112		Negative.................. 48	

Allergen Frequency in Positive Reactors			
Foods		Inhalants	
Egg white................	68	Pollens....................	6
Wheat....................	44	Feathers..................	5
Milk.....................	32	Wool.....................	1
Orange...................	12	Horse dander..............	1
Oats.....................	11	Orris root................	1
Potato...................	9		
Corn.....................	6		
Peas.....................	4		
String beans..............	4		
Rice.....................	3		
Barley...................	3		

of their large series; 32 of the 47 successfully treated cases were from the test-positive group, and 15 from the group with negative skin tests. In 18 additional patients the diet was shown to be decidedly a factor though not the only one—15 gave skin reactions and 3 did not. The degree of reaction is by no means indicative of the part played by the sensitization, for, as Hill (1931) has well remarked, no infant who has the hyperacute type of sensitization is likely to have eczema, for the ingestion of the offending protein makes him so immediately ill that it is quite obvious what is causing his symptoms, and the food is immediately removed from the diet. On the other hand it is quite possible that a sensitization may be too slight to give a positive test and yet be enough to cause eczema-dermatitis; for instance, those cases that give a negative test to cow's milk and clear up nevertheless at once when this is removed from the diet. The large proportion of infants giving positive tests to egg white in all series studied to date has been a puzzling observation, for in most of them egg has usually not yet been included in the diet. Ratner (1931) has obtained some evidence that the fetus can be sensitized *in utero*, but the tentative explanation of Smyth *et al.* is also of speculative interest: They feel that the molecular weight of egg albumin may be the common denominator of all protein molecules, that other proteins are multiples of egg albumin, and that further sensitization depends on combinations or arrangements which follow some law of multiples or factors of digestive change.

Hill and Stuart (1929) have developed an easily available and digestible milk-free food for use in cases of milk sensitiveness. The product, which is known as Sobee, is composed of soy bean flour, barley flour, olive oil, sodium chloride and calcium carbonate. It contains adequate amounts of the necessary minerals and of vitamin B, but must be supplemented by orange juice and cod liver oil for the other vitamins. Six level tablespoonfuls of this food are added to 7 ounces of water, 1 fluidounce of the mixture containing 17 calories. Unless the stools are loose, Hill adds a level tablespoonful of a mixture of maltose and dextrin to this mixture, which raises the carbohydrate percentage to approximately 7. Hill uses the Sobee in all cases in which there is a positive skin test to milk protein or in very severe cases even if the test is negative; in all others evaporated milk is used. He discontinues it if no improvement has occurred in two weeks; he has been successful in about half the cases, but he says (1933): "If the eczema is due to milk, it will be cured with Sobee feeding." Smyth *et al.* have found some infants unable to take Sobee, apparently because of sensitiveness to barley.

Many pediatricians have observed that the boiling of milk for four to six hours, the prolonged boiling of all foods, or the substitution of evaporated or dried milk are often helpful measures. A standard brand of evaporated goat's milk is also used with advantage.

Focal Infection as a Factor.—It is a very definite and probably correct clinical impression that a focus of infection somewhere in the body has a very deleterious influence on eczema-dermatitis. Obviously, every effort should be made to eradicate foci, but bearing in mind the "high-strung" nature of many of these patients, the pursuit of the elusive foe must be made with the utmost calmness and even leisure.

Types of Skin.—The person with the dry, ichthyotic, parchment-like skin will be better in summer or in warm climates because of the increased sweating, but the prognosis in him is unfavorable for the reason that his type of skin is definitely hereditary and so he begins his eczema-dermatitis career with a tendency which is incurable. He needs to avoid soap and to use greases plentifully, tends to become easily infected, and should probably not be given roentgen therapy, "which makes a bad matter worse by causing glandular atrophy." In the opposite type, the person with an oily, seborrheic tendency, Stokes feels that there is a definite indication for reduction of carbohydrates in the dietary, since the process is probably closely bound up with the carbohydrate storage mechanism and metabolism in the skin. In these cases the scalp, which is always concerned in the seborrheic process, must be treated, sulphur will be found to be almost specific when properly used, and there is a definite indication for the use of the roentgen ray to reduce the activity of the sebaceous glands. Prognosis is better than in the ichthyotic type.

A good ointment for use after the bath by persons with excessively dry skin is the following:

℞.	Hydrous wool fat	ʒv	20.0
	Glycerite of boroglycerin	ʒij	60.0
	Petrolatum to make	ʒiv	120.0

Pyogenic and Mycotic Factors.—Pustular complications point to the necessity to employ mild wet antiseptic dressings and later ammoniated mercury ointment, beginning with not above 1 or 2 per cent concentration. x-Rays are to be used cautiously but ultraviolet radiation may be of some value. Those who are investigating the metabolism of the skin feel that here also the carbohydrate intake should be reduced. With regard to the mycotic factor, it can only be said that undoubtedly many cases of so-called "epidermophytosis" (see p. 651) are really eczema-dermatitis, and conversely that some cases of eczema-dermatitis have a mycotic factor which is uppermost. Certainly many cases of epidermophytosis that are resistant to the ordinary treatment will be found upon careful restudy to have become eczematous, particularly beyond the borders of the original mycotic affection, and are being aggravated perhaps by the application of strong karatolitics.

2. Local Treatment

Early Stage.—In the vesicular stage the use of wet dressings is the method of choice. They should not be applied with an occlusive covering, such as oiled silk or paper, but in such way as to gain the additional soothing and antipruritic effect of evaporation. Potassium permanganate is acceptable in 1: 10,000 to 1: 15,000 strength; the prescription contains approximately 1: 8000.

℞.	Potassium permanganate	gr. j	0.06
	Water to make	Ōj	500.00

Of course saturated solution of boric acid may also be used, but the permanganate solution is not apt to become excessively irritating if inadvertently allowed to dry, as the boric acid may occasionally do. Lead or aluminum acetates are also much used because they are astringent and tend to lessen exudation, and are also to some extent antipruritic, but they are often too irritating to be borne by acutely inflamed tissues. The diluted solution of lead subacetate of the N.F. was deleted from the U.S.P. because too weak for most purposes; it is best to write for U.S.P. solution of lead subacetate and direct the patient to dilute it with 10 to 20 parts of water. The solution of aluminum acetate (N.F.) is to be diluted with 5 to 10 parts of water. Abramowitz (1931) calls attention to the undeserved disuse of full-strength alcohol for wet dressings when there are no open lesions.

In excessively itching cases the alkaline colloid bath is often helpful. Fill the tub half full with water just at body temperature, add a cupful of sodium bicarbonate, and then place in a cheesecloth bag 3 cupfuls of previously boiled oatmeal, and squeeze it in the bath until the water becomes opalescent. Such baths may be taken for ten to twenty minutes several times daily. Afterward the patient is to be patted dry and may have a boric acid, or the official rose water, ointment lightly applied; or the body may be powdered. In some patients, 1 quart (1 liter) of vinegar to the tub of water has antipruritic effect.

Some patients do not bear wet dressings well and must be treated with such lotions as will coat the lesions, or perhaps even with powders. The N.F. calamine lotion

℞.	Prepared calamine	℥j℈iiss	40.0
	Zinc oxide	℥j℈iiss	40.0
	Glycerin	℈iiss	10.0
	Solution of calcium hydroxide to make	Ōj	500.0

coats well but will crust if allowed to dry too much between applications; it is to be removed with sweet oil, not water, or with the oil and egg-yolk method of Glaze (1924): Thoroughly and gently work oil into the skin and then add a small quantity of egg yolk (one yolk will serve for twenty or thirty cleansings if used economically), and briskly work up an emulsion; the addition of a few drops of water helps. Rinse in cool water. In some patients the content of inert powder in the calamine lotion is too drying and irritating, but they will often find a mixture of it and sweet oil in equal parts very soothing.

A simple powder for dusting on dry or wet lesions is the following:

℞.	Boric acid	℥ij	8.0
	Zinc oxide	℥j℈iiss	40.0
	Talcum to make	℥iv	120.0

The substitution of salicylic acid for the boric acid, in equal quantity, will make the powder antiseptic, but of course such a mixture must be used with extreme caution on acutely inflamed lesions. A menthol-boric acid combination, with talcum to make it stick, is often remarkably antipruritic:

℞.	Menthol	gr. xl	2.5
	Boric acid	℥ij	60.0
	Talcum to make	℥iv	120.0

Sometimes before using such a powder it is of advantage to sponge the affected area with hot sodium bicarbonate solution and then apply the powder after merely mopping off the solution.

For more active antipruritic effect, 1 to 2 per cent each of phenol and menthol may be added to the calamine lotion, but of course open or very acutely inflamed lesions contraindicate this application.

In some acute cases, particularly of infantile eczema-dermatitis, White's crude coal-tar ointment may be used from the very beginning, taking care that the preparation is made according to the corrected formula, and that a properly prepared tar is used:

℞.			
	Crude coal tar	℥ss	2.0
	Zinc oxide	℥ss	2.0
	Petrolatum	℥j	30.0

The crude coal tar is often used full strength as a paint, particularly for application to the cheeks and the resistant lesions behind the ears. With infants also it is nearly always necessary to prevent scratching; tying the wrists and ankles loosely to the sides of the crib is usually found to be the best method. A light masturbation splint, applied just above the knees, will effectively prevent rubbing with the feet. Wool should not come in contact with the body, and in some cases it is best to dress only in a diaper in a draped crib with an electric bulb to keep it warm. Pilcher (1927) writes as follows of epinephrine to relieve the excessive itching: "The hypodermic dose was from 0.1 to 0.3 cc. of the 1: 1000 solution, seldom more than 0.2 cc., however. This is somewhat large in comparison with the usual adult dose, but harmful effects were not seen. Occasionally pallor of the face and extremities (from vasoconstriction) was noted, of but a few minutes' duration without other signs of toxicity. It is my impression that the relatively large dose is necessary for effective results. The infants varied somewhat in their reaction to epinephrine, for instance, one of 9 Kg. weight was relieved of its suffering with 0.15 cc. and became quite pale with 0.2 cc., while a 5.5-Kg. infant of about the same age required 0.2 cc. for results and showed pallor only with 0.3 cc. The relief is usually striking, is noted promptly, often within two minutes, just as it is in urticaria, and may persist for an hour or more, and not infrequently the patient falls into a restful sleep."

SPECIAL ANTIDOTAL MEASURES IN IVY POISONING.—The vesicles and bullae should be punctured and drained and the parts then thoroughly washed with soap (generous lather) and water. In washing and rinsing it is important to bear in mind that the object is to get rid of the irritant, therefore the soaping and rinsing must be done in the direction away from the unaffected parts; *i. e.*, wash from the elbows down toward the hands and rinse in the same way. If the area is then rinsed or wiped over with alcohol, which is a solvent for the poison, this too must be done in the direction away from the unaffected skin. Gasoline also is a solvent to be used in the same way.

Lead.—Lead preparations, such as the lead and opium wash of the N.F. (lead acetate, 17.5 Gm., tincture of opium, 35.0 cc., water to make 1000 cc.) are not so popular now as formerly; at best they merely precipitate the poison, which must then be washed away.

Sodium Sulphite and Phenol.—Sutton says that a saturated solution of sodium sulphite, to which 0.5 per cent phenol has been added, has served him well; the following should be written:

℞.			
	Exsiccated sodium sulphite (U.S.P. IX)	℥viij	250.0
	Phenol	℥j gr. xv	5.0
	Water to make	Oij	1000.0

Formaldehyde and Phenol.—Hessler has satisfactorily used formaldehyde and phenol; he writes: "My usual formula is: solution of formaldehyde (formalin), 5 cc.; saturated aqueous solution of phenol (1:15), 10 cc.; distilled water to make 100 cc. (to this may be added a drop of methylene blue solution, as blue is a color that leads people to pause about using internally. To disguise the phenol odor, to which some object, a drop of some essential oil may be added). In dispensing I supply a 4-drachm vial with a swab in the cork and with the directions: Apply freely the first time; after that use sparingly every few hours as needed. . . . The hardening and tanning effect of formaldehyde must be considered and explained to patients. The earlier the solution is applied, the better the effect."

Zinc Sulphate.—Irving writes enthusiastically of the use of zinc sulphate. "All irritation and even eruption can be prevented if it is used immediately after exposure. If used within twenty-four hours after exposure or ten hours after the appearance of the vesicles, it will abort the attack. If the case is not seen until the deeper layers of the epidermis are involved, the cure is slower but just as sure. To abort an attack, use 10 grains (0.6 Gm.) of zinc sulphate to 1 ounce (30 cc.) of water. For later treatment, use half strength."

Ferric Chloride and Paraffin.—McNair has championed ferric chloride and paraffin. "The effect of ivy poisoning is much like that of a burn, and the treatment suggested resembles that used successfully during the war in burn cases. The affected parts are first bathed with ferric chloride solution, to neutralize the poison. The skin is dried and melted paraffin is painted over it. A thin sheet of cotton is laid over the wound, and this also is covered with paraffin. The affected area is thus protected from air and from rubbing, and new skin is given a chance to grow." The paraffin may also be swabbed on, as is often done upon the face.

Benzoyl Peroxide.—Lamson (1931) has stated that very great relief follows upon the application to the lesions of benzoyl peroxide as a dusting powder in a considerable proportion of cases, but points out the inadvisability of using the substance in this form because of its high inflammability and explosibility. A paste made from the powder and a lubricating jelly containing glycerin is said by him to be just about as effective and to be nonexplosive and no more inflammable than a bandage.

Whole Blood Injections.—Grimes (1931) has reported a series of 20 cases in which 10 cc. of the patient's own blood was drawn from a vein and immediately reinjected into the gluteal region; the symptoms disappeared so rapidly that he suggests some sort of specific action. It will be interesting to have a further report of the use of the method.

Subacute Stage.—After the more acute symptoms have subsided, the use of creamy pastes and salves may be begun, either for protection from clothing and dirt in the milder cases, or to tide over the period of subsiding inflammation in those cases in which it is apparent that the use of stronger stimulating and keratolytic agents will be later necessary. They are spread over the lesions like butter. Unna's soft zinc paste is much used:

℞. Zinc oxide.................................	℥j	30.0
Precipitated calcium carbonate..................	℥j	30.0
Linseed oil..................................	℥j	30.0
Solution of calcium hydroxide................	℥j	30.0

Lassar's zinc paste has a small amount of salicylic acid (2 per cent), which is slightly stimulating, and it is of such consistency that, if hydrous wool fat is substituted for half the petrolatum, a liberal dusting with talcum powder will form a crust on top of the application that requires little further protection from the clothing.

℞.	Salicylic acid	gr. xl	2.5
	Zinc oxide	℥j	30.0
	Starch	℥j	30.0
	Petrolatum	℥ij	60.0

Another well-known paste is that of Boeck:

℞.	Glycerin	ʒiij	12.0
	Starch	ʒvj	24.0
	Talcum	ʒvj	24.0
	Solution of lead subacetate to make	℥iv	120.0

Some observers of large experience like to use ichthyol in this stage; Becker (1931) favors the following:

℞.	Ichthyol (sulphonated bitumen, N.F.)	ʒj	4.0
	Zinc oxide	℥j	30.0
	Petrolatum to make	℥iv	120.0

In using any of these pastes or salves, water should not be employed for their removal; use sweet oil, or the method of Glaze (see p. 668).

Chronic Stage.—Before applying any of the stimulating and keratolytic agents in effective strength, it is good practice to try out the sensitiveness of the skin with a very mild stimulant; for instance, the ichthyol-zinc paste above, or one can proceed to the use of salicylic acid and the tars by first applying the following, in which each of the active ingredients is present only to the extent of 0.5 per cent (therefore, doubling these two figures would give 1 per cent, tripling 1.5 per cent, quadrupling 2 per cent, etc.).

℞.	Salicylic acid	gr iiss	0.15
	Pine tar	gr. iiss	0.15
	Zinc oxide	ʒij	8.00
	Petrolatum to make	℥j	30.00

The best of the available tar preparations are pine tar, coal tar and oil of cade. For any of them, dosage must be determined in each individual case; as previously stated, the coal tar is often surprisingly well borne in high concentration. The oil of cade, which is prepared from juniper wood, has perhaps the least unpleasant odor, but all of the tars are nasty messes. The prescription on page 669 is a satisfactory basic one for coal-tar therapy, or any of the tars may be combined with salicylic acid, as in the prescription just above on this present page. Perhaps it is of some value to know that the wood tars are acid in reaction and the coal tar alkaline.

Sulphur may also be used in any proportion if the patient's tolerance is first carefully tested; the seborrheic greasy type will bear it best and derive the most benefit from it. In the following, 3 per cent is combined with 1 per cent of salicylic acid, and an ointment instead of paste base is used.

℞.	Precipitated sulphur	ʒss	2.0
	Salicylic acid	gr. x	0.6
	White wax	ʒj	4.0
	Hydrous wool fat	ʒv	20.0
	Petrolatum to make	℥ij	60.0

If greater, cerate-like consistency is desired, paraffin may replace the wool fat and be increased up to 50 per cent.

Resorcinol concentration must also be gauged by each patient's individual reaction; it is best perhaps to begin with 1 or 2 per cent, but less than 5 per cent is rarely effective on thickened areas; it is occasionally carried up to 20 per cent. The prescription contains 5 per cent:

℞.	Resorcinol..	gr. xlv	3.0
	White wax...	℥j	4.0
	Hydrous wool fat......................................	℥v	20.0
	Petrolatum to make...................................	℥ij	60.0

For more prolonged application, the paste base would be substituted.

Ammoniated mercury is also very useful at times; in the following prescription, 5 per cent is combined with 20 per cent of the liquid tar preparation of the N.F.:

℞.	Ammoniated mercury...............................	gr. xlv	3.0
	Solution of coal tar.................................	℥iij	12.0
	Hydrous wool fat....................................	℥j	30.0
	Petrolatum to make.................................	℥i	60.0

There is twice as much wool fat as petrolatum here because of the necessity to incorporate the large amount of fluid; the anhydrous fat would be even better.

Local treatment of some sort is necessary in practically all cases of eczema-dermatitis, but it is by no means certain that in a given case the same preparation will be serviceable for all lesions. At times acute weeping areas on one portion of the body will demand wet dressings while lichenified areas elsewhere are being treated with the tars, salicylic acid, etc. Utmost cooperation on the part of the patient is of prime importance.

BOILS

(Furunculosis)

Boils are acute, deep-seated, circumscribed inflammations of sebaceous glands or hair follicles; the causative organism is probably a staphylococcus. In the beginning the skin is smooth, tense and red, but in a few days the head of the elevation either becomes pustular or the whole mass becomes boggy; at this point the boil either discharges its pus and necrotic tissue or retrogresses without rupture. There may be a great many boils present at one time on various portions of the body surface, and in some cases new "crops" continue to appear for many months. The individual lesions are very painful and the patient is extremely uncomfortable, but the malady is seldom dangerous to life except in the diabetic or nephritic, or if the boils are on the face or upper lip. Of course, a crop of boils superimposed upon an acute infectious disease, such as typhoid, is a very serious matter.

THERAPY

General Measures.—The individual suffering from this affliction should be given a complete physical examination, during which the discovery of some debilitating constitutional disease may furnish the key to the therapy. The elimination of demonstrable foci of infection has sometimes been followed by rapid improvement, but by no means regularly. There is sometimes success, more often failure, with stock or autogenous vaccines. The attempts of Greenbaum and Harkins (1930), and of Weise (1930), to induce immunity by injection of the filtrable products of the staphylococcus, are being watched with interest, but I imagine many observers will agree with me that there is nothing to date in any reports on the use of vaccines or toxins in furunculosis that proves the results to be any different than might be expected from simple nonspecific protein therapy. That the results obtained with bacteriophage are explainable upon any other basis also remains to be shown. The following case report of Cipollaro and Sheplar (1932) will serve to indicate the method and also the results that I am sure everyone is seeing at times. But let us make haste slowly here in the matter of ascribing all credit to the bacteriophage; I have seen even more marvelous results follow the use of sulphuric acid, as in the prescription below, but in neither of the 2 cases could I ever be sure that the water without the drops, or with some other drops, might not have done just as well.

A. H., a man, aged thirty-eight, a tinsmith, had been suffering from recurrent and multiple furuncles for the past six years. He had many furuncular lesions scattered over both arms. A culture of the pus revealed pure *Staphylococcus aureus*, which was readliy susceptible to our bacteriophage.
He received a total of twenty-three injections of phage at daily intervals. These were given into the arm in 1-cc. doses. Locally, the furuncles were given applications of wet dressings of bacteriophage and normal saline solution. One-fourth cc. of bacteriophage was injected into some of the larger lesions. This patient was entirely cured, and no recurrence was reported almost a year later.

The drugs used internally in the attempt to put a stop to the attack are legion, which probably means that none of them are consistently of value. I therefore set down here only those prescriptions that I believe to be most often employed—as to the rationale of their use perhaps the least said the better.

Rumex mixture:
R. Potassium acetate.................................. ℨvj   24.0
     Tincture nux vomica........................... ℨij   8.0
     Fluidextract of rumex to make...................... ℥iv   120.0
     Label: 1 teaspoonful after meals.

or

Startin's mixture:
R. Ferrous sulphate..................................... ℨj   4.0
     Dilute sulphuric acid (U.S.P.)...................... ℨiv   15.0
     Magnesium sulphate............................. ℥j   30.0
     Syrup of ginger..................................... ℥j   30.0
     Water to make.................................... ℥iv   120.0
     Label: 1 teaspoonful after meals and upon retiring, or 4 teaspoonfuls before breakfast.

or

R. Dilute sulphuric acid (U.S.P.)................. .... ℨiij   90.0
     Label: 20 drops in water after meals.

or

R. Calcium sulphide.................................. gr. vj   0.4
     Lactose sufficient to make twenty-four capsules.
     Label: 1 capsule after meals and upon retiring.

Young (1926) has reported 9 cases of boils and carbuncles cured or improved by the intravenous use of mercurochrome-220; for the technic, see page 163.

Local Treatment.—I do not believe that there is any known substance that will abort the lesion when applied locally; the heavy application of full-strength tincture of iodine while the furuncle is still small probably has the best reputation. To hasten its maturation, in order that the contents may be evacuated spontaneously or with the aid of the knife, hot compresses are sometimes of value, though it is often very difficult to accelerate the pace of a boil's development. Certainly linseed or any other kind of special poultice (honey, sugar, bacon, bread and milk, or the what-nots of household medicine) has no advantage over the plain water beyond the requiring of less attention after it is applied, but the addition of an antiseptic, such as 1 teaspoonful of compound cresol solution to the pint of water, is of value in protecting the surrounding skin.   To make a linseed poultice, add 1 part linseed meal with constant stirring to about 3 parts of boiling water to make a thin dough; spread about ½ inch thick on cloth and fold the edges to prevent escape; cover with oiled silk and cotton after applying.   The poultice may be reheated as often as needed.   The body should be kept absolutely clean by a daily bath with hot water and soap; 4 ounces (120 Gm.) of boric acid may be added to the small tub of water. It is well after the bath to pat the body dry with a clean towel rather than to rub it, a procedure that will lessen the liability to spread of the infection by contact, and also protect any small pimples that might be present from abrasion and consequent greater liability to infection.   Underclothing and bedclothing should be changed daily.

ACNE

Acne is an inflammatory skin disease symmetrically involving the face; sometimes, also, the interscapular or sternal regions are involved, and occasionally the whole back.   The skin is greasy, contains many blackheads (comedones), and the acne lesions, which are at first papular, then become pustular, and finally dry up with more or less crusting.   The essential process in the disease is a functional overactivity of the sebaceous glands, combined with a follicular hyperkeratosis; upon this is superimposed pustulation, and, at times, deep-seated granulomatous infiltration.   The causative organism is believed to be *Bacillus acnes*, with the ordinary staphylococci as secondary pyogenic invaders.   Acne is essentially a disease of adolescence, but a considerable proportion of the cases persist well into middle life.   The first appearance of the disease in an individual past twenty-five should cause the physician to enquire into his or her occupation (tar, oils, paraffin, chlorine), search for foci of infection, determine whether iron or cod liver oil are being taken, and question regarding the use of goiter preventives.   Shelmire (1928) has traced a number of late appearing acne cases to the ingestion of iodized table salt.

THERAPY

General Measures.—The acne patient should be given a thorough physical examination, and especially should a careful history of past ailments be taken, for the elimination of chronic foci of infection has occasionally been rewarded by rapid improvement.   Usually, however, the malady responds all too slowly to any type of treatment.   Tonics and laxatives should be given if indicated, but here, as everywhere else, I am opposed to the routine employment of drugs "to keep the bowels open" unless constipation is actually shown to exist.   Startin's mixture is used in nearly every case at some time; cannot someone determine for us how much it is really worth?

Startin's mixture:

℞			
Ferrous sulphate	ℨj	4.0
Dilute sulphuric acid (U.S.P.)	ℨiv	15.0
Magnesium sulphate	℥j	30.0
Syrup of ginger	℥j	30.0
Water to make	℥iv	120.0

Label: 1 teaspoonful after meals and upon retiring, or 4 teaspoonfuls before breakfast.

Yeast should certainly be left to the quacks.

Local Treatment.—The things necessary are to get rid of the blackheads, cleanse and disinfect the skin as much as is possible, and apply a keratolytic agent. The face should be bathed in hot water until it becomes quite red, the blackheads pinched out, or preferably removed with an extractor, all abscesses incised and drained, the face again bathed in hot water to which 1 teaspoonful of the compound solution of cresol has been added to the pint, and then the keratolytic should be applied. At the New York Skin and Cancer Hospital it was formerly, and probably still is, the custom to write for *lotio alba* in strengths designated as "2 ply," "4 ply" and "6 ply." The prescription below is for the 2 ply lotion; the 4 and 6 ply were obtained by keeping the total quantity of the lotion constant but doubling and trebling the two active ingredients.

℞.	Zinc sulphate..	ʒij	8.0
	Sulphurated potassa..................................	ʒij	8.0
	Water to make......................................	℥iv	120.0

This is to be applied at night and washed off in the morning with hot water and some such gritty soap as hand sapolio; it has also been recommended that potassium nitrate be added to the water in the proportions of 30 grains (2 Gm.) to the pint (500 cc.). After drying, talcum powder to which has been added 1 drachm (4 Gm.) of sulphur to the ounce (30 cc.), should be freely dusted on. This treatment, because of its violence, has frequently to be interrupted by periods during which only cold cream is used at night and calamine lotion (see p. 668) during the day.

Vaccine Therapy.—From 1909 to 1913, the vaccine treatment of acne occasioned very considerable interest and was given an extensive trial, especially in England and the United States; then it apparently died the death. In 1923, Howard Fox sent a questionnaire regarding this type of therapy to the seventy-nine members of the American Dermatological Association; of the seventy-one who replied, a trifle over 50 per cent found the acne bacillus vaccines of more or less value, while 75 per cent gave similar answers regarding mixed vaccines. This was surprising until a study was made of the qualifying statements, when it appeared that only "in certain instances" did most of the observers find the vaccines of value. Fox concludes from his study that "the majority of dermatologists have either wholly or partly given up its use. Good results have undoubtedly been obtained by a few investigators after patient efforts with special technic. In the hands of the majority, the results in general have been unsatisfactory. The weight of opinion is that mixed vaccines (of both acne bacillus and staphylococcus) are of more value than those of acne bacillus alone. Stock and autogenous vaccines are considered by the majority to be of equal efficiency. Whatever value these vaccines may possess is restricted to their use in selected cases, chiefly of the pustular type, or as an adjuvant to other methods of treatment. The action of vaccines is slow, and improvement is often temporary."

Sutton writes (1926) that for two years he has been using an autogenous colon vaccine, made from bacilli obtained from the patient's stool, with very encouraging results. "It is probable that the benefit derived is not due to a specific action, however, but is simply dependent upon the injection of a foreign protein, to which the patient is already sensitized."

Ultraviolet Light.—This agent is highly capricious in its effectiveness, just as is natural sunlight. It always seemed to me that the only cases deriving more than a superficial specious benefit from its use were those in which considerable peeling of the skin was induced; but its success even in cases burned to this extent was far from predictable in my day. Dermatologists tell me that its status has not changed in the relatively few years since I have had any intimate experience with this type of therapy. In the literature I have been unable to find a recent study of its use with controls.

Viosterol.—In a preliminary communication, Doktorsky and Platt (1933) record marked improvement in 90 per cent of their series of 35 adult patients given 10 drops of viosterol daily and increasing during two weeks to 20 drops daily; improvement was sustained throughout the period of treatment.

x-Ray Therapy.—It would seem that the *x*-ray is the most valuable agent so far made available for the treatment of stubborn cases of acne, but this has been true only since the relatively recent introduction of the Coolidge tube and the interrupterless transformer. It should be needless to say that the treatments are to be given only by one who is specially trained in this work; every physician who has *x*-ray equipment, and even most of the self-styled *x*-ray specialists, cannot qualify. The indications, as set down by Fox, in 1923, still apply:

"Even if it is admitted that nearly every case of acne can be cured by the roentgen ray, it would certainly not be advisable to use this agent in such a routine manner. There are many cases of a mild type that are amenable to other methods of treatment, both local and general. There is no doubt that improvement may result from surgical measures (such as expressing comedones and opening abscesses), from soap frictions, peeling lotions, the quartz lamps, etc. Most of these methods have their disadvantages, however. Some are disagreeable to the patient, and, at best, their action is much less permanent than irradiation, relapses occurring with discouraging frequency. After considerable experience with such methods . . . I have come to the conclusion that except in mild cases of acne, nothing but time and the roentgen ray will effect a permanent cure. For such cases, I feel that, with carefully controlled modern technic, the roentgen ray can be used as a routine method of treatment."

Fox obtained satisfactory results in about 60 per cent of 191 cases with an average of thirteen treatments; in Michael's (1928) series of 191 patients, 53 per cent were cured by one course of 10 or more treatments, and 12 per cent were greatly improved. Parkhurst (1932) has reported cure in 84 per cent of a series of 335 patients with an average course of thirteen weeks.

WARTS

Warts, as is well known, are seen principally in children, but they may develop for the first time in adults. The most frequently encountered types are: The small, flat, so-called "juvenile" warts, occurring principally on the face and backs of the hands; the larger excrescences, known as verruca vulgaris, with a predilection for the backs of the hands and wrists, but also occurring on all other parts of the body; and the projecting, filiform, narrow-based type, seen principally on the face and scalp. The cause of warts is unknown, though they seem to be auto-inoculable.

THERAPY

Local Treatment.—Perhaps the most valuable method employed at the present time is fulguration; the lesions turn black and drop off several days after treatment. The use of *x*-rays is often enthusiastically lauded, and recently radium also; doubtless the results are excellent in most cases, but it seems to me that warts are very benign affairs in which to use these potent and dangerous agents; certainly only skilled dermatological radiologists should be permitted to give such treatments—most of the self-styled experts cannot qualify. For the treatment of single lesions in which temporary unsightliness and a certain amount of scarring are not objected to, the use of ethyl chloride, the curet, and silver nitrate are quite effective: The site is frozen with the ethyl chloride (which in itself is said to be effective in destroying warts), the lesion is quickly curetted out, and the wound is then thoroughly treated with the silver nitrate stick. Carbon dioxide snow is often effectively used. The following are examples of the great variety of caustics and keratolytics that are applied; they sometimes succeed in accomplishing the removal of the lesions, but the process is usually very tedious.

(a) *Salicylic acid.*

℞. Salicylic acid..................................... ℨiss   6.0
    Collodion....................................... ℥j   30.0
    Label: Touch the wart two or three times daily with the solution, having previously removed the adherent collodion.

℞. Salicylic acid..................................... ℨiss   6.0
    Chloral hydrate.................................. ℨiiss 10.0
    Collodion....................................... ℥j   30.0
    Label: As above.

℞. Salicylic acid..................................... ℨiss   6.0
    Mercurous chloride............................... gr. xv 1.0
    Lanolin... ℥v   20.0
    Label: Apply to wart several times daily.

(b) *Arsenic.*—This drug is usually applied in the form of Fowler's solution (U.S.P. solution of potassium arsenite), first softening the lesions by the use of a 5 per cent solution of potassium hydroxide. A modified Marsden paste (Hare) may also be applied if the warts are few:

℞. Arsenic trioxide................................. gr. lxxv 5.0
    Acacia.. gr. lxxv 5.0
    Cocaine hydrochloride............................ gr. xxx   2.0
    Glycerin.. ♏xxx   2.0
    Water to make a paste.

This is applied on gauze and kept in place for twenty-four to thirty-six hours; the slough is then poulticed away. This is radical treatment.

(c) *Strong Acids.*—Chromic "acid" is applied in 20 per cent solution. Nitric acid is applied full strength with a glass rod and neutralized with salt solution when it has corroded deeply enough. Trichloracetic acid is applied in liquid form with a glass rod.

(d) *Vleminckx's Solution.*—This, the solution of sulphurated lime of the N.F., is made as follows: Mix 165 Gm. of calcium oxide with 250 Gm. of sublimed sulphur and add gradually to 1750 cc. of boiling water; boil, with frequent stirring, to 1000 cc. and maintain this volume by additions of water while boiling for one hour; cool, strain, and decant the clear brownish liquid after standing. Pusey writes that "the solution has served me well in many of these troublesome cases. The method of application that I have found most effective is to put on a small dressing, just a little larger than the wart, wet with full-strength Vleminckx's solution, and held in place by adhesive plaster. This is left on over night, and repeated until irritation is produced; then it is used less frequently until the wart disappears, or until, in case of plantar warts, the desiccated horny mass can be dug out."

Systemic Treatment.—I do not believe that any warts other than those of the so-called "juvenile" flat type ever respond favorably to internal medication; even in this flat type the results are extremely variable, but the following three drugs are worth trying in turn.

(a) *Mercurous Iodide (Protoiodide of Mercury).*—A ¼-grain (0.015 Gm.) tablet is taken after meals three times daily for several weeks; in favorable cases the warts gradually disappear. White introduced the method, in 1925, since when its value has been several times attested.

(b) *Sulpharsphenamine.*—Sutton announced, in 1926, that he had successfully treated 5 cases with this drug. "The average dose has been 0.4 Gm., and only sulpharsphenamine has been employed. The drug is dissolved in a minimal amount of sterile water, and injected directly into the gluteal muscles. In each instance, only one injection was required. Further reports, from other observers, would be of interest."

(c) *Nitrohydrochloric Acid.*—Several years ago, while treating 2 patients with nitrohydrochloric acid for the relief of hay fever, the disappearance of several flat warts was observed in each patient. Thinking that I had stumbled by accident upon something of value, I at once went to the literature and found that the drug had long been used for the purpose. Since that time, I have used it in 2 additional cases; in one it was entirely successful, and in the other a complete failure. In a single case of the vulgaris type of wart it also failed. I used the same prescription that has been advised in the treatment of hay fever:

R̥. Nitrohydrochloric acid (*not* the dilute)............... ℨivss   18.0
  Water to make...................................... ℥iv   120.0
    Label: 1 teaspoonful in water after each meal. (N.B.: Do not permit
      the use of cathartics not prescribed by physician, as there is some
      slight danger of calomel being converted into mercuric chloride by this
      acid.)

Other observers have employed more dilute solutions, but since it has been shown that this strength can be safely taken for a month or more, I believe the percentage of successes with the drug can probably be increased by use of this stronger preparation; the matter should be put to the test.

HERPES ZOSTER
(Shingles)

Herpes zoster is an acute inflammatory skin disease characterized by the appearance of crops of vesicles seated upon erythematous bases along the course of one or more of the peripheral sensory nerves, the sites of predilection being the thoracic, lumbar, brachial and supra-orbital regions. In the average case the lesions dry into crusts and disappear in a week or two with little or no accompanying pain, but in severe cases there may be many successive crops of vesicles that persist for a long time and become pustular, rarely even gangrenous; pain of a neuralgic character is usually severe in these cases, and in the elderly there is often much pain though the eruption be slight. The disease is now generally conceded to be a specific acute infection of the posterior root, gasserian or geniculate ganglia, or paraganglionic tissues, with secondary manifestations in the skin; a few observers, however, maintain that it is an atypical form of chickenpox, but the evidence so far brought forward in favor of such a view is of very doubtful value (see the recent reviews of McCormick, 1931, and Traub and Tolmach, 1931).

THERAPY

The eruption runs a self-limited course that apparently cannot be modified by treatment. Indeed, in most cases the only indication is to protect the lesions from traumatism and subsequent infection. For this purpose it usually suffices to apply a dusting powder of thymol iodide and cover the parts with cotton held in place by adhesive strips. For the relief of moderate pain the usual analgesics are used: Acetylsalicylic acid (aspirin), 5 to 10 grains (0.32 to 0.65 Gm.); acetphenetidin (phenacetin), 5 grains (0.32 Gm.); or amidopyrine (pyramidon), 5 grains (0.32 Gm.). In severe cases the pain is not so easily relieved; resort to the opiates can of course be had, but codeine sometimes does not suffice and the objections to the prolonged use of morphine are obvious. Of the many local applications devised for the relief of this pain, only two are, I believe, of relatively uniform value: The occasional spraying of the skin over the affected ganglion with ethyl chloride; and the application of paraffin as in the treatment of burns (method on p. 723). Sidlick (1930) has reported very successfully upon the use of injections of pituitrin, as suggested some years ago by Vandel. Fifty-four patients were given injections intramuscularly of 0.5 to 1 cc. at twenty-four-hour intervals; most of them required only two injections but a number required three and one as many as six. He found pregnancy the only contraindication to the treatment and occasional momentary faintness the only untoward effect. Niles (1932) has also obtained good results in a smaller series. Ruggles (1931) has reported excellent results in 15 cases from the intravenous administration of sodium iodide; routinely he employed a 20-cc. solution of 30 grains (2 Gm.) on the first, second, fourth and seventh days, but several of the patients did not require the full course. Both Sutton and Stelwagon state that a mild galvanic current (1 to 5 ma.) is often of very great service in persistent neuralgias. The positive electrode is placed over the affected ganglion, the negative drawn along the course of the nerve backward toward the cord; it is recommended that the current be used during ten or fifteen minutes each day. Freude (1931) has resorted to paravertebral novocain injections in several of these cases.

ANAL AND GENITAL PRURITUS

There are many ascertainable causes for itching about the anal and genital regions, such as constipation, anal fissure, hemorrhoids, pinworm infestation, leukorrhea, diabetes mellitus, etc. Removal of the cause will bring complete relief in many instances, but there also exists a class of cases to which the word "idiopathic" can be correctly applied, since they are associated with no demonstrable etiologic factors and respond but poorly to the milder types of treatment.

MILD LOCAL THERAPY

Absolute cleanliness is essential. The parts should be washed after every defecation, and the genitals several times daily. Oftentimes the application of a hot wet pack for a few minutes after washing brings relief which persists for a half hour or more. The following are examples of the antipruritic ointments that are most frequently used:

℞.	Yellow mercuric oxide	gr. xx	1.2
	Hydrous wool fat	℥ij	60.0
	Petrolatum to make	℥iv	120.0

℞.	Ammoniated mercury	gr. xl	2.4
	Hydrous wool fat	℥ij	60.0
	Petrolatum to make	℥iv	120.0

℞.	Crude coal tar	ℨiij	12.0
	Zinc oxide	ℨiij	12.0
	Petrolatum to make	℥iv	120.0

The amount of coal tar contained here, 10 per cent, may be much increased.

℞.	Phenol	gr. xl	2.4
	Zinc oxide	ℨiij	12.0
	Ointment of rose water (U.S.P.) to make	℥iv	120.0

℞.	Phenol	♏xx to xl	1.2 to 2.4
	Menthol	gr. xx to xl	1.2 to 2.4
	Ammoniated mercury ointment (U.S.P.)	℥j	30.0
	Zinc oxide	℥j	30.0
	Anhydrous wool fat	℥ij	60.0
	Lime water to saturate and make ointment.		

℞.	Ethyl aminobenzoate (benzocaine)	ℨiij	12.0
	Salicylic acid	gr. xlv	3.0
	Hydrous wool fat to make	℥iv	120.0

℞.	Benzyl alcohol	ℨiss	6.0
	Hydrous wool fat to make	℥ij	60.0

RADICAL LOCAL THERAPY

(*a*) **Alcohol Injections.**—At the Johns Hopkins Hospital, Stone has been utilizing the destructive effect of alcohol for a good many years; most of his patients are greatly relieved for a relatively long time. The patient is placed under light general anesthesia, and the whole area is prepared as for any other operation. Then, using a *small* syringe with a *small* needle, to avoid placing too much alcohol in one spot or delivering it under too great pressure, 95 per cent alcohol is injected subcutaneously at punctures about ¼ inch apart until the whole field is "stippled." Only 2 to 4 drops are injected at each puncture, and the injections are carried up to about ¼ inch from the anal margin, but they are not made within the anal canal itself. The scrotum, labia majora, and folds of the groins have been injected without resultant trouble. The area is then sponged off with a wet alcohol sponge and no dressing applied. There is only slight after-soreness and the itching is abolished at once. Too large an amount of alcohol injected into any one puncture, or the placing of it *in* instead of *under* the skin, will cause a slough.

In Stone's (1926) more than 200 cases, relief was obtained for from three months to several years, the average being six to twelve months. The treatment may be safely repeated when the symptoms return.

(*b*) **Quinine and Urea Hydrochloride.**—I quote from the paper of Moorer (1924), who developed this method of treatment:

"Under thorough infiltration of the skin and subcutaneous tissue extending ½ inch beyond the area affected, with 0.5 quinine and urea hydrochloride solution, itching is at once arrested; excoriations rapidly heal, and within a few days the skin resumes its normal smoothness and luster.

Anesthesia, however, persists for from several days to as many weeks, and, at the expiration of this period, a second and sometimes a third infiltration is or may be required. It has not been necessary to employ a fourth infiltration in any case thus far treated, as the causative factor is searched for, and, if found, eliminated during the days of freedom from itching produced by this simple measure. Occasionally, one injection suffices, and the patient remains away for months; but he finally returns to have skin tabs removed or other operative rectal procedure which he was told in the first instance would be needed to insure permanent relief, attended to.

"The technic consists in rendering the part clean with water, a good soap, and a soft sponge; application of a solution of mercurochrome-220-soluble as an antiseptic, and the injection of a small area with 1 per cent procaine as a starter. The remainder of the diseased skin is then infiltrated, after which the underlying subcutaneous structure is ballooned out with quinine and urea hydrochloride solution until the patient complains on resuming a chair that he is 'sitting on a cushion.' The precautions to be observed are as follows:

"1. A decided neurotic element exists in all pruritus cases; therefore, it is wise to administer hypodermically ¼ grain (0.015 Gm.) of morphine before beginning this treatment, for the prevention of shock; otherwise, profound depression, resembling greatly the first few hours succeeding a grave surgical operation, is likely to follow.

"2. Not more than 10 cc. of 1 per cent procaine should be used, but quinine and urea hydrochloride solution from 0.25 to 0.5 per cent strength may be used in any necessary quantity, as much as 200 or 300 cc. (quinine and urea hydrochloride solution in greater than 0.5 per cent strength may produce a slough or an unpleasant induration).

"Results in a number of cases have been as good as with a Ball or Lynch operation, and infinitely better than with the cautery. The pressure on the terminal nerves produced by the forcible injection of fluid in large amount brings about a temporary paralysis equal in duration to that produced by severance of their filaments with a knife, and to the mind of the average patient is much more acceptable."

(c) x-Ray and Radium.—Both these agents are of very great value in the treatment of severe cases, but they are not to be carelessly used; at once most valuable and most dangerous agents they are. As I have repeatedly stated in this book, only specially trained radiotherapists should be permitted to use x-ray or radium in treatment; the vast majority of the self-styled "x-ray men" cannot qualify.

SCABIES

Scabies is an infectious disease caused by an animal parasite, *Acarus scabiei*, the female of which incites the itching by burrowing into the skin in order to lay her eggs. These burrows, which are tortuous and marked by a slight elevation at one end and a grayish speck at the other, can be seen with a strong hand lens. The sites of predilection are the dorsal surfaces of the webs between the fingers, the anterior axillary fold, the lower abdomen, the nipple region in the female, and the shaft of the penis in the male. In cleanly individuals the spread is usually not beyond these points, but in dirty individuals and in severe cases the whole body may be involved, though the face and scalp nearly always escape. In children the palms and soles are also often infested; superimposed eczematous and impetiginous lesions are also frequent in young patients and in patients of any age who do not resist the desire to scratch excessively. The disease probably never disappears spontaneously.

THERAPY

The older method of using sulphur to combat scabies is to make an ointment of 20 per cent sulphur, 30 per cent soft soap (or up to 20 per cent potassium carbonate) to facilitate access to the parasites by softening. Fantus (1930) advocates the use of the following formula, in which there is 10 per cent oil of cade for antipruritic effect:

℞.	Oil of cade..	℥iij	12.0
	Precipitated sulphur..................................	℥vj	24.0
	Soft soap..	℥j℥j	36.0
	Petrolatum..	℥iss	48.0

The patient must first take a soaking bath, followed by brisk towelling, then rub the ointment into the body, powder with talcum if desired, and go to bed. Repeat on each of three to five nights, removing the ointment if necessary during the day. The bedclothes should be sterilized by boiling or formalin on the last day. All members of the family must be treated. Soothing ointments and baths will easily control sulphur dermatitis should it appear.

De Mello (1931) has reported the successful use of compound solution of cresol, which is painted over the entire body below the neck. "The treatment is repeated once or twice, and at the end of a week, if any evidence of further trouble is found, the treatment is again repeated." It is looked upon as superior to the older sulphur method in being less "messy"; dermatitis has apparently been no more severe than that following sulphur.

The Danish method of treating scabies has shown itself to be superior to all others. First used in Copenhagen by Ehlers, in 1911, it was described by Lomholt, in 1920, the report being based upon 678 cases treated during the course of the preceding five years. All of these patients were cured in twenty-four hours, without a single relapse. In 1924, Greenwood reported the results in 84 cases treated at the Massachusetts General Hospital; of these, all were cured in twenty-four hours, except 3 who had not followed directions, results which have been obtained very widely since. I quote Greenwood's description of the ointment and the method of employing it:

"1. One Kg. of sublimed sulphur is mixed with 2 Kg. of 50 per cent solution of potassium hydroxide (as free from water as can be obtained). Gentle heat is applied until reaction ceases and the solution becomes clear. When the process is complete, one should be sure that the sulphur is in excess to a slight degree.

"2. Petrolatum, 225 Gm., is mixed with wool fat, 225 Gm., without heat.

"3. To this mixture is added 375 Gm. of the solution of sulphur and potash mentioned above.

"4. To 40 Gm. of 20 per cent sodium hydroxide solution is added 28 Gm. of zinc sulphate. The mixture is agitated thoroughly until reaction ceases, poured on filter paper, and washed thoroughly; then the washed precipitate is added to the foregoing.

"5. Liquid petrolatum is added to obtain a total weight of 1000 Gm.

"6. Five Gm. of oil of bitter almond is added to check the somewhat disagreeable odor of hydrogen sulphide.

"The important elements in the ointment are the sulphides of potassium, on which its activity depends, a production of hydrogen sulphide taking place when the ointment is placed on the skin.

"The directions for use of the ointment as given in the original article are, briefly, as follows: The patient receives an ordinary cleansing bath, dries himself thoroughly, and afterward rubs the whole of his body, except his head, carefully with the ointment. The ointment must cover all the skin, but hard rubbing is neither required nor desirable. The patient ought then to wait for a quarter of an hour to give the ointment time to get into the skin; after this he can go to bed. The next day, at about the same hour, he receives a bath and fresh underclothing, and the treatment is finished. Meanwhile, all his clothes have been disinfected. We have followed these directions in our cases, in addition insisting on the disinfection of the bedding.

"In our experience with scabies we have found it commonly necessary to treat the entire family, and in such cases the three- or five-day treatment is often an almost insurmountable obstacle to a cure because the family will not, or cannot, carry it out thoroughly; and it is in such circumstances that the twenty-four-hour method of treatment is of most value. With the three- or five-day treatment we frequently have a continuation of the itching for one or two weeks after the original disease is cured. This is often from a mild or severe sulphur dermatitis which follows the treatment. With the twenty-four-hour method we have not encountered such cases."

This ointment is now available in the United States in proprietary form under the name of Tilden's Danish Scabies Ointment, manufactured by the Tilden Co., and Scabicide, manufactured by the Upjohn Co. In Lomholt's series there were but 2 cases of induced dermatitis, both traced to some ill-prepared ointment. In Greenwood's series there were also 2 cases, both having used the ointment continuously for five days. He writes: "It is distinctly inadvisable to use it in this way, judging from these cases. We have used it in patients with delicate blond skin, as well as in the pigmented, more resistant types, in children as well as adults, and have had no bad results when it was properly used."

HEAD LOUSE INFESTATION

1. **Kerosene.**—The ordinary grocer's kerosene is usually diluted with equal parts of olive or cotton seed oil to render it less inflammable; the scalp is then thoroughly soaked with this mixture and covered with a loose cloth. The head should be kept covered for twenty-four hours, after which the mixture is to be thoroughly washed out with soap and warm water. The treatment may be repeated as often as is necessary with intermissions of a few days.

This treatment is fairly effective in killing the lice, but it does not destroy most of the nits at the first application. The fine comb should be freely used between treatments.

2. **Xylol.**—The usual mixture used is equal parts of xylol, alcohol and ether; this is of course very inflammable but evaporates quickly. One thorough treatment of the scalp and hair with this preparation usually suffices to kill all the lice and nits, but the latter adhere more tightly to the hairs after being killed in this way than they do while alive. The fine comb must be diligently employed; it is said that vinegar will wash out the nits. The treatment can, of course, be repeated if necessary.

3. **Larkspur.**—This substance (the Delphinium of the N.F.V) is not so much employed nowadays as formerly, either of the two previously listed

mixtures being superior to it in most instances. Of the many formulae for its preparation, the following is perhaps the cheapest and easiest compounded:

Larkspur seed..	100.0
Potassium carbonate....................................	10.0
Alcohol...	500.0
Water to make..	1000.0

Mix the seed and the carbonate with 500 cc. of water; boil the mixture for five minutes; when it has become cold, add the alcohol; strain, and add enough water to make the finished product measure 1000 cc. Filter, if not clear.

4. **Ethyl Acetate.**—Schnell (1921) has very successfully employed this drug. The following description of his method appeared in the correspondence columns of the Journal of the American Medical Association, 78, 371, 1922:

"For the application of acetic ether (ethyl acetate) to rid a subject of head lice, Schnell recommends a special type of hood, which, while fitting the head tightly at the outer border, so as to prevent the escape of vapors, has a roomy crown with sufficient space for the hair to hang loose, thus permitting the fumes of ethyl acetate to penetrate to all parts of the head. On a thin layer of absorbent material (artificial cellulose), from 5 to 10 cc. of ethyl acetate is distributed as evenly as possible over the hairy scalp, whereupon the hood is immediately applied and drawn tight across the forehead by a band of porous material within the hood and tied behind the head, while another band beneath the chin secures the lower portion. The lice are usually all killed at the end of fifteen minutes, but it is safer to leave the hood on for thirty minutes. As a rule, the nits are also killed by one application, but it is not superfluous to give a second application after an interval of a week, when any nits that may have escaped will have hatched out. He warns that in the presence of a perforated tympanic membrane, the ears should be protected by rubber stoppers. When the treatment is given by laymen, it is well that this precaution be always taken."

CRAB LOUSE INFESTATION

In addition to scrupulous cleanliness, accomplished by the frequent and vigorous employment of soap and water, any of the following preparations will usually destroy these parasites, if applied several times daily:

℞.	Mercuric chloride...................................	gr. iv	0.25
	Alcohol..	℥iv	120.0
	Water to make.....................................	℥viij	240.0
℞.	Mercuric chloride...................................	gr. iv	0.25
	Household vinegar..................................	℥iij	90.0
	Water to make.....................................	℥viij	240.0
℞.	Tincture of cocculus (N.F.V)......................	℥ij	60.0
	Alcohol..	℥ij	60.0
	Water to make.....................................	℥vj	180.0
℞.	Ammoniated mercury...............................	℥iss	6.0
	Lanolin..	℥j	30.0
	Petrolatum to make................................	℥ij	60.0
℞.	Ointment of yellow mercuric oxide (U.S.P.).........	℥ij	60.0
℞.	Mild mercurial ointment (U.S.P.)..................	℥ij	60.0
℞.	Xylol..	℥ss	15.0
	Hydrous wool fat...................................	℥j	30.0
	Petrolatum to make................................	℥ij	60.0

BODY LOUSE INFESTATION

Since delousing measures are important in the handling of typhus and relapsing fevers, as well as trench fever, and as these entities are certain to reappear in severe form in the next war, I have thought it advisable to give here the description of delousing procedures that appeared in the report of the British Trench Fever Investigation Committee in 1918 (Byam, W., in the Bibliography):

"It is not enough to allow a man a hot bath and to cleanse his clothing. Eggs are frequently present on the pubic and axillary hair and give at once a new focus of infestation, while the men at present are often returned to untreated beds and billets. Blankets, beds, dugouts, hats and billets should all receive attention. That lice are not seen in these does not necessarily mean that they are not present. While Peacock is doubtless right in his statement that lice spread mainly from person to person, the important thing is to remove every possible source of reinfestation. In a series of experiments carried out at Hampstead Military Hospital, in which the movements of lice on febrile men were being observed, from 6 to 20 per cent of the lice employed disappeared in the course of the various trials, of which each lasted for about twenty-four hours. Careful searching did not discover the wanderers, though they would certainly be still in the room. Lice have a proclivity for wandering, and are able to exist without feeding for a week at ordinary room temperatures, and longer under cooler conditions. Nuttall records ten days at a temperature of 5 C. (41 F.) as the longest period which lice have been known to survive unfed.

"Disinfestation of Troops. For the details and working of the various devices for disinfestation, reference should be made to the writings of Bacot, Nuttall and Peacock. The following notes are the merest summary of what has become a very bulky subject:

"All men from one set of billets, huts or dugouts should be paraded together at the same time for disinfestation, with their blankets and kits if possible. The men should be shaved free of pubic and axillary hair and chest hair if thick. Their heads should be very closely cropped, and they should be given a hot bath. After the bath their underclothing should be smeared over with some louse-destroying grease to render them repugnant for a time to fresh infestation and to destroy any nits still adhering to them. Every care should be taken when removing hair not to abrade the skin, as careless shaving has been found to increase the incidence of other diseases conveyed by the excreta of lice. The shaving or very close cropping of the body hair is essential, as otherwise nits, which are often present there and are not killed by bathing, remain to reinfest the man. The most satisfactory grease for application to the underclothing is one composed of crude unwhizzed naphthalene from the coke oven, 4 parts; soft soap, 1 part (Bacot and Copeman). That the naphthalene should be as specified is of great importance, and a sample of each delivery should be tested by an expert entomologist. Its odor is not unpleasant to most persons and it causes little or no irritation to the skin. Men should be discouraged from using proprietary remedies, as many of these are useless, disheartening the men and making them sceptical about the efficacy of any remedy. The men should be carefully inspected a week after disinfestation and be urged to report immediately on reappearance of any lice. The entire clothing and bedding of men should be treated by heat or some louse-destroying solution.

"Disinfestation by Heat. All clothing should be included in the treatment, blankets and kits, when possible. The heat may be wet or dry; the latter is preferable, as clothing may then be worn immediately after treatment. Moist heat should never be used for leather articles.

"To kill lice and their eggs with certainty, 55 C. (131 F.) for thirty minutes, or 60 C. (140 F.) for fifteen minutes must be attained. Such temperatures will not disinfect the excreta of lice. The necessary temperatures for this purpose have not yet been determined. [A temperature of 100 C. (212 F.) has since been found to be effective—H. B.]

"The heat throughout the chamber should be as even as possible. The garment should be hung on rails or loosely packed to insure the heat's reaching every part. If pegs are used, garments are apt to get torn.

"The heat of the chamber should be indicated by a maximum thermometer placed so that it can be read from the outside. The Grant Peacock hut and the hot chamber adopted by the Canadian army have been found efficient, as also has the Serbian barrel, though the latter is small. The ideal device for regimental use has yet to be invented. It should be as mobile as a field kitchen, capable of dealing with the clothing of twenty men at a time, simple to work, and economical in firing. It should be capable of being easily loaded and unloaded, and attain the requisite temperature quickly. One end of the chamber should open completely, and all material under treatment be on a movable rack running on wheels or slides. When treatment is complete, this rack is drawn out, and a second, already loaded, thrust in. By this means a minimum of heat is lost and a maximum of time is saved. According to Peacock, the time usually occupied in loading, heating up and unloading is about equal to the time of actual disinfestation.

"The ironing of clothing, especially along the seams, with heavy hot irons has been found useful. It is a palliative and not a thorough treatment. In the German army the clothing is pressed against hot iron plates in preference to hand ironing.

"Disinfestation by Solutions. Bacot and Lloyd have found that all lice and eggs on clothing are destroyed by soaking in a 2 per cent solution of either (a) liquor saponatus cresoli fortis, or (b) compound solution of cresol (crude phenol and soft soap in equal parts) at any temperature above 32 F. for twenty minutes. One per cent compound solution of cresol at from 60 to 63 F. was found to be equally effective in twenty minutes, but liquor cresolis less so. The 2 per cent solutions allow a margin for the weakening of the solutions during use. If fuel is scarce, such soaking may be found preferable to heat.

"Fumigation. While the men are undergoing treatment, their billets, dugouts and huts should be fumigated, together with articles of bedding or clothing not treated by heat or solution.

"The best gases to use are sulphur dioxide or hydrocyanic acid gas. The latter is dangerous except in buildings which can be readily ventilated, but it is the more certain of the two. For its production Howard recommends potassium cyanide (from 98 to 99 per cent), 1 ounce; sulphuric acid, $1\frac{1}{2}$ ounces; water, 3 ounces, for every hundred cubic feet of space.

"The percentage of the potassium cyanide should be stated when ordering, as it is sold in three strengths.

"The water and sulphuric acid should be mixed in a large vessel, and the requisite amount of cyanide, wrapped up in paper, dropped in. As the gas is released with violent effervescence at once, the operator should leave the room without delay.

"Formaldehyde is useless, and it must not be thought that any gas which is fatal to man is necessarily so to the louse."

OPIUM AND COCAINE ADDICTION

The drug addict is a constitutional psychopath, whose peculiar weakness lies in the fact that he attempts by use of his drug to smooth out of life the boring, monotonous and fatiguing facts and memories that his normal fellowmen overcome either by a partial immersion of themselves in the struggle itself, or by achieving finally, albeit for the most part unconsciously, a rational stoicism. That is to say, he is told that by this artificial means he can easily make his life more worth living, and thus takes his first dose —and in so doing confesses himself one of the weak-minded, ne'er-do-well sort, for, as Sceleth has well said, there is something wrong in the mental make-up of an individual who will take a sniff of heroin or a shot of morphine merely because someone tells him it will do him good. After the first few doses he continues to take the drug for the maintenance of whatever type of relief it has afforded him, and finally, though he may no longer be obtaining any pleasurable effects, he persists in its use because he is altogether too weak to face the temporary though severe suffering which his puny attempts to stop have shown him will be his lot. Of course there are a few normal individuals who acquire the habit by a too-long indulgence in a drug after the pain for which it was prescribed has ceased to exist as an indication for its use, but the number of these is always small and the probability of their cure so good that they do not essentially form a part of the major problem of drug addiction. In New York, and presumably in other cities of the eastern seaboard, heroin is the drug most employed, while in Chicago and other cities of the middle west, morphine is used because of the scarcity of the other drug. Cocaine would seem to be used in the South more than in other parts of the country. Paregoric habitués are fairly numerous, some using as much as a quart a day. Opium smoking and the practice of taking opium by the mouth have almost disappeared in America.

Drug addiction probably exists to a greater extent in the United States than in any other country, though its prevalence here has been enormously exaggerated. Certainly there can be nothing like the million or more cases vouched for by the type of person who makes it his profession to weep publicly over these matters in the lay and pseudoscientific press. The true number was probably estimated with fair accuracy by Kolb and DuMez, in 1924, to be 110,000, representing in their opinion a decrease of approximately 154,000 since 1900. Sceleth (1924), who is certainly qualified to speak on the subject, has stated his opinion that there have never been more than 5000 addicts in Chicago at any one time. Also it is worthy of note that of the 98,714 patients discharged from the Marine Hospitals, operated by the U. S. Public Health Service, in 1925–26–27, only 55 were classified as drug addicts, though these hospitals undoubtedly get their full share of this class of patients.

Morphine and heroin addiction have always been rare in Great Britain, and apparently have even decreased in recent years; this seems also to be true throughout the Scandinavian countries. In Germany, though addiction increased considerably after the war, the total number of addicts is probably relatively small and is said to be declining, though unfortunately the available statistics are based solely upon the amounts of the drugs supplied by physicians. As to the position in France, Spain, Italy and the Balkan countries there is little information, which is true also with regard to Russia. I have been told that in Mexico, Central and tropical South

America addiction is quite rare, but that in Buenos Aires and Rio de Janeiro there is a major problem such as exists in the large cities of the United States. In Egypt, Russell Pasha, director of the narcotics intelligence bureau, has stated, in 1932, that 282,000 of the male population of 3,137,000 are addicted to hashish, 93,000 to opium and 54,000 to heroin. In British India, opium eating—the capsules of the poppy are macerated with water and the fluid swallowed to produce euphoria—is a widespread practice, but it seems to be rapidly declining; however, the number of persons addicted to cocaine in association with the chewing of betel nut is said to be between one-fourth and half a million. Pfister's picture of the truly terrible victimization of Southern China is given here in my own halting translation of a portion of his *Brief aus China*, in 1932: "Travel in Yunnan, with overnight stops in crowded rural inns, brings the cancer of the land, opium addiction, most impressively before one's eyes. Yunnan is the land of extensive opium culture. At the time of my journey in late autumn the harvest was already over and all of the many fields were otherwise employed, but one came upon opium at every step; it was thrown upon the caravan tracks in heavy bundles by the coolies, openly sold in the stores in every village, and smoked everywhere. The bearers of my expedition smoked it just as did the soldiers who had been given me as military guard from station to station. Rich and poor, priest and coolie, men and women, all smoke opium, but not only, as is still believed in Germany, for sake of the quieting and hypnotic effect, but because they want the stimulating effect. After a wearying march I was often able to observe how the fatigued bearers became fresh and ready again after several pipes. Of course, too much caused the opposite, sleep-producing effect. Opium is so cheap in Yunnan that every coolie can debauch himself in this way for a couple of copper coins." It seems to me a curious, noteworthy thing that in another closely related population, the Japanese, addiction is unknown as a national practice and that the evil is being rapidly uprooted among the Chinese population of Formosa, now under Japanese control.

By the middle of the summer of 1933, the international convention for the limitation of manufacture and the regulation of distribution of narcotics had received the necessary twenty-six ratifications and is now in operation with a central office in Geneva. Illicit traffic will unquestionably be greatly curbed in a few years.

THERAPY

The only legitimate, because the only effective, method of treating drug addiction consists in placing the patient under the absolute control of incorruptible physicians and attendants, who can give their whole time to the prosecution of the cure, of which the following are the principal elements: (a) Rapid withdrawal of the drug, (b) the use of some form of belladonna as a physiologic antidote, (c) the promotion of elimination and the stimulation of the activity of the intestinal glands by the use of cathartics, (d) the employment of as much rest as possible and the use of stimulant drugs to support the patient during the more or less severe symptoms attendant upon the taking away of the drug. The so-called "reductive" dosage ambulatory treatment of addicts, defined by the U. S. Internal Revenue Bureau as the "prescribing or dispensing of a narcotic drug to an addict, for self-administration at his convenience," has been uniformly condemned as a method of treatment by every competent medical authority, is prohibited by law in a number of States, and is also prohibited by implication in the Harrison law and the numerous court decisions relating to it.

The three treatments most often used are known as the Lambert-Towns, the Pettey, and the Sceleth. I shall describe each of them here, but shall institute no comparisons, since each is effective if properly employed. The formulae which form the bases of these methods are certainly open to criticism by pharmacologists, but since the object of this book is to set down a description of the actual uses of drugs and biologicals in practice, quibbling comments would seem to be out of place. Of course the details of the cure must be adjusted somewhat to the patient's idiosyncrasies and must also be considerably modified in the presence of marked cardiovascular or renal disease.

1. **Lambert-Towns.**—Mr. Charles B. Towns, a layman, discovered and offered a treatment for the morphine and alcohol habits in 1904, at which time, however, he did not explain the ingredients of the preparation that he used. Later he did explain this treatment to Dr. Alexander Lambert of New York, who tried it and described it in 1909. Subsequently Lambert and others have published many articles on this treatment. I quote below an adequate description that appeared in the Journal of the American Medical Association in 1915.

"Vigorous elimination is the most important feature of the method, and is secured by the administration of compound cathartic pills and blue mass or some other form of mercury. The other essential measure is the persistent use of the following belladonna mixture:

℞	Tincture of belladonna (15 per cent).................	℥ij	60.0
	Fluidextract of xanthoxylum........................	℥j	30.0
	Fluidextract of hyoscyamus........................	℥j	30.0

"A patient addicted to morphine is given five compound cathartic pills and 5 grains (0.32 Gm.) of blue mass. Six hours later, if the bowels have not moved, a saline is given. After three or four abundant movements of the bowels (and not until then) the patient is given by mouth or hypodermically, depending on his habitual method of taking the narcotic, in three divided doses, at half-hour intervals, two thirds or three fourths of the total daily twenty-four-hour dose of morphine or opium to which he has been accustomed. Observe the patient closely after the second dose, when about half the total twenty-four-hour dose has been taken. A few patients cannot comfortably take more than this amount. Six drops of the belladonna mixture dropped with a medicine dropper are given in capsules at the same time as the morphine or opium, and should be repeated every hour for six hours. At the end of six hours the dose of the mixture is increased 2 drops. This dose is then continued at hour intervals for another six hours, when the dose is increased by 2 drops, and again continued at the same interval, increasing the dose each six hours until it reaches 16 drops. It is then continued in this amount, but is diminished or discontinued at any time if the patient shows belladonna symptoms such as dilated pupils, dry throat or redness of the skin, or mental symptoms. It is begun again at reduced dosage after these symptoms have subsided. Unusual sensitiveness to belladonna will usually be manifest in six or eight hours, when the dose can be cut down 2 to 4 drops and then raised by 1 drop every six hours. On the other hand if after twelve hours the 16 drops have not produced dryness of the throat the dose may be increased to 18 or 20 drops every hour until the dryness occurs, and then the amount may be reduced.

"At the tenth hour after the initial dose of morphine five compound cathartic pills and 5 grains (0.32 Gm.) of blue mass should again be given. If they have not acted in six or eight hours, give some vigorous saline. When the bowels have acted vigorously, which is usually at about the eighteenth hour, give half the original dose of morphine; that is, one half or three eighths of the original total daily dose. The belladonna mixture is

44

still continued, and ten hours after the second dose of morphine, five compound cathartic pills and 5 grains (0.32 Gm.) of blue mass are again given, if necessary followed by a saline seven or eight hours later. After the bowels have acted thoroughly, at about the thirty-sixth hour, the third dose of morphine is given, which should be one sixth or three sixteenths of the original dose. This is usually the last dose of morphine. Ten hours after the third dose of morphine, the forty-sixth hour, again give the five compound cathartic pills and 5 grains (0.32 Gm.) of blue mass, followed seven or eight hours later by a saline. After the bowels have moved thoroughly a bilious green stool should be expected and after its appearance 2 ounces (60 cc.) of castor oil should be given to clear out thoroughly the intestinal tract. It is sometimes found necessary to continue the belladonna mixture over one or two additional cathartic periods before giving the oil. After giving the last dose of compound cathartic pills, and before giving the oil, the patients will have their most uncomfortable time, and may be relieved by 5 grains (0.32 Gm.) of codeine hypodermically. This should not be kept up long after the oil is given. Beginning about the thirtieth hour the patients should be given strychnine or digitalis or both every four to six hours.

"Withdrawal pains can sometimes be relieved by ergot and strychnine, by massage, sodium salicylate or by some salicylic compound combined with coal-tar products such as antipyrine, acetphenetidin or pyramidon. Indiscretions in eating or exercise two or three days after stopping the drug may cause a recurrence of the withdrawal pains, due to exhaustion or indigestion. This trouble will quickly disappear without narcotics.

"Insomnia may be troublesome and may be treated by bromides, chloral or other hypnotic. Lambert's experience is that veronal acts badly in these cases. Muscular fatigue is the best hypnotic, and regular exercise may be carefully taken within a week after the discontinuance of the drug. It is important to build up the patients physically.

"Morphine and alcohol addicts should be treated for the morphine addiction and the alcohol may be tapered off gradually. The gastritis usually found may cause difficulty in retaining medicines or food. Sodium citrate in doses of 5 to 10 grains (0.32 to 0.65 Gm.) every hour will relieve this condition, and if necessary may be supplemented by 10 to 20 grains (0.65 to 1.3 Gm.) of cerium oxalate.

"Cocaine and morphine addiction make a difficult combination to treat, but the procedure should be that for morphine, with plenty of strychnine or other stimulant. The cocaine should be withdrawn at once. The patients may become delirious and unmanageable after the effect of the morphine wears off.

"The cocainist should be treated like the alcoholic, by withdrawing the cocaine, giving the belladonna mixture every hour, increasing as with the morphine patients, and the five compound cathartic pills and 5 grains (0.32 Gm.) of blue mass, the first doses being taken simultaneously. At the end of the twelfth hour repeat the cathartics and the saline, and likewise at the twenty-fourth and thirty-sixth hours. After the last cathartic the bilious stools will appear, and at the forty-fourth or forty-fifth hour the castor oil is given. Unless the bilious stools appear it may be necessary to continue the treatment over one or two more cathartic periods.

"Though each patient presents an individual problem, Lambert insists that the plan must be adhered to closely. The cholagogue action of the mercury is essential and the persistent repetition of the doses of the belladonna mixture so as to produce the physiologic effect is required to prevent the craving for the drug."

2. **Pettey.**—This method was devised by Dr. George E. Pettey, of Mem-

phis, Tenn., in 1909. I quote below the adequate description that appeared in the Journal of the American Medical Association in 1915.

"The method of Pettey in morphine addiction also employs active purgation as one of its principal features, with sedation in the form of scopolamine after the drug is withdrawn, with large doses of strychnine in the purgative to increase peristalsis and also afterward for its supporting effect. The steps in the treatment may be described as follows:

"On the day treatment is begun the patient may take his usual doses of the drug. He is required to abstain from dinner and supper, and at 4, 6, 8 and 10 P. M., he is given the following purgative prescription divided into four capsules:

B.	Calomel	gr. x	0.65
	Powdered extract cascara sagrada	gr. x	0.65
	Ipecac	gr. j	0.065
	Strychnine nitrate	gr. ¼	0.015
	Atropine sulphate	gr. $\frac{1}{50}$	0.0013

"No opiate and no nourishment are to be given the following morning until the bowels have moved thoroughly. In order to insure the movement of the bowels, six or eight hours after giving the last purgative capsule, ½₀ grain (0.003 Gm.) of strychnine should be given hypodermically and a half hour later 2 ounces (60 cc.) of castor oil or a bottle of citrate of magnesia. Both the strychnine and the oil or saline should be repeated every two hours until the intestinal canal has been thoroughly emptied, and no morphine should be given during this time. The thorough elimination will afford relief from the discomfort of abstinence from the drug and this should be taken advantage of to postpone the morning dose of the narcotic. When the demand for the drug becomes insistent it may be given in not more than one half or two thirds the usual dose at the same intervals at which the drug was formerly taken. After the purgation liberal feeding may be allowed until within six or eight hours before the next purgative course. This should be forty-eight hours from the beginning of the first purgative course, and may be more or less active, according to the effect obtained from the first, but none of the purgative ingredients should be left out, and large doses of strychnine are insisted on. The morphine in reduced dose, sufficient to keep the patient comfortable, may be continued until the last dose of the second purgative course, when the drug is to be discontinued and no other opiate should be given. Six or eight hours after the second purgative course has been completed, strychnine hypodermically and the oil or saline should be repeated as after the first course, until free bowel movements occur. The patient will now be able to go longer before feeling the effect of abstinence from his morning dose, especially if he remains in bed, which he should do. Within six or eight hours after the time for the morning dose the patient's demand for relief from discomfort should be met by giving, instead of the opiate, ½₀₀ grain (0.0003 Gm.) scopolamine hypodermically, and this should be repeated in thirty minutes. If the patient has not fallen asleep after the second dose a third may be given in a half hour or hour, which may be of the same size or double the previous dose, depending on the effect. This will produce either sleep or mild intoxication, in either of which conditions the patient will not suffer. Immediately he awakes another dose of scopolamine, ½₀₀ grain (0.0003 Gm.), should be given, and repeated to keep up a mild belladonna intoxication and to maintain the patient free from pain. This impression from the scopolamine should be kept up for thirty-six to forty-eight hours after beginning it, and then should be discontinued. During the scopolamine period and for twenty-four hours afterward, 20-grain (1.3 Gm.) doses of sodium hyposulphite may be given every two hours, which will supplement the effect of the calomel purgative and the patient will have small, bilious stools, unattended by colic or griping.

"Convalescence will be reached on the fifth or sixth day and no further medication is indicated as far as the addiction is concerned and the patient will be comfortable. Deficient heart action during or after treatment may be treated by sparteine sulphate in doses of 2 grains (0.13 Gm.) every four to six hours."

3. **Sceleth.**—This treatment was introduced by Dr. Charles E. Sceleth, of Chicago, in 1915, after a very large experience with it in emergency hospital practice in that city. I quote from his own description of the method:

"Though there are many angles to the plan, its essence rests in the formula:

℞.		
Scopolamine hydrobromide	gr. $\frac{1}{100}$	0.0006
Pilocarpine hydrobromide	gr. $\frac{1}{12}$	0.0054
Ethyl morphine hydrochloride (dionin)	gr. $\frac{1}{2}$	0.032
Fluidextract cascara sagrada	♏xv	1.0
Alcohol	♏xxxv	2.3
Water to make	ʒj	4.0

"The amount prescribed and the indications for its continuance or modification vary with the case. Patients who are addicted to the use of more than 10 grains (0.65 Gm.) of morphine a day are given 60 minims (4 cc.) of the mixture every three hours, day and night, for six days. The dose is reduced to 30 minims (2 cc.) on the seventh day, to 15 minims (1 cc.) on the eighth day, and on the ninth day to 15 minims (1 cc.) three times during the day only. On the tenth day the mixture is discontinued altogether and tonic treatment begun, as outlined below.

"Addicts accustomed to the use of less than 10 grains (0.65 Gm.) of morphine a day and more than 5 (0.32 Gm.) are started with a dose of 45 minims (3 cc.), which is reduced on the seventh day in a manner analogous to that just detailed; while to those who have been taking less than 5 grains (0.32 Gm.), only 30 minims (2 cc.) are given as an initial dose.

"The dangers associated with the use of this combination are trivial. Scopolamine delirium occurs in about 4 per cent of the cases. Should delirium develop, the scopolamine should be omitted for a few doses, and as the condition improves, added once more in smaller quantities. The greatest danger, however, collapse, does not arise from the scopolamine mixture *per se*, but is incidental to the withdrawal of the morphine. The tendency to collapse is undoubtedly favored by the presence of two drugs which act on the vagus—scopolamine, which is vago-inhibitory, and pilocarpine, which is vagotropic. If the pulse falls below 40 or goes above 120 per minute, the mixture is stopped and the patient is given the only drug which can offset the collapse, namely, morphine itself. The latter is injected in ⅓-grain (0.02 Gm.) doses every fifteen minutes until results are obtained. Patients in collapse should not be given too large doses of morphine, or its derivatives, after treatment has been in progress for several days, as the dose to which the addict has been accustomed is likely to be overwhelming. The vomiting and insomnia which occur more or less constantly are not due to the scopolamine mixture, but occur with any treatment, and accordingly are not to be looked on as special complications.

"It may be stated as a safe criterion that if on the third or fourth day of treatment by this method the pupils are dilated and react to light and accommodation, the patient is reacting properly and the outlook is good.

"As regards the other steps in this mode of treatment, a few remarks will suffice. The patient on admission is put to bed, given three compound cathartic pills, followed by a saline cathartic (Epsom salt), and at once started on the scopolamine mixture. During the first few days of the course the diet should be light and easily assimilable, and liquids should be pushed; the patient should drink 3 pints or more of water a day. On the tenth day, at which time the mixture is discontinued, strychnine nitrate, $\frac{1}{30}$ grain (0.002 Gm.), is given for three doses; the following day the amount of strychnine is reduced to $\frac{1}{60}$ grain (0.001 Gm.), which is continued three times a day for a week.

"By the fifth day, as a rule, the patient's desire for morphine is gone. He then manifests a desire for a more substantial diet and begins to put on weight rapidly. When the mixture has been stopped, and the patient's strength permits, graded exercises, in the open if possible, are instituted with the purpose not only of improving his physical condition but of allowing him to acquire a bodily fatigue, which is recognized by all as the best antidote to the insomnia—the abstinence symptom most likely to persist and the most difficult to conquer. A warm bath of 110 F. for ten minutes, or a neutral bath of from 94 to 98 F. for twenty minutes, will often relieve restlessness and insomnia. Carbonated waters are very gratefully received.

"Heroin cases should be treated the same as morphine addicts. For opium addicts 30 minims (2 cc.) of the mixture should be administered every three hours, and the ethylmorphine hydrochloride reduced to $\frac{1}{8}$ grain (0.008 Gm.) per dose. For cocaine addicts, if it is desired to have the patient avoid any discomfort, he should be given 15 minims (1 cc.) of the mixture every three hours without the ethylmorphine hydrochloride for three days; when cocaine is used alone it is always safe to discontinue it abruptly without any treatment, as there is never any danger of collapse. With the morphine addict who is using 10 grains (0.65 Gm.) or more a day, however, if it is abruptly or gradually discontinued, without suitable treatment, there is danger of death from cardiac collapse. I doubt if the system can assimilate more than 10 grains (0.65 Gm.) of morphine at a dose. I make no distinction between the patient using 10 grains (0.65 Gm.) or 60 grains (4 Gm.) per dose."

Codeine Substitution.—Lambert (1931) has recently stated that when a properly trained staff is not available for the carrying out of such detailed treatment schemes as the above three, his new method of codeine substitution may be satisfactorily employed. It is described as follows: "The best method of giving this treatment is to calculate the amount of morphine, in terms of Magendie's solution, that a patient is taking in twenty-four hours, and then for a ten-day reduction, diminish the morphine each day about one tenth. As the morphine is best given at four-hour intervals, and there are six doses a day, the total daily amount is again divided by 6, and the amount of reduction is easily calculated in the number of minims of Magendie's solution [a solution of 16 grains morphine sulphate per 1 ounce of water—H. B.]. For instance, if the patient is taking 4 grains (0.26 Gm.) a day the equivalent to 120 minims a day of Magendie's solution, he is taking 20 minims every four hours; if he is to be reduced 12 minims a day, he is reduced each day at each four-hour dose 2 minims of his Magendie's solution; in this way in the ten days his Magendie's solution is brought down to zero.

"But at the same time that his morphine is reduced, the codeine is increased from the second day beginning at $\frac{1}{2}$ grain (0.03 Gm.) every four hours the first codeine day; then 1 grain (0.065 Gm.) every four hours the second day; then 3 grains (0.2 Gm.) every four hours the third day; 4 grains (0.26 Gm.) given every four hours the fourth day, and 5 grains (0.3 Gm.) every four hours the fifth day, continued at 5 grains every four hours until three days after the last dose of morphine has been given, when it is tapered off as rapidly as the discomfort of the patient permits. It is wise to use the codeine phosphate because of its greater solubility, and if the codeine solution is made up in the same form as Magendie's solution it is easily accessible, and desired amounts can be given every four hours simultaneously in the same syringe as the Magendie's solution. In this way the patient does not know when the morphine ceases to be given to him. If this amount of codeine is not sufficient, extra doses of codeine can be given without harm to the patient or to his reduction treatment. This large amount of codeine is apt to be very constipating, and the patients should receive the amount of cathartic necessary to keep their bowels in good action; severe purging is not necessary under this form of treatment, and it is apt to irritate the gastro-intestinal tract. Of course, the patient's intestinal tract should be thoroughly cleared out before the treatment is begun; it is also wise to test out the patient for the first twenty-four or fory-eight hours of treatment with the amount of morphine that the patient says he is taking, to see whether or not he is comfortable.

"The advantage of this codeine and morphine treatment is that since the patients suffer so little there is no occasion for deception, there is no question of a defense reaction for fear of suffering, they get away from their drug without the irritability and fear of suffering that the abrupt methods and old forms of treatment gave them, and they are quite manageable."

Narcosan, Insulin, Sodium Thiocyanate (Rhodanate).—Narcosan was thoroughly discredited by the studies of the Mayor's Committee in New York City, in 1928–29 (see Lambert, in Bibliography). For the widely published claims of Bancroft regarding the value of sodium thiocyanate (rhodanate) in this condition, I know of no experimental, or satisfactorily controlled clinical, observation in substantiation. Sakel (1930) stated that insulin in large doses is of great assistance in the treatment of addiction. There has been no general confirmation of this claim but Howard (1933) has reported that in 10 cases he found that the withdrawal period was made easier by the use of insulin. If the patient has been taking more than 3 grains (0.2 Gm.) of morphine daily over a period of six months or more, he gradually reduces the dose by half and then substitutes insulin; the following case report is illustrative:

The first patient treated by this procedure was a doctor's wife, aged forty-three, weight 155 pounds, and of normal physique. She has used morphine continuously for twenty-two years. Most of the time she has required 3 grains a day but for the five or six months previous to admission, following the death of her husband, she has been taking 5 grains a day. During the first week of treatment the dosage was gradually reduced to 3 grains a day. This was accomplished with no apparent discomfort. Then insulin was substituted for the morphine without the patient being told of the change. The dose was necessarily arbitrary but 20 units were given as an initial dose at the time that morphine was given. The patient apparently was not aware of the change as she was not uncomfortable but asked if the dosage had been reduced again. At the time the next dose of morphine was due she was again given 20 units of insulin instead. This was eight hours after she had received any morphine and she showed no withdrawal symptoms such as perspiration, diarrhea, nausea, etc. There was some restlessness characterized chiefly by twitching of the legs. The pupils of the eyes were moderately dilated. At bedtime she was given 15 units of insulin and 10 grains of barbital. She went to sleep shortly but awoke during the night and was given an additional 10 units. She slept in all about six hours. During the first twenty-four-hour period she was given 100 units of insulin and the consumption of food was less than usual for her. There was no evidence of hyperinsulinism, the blood sugar varied from 100 to 125 mg. per 100 cc.

During the next forty-eight hours insulin was given in 10-unit doses about every five hours. At the end of this time the blood sugar and blood pressure returned to normal and the patient was told of the procedure. She expressed herself as being quite well satisfied with the treatment and said that she had had no discomfort. The insulin was continued for a week, 5-unit doses being given before meals. She left the sanitorium in very good physical condition.

ACUTE POISONING

THE CORROSIVE AGENTS

The corrosives most frequently swallowed accidentally or with suicidal intent are sulphuric, nitric, hydrochloric and oxalic acids, sodium or potassium hydroxide (lye), sodium or potassium carbonate, ammonium hydroxide, mercuric chloride (corrosive sublimate), and phenol (carbolic acid). The general symptoms of the group are: Corrosion of the mucous membranes from the lips down to the pylorus; extreme pain, soon followed by the vomiting of food, shreds of mucosa, mucus, and blood that is dark brown due to conversion into hematin and other products; profuse bowel movement that is at first normal but later contains blood and shreds of mucosa; respiratory symptoms due to contact of some of the corrosive material with the air passages; and quick shock and collapse. Those escaping immediate death may succumb to perforation of the stomach or the symptoms resultant upon stricture of the esophagus or pylorus. In addition, the victims of phenol and mercuric chloride suffer a very severe nephritis, the takers of concentrated ammonia are subject to early unconsciousness and standstill of the heart, and those having swallowed oxalic acid (much used as a bleaching agent in the household) develop calcium deprivation symptoms, such as cramps, headache, convulsions, etc.

THERAPY

1. **Acids.**—The acid must be quickly diluted with large amounts of water and neutralized with alkalis. Sodium bicarbonate, sodium carbonate, milk of magnesia, chalk, soapsuds, plaster from the wall, or any other alkali at hand will serve; it should be given in relatively weak concentration but in large quantity. Later, milk, egg white, starch mucilage, acacia emulsion, or any bland oily substance such as liquid petrolatum or butter will be soothing. Supportive drugs are indicated: Strychnine sulphate, $\frac{1}{30}$ grain (0.002 Gm.); atropine sulphate, $\frac{1}{60}$ grain (0.001 Gm.); caffeine sodium benzoate, 2 to 5 grains (0.13 to 0.32 Gm.); metrazol, $1\frac{1}{2}$ grains (0.1 Gm.); camphor in oil, 1 to 2 cc.—all to be given intramuscularly; or whisky, 1 ounce (30 cc.), or aromatic spirits of ammonia, $\frac{1}{2}$ to 1 drachm (2 to 4 cc.), by mouth. The value of morphine in decreasing pain and thus perhaps avoiding shock should not be overlooked. Keep the patient warm.

Oxalic acid requires certain special mention, for the reason that the alkalis form salts that are more soluble and more toxic than the acid itself, and therefore cannot be used. Calcium and magnesium salts, however, unite with the acid to form insoluble salts: wall plaster is acceptable, even though it is alkaline, and so too is lime water. It should be noted that patients may experience the calcium deprivation symptoms even though they have taken too small a dose of the oxalic acid to cause the corrosive symptoms; in such cases $\frac{1}{10}$ grain (0.006 Gm.) of apomorphine hydrochloride, administered hypodermically, is indicated as an emetic. Action must be quick in the treatment of these cases for the poison is rapidly absorbed. The intravenous administration of calcium is of course also indicated (see p. 714).

2. **Lye and Other Alkalis.**—The treatment is the same for poisoning with corrosive acids, save that here weak acids are used as antidotes, usually in the form of lemon juice or vinegar, diluted several times with water.

3. Phenol.—Sodium sulphate is the most valuable antidote for phenol poisoning; it should be used by lavage, 4 drachms (15 Gm.) to the pint (500 cc.) of water, the washing to be continued until the phenol odor disappears. Baumann and Preusse suggested this measure many years ago because of the known conjugation of phenol with sulphuric acid arising in metabolism, the products being eliminated as comparatively harmless ethereal sulphates or sulphonates. Latterly, however, the chemistry of this reaction has come to be doubted, but the measure is a very valuable one nevertheless, perhaps due to some hindrance it offers to absorption plus the induced purgation.

Alcohol has been shown by clinical observation and the careful experiments of Macht (1915) to be of no value. The same is true of glycerin. Indeed, alcohol if given as an antidote after the poison has been taken may hasten death, despite the well-known fact that a drunken individual swallowing phenol is not so seriously affected as is a normal person. These apparently contradictory facts are not understood. Gibbs (1931) recommends, very rationally, the administration of as large quantity of liquid petrolatum as the patient can be induced to swallow, the endeavor being to have the phenol taken up by (*i. e.*, dissolved in) this nonabsorbable oil.

Of course the acute nephritis must be given serious attention.

4. Mercuric Chloride.—The treatment of mercuric chloride poisoning is very unsatisfactory for the reason that practically all patients who have taken as many as three of the U.S.P. tablets, containing approximately $7\frac{1}{2}$ grains (0.5 Gm.) of the salt, regularly develop anuria on about the fourth day, and almost as regularly die from lesions of the kidneys, liver, or colon. I do not mean that none are ever saved, because of course they are, but the number saved is pitifully small compared with the number that dies. None of the special types of treatments so far advocated, nor any of the "specifics," have proved their worth. Many men are earnestly engaged in a study of methods of overcoming the vicious effects of this poison when it has gained entrance into the blood stream, but truly helpful suggestions are very slow in forthcoming. I quote below the routine treatment described by Lambert and Patterson (1915) because I believe it to be the one still most closely followed, at least throughout the United States.

"The treatment, as it is formulated at present for cases coming under observation early, is as follows: The first indication is to give the patient the whites of several eggs and then to wash out the stomach thoroughly. This has usually been done before the patients are admitted to the hospital. [Raw eggs and milk precipitate the mercuric chloride about equally effectively. Milk would have the advantage that it would spread more rapidly over the stomach and would therefore act more promptly. It may be best to administer first a glass or two of milk, then several raw eggs, to increase the protein without too much bulk. Egg white does not have any advantage over the whole eggs. If the tablets have been swallowed dry, and if milk is not available, it would be advisable to administer half a glass of water just before the eggs, to prevent the cementing of the tablet by the egg white.—Sollmann *et al.*, 1927.] On admission, the stomach contents are expressed and examined for mercury, the stomach is thoroughly washed, and a pint of milk introduced. If no stomach contents are obtained before lavage, then the lavage water is examined for mercury. The metal appears in the urine in from three to twenty-four hours after it has been swallowed. If more than a day has elapsed since the poisoning occurred, a stool should also be examined for the poison. If the first lavage does not allay the nausea and vomiting, it is repeated after an hour, and the following routine is begun as soon as the stomach will permit:

"(*a*) The patient is given every other hour 8 ounces (250 cc.) of the following mixture: Potassium bitartrate, 1 drachm (4 Gm.); sugar, 1 drachm (4 Gm.); lactose, ½ ounce (15 Gm.); lemon juice, 1 ounce (30 cc.); boiled water, 16 ounces (500 cc.). Eight ounces (250 cc.) of milk are administered every alternate hour.

"(*b*) The drop method of rectal irrigation with a solution of potassium acetate, a drachm to the pint, is given continuously. The amounts of urine secreted under this treatment are very large.

"(*c*) The stomach is washed out twice daily.

"(*d*) The colon is irrigated twice daily, in order to wash out whatever poison has been eliminated in that way.

"(*e*) The patient is given a daily sweat in a hot pack.

"It is imperative to emphasize the necessity of keeping up the treatment with the colonic drip enteroclysis day and night without interruption. It entails discomfort for the patient, but the victims of accidental poisoning are always willing to do anything to recover from their plight, and the attempted suicide usually repents rapidly of his error, and the hope of his life being saved stimulates his patience and desire to cooperate.

"In cases in which one single dose has been taken, after two negative examinations of the urine, on successive days, it seems legitimate to stop the treatment. . . . For the less severe cases, a week may be a sufficient time for treatment. When large or successive doses have been taken, or when there is a preexisting kidney lesion, or when treatment begins several days after the poison is taken, longer periods of treatment, up to three weeks, are necessary.

"Under the treatment detailed above, these patients quiet down to their routine, and, as a rule, do not suffer except from the discomforts of the therapeutic measures. The stomach becomes tolerant of the milk diet and the alkaline drink after from twenty-four to thirty-six hours. The kidney secretion at first is excessive, and may run up to 130 or more ounces in the twenty-four hours. This usually diminishes in spite of the continued exhibition of fluid between the fifth and the tenth day, and may nearly stop altogether. It is at this period that the continuous water cure and the rest in bed must be insisted on. If this period is successfully passed, the secretion of urine again increases often to a higher level than at first. The mercury itself seems to act as a diuretic at this stage of the treatment. The bowels usually show some irritation, but when the treatment is faithfully carried out, the tendency to diarrhea and colitis is regularly controlled by the colonic irrigations, and other medication for this symptom has been rarely necessary."

Sodium Thiosulphate.—This drug has been used very much in recent years upon the theory that it effects the conversion of the poison into the harmless HgS. The results are conflicting—*i. e.*, they are of such nature that some physicians loudly praise the drug and others loudly condemn it as worthless. The usual procedure is to administer intravenously 15 grains (1 Gm.) in 10 cc. aqueous solution, once or twice daily. However, in a very severe case recently, Marchbanks *et al.* gave 10 cc. every eight hours until the patient had five doses, and Blaisdell (1931) states that in his hospital there have been no deaths among the 10 patients treated since the administration of 90 grains (6 Gm.) daily for three to five days became the routine practice. It is strange that it has not been found possible (see Melville and Bruger) to show a prolongation of life in laboratory dogs by this method.

Cecostomy.—A number of pathologists have been impressed by the gangrenous colitis observable oftentimes at autopsy, to which Berger *et al.* (1932) have given some sort of expression by advocating immediate cecostomy as soon as the patient is admitted and then the institution of constant colonic lavage. The discussion of their paper by Krumbhaar and others indicated some reticence in accepting proof of the necessity for this radical step in all cases, but the viewpoint certainly has the merit of being both interesting and new.

GASOLINE AND KEROSENE POISONING

Inhalation of gasoline vapors in sufficient concentration causes headache, inebriation, tremor, cyanosis, dyspnea, convulsions, collapse and death. When the gasoline is swallowed, death may occur in a few minutes, though the fatal dose is extremely variable—1 ounce has killed, ½ pint has been survived. Postmortem findings may be negative or there may be slight hemorrhagic changes in the gastro-intestinal tract, kidneys and lungs. Kerosene, not infrequently swallowed by infants, is upon the whole less toxic than gasoline and extremely variable in its effect, probably due to the variable content of volatile fractions. The most usual symptoms are burning pain in mouth and throat, coughing, thirst, colic, diarrhea and painful micturition. Drowsiness, dyspnea, coma and death may follow but this is rare; one of Price's (1932) 4 cases died in bronchopneumonia, and Waring (1933) has reported the cases of 9 children who developed definite signs of pulmonary involvement.

THERAPY

No distinctive treatment has been developed. The stomach should certainly be washed out at once and a brisk catharsis promoted; the use of stimulants and the application of heat are of course indicated. I find no record of any instance in which the cough required treatment. The colicky pains and diarrhea apparently persist only a short time. Barbour (1926), who feels that the clinical and blood pictures in kerosene poisoning are similar to those in carbon monoxide poisoning, suggests the advisability of bloodletting and transfusion in severe cases.

ARSENIC POISONING

Acute arsenic poisoning is not rare, due to the fact that the arsenical pigments are much used in the arts and industries, rat and some fly and roach poisons contain arsenic, and Paris green is extensively used in rural regions as an insecticide. The symptoms usually come on an hour or more after the poison is swallowed, but may appear in a few minutes if the stomach is empty. There is pain in the mouth and esophagus, then in the stomach and entire abdomen. There is nausea and vomiting, often of blood, and early a profuse watery diarrhea. Paralysis of the splanchnic capillaries causes an immense quantity of fluid to escape into the connective tissues; this raises the mucosa into many large blisters and results in large pieces of it being swept away when the fluid bursts into the lumen of the intestine. The abdomen is greatly distended and the colicky pains so severe that shock is often caused. The stools are of the rice-water type and conceivably might cause some difficulty in differentiating this condition from Asiatic cholera. There is immense thirst, scanty and albuminous urine, and finally suppression of the urine. If death does not come in a few hours to a few days, paralyses of the lower extremities are frequent, as are also fatty degeneration of the liver and kidneys.

THERAPY

The stomach should be washed out with warm water until no more arsenic can be recovered, and then warm milk or other demulcent drink may be given. A large dose of castor oil, or a saline cathartic, is also indicated to flush out the poison perhaps pocketed in the upper part of the gastro-intestinal tract. If no stomach tube is available when the patient is first seen, or if its introduction is impossible or considered to be inadvisable, the emetic drugs should be resorted to, for this stomach must be thoroughly emptied:

Household mustard........ 1 to 2 drachms (4 to 8 Gm.) in water.
Ipecac.................... 1 drachm (4 Gm.) of the powder or 4 drachms
                          (15 cc.) of the syrup, in water.
Copper sulphate........... 7½ grains (0.5 Gm.) in water.
Zinc sulphate............. 30 grains (2 Gm.) in water.
Apomorphine hydrochloride. $\frac{1}{10}$ grain (0.006 Gm.) hypodermically.

The mustard is the least dangerous but also the least effective. The ipecac is uncertain in action and quite depressing. Both copper and zinc sulphates cause vomiting in a very few minutes, and under the conditions obtaining here, i. e., where there are no corrosions of the gastric mucosa, they are not rapidly absorbed and hence are usually not very depressing. However, if they do not cause emesis, further attempt should be made to get them out of the stomach for the reason that they are very irritant. Apomorphine is a very reliable emetic, but it is well known that the after-depression is sometimes very great.

The arsenic antidote is kept by the druggist in two bottles, one containing a solution of ferric sulphate, and the other a suspension of magnesium oxide. These are mixed when needed and the freshly precipitated ferric hydroxide is given. The dose of this precipitate is 4 ounces (120 Gm.), but it may be given 1 ounce (30 Gm.) at a time every few minutes for several doses, as it is not poisonous. Reliance is not to be placed on this antidote, for McGuigan and Atkinson (1923), confirming the earlier work of De Busscher, find that such delay in death as is obtained by its use is slight and unimportant and is probably due to the colloidal nature of the antidote and its effect upon absorption rather than to its chemical neutralization of the poison. Clinical observation and impression amply confirm these experimental results.

The patient should of course be supported, as described under the treatment of acid poisoning, and the dehydration must be combated by all means possible.

CYANIDE POISONING

These patients are practically always in coma when the physician reaches them. There may be muscular spasms with perhaps even moderate opisthotonos. Respiration is by this time usually very shallow and irregular and the pulse of a very poor quality if perceptible at all; cyanosis is usually marked, the pupils often widely dilated. In many cases, the urinary sphincters are relaxed; there may also be froth at the mouth and the odor of cyanide on the breath.

THERAPY

Artificial respiration and oxygen inhalation, gastric lavage with sodium bicarbonate solution, the usual stimulants—sometimes even 1 cc. or more of hydrogen dioxide injected subcutaneously—are tried in most cases and practically always without results. It would seem, however, that Hanzlik and Leake have recently made an excellent contribution to this subject by calling attention to earlier studies of others by which the rationale of the use of methylene blue was indicated. Geiger (1933) has succeeded astonishingly with the drug in the three instances of its use so far recorded. In the first case: Within five minutes of the beginning of the slow intravenous injection of 50 cc. of a 1 per cent sterile aqueous solution of methylene blue (methylthionine chloride, U.S.P.), the patient was conscious and "appeared to be essentially normal except for a severe chill and an apparent flushing." Recovery was complete within fifteen minutes, and within the half hour the patient, a man of some education, was able himself to write a lucid description of his experience.

Cases 2 and 3, while perhaps not quite so spectacularly resuscitated, were also unquestionably restored to life by use of the dye. These 2 cases, in both of which a second injection was given, apparently demonstrate that quantities up to 100 cc. of a 1 per cent solution can be used within a period of one-half hour without untoward symptoms since measurable quantities of methemoglobin did not appear in the blood of these patients.

STRYCHNINE POISONING

The presence of strychnine in some of the vermin exterminators has led to some cases of accidental acute poisoning in rural regions, but most of the recorded cases, except in children, have been suicidal or homicidal, for the dangerous nature of the drug is so well known as almost to preclude its careless handling. The patients usually say that there is a peculiar feeling at the beginning of each attack, like a slow electric shock that starts above and behind the eyes and sweeps over the whole body; then the spasm begins. The usual position is that of opisthotonos. The spasms last from one-half to five minutes with complete relaxation between. Consciousness is not lost and the suffering is excruciating. Between spasms there is a sensation of approaching death and the patient will plead for someone to hold him, seeming to feel that he is being ruthlessly hurled into oblivion. The usual interval between spasms is five minutes or more, most patients not surviving more than five of these full convulsions; death is either due to asphyxia or to exhaustion. This type of poisoning must be differentiated from the following:

Tetanus.—History of antecedent injury, less complete relaxation, trismus (lockjaw) and risus sardonicus earlier, much slower onset and course, much longer interval between paroxysms, absence of opisthotonos.

Epilepsy.—Clonic spasms, bestial sounds, absence of opisthotonos, unconsciousness.

Eclampsia.—Complete unconsciousness during and between spasms, absence of complete opisthotonos.

THERAPY

Nota bene: What follows is the older type of therapy which seems now to have been completely outmoded by the use of barbiturates, particularly amytal (see next page).

Keep the room as quiet and dark as possible and do not touch the patient unless he expects the contact. Anesthetize with chloroform or ether (but not with nitrous oxide, which exaggerates the reflex excitability and the asphyxia), and while unconscious introduce 30 to 45 grains (2 to 3 Gm.)

of chloral hydrate into the rectum in a retention enema. Also while still anesthetized introduce the stomach tube, sacrificing teeth if necessary to prevent its occlusion when patient returns to consciousness. Wash out the stomach at intervals of a few minutes with potassium permanganate, 15 grains (1 Gm.) to the quart of water; this destroys the poison by oxidation. The following precipitate the poison in a relatively insoluble form: Tincture of iodine, 15 minims (1 cc.) in a glass of water; tannic acid, 1 drachm (4 Gm.) in a glass of water; these two substances may be repeatedly given if washed out after a few moments. Satisfactory forms of charcoal or of fullers' earth are too infrequently available to be of practical value as adsorbents.

Morphine should be very cautiously used if at all, since it may dangerously add to the respiratory difficulty. Artificial respiration is a most valuable measure; tirelessly persisted in by relays of workers it has saved many lives. During the convulsion an amyl nitrite pearl crushed under the nose may hasten relaxation; or, if the patient does not breathe, 5 to 10 minims (0.32 to 0.65 cc.) may be injected subcutaneously.

Barbiturates.—Based upon Haggard and Greenberg's (1932) experimental studies, Wheelock (1932) has very successfully used these drugs in one case. Five grains (0.3 Gm.) of phenobarbital sodium given hypodermically did not prevent the precipitation of a severe convulsion when attempt was made to raise the patient from the floor; a 5-grain (0.3 Gm.) ampule of the same drug given intravenously also did not produce complete relief. She was then given intravenously 15 grains (1 Gm.) of sodium amytal in 10 cc. of water, 1 cc. per minute. About the fourth minute the patient dosed, and at the end of the injection she was snoring. Further therapy consisted in the use of a mixture of three bromides by mouth. There were no further spasmodic symptoms and recovery was complete. A number of similar reports are already on record so that it seems we now have at hand practically a specific remedy in strychnine poisoning. Kempf, McCallum and Zerfas (1933) have reported 11 cases all treated with success; one of their case reports illustrates both the method of using the amytal and its astonishing efficiency (in 1 case 7½ grains (0.5 Gm.) of pentobarbital sodium was used with equal success):

CASE 6.—M. D., a white woman, age thirty years, well developed and well nourished, apparently in good physical condition, took a quantity known to be more than 8 and less than 12 grains of powdered strychnine sulphate at about 2.30 A. M., May 27, 1930. About 2.45 she began to have twitchings and mild convulsions, and she was brought into the hospital at 3.20 in complete convulsions with opisthotonos and cyanosis. Seven and one-half grains of sodium amytal given intravenously at 3.30 was sufficient to quiet her, but not enough to allow a gastric lavage. At 3.40, after another 7½ grains of sodium amytal had been given intravenously, a gastric lavage was done and the stomach found empty. The patient was partly awake and attempted to vomit after the lavage. She remained quiet until about 4.15, when she began groaning and having muscular twitchings. Six grains (0.4 Gm.) of sodium amytal intravenously at 4.20 was sufficient to keep her asleep until we attempted to give her an intravenous injection of physiologic solution of sodium chloride at 5.30. She was given 7½ grains of sodium amytal followed by 750 cc. of physiologic solution of sodium chloride intravenously with the idea of increasing diuresis. In spite of the fact that she had had 28½ grains (1.8 Gm.) of sodium amytal intravenously between 3.30 and 5.30, she was awake at 7.30. She was very groggy from the sodium amytal but did not show hypersensitivity from strychnine. At 9 o'clock she was given a high colonic flushing with a gallon of tap water and did not show any signs of strychnine poisoning during the process. During the morning she was awake and restless but slept at intervals, and during the afternoon and that night she slept very well. The next day she was awake and rational but complained of some gastric pain and of sore muscles, which disappeared during the day. She was released the following day, May 29th, in good condition and apparently fully recovered.

Apomorphine.—Haggard and Greenberg have reported the cases of three individuals taking fatal doses in which this drug, given hypodermically in a single dose of $\frac{1}{10}$ grain (0.006 Gm.) to the two children, $\frac{1}{5}$ grain (0.012 Gm.) to the adult, was apparently life-saving. In each instance the injection precipitated a convulsion, but shortly there was relaxation and sweating and no more convulsions, though some amount of spasmodic movement continued for awhile.

MORPHINE POISONING

Accidental, and more often suicidal, morphine poisoning is of relatively frequent occurrence. The patient progresses gradually from an overpowering sleepiness into a deep coma from which it becomes finally impossible to waken him. The respirations become slower and slower, finally becoming irregular and stertorous, and then they stop; usually the heart has been relatively little affected and continues to beat for some time after respiration has entirely ceased. In the beginning the skin is warm and moist, but later becomes cold, clammy and cyanotic; the pupils are constricted to the so-called "pin-point dimension," but they undergo a terminal dilation. As death approaches the sphincters relax. Convulsions are rare in adults but are sometimes seen in infants.

THERAPY

If the drug has been taken by mouth the stomach should at once be washed out, and the washing several times repeated, with 15 grains (1 Gm.) of potassium permanganate to the quart of water; this destroys the morphine. Hatcher's (1925) experimental studies in both man and animals indicate that the drug is not excreted into the stomach in amounts that can possibly be of any importance; hence the stomach washing is probably of no value when the drug has been taken by the needle. Emetics (see p. 699) act very slowly in the presence of morphine and should not be relied upon.

The patient must be kept awake and preferably in motion. Walk him between two attendants and annoy him into defensive movements by dashes of cold water upon the face, etc.; but keep him warm. Try in every way to make him talk. Employ artificial respiration if breathing becomes dangerously infrequent. McCurdy (1929) has recorded the successful employment, during many hours, of the routine hospital mixture of carbon dioxide-oxygen. Use caffeine, preferably as strong black coffee, or as caffeine sodium benzoate, 5 grains (0.32 Gm.) or more hypodermically.

Regarding the use of atropine, Sollmann writes (1932) as follows: "Atropine has been used extensively and somewhat indiscriminately in the treatment of morphine poisoning. It may be a dangerous remedy. The most conspicuous antagonistic actions of these two poisons are on the pupil, heart rate, psychic processes, secretions, etc.—*i. e.*, upon functions which are of subordinate importance in dangerous cases of poisoning. Any useful antagonisms must be sought in their actions on the circulation, respiration and metabolism. The effects of morphine and atropine on these functions are antagonistic only with certain stages; whilst more severe grades are actually synergistic. The later paralytic effects of atropine coincide with those of morphine; whilst in the last stages of morphine poisoning the centers are too greatly depressed to respond to the slow and weak stimulation of atropine. The usefulness of this antidote exists therefore only if moderate doses of atropine are given in moderate morphine poisoning (or *vice versa*). This conclusion is supported by several series of experiments on animals. As a practical deduction, the atropine should be given hypodermically in the dose of $\frac{1}{40}$ grain (0.0015 Gm.) and this should not be repeated. It is fair to state, however, that this is not the universal opinion. For instance, Roch (1907) advises $\frac{1}{30}$ grain (0.002 Gm.), frequently repeated, until the pupils begin to dilate."

When the patient is out of danger the attempt must be made to break through the peristaltic depression by enemas and cathartics. Watch these patients for a long time; fatal relapses have been known to occur after several hours of apparent return to normality.

***

CHLORAL HYDRATE POISONING

These cases are nearly all seen in individuals who have taken an overdose of a physician's prescription, either accidentally or with suicidal intent. There is deep narcosis with constricted pupils, complete muscular relaxation, very slow and shallow respiration, barely perceptible pulse, cold clammy, skin, rapid fall of temperature and blood pressure.

THERAPY

Wash out the stomach by the use of the pump as soon as possible. The emetics (see p. 699) are doubtfully advisable here for two reasons: First, they are much reduced in effectiveness because of the central depression; and, second, the patient's heart should not be subjected to the strain of retching and vomiting. Raise the foot of the bed to bring as much blood as possible to the medulla. The following stimulants may be tried: Whisky, 1 ounce (30 cc.) at intervals; aromatic spirits of ammonia, $\frac{1}{2}$ to 1 drachm (2 to 4 cc.); hot black coffee, by mouth or rectum, or caffeine sodium benzoate, 5 grains (0.32 Gm.) intramuscularly; strychnine sulphate, $\frac{1}{20}$ grain (0.003 Gm.) to $\frac{1}{10}$ grain (0.006 Gm.); atropine sulphate, $\frac{1}{40}$ grain (0.0015 Gm.), to be given intramuscularly but not to be repeated; metrazol, $1\frac{1}{2}$ grains (0.1 Gm.) intramuscularly; camphor in oil, 1 to 2 cc., intramuscularly. Artificial respiration is indicated when the respirations become dangerously slowed. *Keep this patient warm.*

***

BARBITURATE POISONING

These drugs have become rather popular for suicidal purposes, being obtainable in relatively tasteless tablets that are sure in their effect if enough of them are taken. The symptoms are deep narcosis with constricted pupils, slow and shallow respiration, feeble pulse, pronounced fall in blood pressure and temperature, increased reflexes, and sometimes suppression of the urine and also convulsions.

THERAPY

The emergency treatment is about the same as for chloral poisoning (see above). Arnett (1933) has been the first to act upon the suggestions of pharmacological experimentation in his employment of ephedrine and picrotoxin in a child of three and three-quarter years who was seriously poisoned with amytal. Five-sixths grain (0.05 Gm.) of ephedrine sulphate was introduced through the stomach tube and $\frac{1}{100}$ grain of picrotoxin given hypodermically; the latter was repeated after one and three-quarter hours. Routine eliminative treatment was also employed but the rapidity of the recovery was certainly surprising.

Since the barbiturates vary considerably in their rate of destruction and elimination, fluids should be pushed for several days as a safeguard against relapse. The experimental studies of Johnson *et al.* (1930) suggest that glucose might well be administered intravenously for the promotion of diuresis. Great weakness and ataxia persist for many days in most instances.

ATROPINE POISONING

Rather mild degrees of poisoning with members of the belladonna group are frequently seen in practice; occasionally, also, serious poisoning occurs either in an individual with an idiosyncrasy for the drug or in one to whom an overdose has been given. Where the various plants having this type of action grow wild, or are much used for ornamental purposes, children are now and then poisoned by eating the berries. The symptoms are very violent, but the prognosis as to life is good because of the rapid excretion of the poison. In fully developed cases the symptoms are exhibited in two phases; first, difficulty in swallowing, pain in the throat, great thirst, visual disturbances, nausea, redness of face and neck, rise in temperature, rapid pulse, and excitement that goes into delirium and often into mania; second, giddiness, staggering, stupor, respiratory and circulatory collapse.

THERAPY

If the poison has been swallowed, lavage the stomach with potassium permanganate, 15 grains (1 Gm.) to the quart of water, or the tincture of iodine, 15 minims (1 cc.) to the glass of water. Give the physiologic anti-dote, pilocarpine nitrate, in doses of $\frac{1}{6}$ grain (0.01 Gm.) repeated until the mouth becomes moist. Morphine sulphate, $\frac{1}{4}$ grain (0.015 Gm.), combined with sodium bromide, 15 grains (1 Gm.), may be given several times at four-hour intervals in the attempt to control the excitement, but this sedative medication should be stopped as soon as the picture changes. For the final depression, treat practically as a case of chloral poisoning (see p. 703).

In Comroe's (1933) case—a patient who had swallowed $7\frac{1}{2}$ grains (0.5 Gm.) of atropine sulphate in solution one and one-half hours before being seen—gastric lavage with large quantities of sodium bicarbonate was per-formed in the receiving ward and 50 cc. of a saturated solution of mag-nesium sulphate was placed in the stomach. In the ward it was discovered that paradoxically the patient was suffering from acute pulmonary edema. After phlebotomy of 500 cc. an indwelling catheter was inserted and 400 cc. of urine obtained. When respiration became shallow, carbon dioxide and oxygen were administered. A Jutte tube was passed and 5000 cc. of water given within forty-five minutes, over half of which was vomited; continuous hypodermoclysis of saline solution was begun and cold sponges given in an attempt to reduce the fever. Maniacal outbursts were controlled with 2-grain (0.12 Gm.) doses of phenobarbital. Morphine was not given because of the danger of deepening the late depression; pilocarpine was also withheld in the belief, probably correct, that myoneural junctions poisoned by atropine would not respond to it. The recovery of this patient, after ingestion of $7\frac{1}{2}$ grains of atropine, probably establishes a record.

IODINE POISONING

Accidental and suicidal poisoning with this substance is not rare. It is usually swallowed in the form of the official tincture. There is severe gastro-intestinal pain, vomiting, diarrhea, hemorrhagic nephritis, and depression and collapse.

THERAPY

Use the emetics (see p. 699) if necessary, but attempt to introduce the stomach tube as soon as possible and wash out with a starch decoction (obtained by boiling in water either laundry starch, rice or barley) until the washings no longer come away blue. The boiled starch is preferable because it combines more actively with iodine, but lacking it in an emergency, the raw article may be used; try to get some of it down even before the passing of the tube. Sabbatani (1913) advises the employment of a 5 per cent solution of sodium thiosulphate (the plain "hypo" bath employed by photographers is usually a 20 per cent solution) to fix the iodine as sodium iodide. At intervals introduce a demulcent to lessen the gastric irritation, such as eggs, milk, butter, liquid petrolatum. Treat the final depression as for chloral poisoning (see p. 703).

ALCOHOL POISONING

We are concerned here only with the final anesthetic stages of exceptionally severe acute alcoholism, since the hilarious and stuporous stages of an ordinary intoxication rarely come under observation for treatment as poisoning. The patient is in as deep coma as though chloral had been taken; the pupils are normal or dilated, never contracted. The skin is cold, clammy and pale, the respirations are somewhat slow and stertorous, the pulse is rapid and becomes increasingly weak, reflexes are lost, and the temperature is considerably below normal.

THERAPY

Apply external heat to this patient and stimulate him as much as possible: Atropine sulphate, $\frac{1}{40}$ grain (0.0015 Gm.), not to be repeated; strychnine sulphate, $\frac{1}{30}$ grain (0.002 Gm.); metrazol, $1\frac{1}{2}$ grains (0.1 Gm.); camphor in oil, 1 to 2 cc.—all to be given intramuscularly. It would seem, from the work of Pilcher (1912), that strong black coffee, or caffeine sodium benzoate, 5 grains (0.32 Gm.), may be safely given in poisoning of moderate degree, but that in cases in which a fatal issue is probable the drug would only be detrimental; aromatic spirits of ammonia, $\frac{1}{2}$ to 1 drachm (2 to 4 cc.), may be given at intervals if the patient can be made to swallow. It is usually advised that the stomach be emptied by a hypodermic dose of $\frac{1}{10}$ grain (0.006 Gm.) of apomorphine hydrochloride, but I doubt the advisability of this in view of the after-depression of this drug. Later, when the patient has been somewhat revived and if the stomach does not empty itself, then the drug may be used, but even here the stomach tube would seem to be preferable. For the subsequent gastric symptoms, starvation plus a gradual return by way of soft foods to the full diet, is the best remedy. The wracking headache will be relieved by 2 grains (0.13 Gm.) of caffeine citrate combined with 5 grains (0.32 Gm.) of phenacetin or pyramidon, or 3 grains (0.2 Gm.) of acetanilid, the dose of either of these combinations to be

45

repeated three or four times in the twenty-four hours. Larger doses than these of the coal-tar antipyretics (acetanilid, phenacetin), or of pyramidon, are seldom more effective and are more likely to cause the undesirable side-effects of this group; sweat and chills, gastric disturbances, skin eruptions, renal irritation, methemoglobin cyanosis and collapse. In some instances a dose of codeine sulphate, ½ to 1 grain, is necessary; it is best to give it in solution, for, though the codeine is not itself habit-forming, persons addicted to habitual alcoholic debauching are considered to be fair candidates for the acquisition of the more sinister habits that might be suggested to them by the complete relief afforded by this use of the needle.

WOOD (METHYL) ALCOHOL POISONING

This type of poisoning, that increased so much in incidence in the United States during the first years following the introduction of so-called "prohibition," markedly declined as relatively safe contraband liquor became available and now that prohibition has been officially abandoned will probably be seen with great rarity. It is characterized by a state of alcoholic inebriety, partially induced by the wood alcohol but largely by the ethyl alcohol also present in the ingested liquor, violent gastric pain and vomiting, disturbances of vision with dilated irresponsive pupils, dyspnea, cyanosis, rapid weak pulse, and a period of delirium followed by collapse. If death does not occur in twenty-four to forty-eight hours, there will be partial blindness, which may clear up for a while but is again followed in many cases by total optic atrophy.

THERAPY

The stomach should be washed out frequently by use of the stomach pump, though in the beginning it may be necessary to give a dose of apomorphine hydrochloride, $\frac{1}{10}$ grain (0.006 Gm.). This will empty the stomach and somewhat subdue the patient in order that the tube may be introduced. Then as soon as possible give a dose of morphine sulphate by the needle, $\frac{1}{4}$ grain (0.015 Gm.), in order to lessen the patient's suffering and make cooperation more perfect; if the delirium is wild, $\frac{1}{300}$ to $\frac{1}{200}$ grain (0.0002 to 0.0003 Gm.) of scopolamine hydrobromide (hyoscine) may be combined with the morphine. The lavage is to be done with 4 per cent sodium bicarbonate solution, and as soon as possible some of this solution should be introduced into the rectum; thus the stomach is emptied repeatedly and the acidosis is combated at one and the same time. Much of the methyl alcohol is burned into formic acid, and, while it is not known that this substance causes the chief symptoms, i. e., visual disturbances, delirium, respiratory and circulatory collapse, yet it very probably contributes much toward the acidosis that is known to be present. We know of no means of destroying nor of hastening the elimination of this formic acid, but the acidosis we can treat. Keep the patient warm and support him: Atropine sulphate, $\frac{1}{40}$ grain (0.0015 Gm.), not to be repeated; strychnine sulphate, $\frac{1}{30}$ grain (0.002 Gm.); metrazol, 1½ grains (0.1 Gm.); camphor in oil, 1 to 2 cc.; caffeine sodium benzoate, 5 grains (0.32 Gm.)—all to be given intramuscularly; or aromatic spirits of ammonia, ½ to 1 drachm (2 to 4 cc.) by mouth. Before bringing the tube out of the stomach for the last time leave a large dose of a saline cathartic there to flush out the bowel.

ACETANILIID, ANTIPYRINE AND PHENACETIN POISONING

Acute cases of poisoning with any one or a combination of these drugs are rather frequently seen due to the injudicious use of headache powders by the laity. The symptoms appear somewhat suddenly and consist of depression and confusion, dyspnea, rapid weak pulse, methemoglobin cyanosis, clammy sweat, cold extremities, and a subnormal temperature.

THERAPY

This stomach should be washed out for some time with warm water, and a dose of a saline cathartic should be left in the stomach before withdrawing the tube. Meanwhile try to get the patient warm and support him with one or more of the following drugs: Atropine sulphate, $\frac{1}{40}$ grain (0.0015 Gm.), not to be repeated; strychnine sulphate, $\frac{1}{30}$ grain (0.002 Gm.); metrazol, $1\frac{1}{2}$ grains (0.1 Gm.); camphor in oil, 1 to 2 cc.; caffeine sodium benzoate, 5 grains (0.32 Gm.)—all to be given intramuscularly; or whisky, 1 ounce (30 cc.), or aromatic spirits of ammonia, $\frac{1}{2}$ to 1 drachm (2 to 4 cc.), by mouth. There is no specific antidote.

ACETYLSALICYLIC ACID (ASPIRIN) POISONING

More and more cases of idiosyncrasy for this drug are being recorded. Perhaps the most frequent symptom is severe dyspnea but a picture similar to that of the nitritoid reaction to arsphenamine is also seen; in these latter cases, epinephrine would seem to be indicated. In other cases there is simply headache, ringing in the ears, dizziness and collapse. All the supportive drugs are of course used here. In a case seen shortly after a large dose has been taken, the use of the stomach tube may seem advisable; in any case thorough catharsis should be promoted. In protracted cases the patient is very thirsty and highly acidotic; much fluid should be given, and sodium bicarbonate by mouth and rectum.

COCAINE POISONING

The number of fatalities from the use of cocaine is small in comparison with the large number of cases in which the drug is used, even granting that many of the fatalities are not reported; but the number of moderately severe reactions is quite large. Serious cases are of two types: (*a*) The patient seems suddenly to absorb the drug all at once, he gasps, clutches himself frantically, becomes very pale, falls over in a convulsion, and is dead almost before one realizes what is transpiring; (*b*) the events take place somewhat more slowly; the patient becomes very talkative, laughs and cries unnaturally, wants to move about; there is dizziness, irregular pulse and respiration, nausea and vomiting, great abdominal pain, delirium, convulsions, and finally coma and death; the entire process requires several hours. Nowadays of course most of the cases follow the application of cocaine to the mucous membranes, but occasionally they follow upon the accidental use of cocaine instead of procaine in infiltration, and rarely the use of procaine or some of the other synthetic substitutes for cocaine.

Prevention of Absorption.—If cocaine has accidentally been injected subcutaneously, the quick application of a tourniquet above the site of injection, if this has been in one of the extremities, may be life-saving; the pulse should not be completely obliterated.

THERAPY

Stimulants.—Cocaine is relatively rapidly destroyed, or at least rendered innocuous, by contact with the tissues, therefore anything that will keep the patient alive for a few minutes is of value. Actually, however, the stimulant drugs have not saved many lives, though whatever is at hand should be used: Whisky, 1 ounce (30 cc.); aromatic spirits of ammonia, 1 drachm (4 cc.); metrazol, 1½ grains (0.1 Gm.) intramuscularly; camphor in oil, 1 to 2 cc.; strychnine sulphate, $\frac{1}{30}$ grain (0.002 Gm.); atropine sulphate, $\frac{1}{40}$ grain (0.0015 Gm.). Herzfeld reported some years ago that the ingestion of 1 to 2 ounces (30 to 60 cc.) of whisky or brandy, ten to thirty minutes before the administration of the cocaine, was very effective in preventing unpleasant occurrences.

Barbital and Phenobarbital (Veronal and Luminal).—Based upon the laboratory experiments of Tatum, Atkinson and Collins (1925), the use of the barbituric acid derivatives both in prophylaxis and treatment of cocaine poisoning has become quite general. Leshure (1927) administers sodium barbital (soluble veronal), 6 to 12 grains (0.4 to 0.8 Gm.) by mouth, one-half hour before inducing anesthesia; he reports 100 cases so treated that have not manifested any of the symptoms of cocaine intoxication. Guttman has used phenobarbital (luminal) in prophylaxis; among 391 individuals given the drug before operation under cocaine anesthesia there was but one instance of intoxication, and that occurred in a patient who had not been given the phenobarbital until just before the application of the cocaine; during the previous year, 416 operations had been performed under cocaine anesthesia, with some signs of intoxication occurring in 19 per cent of the patients. He also reports several cases in which barbital sodium was successfully used in treatment. The details of administration are as follows: (a) As a prophylactic, 3 grains (0.2 Gm.) of phenobarbital should be given thirty minutes before operation so as to assure plenty of time for absorption; (b) in cases of mild intoxication, 3 grains (0.2 Gm.) of soluble barbital may be given hypodermically, or 1½ grains (0.1 Gm.) may be added to a hypodermic injection of 5 cc. of a saturated physiologic saline solution of paraldehyde; (c) in severe intoxications, 5 cc. of the paraldehyde-soluble barbital mixture may be given intravenously.

Morphine is contraindicated by reason of adding to the respiratory depression.

CARBON MONOXIDE POISONING

Carbon monoxide poisoning is of frequent occurrence, most of the cases being due either to accidental or deliberate inhalation of the concentrated fumes of artificial illuminating gas or the exhaust of an automobile. The patient is comatose and has a peaceful expression, though there is often twitching of the facial muscles; the temperature is usually above normal; the skin is pale, but the lips are nearly always scarlet red and there is a scarlet blush on the cheeks and sometimes over the whole body; a brownish-red stippling, much resembling hemorrhagic purpura, is sometimes seen, particularly on the arms. The early symptoms are entirely due to the fact that hemoglobin has a much greater affinity for carbon monoxide than for oxygen, so that the patient is maintained in a state of partial asphyxia. If rescue is effected after only a short exposure (the degree of poisoning depending of course upon the concentration of the gas, the drafts in the room, and many other variable factors), the prognosis for recovery is good, but if profound asphyxia has persisted for very long, recovery does not take place even after all of the carbon monoxide has been released and eliminated; in these cases there has been irremediable brain injury. Many of the late deaths are also due to pneumonia.

THERAPY

Artificial respiration must be started at once and continued until the breathing becomes spontaneous. Henderson and Haggard have conclusively shown the value of the inhalation of oxygen plus carbon dioxide. In the beginning, 5 per cent of the latter was advocated, later 7 per cent, and now the studies of Murphy and Drinker (1930) indicate that 10 per cent is probably the ideal concentration. Continuance of this gas treatment beyond one and one-half hours is useless, since by that time practically all the carbon monoxide will have been eliminated. The introduction of a 4 per cent sodium bicarbonate solution by vein or rectum is indicated by reason of the acidosis that is present. Blood transfusion in the first hour or two is tempting and is nearly always performed in serious cases, but on the whole the results have been disappointing. The patient should be kept warm. Permitting exertion of any sort before complete restoration to normal is dangerous. Henderson (1931) trenchantly remarks: "The less the ambulance surgeon uses his hypodermic syringe on patients with carbon monoxide asphyxia, the better." Reports have come out of France of the successful use of sodium thiosulphate by stomach and vein, but neither the rationale nor value of this method has been established.

Following the report of resuscitation of patients poisoned with cyanide with methylene blue (see p. 700) it was to be expected that reports of the drug's employment in gas poisoning would follow. Several have, indeed, but up to the time of writing the evidence that methylene blue was the agent responsible for the recovery seems to me to be unmistakable only in the case of Nass (June 10, 1933), whose patient seems to have been saved by the intravenous administration of about 45 cc. of a 1 per cent solution; other routine treatment was subsequently employed.

METHYL CHLORIDE POISONING

Poisoning by methyl chloride has been of infrequent occurrence until recently, when, during 1928–29, there were reported 29 cases with 13 deaths, in Chicago—all in kitchenette apartments in which there was discovered a leak in the multiple unit refrigerator system. The onset of symptoms, according to the careful report of Kegel *et al.* (1929) is generally marked by progressive drowsiness, mental confusion, stupor, weakness, nausea, colic and vomiting; some patients experience tremor, hiccup, headache and visual disturbances. The pulse, temperature and respiration are all increased, the pupils are widely dilated, there is anuria and a blood picture suggestive of a primary anemia. Prolonged coma is of common occurrence. Death is always preceded by severe opisthotonic convulsions accompanied by profound cyanosis. A peculiar musty, sweetish odor of the breath is a diagnostic aid.

The gas is colorless and of such faint odor as to be undetectable in even very poisonous concentration; in two instances in Chicago, open windows in the apartment did not protect against lethal doses.

THERAPY

Kegel *et al.* state that after removal of the patient from exposure, the gas is quickly eliminated, and that progressive symptoms in the more severe cases are due to continued injury from oxidation products of the gas until they are eliminated, and to degeneration of nerve cells. In the acute stage, oxygen must be administered until the peculiar odor disappears, even though the patient has to be restrained for the purpose. It is also considered imperatively necessary that sodium bicarbonate be gotten into the system in any way possible; 500 cc. of Ringer's solution (sodium chloride, 4.5 Gm., calcium chloride, 0.12 Gm., potassium chloride, 0.21 Gm., sodium bicarbonate, 0.15 Gm., distilled water, 500 cc.) given intravenously will further combat dehydration and acidosis. Convulsions may be allayed by potassium bromide, 1 drachm (4 Gm.) in 4 ounces (120 cc.) of water, given as a retention enema, *but under no conditions should chloral or chloroform be given.* Stimulants as indicated. In the subsequent treatment, anemia must be combated.

FOOD POISONING
(Acute Diarrhea)

Most individuals poisoned by the ingestion of spoiled food or of contaminated water manifest the following symptoms: Gastric pain, nausea and perhaps vomiting, vertigo and cold clamminess of the skin, and diarrhea often accompanied by considerable tenesmus. I have used the words "acute diarrhea" in the title because it is this symptom that causes the most discomfort to the patient after the first shock of the attack has passed.

THERAPY

The patient's stomach should be completely emptied at once. If he is much nauseated, or has already been vomiting, the introduction of several glasses of warm water into the stomach and then the stroking of the posterior pharyngeal wall with the finger, usually suffices to produce satisfactory emesis; however, one should not hesitate to use the emetic drugs (for a list see p. 699). As soon as the stomach is emptied a cathartic should be introduced: Castor oil, 1 ounce (30 cc.); or calomel, 3 grains (0.2 Gm.), to be followed after six to eight hours by a saline cathartic; or magnesium sulphate, or any other saline, in full dose. The patient should be absolutely at rest, take no food, and drink freely of water, hot tea or lemonade. Two hours after the cathartic has been given the administration of bismuth may be begun: 15 grains (1 Gm.) of bismuth subcarbonate combined with 5 grains (0.3 Gm.) of phenyl salicylate (of doubtful value) every two hours for ten doses. The suspension may well be made as follows:

℞. Bismuth subcarbonate.............................. ℨiv   15.0
    Phenylsalicylate.................................. ℨj gr. xv   5.0
    Glycerin.. ℥j   30.0
    Syrup of tolu to make............................. ℥iv   120.0
       Label: 2 teaspoonfuls every two hours for ten doses.

Colicky pain is usually controlled by 2 drachms (8 cc.) of paregoric every two hours for two or three doses; occasionally it will be necessary to give a single hypodermic of ⅛ grain (0.008 Gm.) of morphine sulphate combined with ¹⁄₁₂₀ grain (0.0005 Gm.) of atropine sulphate.

These patients are often very much depressed and need support; the following drugs may be used with discretion: Whisky, ½ to 1 ounce (15 to 30 cc.) to be sipped well diluted; strychnine sulphate, ¹⁄₃₀ grain (0.003 Gm.), hypodermically; caffeine sodium benzoate, 5 grains (0.3 Gm.), intramuscularly; metrazol, 1½ grains (0.1 Gm.), intramuscularly; camphor in oil, 1 to 2 cc., intramuscularly; aromatic spirits of ammonia, ½ drachm (2 cc.).

Feeding with soft foods may be cautiously begun within twelve to twenty-four hours. It is usually advisable to continue the bismuth subcarbonate (without phenyl salicylate) in doses of 15 grains (1 Gm.) three times daily for several days. The reader is also referred to the description of the apple diet on page 60.

BOTULISM

Botulism is acute poisoning caused by the toxin of *B. botulinus,* an organism whose spores are widely distributed in nature, being found in the soil, on fruit and vegetables, in dust, in the intestinal tract of herbivorous animals, and in the larvae of worms. The disease is caused by the ingestion of a great variety of contaminated animal and plant foods; in the United States principally plant products, in Europe principally meats. Both the bacilli and the toxin are readily destroyed by boiling, but the spores resist boiling for five hours and are only killed by temperatures above 230 F. (110 C.). Eight per cent brine, or 50 per cent sugar concentration, inhibit the growth of the bacillus and prevent the formation of the toxin. In the United States and Canada, from 1899 to August 13, 1932, 193 outbreaks of botulism have been reported, a total of 645 cases with 428 deaths, giving a case mortality of 66.3 per cent (in the most recent of these reports, there were 13 deaths in the afflicted group of 16). A very large percentage of the outbreaks is due to foods preserved at home without sufficient sterilization, though some have been caused by commercially canned products.

Symptoms do not usually appear until eighteen to thirty-six hours have elapsed. At first there is malaise associated with constipation and subnormal temperature. Gastro-intestinal symptoms are unusual and when they occur are seldom violent. Then dizziness, headache, and disturbances of vision appear: Scintillation, diplopia, mydriasis, blepharoptosis and loss of the light reflex. Swallowing becomes extremely difficult, the tongue and breath foul and the mouth excessively dry, and general muscular weakness comes on. In some cases the patient appears to be completely paralyzed, but in others there are violent paroxysms induced by the attempt to swallow. The pulse is slow, then becomes rapid; breathing becomes labored and death follows from respiratory failure. Most of the victims die within three to six days, but in those who recover there are no permanent sequelae though convalescence is very slow.

THERAPY

The indications here are to empty the gastro-intestinal tract, support the patient, relieve the discomfort, and administer the antitoxin.

Emesis and Lavage.—The stomach should be emptied by the use of any of the emetics listed on page 699. Then a full dose of castor oil or one of the saline cathartics should be administered. This treatment is rational, since the poison has been taken by the mouth, but what can be expected from it is sufficiently indicated in the fact that the symptoms usually do not appear until eighteen to thirty-six hours after the food has been ingested.

Support and Stimulation.—Keep this patient warm. Any of the following stimulant drugs are indicated: Whisky, $\frac{1}{2}$ to 1 ounce (15 to 30 cc.) at intervals; aromatic spirits of ammonia, $\frac{1}{2}$ to 1 drachm (2 to 4 cc.); strychnine sulphate, $\frac{1}{30}$ grain (0.002 Gm.); metrazol, $1\frac{1}{2}$ grains (0.1 Gm.), intramuscularly; camphor in oil, 1 to 2 cc.; caffeine sodium benzoate, 5 grains (0.32 Gm.). Atropine would only add to the discomfort.

Relief of Discomfort.—The excessive dryness in the mouth and throat can sometimes be lessened by the administration of pilocarpine nitrate, the dose of which is $\frac{1}{12}$ grain (0.005 Gm.) hypodermically; but the advisability of employing this drug, in view of the sweat and depression that it causes, must be carefully weighed in each case.

Antitoxin.—It has been repeatedly shown by animal experiments that the specific antitoxin is capable of neutralizing *B. botulinus* toxin, but the relative infrequency of outbreaks of botulism does not warrant the distribution of this antitoxin throughout the country by commercial firms on the same scale as in the case of other therapeutic sera; a supply can always be had, however, at the Hygienic Laboratory, Washington, D. C., and at the Department of Health of the City of New York. According to Allen and Ecklund (1932), Jensen and Salisbury, Inc., Kansas City, Mo., are the sole commercial manufacturers of the product in the United States. Another factor that has prevented the control of outbreaks by the use of this serum is its relative inefficiency if not employed soon after the poison has been ingested, *i. e.*, by the time most of the cases are diagnosed it is already too late for the antitoxin to be of much value.

Sedatives and Anesthetics.—In the course of a series of animal experiments designed to investigate the path of absorption of *B. botulinus* toxin, Bronfenbrenner and Weiss (1924) made the accidental discovery that prolonged ether anesthesia delayed the onset of symptoms. Further studies showed that the same results could be obtained when luminal sodium, nitrous oxide-oxygen, or morphine were substituted for the ether. It has been suggested that these observations be utilized in practice to keep the patients alive and relatively atoxic until a supply of antitoxin can be obtained.

MUSHROOM POISONING

In practically all cases of mushroom poisoning there are variable degrees of gastro-intestinal disturbance: Nausea, vomiting, gastric pain, diarrhea. In addition, depending upon the species of mushroom ingested, there may be any of the following symptoms: Nephritis with anuria or hemoglobinuria; jaundice; excessive perspiration, salivation and lacrimation; dilatation of the pupils, mental confusion, excitement, convulsions, coma and death.

THERAPY

The stomach should be emptied by the use of any of the emetics listed on page 699. Then a full dose of castor oil or one of the saline cathartics should be administered. Keep the patient warm. Any of the following stimulant drugs may be used if indicated by the state of the patient's pulse or respiration: Whisky, 1 ounce (30 cc.); aromatic spirits of ammonia, $\frac{1}{2}$ to 1 drachm (2 to 4 cc.); strychnine sulphate, $\frac{1}{20}$ grain (0.003 Gm.); metrazol, $1\frac{1}{2}$ grains (0.1 Gm.), intramuscularly; camphor in oil, 1 to 2 cc.; caffeine sodium benzoate, 5 grains (0.32 Gm.). Atropine sulphate, $\frac{1}{100}$ to

$\frac{1}{40}$ grain (0.0006 to 0.0015 Gm.), will act as physiologic antidote if there is sweating, salivation and lacrimation. For the nephritis or jaundice nothing specific can be done. To quiet the excited patient, morphine sulphate, $\frac{1}{8}$ grain (0.008 Gm.), may be given, or the following may be used: Barbital (veronal), 2 grains (0.13 Gm.) every four to six hours; phenobarbital (luminal), $\frac{1}{2}$ grain (0.03 Gm.) every four to six hours; amytal, $\frac{3}{4}$ grain (0.045 Gm.) every four to six hours; sodium bromide, 10 to 15 grains (0.6 to 1 Gm.) every four to six hours.

LEAD POISONING

The first symptoms of lead poisoning are usually abnormal fatigue accompanying irritability and sleeplessness, headache, loss of appetite and vague nausea and body pains. Constipation and increasing muscular weakness, especially of the extensors of the right hand, become marked, and then there appears tremor of the mouth and eye muscles, the latter detectable when the patient lowers the lids. Tremor of the extended fingers usually appears somewhat late, as do also actual radial paralysis and colic. During the colic—which is caused by tonic stimulation of the intestinal musculature by the direct action of the lead so that there is a contraction ring with an area of high pressure due to increased peristalsis above—the severe pains are located below the umbilicus in a scaphoid abdomen, and in contrast to appendicitis and peritonitis there is no tenderness and the suffering is relieved by pressure. The writhing of the intestines is often clearly to be felt. Frequently there is a desire to vomit and to defecate, but very little comes of this; obstinate constipation is certainly the rule, though diarrhea is on record. The patient sweats and the temperature and pulse rate are much decreased; a rise in blood pressure and blood sugar is usual but not invariable. There is also an apparent inability of the vessels to relax, which accounts for the marked pallor and the slow hard pulse as well as the hypertension; this may also give rise to sudden but usually temporary attacks of blindness (the contractions can sometimes be seen in the retinal and conjunctival vessels), occasionally to contracted kidney in protracted cases, to angina pectoris and gangrene of the extremities, and, together with a direct poisoning of the brain cells, to encephalopathy, manifested in hallucinations, babbling, delirium or stupor. Whether the peripheral paralyses due to lead are of neuritic, muscular, spinal or vascular causation is not known. Sterility and miscarriage as accompaniments of the malady were recognized many years ago. Death is nowadays unusual but there may be degenerate neurological sequelae of a most distressing sort, particularly in children, probably as a result of prolonged increase in intracranial pressure. The roentgenological diagnosis in children is now recognized as possible, but it is my understanding that all pediatricians and roentgenologists are not at one regarding some differential points.

Pallor in this disease is not a direct expression of the anemia, for even in severe cases the red cells rarely fall below 3.5 million and the hemoglobin below 65 per cent. With regard to stippling of the red cells, one may say: (a) There is no lead poisoning entirely without stippling, but there may be stippling which indicates only absorption of lead without clinical poisoning. (b) The proportion of 100 or even more stippled cells per million may be seen in lead workers without symptoms, but the proportion of 500 or more is considered of great diagnostic importance. (c) Stippling is not entirely pathognomonic since it may also follow ingestion of silver or zinc and is promoted by potassium iodide. (*d*) If there is also leukocytosis, the other types of metallic poisoning, benzene poisoning, diseases of the blood-forming tissues and malaria must be ruled out. A moderate lymphocytosis is seen in some cases, perhaps a slight increase in monocytes also. Both the lead line on the gums, which depends much upon the state of the mouth, and the presence of lead in the urine indicate absorption but tell little about the degree of clinical involvement. The lead content of the blood may be 0.36 mg. per cent as against the normal 0.005 to 0.035 mg. per cent. Lead storage takes place principally in the calcareous portions of the bones, only secondarily in the liver and kidneys. Jaundice is due to blood disintegration and not to liver damage. A diagnostic point apparently more often resorted to abroad than in this country is the observation of a much increased coproporphyrin content in the urine. So far as absorption, storage and elimination are concerned, it has been shown that the metabolism of lead and calcium are closely related, but the minutiae of these processes are not yet understood. The question of delayed callus formation in lead-poisoned individuals suffering fracture has been raised, and one school believes that there is injury to the calcium-secreting osteoblasts with actual bone necrosis as a possibility. The high incidence of arthritis and analogous conditions is also believed to reflect bone injury.

There is much of lead poisoning in the literature of recent centuries. Major, indeed, makes it a truly venerable disease in a delightful historical study in which he proposes one Nikander (second century, B. C.) as "poet laureate of lead colic." Not until the eighteenth century was the entity given scientific status, however, a service performed by Sir George Baker (1722–1809), who got himself denounced as a faithless son of his county for showing that Devonshire colic was due to the lead in Devonshire cider. Today, lead poisoning ranks first among the industrial diseases, and epidemics are not of infrequent occurrence as well; in 1930, there were serious outbreaks in two Continental cities whose water is conveyed in lead pipes. Bizarre, indeed, are some of the ways in which we can take harmful amounts of lead into the body, but there is no space here for the list. In infants, the chewing upon painted toys, the crib, etc., is probably the most frequent source.

THERAPY

After prevention of the possibility of further absorption of lead by whatever means are required in the individual case, the treatment is divided into two periods: The mobilization of the lead outside of the blood stream in order to bring about subsidence of acute symptoms, and the promotion of lead elimination.

Mobilization of Lead in Acute Cases.—In the presence of colic or other severe acute manifestations calcium is given because as calcium is stored in the bones lead is stored also, as was shown by Aub, Hunter and their associates, in 1925. Practically instant relief is brought by the very slow intravenous injection of 20 cc. of a sterile 5 per cent solution of calcium chloride; in the series of 24 cases reported by Bauer *et al.* (1931) the patients almost invariably went to sleep, though some slight abdominal soreness remained. Evidently there is some antispasmodic action here also. During the period of freedom from pain a full dose of magnesium sulphate is usually given to sweep out the relaxed bowel. The calcium injection may be safely repeated in four hours if the spasm returns, as it usually does several times in the more severe cases. These injections must be given with the greatest possible care, for if the solution is introduced more rapidly than at the rate of 2 cc. per minute severe nausea and vomiting are practically certain to occur; furthermore, rapid administration may cause acute paralysis of respiration and circulation. Even at best there is usually a fall of 10 to 40 mm. in the blood pressure due to peripheral vasodilatation, and the patient feels as though his entire body were on fire. Another precaution: Be sure that the needle is in the vein, for calcium injected into the adjacent tissues causes slough. Failing the facilities for giving the calcium chloride intravenously, morphine and atropine must be employed, ¼ grain (0.015 Gm.) and ¹⁄₁₀₀ grain (0.0006 Gm.) respectively, or perhaps even higher doses; these drugs are slower but relatively sure in their action. The nitrites, as used in angina pectoris (see p. 542), are also of value.

After the more acute symptoms are controlled, the usual practice is to continue calcium therapy at a more leisurely pace for a few days to assure maximum storage before elimination is begun. This is best accomplished through an alkaline diet in the form of milk, green vegetables and potatoes, and the additional administration of calcium by mouth. Leschke (1931) has found calcium gluconate, which is soluble and readily absorbed, the best drug in his large experience; he gives 7½-grain (0.5 Gm.) doses in milk at three-hour intervals, so that the patient obtains five or six doses daily.

Elimination of the Lead.—After several days of the above mobilization therapy, the treatment is swung around in the opposite direction, and eliminative procedures are begun; that is to say, a régime of calcium starvation is instituted. This is best accomplished by giving a calcium-poor diet consisting of much meat, fish, eggs or cheese, and no green vegetables; a very small amount of potatoes and some milk are permissible—but very little of these. In addition acids are given to promote the abstraction of calcium from the bones; 20 to 30 grains (1.3 to 2 Gm.) of ammonium chloride four to six times daily, or hydrochloric acid, 30 minims (2 cc.) of the U.S.P. dilute if the patient can be gotten to take so much—administering in weak lemonade will help. Leschke believes that the cure works better if applied in a stop-and-go manner. He prescribes four days of cure and three days of pause, permitting on the latter a more varied though still calcium-poor diet and reducing the acid considerably; he also favors the taking of coffee and tea for their diuretic effect. He likes also during the entire period of de-leading to give a pill of atropine and papaverine; some such combination as the following might be written:

℞. Atropine sulphate.................................. gr. ½   0.03
    Papaverine....................................... gr. xxx   2.0
    Make 60 pills.
    Label: 1 pill after meals.

Some physicians like the use of iodine instead of acids to hasten elimination, as suggested by Melsens as long ago as 1849. Five to 10 grains (0.3 to 0.6 Gm.) of potassium iodide, well given in milk, three times daily is probably a good starting dose, but this is often considerably increased if well borne by the stomach. Sodium bicarbonate is also effective, probably by converting the insoluble tribasic lead phosphate into the soluble dibasic salt. Large doses are given, 5 to 8 drachms (20 to 30 Gm.) daily, divided into five or six portions. Leschke considers it less dangerous to use the iodide first and then, when it is felt that most of the lead has been eliminated, change to the sodium bicarbonate, his fear being of course that the promotion of too rapid streaming out of the lead will give rise to further cell injuries. It is indeed an astonishing fact, and one that to me is wholly inexplicable, that we practically never see such damage occurring as the lead comes out, though we assume that the inward passage is the cause of the severe symptoms.

Instead of any of the above medicaments, parathyroid extract has been injected intravenously with excellent results; 40 to 80 units daily in one or two doses. However, as this necessitates frequent blood-calcium determinations as a safeguard against hypercalcemia and possible renal injury, it seems to me to be needlessly drastic therapy.

As most of the lead is eliminated through the bowel, the giving of saline cathartics, particularly magnesium sulphate, is considered to be especially important; senna, cascara and other drugs which may cause a more spasmodic type of movement are contraindicated, but later in the treatment mineral oil may be substituted for the salines.

The anginal symptoms and the peripheral vascular spasmodic disturbances are treated with the xanthine diuretics as usual. In the treatment of the paralyses, months of patient massage, active movement and perhaps the application of the galvanic current are needed. Some physicians also favor the use here of large doses of strychnine sulphate, $\frac{1}{20}$ grain (0.003 Gm.) or more three times daily.

SNAKE BITE

The total number of deaths annually throughout the world from the bites of poisonous snakes is probably between 25,000 and 35,000, of which 20,000 to 25,000 occur in India alone. The other cases are scattered throughout all the rest of the world, few regions being without one or more dangerous families of snakes; Europe, however, is relatively free, perhaps no more than 2 or 3 fatal cases occurring there each year. The chief snakes according to their distribution are: Asia, the several vipers, the daboia, the habu, the cobra, the king cobra, the krait; Africa, the vipers, the puff-adder, the asp; Oceania, brown snake, black snake, copperhead, tiger snake, death-adder; Europe, the vipers; North America, the vipers, the water moccasin, the copper head, the rattlesnakes, the harlequin snake (southeastern United States and Central America); South America, the vipers, the copperhead, the water moccasin, the rattlesnakes, the fer-de-lance, the bushmaster, the coral snake (also occurs in the West Indies), the caiaçaca, the jararacussú, the jararaca, the surucucú de patioba, and the yarará ñata.

The symptoms of poisoning vary with the different snakes; I have drawn freely upon Amaral for the following descriptions. *Cobra:* Local burning, edema and congestion; prostration; nausea, vomiting, salivation, cold sweats; rapid and weak pulse, rapid and later slow and weak respiration; difficulty in speech and progressive muscular paralysis; respiratory death. *King cobra:* Little or no local reaction; difficult and stertorous respiration; patient remains in a semiconscious state until death from respiratory paralysis. *Krait:* Rapid emaciation, progressive muscular weakness and other symptoms of slow intoxication; death after six or more days from respiratory paralysis. *Daboia:* Intense local reaction, ecchymosis and hemorrhages; nausea, vomiting and collapse with rapid weak pulse; if death is not immediate, hematuria and albuminuria, anemia, intense emaciation, and then death. *Jararaca, jararacussú, fer-de-lance, caiçaca, habu:* Immediate local edema which spreads rapidly, ecchymosis, severe pain and hemorrhage at site of bite; parched throat, thirst, congestion, hemorrhages (except following the bite of the habu) into the mucous membranes and even through the skin, albuminuria, death in toxic exhaustion (habu causes respiratory paralysis and jararacussú visual impairment). *Rattlesnake:* Local pain, hemorrhage, ecchymosis, gangrene; rapid general symptoms (I once saw a young negro lad vomiting and profusely sweating twenty minutes after I had seen him bitten by a large diamond back) consisting of rapid and weak pulse, nausea and vomiting, sometimes diarrhea, cold sweats, and a series of collapses until early death takes place. The pigmy rattler and the American copperhead do not seem to be among the most poisonous snakes; also a bite by the true water moccasin (not the maligned, though vicious, common water snake) is quite rare. *Harlequin and coral snakes:* No local evidences except intense pain; depression, somnolence, convulsions, death in collapse; the coral also causes salivation and lacrimation.

THERAPY

Immediate Surgical Treatment.—Apply a tight bandage proximal to the bite and leave it in place for about twenty minutes, after which it may be partially loosened at intervals to relieve the congestion but permit only gradual absorption. Enlarge the wound with crucial incisions ¼ inch deep and suck out the venom; then apply any of the following: Strong acids, phenol, tincture of iodine, bichloride of mercury (dangerous if too much is absorbed), tincture of ferric chloride, alcohol, potassium permanganate. The rubbing of crystals of this latter substance into the wound, and the injection into and around it of a 2 per cent solution, was formerly looked upon as very valuable, but the injections at least seem now to be discredited. Intravenous injections of potassium permanganate are very dangerous; I once saw a patient thus killed who might otherwise have survived the bite, as the rattler was small. Hutchison (1929) says that suction should be continued for twenty minutes out of each hour for fifteen hours.

General Supportive Measures.—Use the stimulants as indicated: Aromatic spirits of ammonia, ½ drachm (2 cc.) at intervals of ten to fifteen minutes; caffeine sodium benzoate, 5 grains (0.32 Gm.) intramuscularly, or caffeine as strong hot black coffee; metrazol, 1½ grains (0.1 Gm.), intramuscularly; camphor in oil, 1 to 2 cc.; strychnine sulphate—large doses of this drug are used, ⅟₁₅ to ⅛ grain (0.004 to 0.008 Gm.), at fifteen-minute intervals until slight spasms occur; whisky, ½ to 1 ounce, so long as it is acting only as a stimulant and not as an intoxicant. The popular belief that to get maudlin and even "dead" drunk is the best treatment for snake bite has no basis in actual fact; indeed, it would seem that such treatment lessens the patient's chance of recovery.

Specific Antisera.—(*a*) *In India.*—Despite the fact that Calmette's serum, made by immunizing the horse, seems to be absolutely antidotal to cobra venom, its use can hardly have made even a faint impression on the mortality record in India. The working people, scattered in isolated villages over an enormous territory, often sleep out at night and thus fall easy victims to the wandering cobra that, seeking its meal of snakes, finds the sleeping native and wantonly bites him. There is little hope that the serum will ever be sufficiently well distributed that its administration will become possible to many of these unfortunates soon enough to save their lives.

(*b*) *In South America.*—We know practically nothing, of course, of the incidence of fatal snake bite in the wilds of this continent, but on the large estates and industrial workings the conditions are more favorable for treatment than in India. The working population, while scattered through the forests, particularly in the north, are more or less concentrated about the haciendas, making it easy to see the victims promptly and provide efficient care: It has been stated that the antivenins are being used successfully under these circumstances.

(*c*) *In North America.*—Amaral, formerly head of the Institute of Butantan São Paulo, and at present director of the Antivenin Institute of America, has devised a polyvalent serum against the venoms of the rattlesnake, water moccasin and copperhead. It is manufactured by Mulford (Antivenin Nearctic Crotalidae, N.N.R., 1933). The contents of one syringe should be injected as soon as possible and the dose repeated every one or two hours unless and until symptoms are markedly diminished; intramuscular injections are advised, in severe cases, intravenous. The doses are doubled for children, because the smaller the body the greater the proportionate amount of venom in the tissues. The problem of getting this antidote to the victim, who has probably limped into some isolated village, is of course a difficult one; however, it is believed that in time numerous stations will be established, which, when reached by telephone, will send out a supply of the serum in an airplane and drop it over the place from which the call was sent. The feasibility of this plan has already been shown in the region around San Diego, California, the point of telephone call being the zoological garden in that city.

(*d*) *In Central America.*—The Mulford antivenin (Antivenin (Bothropic), N.N.R., 1932) is being extensively and effectively used in Central America since the development of the snake farm for collection of venoms at Tela, Honduras. It is used, it seems, against bites of the *fer-de-lance*, hog-nosed snake, Tamagás verde, timbo, and eye-lash viper. George (1929) has stated that an antivenin against cascabel, the tropical rattlesnake, is also now available, but I find no record of the production of a specific anticoral venom.

SPIDER BITE

In the United States all of the authenticated cases of arachnidism have been due to the bite of *Lactrodectus mactans,* commonly known as black widow, shoe-button spider, hourglass spider and T-dot spider. To Bogen is due great credit for reawakening interest in this subject. At the time of his last report, September, 1932, there were available records of 380 cases with 17 deaths in 18 states; add to this the many hundreds of unrecognized or unreported cases and it will be seen that this type of poisoning deserves serious attention. Most of the victims have been males who were bitten on the penis or adjacent parts while sitting in an outdoor privy. The stinging pain of the bite soon subsides and there is usually little or no visible lesion; then, fifteen to thirty minutes later, pain reappears, usually at the site of the bite and spreads all over the body, reaching its maximum about an hour after the bite. There is generalized muscle spasm and very often a boardlike rigidity of the abdominal wall. The pain is agonizing but local tenderness is usually entirely absent; the patient usually sweats profusely, is restless and anxious, and may exhibit spasmodic twitching of the muscles of the extremities, priapism, localized edema and urinary retention. There may be a mild rise in temperature accompanied at times by a slow pulse; the blood and spinal fluid pressures are usually above normal.

THERAPY

Of course the vast majority of the victims of this spider recover in a few days, but the acute symptoms are so severe as to necessitate immediate efforts at alleviation. Resort is practically always had to the opiates, though all observers agree that these patients can tolerate very large amounts without deriving much relief from them. Browning's (1930) patient was considerably relieved by nitroglycerin. Hot baths or hot applications are sometimes helpful. Bogen has performed spinal puncture in a few cases with striking immediate relief and he highly recommends the procedure.

Intravenous injection of 10 per cent magnesium sulphate solution gave only "some apparent relief" in the one case in which it was tried. Blood taken from recovered victims, from one to ten weeks after the bite, was given to 24 patients soon after admission to the hospital, the injection being repeated in three instances. From 2 to 35 cc. of the serum, given intramuscularly, has produced substantial relief in each instance. Bogen feels, and others are in agreement with him, that the stimulant drugs and alcohol should not be used, and furthermore that there is no rational indication for local treatment of the site of the bite other than the simple application of an antiseptic such as tincture of iodine.

BURNS

MILD BURNS

First degree burns, or second degree burns of only small areas, are usually treated by any one or a combination of several of the following methods.

1. **Carron Oil.**—This substance, which is a mixture in equal parts of linseed oil and lime water, is soothing to burned areas, like all oily and alkaline applications. Gauze soaked in the mixture should be very liberally applied and held in place by dry bandages. It is not antiseptic, however, and is therefore best not used on blistered areas.

2. **Picric Acid.**—A 1 per cent aqueous solution of picric acid is both analgesic and antiseptic and is therefore much used; its principal undesirable feature is the fact that it stains everything with which it comes in contact. Small gauze compresses should be soaked in the solution and gently placed so as to thoroughly cover the affected area; rather loose bandages are then employed to hold the dressing in place. Any distended blisters should have been aseptically opened beforehand. After two or three days the dressing may be soaked in picric acid solution to soften it and then it may be removed and replaced with a fresh one; in very mild burns it is usual to leave the original dressing in place until the area is completely healed.

A 5 per cent alcoholic solution may be substituted for the weaker aqueous solution, but the danger of absorption of the poisonous substance is greater in the presence of alcohol, and such a solution should certainly not be used over large areas.

3. **Aluminum Subacetate.**—Both Ravogli and Pusey have highly commended this substance in 2 to 5 per cent solution as both an analgesic and antiseptic of considerable value. The former writes: "When the blisters are distended with serum they are opened, draining the fluid and leaving the epidermis in place to protect the denuded papillary layer. . . . Compresses of sterile gauze are applied on the burned surface and kept continually moist with the aluminum solution, and the whole is bound with a piece of oiled silk, so cut as to hold the dressing in place."

4. **Ethyl Aminobenzoate (Benzocaine, Anesthesin).**—Ten per cent of this substance, which is a local anesthetic, may be applied in lanolin ointment, the whole to be covered with gauze; the treatment is of doubtful value if there are blisters and danger of infection.

5. **Butesin Picrate.**—This substance combines the anesthetic properties of butesin with the antiseptic properties of picric acid and is an excellent dressing for first and mild second degree burns. It is usually applied in the form of the N.N.R. Butesin Picrate Ointment, which contains 1 per cent of the drug in a suitable ointment base. Before applying the dressing, all distended blisters should be aseptically drained.

SEVERE BURNS

All extensive first degree burns, all second degree burns unless only a very small area is involved, and all third degree burns of whatever extent, are to be considered as serious. The treatment resolves itself into the following elements: (a) The combating of shock and fluid deprivation, (b) the prevention and treatment of toxemia, (*c*) the protection of the denuded areas, (*d*) the application of antiseptics to prevent or combat infection, and (*e*) the prevention of contractures and the replacement of tissue by grafting. This last matter lies entirely within the realm of surgery, but the other items will be given further consideration here.

(*a*) SHOCK AND LOSS OF FLUIDS

The treatment of shock cannot be fully considered here. It should be particularly noted, however, that the blood becomes very concentrated after a severe burn. Indeed, it has been maintained by Underhill (1930) that blood concentration is the cause of most of the toxic symptoms of burns, but to most observers it seems more likely that the anhydremia is merely one of the manifestations of a profound toxemia, the true nature of which is as yet unexplained. Still, it is recognized that if a burn involves one sixth of the body area, the loss of fluid in twenty-four hours may equal 70 per cent of the total blood volume, resulting in great blood concentration, slowed circulation, partial asphyxiation, alteration in metabolic processes, impairment of the heat-regulating mechanism with fall in temperature, and suspension to a considerable degree of the vital activities. The call for fluid in large quantities is therefore imperative, and is best answered by the immediate administration of 1000 cc. of physiologic saline at a rate not to exceed 25 cc. per minute, and thereafter fluids by every available channel in the amount of 4 to 8 liters in twenty-four hours—that is until the capillaries have lost their abnormal permeability, fluids are retained, and the concentration of the hemoglobin and blood chlorides approaches normal; this critical period is usually passed in twenty-four to forty-eight hours. Some observers give part of this fluid in the form of glucose solution. There has been occasional mention in the literature of generalized edema following such heroic introduction of fluids, which is thought to be due to renal depression consequent upon edema of the tubules. Permanent renal damage does not result from burns.

Many men of large experience are now quite in agreement with Riehl that early blood transfusion is an adjuvant measure of great value. The late Dr. Davidson, it seems, transfused on admission any patient with a possible lethal burn, and repeated in less than twenty-four hours if shock developed. Seeger (1932) writes me: "We make it a rule to transfuse every child with a burn involving 20 per cent or more of the body surface, regardless of how good the patient's condition may appear to be."

(*b*) TOXEMIA

The toxemia that appears usually several days after the patient was burned is treated by the measures just described, save that they must be continued over a longer period of time. The prevention of toxemia is, however, another matter.

1. **Débridement.**—This procedure comprises the surgical excision, as completely as is possible under the existing circumstances, of all the burned tissue, the patient being under a general anesthetic. While this treatment prevents toxemia by removing the principal source of the toxins, and has undoubtedly saved many lives, it is open to the following objections, as made by Bancroft and Rogers (1926):

"It is a radical procedure with considerable operative risk to a devitalized patient. Islands of epithelium in the hair follicles, sweat and sebaceous glands may be sacrificed that might be saved.

"The after-treatment is extremely painful and infection is very apt to follow.

"Skin grafting must usually be performed to cover the defect. If the condition of the patient is poor and infection present, skin grafting may be so long delayed that a scar tissue base may form beneath the granulation tissue and a second extensive débridement must be performed to make a satisfactory field for the grafts."

2. **Tannic Acid.**—In 1925, Davidson, while investigating the possibility of preventing toxemia by the use of local coagulants, was advised by E. C. Mason that the phosphotungstic acid that he was studying at the time might well be replaced by tannic acid; it is no exaggeration to say that Davidson's subsequent studies of this latter drug have quite revolutionized the treatment of severe burns. In the beginning, he applied a gauze dressing and then soaked it with 2.5 per cent aqueous solution of tannic acid (the solution must be freshly made as it completely deteriorates during a few days' exposure to light and air) and kept the compresses wet with the same until tanning was complete. The technic of Beck and Powers (1926) has, however, completely replaced this method. All clothing and dressings are removed, the patient is placed under a cradle tent on sterile sheets, an electric bulb maintains warmth and dryness, and the tannic acid solution (5 per cent is now universally employed, occasionally raised to 10 per cent) is sprayed on to the burned area from an atomizer every thirty, sometimes every fifteen, minutes until a fine mahogany brown membrane is formed, which usually requires from fifteen to eighteen hours. Thereafter the entire burned area, which is now insensitive, remains exposed to the warm air and the coagulum is left undisturbed until it separates—after ten days or more in deep burns. Experience with tannic acid ointments or jellies about the face and eyes has not been entirely satisfactory, and it is now the usual practice to use the spray here too since the injurious effects to the eyes which were earlier feared have not been found to occur.

In deep burns, infection sometimes occurs beneath the membrane. Seeger (1932) has found that the removal of tanned membrane should suppuration begin beneath it is greatly facilitated by checker-boarding the area with incisions during the tanning process so that 2-inch squares are formed, or the same thing may be accomplished by laying very narrow strips of adhesive across the burned area and tanning the squares between them. It is agreed that boric acid dressing should not be applied because of the danger of poisoning. Glover (1932) finds it advisable to apply continuous Dakin's solution dressings to hasten the separation of the coagulum when fluctuation appears; the normal skin must of course be adequately protected with petrolatum.

Unfortunately, the tannic acid method of treatment is not effective if ointments have been previously applied. In such cases the ointment must be removed (usually with xylol) under heavy morphine dosage or even general anesthesia before the spraying can be begun. It has not been found that burns with chemicals require any special neutralization treatment, such as counteracting acids with alkalis, for all possible damage has already been done and excess of the material can be got rid of by liberal flushing with water or saline solution.

The pH of the Solution.—Seeger (1932) feels that the observations of the action of tannic acid which have been made by chemists in the tanning industry, though bearing directly only upon the responses of nonviable tissues, might well be studied for what clinical applications may be gleaned from them. Wilson (1928) has stated that such acid tannin solutions as are used medically would ruin skins in the ordinary production of leather due to excessive swelling of the tissues. In Seeger's experimental studies with rabbits he has found that when one proceeds from a neutral to an acid range in the solutions a point is quite suddenly reached—pH 6— at which a great degree of edema is produced in the tissues; usually employed solutions are much more acid even than this. The least edematous disruption of tissues he found to occur with solutions nearest the hydrogen ion concentration of 7.4. For clinical use he prepares a solution of this acceptable concentration, as follows: Tannic acid, 25 Gm.; pure anhydrous sodium carbonate, 3.975 Gm.; water, 500 cc. Apparently this neutralization is not accompanied by any loss of tanning power. Dr. Seeger informs me (December, 1933) that experience in approximately 50 cases has shown that the membrane is more pliable when this new solution is used; he also has the impression that healing occurs more rapidly beneath it.

3. Continuous Bath.—The continuous bath treatment is infrequently used because of the special apparatus necessary, under the constant supervision of a specially trained attendant. It is of decided value for the first few days in extensive second and third degree burns of the body, especially when the patient is in coma, with a small rapid pulse, dyspnea and anuria. The continuous bath relieves pain, is sedative, and improves the circulation of the skin; to some extent the absorption of toxic products is prevented. It is difficult to give the continuous bath without a special large tub provided with temperature regulators, large outflow pipes, and rims supplied with hooks for the attachment of supporting sheets and pillows.

The following rules should be followed: (1) First fill the tub with hot water to warm it. (2) Regulate the temperature to 98 F. (37 C.) before placing the patient in the water. (3) Test the temperature every few minutes, and keep it at 98 F. (37 C.). (4) After the temperature is adjusted, shut off the intake. Do not permit a continuous flow. (5) Keep the ears dry. (6) A trained attendant must not leave the room while the patient is in the tub. (7) Avoid exposure on removal from the bath.

(c) PROTECTION OF THE DENUDED AREAS

1. Paraffin Treatment.—In the investigations undertaken by clinicians and pharmacologists as a result of the sensational exploitation of a French nostrum during the early years of the World War, the paraffin dressing of recent burns was found to have the following advantages over all other dressings that had hitherto been devised: (*a*) The wound is protected from the air, which is not only very irritating to the surface but may carry pathogenic organisms; (*b*) the damaged tissues are held somewhat immobile and at rest by the splintlike effect of the wax; (*c*) the heat of the applications perhaps encourages the establishment of new blood supply; (*d*) the paraffin film does not adhere to the injured area, and therefore at the redressings the granulation tissue and the epithelium that is attempting to cover in the denuded area is not injured; and (*e*) redressing is much less painful than with the earlier methods for the reason that granulations have not grown into the dressing. Repair of deep burns is no more rapid with this than with any other method, nor is there any less scarring. Indeed, in most respects this method of treatment is inferior to the tannic acid treatment. Where still used, the usual practice is to apply first a coat of liquid petrolatum, which is painless and protects against the heat of the paraffin, then a thin layer of cotton, then the melted paraffin is applied, and perhaps additional layers of cotton and paraffin. Special spraying apparatus may of course be used, but the ordinary sprinkling can is satisfactory and indeed so is painting. Sollmann has described the two following methods of melting the paraffin and maintaining it at proper fluidity:

"*Food Warmer.*—This is the pint size sold in the stores for warming of babies' milk bottles. When filled one half or two thirds with paraffin of melting point, 47.5 C., it can be used in three minutes after the current is turned on. If the current is then turned off for two minutes, it will have just the right temperature. It will remain usably melted for ten minutes without current, when a crust begins to form; it can then again be made usable by turning on the current for a few moments.

"This should be particularly useful when the paraffin is used only occasionally, as in ordinary office practice.

"*Acetate Thermostat.*—Sodium acetate has the curious property of melting and congealing at just about the temperature that is needed for the application of the paraffin. It retains this temperature constant for a long time while passing from the liquid to the solid state. When sodium acetate is used to fill a pot surrounding a vessel containing paraffin, it keeps the paraffin melted at just the right temperature for application for three hours after the pot has been removed from the fire. If in the meantime it has been set into a fireless cooker, the time could of course have been further prolonged.

"The advantages of this will be appreciated at once: The paraffin needs no further attention after it has been melted, until three hours afterward, and then it can be quickly reheated. The paraffin pot can be carried to any part of the shop, or in an ambulance to the dressing station. The sodium acetate is syrupy, and does not easily spill; it does not evaporate, so that no attention is required in this direction; indeed, the outer and inner vessels could probably be joined by solder.

"The device that I am using, which appears especially practical, consists of an ordinary glue pot of size O. The outer pot is filled two thirds with official sodium acetate (requiring probably something over a pound). The inner vessel holds about a pound of paraffin."

Mummery (1933) has surprisingly advocated the desertion of the newer tannic acid treatment except for the most serious types of burns and the return to the use of paraffin containing acriflavine, in the proportions of 1:1000. Most experienced observers had omitted antiseptics from their paraffins, however, before the method lost its vogue.

2. Gelatin and Formaldehyde.—Fist has offered the following modification of the paraffin treatment:

"A dressing that presents several advantages may be prepared by dipping gauze into a hot, dilute, aqueous solution of pure gelatin, drying it, and then treating with solution of formaldehyde U.S.P. of half strength, and finally washing and drying. The result is a gauze that is unaffected by moisture; it will not stick to a granulating surface, and may be kept in a warm climate or sterilized in an autoclave.

"When this prepared gauze has been used as a dressing, granulation has proceeded with great rapidity. Just how much of the stimulation is due to the formaldehyde in the compound is a matter that will bear investigation.

"The gauze, when dry, is slightly stiffer than paraffined gauze but softens somewhat when moistened. If well-diluted gelatin solution is used, the dressing is not too stiff for application to raw surfaces.

"Before the gauze is applied the surface should be well cleansed and then dried, preferably by means of hot air. The dressing should be removed daily, the wound cleansed and dried, and a new dressing applied. Pure gelatin is easily obtainable and should always be used. Four ounces of pure gelatin dissolved in 1 gallon of water will moisten quite a quantity of gauze. After the gauze is dried, it is immersed for a few minutes in solution of formaldehyde U.S.P., diluted to half strength, to fix the gelatin. The gauze is then washed, dried, packaged and sterilized. Any good hospital can sterilize the gauze, as it is not injured by autoclaving."

(d) THE APPLICATION OF ANTISEPTICS

Aldrich and Firor (1933) challenge the hypothesis that absorption of noxious materials and the abnormal concentration of the blood are the causes of severe toxemia. Instead, they feel that the entire symptomatology can be accounted for on the basis of infection alone. In their investigations they found that all cultures taken from the burned areas in the first twelve hours are sterile, save for the occasional occurrence of *Staphylococcus aureus* and *albus* and *B. coli*, but that thereafter streptococci grow in the cultures in all severely burned patients, the concentration of the organisms increasing with the signs of increasing toxicity in the patient. They have therefore begun treating their patients by the application of gentian violet in 1 per cent solution, without preliminary cleansing of the burned area unless it is covered with oils or grease, and with the patient under a cradle maintained just warm enough for comfort. The solution is sprayed on every two hours in the beginning while the sterile eschar is rapidly forming and the wet oozing areas are becoming dry and tough; blebs are then opened and the sprayings continued at four- to six-hour intervals during the day until healing is complete. Pain has usually ceased by the time the effect of the preliminary narcotic has worn off. Areas of softening from accumulation of secretions, liquefaction of fat or invading infection are carefully removed with forceps and the exposed surfaces sprayed. Unless actual charring has occurred, it is said that islands of epithelium spread rapidly under the scaffolding of the eschar, which is kept trimmed on the periphery as healing progresses. If grafting is to be done the eschar is removed after about three weeks by the application of warm sterile saline compresses.

A patient presenting with an old burn already septic is treated in the same way without preliminary clean-up, but the eschar formed of the necrotic matter and pus is usually removed every day and the area sprayed immediately afterward.

Aldrich states that in his patients thus treated there is no great amount of prostration after the preliminary shock; that they lie quietly in no apparent pain, are cooperative in the matter of taking food and drink so that intravenous supportive measures can be dispensed with, there is little fever and that not of the septic type, and that there are no indications of nephritis or increasing anemia and no fall in chlorides or rise in nonprotein nitrogen.

Connell *et al.* (1933) have used 1 per cent of the dye in a tragacanth jelly base which they place in a thick layer on four or five sheets of gauze and apply to the burned area, repeated applications being unnecessary except in severe cases. To make the 1 per cent jelly add 1 ounce (30 Gm.) of tragacanth to 1000 cc. of 1 per cent aqueous solution of gentian violet. Robertson (1933) apparently proceeds in about the same way as Aldrich in his cases, using however a 1:800 solution of acriflavine.

The following is a list of the principal preparations in use in the treatment of burns in which infection has already occurred:

Picric Acid.—A 1 per cent solution is used; for details, see page 720.

Butesin Picrate Ointment.—The ointment contains 1 per cent of butesin picrate, which combines the anesthetic properties of butesin with the antiseptic properties of picric acid. It is probably of more value in the treatment of mild uninfected burns.

Hydrogen Peroxide.—Diluted with several parts of water, this drug is used several times daily to wash the burned area.

Boric Acid.—Used as the saturated aqueous solution (4 per cent), either as a wash or for compresses.

Resorcinol.—May be used in 1 per cent aqueous solution, or in the same proportion in olive oil (it is nearly insoluble in liquid petrolatum).

Betanaphthol.—This drug is only slightly soluble in water; however, it may be dissolved in a little alcohol and shaken with olive oil or liquid petrolatum in the proportions of 1 part of the betanaphthol to 400 of the oil.

Basic Fuchsin.—Used in 1 per cent aqueous or oily solution, or in an ointment.

Scarlet R.—Used as a 4 to 8 per cent ointment, or in solution in oil.

Gentian Violet.—Used as a 1:5000 solution in water, or a suspension in olive oil or liquid petrolatum, first dissolving the drug in a little alcohol and then shaking with the oil (see, however, the Aldrich method of using the dye in the primary treatment, p. 725).

Acriflavine.—Used as a 1:5000 solution in water, or a suspension in olive oil or liquid petrolatum, first dissolving the drug in a little alcohol and then shaking with the oil. Robertson uses 1:800 in the Aldrich method.

Dichloramine.—Used in 2 per cent solution. Ordinary petrolatum, irrespective of its color, is very destructive of dichloramine, and cannot be used effectively in connection with it. Liquid petrolatum can be used as a vehicle for the dichloramine in emergencies, but the best vehicle is chlorcosane (chlorinated paraffin of the U.S.P. X). Sollmann (1919) has shown that an ointment of 3 parts of ordinary surgical paraffin and 7 parts of liquid petrolatum has relatively little destructive action on dichloramine and can be used as a protective dressing on burns treated with dichloramine-chlorcosane solution, or even as a basis for dichloramine ointment.

Mercurochrome Ointment.—An ointment of the following proportions has been found useful, but Christopher (1932) feels that one should be on guard against possible mercury poisoning if continuous application is made over a long period of time.

℞.	Mercurochrome–220 soluble	gr. x	0.6
	Hydrous wool fat	ʒj	4.0
	Petrolatum to make	ʒj	30.0

LIME BURN OF THE EYE

The first step in the treatment is to drop into the conjunctival sac a few drops of a 1 per cent solution of holocaine, or of a 4 per cent solution of cocaine, in order to relieve the intense pain and to facilitate the manual removal of remaining particles of lime as quickly as possible. The irrigation should be begun at once with a stream of cold water. A weak solution of vinegar, or a sucrose solution, have been often used in the belief that they would neutralize the lime; or milk or olive oil are instilled, after thorough washing, for their soothing effect. Subsequently, cold applications should be made to the closed lids and a boric acid solution dropped into the eyes every two or three hours. I believe it is also considered good practice by some ophthalmologists to fill the conjunctival sac with an antiseptic ointment, such as 1:10,000 mercuric chloride in petrolatum, or 0.5 per cent of the yellow oxide of mercury in the same base.

Neutral Ammonium Tartrate.—In 1905, Zur Nedden showed that a solution of this drug is remarkably efficacious in removing the opacities of the cornea that are the most dreaded of the sequelae of lime burns. Barkan and Barkan (1924) have amply confirmed the findings. The thoroughly cocainized eye should be immersed in a 4 per cent solution for from one-quarter to one-half hour twice daily, within a few days increasing to 10 or 20 per cent, according to the sensibility of the patient. If the burning sensation interferes with the treatment, a drop of cocaine may be instilled and the bath continued. It is of the utmost importance that the solution be freshly made of *neutral* ammonium tartrate (the commercial product usually is slightly acid). Barkan and Barkan also recommend this as emergency treatment, but only provided every particle of the lime has first been washed out of the eye.

WAR GAS BURNS

(See the Chapter on Diseases of the Respiratory Tract, p. 456)

WHITE PHOSPHORUS BURNS

Although white phosphorus has been largely replaced by various substitutes in the industries, this is not true in military practice. During the late World War enormous quantities were used as a smoke screen producer, as an incendiary agent, and above all for its burning and terrorizing effect on hostile troops, when used in Stokes mortar shells, Livens projectors and hand grenades. During the interval between wars it is also being used in troop maneuvers, and a number of serious accidents have occurred, both in filling plants and in the field, as a result of premature bursts of grenades and shells. A great difficulty in the treatment of these burns is that the phosphorus adheres to the flesh, where it continues to fume and occasionally bursts into flame again. The smoldering and fuming is sometimes even resumed after removing the patient from the continuous bath (described on p. 723).

Copper Sulphate.—In recent experimental studies of the various agents available for neutralization of the phosphorus, conducted by Walton in the United States, it was found that this drug is most efficacious as an antidote. He writes as follows:

"As the result of these experiments, a 1 per cent copper sulphate solution is recommended as a treatment for white phosphorus burns, and a 1 per cent solution of copper sulphate should be kept on hand at all shell and grenade filling stations, at Stokes mortar batteries when white phosphorus shells are being used, and at first-aid stations. Large pads of absorbent cotton should also be at hand. Whenever a phosphorus burn is received, a large sponge of absorbent cotton should be saturated with a 1 per cent copper sulphate solution, and applied to the burning phosphorus. Within two or three minutes, it will be possible to remove the sponge. The copper-coated phosphorus should then be removed by forceps or by irrigation, and the case then treated like any other burn."

OBSTETRICS

THE INDUCTION OF LABOR WITH CASTOR OIL, QUININE, AND PITUITRIN (OR PITOCIN)

The method of inducing labor for the relief of distress or undue discomfort at term, or in cases of pregnancy prolonged beyond term, was introduced by Watson, of Toronto, and has come to be quite widely used. Of course, as Watson pointed out, to give pituitrin to a patient with a rigid cervix, or in a case of delay due to a small pelvis, large head, malposition of the head or rigid pelvic floor, is to court disaster, but experience has shown that when smaller doses of pituitrin are used than were originally recommended, and if there is no possible obstruction to the passage of the child, the method properly employed has not been shown to be dangerous either to mother or child. The question of true postmaturity is of course open to discussion, for, as R. W. Holmes well said once before the American Gynecological Society, "We know not when pregnancy begins, therefore we cannot definitely fix the day of confinement. In the classroom this graphic illustration is given: it takes twenty-four hours for a train to go from Chicago to New York. What time does it arrive? The astute student demands the time that it left the first city." However, the condition is undoubtedly seen. Other less frequent indications are found in women whose obstetrical history indicates that they will likely suffer a precipitate labor while en route to the hospital if allowed to go too long, women with ruptured membranes near term, and in instances of progressive toxemia at term. The technic employed by Mathieu and Sichel (1932), who report 96.6 per cent of successful inductions in 320 consecutive cases, is here set down:

"The method is as follows: In the hospital, the patient is given 2 ounces of castor oil and 10 grains of quinine sulphate and exactly two hours afterward, a hot soapsuds enema. As the enema is about to be expelled, 3 minims of pituitary extract are given hypodermically. This same dose of pituitary extract is repeated every thirty minutes until labor starts and *no longer*. From then on, the labor is conducted as though the onset has been normal. Failure is admitted and the procedure stopped if eight hours pass without labor being started or if there is absolutely no sign of any effect toward induction or if the continued use of the injections is too trying to the mother. In such cases the procedure is stopped, the mother is given an hypnotic or sedative and after twenty-four or forty-eight hours, the induction is again attempted.

"During the entire induction the gravida should be flat on her back with only one pillow for her head; failure might follow if she is allowed to walk about." The number of attempts necessary was as follows:

Number of attempts.	Cases.
One	216
Two	62
Three	24
Four	4
Five	3

Nasal Use of Pituitrin.—Hofbauer, Hoerner and Oliver (1927) have reported their attempts to induce labor with the castor oil-quinine-pituitrin combination, applying the latter to the nasal mucous membrane in the hope of accomplishing slower and more even absorption, combined with the ability to stop the action when active labor has been induced. Many physicians have found the method entirely satisfactory. Pitocin may of course be substituted for whole pituitrin.

Technic.—A pledget of cotton, on which has been dropped 20 minims (1.3 cc.) of pituitrin, is placed between the inferior turbinate (absorbing surface) and septum of a previously thoroughly cleansed nostril. After an hour, or at most two hours, it is removed and a similar one placed in the other nostril.

Quinine Idiosyncrasy.—There are a few cases reported in the literature in which children died after the administration of quinine and it was felt that no other explanation than quinine poisoning could account for their death, and there is experimental evidence that the drug may produce intra-uterine death, but the statistics of Sadler, Dilling and Gemmell (1930) show that this risk is not greater than that of stillbirths from undiscovered causes in otherwise normal labors. It is worthy of note, however, that in the last 120 cases of Mathieu's series, cited above, the quinine was omitted because it was found that the method was just as successful without it.

Thymophysin (Thytuitary).—This preparation is a combination of the extracts of thymus and posterior pituitary lobe. It has been much extolled, particularly in the German literature, but I find no evidence, whether pharmacological or clinical, which unequivocally shows its superiority to pituitary substance or pitocin alone.

ANTISEPTIC PREPARATION OF THE VULVA

It is only comparatively recently that the presence of pathogenic bacteria in the vagina has come to be generally recognized, for Williams, in 1893, and again in 1898, confirmed the earlier findings of Krönig that the vagina was sterile or contained only nonpathogenic bacteria. However, in 1912, Jötten examined 100 cases and found streptococci, which were frequently hemolytic, in 67 per cent of the vaginal secretions; Fricke, too, working under Williams, examined 47 patients in their homes, and in this series the vulva contained streptococci in 75 per cent and with the Menge tube the vaginal vault was found to contain the organism in 55 per cent of the cases. The reason for not obtaining growths of organisms in the earlier work was probably the use of improper media. It is now agreed that the organisms do exist in the lower birth canal but that auto-infection does not take place as a usual thing because of the immunity of the woman to the strains of organisms there present. However, the local use of antiseptics to make assurance doubly sure is coming into what seems to me a deserved popularity.

Scrub and Flush.—Perhaps the most usual procedure employed is the following: At the onset of labor the pubic hair is shaved, the patient is given an enema, the bladder is emptied, and finally a bath is taken. With regard to the bath, both Stroganoff in Petrograd and DeLee in Chicago have found that the substitution of the shower for the tub bath has reduced the morbidity of maternity because the soiled water in the tub is bound to get into the vagina to some extent, especially in multiparae; in the average home, however, the shower apparatus is not available. At the time of delivery or of vaginal examination, the vulva, inner thighs, and lastly the anal region are washed carefully with soap and sterile warm water; the patient is to be dried with a sterile towel. Then one of two procedures is followed:

either (*a*) the entire region from the ensiform to the knees is liberally sponged with 1:1500 bichloride of mercury solution, or (*b*) the vulva and thighs alone are irrigated from above with this solution, using about 2 quarts, warmed to body temperature and poured from a pitcher. If delivery is not to follow immediately, a sterile towel is wrung out in the solution and folded over the vulva.

Iodine.—Siddall (1925) has shown that there is some reason to doubt that the usual scrub and flush of the perineum and vulva prior to delivery is as satisfactory as it has been thought to be, and that, indeed, the incidence of puerperal sepsis may be higher where these procedures are employed than in cases in which all predelivery attention, save hair-clipping, is omitted. He then describes the use of 2 per cent iodine solution in labor, painting the vulva, perineum, lower part of the abdomen, inner sides of the thighs, and the part of the head in view just after a pain. Anesthesia must be instituted or continued for a few moments until the burning pain of this application has passed. In a series of 229 spontaneous deliveries he is able to show a puerperal sepsis incidence of only 3.9 per cent as compared with 16.3 and 12.4 per cent for the usual clean-up and for nonpreparation, respectively. Unfortunately, little reliance can be placed upon these figures for the reason that the iodine cases were all delivered by trained obstetricians, the others by interns.

The U.S.P. tincture of iodine diluted with 2 to 3 parts of 70 per cent alcohol may also be used. It is well to bear in mind that in applying iodine after the mercuric chloride solution has been used there is some danger of setting up a severe dermatitis, due to the formation of red mercuric iodide.

Mercurochrome.—Mayes prefers mercurochrome to iodine because (*a*) it can be applied without an anesthetic, is painless, and there is no danger of irritation or blistering of the skin or mucous membrane or vagina or rectum, (*b*) repeated applications can be made during labor and delivery, (*c*) it can be used in large amounts, (*d*) it is apparently harmless to the baby, (*e*) it is not incompatible with the bichloride of mercury, which may have been used in the earlier scrub and flush, and is often used by nurses during catheterization, (*f*) the skin and mucous membranes, although stained, are still soft and pliable, (*g*) it does not coagulate protein, and can be applied to lacerated tissue without injuring the exposed structures. Mayes has been engaged for a number of years in a most careful study of mercurochrome antisepsis in labor; the present technic is here summarized.

Preparation on Admission.—The pubic hair is shaved off and the perineum and surrounding field cleansed with green soap and water, making sure of the removal of all sebaceous material from the labial folds. The external genitalia and surrounding area are sprayed with a 4 per cent aqueous solution of mercurochrome, using a stick sponge if the atomizer does not work properly. The vaginal syringe used, Asepto No. 1 (B.-D. and Co.), has an outside diameter of ⅞ inch, a 7-inch barrel, and is marked for 3 cc. "The syringe should be filled with mercurochrome to this point. Then the labia separated and the point of the syringe is passed along the vaginal floor until it reaches the vault. After the syringe is inserted properly, the labia should be held close together around the syringe with the thumb and finger of a gloved hand. This keeps the fluid from leaking when the bulb is pressed, causes the fluid to enter the vagina under slight pressure and insures its coming in contact with the entire vaginal mucosa. . . . If the labia are not held closely together, or if the instillation is done when the cervix is fully dilated and retracted past the presenting part, it is evident that it is impossible to instill the vagina properly. This is the reason why we insist that the instillation be started as near the beginning of labor as possible. Two small sponges, held one on either labium, will keep the

gloved hand from slipping, and as the syringe is withdrawn and the excess
fluid starts to escape, it may be collected in the syringe by releasing the
bulb and moving the syringe from side to side. Any fluid not taken up by
the syringe is absorbed by the sponges. If the labia are not held closely
together around the syringe, the barrel tends to keep the mercurochrome in
the vagina, but even in spite of this a large part of the fluid will escape
without ballooning the vaginal vault." A thick pad under the patient ab-
sorbs spill from the vagina and saves staining the bed-linen.

Care of the Perineum During Labor.—The perineum is cleansed with
three moist sterile sponges, and the spraying and instillation repeated every
twelve hours. Every two or three hours during active labor all dried blood
and mucus is removed from the perineum; this is considered important.

Vaginal Examination.—The perineum is thoroughly cleansed and
sprayed, the labia separated with the gloved hand and the introitus sprayed.
After inserting two fingers into the vagina and depressing the pelvic floor,
2 drachms (8 cc.) of mercurochrome solution is put into the vagina from
the syringe, the separating and withdrawing of the fingers allowing the
mercurochrome to reach the upper part of the vagina. When vaginal examination is made on admission, vaginal instillation, as above, is made
immediately after.

Preparation for Delivery.—The perineum and surrounding areas are
cleansed, all dried blood and mucus being removed, then dried with a sterile
towel and sprayed with a 4 per cent aqueous, alcohol, acetone, mercurochrome solution (see p. 774). This is done systematically, beginning over
the pubes and moving the atomizer back and forth across the field until
the whole area is covered. *The above acetone solution is never to be used
for the vaginal instillations.* After the pelvic floor is depressed, 2 drachms
of the aqueous solution are put into the vagina. If the delivery is a long
one, or if forceps are applied, more is introduced. If the perineum becomes
soiled with feces, it is cleansed with a moist sponge, more mercurochrome is
instilled or the perineum is sprayed with it. After delivery if there is
laceration or an episiotomy wound to be sutured, the blood is cleared away
and more mercurochrome put into the wound before suturing.

Postpartum Care.—The perineum is sprayed at least once daily with
the aqueous solution. If there has been bad laceration, a previous vaginitis,
or if the patient is a poor risk, 2 drachms of the solution is instilled daily
into the vagina, using Asepto syringe No. 2, which has a diameter of only
½ inch.

In 1932, Mayes stated that at his hospital there were as many maternal
deaths in the 5000 deliveries before the use of mercurochrome as there were
in the 10,000 following its use. Morbidity, computed according to the
standard of the American College of Surgeons and the Congress of Vienna
(a rise in temperature to 100.4 F. on two consecutive days, not including
the first twenty-four hours and occurring on or before the tenth day) has
also steadily declined as the mercurochrome technic has been perfected.

QUININE IN THE FIRST STAGE OF LABOR

Perhaps none of our present-day therapeutic procedures has been so
unfairly treated as the truly valuable use concomitantly of castor oil and
quinine in the attempt to convert a nonproductive into a productive labor.
One cannot escape the impression that prejudice has at least in some instances smothered the evidence. Who has not heard in some northern or

eastern clinic, "Oh, that's alright down South, but it won't work up here"—
the obvious inference being that southern women are more or less attuned
to the action of quinine, all residents of that benighted region having malaria, of course! The Watson method of inducing labor that has not yet begun
is described elsewhere (see p. 728); here we are concerned solely with the
use of quinine and castor oil in patients, usually primiparae, in whom the
head is fixed and there is some dilatation of the cervix, and then productive
labor pauses for many hours. The oil by stimulating peristalsis in the
intestine probably induces a sympathetic muscular action in the uterus, or
perhaps only renders the latter more susceptible to the quinine, which increases the force of the intermittent uterine contractions by direct action
upon the organ.

Method.—In primiparae 1½ ounces of castor oil should be given at
midnight, in multiparae at about 7 o'clock in the morning, the object being
to revive the labor during seasonable daylight hours. As soon as the oil
has acted a hot cleansing enema is given, and immediately thereafter the
first 5-grain (0.32 Gm.) capsule of quinine sulphate; the dose of the latter
to be repeated every half hour until 20 grains (1.3 Gm.) have been taken.
In Germany (Muschallik, 1920), and perhaps elsewhere on the Continent,
the quinine is frequently given intramuscularly or intravenously. The drug
should be stopped if there is complaint of visual or aural symptoms or of
nausea, and the operator must be prepared to terminate the labor if there is
real fetal or maternal distress. It should be further noted that many obstetricians feel that labor after quinine is more painful than it would otherwise have been, and that the tendency toward severe postpartum hemorrhage
is perhaps somewhat increased.

Results.—In Pittsburgh, Williamson (1922) reported on 300 cases, in
which he was successful in inducing labor in 46.6 per cent, divided as follows: Primiparae, aged eighteen to thirty-nine, successful cases, 60, unsuccessful cases, 80; multiparae, aged twenty-one to forty-three, successful
cases, 80, unsuccessful cases, 80.

PITUITRIN (OR PITOCIN) IN THE SECOND STAGE OF LABOR

Immediately after Blair Bell's first report of the use of pituitrin in obstetrics, in 1909, the drug leaped into an immense popularity. In Germany
particularly, during 1911 and 1912, medical journals were filled with eulogis-
tic accounts of its marvelous actions. According to these early reports the
use of the drug was devoid of all danger; forceps were relegated to the
limbo of obsolete things; and the obstetrician, armed with this wondrous
pituitrin and a hypodermic syringe, was easy master of all that might befall
in the course of labor. From the outset its use was resisted in a few centers,
but over most of the world it came very rapidly to be employed almost as a
routine, especially where German influence was strongest. Rucker and
Haskell relate that in certain parts of Cuba, Porto Rico and South America
its use became so common that it was adopted by the midwives. In all of
the United States and Canada only a few leaders were holding out against
it from the very beginning. Then came the reaction. Beginning with the
paper of Edgar, in 1913, there appeared during the next few years so many
reports of the serious occurrences associated with the use of this drug, such
as fatal compression of the fetus, premature separation of the placenta,
tetanic uterine contraction, fetal asphyxia, deep laceration of the cervix,
and fatal rupture of the uterus, that the pendulum noticeably lagged in its

course and those opposed to the drug found the courage to openly advocate its total desertion. And, finally, out of all this great stir in the obstetrical world, it became possible to sort out truth from untruth in regard to the indications, dosage and dangers of this new agent. Pitocin is nowadays of course often substituted for the original pituitrin.

Indications.—I quote the statement of Mundell (1917), which some practitioners look upon as too conservative:

"Its field of usefulness is in secondary inertia during the late stages of the second stage of labor in multiparae. Used here in properly selected cases, after due consideration by one who has good obstetric judgment, its results are usually happy, and it is a boon to the tired mother and her attendants. An ideal case for its use would be a healthy multipara with a history of previous normal labors, late in the second stage of labor, when the pains have become slow and weak, owing to uterine inertia, with a normal presentation and with the bag of waters ruptured, with the cervix fully dilated, and with the head molded and through the brim just above a relaxed perineum. In such a case the baby will usually be born in a remarkable manner after its administration. This may seem to be a narrow field, but we frequently run across just such cases. It is in this type of case that pituitary extract frequently replaces the low forceps operation. The placenta, as a rule, is detached more quickly than usual, and not quite so much blood is lost.

"The administration of an anesthetic when the extract begins to act is a wise measure, and it is well to be always prepared to deliver with forceps. Occasionally, even in these well-defined cases, delivery may not be immediate, and in such cases the result may be bad for the baby. To step beyond these narrow confines of indications is indeed entering on dangerous territory. Especially is this true as regards the life of the baby. It is recommended in small doses by some good authorities and is frequently used in cases of slight contraction at the brim with sometimes very good results if the birth occurs within a few minutes, but frequently with disastrous results to the baby if delivery is delayed. In such cases, forceps are urgently indicated. Its use in such cases is risky beyond question."

Dosage.—It is now fully agreed by all observers that the doses recommended when the drug was introduced are much too large. Where all indications for its use exist, obstetricians are now giving a dose of 3 to 5 minims (0.2 to 0.3 cc.) subcutaneously or preferably intramuscularly. The effect generally appears in ten to twenty minutes (occasionally much sooner and with great violence) and lasts from one-half to one hour; this dose may be cautiously repeated several times at thirty- to sixty-minute intervals. Mundell writes: "I have observed that the first dose usually produces the best reaction, and, when succeeding doses have been required, the results have not been so good."

Dangers.—The great majority of the unfortunate accidents with this drug have resulted from its injudicious use: Either using it when it was contraindicated, or using too much when it was actually indicated. However, the reader is here informed that its use may result in most undesirable consequences even when most properly employed. Cases of rupture of the uterus in the practice of expert obstetricians, using the drug in small dose in the presence of a completely dilated cervix and an unobstructed birth canal, have been reported. Also fetal asphyxia and intracranial hemorrhage, and the incidence of cervical and perineal tears, are certainly higher when it is used. Of course it would be absurd to say that the drug should never be employed in the second stage, for in its proper place and dosage it is a most valuable addition to our armamentarium; but it is a tricky drug, and therefore "safe" doses are not always safe.

ERGOT AND PITUITRIN (OR PITOCIN) IN THE THIRD STAGE OF LABOR

Ergot.—There is little to write regarding the use of this drug save to say that it is the routine practice with many physicians to give by mouth 1 drachm (4 cc.) of the fluidextract at once upon the delivery of the placenta. The effect comes on in fifteen to thirty minutes and lasts from thirty to ninety minutes; the uterus becomes harder under this medication and thus the tendency to postpartum hemorrhage is lessened; perhaps also involution is promoted. The following N.N.R. preparations are sometimes used in place of the fluidextract:

(*a*) Ergot aseptic, 15 to 30 minims (1 to 2 cc.) by intramuscular injection.

(*b*) Gynergen (ergotamine tartrate), one-half to one ampule, containing 8 to 15 minims (0.5 to 1 cc.) intramuscularly; by mouth, 1 tablet (containing 1 mg.) two to four times daily.

Sühs (1930), using small doses of ergot three times daily for the first three or four days postpartum, observed disturbances in the discharge of the lochia and the involution of the uterus with only half the frequency seen in an untreated group of cases; the number in the treated and control groups was fifty-three each.

Ergotole; Extract of Ergot, Purified; Ergotin-Merck; Liquid Ergot-Mulford; and Secacornin have been dropped from N.N.R. until satisfactory methods of assay and satisfactory standards to insure uniform potency are adopted.

Pituitrin (or Pitocin).—A few obstetricians give pituitrin (or pitocin) instead of ergot at once when the placenta has been delivered, and a few careful workers have been studying the use of the drug before the expulsion of the placenta and membranes. Seides (1923) reports on its routine use in this way in 500 cases, taken just as they came: Primiparae, 156; multiparae, 344; spontaneous births, 450; breech cases, 11; transverse, 1; face, 5; brow, 1; twins, 8; hydramnios, 2; prolapsed cord, 3; versions, 7; forceps, 33; anesthesia, 42.

Procedure.—As soon as the fetal head emerged from the vulva, the patient was given 8 minims (0.5 cc.) of pituitrin hypodermically. As soon as signs that the placenta had left the uterus were observed, the attendant placed his hand on the abdomen, spanning the recti muscles, and instructed the patient to bear down. This brought about expulsion of the placenta and terminated the third stage.

Seides gives the following comparison as to time relations: "Normally, after expulsion of the fetus, the unaided uterus remains quiescent for from five to twenty minutes before it begins to contract again. The contractions occur at intervals of four or five minutes. On the average it takes about twenty-five minutes for the placenta to be completely separated. In the 500 consecutive cases in which we used pituitrin in the beginning of the third stage, the average period of rest of the uterus was three minutes. The contractions came on at intervals of two to three minutes. The average number of uterine contractions preceding the signs of placental expulsion from the uterus was two. The average duration of the third stage was seven minutes."

In only 1 case was the placenta retained due to a spasmodic contraction of the internal os; it was relaxed by anesthesia. Manual removal of the placenta was done three times, after the lapse of four, six, and one hours respectively, but in all 3 cases the cervix was found to be open and the hand could easily pass up into the uterus. Immediately after expulsion of the placenta the uterus contracted firmly and stood out prominently; in only 15 cases this contraction was not well maintained, ergot being given then in addition. In no case was there sufficient blood loss to be termed post-partum hemorrhage. During the first period after delivery, ranging from six to twelve hours, after-pains occurred more frequently than is usual, occurring even among primiparae. Subsequently the after-pains were in-frequent and mild. Involution of the uterus progressed so satisfactorily that a great number of the patients were allowed out of bed as early as the fifth day. When discharged on the tenth day, in 473 cases the uterus was well down in the pelvis, and in only 27 was the fundus above the symphysis.

POSTPARTUM HEMORRHAGE

Serious or fatal postpartum bleeding may be due to any of the following causes: Lacerations somewhere along the tract; abnormal placenta; retained placenta; uterine atony, the causes of which are many; constitutional dis-ease; retained placental fragments or blood clots; subinvolution; neoplasms. The measures employed in checking the hemorrhage are merely mentioned here, the reader being advised to consult a text-book on obstetrics for a detailed description of their use: Massage of the uterus through the abdomen to facilitate the separation of the placenta; compression of the uterus through the abdomen to facilitate expression of the placenta; manual re-moval of the placenta; hot or cold douching of the uterine cavity; com-pression of the uterus in anteflexion; packing of the uterus with sterile gauze; repair of lacerations; administration of ergot (see p. 734) and pitu-itrin (see p. 734); saline solution by hypodermoclysis and proctoclysis; blood transfusion; compression of the abdominal aorta.

OBSTETRICAL ANESTHESIA

The indications for anesthesia in labor are the following: (*a*) The relief of excessive pain in the first stage after the pains have become frequent and regular; (*b*) the relief of excessive pain in the second stage; (*c*) the relief of great excitement in the first or second stage; (*d*) to check the patient's refusal to bear down because of pain in the second stage; (*e*) to decrease the force of excessive contractions of the uterus at either the end of the first or during the second stage in order to lessen the likelihood of uterine rupture or cervical or perineal tears; (*f*) to protect the infant from harmful pressure when the uterus is excessively contracting; (*g*) to facilitate surgical repair of injured tissues; (*h*) and in general to protect the woman from the un-necessary and profound physical and psychic shock of labor.

CHLOROFORM AND ETHER IN THE SECOND STAGE

It is the practice of most physicians to give a few whiffs of chloroform or ether to dull the worst of the pains when the effacement of the cervix is being completed, and to anesthetize the patient to whatever extent is neces-sary to relieve most of the final agony when the head is emerging from the vulva. In what follows I shall attempt a comparison of ether and chloro-form for these purposes.

Method and Dosage.—Regarding ether, I quote DeLee: "Any simple inhaler, or even a handkerchief held in the hand, will suffice. The open method is preferred, because in obstetrics the carbonization of the blood, so common in general anesthesia, must be avoided in the interests of the child. When the pain begins, 45 drops [about 3 cc.] of ether are poured on the mask, and the patient takes deep breaths of the vapor; as the pain increases a few drops more are given; as the pain subsides, the mask is removed. The patient obtains relief from pain, but consciousness is not abolished. This procedure is repeated until the head is just about to escape from the vulva, when the ether is poured on frequently, and the first stage of surgical anesthesia is reached, consciousness being abolished for a few minutes, during which time the infant is delivered. Administration begins at the end of the first stage."

The usual method of using chloroform is to apply to the mask, or to a bit of cotton held in the hand, 5 to 10 drops (about 0.3 to 0.6 cc.) of the drug to be inhaled during the twenty to thirty seconds of the height of each severe pain. During the last expulsive pains the number of drops may be increased to 15 (1 cc.) for each pain, or, if considered necessary, the rate of dropping may be maintained at 5 to 10 for every ten seconds in order to insure a brief period of complete analgesia during the last agony.

In England at present, extensive trial is being made of small ampules, much like those used for amyl nitrite, each containing 20 minims of chloroform and intended to be crushed in a bit of gauze by the patient herself and held over the nose. It is hoped that by this means an effective method of bringing an analgesic measure into the hands of midwives will be developed. Rivett (1933) has analyzed the records of nearly 4000 cases in which the capsules were used at Queen Charlotte's and the Middlesex Hospitals. In over 90 per cent of instances the patient obtained relief from pain, great relief in more than 50 per cent. In over 60 per cent the course of labor was not altered; in about 15 per cent progress seemed to be assisted by abolishing the restraining efforts of the patient. Occasionally labor was prolonged but never seriously; the number of cases in which instruments were used was below the average but probably because the capsules are employed only in normal cases.

A rather satisfactory method of enabling the woman to administer her own anesthetic at times is to stuff a large piece of blotting paper in an ordinary glass tumbler, pour a few drops of chloroform on it, and direct the patient to hold it an inch above her mouth and inhale during the height of each severe pain; as she becomes narcotized the hand falls away from its strained position and the anesthetic is thus withdrawn. Unfortunately, the glass often falls from the hand and may roll away out of reach. I have also read of a device by which the cone was suspended on a rubber band just above the head but high enough that it had to be reached for and held over the mouth and nose by the patient; when relaxation came, she of course released her hold on the cone, which was then drawn up out of respiratory range. Brown (1933) is employing the inhaler shown in the accompanying illustration, which embodies the principle of the unspillable inkwell; if made of metal, or preferably heavy glass, the inhaler will not break if dropped. Dimensions 3 x 1½ inches over all; distance between the two open ends, ¾ inch.

Efficiency.—From the standpoint of efficiency in producing these brief periods of analgesia, chloroform has the following advantages: (*a*) It is quicker in action than ether, (*b*) the dose is smaller, therefore it is less bulky to carry in the satchel, (*c*) it is pleasanter to take and causes less suffocation and excitement in the patient.

Effect on Labor.—It is generally held that both drugs diminish the pains and thus delay labor somewhat, and that chloroform is the worse offender in this regard; but it is extremely probable that, in the small doses used by careful physicians, neither drug very materially lessens the uterine activity.

Also it is well to bear in mind that either of them may actually hasten labor by checking the patient's unwillingness to completely bear down because of pain.

Effect on Hemorrhage.—Both drugs are held to increase hemorrhage by producing relaxation of the uterus, chloroform certainly to a greater extent than ether.

Deleterious Effects on Mother (Acute).—Acute death of the mother under either ether or chloroform, when properly used in obstetrics, is so very rare that many observers believe the pregnant woman to be peculiarly resistant; however, it seems much more likely that the low mortality is due to the small doses employed.

Deleterious Effects on Infant (Acute).—These are practically nil when the drugs are properly used, though it is unquestionably a fact that chloroform diminishes the oxygen capacity of the blood.

Deleterious Effects on Mother (Delayed).—Ether is irritating to the mother's respiratory tract, and if much has been administered there will be nausea and postpartum vomiting; chloroform escapes both these charges. In general surgery, where full anesthesia is established and maintained for a variable time in all cases, postanesthetic albuminuria occurs in about one fourth of the ether cases and one third of the chloroform cases; in the light grades of anesthesia employed in obstetrics the occurrence of this symptom is relatively rare, but the proportions between ether and chloroform probably still obtain. Aspiration pneumonia is more frequent after ether than chloroform, but at most its occurrence is very rare following obstetrical anesthesia. Ether is contraindicated in the presence of acute respiratory disease, but actually it is often employed without damage; in chronic respiratory affections it is not contraindicated.

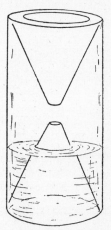

Chloroform is especially harmful in the presence of .hepatic disease, pregnancy toxemia, eclampsia, nephritis, heart disease, toxic goiter, sepsis diabetes mellitus, and the other chronic wasting diseases. With late, or "secondary" chloroform death, due to the toxic effect of the drug upon the liver during surgical anesthesia, all are familiar, but it is perhaps not so well known or

Chloroform inhaler of R. Christie Brown (Lancet, February 18, 1933).

admitted that this occurrence sometimes follows light and intermittent obstetrical anesthesia.

Deleterious Effects on Infant (Delayed).—It is all but universally admitted that even small amounts of chloroform administered during the course of labor may cause marked fatty degeneration in the livers of the newborn.

Danger from Decomposition of the Drugs.—Ether is inflammable and explosive and cannot be safely used near an open flame, but as a matter of fact accidents with it are very rare. Chloroform, under the same circumstances, is decomposed into hydrochloric acid, chlorine, and carbonyl chloride (phosgene gas), which are not only very irritating to the respiratory tract of all persons present and toxic as well, but greatly increase the incidence of postpartum pneumonia in the mother.

For Physician Working Alone.—From the foregoing comparison it is apparent that ether is superior on most counts, and it is certainly used almost exclusively in hospitals or private practice in the cities where trained assistance can be easily obtained; but I cannot agree with the metropolitan obstetricians, many of whom maintain that chloroform has no longer any place in obstetrics and should be abandoned even in country practice. Let us not forget that all over the world are many doughty physicians who are forced by circumstances to practice in a rough and ready manner; keen observers of fact, who scorn the notion that chloroform can at present be dispensed with by them. Witness Simpson, before a relatively recent session of the American Medical Association: "I am in country practice and often deliver women without any assistance. I have to use chloroform. All other anesthetics are out of the question when one man does the operating and gives the anesthetic at the same time." And Carstens: "If you are out in the country, five miles from nowhere, with nobody in the house but the husband, and he faints and you have to take him by the collar and put him out in the snow and then come back into the house and give that woman an anesthetic all alone, and put on forceps—I would like to see anybody do it and give ether. I uphold everything that is said about ether when you have all the facilities, the anesthetist, and the assistants in the hospitals, but leave chloroform to the general practitioner who has to do the whole work."

It is worthy of note that recently (1932) the announcement that chloroform would be replaced by ether at the famous Rotunda Hospital, in Dublin, because of the greater danger of the former, provoked a large number of adverse comments in the British medical journals, all to the effect that the general practitioner finds chloroform much more valuable for the reasons above stated.

NITROUS OXIDE-OXYGEN IN THE SECOND STAGE

The delivery room studies of Lynch, Skeel, C. H. Davis, Danforth and others during the past few years have popularized the use of gas-oxygen analgesia.

Method and Efficiency.—Danforth and Davis write as follows:

"Nitrous oxide is the one thing yet thoroughly tested which will relieve the pain of labor without at the same time diminishing the force and frequency of the uterine contractions, and which may be used for periods up to several hours without appreciable loss in the force of the uterine contraction.

"We have felt that, as a general thing, it is wise to restrict the giving of gas to periods not exceeding three hours. We have both, on rare occasions, extended its use over much longer periods without untoward results, but believe that very extended periods of administration may produce some fetal asphyxiation. A two-hour period will include the great majority of cases.

"The gas may be given pure or mixed with oxygen. In cases in which a small number of breaths suffice to control the pain of a contraction, the nitrous oxide alone will do. In others, oxygen may be combined in varying proportion as the individual patient may need.

"One most essential point to which we have both drawn attention in previous communications is the necessity of commencing the giving of gas for each pain immediately on the onset of the contraction. When it is not begun till after the pain is well started, it is not possible to obtain the maximum relief, and in many cases there is but little or no benefit. Failure to pay attention to this point has been responsible for most poor results.

"The number of breaths of the gas or mixture varies from three to six in the majority of cases. It is necessary to ascertain in each case what dosage is needed, and to increase it as needed. This is not difficult, and a little experience renders it easy. We may mention also that use of hypodermic medication in the first stage often renders the giving of gas in the second stage easier.

"The intermittent administration of gas may be continued, as we have indicated, through the second stage till near its end, when light anesthesia is needed. As the head distends the perineum and delivery is evidently at hand, we have found it to be of decided advantage in most cases to add a little ether, which may be done by means of the ether attachment with which most gas machines are equipped. As delivery is actually to be accomplished, the patient is told to breathe rapidly and deeply so that a brief unconsciousness is produced, during which delivery occurs. A method which in our work has been very satisfactory is as follows: After the head has advanced till delivery is imminent and the woman is taking the gas-ether combination, we rapidly deepen the anesthesia to unconsciousness, and then by a Kristeller expression cause the child to be delivered. As the head emerges, the ether is turned off, and, as the delivery is completed, the anesthetist rapidly empties the bag of the gas apparatus, and then allows the mother to breathe pure oxygen. This, we have thought, helps the child rapidly to attain a normal pinkness. If the cord is not pulsating, oxygen may be given directly to the baby by means of the ordinary nasal inhaler. This is very important in all cases in which there is any evidence of fetal asphyxia or delayed breathing. In many cases the mother will be wholly unaware of the delivery."

Gas in Operative Obstetrics.—"When it is desired to do an episiotomy, if the gas is continued from one pain through the interval between pains and into the next pain, as a rule the incision may be made without pain and often without the mother's knowledge.

"While we desire particularly to emphasize the value of this mode of pain relief in spontaneous labor, as it is in these that effective analgesia is most frequently lacking, we have found that nitrous oxide-oxygen is applicable to the majority of obstetrical operations. Here, however, the problem becomes one of proper administration of surgical anesthesia. This is a little more difficult, but is entirely possible and practicable and quite within the power of any reasonably well-trained anesthetist.

"The most frequent obstetrical operation is the outlet forceps operation. This, in the majority of cases, may be done under gas-oxygen with entire satisfaction. The anesthetic is carried to the point at which voluntary motion does not occur when instrumentation is begun, but it is not necessary or desirable to push it to the point of complete relaxation. The operation is then carried out in the usual way. We have found that with an anesthesia so light that uterine contractions continue, the expenditure of tractive force on the forceps is less than is otherwise needed, with a correspondingly lessened amount of operative trauma on the fetal head. The amount of tractive force needed may be still further reduced by using (Kristeller) pressure on the fundus of the uterus.

"The ordinary perineal repair is done with ease under a properly given gas anesthetic. There is usually no objection to ether for the repair.

"The more difficult forceps extractions, those done on the head lying in the midplane or engaged in the pelvic inlet, may also be carried out satisfactorily under gas. We would here, however, voice the caution that when deep narcosis is to be maintained for a protracted period prior to delivery, ether be used, as prolonged administration of gas experimentally has been shown to produce tissue change in the young of laboratory animals, comparable to asphyxiation.

"Operations that require marked uterine relaxation for their safe carrying out are better done under ether. Version and manual rotation of the head are the outstanding exceptions to the use of gas. Those who desire to use the method described by Kielland for the introduction of his forceps on a head in the transverse or occiput posterior position, with the intra-uterine rotation of the anterior forceps blade, should use ether to avoid wounding the unrelaxed uterine wall. We believe, therefore, that nitrous oxide-oxygen may be applied to almost all obstetrical operations, the only exceptions being those requiring marked uterine relaxation. During analgesia while the child is in the uterus we believe that rebreathing should be avoided, and it is better that the intermittent administration of gas should not exceed three hours."

Dangers and Objections.—A properly given gas analgesia carries with it practically no risks for either mother or child, but I believe the fact cannot be too strongly stressed that if carried to the point of anesthesia it does become quite dangerous. In all but the specialty hospitals most of the obstetrical anesthetics are given by nurses or untrained interns; which, in the nature of things, is quite alright unless the obstetrician yields to the temptation to allow this amateur anesthetist to push the gas to the point of complete anesthesia for perineal repair—to do this is to court disaster!

Regarding the effect of this anesthetic on bleeding, Danforth and Davis confirm the experience of all observers when they say: "A very definite advantage which the use of gas for operative work possesses is the increased activity of uterine muscle after anesthesia. This to a considerable degree diminishes bleeding, and measures for the control of blood loss are needed much less frequently than when working with anesthetics which cause a more marked muscular relaxation."

Of course the principal objection to the use of gas-oxygen is the fact that it is not available for use outside of hospitals or the homes of the financially more fortunate classes, for not only must the tanks and apparatus be transported, but a person qualified to operate the same must be provided.

ETHYLENE-OXYGEN IN THE SECOND STAGE

Ethylene is preferred in a number of hospitals for the reason that analgesia can often be obtained with weaker mixtures of it than of nitrous oxide; also it has a shorter induction period than the latter gas. However, it seems that most obstetricians are in agreement with Plass and Swanson (1926), in whose report of its use in 592 women in labor is the statement, "We have made no attempt to develop the full anesthetic effect of the gas and have preferred to add ether rather than to lower the percentage of oxygen to the point at which cyanosis became evident. The addition of small amounts of ether over short periods has been looked on as not essentially undesirable." In other words, ethylene is being used just as is nitrous oxide: to take the worst edge off the pains of the latter part of the first stage and those of the second stage, perhaps even to abolish them altogether; but when anesthesia is wanted for the final expulsive period, then ether is added. It should be noted that relaxation is perhaps on the whole better with this new gas, so that the use of ether is not so often necessary as with nitrous oxide.

The gas has the same objections as apply in the case of nitrous oxide; namely, that it is ill suited for home use, especially in the country, as it requires much apparatus and the services of a trained anesthetist. In addition it is highly explosive, and its use is very dangerous except in operating rooms in which every chance of ignition has been carefully eliminated. It does not seem to delay labor any more than does nitrous oxide, but it does increase bleeding slightly more than the other gas; Sanford (1926) has shown that this is also true of the bleeding time in the newborn. Neither ethylene nor nitrous oxide, however, increases the bleeding as do ether and chloroform. A number of observers have remarked the fact that vomiting is more frequent after ethylene than after nitrous oxide; also a few patients find the "molasses" or "phosphorus matches" odor of ethylene objectionable.

SPINAL ANESTHESIA

The various methods are being studied in several centers both in this country and abroad, but it seems to me that the subject is still too entirely in the experimental stage to warrant description here. Two principal objections to the employment of any of these methods have in no wise been overcome as yet: First, the fact that the period of anesthesia lasts only from forty-five minutes to two hours; and second, that very great skill and special technical knowledge are required in those who introduce dangerous drugs by this route.

ETHER-OIL ANESTHESIA

Since 1923, Gwathmey, of New York, and his associates have been studying what they chose to call in the beginning "painless childbirth by synergistic methods," the thesis being that the intramuscular injection of magnesium sulphate synergizes (*i. e.*, potentiates or increases) the analgesic power of the morphine with which it is injected, and also the ether subsequently used, to such extent that it is possible to carry a woman through a relatively painless labor by the use of an otherwise ineffective amount of ether-oil by rectum. Quinine, and alcohol for its solution, is added to the ether-oil retention enema in order to overcome the delay in labor that the mixture admittedly might otherwise cause. My own studies have perhaps established a basis in animal experimentation for the great efficiency claimed for the method, but upon the point of the actual occurrence of synergism between magnesium sulphate and morphine I have never been able to agree; however this is probably largely an academic point, and can certainly be allowed to rest for the moment. In recent years I have made a thorough study of the literature of the subject and have become firmly convinced that this method of lessening the suffering of childbirth is the simplest, safest, and most effective for wide and general application that has been devised to date.

Technic.—The following is Harrar's description of the technic employed at the New York Lying-in Hospital, where the method has been largely developed. I have employed italics to bring out sharply the points of drug administration.

"The treatment should not be started until the woman is in active labor. The pains should be at least at five-minute intervals and lasting at least forty seconds. The length of the contractions are best judged by placing the hand on the abdomen and timing them with the watch, as the outcry of the woman is often a poor index of the strength of the pain. Waiting for the labor to be well-established thus at once eliminates cases of so-called 'primary inertia' from treatment. In a primipara it is best to wait until the cervix is fairly well effaced and dilated to a diameter of at least two fingertips; in a multipara it can be started before this degree of cervical dilation is reached, if the pains are of the proper length and interval as described. *At this time a cleansing soapsuds enema is given, and this is followed by the primary, intramuscular injection of ⅙ or ¼ grain (0.01 or 0.015 Gm.) of morphine and 2 cc. of 50 per cent solution of magnesium sulphate deep into the gluteal region.* Judgment must be used as to the soapsuds enema, as it may not be required, if the customary soapsuds enema at the onset of labor has been recently given. The rectum must be both empty and quiescent to retain properly the instillation of ether in oil that is to follow the primary morphine and magnesium sulphate intramuscular injection. Experience has shown that ¼ grain (0.015 Gm.) of morphine is usually the proper dose, but in a small woman ⅙ grain (0.01 Gm.) will be sufficient. Labor should be well under way as previously stated, so that the morphine will not stop the uterine contractions altogether. Tell the patient the object is to relieve her pain, but do not promise her a painless labor.

"After this primary intramuscular injection of morphine and magnesium sulphate the patient is to be kept quiet, oiled cotton is placed in the auditory canal, and the room is darkened. These attentions are reminiscent of the scopolamine amnesia suggestions, but they are of undoubted value in the proper induction of any seminarcosis. *Twenty minutes after the primary morphine and magnesium sulphate injection we give a second intramuscular injection consisting of 2 cc. of 50 per cent solution of magnesium sulphate alone. This is given no matter whether the effect of the primary injection is sedative or not, as it tends to prolong the action of the morphine.*

"We now come to the manner of giving and the time of the rectal instillation. It must not be used too soon. If the effect of the morphine and magnesium sulphate is sedative, withhold the instillation until the effect of the former is almost worn off. It is easier to give when the patient is still somewhat under the effect of the morphine; however, three- to five-minute intervals between uterine contractions should be present. For the beginner it is better to let the morphine and magnesium sulphate wear off entirely and to withhold the instillation until the patient is again complaining and the pains, at three- to five-minute intervals, are good and strong. *If there is no relief from the morphine and magnesium sulphate within one-half hour after the second injection, which consisted of 2 cc. of 50 per cent magnesium sulphate alone, proceed with the ether instillation.* The ether instillation thus rarely should be given within an hour after the first injection of morphine and magnesium sulphate. It may be from one to three hours before it is needed, depending on the patient's distress. The ideal time in a primipara is at about three fingertips' dilation of the cervix.

"The retention enema which can readily be prepared by any druggist, consists of:

R.	Quinine alkaloid	gr. xx	1.2
	Alcohol	ℳxl	2.4
	Ether	ℨiiss	75.0
	Olive oil to make	ℨiv	120.0

"It is given as follows: The contents of the bottle containing the ether mixture and the bottle containing 2 ounces of plain olive oil are warmed by letting them stand for a few minutes in warm water, first loosening or removing the corks. The patient is then placed on her left side and vaseline is liberally applied around the anus so that the ether mixture if expelled will not irritate. State to the patient, just before beginning the instillation, that its object is to relieve her pain, and thus secure her cooperation. Tell her that during the instillation she is not to press down during pains, but to breathe deeply with her mouth open, and at all times to 'draw up' with her sphincter as if she were trying to avoid expelling gas. This will tend to induce reverse peristalsis and permit the fluid to run in more readily.

"The apparatus consists of a 4-ounce funnel attached to a 20-inch length of rubber tubing, which is in turn connected by a glass connecting tip to a red rubber catheter, size 20 or 22 French. A rectal tube is too large.

"Pour into the funnel 1 ounce of warm, plain olive oil. Just as the oil runs out of the catheter pinch the latter near the glass connecting tip with an artery clamp. In this way all the air will be expelled from the tubing. Some of the 1 ounce of oil should still remain in the funnel. The catheter is now introduced into the rectum for about 4 inches. If the fetal head is well down in the pelvis, the gloved finger must be inserted into the rectum along with the catheter to insure its passage past the head. A little of the warm ether mixture is added to the oil in the funnel, the clamp released and the contents of the funnel slowly permitted to run into the rectum. The remainder of the ether mixture is gradually added, at no time permitting the funnel to become entirely empty. Just as the last of the ether mixture is about to leave the funnel, add the remaining ounce of the warm plain olive oil. Allow this to start running into the rectum and clamp the tube. It is important in order to avoid the expulsive desire that we prevent the entrance of any air bubbles into the rectum. Now make pressure on the anus with a towel during two or three contractions, leaving the pinched catheter in place meanwhile, then gently withdraw the catheter. Should a uterine contraction intervene during the instillation simply make pressure against the anus with a folded towel and let the funnel act as the escape reservoir. Continue to make pressure over the anus during three or four contractions after the catheter is removed. All these details are important and the successful retention of the instillation largely depends on the meticulous care with which it is given.

"*A third intramuscular injection of 2 cc. of a 50 per cent solution of magnesium sulphate alone is then given immediately to prolong the action of the ether.* The patient may now turn upon her back or assume whatever position is most agreeable to her. The same quiet is maintained as before. Do not make a vaginal or rectal examination too soon after the instillation or the instillation will be expelled. Do not be misled by the quiet behavior of the patient into thinking she is having very slight contractions or none at all. Within fifteen or twenty minutes you can smell ether on her breath, she becomes flushed, and occasionally has a little of the excitability of the first stage of ether anesthesia, but rarely to the extent of requiring restraint.

"The patient is drowsy and sleeps lightly between the pains, but consciousness is not entirely lost. She responds somewhat tardily to questions and usually obeys commands as to change in posture. When a uterine contraction occurs she manifests her suffering to a greater or lesser degree and again dozes. Occasionally the casual observer would have the impression that there was very little amelioration of the pain, the patient complaining and restless during the contractions, and yet afterward we find the amnesia secured to have been as definite as that after scopolamine. Frequently the patient confesses of her own volition that she remembered very little after the rectal instillation was given.

"The obstetrical side of the case and the progress of labor must be closely watched. Functional abnormalities must be discovered and corrected as they arise, and the mechanism of labor followed and managed as thoroughly as though no analgesia were being employed.

"*When the effect of the first ether instillation has worn off; that is, when the patient again complains of pain, which is usually in from two to three hours, a second, or even a third, rectal instillation may be given at intervals of three hours or more. The first instillation given contains 20 grains (1.2 Gm.) of quinine alkaloid; in subsequent instillations only 10 grains (0.6 Gm.) are used. Each subsequent instillation is accompanied with one intramuscular injection of 2 cc. of a 50 per cent magnesium sulphate solution.* Contrary to some authorities we are convinced that the quinine is absorbed by the rectum, as evidenced by the occasional complaint of buzzing and ringing in the ears or slight deafness after the labor. We tried 30 cases, omitting the quinine entirely and found the omission of the quinine caused definite second stage and perineal delay. Dr. Losee, of the hospital laboratory, has now definitely proved the rectal absorption of quinine by its qualitative recovery from the urine in 92 out of 100 parturients.

"A minimum of inhalation ether is needed for the delivery, and the anesthetist must be cautioned about this. Frequently no additional anesthesia is needed even for a perineorrhaphy. Chloroform should never be used with the ether rectal instillation. Gas, if desired, is safe and very satisfactory as an adjuvant anesthetic for the delivery."

Efficacy.—In Gwathmey's report of 1930, the following statistics from several hospitals are offered; the reports of many physicians whose individual experience runs only into one or several hundreds of cases would in the aggregate add many thousands of cases to this list, but it seems to me that the compilation of such a table would be little more impressive than the fact that such hospitals as Gwathmey lists have continued to employ the method with satisfaction for what has now become much more than an experimental period.

STATISTICS OF OBSTETRICAL ANALGESIA (GWATHMEY METHOD)

	Cases.
Lying-in Hospital, New York	
The "Analgesic Record" charts for two years show that the method is used on an average of 240 times each month (approximately 68 per cent of all cases), or 2880 times per year; and that for the five years since the method was introduced it has been used in	14,000
(This does not include the private cases, which are not charted.)	
New York Nursery and Child's Hospital, New York	
Between 500 and 600 obstetrical analgesias per year are given, a total for five years of over	2,500
Manhattan Maternity Hospital, New York	
Four hundred cases a year, or, for five years	2,000
Cincinnati General Hospital, Cincinnati, Ohio, and private cases of Drs. Crudington, Beatty, and others	2,000

It has been the practically universal experience that partial or complete relief from pain results in from 80 to 90 per cent of instances, often with the added advantage of amnesia, as pointed out above by Harrar. The progress of labor is not delayed, rotation occurs in about the same proportion as otherwise, and postpartum hemorrhage is said to occur with less frequency than with any inhalation method. The incidence of forceps delivery seems to have been markedly decreased. No fetal deaths attributable to the method have been recorded, the baby usually being born crying, the patients go through labor with less postpartum fatigue, and the careful follow-up studies at the New York Lying-in Hospital have found no contraindications with regard to after-effects. The applicability of the method to the conditions of general practice is amply testified to by many physicians. Gwathmey (1930) writes:

"The house surgeons of the Lying-in Hospital are changed every four months, as are also their associates and assistants. Since starting this method it has been in the hands of over 200 inexperienced men, none of whom knew anything of either colonic anesthesia or obstetrical analgesia before coming to the hospital. The method has been employed over three thousand times in the Out-patient Department of the hospital, in the homes of the patients, where it is given under the most trying conditions imaginable, but even under these circumstances it is successful in over 80 per cent of the cases, and no fatalities attributable to the method have occurred. We are justified in stating that it is simpler than any other method, and can be used anywhere. In not a single instance has an anesthetist been used with the method, even in its initial development. The ingredients are cheap, and the mixture can be prepared easily by any pharmacist, or by physicians who are accustomed to prepare their own medicines."

Preparations said to contain the proper mixture in an ether-tight and catalytically inert container are now commercially available but I do not know to what extent they fulfill all the requirements.

Objections to the Method.—(a) *Synergism.*—My quarrel with the use of this term has been referred to earlier.

(b) *Magnesium Sulphate.*—It would seem to be without point for me longer to hold out against the use of so much of this drug, as I did in the first edition of this book. The practical experience of a large number of physicians in many thousands of cases shows that respiratory embarrassment whether to mother or child does *not* occur.

(c) *Excitement*—The only reports of an initial period of very annoying excitement have come out of central Europe, where the method is much employed; but in recent years there has been no mention of such occurrences, which strongly indicates that increased experience has shown where the fault lay.

Local Effects in Anal Region.—Writing on this point, Harrar says: "Close attention to all the details of giving the retention enema will obviate its loss in bulk. The frequent extrusion of small quantities of light yellow, sour-smelling, liquid fecal matter, making it more difficult to keep the field clean in the perineal stage, will not occur if the cleansing soapsuds enema is completely expelled before giving the rectal instillation. In some cases nausea is present, but not as commonly as after inhalation etherization. Patients will at times complain of a slight burning sensation in the anal region immediately after the rectal instillation. The liberal use of vaseline will prevent this, though it sometimes may be due to an unrecognized fissure. Now and then there is some distention of the colon with gas but not to any serious degree. Rarely the patient has diarrhea during the first twenty-four hours postpartum." McCormick (1932) feels that so far as colitis, hemorrhoids, fissure, fistula and gross rectal pathology are concerned, the reaction from the ether-oil mixture is perhaps no more pronounced than the proctoscopically proved irritation of the cleansing soapsuds enema, which in itself he considers a very likely factor in the occasional instillation burning. For my own part I do not see why sodium bicarbonate enemas (see p. 434) should not be routinely substituted. Emge and Cooley (1929) had six quite distressing irritations in their series of 200 deliveries, but not of sufficient seriousness to check their enthusiasm for the method. Most other reports, however, hardly mention the subject at all; for instance, Stevens (1932), whose series comprised 540 cases, merely says, "if the technic is followed no inflammation of even a mild type occurs."

Other Objections.—An occasional instance of mild idiosyncrasy to quinine on the part of the mother is recorded, but I find no report of lasting or even acutely dangerous symptoms in either mother or child. Most observers believe that, because of the quinine, the method should not be employed in a woman having any preexisting auditory disturbances, but of other marked contraindications there seem to be none save such as are indicated in the discussion above. Apparently the method can be used with safety in all normal cases, in dystocia, in toxemias, in cardiac and nephritic cases, and in tuberculous conditions.

"Fool-proof" this method certainly is not, and with it as with any other technical procedure practice tends toward perfection; still, I feel that its rules are simple and easily learned and that this practical aid in obstetrics could probably be acquired very profitably by many more practitioners than have as yet familiarized themselves with it.

Modification in Technic.—Of numerous modifications proposed from time to time, that of McCormick is the only one which seems particularly attractive. He makes the point that the average practitioner does not perhaps always make the injection of the magnesium sulphate into the buttock correctly, as shown in the sketch on the next page, and therefore at times has an abscess to deal with. He is therefore studying the substitution of barbiturates, finally settling upon pentobarbital sodium, which he gives orally in a dose of 3 grains (0.2 Gm.) and 1½ grains (0.1 Gm.), respectively, in place of the first two magnesium sulphate injections. The morphine is given with the second dose if the patient is a primipara and the labor active, but if the labor is of the prolonged sort, the second dose of the pentobarbital is repeated once or oftener before giving the morphine. His results, so far in every way satisfactory, will be interesting to watch. Sodium amytal he had discarded after trial in 200 cases because of the restlessness it caused. McNeile and Vruwink (1927), however, were satisfied with the effect of substituting the hypodermic injection of 3 grains (0.2 Gm.) of sodium

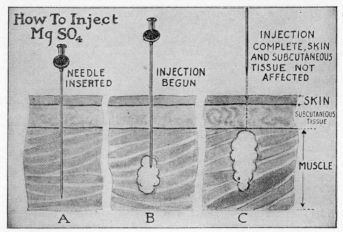

Magnesium sulphate injection (New York Lying-in Hospital).

barbital (veronal) for the magnesium sulphate in their first 200 cases; I do not know what their subsequent experience has been.

BARBITURATE ANESTHESIA

Under this head will be discussed briefly those barbiturates which have been principally used by mouth, sodium amytal and pentobarbital sodium (nembutal). The intravenous use of sodium amytal will not be discussed for the reason that the vast majority of physicians in this country concur in the opinion of the Council on Pharmacy and Chemistry (Jour. Amer. Med. Assoc., 97, 1886, 1931; ibid., 101, 208, July 15, 1933) that any advantages that may exist in the choice of barbiturates as aids in anesthesia can be easily procured by giving the drugs by mouth, thus avoiding the obvious disadvantages of employing the intravenous route. (The intravenous administration in eclampsia—where tradition at least has hallowed an abandonment to heroic measures—is perhaps another matter. See p. 755.)

Sodium Amytal.—A quite large literature has appeared on this subject, the typical methods and results being such as reported by Van Del (1933), who gave the drug by mouth to 150 patients when regular pains occurred accompanied by cervical dilatation. To 75 of these patients an initial dose of 9 grains (0.6 Gm.) was given, and in about three hours, as labor advanced, a second dose of 6 grains (0.4 Gm.). The initial dose in the other 75 patients was 15 grains (1 Gm.) followed by a second dose of 6 grains (0.4 Gm.). Using complete amnesia within one hour after administration of the drug as the criterion of efficiency, results were only fair with the initial 9-grain dose but very good with the dose of 15 grains. The sedative action was noted in about twenty-five minutes, the patient going to sleep; during contractions she became restless and cried out, but as the pain receded became somnolent again. Physically the patients passed well through labor but they did not cooperate well in "bearing down"; however, it seems that labor was not prolonged. No deleterious effects were noted in the babies and the postpartum periods were passed without unusual incidents. Immediately following delivery the patients usually slept for six hours and usually had only a slight recollection of the labor. •

About 10 per cent of Van Del's patients became quite restless as a result of the drug, moving about and disarranging the sterile field. This is a complaint against the drug by nearly all who have used it. Another objection often heard is that the number of instrumental deliveries is increased. Whether the incidence of apneic or narcotized babies is somewhat above the normal figure is a matter over which there is some wrangling at the present time, but I suspect that as the reports accumulate general acknowledgment of such increase will be necessary.

Sodium Amytal and Morphine.—In a group of 50 patients, Van Del (see above) used a single dose of only 6 grains of sodium amytal and followed it by ⅙ grain (0.01 Gm.) of morphine when the pains became more severe. He felt that the results in this group were excellent in that even severe pains did not arouse the patient, restlessness was rare, amnesia was more prolonged, and there was no greater loss in cooperation than was characteristic of the cases in which amytal was used alone.

Sodium Amytal and Scopolamine (Hyoscine).—Nelson (1932) has used this combination in 100 cases with a standard initial dosage of 9 grains (0.6 Gm.) of sodium amytal followed in one-half hour by $\frac{1}{100}$ grain (0.0006 Gm.) of scopolamine for patients of 130 pounds; for patients weighing less, 6 grains (0.4 Gm.) of amytal were used, and for those over 190 pounds, 12 grains (0.75 Gm.). In patients who were in labor over three hours and seemed too rational for perfect amnesia, an additional dose of sodium amytal, 3 grains (0.2 Gm.), and scopolamine, $\frac{1}{150}$ grain (0.0004 Gm.), was given, but it was difficult to determine the relationship between rationality and amnesia.

Eighty-four per cent of the patients in this series experienced complete amnesia and there was the usual observation of great restlessness in a certain proportion of the cases. Only 6 patients, being under 130 pounds, were given the smaller amytal dosage and the results in them were not entirely satisfactory. Nelson observed that in patients seen early in labor and treated at once the best effect was obtained, though of course in many of these cases the second dose of amytal had to be given.

Amytal Idiosyncrasy.—Individual susceptibility to amytal's effects varies considerably, though with the present tendency toward conservatism in dosage, as noted in the above accounts, these differences are not often likely to furnish matter for much concern as regards life of patient and baby, however much the amnesia may be affected by the unusual responses. The most marked instances of idiosyncrasy which I have noted are 2 cases of Hamblen and Hamblin (1931): One patient who remained fully conscious after 30 grains (2 Gm.) and described the labor as the most painful she had ever had, another who went into serious vasomotor collapse after a total of 21 grains (1.2 Gm.).

Pentobarbital Sodium (Nembutal) and Chloral Hydrate.—The first report of the routine use of pentobarbital sodium in labor—that of O'Sullivan and Craner (1932)—described its combination with chloral hydrate in a technic which has since been quite satisfactorily used by others; witness Riggall's (1932) enthusiastic endorsement from the standpoint of a practitioner in a remote region where confinements often take place under very primitive conditions. In the judgment of O'Sullivan and Craner, observance of the following points make for best success: (*a*) An initial dose of pentobarbital sodium of 3 grains (0.2 Gm.) in primiparae when pains are occurring regularly and the os is dilated two to three fifths, in multiparae, one to two fifths; (*b*) ten minutes later (to avoid vomiting), 30 grains (2 Gm.) of chloral hydrate in freshly prepared lemonade sweetened with 3 or 4 teaspoonfuls of sugar, to be sipped slowly; (*c*) subsequent doses of 1½ grains (0.1 Gm.) pentobarbital and 30 grains (2 Gm.) chloral, given in same order as before; (*d*) the first "repeat" dose to be given two hours after the initial dose, subsequent doses every three hours; (*e*) a total dosage of 7½ grains (0.5 Gm.) pentobarbital and 120 grains (8 Gm.) chloral not to be exceeded in twelve hours.

In their 60 consecutive cases they had painless labors in 62 per cent, very good results ("vague recollection of a few incidents, such as the birth of the head") in an additional 21 per cent. There were no ill effects to the mothers or children. In 40 per cent of the cases there was slight prolongation in the first stage and in 50 per cent in the second stage, bearing-down efforts being impaired in these latter instances also; no delay in the third stage. Against the forceps rate in their hospital for the preceding two and one-half years, there was an increase of 3.2 per cent in these 60 cases, hardly a fair comparison, however; most patients slept for one to eight hours after delivery and awakened fresh and well, though transient nystagmus was noted in four instances and one patient had double vision for five hours. Restlessness of varying degree occurred in 12 cases; in 2 it was severe. An injection of morphine, $\frac{1}{12}$ to $\frac{1}{6}$ grain (0.005 to 0.01 Gm.) with the initial dose of nembutal, was given in 10 cases of heart disease to prevent the restlessness, but it is difficult to determine from the report how successful this additional measure proved to be.

Avertin (Tribrom-ethanol) Anesthesia.—I do not feel that there is as yet any pronounced indication that this drug, given by rectum for "basal" anesthesia, will make a lasting impression in the practical obstetrical field. The margin of safety in dosage is very narrow, the solutions decompose rapidly into an irritating and nocuous substance, excitement is induced at least as often as with the barbiturates, supplemental administration of an inhalation anesthetic is nearly always necessary, and prolongation of labor with a consequent increase in instrumental delivery is evident in many reports. The Council on Pharmacy and Chemistry has not yet accepted the drug for inclusion in N.N.R.

TWILIGHT SLEEP

Twilight sleep, the so-called "Freiberg Dämmerschlaf" consisting in a single injection of morphine and numerous subsequent injections of hyoscine, plus measures designed for psychic effect upon the patient, has been practically abandoned (save for the modified forms described below) because of the prolongation of labor, frequency of fetal asphyxia, excessive thirst and intense headache; infection through soiling, blurred vision, delirium often lasting well into the puerperium, difficulty in recognition of the onset of the second stage and of complications, and the violence and uncertainty of the whole procedure. Latterly, Van Hoosen (1928) has modified the technic by omitting the morphine and giving at the onset of active labor $\frac{1}{100}$ grain (0.0006 Gm.) of hyoscine at half-hour intervals for two or three doses and then every two hours as needed. Her report and those of several others indicate that most of the above objectionable features have been eliminated—there is good pain with apparently good analgesia, the babies are pink and postpartum hemorrhage is reduced—but the sphincters are still relaxed and the patients must be watched closely and are kept with hands fastened above the head during delivery to avoid contamination of the field. Fist (1930) believes that he improves on this, that is, converts the scene from a very noisy into a quiet calm one, by giving intramuscularly 2 cc. of 50 per cent magnesium sulphate solution and $\frac{1}{200}$ grain (0.0003 Gm.) of hyoscine, repeating the former every half hour until pain is relieved, and the latter every hour if necessary to obtain relief. Adams (1924) combines morphine and magnesium sulphate, $\frac{1}{6}$ grain (0.01 Gm.) of the former in 2 cc. of a 25 per cent solution of the latter, repeating once if necessary.

The opiates may be safely used in the first stage only if the labor is expected to last two, or preferably, three hours longer, the effect upon the baby of reasonable amounts of this respiratory depressant being negligible during this period while its oxygen supply is secured by the placental-fetal circulation; but there must be little or no opiate in the blood at the time of birth, for the reason that the carbon dioxide that has accumulated during the compression of the placenta by the vigorous and prolonged terminal contractions of the uterus must have a thoroughly receptive respiratory center upon which to operate, if the baby is to take its first spontaneous breath.

HYPEREMESIS GRAVIDARUM
(Pernicious Vomiting of Pregnancy)

Ordinary "morning sickness" occurs in about 50 per cent of pregnant women, but the severe form with which we are here concerned is relatively rare. It usually begins between the third and sixth week and lasts several weeks to months; the course may be continuous or intermittent. The symptoms are loss of appetite, nausea, persistent vomiting, foul breath, emaciation, intolerable thirst, mental aberration, headache, delirium, coma and death. The pathologic findings in the urine and blood are entirely the result of the starvation and dehydration. Many cases recover spontaneously, either quickly or slowly, but a few go on to death; before this final event the patient usually miscarries and the stomach suddenly becomes retentive of food.

While there is as yet no proof positive of the actual cause of this malady, the theory that it is due to a metabolic disturbance in the mother resulting in severe carbohydrate deficiency is at present serving very well as a point for therapeutic departure.

THERAPY

Abortion.—Therapeutic abortion will cure all cases if the mother is not already too near death from starvation and exhaustion to stand the operation. But of course this is not advocated as a routine measure by any one; indeed, when to empty the uterus is an obstetrical point of such nicety that its discussion has no place in a book of this sort. Certainly, under the newer treatment, this radical procedure is being resorted to much less frequently than was formerly the case.

Diet, Sedatives and Glucose.—The theory of carbohydrate deficiency or glycogen deficiency of the liver as the etiologic factor in the nausea and vomiting of pregnancy was apparently first stated by Duncan and Harding, in 1918, and extensively developed independently by Titus and his associates, in 1920, and Harding, in 1921. I believe that Titus' (1925) description of the procedure is representative of the method as now employed.

Treatment of Mild Cases.—"It is sufficient to say that the patients should be given precise directions as to when and what to eat. They should be told to eat a total of at least seven small meals a day at definite intervals, beginning before arising in the morning and ending at bedtime in the evening. Carbohydrate foods of all kinds should be chosen, and the physician should particularly specify such articles as cooked fruits, dates and raisins, green vegetables, crackers and cookies, honey, sugar, and such desserts as puddings, custards and ices.

"A formula may be given the patient to prepare as follows: 1½ ounces of lactose, 2½ teaspoonfuls of sodium bicarbonate, dissolved in 1 pint of water, this being approximately 10 per cent of lactose and 2 per cent of soda in solution. Two ounces of this is to be taken every two hours."

Treatment of Moderately Severe Cases.—"Isolation in the hospital is advisable wherever possible, and to simplify the treatment it is well to have a typewritten, detailed outline of a general course of management to attach to the patient's chart. This routine form is to be varied, however, according to individual needs.

"Beginning the treatment in the evening if possible, she should fast completely for a few hours, then be given only water in small amounts by mouth until morning. At this time easily assimilated liquids such as sweetened orange albumin, glucose solution, or broth are begun and given at hourly intervals until the patient goes to sleep at night.

"She receives two daily enemas (morning and evening) each followed by a dose of chloral, 10 grains (0.65 Gm.), and bromides, 30 grains (2 Gm.), by bowel, proctoclysis of glucose and soda solution being given as constantly as possible. Intravenous injections of glucose should be begun promptly, especially if vomiting does not cease at once, and are repeated once or twice daily, depending on indications and response to the treatment. [Veronal (barbital), in doses of 2 grains (0.13 Gm.) every six hours, or luminal (phenobarbital), in doses of ½ grain (0.03 Gm.) at the same intervals, may be substituted for the bromide and chloral. If the veronal sodium is given hypodermically, the same dose as above stated should be used, but if luminal sodium is given by the needle, an increase of 10 per cent over the above-stated per orum dose is permissible. The latter drug has been successfully used by Dieckmann and Crossen (1927), who, however, employed 75 to 90 grains (5 to 6 Gm.) of sodium bromide once or twice daily by rectal tap until the luminal had time to act (eight to twelve hours).—H. B.]

"Usually by the third day small and frequent 'doses' of soft nourishment will be retained, and this improvement is followed by a gradual daily increase in both quantity and variety of food. Both the nausea and the vomiting have usually disappeared entirely by the end of a week's treatment, although a few more days may occasionally be necessary for the return to general diet.

"Kosmak has formulated an absolutely fundamental rule in the treatment of these patients. He says, 'The cardinal fact to be borne in mind is that no routine method applicable to all classes of cases can be recommended, and that in each instance, particularly in the severer types, consideration must be given to the individual patient. While we can follow certain general routine procedures in certain groups of cases, they must be changed as circumstances dictate.' "

Treatment of Patients in the Serious or Pernicious Group.—This consists in the more vigorous application of the treatment employed in the moderately severe cases.

Method of Giving Glucose.—Titus feels that the glucose should be given in 25 per cent aqueous, not saline, solution, 75 Gm. for the initial dose and 50 Gm. for the subsequent doses, but many observers disagree with him. Dieckmann and Crossen give 1000 cc. of a 10 per cent solution three times daily, as do also Harding and Van Wyck and their associates, and Thalhimer says, "The initial treatment consists of 100 Gm. of glucose given intravenously in as much water as the dehydrated condition of the patient indicates (1 to 2 liters)." Among Hendon's large series of cases of all sorts treated with his venoclysis, a method of continuously administering glucose by the vein (see p. 164), there have been 14 cases of hyperemesis gravidarum "upon whom some of our best obstetricians had used all the known methods of treatment except the induction of abortion." These women, one of whom was unconscious when the treatment was begun, all recovered in from three to five days.

It is now the consensus of opinion that the concomitant use of insulin is unnecessary since there is no evidence of a lack of this hormone.

The Importance of Fluids.—Harding and Van Wyck have for some time been stressing the fact that the best laboratory guide for treatment is the observation of the daily excretion of urine. Cases that respond successfully to this therapy show, coincident with improvement in clinical condition, a greatly increased volume of urine with a lowered specific gravity. They continue the intravenous administration of glucose solution until diuresis is obtained, meaning by diuresis that the twenty-four-hour output of urine shall reach at least 1000 cc. and shall have a specific gravity of 1.010 or less. No attempt is made to feed solids by mouth, but the patient, even if vomiting freely, is urged to drink any liquid she may fancy except tea, coffee, milk or cocoa. They state: "The use of glucose, though important, has thus become secondary to the use of fluids in treating a severe case of pernicious vomiting of pregnancy. . . . The successful treatment of hyperemesis gravidarum depends upon the use of fluids."

Miscellaneous Measures.—(a) *The Nervous Element.*—This must not be overlooked. Sometimes the severe symptoms will almost miraculously vanish when an obnoxious person, not infrequently the husband, is entirely banished from the presence of the patient; or she will suddenly recover when threats to employ the actual cautery or some other severe form of therapy are seriously made. A few observers believe that there is a psychopathic factor underlying all cases.

(b) *Duodenal Tube Feeding.*—Van Wyck (1931) has recently put the additional feeding by duodenal tube on a more definite basis by recording his observation that those who respond slowly or not at all to the intravenous administration of glucose show a persistent urobilinuria (in the absence of adequate laboratory facilities, urobilinuria may be assumed to be present when the urine has a characteristic orange-red color). This he interprets as evidence of a gravely disordered liver function which calls for the administration through the duodenal tube of additional calories. The method is to give 3 ounces (90 cc.) of skimmed milk and the same quantity of 10 per cent glucose solution every two hours throughout the twenty-four; this gives the patient 780 additional calories as well as 2000 cc. more water.

Luikart (1933) believes that the exclusive employment of glucose and large amounts of fluid may wash out considerable amounts of vitamin B complex (vitamin B_1, the antineuritic vitamin; vitamin B_2, the antipellagra vitamin), which may indeed already have been lowered by the pregnancy itself. He adds orange juice, broth, lactic acid milk and cream to the glucose solution given through the duodenal tube.

(c) *Rectal Feeding.*—In some cases it seems advisable to feed by the rectum during the time that food is being kept out of the stomach. Bacon (1918) describes the procedure as follows: "The cleansing enema may be given early in the morning, at 7 or 8 A. M. Then the nutrient enemas would start at about 9 A. M., 2. P. M., and 7 P. M. Sometimes it will be found desirable to add 10 drops of tincture of opium to the evening enema. The composition of the rectal feedings will have about the following proportions: Glucose, 50; alcohol, 50; calcium chloride, 0.3; sodium bicarbonate, 3;

sodium chloride or bromide, 4; vitamin, as much as it sufficient; distilled water, enough to make 1000. This mixture has an energy value of about 550 calories. From 300 to 500 cc. are to be given three times a day. If 1500 cc. are given each day, the patient will receive 825 calories. . . . Rectal feedings are discontinued gradually and not until the stomach feeding is reestablished."

(d) *Acids or Alkalis.*—Dieckmann and Crossen (1927) have found that dilute hydrochloric acid, in a dose of 10 to 15 minims (0.6 to 1 cc.) three or four times daily, is more efficacious than sodium bicarbonate. This is in line with their finding that there is either a normal acid-base balance, a compensated alkali excess (normal pH and high CO_2), or a compensated alkali deficit (normal pH with low CO_2), the latter occurrence being rare.

ECLAMPSIA

Eclampsia is a child-bed malady characterized by convulsions, coma and a high death rate, but nearly always preceded by certain symptoms that should be recognized for what they are by the competent physician. These prodromal symptoms are: Systolic blood pressure of 140 mm. or above; any sudden rise from the patient's normal blood pressure; albuminuria with a high globulin ratio (Eastman, 1931), casts, or both, in the urine; headaches with sudden onset; epigastric pain; edema; diminished urinary output; ocular symptoms, eyeground abnormalities; nervous irritability. In the acute attack itself the patient falls over unconscious, and passes from a rigid spasm with opisthotonos, flexed arms, clenched fists, distorted features and dilated pupils into a clonic convulsion, during which the whole body twitches very violently, the tongue is protruded and often severely mutilated by the champing jaws, the eyes are bulging and bloodshot, the face is swollen and cyanosed, blood-tinged foam comes from the mouth, and the pulse is rapid and pounding. The chest is rigidly fixed. After from thirty seconds to a minute and a half or two minutes, relaxation takes place and the patient may wake up very exhausted and bewildered; or in the most severe cases, she remains in coma between spasms. Sometimes there is delirium between attacks. A few cases of "eclampsia without convulsions" are on record.

At autopsy the characteristic lesions are found in the liver: Necroses beginning in the periportal spaces and encroaching on the periphery of the lobules, but Rowe (1932) has shown that it is not always possible to demonstrate an "hepatic factor" during life. It has now become apparent that the antemortem changes in the blood do not bear out the original supposition that the malady is associated with nitrogenous retention, but Bell (1932) states that in fatal cases there is to be found a characteristic glomerular lesion. Titus and his associates believe that the convulsions appear coincident with hypoglycemic levels during a profound disturbance in carbohydrate metabolism which characterizes the disease, a position which is denied by Stander *et al.* The latter group also maintains that the acidosis which they observe at the time of the convulsions is due to an uncompensated alkali deficit and is not to be regarded as a causal factor in the fits. In explanation of the water retention and edema, capillary spasm and hypertension, Anselmino *et al.* propose the hypothesis that eclampsia is an endocrine disturbance probably of pluriglandular nature but in which great overproduction of the hormones of the posterior pituitary dominates the picture. Dieckmann (1931), while admitting the tissue water-logging, feels that the principal change in the blood is a concentration.

The disease is more common in cold than in warm climates. Baker (1927) states that about 27 per cent of obstetrical deaths are due to eclampsia. It would seem that in about 60 per cent of the cases convulsions begin during labor, with 20 per cent before labor and 20 per cent after delivery. Primiparae are more often affected than multiparae.

THERAPY

The subject will be dealt with under the followings heads: (1) Stroganoff, (2) Rotunda, (3) Magnesium Sulphate, (4) Sodium Amytal, (5) Glucose, (6) Combination "Conservative" Therapy, (7) Dehydration, (8) Management of the Convulsion, (9) Miscellaneous Measures, (10) Diet, (11) Operative Interference.

1. **Stroganoff.**—This method of treatment was devised by Prof. V. V. Stroganoff, in Leningrad. In its description I am following Stander's report of his visit to Stroganoff's hospitals, in 1925.

(*a*) Upon admission: (1) Dark room with a minimum of noise. (2) Special nurse. (3) Examination or disturbance of patient only when absolutely necessary, and then usually under chloroform. (4) Morphine sulphate, ¼ grain (0.015 Gm.) hypodermically, while under chloroform narcosis, usually about 10 to 15 Gm. of chloroform being employed.

(*b*) One hour after admission: Chloral hydrate, 30 grains (2 Gm.), per rectum with 100 cc. physiologic saline and 100 cc. milk. Should the patient be conscious, the chloral hydrate can be administered by the mouth with 100 cc. of milk. (Note: Chloral hydrate is always administered without the use of chloroform except where the patient has had one or more convulsions after admission; then about 10 Gm. of the anesthetic are used with each dose of chloral hydrate.)

(*c*) Three hours after admission: Morphine sulphate, ¼ grain (0.015 Gm.), hypodermically, under 10 to 15 Gm. of chloroform.

(*d*) Seven hours after admission: Chloral hydrate, 30 grains (2 Gm.), as above.

(*e*) Thirteen hours after admission: Chloral hydrate, 22 grains (1.5 Gm.), as above.

(*f*) Twenty-one hours after admission: Chloral hydrate, 22 grains (1.5 Gm.), as above.

(*g*) After each convulsion: Oxygen is administered as quickly as possible. This is kept up until the breathing improves, usually about five minutes.

(*h*) After three convulsions in the clinic: Venesection of not more than 400 cc. is resorted to.

(*i*) In case of frequent convulsions: Chloroform and chloral hydrate to be used more energetically than outlined above.

(*j*) No convulsions for twenty-four hours: If patient has been free from convulsions for twenty-four hours or longer after admission, and has not yet been delivered, she should be given about 8 grains (0.5 Gm.) of chloral hydrate every eight hours for about three days.

(*k*) Child: Operative delivery is resorted to only when intervention becomes absolutely necessary for the sake of the child.

In the hands of Stroganoff this method has produced the astonishingly low maternal mortality of 7.7 per cent in 390 cases; indeed, if certain cases are ruled out in which the technic was not rigidly followed, the maternal mortality is only 2.84 per cent! Stander says that a study of Stroganoff's statistics leads him to believe that on the whole he has been dealing with much milder types of eclampsia than commonly concern us in the North American clinics. The two outstanding objections to the Stroganoff method

48

are the routine use of relatively large amounts of chloroform at frequent intervals and the employment of venesection. Regarding the first, it is the consensus of opinion in America that chloroform is too hepatoxic for employment in this malady, and that, furthermore, the attempt to control the convulsions by the use of general anesthetics is unsatisfactory, for, as Speidel says (1925), "when the initial twitch has begun, the patient goes through the entire procedure, opisthotonos, cessation of breathing, etc., regardless of what anesthetic is administered. With the spasmodic contraction of the diaphragm that is incident to the convulsion, it is questionable whether the patient inhales at all." As to the venesection, many observers are of opinion that it should not be employed—but certainly if it is used routinely as an integral part of the treatment, one would think that much more than 400 cc. of blood should be withdrawn if any considerable drainage of toxins is to be accomplished.

2. **Rotunda.**—This method of treatment was developed by Fitzgibbon (1923) at the Rotunda Hospital, Dublin, and was remarkable for the fact that neither morphine nor any other sedative or antispasmodic drug was employed, the treatment consisting of starvation, gastric and colonic lavage with sodium bicarbonate solution, the introduction of purgatives at frequent intervals, water by the mouth, and hypodermoclysis of bicarbonate solution. Extensive trial has shown that the results are not satisfactory, and the method has been modified considerably. *Glucose and venesection.*—Glucose is given either by mouth or rectum, rarely intravenously. Regarding venesection, Solomons, Master of the Hospital (1933), writes: "Although brought up on the dangers of this procedure, I have been converted to it as a valuable aid in treatment." Eight ounces (250 cc.) of blood are withdrawn if the systolic pressure exceeds 160 mm. Hg and is repeated daily if necessary. *Morphine.*—Half a grain (0.03 Gm.) with the first fit and ¼ grain (0.015 Gm.) with each subsequent fit, but not to exceed 2 grains (0.12 Gm.) in the twenty-four hours and with the injections spaced at least two hours apart. *Colon lavage.*—At once and repeated if the bowels do not move satisfactorily in six hours; occasionally repeated again ("the bowels should move four or five times daily"). Anuria also calls for repetition of the lavage as it is felt that the toxemic state prevents the kidneys from functioning. Linseed poultices are applied to the loins at two-hour intervals to favor urinary secretion. *Gastric lavage.*—This is performed now only when urgent symptoms, such as excessive vomiting, demand it; a purgative is left in the stomach (if conscious when admitted a purge is given at that time). *Hypodermoclysis.*—If the patient is not improving, the pulse is weak and thready and there is insufficient secretion of urine, a solution of sodium bicarbonate —1 drachm (4 Gm.) to the pint (500 cc.)—is infused under each breast and repeated if improvement does not follow. "No matter what theoretical objections are advanced to the administration of fluids under the breasts, we still persist and believe in it as a valuable adjunct in treatment."

3. **Magnesium Sulphate.**—As long ago as 1907, Einer reported 2 cases of eclampsia treated with magnesium sulphate, and a few scattered cases later appeared in the German literature, but the profession as a whole was perhaps first attracted to the use of the drug by the report of Fischer, in 1916. He believed the convulsion to be the expression of an acute acid intoxication with edema of the central nervous system, and used 250 cc. of a 2 per cent solution of magnesium sulphate to further dehydration. In the same year, Loomis and Sherrick, and McNeile, all of California, employed it in the same way. At the present time it is widely used in combination with other measures, both for its antiedemic and anticonvulsant properties. Twenty cc. of a 10 per cent solution is given intravenously on admission and repeated every hour in full or half doses until convulsions cease; another

much employed method is to give 10 cc. of a 25 per cent solution intramuscularly on admission and half the dose each hour until convulsions cease (some observers preferring to give the subsequent doses only after each convulsion instead of routinely each hour to cessation of the fits).

4. **Sodium Amytal.**—As was to have been expected, the barbiturates are now having their turn, in Germany pernocton, in America and England sodium amytal. Experimental studies apparently indicate that the latter has no harmful effect on the fetus, on liver function, alkali reserve or the secretion of urine. Hamblen and Hamblin (1932) give 15 to 18 grains (1 to 1.2 Gm.) in capsules on admission; if the patient is unable to swallow, the dose is introduced through the nasal catheter. Subsequently, 3 to 6 grains (0.2 to 0.4 Gm.) is given approximately every four hours, the indication being restlessness or a rise in blood pressure. After 30 to 45 grains (2 to 3 Gm.) have been given they find that a deep sleep can be maintained by 3-grain (0.2 Gm.) doses at increasingly long intervals. In their 6 cases, convulsions were controlled immediately with the initial dose; no other sedatives were employed, nor was any inhalation anesthesia required for delivery. In the hands of most other observers, the drug has been given intravenously, but this oral method seems to me a distinct advance, though Watt (1932) failed to control the fits in one of his 2 cases, succeeding always when he gave the drug intravenously. Much more experience is needed before we can consider that the worth of this treatment has been established. The intravenous method is described on page 756.

5. **Glucose.**—Following the development of the theory that the eclamptic convulsions are due to hypoglycemic states, the administration of glucose began and has won a distinct place for itself, though whether for the above reason or for its eliminative (diuretic) effect has now become a matter of individual opinion; the furnishing of nourishment and water to the tissues, and the liver-sparing effect, are also not overlooked. It is now the consensus of opinion that insulin should not be concomitantly employed as we are not dealing here with a lack of this hormone. Regarding the method of giving glucose, Titus *et al.* write:

"The intravenous administration of hypertonic glucose solution in single doses of 75 Gm. in 300 cc. of water (25 per cent solution) at the rate of not more than 1 Gm. per minute, or from an hour and a quarter to an hour and a half for the entire injection. This should be repeated after intervals of four or five hours during the attack and for a time following cessation of the convulsions (three or four times in twenty-four hours, according to the needs and response of the patient) until fluids can be taken freely by mouth."

My belief is that the venoclysis method of Hendon (see p. 164), by which glucose solution is administered continuously, will ultimately be given extensive, and probably successful, trial in eclampsia as well as hyperemesis.

6. **Combination "Conservative" Therapy.**—The call has been sounded repeatedly in the literature of the past few years for the establishment of a conservative therapeutic approach which shall incorporate in due proportions the best of the eliminative and sedative features of all of the "single-track" types of treatment. With the first of the two routine conservative methods cited below the mortality in 100 cases was 5.4 per cent; the second method had been used at time of publication in only 30 cases, but it is included here to indicate how sodium amytal is being employed in a definite plan of this sort.

(A) *First Conservative Method.*—Upshaw (1932) writes: "A systematic routine has been followed, with little variation. The management is, briefly, as follows: A patient entering the hospital in a state of convulsions is first given a hypodermic injection of morphine sulphate, ¼ grain (0.0162 Gm.). Then 20 cc. of 10 per cent magnesium sulphate is given intravenously and repeated every hour until convulsions are controlled or until four or five injections have been given. Often the magnesium sulphate is give intramuscularly after the first injection. Next, 300 cc. of 25 per cent glucose in freshly distilled water is given intravenously. The glucose solution is repeated every eight hours until after delivery or until full control of convulsions, and then every twelve hours for two days following delivery in severe cases. It is reasonable to assume that the magnesium sulphate quickly relieves the intracranial pressure by reducing the edema of the brain. In a large service where this drug is used extensively in preeclampsia as well as in eclampsia, we have observed no appreciable respiratory or circulatory embarrassment. By immediately following the intravenous injection of magnesium sulphate with concentrated glucose solution and by repeating at regular periodic intervals, diuresis is readily established and maintained. It is also believed that glucose prevents a recurrence of the cerebral edema, because once the convulsions have been controlled it has been rare that we have had to resort again to magnesium sulphate or to other sedatives. The morphine is not repeated except as indicated for relief in labor.

"Labor is not induced until the convulsions are controlled and dehydration at least partially overcome. For the past three years we have induced labor by rupturing the membranes and allowing a large amount of the amniotic fluid to drain away. This is done by careful technic, the dangers of infection always being kept in mind. We believe that the larger the amount of amniotic fluid allowed to escape, the more quickly and surely will labor be established. So successful has this method been that a Voorhees bag or a catheter has not been used in the past eighteen months to induce labor. Occasionally one or two 2-minim (0.12 cc.) doses of solution of pituitary have been given after rupture of the membranes when there has been a delay in the onset of labor.

"Inhalation ether anesthesia for labor by open drop method is used exclusively in our service. In patients with eclampsia this is given guardedly and only at the time for expulsion of the child's head. We believe with Stander that anesthesia in eclampsia should be reduced to a minimum, and that patients in semicomatose or comatose states should receive no anesthesia at all."

(B) *Second Conservative Method.*—The treatment used by King *et al.* (1932) may be described as follows:

1. On admission morphine sulphate, ¼ grain, is given hypodermically, this dose being repeated if necessary in case of slight or moderate restlessness.

2. Sodium amytal, 7½ grains, is given intravenously. If the convulsions recur, or if there is marked nervous irritability, this dose too may be repeated as often as required.

3. As soon as the full effect of the amytal is obtained the stomach is washed out, and 2 ounces of 50 per cent magnesium sulphate is given through the stomach tube.

4. If there is marked hypertension, 300 to 400 cc. of blood is drawn off from a vein, and through the same needle 1000 cc. of 10 per cent solution of glucose is administered without insulin; this treatment is usually repeated in twenty-four hours.

5. At a convenient time a soapsuds enema is given—more than once if need be. This is eliminative, and prepares the rectum for the rectal administration of more sodium amytal if thought proper.

6. Thereafter, sodium amytal in 3-grain doses is given by mouth or by rectum every four hours. Its administration is continued until it is felt that all danger of recurrence of the convulsions is past, usually in thirty-six to forty-eight hours.

7. Only water or a glucose and water mixture is given by mouth or by stomach tube until the patient is fully conscious, after which a light diet rich in carbohydrates is allowed.

8. If there is edema of the lungs, atropine sulphate, $\frac{1}{50}$ grain, is given hypodermically and repeated as necessary.

9. If labor does not supervene spontaneously it is induced by catheter or bag. This proved necessary eight times.

10. Labor is usually allowed to terminate spontaneously, but low forceps is used occasionally.

Particular warning is given against injecting an amytal solution that is not absolutely clear for four or five minutes after its preparation, and also against injecting faster than at the rate of 1 cc. per minute. Transient depression in blood pressure and also in respiratory rate accompanies the injections; the reader is advised to try the oral method of using the drug, described on page 755.

7. **Dehydration.**—Arnold and Fay (1932), accepting the water-intoxication theory of the disease, urge a remodelling of the present type of treatment which consists among other things (as seen above) in the administration of large amounts of fluid to flush out hypothetical toxins. Instead, they advocate extreme fluid limitation and drainage, combined with the use of sedatives, about as follows: (a) Immediate administration of 2 to 3 grains (0.12 to 0.2 Gm.) of sodium luminal hypodermically, repeating in two hours if need be, but no morphine to be given unless absolutely necessary after the administration of glucose and the spinal drainage. (b) Fifty cc. of 50 per cent glucose solution intravenously at once. (c) Drainage of the spinal canal as completely as possible (45 to 100 cc.), preferably with the head raised to an angle of 30 degrees; when impracticable, venesection until systolic pressure falls 30 to 50 points. (d) Glucose administration repeated in three to four hours and spinal drainage in four to six hours unless there is marked improvement. (e) Magnesium sulphate by mouth or bowel in effectual doses. (f) Absolutely no fluid, except the magnesium sulphate cathartic, for at least twenty-four hours. (g) A continuance of mild dehydration by purgation for several days, combined with a fluid restriction to little more than the quantity of fluid passed as urine. Apparently the method is productive of good results in the hands of these observers. However, one must remark in passing that while concentrated glucose may serve well as a dehydrating agent, and that perhaps one of the important services of the magnesium as parenterally given in the other schemes of treatment is just that, still not all hypertonic solutions can be so used; in the experience of Harding and Van Wyck (1930) the intravenous administration of hypertonic saline solution was disastrous, indicating that the water intoxication in eclampsia, if it exists, is not entirely the same as that so easily produced experimentally in dogs.

8. **Management of the Convulsion.**—Solomons (1933) writes: "Everything must be ready, the gag, the bullet forceps to catch the tongue, the mucus extractor, the spoon with handle bound, or the toothbrush to slip in between the teeth. During a fit mucus pours from the mouth like water from a tap, and during a fit the patient must be brought over with her face to the ground, the tongue brought forward, and the mucus removed or she will surely die. She is placed in a quiet room, *not dark*. . . . She lies on the side."

9. **Miscellaneous Measures.**—Veratrum viride has died the death it seems; calcium has been shown to have no value; the evidence with regard to hepatic extract is too conflicting to indicate its long survival. Dieckmann, consistently with his stress upon the matter of blood concentration, has administered gum acacia solutions intravenously with apparently good

success, but has reported a quite insufficient number of cases to give much value to the observation as yet. In passing, mention might be made of the reported administration of a few injections of apomorphine; simple and interesting, it seems to me, in view of the results in strychnine poisoning (see p. 701).

10. **Diet.**—The advantages of the low-salt diet as used in nephritis have been accepted as fairly well established; it is extremely doubtful if the rigid protein restriction still practiced by so many physicians is of any more advantage in eclampsia than in nephritis, in which disease it is already discountenanced (see p. 471).

11. **Surgical Intervention.**—In the first edition of this book, I attempted to present both sides of this question in the words of the recognized authoritative advocates of both interference and noninterference. It seems to me that the result was a very wordy stalemate which in several pages expressed no more than I can right here by saying that there is complete disagreement on the point. Certainly, however, the student of obstetrical literature in recent times cannot fail to mark the very decided trend toward the more conservative position which favors interference only when driven to it by necessity.

<hr />

PUERPERAL SEPSIS

In 1847–49, Semmelweis, in Vienna, recognized puerperal fever as being a true sepsis, but his greatest treatise on the subject was not published until 1861, long years after disgust with the persecution of his colleagues had caused him to leave Vienna for Budapest. O. W. Holmes had reported (and been also bitterly opposed) on the contagiousness of the disease in 1842, but his studies had not been as clinchingly final as those of the Hungarian.

The treatment of puerperal sepsis will not be separately discussed here, the subject having been covered under the title "Sepsis," on page 159.

<hr />

PHLEGMASIA ALBA DOLENS
(Milk-leg)

This malady usually makes its appearance between the eighth and twentieth days after delivery, usually as a thrombophlebitic complication of a general septic process, but sometimes apparently independently. The local signs and symptoms are: Pain in the groin and calf; the upper thigh becomes rapidly swollen, hot, extremely sensitive, and peculiarly white or yellowish white in appearance; and later the lower leg may swell also. The general symptoms are those of sepsis. The affection may spread to the other leg, and the arteries may also become involved, with resultant serious gangrene. The attack being protracted, and the great pain and the danger of embolism preventing the movement of the body, bed sores often complicate the picture.

Other types of this malady are the simple thrombosis of the saphenous and femoral or iliac veins, which is milder and has a very good prognosis, and cellulitis of this region (the effected area is *red*), which is very often fatal.

THERAPY

The treatment of the sepsis is of the utmost importance (see p. 159). In addition, the limb must be kept absolutely quiet to prevent pulmonary embolism, and precautions must be taken, by proper padding and the local use of alcohol, to prevent bed sores. Either moderately hot or cold applications are gratefully received in most cases. There is no need to deny these patients the relief obtainable from the opiates, but codeine should be preferred to morphine as it is often necessary to repeat the dose many times. Some physicians favor the slight elevation of the leg to favor return circulation. Of course surgical indications must be met as they arise.

The patient must be kept in bed for several weeks after the temperature has become and remained normal, and then the return to active life is to be made *very* gradually. However, mention must be made of Kappis' (1930) report: In 100 cases his treatment consisted in strapping from toes to thigh with an elastic bandage and permitting the patient to become ambulatory—with a percentage of infarcts and fatal emboli no greater than occurs in immobilized cases.

BREAST ABSCESS

The symptoms are chill and fever and the signs those of local inflammation in the breast. When abscess forms, the treatment is entirely surgical, which of course will not be described in this book. In a few cases with premonitory symptoms it is possible to abort the abscess by taking the infant away from the affected breast, putting on a binder, and applying ice-bags; if this treatment is successful, the infant can sometimes be returned in twenty-four hours. This seems to be largely a disease of the primipara and of the blond, and to occur much more often in private than in hospital practice.

Prevention.—The practice since time out of mind has been to wash both breast and baby's mouth with boric acid solution before and after nursing in the attempt to prevent abscess—this, it seems, without adequate proof that the boric acid was effective. However, Van Dolsen (1927) has recently studied the matter and has determined by cultural means that the mouths of babies are almost entirely free from streptococci and staphylococci, both of which he found in abundance on 30 out of 50 cultured breasts. He then determined that the boric acid treatment does not appreciably alter this flora. He is now using 0.1 per cent sodium hypochlorite solution, which he finds will kill all surface bacteria if a bit of gauze soaked in it is allowed to lie for one minute on the nipple region. There is no irritation either to breast or mouth of baby. Van Dolsen has thus successfully prevented abscess for six months on an active obstetrical service. He makes the point that of course no baby is ever allowed to nurse a fissured breast, which "is to invite an abscess." Regarding the use of the Dakin's solution, however, Smith (1932) remarks that it has been just about as effective a preventive in his experience as water would have been.

MISCELLANY

CHRONIC NONSPECIFIC ARTHRITIS

Chronic arthritis has not escaped the common fate of all diseases about which we know very little, namely, a reclassification of the types about every fortnight. However, increasingly in recent years, it has come to be recognized that the cases can be placed with rather good assurance in one or the other of two groups, as follows. *Rheumatoid arthritis:* This is the chronic infectious type which is seen in individuals in the twenties, thirties and forties more often than at any other age, and is thought to be due to some primary focus of infection, such as in the teeth, tonsils, sinuses, gallbladder, cervix, prostate, colon, etc. The first attack is often acute, but the onset may also be very gradual. There are local inflammatory and proliferative changes in the joints, great pain and tenderness and limitation of motion, migration from joint to joint, and enough new growth of fibrous tissue about the joints to cause persistent periarticular swelling. Ankylosis, which is very common in this type of arthritis, usually does not appear until after the patient has suffered several attacks. The microscopical changes in the subcutaneous nodule are looked upon as highly characteristic. The form of the malady earlier known as arthritis deformans or atrophic arthritis, in which there is thickening of the capsule and marked destruction of the articulating surfaces with telescoping of the joints and ulnar deviation of the hands and fingers, is now included as merely a very severe grade of rheumatoid arthritis, which, as expressed by Cecil (1933), "is primarily a disease of the synovial membrane and other soft parts of the joint." *Osteoarthritis:* This is degenerative arthritis of the senile type, in which the onset of pain and stiffness in the joints is usually insidious (the "menopausal" type is no longer differentiated) ; there is degeneration and thinning of the cartilage with new growth of bone around the edges of the joints involved, principally the spine, knees, knuckles, feet and shoulders, but without fusion of the articular surfaces. This affection, which is a disorder of cartilage and bone, is not thought to be infectious in origin—indeed it may be just one of the manifestations of senescence, though it seems to me that any dogmatic statement that this *is* so is not yet justified.

Arthritis is the oldest disease entity of which there is historical and authentic record, for prehistoric man, and even reptiles of geological periods which antedated the appearance of man, were ravaged by this malady. All of the enlightened nations are now alive to the appalling toll in suffering and disability taken by this disease, and it is ardently hoped that preventive and remedial measures of value will soon be evolved by the national and international committees that have devoted themselves to this subject since the World War.

THERAPY

The history of the treatment of arthritis is marked by the grave stones of discarded specifics almost without number. Space does not permit the listing of even the majority of the agents that are today being urged as of some value in this condition; I therefore set down here only those that are most frequently used, cautioning the reader that at best the results of his utmost endeavors will be but poor in the present state of our knowledge of this malady.

Eradication of Foci of Infection.—This is the most important feature of the treatment of rheumatoid arthritis, and is of very doubtful value in the other type.

Nonspecific Proteins.—The methods of obtaining the foreign protein type of response are described on page 327. An occasional case of rheumatoid arthritis· responds well, but there is no convincing evidence that this happy result is obtained more often with the streptococcic vaccines which have been recently championed, or with the new Ponndorf vaccine containing tubercle bacilli, tuberculin, staphylococci, streptococci and pneumococci, than with any of the other methods.

Salicylates and Cinchophens.—The drugs of these two groups are used much as in the treatment of acute rheumatic fever (see p. 149); unfortunately, the relief afforded is in many cases very slight.

Iodides.—The iodides are usually used in the form of either the syrup of hydriotic acid, 1 drachm (4 cc.) in water after meals, or 10 minims (0.65 cc.) of the saturated solution of potassium iodide at the same intervals. The best results follow iodide therapy in the osteo-arthritis (senile) type, but the best is certainly none too good.

Alkalis.—There is a firmly entrenched clinical impression that alkalis are helpful in some of these cases. They may be employed in the form of the well-known hospital A.B.C. mixture, each teaspoonful of which usually contains 5 grains (0.32 Gm.) of potassium acetate, bicarbonate and citrate; or some such prescription as the following may be employed, in which the potassium citrate has a dose of 15 grains (1 Gm.).

℞.	Potassium citrate	℥ij	60.0
	Peppermint water to make	℥viij	250.0

Label: 1 teaspoonful in water after meals.

There is also an official effervescent potassium citrate, the dose of which is 1 teaspoonful (5 cc.) in water, to be drunk while effervescing.

The fruit juices, in the form of limeade, lemonade or orangeade, are also used to "alkalinize the system."

Ortho-iodoxybenzoic Acid.—Unfortunately the early claims made for this drug have failed of confirmation; it has been dropped from the N.N.R. as being of no value in arthritis.

Tonics.—Both arsenic and cod liver oil are felt to be of value in building up and maintaining the strength and nutrition of the unfortunates afflicted with rheumatoid arthritis. The former is used as Fowler's solution (solution of potassium arsenite) in 3-minim (0.2 cc.) doses three times daily and very gradually built up; the cod liver oil should be given just as in the treatment of tuberculosis (see p. 240).

Diet.—As in all other chronic diseases for which we have as yet no specific remedy, the virtues of special diets have been repeatedly urged; but it has not been shown that the routine employment of any of these diets is uniformly successful, except that most observers are in agreement that the reduction of weight in obese elderly patients is of considerable importance; for methods, see page 392. It is to be ardently hoped that the recently reported excellent results of Martin (1933), who used low-purine or low-carbohydrate diets (see the articles on gout and diabetes mellitus), will prove to be more than one of the many flashes in the pan. Of course his therapy was instituted only when careful studies of the blood indicated a low purine or carbohydrate tolerance.

Physiotherapy.—Baking, massage, light therapy, passive movement, regulated exercise, diathermy, colonic irrigation—various combinations of these measures are employed in practically all cases with very indifferent results.

Surgical.—Good results sometimes follow the performance of a sympathetic ganglionectomy and ramisectomy in selected cases.

Orthopedic.—The special methods of extension, fixation, etc., also of great importance in many cases, are entirely surgical matters.

Spa and Climatic Treatment.—There comes a time in the course of most cases of chronic arthritis when the patient will be benefited by a trip to a spa, but unfortunately the economic strain of such a sojourn cannot be borne by the majority of individuals. Likewise, those who can move permanently into a warm climate, not necessarily dry, will often be greatly benefited if the malady is not too far advanced.

L'Envoi.—Need I point out that, contrary to the views held by some of the foremost students of arthritis, I look upon our present grasp of its therapy with a most rheumy, gloomy eye. The *cause* must be found—*and in both types it probably lies somewhere hidden among the metabolic dyscrasias!*

ESSENTIAL DYSMENORRHEA
(Painful Menstruation)

Perhaps more than 50 per cent of women suffer from dysmenorrhea, the severity of the cases varying from a mild physical and mental discomfort, that is little greater than the normal depression during the period, to severe attacks of pain that wrack the patient's back, head, legs, and lower abdomen for several days and leave her in a state of great fatigue during the early part of the intermenstrual period. Grant that dysmenorrhea is only a symptom and not a disease, and classify the various types on an alleged causative basis, the fact will still remain that there is a constitutional something underlying all the cases; that is to say, that the dysmenorrheic woman differs in some essential way from the nondysmenorrheic. This position is of course challenged, and the attempt is made to find a "neuralgic," "ovarian," "congestive," "obstructive," "inflammatory," or "mechanical" cause in all cases—which would all be very fine were it not for the fact that the very same *causes* are found in many individuals who do not have dysmenorrhea. Therefore, in the present state of our knowledge, the term "essential dysmenorrhea" would seem to be permissible.

THERAPY

1. **Surgical Measures.**—Various surgical measures are employed, of which perhaps the soundest theoretically is dilatation of the cervix in the attempt to convert the nulliparous uterus into a similar condition to that of the parous uterus, for it is noteworthy that women who have suffered from dysmenorrhea rarely continue to do so after they have borne a child. This dilatation, however, oftentimes gives only temporary relief, in which cases the use of pessaries is then advised in the hope of prolonging the asymptomatic period—a practice that many physicians look upon as vicious. It is also claimed that if the internal os is severed in addition to the dilatation, the percentage of permanent cures is greatly increased. This may be true, but since most of these cases will not consent to operation (even were it advisable to urge it, which is questionable), the method is of relatively little use. Dilatation does not seem to be as popular with surgeons now as it was a few years ago; the controversial point is indicated in Moench's statement (1927) that "many men will ardently defend the theory that an even moderately constricted ureter will give rise to severe pains and colic and

then deny absolutely that a narrowed cervix causes dysmenorrhea, and this despite the fact that the ureter has to conduct practically only water, whereas the cervix must allow blood and small bits of tissue to pass."

Carbon dioxide insufflation of the fallopian tubes has been advocated of late, but has not been effective in the hands of all workers.

I believe that all but a relatively few enthusiastic gynecologists have given up the routine suspension of retroverted uteri, a truly heinous anatomical abnormality that has at one time or another been held responsible for one and all of the ailments of the daughters of Eve.

2. Exercise.—In America, Miller (1930) and Ewing (1931), and in England, Clow (1932), have felt that correction of faulty posture and the regular performance of certain simple exercises have been helpful measures in a rather considerable proportion of the large number of young women examined by them in industry. Clow's exercises follow; of course they are to be prescribed only for women otherwise healthy:

TABLE OF EXERCISES FOR HEALTHY DYSMENORRHEIC WOMEN

1. *Floor Polishing.* Kneel on "all fours." Swing right arm, with elbow stiff, through a semicircle, as if polishing the floor, reaching as far forward and as far back as possible. Repeat swing ten times with each arm.
2. (*a*) *Bending.* Stand with feet apart. Stretch arms above head, bend forward and touch ground with knees straight. Return to first position. Repeat slowly eight times.
   (*b*) *Twisting.* Stand with feet apart. Stretch arms to side on level with shoulders. Twist trunk round until right arm points directly backward. Twist again until left arm points directly backward. Repeat vigorously ten times.
   (*c*) *Swaying.* Stand with feet apart. Stretch arms above head. Sway body and arms to right then left. Repeat slowly ten times.
3. *"Rowing."* Sit on floor with knees straight and feet pressed against wall. Lean forward and touch wall with knuckles, allowing knees to bend slightly. Repeat rhythmically twenty times.
4. *Right to Left and Left to Right.* Stand with feet apart. Swing right arm up as far as possible. Bend down bringing right arm over and touch left foot. Repeat six times. The same with the left arm and right foot.
5. *Floor Patting.* Kneel, sitting back on heels. Twist body and tap floor with both hands four times on left side. Kneel upright. Twist body and repeat tapping on right side. Repeat eight times each side.
6. *Bean Picking.* Throw 20 small objects, such as beans, on the floor. Pick up one at a time and place on a shelf above the head using hands alternately. Do it as quickly as possible.

3. Intranasal Therapy.—The question of the interrelationship between the nose and the uterine organs was first raised by Fliess, in 1897, and in the years immediately succeeding gave rise to a considerable controversy among German otolaryngologists and gynecologists; a writer in 1912 was able to list 296 articles. The "genital spots" in the nose are the tuberculum septi and the anterior portion of the inferior turbinate on either side. It is claimed that at menstruation these areas swell, become sensitive, and bleed easily. Leaving aside the controversial matter, which has no place here, it would seem that treatment of these areas does deserve some consideration, for Mayer, in 1914, was able to report 81 cases, of which 60 per cent were permanently cured and a total of 75 per cent obtained considerable relief, and Crossen, in 1926, has collected the reports of 81 cases treated by three physicians, with success in 63 cases, or 77 per cent. The method is laughed at too much and tried too little.

Method.—Apply 20 per cent solution of cocaine to the genital spots during the height of the pains; if they cease, the case is likely to respond favorably to the treatment which aims at permanent ablation of these spots and is instituted between periods. This consists of the application of trichloracetic acid to the spots four times at intervals of about five days, allowing time between treatments for the disappearance of the slough that forms. The applications are painful and may be preceded by cocainization.

4. Sedatives.—It is the rare and fortunate case that responds favorably to the sedatives alone. The following are the most frequently employed drugs: (a) Sodium bromide, 10 to 20 grains (0.65 to 1.3 Gm.), after meals and again upon retiring; (b) sodium bromide and chloral hydrate, 15 grains (1 Gm.) of each upon retiring; (c) barbital (veronal), 2 grains (0.13 Gm.), after meals and again upon retiring, or 7½ to 10 grains (0.5 to 0.65 Gm.) upon retiring; (d) phenobarbital (luminal), ½ grain (0.032 Gm.) after meals, or 1½ grains (0.1 Gm.) upon retiring. Paraldehyde is preferred by some physicians because it is not depressing to the heart, though I believe the danger of serious depression from any of these other drugs in the doses advised is nil; it is given in a dose of 1 to 4 drachms (4 to 16 cc.), on crushed ice or in one of the higher alcoholic vehicles (see p. 785). Small doses of scopolamine hydrobromide (hyoscine), $\frac{1}{300}$ to $\frac{1}{200}$ grain (0.0002 to 0.0003 Gm.), at six-hour intervals, are not contraindicated, though one should always bear in mind the uncertainty and irregularity in action of this drug.

5. Analgesics.—It is unusual for a patient with severe dysmenorrhea to obtain complete relief from drugs of this class, but many patients do have the worst edge taken off their pain by them. The following are the most frequently used:

(a) *Alcohol.*—This is the analgesic par excellence here, as many patients know without being so instructed by the physician. I am of course well aware of the danger of habit formation with this drug, but to cry fie upon its use as do nearly all of the gynecologists, is going too far in my opinion. Certainly not all our patients are so poorly balanced that they will become habitual tipplers if we advise them to take a whisky toddy two or three times daily for two days once each month. In the days before prohibition descended upon us it was possible to prescribe some innocuous drug in alcoholic menstruum without the patient knowing what it was that really accomplished the relief. If all the smoke of loose talk could be blown aside, I wonder how much real proof that these prescriptions were abused would be disclosed? I believe that there are plenty of women capable of taking alcohol in small amounts and at long intervals as a medicine. That the gynecologist fears this type of therapy more than does the general practitioner is probably due to the fact that the gynecologist, like all other specialists, knows his patient too little to have a valid opinion of her stability.

(b) *Opium.*—Opium will of course relieve this pain, but its use is very dangerous because of the great likelihood of inducing the habit. There are some cases, however, in which respite can be obtained by no other agent. Codeine is preferable to morphine; the ½-grain (0.032 Gm.) dose twice a day, or the ¼-grain (0.015 Gm.) dose at more frequent intervals is less completely analgesic than the stronger drug, but it is also less constipative, less nauseant, and less depressant to the general metabolism. The danger of codeine habituation is practically nil.

(c) *Pyramidon, Phenacetin and Acetanilid.*—Amidopyrine (pyramidon) is well given in a capsule containing 5 grains (0.32 Gm.) plus 2 grains (0.13 Gm.) of caffeine citrate, three or four times in the twenty-four hours. It should be given alone of course to those patients who are made sleepless by the caffeine. Phenacetin (acetphenetidin) may also be given with or without the caffeine, both drugs in the same doses as above. Acetanilid is given in 3-grain (0.2 Gm.) doses, several times at intervals of three hours; larger doses are seldom more effective and are more likely to cause the undesirable side-effects of this group: Sweat and chills, gastric disturbances, skin eruptions, renal irritation, methemoglobin cyanosis and collapse.

(d) *Salicylates.*—Few patients are relieved by these drugs. Either sodium salicylate or acetylsalicylic acid (aspirin) are used in doses of 5 to 15 grains (0.32 to 1 Gm.) every three hours. The more expensive cinchophen and neocinchophen are not needed here, since the gastric irritation caused by the salicylates is not seen in this short time.

6. **Antispasmodics.**—(*a*) *Atropine.*—In 1911, Novak, of Vienna, being struck by the fact that many women with increased irritability of the autonomic nervous system suffer with dysmenorrhea, began the treatment of the condition by the oral administration of atropine, Drenkhahn having been applying the drug directly in the cervical canal for a number of years. In the experience of most physicians who continue to use the drug—and nearly all do, for there is occasionally a strikingly good result—the colicky pains are much more relieved than are the backache, bearing down in the lower abdomen, lassitude, etc. Ordinarily, $\frac{1}{100}$ grain (0.0006 Gm.) is given three times daily, beginning two days before expected onset and continuing until the second or third day of menstruation.

(*b*) *Benzyl Benzoate.*—This drug and the similar compounds, benzyl fumarate and benzyl succinate, have failed to prove their worth. They have been dropped from N.N.R. and their day is probably done.

7. **Combined Use of Sedatives, Analgesics and Antispasmodics.**—I wish to set down here a prescription that has served well so many practitioners that it deserves a place in any treatise on the therapy of dysmenorrhea. I refer to the following combination of luminal, pyramidon, and a drug of the atropine group—first recommended, I believe, by Fantus, of Chicago:

R̸. Phenobarbital (luminal)............................ gr. vi   0.4
     Extract of hyoscyamus............................ gr. x   0.6
     Amidopyrine (pyramidon)......................... ℨj   4.0
     Make twelve capsules.
     Label: One capsule every four hours, not to exceed four doses in one day.

Each capsule contains $\frac{1}{2}$ grain (0.03 Gm.) of luminal, $\frac{5}{6}$ grain (0.05 Gm.) of the extract of hyoscyamus, and 5 grains (0.3 Gm.) of pyramidon. The backache as well as the colicky pain is not infrequently much relieved by this combination of drugs.

8. **Ovarian Therapy.**—I suppose that one has definitely and finally to admit that whatever of success has been achieved in the past with ovarian extracts was explainable on the grounds of coincident or psychic effect— bought at a too high figure for these times. At present there is a considerable stir in the investigational field, but the results insofar as they apply directly to dysmenorrhea are still only of experimental value; no new therapy, even tentatively proved, has yet resulted from this work.

DELIRIUM TREMENS

This is a type of acute insanity that develops in a relatively large proportion of heavy drinkers of alcohol under any of the following circumstances: (*a*) After a particularly heavy or prolonged bout of drinking; (*b*) during the first few days of an acute infectious disease; (*c*) following trauma, particularly fractures and injuries to the respiratory tract; (*d*) following the sudden withdrawal of liquor. After one or more days of prodromal uneasiness and insomnia, the patient begins to tremble and becomes actively delirious, in which state he remains without sleep for an average period of five or six days and then slowly recovers or dies. The outstanding features of the delirium in typical cases are: First, the fact that the patient is aware of his own personality but is disoriented as to time and the outside world;

second, that he is in a state of great fear; and, third, that the hallucinations are of sight almost exclusively. The temperature remains normal in uncomplicated cases unless the muscular activity is very great; the heart rate and force also correspond directly to the patient's activity except insofar as they are altered by previously existing cardiovascular disease. In the most serious cases, the state of postdelirious stupor known as "wet brain" supervenes: Delirium gives way to semicoma and tremor to immobility, and the patient lies upon his back making "rope-climbing" movements with his hands above his head. In fatal cases the body becomes rigid and the coma deepens into death. In the less serious cases, delirium is superseded by heavy sleep of several days' duration and ultimate recovery.

The mortality in uncomplicated cases of delirium tremens is about 15 per cent; it is much higher in traumatic and infectious cases.

THERAPY

Purgation.—It is routine practice in practically all emergency or general hospitals where the cases are frequently seen to administer a brisk cathartic at once; either a large dose of the salines (see list and dosage on p. 477), or 3 grains (0.2 Gm.) of calomel, followed in four to six hours by a saline.

Sedation.—To produce sleep is of the utmost importance; indeed, if the patient is seen before the delirium is fully developed its occurrence may be prevented by the judicious use of the sedatives. The following drugs or combinations are employed; it is well to alternate any of them with the following carminative mixture designed to overcome the stagnation of the gastric contents that is a frequent feature of these cases.

℞.	Tincture of capsicum	℥ss	2.0
	Spirits of peppermint	℥ij	8.0
	Tincture of ginger	℥ij	60.0
	Alcohol to make	℥iv	120.0

Label: One teaspoonful well diluted.

(*a*) *Paraldehyde.*—Two to 4 drachms (8 to 15 cc.), to be repeated in one hour if necessary. The excitability of a few patients will be increased by this drug.

(*b*) *Chloral Hydrate.*—Thirty to 45 grains (2 to 3 Gm.), not to be repeated in full dose under several hours.

(*c*) *Codeine Sulphate.*—One to 2 grains (0.06 to 0.12 Gm.) by mouth.

(*d*) *Paraldehyde, Chloral and Codeine.*—In some institutions the above three drugs are combined in the following proportions and given at once in one dose: Paraldehyde, 2 Gm. (8 cc.), choral, 30 grains (2 Gm.), codeine, 1 grain (0.06 Gm.).

(*e*) *Morphine and Scopolamine.*—Morphine sulphate, ¼ grain (0.015 Gm.), and scopolamine hydrobromide (hyoscine), $\frac{1}{100}$ grain (0.0006 Gm.), the latter to be repeated in doses of $\frac{1}{200}$ grain (0.0003 Gm.) at intervals of six hours. This treatment is not as popular as it once was: It is often not as effective as the other sedatives in combination; the hyoscine sometimes increases instead of decreasing the delirium, especially in women; the two drugs together occasionally produce an alarming respiratory depression; and there is the chance of inducing the morphine habit.

(*f*) *Apomorphine.*—Apomorphine hydrochloride, $\frac{1}{10}$ grain (0.006 Gm.), combined with strychnine sulphate, $\frac{1}{30}$ grain (0.002 Gm.), often acts excellently as a sedative. Lambert writes: "This does not produce as much emesis as one would expect, but it quiets the most profane and belligerent patient with surprising rapidity."

(*g*) *Intravenous Injection of Hypertonic Solutions.*—Hogan, in 1916, reported excellent results following the intravenous injection of 1000 cc. of a solution containing 5.8 Gm. of sodium chloride, 8.4 Gm. of sodium bicarbonate, 10.2 Gm. of sodium bromide, and water to make 1000 cc. In some instances he also gave in addition 250 cc. of a 30 per cent glucose solution. I am unable to find any further references to this method of treatment in the subsequent literature of the subject.

Control of Tremor.—Again I quote Lambert: "The marked tremor is best controlled by administration of strychnine and ergot; or, in some cases, by giving nux vomica, ½ grain (0.03 Gm.), ergot, ½ grain (0.03 Gm.), and extract of gentian every two hours."

Wet Brain.—In the treatment of this condition the stimulants are indicated, but it is not a matter of record how much good they actually accomplish: Atropine sulphate, $\frac{1}{40}$ grain (0.0015 Gm.), not to be repeated under six hours; strychnine sulphate, $\frac{1}{30}$ grain (0.002 Gm.); metrazol, 1½ grains (0.1 Gm.), intramuscularly; camphor in oil, 1 to 2 cc., intramuscularly. Aromatic spirits of ammonia, ½ to 1 drachm (2 to 4 cc.), is a reflex stimulant of some value, but usually these patients cannot be gotten to swallow anything. Alcohol is contraindicated.

SEASICKNESS

There are some individuals who suffer from loss of appetite and low-grade nausea, but without actual vomiting, throughout the first few days of a voyage and then recover their normal feeling of well-being; others there are who experience only an excruciating headache without the least gastrointestinal symptoms; but the symptoms in the most frequent type of the malady have been listed by Desnoes as follows: "Discomfort in the epigastric region, varying with the rise and fall of the ship; anorexia, salivation, with frequent swallowing movements; headache; dizziness, weakness, progressing to faintness; cold perspiration of the skin, and pallor of the face, with the oft-described greenish hue. The facial expression, which is one of great dejection and apathy, faithfully records the internal feelings. Waves of nausea finally get so strong that the desire to vomit is overwhelming, and after that act is consummated great relief is experienced. The vomiting is very often projectile in character, and there may be little or no nausea preceding." Most cases terminate spontaneously after a few days at sea, but there are a few individuals who suffer continuously throughout an entire voyage. Even professional seafaring men are occasionally made slightly ill when the ship begins to pitch or roll in an unusual fashion, particularly if they walk to a part of the vessel which they are not in the habit of visiting.

Despite the respectable antiquity of this malady we are still without an entirely satisfactory explanation of its etiology. Each of the following factors has at some time been urged as the sole cause, but it is more probable that all of them operate to some extent in varying proportions in each case. (a) The labyrinthine theory suggests that the upset is caused by overstimulation of the equilibratory organs in the internal ear, with resultant overflow of stimuli from these to other centers, such as the vagus. (b) The theory that confusion results from the multiplicity of unusual stimuli coming along those sensory nerves that ordinarily have to do with the adjustment of our bodies in space. (c) The theory that eyestrain caused by the glare of the sea and sky, and the unusual fixation upon moving objects, reflexly causes the symptoms. (d) The theory that the wide excursions made by the freely movable organs of the abdominal cavity unduly irritate the vagus nerve. (e) The theory that autosuggestion is causative. (f) The theory that the malady is an acidosis.

THERAPY

Postural Treatment.—Unless the psychic element is uppermost, the patient probably profits most by lying in the prone position with the head very little, if at all, raised. The nearer the center of the ship he stays the better. Sudden movements should be avoided, such as bending forward or getting up rapidly, or hurriedly ascending or descending the companionway.

Value of Fresh Air.—The patient should recline on deck, if possible; however, many patients are embarrassed by their illness in the presence of others, and can relax freely only in the privacy of their cabins, in which cases all facilities for maintaining the circulation of the air in the room must be utilized.

Prevention of Eyestrain.—The seasick individual should lie facing the deckhouse and not the sea and should avoid using the eyes as much as possible, reading only for brief periods and keeping the eyes closed at other times. Some persons immure themselves in a darkened cabin as soon as they board ship and leave it only when the port of destination has been reached. Perhaps a few thus avoid illness, but the fact should not be overlooked that blind persons also suffer from seasickness.

Plugging of the Ears.—The simple procedure of plugging the ears with cotton is said to greatly relieve the symptoms in some instances. It is very likely that whatever relief the late President Coolidge obtained from the application of local anesthetics to the ear canal was ascribable to the effect of plugging the canals with the cotton pledgets on which the solutions were placed. Just why such plugging should occasionally be effective is unknown—perhaps we must say again, psychic effect!

Abdominal Binder.—The use of a tight binder across the lower abdomen has many staunch supporters among experienced travelers; most physicians believe that only those who suffer from visceroptosis are thus relieved. However, during my own brief experience as a ship surgeon one of my fellow officers repeatedly demonstrated to me that he became quite ill whenever he removed his binder in a heavy sea. This man was apparently not visceroptotic, though of course x-ray studies were not made, nor do I believe that he was under any psychic thralldom to his belt, for he had followed the sea for many years and had only recently discovered that he could pass unscathed through storms in this way.

Diet.—On this head Oriel (1927) writes: "One finds that if passengers can be persuaded to eat plenty of fruit and carbohydrates and to avoid fats that they are never violently sick. The common error is to avoid food, which, of course, leads to early exhaustion of the glycogen reserve. Acidosis is the inevitable sequel. Once this train of events is in progress other factors, such as inability to take food and constant vomiting, tend to make the acidosis more severe." Seasick persons should eat, no matter if they lose one meal after another, for vomiting something is easier than the endless retching of an empty stomach. Swallowing small chunks of ice, or sipping cold ginger ale or champagne, are often helpful measures in dispelling nausea.

Certainly the excessive smoking and drinking in which many individuals indulge while at sea cannot but aggravate the bout of illness when heavy weather comes.

The following carminative mixture will hasten the passage of the stomach contents into the duodenum, and may prevent the onset of the complete syndrome in an individual who is only slightly nauseated:

℞.	Tincture of capsicum	℥ss	2.0
	Spirits of peppermint	℥ij	8.0
	Tincture of ginger	℥ij	60.0
	Alcohol to make	℥iv	120.0

Label: One teaspoonful well diluted after meals; may be repeated if desired.

Glucose.—Sidney Jones (1925), surgeon of the *Aquitania,* has suggested that seasickness is an acidosis, and is curable by the administration of glucose. Oriel (1927) has studied the matter as thoroughly as would seem possible at sea and has presented findings, as follows:

(*a*) That labyrinthine disturbances, if present, do not give rise to nystagmus or to alternation in labyrinthine tests.

(*b*) That autosuggestion is not wholly responsible, as there is a distinct metabolic upset found in the prevomiting stage, as shown by (1) hyperglycemia followed by hypoglycemia; (2) increased ammonia excretion; and (3) the presence of acetone in the urine.

(*c*) That when vomiting is established there is a very severe acidosis, as indicated by excretion of ammonia up to 265 mg. per cent, and the presence of much acetone and diacetic acid in the urine.

(*d*) That the administration of glucose causes diuresis, abolition of acetonuria, and a fall in the ammonia excretion, resulting clinically in the relief of symptoms.

"Glucose was given in doses of 3 drachms (12 Gm.) to more than 1000 patients with seasickness, and the following results were noted. The effect observed in well-established cases was much superior to that obtained by the exhibition of other remedies such as atropine and strychnine, belladonna, chloral, bromides, alkalis, and the various patent remedies. When glucose is administered to a well-established case acetone disappears from the urine, diuresis takes place, and ammonia excretion is lowered, with a corresponding increase in total acidity in the urine. *Pari passu* with the metabolic change there is an improvement in the general condition, and headache is abolished. The occurrence of diuresis is interesting and similar in nature to that which occurs after the other acidoses such as postanesthetic vomiting and cyclic vomiting. The effect of giving glucose is also good in the prevomiting stage, and here again acetone is abolished. It is an undoubted fact, however, that glucose administered to a well-established case is much more dramatic in its effect than in the prevomiting stage. . . . If the vomiting is severe and glucose cannot be retained for fifteen minutes (in which time a large portion is absorbed) it has been given with success both intravenously and rectally."

Both Marrack (1931) and Maitland (1932), on the basis of much experience, have questioned this opinion that there is a distinct metabolic upset as a contributory antecedent of the actual bout of sickness, though not denying that glucose is at times helpful in its treatment.

Cathartics.—The normal individual should be warned that he is liable to become somewhat constipated during the voyage and will do well to employ a simple cathartic on any day that he has not gone to stool. Constipated individuals should by all means try to have their condition corrected (see p. 432) before they go to sea. I think the drastic catharsis induced by many voyagers before they board ship is unnecessary.

Belladonna, Hyoscine and Strychnine.—Girard many years ago advocated the use of atropine sulphate, $\frac{1}{120}$ grain (0.0005 Gm.), combined with strychnine sulphate, $\frac{1}{60}$ grain (0.001 Gm.), subcutaneously, at the beginning of a voyage, during rough weather, or on the advent of a storm; this dose to be repeated twice, at hourly intervals, or until incipient dryness of the throat and disturbance of vision indicate its discontinuance. I believe that the attempts to prove the rationale of this combination, based upon the pharmacological actions of its components, have not been fortunate; but it is certainly a clinical fact that the mixture does often relieve seasickness. Desnoes (1926), a medical officer of the United Fruit Company, writes:

"In our experience we have secured better results with scopolamine hydrobromide (hyoscine), a close relative of atropine. It is given in small

49

doses and is frequently repeated, in order to discover the idiosyncratic patient before much of the drug has been taken, and to secure maximal sustained effect with the minimal amount of medication. Our routine drug treatment in mild cases of seasickness is $\frac{1}{400}$ grain (0.00016 Gm.) scopolamine hydrobromide, by mouth every hour until the patient is relieved or until the physiologic effects are obtained. A simple way to give this is 1 teaspoonful every hour of a mixture containing scopolamine hydrobromide, $\frac{1}{50}$ grain (0.0013 Gm.), spirit of peppermint, 3 minims (0.2 cc.) elixir of lactated pepsin, sufficient to make 1 ounce (30 cc.). In cases with much depression, strychnine sulphate, $\frac{1}{60}$ grain (0.001 Gm.), is added to the mixture, and for severer cases with much vomiting scopolamine and strychnine are given by hypodermic injection."

Hirsch (1931) has also recently testified to the usefulness of scopolamine.

Sedatives.—Desnoes, above quoted, continues: "As the psychic element enters into nearly every case, a centrally acting hypnotic is usually necessary; for this we use chlorbutanol (chloretone), from 5 to 10 grains (0.32 to 0.65 Gm.) in capsules, repeated in six hours if necessary. Besides inducing sleep, this remedy has an anesthetic action on the gastric mucosa. A convenient way of dispensing chlorbutanol, together with the previously mentioned drugs, is to place the tablets in the capsule with the chlorbutanol, and all three may be taken together." For a list of other sedatives that might be used with advantage see page 578. In my own brief experience I several times saw chloretone succeed when other sedatives had failed.

Morphine and Rectal Feeding in Excessive Vomiting.—Desnoes describes his handling of these cases as follows:

"Cases of excessive vomiting that tax our efforts at control are occasionally encountered. After the usual remedies are tried, including the mustard plaster applied to the epigastrium, from $\frac{1}{8}$ to $\frac{1}{4}$ grain (0.008 to 0.015 Gm.) of morphine sulphate, administered hypodermically, combined with from $\frac{1}{200}$ to $\frac{1}{150}$ grain (0.0003 to 0.0004 Gm.) of atropine sulphate, is the court of last resort. Provision must be made for the curious fact that the drug most potent in checking vomiting is followed by vomiting as a common after-effect. After the patient awakes from the sleep induced by the drug, he should be directed not to raise his head from the bed for several hours. Iced brandy, champagne or strong coffee may be given through a drinking tube, but if nausea reasserts itself it is best to continue the administration of morphine, combined with atropine, in progressively descending dosage, using perhaps every four hours half the previous dose. If neither food nor water can be retained in the stomach for twelve hours or so, no time should be lost in resorting to rectal alimentation. The only substances of food value that can be absorbed from the lower intestine are amino-acids, simple sugars and alcohol. The old method of trying to maintain nutrition by the introduction of ordinary foodstuffs through the rectum has been shown to be inefficacious. Skimmed and pancreatinized milk may be used, or the clysma suggested by Smithies: Alcohol, 50 per cent, 1 ounce (30 cc.); glucose, 1 ounce (30 cc.); physiologic sodium chloride solution, sufficient to make 8 ounces (240 cc.). Karo corn syrup is a concentrated solution of practically pure glucose and is easily obtainable. This injection should be administered at body temperature by the drop method, with the patient on his back and the hips elevated; it should be repeated two or three times during the day. A bulk of 10 ounces (300 cc.) should not be exceeded. Needless to say, feeding by mouth should be resumed as soon as possible, commencing with such easily digestible articles as milk, bouillon tea, ice cream and arrowroot crackers."

Nitrites.—Pearcy and Hayden (1928) stated that 3 to 5 grains (0.2 to 0.3 Gm.) of sodium nitrite every two hours relieved eight persons of seasickness within four hours; the symptoms did not recur in any of these patients. Sellheim (1928) also independently reported that several persons were protected from the malady or cured of it by one dose of two drops of a 0.5 per cent solution of nitroglycerin placed directly on the tongue. According to Lebensohn (1930), British investigators have been unable to confirm these observations.

Psychotherapy.—Many individuals, especially first-trippers, agitate themselves into a very nervous state before they board ship and are almost certain to develop seasickness as soon as the ground swell is felt. In these cases it is perhaps advisable to use small nonnarcotic doses of the sedatives for several days before the voyage is begun, advising the ship surgeon when possible what has been done in order that he may be guided in his medication during the first few days at sea; indeed, the carrying of a note to this officer, with a request for what is looked upon as "special care," often has a profoundly helpful effect upon nervous individuals who dread the ordeal of a bout of seasickness alone on a large ship; upon the reaction of the plagued surgeon let us draw the charitable curtain!

Helpful admonitions regarding conduct during the voyage are the following: (*a*) Divert yourself in the company of others as much as possible, but do not plunge too strenuously into unwonted exercise; (*b*) look shipward instead of seaward for the first few days, but do not "strain" yourself to do this else it will only serve as a reminder of the ever-lurking illness; (*c*) avoid the sight of sick individuals as much as possible; (*d*) go in jauntily to meals as soon as they are announced for procrastination often spells disaster at this juncture; (*e*) if on a small ship, keep to windward of the deckhouse in order to avoid the odor of cooking food.

HEAT STROKE
(Sunstroke)

The most common form of heat stroke is that known in the South as "a touch of the sun" or "overcome by the heat." The individual suddenly becomes acutely sensitive to the oppressive atmospheric conditions, grows pale with a clammy skin, has disturbances of vision, feels very weak and perhaps nauseated, and either crumples down in the sun or manages to drag himself into the shade before collapsing; the pulse is fast and weak, the respirations rapid and shallow, the pupils dilated, temperature normal or subnormal. The mortality from this type of heat stroke is practically nil, but the patient often recovers very slowly and is ever after unusually sensitive to high temperatures.

The severe and frequently fatal form of heat stroke is characterized by a brief prodromal period not easily distinguishable from that described above, but consciousness is early lost, and it is noticed that the skin, instead of being clammy, is dry and hot and that the temperature is very high. The pupils are usually dilated in the beginning as in the milder form, but the pulse is rapid and full and the breathing deep. It is only later that the pulse becomes irregular and feeble and the respirations become shallow and finally of the Cheyne-Stokes type; at this stage the pupils are found to be contracted and the conjunctivae injected. In many cases involuntary passage of characteristically foul feces takes place and the patient's body odor also becomes offensive. Muscular twitchings and rolling of the head are common; sometimes epileptiform convulsions take place. As death approaches evidences of pulmonary edema are often to be found.

THERAPY

In the mild cases, the patient must be made to lie in the coolest place available, his clothing should be opened, and he should be given water to drink if he desires it. If the pulse remains rapid and weak for long, one of the following stimulants may be advantageously used: Caffeine sodium benzoate, 2 to 5 grains (0.13 to 0.32 Gm.), intramuscularly; metrazol, 1½ grains (0.1 Gm.), intramuscularly; camphor in oil, 1 to 2 cc., intramuscularly; aromatic spirits of ammonia, ½ to 1 drachm (2 to 4 cc.), in water by mouth. Occasionally in these cases the temperature falls quite far below normal and it becomes necessary to apply external heat and administer hot drinks; one should be careful here as a sudden high rise of temperature may be induced. The treatment is also at times complicated by the necessity of administering chloral and bromide by rectum to control the convulsions.

In the hyperpyrexia cases attempt must be made to stimulate the heart by means of the above stimulants, but the most imperative need is to reduce the temperature. The following methods are employed:

(*a*) Place the patient in water cooled to 50 F. (10 C.) by floating a cake of ice in it, and keep him there until the rectal temperature falls to 102 F. (38.8 C.). After this temperature is reached the body will continue to lose heat in favorable cases even after removal from the water; sometimes the fall will go below the normal line. It is imperative that vigorous manual friction of the skin be made continuously while the patient is in the tub, for unless hyperemia of the skin capillaries takes place the overheated blood will only be driven in instead of being cooled at the surface.

(*b*) Injection of 1000 cc. or more of ice water into the rectum. This method is very little employed in the large clinics where many of these cases are seen each summer.

(*c*) Rubbing the body with ice, or placing the patient in sheets wrung out of ice water. These methods also are looked upon as less efficient than the following:

(*d*) The abstraction of heat by evaporation of water from the body surface. This is best accomplished by spraying water onto the stripped body from a fine nozzle, meanwhile maintaining a constant current of air either by means of hand or electric fans. There is no advantage in using ice water as tepid water will remove practically as much heat. This method has replaced all others in most hospitals, and has the added advantage that it can be utilized anywhere since it does not depend upon the use of ice. When the rectal temperature reaches 102 F. (38.8 C.) the evaporation may be stopped during a period of observation. Hearne, with the British troops in Mesopotamia, found that the cessation of sweating, once it has been established, is a valuable sign of impending recurrence, and that if these patients are covered with a moist sheet and the fanning resumed, artificial perspiration will be established and recurrence sometimes averted.

STOKERS' CRAMPS

This is a type of heat exhaustion seen frequently in those who labor in the heat of fire-rooms, in deep mines, etc. Following a period of muscular twitching, the patient is seized with violent cramps principally of the abdominal groups; sometimes, however, the spasm is so general as to resemble an epileptic attack. The patient is nauseated, dizzy, stuporous, and usually pallid and perspiring; the pulse is rapid but strong and the temperature little if at all above normal. Urine is scanty and the patient is usually very thirsty. These attacks are believed to be due to the fact that in the excessive ingestion of water and its elimination through the skin abnormal quantities of chlorides are lost, though just why this loss of chlorides should cause the cramps is not clear.

THERAPY

The sufferer must be removed to the coolest place available and his desire for fluids should be satisfied. In those cases that are hospitalized, which is rare, the slow rectal injection of 2 or 3 quarts (liters) of very slightly hypertonic saline solution, has been found to be of advantage. Talbott and Michelsen (1933), in their studies during the construction of Hoover Dam, gave 1000 to 1500 cc. of physiologic saline solution subcutaneously or intravenously, sometimes repeated; when given by vein adding 5 per cent of glucose. They felt an exclusive milk diet (*ad libitum*) to be advisable for the first twenty-four hours.

The addition of salt to the drinking water has been tried with apparently good results in preventing the attacks. I quote Davis' abstract of Court's paper published in the Colliery Guardian, a British coal journal, in October, 1924.

"A few colliers were therefore chosen to test the effect of drinking a weak solution of salt in water, the proportion first tried being about 0.25 per cent, or 10 Gm. per gallon of water. Such promising results were obtained that more men were prevailed on to put salt in their daily drinking water. Each collier carried a daily supply of 2 quarts, to which was added at home 1 teaspoonful to each quart of water.

"The results were most gratifying. Six miners after a month's trial declared themselves to be less tired each day after work, and one no longer took his customary nap after reaching home. Another no longer had leg cramps and the families of all reported greater energy evident at home.

"Similar experiments on boiler stokers working at 96 F. in very dry air, in which ½ teaspoonful of salt was added to each quart of their daily ration of 2 quarts, showed that the workers all felt less tired on reaching home."

Further experience has amply proved the worth of the salt addition but the practical difficulty of getting the objectionable salt water drunk is of course great. Glover (1931) has recently advised the providing of 16-grain (1 Gm.) tablets of sodium chloride at the drinking tap, one such tablet, which is only slightly larger than the ordinary aspirin tablet, to be swallowed each time the tap is visited. He was unable to supply convincing evidence of freedom from cramps afforded by this simple measure, but felt it worthy of trial in industrial plants, mines, ships, etc. It has been stated that the local action of this concentrated salt solution might be undesirable, but for my part I fail to see why this should be so.

SKIN DISINFECTION

Practitioners in all branches of medicine find themselves frequently under the necessity of applying antiseptics to the skin, whether in preparing the field for hypodermic, intramuscular or intravenous therapy or for the diagnostic puncture, for sterilization of superficial wounds, or in pursuance of the more specialized activities of the surgeon or obstetrician. I have therefore included in this book a list of the various drug combinations in use for disinfection of the skin, together with comments on the methods of their employment, but shall not at this time institute comparisons of their relative efficiency because it has become apparent that in the present state of our knowledge control is very difficult in the experimental study of antiseptic and disinfectant substances. The observations of Arnold *et al.* (1930) and of Bryan and Mallmann (1933) that the intact outermost layer of the skin of man and of dogs possesses an amazingly efficient self-disinfecting power, has not lightened the burden of investigators in this field.

The Preliminary Use of Soap.—The vigorous scrubbing of the skin with soap and moderately hot water for about five minutes undoubtedly softens and removes a considerable part of the superficial epithelium and thus presents a cleaner field for subsequent application of the antiseptic solution. In the early days of bacteriology, Koch (1881) asserted that the soaps did more than this, *i. e.*, that they were actually germicidal; this belief has been thoroughly overthrown, but unfortunately it seems that many surgeons nowadays are also overlooking the above-mentioned very valuable cleansing effect of soap and water. The addition of small amounts of antiseptic substances to form the so-called "germicidal" soaps has been many times shown to be of no value.

Tincture of Iodine.—The U.S.P. tincture of iodine contains 7 per cent of iodine and 5 per cent of potassium iodide in 95 per cent alcohol. This preparation, or one of the modifications of it below, is perhaps more used than any other substance for skin disinfection. It must be removed with alcohol, however, for otherwise it is very prone to blister the skin, especially where it collects at the margins of the area painted. Of course this cleansing with alcohol is also of value, but it has the additional disadvantages of being time-consuming and of rendering doubtful the exact extent of the operative field when unforeseen additional incisions become necessary. The objection is also sometimes raised against iodine that it may cause intraperitoneal adhesions after laparotomies in which the viscera are brought out on the abdominal wall.

Tincture of Iodine (Diluted).—Three and one-half per cent tincture of iodine, made by diluting the official tincture with an equal quantity of 95 per cent alcohol, is much used in genito-urinary work, where the stronger tincture cannot be employed.

Iodine in Diluted Alcohol.—Two per cent iodine in 70 per cent alcohol is used by many surgeons; here the alcohol, which is used at its optimum strength, also contributes toward the disinfection.

Potassium Mercuric Iodide.—The tablets (or disks) of this salt described in the N.N.R. contain sufficient potassium iodide so that they may be easily dissolved in water; a 0.5 to 1 per cent solution may be used. More often, however, a 1 per cent solution of the drug is made in 80 per cent acetone; this is less irritating than the tincture of iodine but not infrequently causes a marked dermatitis, especially when used in the genital region; here its application is often quite painful as well. The solution is also very pale in color and thus but poorly outlines the operative field. The name "Kalmerid" is sometimes erroneously applied to this solution in acetone, whereas actually Kalmerid is the proprietary name of one of the tablets of potassium mercuric iodide plus potassium iodide just mentioned above.

Picric Acid (Trinitrophenol).—A 5 per cent solution of picric acid in alcohol is used. It is an efficient disinfectant and penetrates well, but it seems not infrequently to irritate the skin of tender regions, despite the paucity of reports to this effect in the literature. It dries slowly and tends to crystallize; also it continues to stain the clothing and bedding for several days after the operation. One should also remember that dressings, towels, etc., near the field of operation, which have been soaked in picric acid and allowed to dry, are quite inflammable—an important matter if the actual cautery is being used.

Mercurochrome Alone and with Alcohol and Acetone.—A 2 per cent aqueous solution of mercurochrome has been widely used but some investigators believe that antiseptic efficiency is increased by the addition of alcohol and acetone. Scott and Hill (1925) advocate the following mixture: 2 Gm. of mercurochrome-220-soluble are dissolved in 35 cc. of distilled water and then 55 cc. of 95 per cent alcohol and 10 cc. of acetone are added while stirring. The mixture must be compounded in this order because of the difficulty of getting the mercurochrome into alcoholic solution, alcohol being desired because of its bactericidal and drying properties. Acetone is used because of its solvent and drying properties and its ability to reduce surface tension and thus to permit quicker and deeper penetration of tissues and bacteria. The preparation goes on very evenly, dries in less than two minutes, is not irritating either at time of application or afterward, and colors the operative field beyond peradventure of a doubt. In the work of Scott and Hill it appears that the mixture had not lost any of its strength forty-six days after making.

Solution S.T. 37 (hexylresorcinol) has come to be much used of late, but Leonard (1930), who devised the preparation, has pointed out that it is suitable only for use on wounds and mucous membranes, lacking as it does the fat-dissolving, staining and quick drying properties desirable in skin disinfectants.

Acriflavine-alcohol-acetone.—Tinker and Sutton (1926) have found a mixture of these ingredients experimentally satisfactory. They advise proceeding as follows to make 100 cc. of solution: Add 10 cc. of acetone and 37.5 cc. of distilled water to 52.5 cc. of 95 per cent alcohol, then dissolve in this 5 Gm. of powdered acriflavine. This solution then contains 5 per cent acriflavine, 10 per cent acetone and 50 per cent alcohol. It should be kept in dark colored bottles and should not be relied upon if more than a week old or if any precipitate has formed. These workers emphasize the following points as being of especial importance:

1. Thorough mechanical cleansing of the skin with soap and water.

2. Liberal use of alcohol and ether or other efficient fat solvents with gauze and friction.

3. The last gauze sponge used before the application of acriflavine to come away from the skin without discoloration.

4. All sponging to be done away from the center of the field toward the periphery.

5. All acriflavine to be left on the skin and not washed away with alcohol as is done with iodine.

The acriflavine-alcohol-acetone mixture is nonirritating to the skin.

Metaphen.—The most effective preparation is probably the following: Dissolve 0.5 Gm. crystalline metaphen in a mixture of 10 cc. acetone and 50 cc. full-strength alcohol; to this solution add slowly, while stirring, a mixture of 1 cc. of a 1 per cent aqueous solution of eosin and 39 cc. of distilled water. This preparation dries in about three minutes, does not burn even on the genitalia, and colors the painted area a delicate pink. The stains to linen and clothing are said to be readily removable with ordinary soap and water; metallic instruments and rubber are apparently not harmed by the solution. Its stability in amber-colored bottles is only about a month, but Scott and Birkhaug (1931) have apparently removed this objectionable feature of instability by adding to 100 cc. of the formula 2.5 cc. of normal sodium hydroxide.

Sterilization of the Hands.—The following is a practical and economical method in use in many hospitals (Jour. Amer. Med. Assoc., 94, 1341, 1930): The usual washing of the hands and forearms for about 2 inches above the elbows is done thoroughly, each part being gone over at least three times with a bland soap (such as ivory) and running water. Nail sticks and brushes are sterilized in the autoclave. Solution of hydrogen peroxide is used for cleaning the nails. The hands are then placed in a 70 per cent alcohol solution and washed, including the forearms, for from one to three minutes. They are then dried with sterile towels, and gloves are put on. The gloved hands are washed from time to time in a solution of 1: 1000 corrosive mercuric chloride and rinsed in sterile water. In making up the alcohol solution, the hospital druggist medicates it with phenol and oil of wintergreen. Two drachms of phenol and 20 drops of oil of wintergreen are added to each gallon of alcohol, U.S.P. The alcohol is then diluted to 70 per cent for use in the operating room. After it is used for washing the hands it is filtered, tested with a hydrometer, and, if necessary, brought up to a 70 per cent solution by the addition of the alcohol solution. It is then used again just the same as the fresh solution. Round bottom shallow basins are used for the alcohol solution and the deep basins for the other solutions.

PARENTERAL ADMINISTRATION OF GLUCOSE

The injection in one way or another of glucose (dextrose) solution has now attained a position of considerable importance as a rational therapeutic measure in general medicine, obstetrics and surgery, notwithstanding the fact that at times unpleasant reactions follow. These reactions are usually characterized by a sharp chill, considerable rise in temperature, and shock and collapse which may be quite serious; exceptionally a death has been reported. However, close attention to the technic of preparation and administration of the solution practically eliminates the possibility of such occurrences.

1. PREPARATION OF SOLUTION

The usual procedure has been to dissolve 25 Gm. of chemically pure glucose in 100 cc. of freshly double distilled water, sterilizing then in cotton-plugged, leadfoil-sealed flasks in a steam sterilizer at 100 C. for one-half hour on three successive days, or in emergencies under 15 pounds pressure in an autoclave for twenty minutes, solutions showing caramelization or sediment after sterilization being discarded. It is probably advisable to filter the solution several times before sterilizing. However, Williams and Swett, and Mellon *et al.* having shown that the glucose solution was changed to an acid pH on sterilizing, the addition of a buffer solution to these solutions was advocated and indeed has been shown to prevent the reactions; but the preparation of these buffer salts is very tedious and time-consuming work and has now practically been relegated to the commercial laboratories, who supply a number of N.N.R.-accepted concentrated solutions, either buffered or accompanied by a buffer solution to be added at the time of diluting with sterilized distilled water. The method of Sanford and Heitmeyer (1928), later somewhat simplified by others, in which dry sterilization of the glucose over calcium chloride and dissolving just before use is employed, was an advance in that it made possible the free use of glucose solutions for intra-peritoneal injections without fear of the reactions which sometimes followed the use of solutions prepared in the more usual way. But the simplest method of all seems to be that of Schwentker, which has been used satisfactorily for the preparation of solution intended for introduction by all the routes:

"Test tubes 6 by ¾ inches (15.2 by 9.5 cm.) are heated near the open end in a Bunsen flame and drawn out so that they present a constriction near the mouth. Into these, 10 Gm. of chemically pure glucose is poured and allowed to run through the constriction into the tube. The constricted part is then sealed off in the Bunsen flame, so that the glucose is hermetically sealed in an ampule. Ampules so prepared are sterilized by boiling in the water bath for thirty minutes on each of three consecutive days. When sterile, the ampules may be kept indefinitely, and are made into solution for use simply by dissolving the contents of one ampule in a flask containing the required amount of sterile distilled water. In practice, I have found it advantageous to keep on hand a supply of flasks containing 200 cc. of sterile distilled water. The contents of an ampule dissolved in one of these yields 200 cc. of 5 per cent glucose solution ready for use; two ampules are dissolved if a 10 per cent solution is required. The glucose dissolves almost immediately."

These ampules have been found to be uniformly sterile even by the most rigid tests. The glucose undergoes no change during this sterilization and therefore the pH of the solution made from the contents of such an ampule is the pH of the water in which the solution is made. It has been the experience of many observers that distilled water boiled in a flask for five minutes is just as satisfactory as autoclaved water, indeed perhaps better because the reaction of distilled water which has had its pH lowered by absorption of carbon dioxide while standing becomes neutral again upon boiling. It would seem that the development of this simple method of sterilizing a measured quantity of glucose in a form which enables it to be easily transported in a hermetically sealed ampule, protected from atmospheric changes and probably indefinitely stable (Schwentker has used ampules three months old), is a distinct advance.

2. PREPARATION OF THE TUBING

The following is the way in which new rubber tubing should be treated before use in order to prevent reactions: (*a*) Soak in soap and water for one hour. (*b*) Wash well with soap and water. (*c*) Wash in running water. (*d*) Soak for six hours in 4 per cent solution of sodium hydroxide. (*e*) Wash well in running water. (*f*) Wash well in distilled water.

3. INTERMITTENT INTRAVENOUS ADMINISTRATION

Perhaps the most usual practice is to give 300 cc. of a 25 per cent solution at the rate of 4 cc. per minute, repeating several times as felt necessary in the twenty-four hours. The usual arsphenamine type of tube and a small caliber needle are used, the tube, tubing and needle having been first thoroughly washed and sterilized, and finally rinsed through with sterile distilled water, before using. The injection is to be made at body temperature, which is insured either by employing one of the special pieces of apparatus, as that of Titus (sold by the Feick Bros. Co., Pittsburgh), or by placing hot-water bags or the electric pad about the lower end of the tubing, or by coiling the tubing through a basin of water at 100 F. or slightly above. As the injection will take about an hour and a quarter, it is well to fix the needle in place at the proper angle with adhesive tape.

4. CONTINUOUS (VENOCLYSIS) INTRAVENOUS ADMINISTRATION

In this method, 10 per cent glucose solution is given continuously during many hours or days; the rate of 200 cc. per hour has been found optimum for the adult (further details on p. 164). In children in a state of dehydration, Karelitz and Schick (1932) have felt that 5 per cent concentration is preferable since the 10 per cent solution caused the excretion of an amount of urine in excess of the amount of fluid consumed, with a resultant increase in dehydration. Hendon, the originator of the method, describes his technic as follows:

"The apparatus consists essentially of a silver and gold plated cannula. Any size required may be obtained, but the 12 gauge is found most frequently useful. Two vacuum bottles suspended from a stand 6 feet high act as reservoirs to contain the fluid and maintain its temperature [Theo. Tafel Co., Louisville]. A visible rectal dripper is joined in the delivery tube. The rubber tubing used must be of the thick-walled stethoscopic variety except for the piece that fits over the cannula. This should be thinner so as to be easily slipped on and off.

"I endeavor to deliver the fluid into the vein at 100 F. It is placed in the container at from 120 to 130, thus allowing for a loss of from 20 to 30 degrees in transit. Recent experience seems to indicate that temperature is not of as much importance as I formerly believed it to be.

"Any conveniently situated vein will do, but I prefer the basilic or cephalic because, for one reason, they lack tributaries. The vessel is exposed above the elbow by a horizontal incision after a tourniquet has been applied. With an aneurysm needle a convenient length of umbilical tape is carried beneath it. The vein is then ligated with catgut distal to the tape. It is now picked up with mosquito forceps and the tourniquet removed. The portion in the grasp of the forceps is snipped with a manicurist instrument known as a cuticle nipper. This enables one to lift up a tongue of triangular-shaped tissue composed of vessel wall. Through the opening thus made the specially devised cannula is introduced beyond its shoulder and the tapes encircling the vessel are tied, one proximal and the other distal to the shoulder. The cannula thus secured is then connected by a piece of rubber tubing and a glass irrigating nozzle to the delivery tube and the flow is started at a rather rapid dropping rate and immediately throttled down to about 40 drops a minute. The rectal dripper serves to permit one to count the drops and register the amount. When I am assured that the connections are patent and the flow established, the tubing is bound to the forearm with encircling strips of adhesive plaster to the wrist. No splints are either desirable or necessary; the patient may assume any position he finds most comfortable. Two vacuum bottles to act as reservoirs are provided so that there need be no interruption in the supply. As soon as one becomes empty the alternate is turned on and the exhausted flask is refilled immediately."

5. INTRAPERITONEAL ADMINISTRATION

When intravenous introduction of the solution is impossible, as is often the case in infants, the intraperitoneal route may be used. Five per cent concentration is employed because it has been found by several observers that a higher concentration tends to attract fluid into the abdominal cavity. Sanford and Heitmeyer write: "The usual sterile procedure is used and the injection into the abdomen is made at the usual point [midline below the umbilicus—H. B.]. To be effective, the glucose should be given in 100-cc. quantities, repeated frequently." This relatively simple procedure is of great value in pediatric practice, but has its definite limitations; it is contraindicated in preoperative and postoperative conditions and in many other pathologic states of the abdominal cavity and its contents, such as distention unless it be only very slight, and particularly in the tympanites of pneumonia. Ravenel (1933) has shown that in premature and very young infants the danger of producing serious hemorrhage by wounding the "obliterated" hypogastric artery is a very real one.

6. SUBCUTANEOUS ADMINISTRATION

It is the general impression that the subcutaneous administration of glucose is too painful to be borne for very long by older individuals but the method is not infrequently resorted to in infants, particularly the newborn. Moore (1932) advises 10 per cent concentration, about 200 cc. being given two to four times daily "or as often as may be necessary."

7. INTRAMUSCULAR ADMINISTRATION

The intramuscular method of introducing glucose in children apparently originated in Nassau's clinic in Berlin. Glaser (1928) has reported favorably in the United States. In a series of more than a hundred cases, which included premature infants as well as older children and an occasional adult, the only ill results noted from the injection of a 10 per cent solution were in 3 cases in which indurated areas, persisting for one or two weeks, appeared deep in the muscles. It was suspected that these were hematomas secondary to blood vessel injury, but this could not be verified because the patients survived. The method of injecting into the muscles of the lateral anterolateral surfaces of the thighs is described as follows:

"A syringe of at least 20-cc. capacity and fairly fine needles (20 gauge) should be used. The solution usually enters the tissues with great ease, particularly in markedly dehydrated patients, and in those instances in which the needle point happens to lie in a fascial plane. The fluid should not be delivered more rapidly than at the rate of fifteen minutes for 100 cc. The amount of solution that may be given depends on the ease with which the muscles become distended, the injection being stopped or the position of the needle changed as soon as the tissues feel tense. In the case of very small infants, particularly premature infants, care should be exercised to avoid overdistention of the tissues as this has caused compression of the veins in several instances, with temporary embarrassment to the venous return and consequent cyanosis of the extremity. From 20 to 40 cc. may be given into the thigh of an infant, and up to 100 cc. or more into the thigh muscles of older children or adults. Absorption of the glucose is usually complete within an hour. In inserting the needles care should be taken to avoid the femoral artery, which lies in a line joining the middle of the inguinal ligament with the internal condyle of the femur. This line may be conveniently marked out with mercurochrome. . . .

"In those instances of infections in premature infants or other infants having a lowered resistance in which blood from the father or other donor was mixed with the glucose, this was usually in the proportion of one fourth or one fifth of whole uncitrated blood to three fourths or four fifths of glucose solution. The mixture of blood and glucose is more rapidly absorbed than whole blood injected intramuscularly but less rapidly than the glucose when it is given alone.

"At this point a word might be said with regard to the advantages of using the thigh muscles for injection instead of the time-honored muscles of the buttocks. Injection of any amount of fluid into the gluteal muscles must necessarily cause pressure, which may be painful, on the ilium, particularly when the patient is in the usual supine position, because these muscles are broad and relatively thin and closely applied to the bone. Moreover, the muscles are closely covered by thick fascia, limiting the amount of fluid which may be given without causing undue distention. In this region, also, unless a real degree of care is taken, certain important structures, as the sciatic nerve or rectum, may be injured, or the pelvis may be entered through the sciatic notch. If the thighs are used according to the preceding directions, these objections are obviated."

SERUM SENSITIVENESS AND DESENSITIZATION

Before the injection of any serum by any route, but particularly if intravenous injection is contemplated, the patient should be carefully questioned regarding a history of asthma, hay fever or hypersensitiveness of any sort, and especially as to hypersensitiveness to horse dander or serum. Serum should be given only very warily, if at all, to those having a positive history unless desensitization is carried out. Patients with a negative history may be tested for hypersensitiveness by dropping into the conjunctival sac 1 drop of the serum or of a dilution of serum and physiologic saline, 1: 1 (as high as 1: 10 for children); the positive reaction, occurring within ten to thirty minutes usually, consists in diffuse reddening and watery discharge. The usually employed epinephrine solution dropped into the eye will control the discomfort of the reaction after its extent and significance have been duly remarked. Such persons as react positively to this test should also be desensitized if it is felt to be imperatively necessary to administer the serum to them.

Cole describes the method of desensitization as follows: "This is effected by injecting small amounts of the serum, at first subcutaneously, beginning with 0.025 cc. and doubling the dose every half-hour until 1 cc. is given; then injecting 0.1 cc. intravenously and doubling the dose every half-hour until 25 cc. can be given without untoward reaction. Four hours later, 50 cc. may be given; and finally after an interval of eight hours, treatment may be continued in the usual manner." It is fortunately not often necessary to resort to this tedious procedure, but it is wise in all patients to inject from 0.5 to 1 cc. of the serum subcutaneously a few hours before the intravenous injection, if time permits; this, together with a very slow rate of injection, will serve as a desensitizing measure.

VEHICLES AND INCOMPATIBILITIES

The following is a list of the principal drugs commonly dispensed in solution in a bottle for administration by mouth, together with a list of the incompatibilities of each with regard to the other drugs in the list. The compilation is the result of an experimental study in my laboratory and its aim is to supply the needed information in a usable form; therefore, where this list does not entirely agree with some others available it is because many of the alleged incompatibilities in the text-books are of no practical importance under the conditions in which the combinations are made in prescribing and dispensing. All the drugs were combined with each other in solution in full therapeutic doses, and the criteria of compatibility were that during four days at room temperature the solutions remained (a) practically transparent, (b) free from objectionable color changes, (c) free from suspensions or precipitates, (d) free from effervescence, and (e) free from visible or invisible deleterious chemical reactions.

For each drug there is also a statement of the vehicles in which it may be prescribed in order to obtain a clear and permanent solution of pleasing appearance.

The use to which the table may be put by each physician in developing his own list of permissible combinations may best be indicated by an example. Let us suppose our patient is being given iron in some form for the correction of a secondary anemia and that from some other cause he develops an intercurrent cystitis. We now wish to give him some potassium acetate in order to lessen the discomfort upon urination; how shall we write our prescription so that he can obtain the two drugs at one time and in a pleasing form? Finding potassium acetate, we see in the list of its incompatibilities only iron and ammonium citrate, syrup of ferrous iodide and the tincture of ferric chloride; the drug is therefore not incompatible with either of the other of our soluble iron preparations, *i. e.*, soluble ferric phosphate and the tincture of ferric citrochloride, and therefore may be combined with either. Turning then to the matter of vehicles, we see that potassium acetate may be prescribed in any of them but that if we are combining it with the soluble ferric phosphate the higher alcoholic vehicles must not be used, or that if the tincture of ferric citrochloride has been chosen the vehicle should not be a syrup.

ACETANILID
  Spirits of ethyl nitrite
Vehicles: Tincture of sweet orange peel; if combined with chloral hydrate it can be gotten into the lower alcohols and even water.

AMMONIUM CARBONATE
  Cascara
  Calcium chloride
  Chloral hydrate
  Hydrochloric acid
  Lime water
  Mercuric chloride
  Morphine salts
  Quinine salts
  Sodium biphosphate
  Sodium and other bromides
  Sodium salicylate
  Strychnine salts
  Syrup ferrous iodide
  Syrup of ipecac
  Tincture ferric chloride
  Tincture ferric citrochloride
  Tincture opium
Vehicles: All except higher alcohols, syrup citric acid, and syrup orange.

AMMONIUM CHLORIDE
  Methenamine
  Sodium nitrite
  Sodium salicylate
  Syrup senna
Vehicles: All.

ANTIMONY POTASSIUM TARTRATE
  Hydrochloric acid
  Iron ammonium citrate
  Lime water
  Mercuric chloride
  Spirits ethyl nitrite
  Tincture ferric chloride
  Tincture opium
Vehicles: All.

ANTIPYRINE
  Chloral hydrate
  Iron ammonium citrate
  Mercuric chloride
  Soluble ferric phosphate
  Spirits ethyl nitrite
  Syrup ferrous iodide
  Syrup hydriotic acid
  Tincture ferric chloride
  Tincture ferric citrochloride
Vehicles: All.

AROMATIC FLUIDEXTRACT CASCARA SAGRADA
  Ammonium carbonate
  Calcium chloride
  Hydrochloric acid
  Mercuric chloride
  Quinine salts
  Sodium biphosphate
  Tincture ferric chloride
Vehicles: All except higher alcohols.

AROMATIC SPIRITS AMMONIA
  Chloral hydrate
  Tincture ferric chloride
  Tincture ferric citrochloride
Vehicles: Higher alcohols.

ATROPINE SULPHATE
  Iron ammonium citrate
  Lime water
  Mercuric chloride
Vehicles: All.

CAFFEINE SODIUM BENZOATE
  Calcium chloride
  Hydrochloric acid
  Mercuric chloride
  Potassium acetate
  Potassium citrate
  Quinine salts
  Sodium salicylate
  Syrup ferrous iodide
  Tincture ferric chloride
  Tincture ferric citrochloride
Vehicles: All.

CALCIUM CHLORIDE
  Ammonium carbonate
  Cascara
  Caffeine citrate
  Codeine salts
  Ephedrine
  Iron ammonium citrate
  Morphine salts
  Potassium citrate
  Quinine salts
  Sodium biphosphate
  Sodium (or potassium) bicarbonate
  Sodium salicylate
  Soluble ferric phosphate
  Strychnine sulphate
Vehicles: All.

CAMPHORATED TINCTURE OPIUM
Tincture ferric citrochloride
Vehicles: Higher alcohols.

CHLORAL HYDRATE
Ammonium carbonate
Antipyrine
Aromatic spirits ammonia
Methenamine
Potassium iodide
Quinine salts
Sodium (or potassium) bicarbonate
Vehicles: All except not in alcoholics with sodium bromide.

CODEINE PHOSPHATE
Calcium chloride
Lime water
Syrup ferrous iodide
Syrup senna
Vehicles: All.

EPHEDRINE HYDROCHLORIDE
Calcium chloride
Sodium (or potassium) bicarbonate
Vehicles: All.

FLUIDEXTRACT ERGOT
Tincture ferric chloride
Tincture ferric citrochloride
Vehicles: Higher alcohols.

GLYCERIN
Paraldehyde
Vehicles: All.

HYDROCHLORIC ACID
Ammonium carbonate
Antimony potassium tartrate
Cascara
Caffeine citrate
Paraldehyde
Potassium acetate
Potassium iodide
Sodium (or potassium) bicarbonate
Sodium nitrite
Sodium salicylate
Spirits camphor
Syrup senna
Tincture colchicum
Tincture digitalis
Vehicles: All.

IRON AND AMMONIUM CITRATE
Antimony potassium tartrate
Antipyrine
Atropine sulphate
Calcium chloride
Mercuric chloride
Potassium acetate
Quinine salts
Sodium salicylate
Syrup ferrous iodide
Syrup ipecac
Tincture ferric chloride
Tincture opium
Vehicles: All except higher alcohols.

LIME WATER
Ammonium carbonate
Antimony potassium tartrate
Atropine sulphate
Codeine salts
Mercuric chloride
Morphine salts
Quinine salts
Sodium (or potassium) bicarbonate
Sodium biphosphate
Sodium salicylate
Solution arsenous acid
Strychnine salts
Syrup ferrous iodide
Tincture opium
Vehicles: All except higher alcohols.

MERCURIC CHLORIDE (BICHLORIDE)
Ammonium carbonate
Antimony potassium tartrate
Antipyrine
Atropine sulphate
Caffeine citrate
Cascara
Iron ammonium citrate
Lime water
Methenamine
Sodium acetate
Potassium citrate
Sodium (or potassium) bicarbonate
Soluble ferric phosphate
Spirits ethyl nitrite
Strychnine sulphate
Tincture ferric citrochloride
Tincture opium
Vehicles: All.

METHENAMINE
Ammonium chloride
Chloral hydrate
Mercuric chloride
Quinine salts
Sodium biphosphate
Syrup ferrous iodide
Tincture ferric chloride
Vehicles: All.

MORPHINE SULPHATE
Ammonium carbonate
Calcium chloride
Lime water
Potassium iodide
Sodium (or potassium) bicarbonate
Sodium nitrite
Spirits ethyl nitrite
Vehicles: All.

PARALDEHYDE
Glycerin
Hydrochloric acid
Vehicles: Higher alcohols.

PHENOBARBITAL

Quinine salts
Tincture ferric citrochloride

Vehicles: ½ grain can be gotten into a teaspoonful dose of the higher alcohols.

POTASSIUM ACETATE

Caffeine citrate
Hydrochloric acid
Iron ammonium citrate
Mercuric chloride
Quinine salts
Spirits ethyl nitrite
Syrup senna
Syrup ferrous iodide
Tincture ferric chloride
Tincture opium

Vehicles: All.

POTASSIUM CITRATE

Caffeine citrate
Calcium chloride
Mercuric chloride
Quinine salts
Syrup senna
Tincture opium

Vehicles: All except higher alcohols.

POTASSIUM IODIDE

Chloral hydrate
Hydrochloric acid
Morphine salts
Quinine salts
Sodium biphosphate
Sodium nitrite
Spirits ethyl nitrite
Strychnine sulphate
Tincture ferric chloride

Vehicles: All except syrup citric acid and
syrup orange.

POTASSIUM SULPHOCYANATE

Quinine salts
Spirits ethyl nitrite
Strychnine sulphate
Syrup ferrous iodide
Tincture ferric chloride

Vehicles: All.

QUININE BISULPHATE

Ammonium carbonate
Cascara
Caffeine citrate
Calcium chloride
Chloral hydrate
Iron ammonium citrate
Lime water
Methenamine
Phenobarbital
Potassium acetate
Potassium citrate
Potassium iodide

QUININE BISULPHATE (*Continued*)

Potassium sulphocyanate
Sodium (or potassium) bicarbonate
Sodium biphosphate
Sodium nitrite
Sodium salicylate
Soluble ferric phosphate
Syrup ferrous iodide
Syrup senna

Vehicles: All except syrup citric acid and
syrup orange.

SODIUM (OR POTASSIUM) BICARBONATE

Calcium chloride
Chloral hydrate
Ephedrine
Hydrochloric acid
Lime water
Mercuric chloride
Morphine salts
Quinine salts
Sodium biphosphate
Soluble ferric phosphate
Syrup ferrous iodide
Syrup senna
Tincture ferric chloride
Tincture ferric citrochloride
Tincture opium

Vehicles: All except syrup citric acid and
syrup orange.

SODIUM BIPHOSPHATE

Ammonium carbonate
Cascara
Calcium chloride
Lime water
Methenamine
Potassium iodide
Quinine salts
Sodium (or potassium) bicarbonate
Sodium nitrite
Syrup ferrous iodide
Syrup senna
Tincture ferric chloride
Tincture opium

Vehicles: All except higher alcohols.

SODIUM BROMIDE

Ammonium carbonate
Syrup senna
Tincture ferric chloride

Vehicles: All.

SODIUM NITRITE

Ammonium chloride
Hydrochloric acid
Morphine salts
Potassium iodide
Quinine salts
Sodium biphosphate
Sodium salicylate
Syrup ferrous iodide
Tincture ferric chloride
Tincture ferric citrochloride
Tincture opium

Vehicles: All.

Sodium Salicylate
  Ammonium carbonate
  Ammonium chloride
  Caffeine citrate
  Calcium chloride
  Hydrochloric acid
  Iron ammonium citrate
  Lime water
  Quinine salts
  Sodium nitrite
  Soluble ferric phosphate
  Spirits ethyl nitrite
  Syrup ferrous iodide
  Tincture ferric chloride
  Tincture ferric citrochloride
Vehicles: All.

Soluble Ferric Phosphate
  Antipyrine
  Calcium chloride
  Mercuric chloride
  Quinine salts
  Sodium (or potassium) bicarbonate
  Sodium salicylate
  Tincture ferric chloride
Vehicles: All except higher alcohols.

Solution of Arsenous Acid
  (This is *not* Fowler's solution, which has
    more incompatibilities.)
  Lime water
  Tincture opium
Vehicles: All.

Spirits Camphor
  Hydrochloric acid
Vehicles: Higher alcohols.

Spirits Ethyl Nitrite
  Acetanilid
  Antimony potassium tartrate
  Antipyrine
  Mercuric chloride
  Morphine salts
  Potassium acetate
  Potassium iodide
  Potassium sulphocyanate
  Sodium salicylate
  Tincture ferric citrochloride
Vehicles: Higher alcohols.

Spirits Peppermint
Vehicles: Higher alcohols.

Strychnine Sulphate
  Ammonium carbonate
  Calcium chloride
  Lime water
  Mercuric chloride
  Potassium iodide
  Potassium sulphocyanate
  Syrup senna
Vehicles: All.

Syrup Ferrous Iodide
  Ammonium carbonate
  Antipyrine
  Caffeine citrate

Syrup Ferrous Iodide (*Continued*)
  Codeine salts
  Iron ammonium citrate
  Lime water
  Methenamine
  Potassium acetate
  Potassium sulphocyanate
  Quinine salts
  Sodium (or potassium) bicarbonate
  Sodium biphosphate
  Sodium nitrite
  Sodium salicylate
  Syrup senna
Vehicles: All.

Syrup Hydriotic Acid
  Antipyrine
Vehicles: All except alcohols.

Syrup Ipecac
  Ammonium carbonate
  Iron ammonium citrate
  Syrup senna
Vehicles: All.

Syrup Senna
  Ammonium chloride
  Codeine salts
  Hydrochloric acid
  Potassium acetate
  Potassium citrate
  Quinine salts
  Sodium (or potassium) bicarbonate
  Sodium biphosphate
  Sodium and other bromides
  Strychnine sulphate
  Syrup ferrous iodide
  Syrup ipecac
Vehicles: All except syrup citric acid and
  syrup orange.

Tincture Belladonna
  Tincture ferric chloride
  Tincture ferric citrochloride
  Tincture opium
Vehicles: Higher alcohols.

Tincture Colchicum
  Hydrochloric acid
Vehicles: Higher alcohols.

Tincture Digitalis
  Hydrochloric acid
  Tincture ferric chloride
  Tincture ferric citrochloride
Vehicles: Higher alcohols.

Tincture Ferric Chloride
  Ammonium carbonate
  Antimony potassium tartrate
  Antipyrine
  Aromatic spirits ammonia
  Caffeine citrate
  Cascara
  Ergot
  Iron ammonium citrate
  Methenamine
  Potassium acetate
  Potassium iodide
  Potassium sulphocyanate
  Sodium (or potassium) bicarbonate

TINCTURE FERRIC CHLORIDE (*Continued*)
Sodium biphosphate
Sodium and other bromides
Sodium nitrite
Sodium salicylate
Soluble ferric phosphate
Tincture belladonna
Tincture digitalis
Tincture hyoscyamus
Tincture opium
Vehicles: All.

TINCTURE FERRIC CITROCHLORIDE
Ammonium carbonate
Antipyrine
Aromatic spirits ammonia
Caffeine citrate
Ergot
Mercuric chloride
Phenobarbital
Sodium (or potassium) bicarbonate
Sodium nitrite
Sodium salicylate
Spirits ethyl nitrite
Tincture belladonna
Tincture camphorated opium
Tincture digitalis
Tincture hyoscyamus
Vehicles: All.

TINCTURE HYOSCYAMUS
Tincture ferric chloride
Tincture ferric citrochloride
Vehicles: Higher alcohols.

TINCTURE NUX VOMICA
Vehicles: Higher alcohols.

TINCTURE OPIUM
Ammonium carbonate
Antimony potassium tartrate
Aromatic spirits ammonia
Ergot
Iron ammonium citrate
Lime water
Mercuric chloride
Potassium acetate
Potassium citrate
Sodium (or potassium) bicarbonate
Sodium biphosphate
Sodium nitrite
Solution arsenous acid
Tincture belladonna
Tincture digitalis
Tincture ferric chloride
Tincture hyoscyamus
Tincture nux vomica
Vehicles: All.

VEHICLES
WATERS

Orange flower water
Anise water
Fennel water
Chloroform water
Peppermint water
Spearmint water
Cinnamon water

Mistura glycyrrhizae composita (compound licorice mixture—brown mixture), not strictly a "water" by definition but conveniently included here; it is much used as a vehicle for cough mixtures.

The following may also be included for the reason that the small amount of alcohol they contain—no more than some of the syrups—need not be considered in regard to solubilities and incompatibilities.

Elixir of anise
Aqueous elixir glycyrrhiza
Compound elixir cardamom
Compound elixir vanilla
Compound elixir almond

ALCOHOLS

LOWER ALCOHOLS (20 to 25 per cent)
Aromatic elixir
Elixir glycyrrhiza
Red aromatic elixir

HIGHER ALCOHOLS (45 to 75 per cent)
Elixir terpin hydrate (45 per cent)
Compound tincture gentian (45 per cent)
Compound tincture cardamom (45 per cent)
Tincture krameria (45 per cent)
Tincture bitter orange peel (55 per cent)
Compound tincture cinchona (60 per cent)
Tincture sweet orange peel (75 per cent)

SYRUPS

Syrup (sometimes called simple syrup)
Syrup citric acid
Syrup orange (also contains citric acid)
Syrup orange flowers
Syrup raspberry
Syrup tolu
Syrup cinnamon

The following are of a strong distinctive taste:
Syrup pine tar
Syrup wild cherry
Syrup ginger
Syrup glycyrrhiza
Syrup cacao
Syrup thyme
Syrup senega
Compound syrup wild ginger
Aromatic syrup eriodictyon (yerba santa)

50

BIBLIOGRAPHY

Abraham, G.: Thrush, Arch. f. Kinderh., 80, 26, 1926.
Abrami and Brissaud: Asthma, Presse méd., 29, 181, 1921.
Abramowitz, E. W.: Impetigo, eczema-dermatitis, Arch. Dermat. and Syph., 23, 644, 1931.
Abt, A. F., and Feingold, B. F.: Diphtheria, Amer. Jour. Dis. Child., 41, 8, 1931.
Abt, A. F., and Traisman, A. S.: Syphilis, Jour. Pediat., 1, 172, 1932.
Abt, I. A.: Urinary infections, Jour. Amer. Med. Assoc., 68, 1100, 1917. Chorea, Jour. Amer. Med. Assoc., 67, 1342, 1916 (discussion).
Abt, I. A., and Levinson, A.: Chorea, Jour. Amer. Med. Assoc., 67, 1342, 1916.
Acton, H. W., and Chopra, R. N.: Amebic dysentery, Ind. Med. Gaz., 64, 481, 1929.
Adams, J. E.: Erysipelas, Brit. Med. Jour., 1920, 2, 779.
Adams, T. W.: Obstetrical anesthesia, Amer. Jour. Obst. and Gyn., 8, 266, 1924.
Addis, T.: Nephritis, Jour. Clin. Invest., 2, 409, 1926.
Adlersberg, D.: Diabetes, Fettreiche odor fettarme Ernährung des Diabetibers, 1932.
Adlersberg, D., and Porges, O.: Diabetes, Med. Klin., 27, 1783, 1931.
Adson, A. W., and Brown, G. E.: Buerger's disease, Jour. Amer. Med. Assoc., 99, 529, 1932.
Ahmen, G.: Syphilis, Hygiea, Stockholm, 86, 482, 1924.
Alajovanine, T., and Horowitz, A.: Syphilis, Bull. et mém. Soc. med. d. hôp. de Paris, 48, 178, 1932.
Aldrich, R. H.: Burns, New England Jour. of Med., 208, 299, 1933.
Alissow, P. A., and Morozkin, N. I.: Typhoid, Compt. rend. Soc. de biol., 97, 1217, 1927
Alivisatos, G. P.: Bacillary dysentery, Deutsch med. Wchnschr., 51, 1728, 1925.
Allan, W.: Amebic dysentery, Boston Med. and Surg. Jour., 183, 545, 1920.
Allen, F. M.: Diabetes mellitus, Jour. Metab. Res., 3, 61, 1923; Jour. Amer. Med. Assoc., 82, 1937, 1924; ibid., 89, 1577, 1927.
Allen, R. W., and Ecklund, A. W.: Botulism, Jour. Amer. Med. Assoc., 99, 557, 1932.
Alloway, F. L., and Lebensohn, J. E.: Tuberculosis, Jour. Amer. Med. Assoc., 79, 462, 1922.
Althausen, L. T., and Kerr, W. J.: Hypertension, Amer. Jour. Med. Sci., 178, 470, 1929.
Althausen, T. L.: Cirrhosis, Jour. Amer. Med. Assoc., 100, 1163, 1933.
Althausen, T. L., and Schumacher, I. C.: Asthma, Arch. Int. Med., 40, 851, 1927.
Alvarez, W. C.: Nervous indigestion, Jour. Amer. Med. Assoc., 89, 440, 1927. Constipation, Jour. Amer. Med. Assoc., 72, 8, 1919; Physiol. Rev., 4, 352, 1924. Peptic ulcer, Jour. Amer. Med. Assoc., 87, 2086, 1926.
Alvarez, W. C., McCalla, R. L., and Zimmermann, A.: Hypertension, Arch. Int. Med., 38, 158, 1926.
Amaral, A.: Poisoning, Nelson Loose-Leaf Med., 2, 683.
Amberson, J. B., McMahon, B. T., and Pinner, M.: Tuberculosis, Am. Rev. Tuberc., 24, 401, 1931.
Amoss, H. L.: Erysipelas, Ann. Int. Med., 5, 500, 1931.
Anderson, H. H., et al.: Obesity, Jour. Amer. Med. Assoc., 101, 1053, 1933.
Anderson, J. M.: Cerebrospinal fever, Jour. Amer. Med. Assoc., 93, 1613, 1929
Anderson, Wm. D., and Homan, C. E., Jr.: Whooping cough, Amer. Jour. Med. Sci., 174, 738, 1927.
Andresen, A. F. R.: Peptic ulcer, Jour. Amer. Med. Assoc., 89, 1397, 1927. Amebic dysentery, Amer. Jour. Trop. Med., 6, 119, 1926.
Andreus and Schlegel: Diabetes mellitus, Arch. Int. Med., 40, 637, 1927.
Andrews, E., and Thomas, W. A.: Nephritis, Jour. Amer. Med. Assoc., 90, 539, 1928.
Andrews, E., et al.: Nephritis, Arch. Int. Med., 43, 139, 1929.
Angle, F. E.: Undulant fever, Jour. Kansas Med. Soc., 30, 323, 1929.
Anselmino, K. J., et al.: Eclampsia, Edinburgh Med. Jour., 39, 376, 1932.
Antonovsky, A.: Bacillary dysentery, Compt. rend. Soc. de biol., 90, 564, 1924.
Aragão, H. de B.: Granuloma inguinale, New Orleans Med. and Surg. Jour., 70, 369, 1917. Yellow fever, Brasil-Medico, 47, 75, 1933.
Aragão and Vianna: Granuloma inguinale, Mem. do Inst. Oswaldo Cruz, 5, 221, 1923 (see also Aragão).
Archibald, R. G.: Kala-azar, Amer. Jour. Trop. Med., 3, 307, 1923. Sickle cell anemia, Trans. Roy. Soc. Trop. Med. and Hyg., 19, 389, 1926.
Archibald, R. G., Hadfield, G., Logan, W., and Campbell, W.: Amebic dysentery, Jour. R. A. M. C., 26, 675, 1916.
Armengol, R. P.: BCG, La Clinica, November, 1928, 321.
Arnett, J. H.: Barbiturate poisoning, Jour. Amer. Med. Assoc., 100, 1593, 1933.
Arnold, Gustafson, Hull, Montgomery, and Singer: Skin disinfection, Amer. Jour. Hyg., 11, 345, 1930.

Aschoff, L.: Nephritis, Deutsch med. Wchnschr., 43, 1345, 1917.
Asheshov, J. N., Khan, S., and Lahiri, M. N.: Asiatic cholera, Indian Med. Gaz., 66, 179, 1931.
Ashford, B. K.: Sprue, Cecil's Textbook of Medicine, Phila., W. B. Saunders Co., 1933, p. 390; Amer. Jour. Trop. Med., 8, 507, 1928.
Ashford, B. K., *et al.:* Hookworm disease, Jour. Amer. Med. Assoc., 101, 843, 1933.
Ashhurst, A. P. C.: Tetanus, Jour. Amer. Med. Assoc., 87, 289, 1926.
Askanazy, S.: Angina pectoris, Deutsch. Arch. f. klin. Med., 56, 209, 1895.
Atchley, Loeb, and Benedict: Diabetes, Jour. Amer. Med. Assoc., 80, 1643, 1923.
Atkey, O. P. H.: Relapsing fever, Bull. Office Internat. d'Hyg. Publique, 24, 1861, 1932; Report on Medical and Health Work in the Sudan for 1931, Khartoum, 1932.
Atkinson, A. J.: Peptic ulcer, Med. Clin. N. A., 16, 493, 1932; Jour. Amer. Med. Assoc., 98, 1153, 1932.
Attlee, W. H. W.: Measles, Brit. Med. Jour., 2, 996, 1930.
Aub, J. C.: Tetany, The Harvey Lectures, Harvey Soc. N. Y., 24, 151, 1928–29.
Aub, J. C., *et al.:* Tetany, Jour. Clin. Invest., 7, 97, 1929. Lead poisoning, Medicine, 4, 1, 1925.
Audrain, J.: Whooping cough, Bull. et mém. Soc. med. d. hôp. de Paris, 44, 795, 1920.
Auld, A. G.: Asthma, Brit. Med. Jour., 1920, 1, 567; ibid., 1, 448, 1925; ibid., 1, 171, 1928; Lancet, 1, 804, 1931.
Avata, A. A., and Woodyatt, R. T.: Erysipelas, Jour. Amer. Med. Assoc., 71, 900, 1918.
Ayman, D.: Hypertension, Arch. Int. Med., 48, 89, 1931; Jour. Amer. Med. Assoc., 98 545, 1932; ibid., 96, 2091, 1931; ibid., 96, 1852, 1931.
Ayman, D., and Pratt, J. H.: Hypertension, Arch. Int. Med., 47, 675, 1931.
Babcock, R. H.: Angina pectoris, Jour. Amer. Med. Assoc., 82, 193, 1924.
Bacon, C. S.: Hyperemesis, Jour. Amer. Med. Assoc., 70, 1750, 1918.
Bacot, A. W.: Trench fever (delousing), Brit. Med. Jour., 2, 447, 1916.
Bader, G. B.: Measles, Jour. Amer. Med. Assoc., 93, 668, 1929; Med. Clin. N. A., 6, 1475, 1931.
Bahr, M., and Breutsch, W. L.: Syphilis, Amer. Soc. Hyg. Assoc., Exhibit, A. M. A., Portland Meeting, 1929.
Baigue: BCG, Réunion Méd., Besançon, April 2, 1928.
Baker, S. J.: Eclampsia, Jour. Amer. Med. Assoc., 89, 2016, 1927.
Baldwin, H. S.: Pneumonia, Amer. Jour. Med. Sci., 181, 788, 1931.
Balyeat, R. M.: Asthma, Jour. Lab. and Clin. Med., 13, 1019, 1928.
Balyeat, R. M., and Rinkel, H. J.: Asthma, Jour. Amer. Med. Assoc., 98, 1545, 1932.
Bamberger, P.: Syphilis, Münch. med. Wchnschr., 128, 1796, 1931.
Bancroft, F. W., and Rogers, C. S.: Burns, Ann. Surg., 81, July, 1926.
Bandmann, M.: Angina pectoris, Ztschr. f. klin. Med., 124, 1, 1933.
Bang, O.: Tuberculosis, Ztschr. f. Tuberk., 44, 298, 1928. Measles, Nordisk Med. Tidsk. 146, March 8, 1930 (through Brit. Med. Jour., 1, 100, 1930).
Banting, F. G., and Best, C. H.: Diabetes mellitus, Jour. Lab. and Clin. Med., 7, 251, 1922.
Banus, M. G.: Typhoid, Internat. Jour. Pub. Health, 2, 164, 1921.
Banyai, A. L.: Tuberculosis, Amer. Rev. Tuberc., 23, 546, 1931.
Barach, A. L.: Pneumonia, Jour. Amer. Med. Assoc., 79, 693, 1922; ibid., 78, 334, 1922; Arch. Int. Med., 37, 186, 1926; Jour. Amer. Med. Assoc., 97, 390, 1931; New York State Jour. Med., October 15, 1931; Anesthes. and Anal., March–April, 1932. Coronary occlusion, Anesthes. and Anal., March–April, 1932.
Barach, J. H.: Diabetes, Jour. Amer. Med. Assoc., 98, 1265, 1932; Ann. Int. Med., 4, 593, 1930; also personal communications to the author.
Barber, H. W.: Lupus erythematosus, Brit. Jour. Dermat., 41, 17, 1929.
Barber, M. A., Komp, W. H. W., and Newman, B. M.: Malaria, U. S. P. H. Rep., 44, 1409, 1929.
Barborka, C. J.: Epilepsy, Jour. Amer. Med. Assoc., 91, 73, 1928; Arch. Neurol. and Psychiat., 23, 904, 1930.
Barbour, H. G., and Winter, J. E.: Rheumatic fever, Jour. Pharm. and Exp. Ther., 35, 425, 1929.
Barclay, A. E.: Thyrotoxicosis, Radiology, 6, 14, 1926.
Barenberg, L. H., and Ostroff, J.: Mumps, Amer. Jour. Dis. Child., 42, 1109, 1931.
Barenberg, L. H., Lewis, J. M., and Messer, W. H.: Measles, Jour. Amer. Med. Assoc., 95, 4, 1930.
Bargen, J. A.: Ulcerative colitis, Jour. Amer. Med. Assoc., 91, 1176, 1928.
Bargen, J. A., *et. al.:* Colitis, Arch. Int. Med., 46, 1039, 1930; The Practitioner, 127, 235 1931.
Barkan, O., and Barkan, H.: Burns, Jour. Amer. Med. Assoc., 83, 1567, 1924.
Barker, C.: Vincent's angina, Nelson Loose-Leaf Med., 2, 34 A.
Barker, L. F.: Thyrotoxicosis, Internat. Clin., 1, 1, 1924.
Barker, L. F., and Sprunt, T. P.: Syphilis, Ther. Gaz., 38, 539, 1922.
Barker, M. H.: Nephritis, Jour. Amer. Med. Assoc., 98, 2193, 1932.
Barker, M. H., and Kirk, E. J.: Nephritis, Arch. Int. Med., 45, 319, 1930.

Barker, M. H., and O'Hare, J. P.: Nephritis, Jour. Amer. Med. Assoc., 91, 2060, 1928.
Barker, N. W.: Buerger's disease, Jour. Amer. Med. Assoc., 97, 841, 1931.
Barksdale, T. S.: Hypertension, Amer. Jour. Med. Sci., 171, 111, 1926.
Barlow, C. H.: Intestinal flukes, Amer. Jour. Hyg., Monograph Series, No. 4, 1925.
Barnes, M. E.: Hookworm, Jour. Amer. Med. Assoc., 79, 964, 1922.
Barnes M. E., and Cort, E. C.: Amebic dysentery, Jour. Amer. Med. Assoc., 71, 350, 1918.
Barney, J. D.: Urinary infections, Jour. Amer. Med. Assoc., 71, 1642, 1918.
Báron: BCG, Wien. klin. Wchnschr., 41, 1167, 1928
Barrier, C. W.: Arhythmia, Jour. Amer. Med. Assoc., 89, 742, 1927.
Bartlett, W. M.: Epilepsy (cited by Peterman, M. G., Jour. Amer. Med. Assoc., 88, 1868, 1927).
Basch: Diabetes mellitus, Klin. Wchnschr., 3, 1861, 1924.
Bass, C. C.: Malaria, Jour. Amer. Med. Assoc., 95, 988, 1930.
Bass, M. H.: Anemia of infancy, Amer. Jour. Dis. Child., 29, 318, 1925.
Bass, M. H., and Denzer, B. S.: Anemia of infancy, Jour. Amer. Med. Assoc., 86, 938, 1926.
Bass, M. H., and Karelitz, S.: Tetany, Jour. Amer. Med. Assoc., 97, 1372, 1931.
Bass, M. H., Denzer, B. S., and Herman, H.: Anemia of infancy, Amer. Jour. Dis. Child., 27, 433, 1924.
Bassett-Smith, P. W.: Undulant fever, Jour. Trop. Med. and Hyg., 24, 173, 1921.
Bastedo, W. A.: Tapeworm, Materia Medica, Pharmacology and Therapeutics, Phila., W. B. Saunders Co., 1932, 162. Achylia, Jour. Amer. Med. Assoc., 85, 743, 1925. Colitis, Jour. Amer. Med. Assoc., 74, 240, 1920, ibid., 98, 734, 1932. Constipation, Jour. Amer. Med. Assoc., 64, 808, 1915. Migraine, Jour. Amer. Med. Assoc., 77, 1396, 1921 (discussion). Sprue, Jour. Amer. Med. Assoc., 95, 1961, 1930 (discussion).
Bauer, E. L., and Wilmer, H. B.: Diphtheria, Jour. Amer. Med. Assoc., 86, 942, 1926.
Bauer, J., and Aschner, B.: Diabetes insipidus, Zentralbl. f. inn. Med., No. 34, 682, 1924
Bauer, J. H., and Meyer, K. F.: Tetanus, Jour. Infec. Dis., 38, 295, 1926.
Bauer, W., et al.: Calcium therapy, Jour. Amer. Med. Assoc., 96, 1216, 1931.
Bauman, L.: Obesity, Jour. Amer. Med. Assoc., 90, 22, 1928.
Bayam and Alves: Hookworm, Pub. do Serv. San. do Est de São Paulo, N. S., 1, 65, 1918.
Bayer: Whooping cough, Med. Klin., 28, 1459, 1932.
Bazy: Tetanus, Bull. et mém. Soc. de chir. de Paris, 42, 2919, 1916.
Beams, A. J.: Pylorospasm, Jour. Amer. Med. Assoc., 97, 907, 1931.
Beck, C. S., and Powers, J. H.: Burns, Ann. Surg., 81, July, 1926.
Becker, S. M., and Ritchie, E. B.: Syphilis, Jour. Amer. Med. Assoc., 97, 389, 1931.
Becker, S. W.: Eczema-dermatitis, Jour. Amer. Med. Assoc., 97, 983, 1931
Beckman, H.: Obstetrical anesthesia, Jour. Lab. and Clin. Med, 10, 189, 1924; Jour. Amer. Med. Assoc., 85, 332, 1925; Amer. Jour. Obst. and Gyn., 15, 72, 1928; ibid., 17, 735, 1929; Jour. Lab. and Clin. Med., 14, 1050, 1929. Allergy, Amer. Jour. Med. Sci., 174, 525, 1927; Wisconsin Med. Jour., 27, 253, 1928; ibid., 31, 533, 1932; Med. Jour. and Rec., 133, 9, 1929; J. Allergy, 1, 496, 1930; Jour. Amer. Med. Assoc., 95, 1582, 1930; Lancet, 1, 1227, 1933.
Beebe, R. T., and Lewis, G. S.: Pernicious anemia, Amer. Jour. Med. Sci., 181, 796, 1931.
Beeson, B. B.: Syphilis, Amer. Jour. Syph., 3, 192, 1919.
Begbie, R. S.: BCG, Edinburgh Med. Jour., N. S.., 38, 174, 1931.
Behrman, S.: Asthma, Lancet, 2, 1433, 1931.
Bell, A., and Pardee, H. E. B.: Stokes-Adams disease, Jour. Amer. Med. Assoc., 94, 1555, 1930.
Bell, B.: Pituitrin in labor, Biochem. Zentralb., 9, 631, 1909.
Bell, E. T.: Nephritis, Amer. Jour. Path., 5, 587, 1929. Eclampsia, Amer. Jour. Path., 8, 1, 1932.
Benedict, et al.: Essential hypertension, Pub. 281, Carnegie Inst. of Washington, 1919.
Benn, E. C., Hughes, E., and Alstead, S.: Diphtheria, Lancet, 1, 281, 1932.
Bennett, J. E., Polozsker, I. L., and Altshuler, I.: Syphilis, Jour. Michigan Med. Soc., 28, 241, 1929.
Benson, W. T.: Erysipelas, Lancet, 2, 1286, 1930.
Benson, W. T., and Rankin, A. L. K.: Sepsis, Lancet, 1, 848, 1933.
Berger, S. S., et al.: Bichloride poisoning, Jour. Amer. Med. Assoc., 98, 700, 1932.
Berljand, A. S., and Weinstein, C. J.: Hypertension, Münch. med. Wchnschr., 35, 1468 1931.
Bernard, N.: BCG, Ann. de l'Inst. Past., 41, 284, 1927.
Bernhardt: Sickle cell anemia, Deutsch. med. Wchnschr., 53, 1161, 1927.
Bernstine, J. B.: Sepsis, Amer. Jour. Obst. and Gyn., 25, 849, 1933.
Bernton, H. S.: Hay-fever, Jour. Amer. Med. Assoc., 80, 1301, 1923.
Berntsen, A.: Varicose veins, Acta clin. Scandinav., 62, 61, 1927.
Bezancon, F., and Jacquelin, A.: Asthma, Presse méd., 39, 1685, 1931.
Bieber, W.: Toxin-antitoxin, Deutsch. med. Wchnschr., 46, 1184, 1920.
Bigelow, G. H., and Anderson, G. W.: Typhoid fever, Jour. Amer. Med. Assoc., 101, 348 1933.

Biggam, A. G., and Arafa, M. A.: Amebic dysentery, Lancet, 1, 1335, 1930.

Bilharz, T.: Blood flukes, Ztschr. f. wiss. Zool., 4, 53, 1852; ibid., 4, 72, 1852.

Billings, W. C., and Hickey, J. P.: Hookworm, Jour. Amer. Med. Assoc., 67, 1908, 1916.

Binger, C. A. L., and Christie, R. V.: Pneumonia, Jour. Amer. Med. Assoc., 91, 367, 1928.

Biraud, Y.: BCG, Ann. de l'Inst. Past., 41, 217, 1927.

Birch, C. L.: Hemophilia, Proc. Soc. Exper. Biol. and Med., 28, 752, 1931; Jour. Amer. Med. Assoc., 97, 244, 1931; Med. Clin. N. A., 17, 351, 1933.

Birkhaug, K. E.: Erysipelas, Jour. Amer. Med. Assoc., 86, 1411, 1926; ibid., 88, 888, 1927.

Bishop, S. S.: Hay-fever, Diseases of Ear, Nose and Throat, F. A. Davis Co., 1897.

Bishop, W. A., and Brosius, O. T.: Hookworm, Jour. Amer. Med. Assoc., 65, 1610, 1915; ibid., 74, 1768, 1920.

Blackfan, K. D.: Meningitis, Jour. Amer. Med. Assoc., 76, 36, 1921. Eczema-dermatitis, Amer. Jour. Dis. Child., 11, 441, 1916.

Blackfan, K. D., and McKhann, C. T.: Nephritis, Jour. Amer. Med. Assoc., 97, 1052, 1931.

Blackfan, K. D., Peterson, M. F., and Conroy, F. C.: Measles, Ohio State Med. Jour., 19, 97, 1923. Chickenpox, Ohio State Med. Jour., 19, 97, 1923.

Blackford, J. M., and Willius, F. A.: Stokes-Adams disease, Amer. Jour. Med. Sci., 154, 585, 1917.

Blackford, L. M., and Boland, J. H.: Syphilis, Jour. Amer. Med. Assoc., 99, 1902, 1932.

Blacklock, B., and Yorke, W.: Trypanosomiasis, Byam and Archibald, Practice of Medicine in the Tropics, 2, 1386.

Blacklock, D. B., and Gordon, R. M.: Malaria, Amer. Trop. Med. and Parasit., 9, 37, 1925.

Blaisdell, E. R.: Bichloride poisoning, Jour. Maine Med. Assoc., 23, 3, 1932.

Blake, F. G.: Tetanus, Surg., Gyn., and Obst., 2, 541, 1906.

Blake, F. G., and Trask, J. D.: Scarlet fever, Boston Med. and Surg. Jour., 193, 659, 1925.

Blanc, G.: BCG, Ann. de l'Inst. Past., 41, 277, 1927.

Blanchard and Laigret: Trypanosomiasis, Ann. de l'Inst. Past. Paris, 38, 460, 1924.

Blanchod, F.: Varicose veins, Rev. Méd. de la Suisse Rom., 43, 155, 1923.

Bland, E. F., and White, P. D.: Nephritis, Jour. Amer. Med. Assoc., 95, 1489, 1930.

Blankenhorn, M. A.: Rheumatic fever, Jour. Amer. Med. Assoc., 66, 331, 1916.

Blatt, M. L., and Dale, M. L.: Scarlet fever, Jour. Amer. Med. Assoc., 98, 1437, 1932.

Blatt, M. L., and Saffro, L. B.: Rickets, Arch. Ped., 49, 109, 1932.

Blauner, S. A., and Goldstein, H.: Measles, Amer. Jour. Dis. Child., 42, 803, 1931.

Block, J. H., and Moore, M. C.: Allergy, Jour. Amer. Med. Assoc., 86, 324, 1926.

Bloedorn, W. A., and Houghton, J. E.: Urinary infections, Jour. Lab. and Clin. Med., 7, 514, 1922.

Bloodgood, J. C.: Vincent's angina, Jour. Amer. Med. Assoc., 88, 1142, 1927.

Bloom, C. J.: Whooping cough, Arch. Ped., August, 1925.

Bloomberg, M. W., and Fleming, A. G.: Diphtheria, Canad. Med. Assoc. Jour., 17, 801, 1927.

Blotner, H.: Malnutrition, Med. Clin. N. A., 15, 991, 1932; Jour. Amer. Med. Assoc., 100, 1235, 1933.

Blum, J.: Diphtheria, Jour. Amer. Med. Assoc., 98, 1627, 1932.

Blum, Grabar, and Thiers: Diabetes mellitus, Compt. rend. Soc. de biol., 96, 643, 1927.

Blumer, G.: Trichinosis, Nelson Loose-Leaf Med., 2, 453.

Blumgart, H. L.: Diabetes mellitus, Arch. Int. Med., 29, 508, 1922. Diabetes insipidus, Med. Clin. N. A., 15, 895, 1932.

Blumgart, H. L., and Weiss, S.: Hypertension, Jour. Clin. Invest., 6, 103, 1928.

Blumgart, H. L., et al.: Heart failure, Arch. Int. Med., 52, 165, 1933.

Blümel: BCG, Münch. med. Wchnschr., 77, 1978, 1930.

Boas, E. P., and Donner, S.: Angina pectoris, Jour. Amer. Med. Assoc., 98, 2186, 1932.

Boas, H.: Syphilis, Acta Derm.-Vener., 3, 559, 1922.

Boas, T.: Hemorrhoids, Deutsch. med. Wchnschr., Nr. 6, 1931.

Boase, A. J.: Bacillary dysentery, Kenya Med. Jour., 2, 245, 1925.

Bock, A. V., Field, H. and Adair, G. S.: Diabetes mellitus, Jour. Metab. Res., 4, 27, 1923.

Bockus, H. L., and Bank, J.: Peptic ulcer, Med. Clin. N. A., July, 143, 1932.

Bogdanovic, P.: Dysentery, Münch. med. Wchnschr., Nr. 31, 1217, 1933.

Bogen, E.: Spider bite, Jour. Amer. Med. Assoc., 86, 1894, 1926; Ann. Int. Med., 6, 375, 1932.

Boles, R. S.: Constipation, Jour. Amer. Med. Assoc., 89, 1766, 1927. B. acidophilus, Jour. Amer. Med. Assoc., 89, 1766, 1927.

Bongenault, R.: Blood flukes, Bull. Soc. de Path. Exot., 20, 285, 1927.

Boone, F. H., and Weech, A. A.: Syphilis, Amer. Jour. Dis. Child., 27, 39, 1924.

Boothby, W. M.: Oxygentherapy, Jour. Amer. Med. Assoc., 99, 2026 and 2106, 1932.

Boots, R. H., and Miller, C. P.: Rheumatic fever, Jour. Amer. Med. Assoc., 82, 1028, 1924.

Borchers, E.: Tetany, Münch. med. Wchnschr., 68, 1609, 1921.

Borovsky, M. P., and Steigmann, F.: Measles, Jour. Amer. Med. Assoc., 100, 1859, 1933.

Boudreau: Thyrotoxicosis, Jour. d. Méd. de Bordeaux, 104, 444, 1927.

Bowditch, H. I., and Leonard, R. D.: Whooping cough, Boston Med. and Surg. Jour., 188, 312, 1923.

Boyd, G. L.: Diabetes mellitus, Amer. Jour. Dis. Child., 29, 329, 1925.
Boyd, J. D., and Nelson, M. V.: Diabetes mellitus, Amer. Jour. Dis. Child., 35, 753, 1928.
Boyd, M. L.: Gonorrhea, Jour. Urol., 19, 89, 1928.
Braasch, W. F.: Urinary infections, Jour. Amer. Med. Assoc., 65, 1769, 1915 (discussion). Essential hematuria, Jour. Amer. Med. Assoc., 61, 39, 1913.
Braasch, W. F., and Bumpus, H. C.: Urinary infections, Tr. Am. Assn. Gen.-Urin. Surg., 18, 281, 1925.
Bradbury, S.: Stomatitis, Cecil's Textbook of Medicine, Phila., W. B. Saunders Co., 1933, p. 677.
Brady, L.: Gonorrhea, Bull. Johns Hopkins Hosp., 37, 400, 1925.
Brahmachari, P., and Brahmachari, U.: Kala-azar, Jour. Trop. Med. and Hyg., 34, 263, 1931.
Bram, T.: Thyrotoxicosis, Med. Jour. and Rec., September 4, 1929; Endocrinology, 16, 157, 1932.
Braslawsky, P. J.: Trench fever, Paris méd., January 14, 1933 (Lancet, 1, 262, 1933).
Brem, W.: Blackwater fever, Arch. Int. Med., 7, 153, 1911.
Breuer, R.: Angina pectoris, Münch. med. Wchnschr., 49, 1604, 1902.
Brill, I. C., and Myers, H. B.: Sepsis, Jour. Amer. Med. Assoc., 84, 879, 1925.
Brindley, P., and Howell, W. L.: Madura foot, Southern Med. Jour., 25, 1022, 1932.
Brody, W., and Crocker, W. J.: Sepsis, Jour. Amer. Med. Assoc., 98, 2191, 1932.
Bromer, A. W., and Blumgart, H. L.: Heart failure, Jour. Amer. Med. Assoc., 92, 204 1929.
Bronfenbrenner, J. J., and Straub, E. L.: Tuberculosis, Jour. Exp. Med., 41, 257, 1925.
Bronfenbrenner, J. J., and Weiss, H.: Poisoning, Jour. Exper. Med., 39, 517, 1924.
Bronfin, I. D., and Singerman, I.: Syphilis, Jour. Amer. Med. Assoc., 98, 1725, 1932.
Brooke, R.: Amebic dysentery, Jour. Amer. Med. Assoc., 62, 1009, 1914.
Brooks, C.: Agranulocytosis, Jour. Amer. Med. Assoc., 99, 1132, 1932 (discussion).
Brougher, J. C.: Thyrotoxicosis, Jour. Amer. Med. Assoc., 94, 471, 1930. Tetany, Clin. Med. and Surg., 38, 167, 1931; Jour. Amer. Med. Assoc., 94, 471, 1930.
Brower, A. B., and Simpson, W. M.: Pernicious anemia, Amer. Jour. Med. Sci., 182, 319, 1931.
Brown, C. F. G.: Peptic ulcer, Med. Clin. N. A., 16, 501, 1932.
Brown, C. F. G., et al.: Peptic ulcer, Jour. Amer. Med. Assoc., 99, 98, 1932.
Brown, E. W.: War gas, U. S. Nav. Med. Bull., 26, 217, 1928.
Brown, H. W.: Worms, Amer. Jour. Hyg., 16, 602, 1932; Proc. Soc. Exper. Biol. and Med., 30, 221, 1933.
Brown, L., Heise, T. H., Petroff, S. A., and Wilson, G. E.: Typhoid, Amer. Rev. Tuberc., 11, 717, 1911.
Brown, O. H.: Urticaria, Southwestern Med., June, 1931.
Brown, P. W.: Amebic dysentery, Jour. Amer. Med. Assoc., 86, 457, 1926.
Brown, P. W., and Osterberg, A. E.: Amebic dysentery, Amer. Jour. Med. Sci., 182, 257, 1931.
Brown, R. C.: Obstetrics, Lancet, 1, 383, 1933.
Brown, T. R.: Sprue, Bull. Johns Hopkins Hosp., 26, 289, 1916.
Browning, W. H.: Spider bite, New Orleans Med. and Surg. Jour., 82, 873, 1930.
Brownson, W. C.: Impetigo, Jour. Amer. Med. Assoc., 69, 176, 1917 (discussion).
Bruce, T.: Tetanus, Lancet, 1917, 1, 680; Trans. Soc. Trop. Med. and Hyg., 11, 1, 1917–18; Brit. Med. Jour., 1917, 1, 118; ibid., 1919, 2, 16; Jour. Hyg., 19, 1, 1920.
Bruen, C.: Hypertension, Jour. Lab. and Clin. Med., 18, 138, 1932.
Brugger: Measles, Münch. med. Wchnschr., 71, 858, 1924.
Brugsch, T., and Horsters, H.: Catarrhal jaundice, Med. Klin., 20, 661, 1924.
Bryan, C. S., and Mallmann, W. L.: Skin disinfection, Jour. Lab. and Clin. Med., 18, 1249, 1933.
Buchanan, G.: Infectious jaundice, Brit. Med. Jour., 2, 990, 1924; BCG, Lancet, 1, 653, 1933.
Buchanan, J. O.: Migraine, Jour. Nerv. and Neur. Dis., 54, 406, 1921; Amer. Jour. Med. Sci., 165, 675, 1923.
Bueermann, W. H.: Peptic ulcer, West. Jour. Surg., Obst., and Gyn., 38, 680, 1930.
Buerger, L.: Thrombo-angiitis obliterans, Circulatory Diseases of the Extremities, Phila., W. B. Saunders Co., 1924.
Bulger, H. A., Smith, F. M., and Steinmeyer, A.: Milk sickness, Jour. Amer. Med. Assoc., 91, 1964, 1928.
Bull, H. G.: Scarlet fever, Jour. Amer. Med. Assoc., 101, 363, 1933.
Bullowa, J. G. M.: Pneumonia, Med. Clin. N. A., March, 1932.
Bunim, J. J., and Wies, F. A.: Cerebrospinal fever, Jour. Amer. Med. Assoc., 100, 178, 1933.
Bunker, H. A., Jr.: Syphilis, Jour. Amer. Med. Assoc., 86, 1815, 1926; Amer. Jour. Psych., 8, 681, 1929.
Burke, C. F., and Meyerding, H. W.: Buerger's disease, Surg., Gyn., and Obst., 80, 389, 1931.
Burn, M.: Measles, Lancet, 1, 1135, 1931.

Burnam, C. F.: Urinary infections, Arch. Int. Med., 10, 324, 1912.
Burnet, F. M., McKie, M., and Wood, I. J.: Bacillary dysentery, Med. Jour. Australia, 2, 714, 1931.
Burnham, A. C.: Poliomyelitis, Med. Rec., 84, 15, 1913. Gallbladder disease, Med. Rec., 84, 15, 1913.
Burrows, M. T.: Poliomyelitis, Arch. Int. Med., 48, 33, 1931.
Burton, A. H. G., and Balmain, A. R.: Sepsis, Lancet, 2, 72, 1931. Diphtheria, Lancet, 2 1401, 1931.
Burt-White, H.: Sepsis, Lancet, 1, 16, 1930.
Bustillo, U.: Malaria, Med. Dept. United Fruit Co. (19th Ann. Rep.), 1930.
Butler, C. S.: Yaws, U. S. Nav. Med. Bull., 30, No. 1, 1932; Lancet, 1, 937, 1931; Ann. Int. Med., 5, 1033, 1932; Amer. Jour. Clin. Path., 2, No. 3, 1932; Internat. Clin., 1930.
Butler, C. S., and Parson, R. P.: Yaws, Amer. Jour. of Syph., 11, 228, 1927.
Butler, C. S., and Peterson, E.: Yaws, Jour. Lab. and Clin. Med., 12, 670, 1927.
Buttiaux, R., and Sévin, A.: Colitis, Ann. de l'Inst. Past., August, 1931, p. 173.
Buylla, P., Parreño, C., and Coronado, C.: Peptic ulcer, Arch. de med. Cirugia y Espec., 34, 804, 1931.
Byam, W.: Delousing (Brit. Trench Fever Inves. Comm.), Jour. Amer. Med. Assoc., 71, 21, 1918.
Cabot, R. C.: Rheumatic fever, Boston Med. and Surg. Jour., 192, 1122, 1925.
Cadham, F. T.: Hiccup, Jour. Amer. Med. Assoc., 84, 580, 1925. Sepsis, Brit. Med. Jour., 2, 460, 1930.
Cady, L. D., and Alvis, B. Y.: Syphilis, Jour. Amer. Med. Assoc., 86, 184, 1926.
Caldwell, W. A.: Syphilis, London C. C. Rep., No. 2821, 1931.
Calmette, A.: BCG, Presse méd., 36, 35, 1928; Ztschr. f. Tuberk., 50, 38, 1928; Rev. de l'Tuberc., 11, 985, 1930; Bull. de l'Acad. de Méd., 105, No. 8, 1931; Jour. Amer. Med. Assoc., 96, 58, 1931; Lancet, 1, 653, 1933.
Calmette, Guérin, Nègre, and Boquet: BCG, Ann. de l'Inst. Past., 40, 89, 1926.
Calvin, J. K., and Goldberg, A. H.: Tetanus, Jour. Amer. Med. Assoc., 94, 1977, 1930.
Cambessédès, H., and Garnier, G.: Undulant fever, Paris méd., 1, 281, 1929.
Cameron, H.: Hyperinsulinism, Brit. Med. Jour., 2, 717, 1930.
Cammidge, P. J., and Poulton, E. P.: Hyperinsulinism, Lancet, 1, 520, 1933.
Campanacci, D.: Nephritis, Wien. klin. Wchnschr., 37, 257, 1924.
Campbell, H. B., and Kieffer, J.: Tuberculosis, Amer. Rev. Tuberc., 6, 938, 1922.
Campbell, M. F.: Epididymitis, Jour. Amer. Med. Assoc., 89, 2108, 1927. Granuloma inguinale, Amer. Jour. Med. Sci., 174, 670, 1927. Urinary tract infection, Jour. Amer. Med. Assoc., 99, 2231, 1932.
Campbell, W. R., and Macleod, J. J. R.: Hyperemesis, Med., 3, 284, 1924.
Cannon, A. B.: Syphilis, Jour. Amer. Med. Assoc., 89, 666, 1923.
Cannon, A. B., and Karelitz, M. B.: Syphilis, Jour. Amer. Med. Assoc., 97, 1523, 1931.
Cantacuzène, J., and Panaitescu, V.: Typhoid, Compt. rend. Soc. de biol., 92, 1138, 1925.
Cantarow, A.: Peptic ulcer, tuberculosis, tetany, Calcium Metabolism and Therapy, Phila., Lea and Febiger, 1931.
Cantlie, N., and Moubarak, S. Y. E.: Malaria, Jour. Trop. Med. and Parasit., 27, 37, 1924.
Cardamatis, J. P.: Blackwater fever, Grèce Médicale, 28, 9, 1926.
Carey, J. B.: Pernicious anemia, Arch. Int. Med., 47, 893, 1931.
Carlson, A. F.: Gallbladder disease, Jour. Amer. Med. Assoc., 85, 1541, 1925 (discussion).
Caronia, G.: Measles, Pediatria, 31, 801, 1923.
Caronia, G.: Kala-azar, Pediatria, 24, 65, 1916; Amer. Jour. Trop. Med., 10, 261, 1930.
Carstens, J. H.: Obstetrical anesthesia, Jour. Amer. Med. Assoc., 67, 559, 1916 (discussion).
Carter, H. R.: Yellow fever, Nelson Loose-Leaf Med., 2, 113.
Carvill, M.: Syphilis, Jour. Amer. Med. Assoc., 96, 1936, 1931.
Cary, W. E., and Day, L. A.: Measles, Jour. Amer. Med. Assoc., 89, 1206, 1927.
Castellani, A.: Yaws, Brit. Med. Jour., 1905, 2, 1280; Nelson Loose-Leaf Med., 2, 339. Sprue, Jour. Trop. Med. and Hyg., 33, 126, 1930. Malaria, Lancet, 1, 1364, 1932 (Report of meeting of Roy. Soc. Trop. Med. and Hyg.).
Castellani and Chalmers: Quinine desensitization, Manual of Trop. Med., 3rd Ed., p. 1192.
Castle, W. B.: Pernicious anemia, Amer. Jour. Med. Sci., 178, 748, 1929.
Castle, W. B., et al.: Pernicious anemia, Amer. Jour. Med. Sci., 180, 305, 1930.
Castle, W. B., and Taylor, F. H. L.: Pernicious anemia, Jour. Amer. Med. Assoc., 96, 1198, 1931.
Castorina, G.: Whooping cough, Pediatria, 31, 151, 1923.
Caulfeild, A. H. W.: Hay-fever, Jour. Amer. Med. Assoc., 79, 125, 1922.
Cavett, J. W.: Nephritis, Jour. Biol. Chem., 87, 16, 1930.
Cecikas, I.: Amebic dysentery, Jour. Amer. Med. Assoc., 72, 213, 1919.
Cecil, R. L.: Arthritis, Jour. Amer. Med. Assoc., 100, 1220, 1933.
Cecil, R. L., and Plummer, N.: Pneumonia, Jour. Amer. Med. Assoc., 95, 1547, 1930; ibid., 98, 779, 1932.
Cecil, R. L., and Vaughan, H. F.: Pneumonia, Jour. Exper. Med., 29, 457, 1919.
Chagas, C., and Villela, E.: Trypanosomiasis, Mem. Inst. Oswaldo Cruz, 14, 3, 54.

Chambers, S. O., and Koetter, G. F.: Syphilis, Arch. Derm. and Syph., 25, 1065, 1932.

Chandler, G. F.: Hay-fever, Med. Jour. and Rec., 136, 337, 1932.

Chantriot: Flagellate dysentery, Clinique, 27, 29, 1932.

Chapman, C. B., Snell, A. M., and Rowntree, L. G.: Cirrhosis, Jour. Amer. Med. Assoc., 97, 237, 1931.

Chase, A. F., and Tasker, A. N.: Flagellate dysentery, Jour. Amer. Med. Assoc., 68, 1528, 1917.

Chase, A. F., Myers, V. C., and Killian, J. A.: Rheumatic fever, Jour. Amer. Med. Assoc. 77, 1230, 1921.

Chatard, J. A.: Pneumonia, Johns Hopkins Hosp. Rep., 15, 155, 1910 (cited by Cole, R.).

Chatin, A.: Simple goiter, Compt. rend. Acad. de Sc., 1850; Gaz. de Hôp., 14, 25, 38, 50, 86, 94, 1852.

Chen, K. K., and Schmidt, C. F.: Asthma, Jour. Pharm. and Exp. Ther., 24, 339, 1924.

Chen, S. M., van Gorder, and Yuan, Y. K.: Amebic dysentery, Natl. Med. Jour. China, 17, 393, 1931.

Chenard and Ferrier: BCG, Bull. Soc. Scient. de Bretagne, January 5, 1929.

Cheney, G., and Niemand, F.: Anemia, Amer. Jour. Med. Sci., 184, 314, 1932.

Chesterman, C. C.: Leukemia, Brit. Med. Jour., 1925, 1, 694. Trypanosomiasis, Trans., Roy. Soc. Trop. Med. and Hyg., 16, 394, 1922; ibid., 18, 311, 1924; ibid., 18, 131, 1924; Lancet, 2, 965, 1925.

Chiari, H., Nobel, E., and Sole, A.: BCG, Ztschr. f. Tuberk., 50, 24, 1928; Bull. Soc. Scient. de Bretagne, 51, 354, 1928; Wien. klin. Wchnschr., 41, 798, 1928.

Choksy, K. B.: Plague, Brit. Med. Jour., 1, 1282, 1908.

Chopra, R. N., Gupta, J. C., Mullick, M. N., and Gupta, A. K. D.: Kala-azar, Ind. Med. Gaz., 63, 252, 1928.

Christian, H. A.: Heart failure, Billings-Forchheimer's Therapeusis, New York, D. Appleton, 5, 254, 1924. Myxedema, Rhode Island Med. Jour., 8, 109, 1925. Chronic nonvalvular heart disease, Jour. Amer. Med. Assoc., 91, 549, 1928. Nephritis, Jour. Amer. Med. Assoc., 93, 23, 1929. Heart disease, Jour. Amer. Med. Assoc., 100, 789, 1933.

Christiansen, M.: Diphtheria carrier, Acta med. Scandinav., 58, 201, 1923.

Christie, W. F.: Roundworms, Jour. Roy. Army Med. Corps., 23, 201, 1914.

Christopher, F.: Burns, Minor surgery, Phila., W. B. Saunders Co., 1932, p. 47.

Christopherson, J. B.: Blood flukes, Lancet, 1918, 2, 325; Brit. Med. Jour., 1927, 1, 418.

Christopherson, J. B., and Newlove, J. R.: Blood flukes, Jour. Trop. Med. and Hyg., 22, 129, 1919.

Churchill, F. S., Landis, E. M., and Glusker, S. D.: Epidemic pleurodynia, Jour. Amer. Med. Assoc., 87, 821, 1926.

Churchman, J. W.: Dyes, Jour. Urol., 11, 1, 1924. Sepsis, Jour. Amer. Med. Assoc. 85, 1849, 1925.

Cipollaro, A. C., and Sheplar, A. E.: Boils, Arch. Dermat. and Syph., 25, 280, 1932.

Claude, H., and Coste, F.: Syphilis, Bull. de l'acad. de méd., Paris, 106, 266, 1931.

Clelland, J. B., and Bradley, B.: Dengue, Jour. Hyg., 16, 317, 1918.

Clemesha, W. W.: Malaria, Lancet, 1, 750, 1932.

Clemesha, W. W., and Moore, J. H.: Malaria, Ind. Med. Gaz., 65, 671, 1930.

Clough: Foot and Mouth Disease, Bull. Johns Hopkins Hosp., 26, 351, 1915.

Clovis, E. E., and Mills, G. E.: Typhoid, Jour. Amer. Med. Assoc., 74, 297, 1920.

Clow, A. E.: Dysmenorrhea, Brit. Med. Jour., January 2, 1932.

Clute, H. M., and Daniels, D. H.: Thyrotoxicosis, Amer. Jour. Med. Sci., 179, 477, 1930.

Coca, A. F., Walzer, M., and Thommen, A. A.: Allergy, Asthma and Hay-fever in Theory and Practice, Baltimore, Chas. C. Thomas, 1931.

Cochrane, R. G.: Leprosy, Lancet, 1926, 2, 95.

Coffey, W. B., and Brown, P. K.: Angina pectoris, Arch. Int. Med., 31, 200, 1923.

Cohn, A. E., and Levine, S. A.: Heart block, Arch. Int. Med., 36, 1, 1925.

Cohn, D. J., Katz, L. N., et al.: Heart failure, Amer. Jour. Med. Sci., 184, 818, 1932.

Cohn, E. J., et al.: Pernicious anemia, Jour. Biol. Chem., 77, 325, 1928; Proc. Soc. Biol. Chem., 7, 49, 1930.

Cole, D. B., and Harper, E. C.: Asthma, Jour. Lab. and Clin. Med., 18, 704, 1933.

Cole, H. N.: Syphilis, Arch. Dermat. and Syph., 13, 219, 1926 (discussion); New York State Jour. Med., 30, 638, 1930. Chancroid, Ven. Dis. Inform., 10, 1, 1929. Eczemadermatitis, Jour. Amer. Med. Assoc., 98, 1521, 1932.

Cole, H. N., and Littman, S.: Syphilis, Jour. Amer. Med. Assoc., 73, 1409, 1919.

Cole, H. N., DeWolf, H., et al.: Syphilis, Jour. Amer. Med. Assoc., 97, 898, 1931.

Cole, H. N., Driver, J. R., and Hutton, J. G.: Syphilis, Jour. Amer. Med. Assoc., 79, 1821 1922.

Cole, H. N., Gericke, A. J., and Sollmann, T.: Syphilis, Arch. Dermat. and Syph., 5, 18, 1922.

Cole, H. N., Hutton, J. G., and Sollmann, T.: Syphilis, Jour. Amer. Med. Assoc., 82, 199 1924.

Cole, H. N., Littman, S., and Sollmann, T.: Syphilis, Jour. Amer. Med. Assoc., 75, 1559 1920.

Cole, H. N., Henderson, K. I., Von Oettingen, W. F., and Sollmann, T.: Syphilis, Arch. Dermat. and Syph., 24, 739, 1931.

Cole, H. N., Hutton, J. G., Rauschkolb, J., and Sollmann, T.: Syphilis, Jour. Amer. Med. Assoc., 83, 593, 1924.

Cole, H. N., Moore, J. E., O'Leary, P. A., Parran, T., Jr., Stokes, J. H., and Wile, V. J.: Syphilis, Ven. Dis. Inform., 12, 145, 1931.

Cole, R.: Pneumonia, Jour. Amer. Med. Assoc., 76, 111, 1921; Nelson Loose-Leaf Med., 1, 203.

Cole, W. H., and Womack, N. A.: Adenoma, Arch. Surg., 23, 466, 1931.

Cole, Avery, Chickering and Dochez: Pneumonia, Monograph No. 7, Rockefeller Inst. for Med. Res. (1917).

Colegate, C. E., and McColloch, H.: Arrhythmia, Amer. Heart Jour., 2, 160, 1926.

Coleman, W.: Typhoid, Jour. Amer. Med. Assoc., 69, 329, 1917; Nelson Loose-Leaf Med., 1, 131, 181. Peptic ulcer, Jour. Amer. Med. Assoc., 83, 885, 1924; ibid., 84, 697, 1925.

Collier, J.: Epilepsy, Lancet, 1, 687, 1928.

Collin, L.: Yaws, Bull. Soc. Path. Exot., 7, 180, 1914.

Collis, W. R. F., and Sheldon, W.: Rheumatic fever, Lancet, 2, 1261, 1932.

Comber, V. H.: Sepsis, Lancet, March 28, 1931, p. 698.

Comroe, B. I.: Atropine poisoning, Jour. Amer. Med. Assoc., 101, 446, 1933.

Connal, A.: Blackwater fever, West African Med. Jour., 4, 32, 1930.

Connell, J. H., et al.: Burns, Jour. Amer. Med. Assoc., 100, 1219, 1933.

Conner, H. M.: Pernicious anemia, Jour. Amer. Med. Assoc., 96, 500, 1931; ibid., 99, 614, 1932; Med. Clin. N. A., June 15, 1932, 1463.

Conner, L. A., and Holt, E.: Coronary occlusion, Amer. Heart Jour., 5, 705, 1930.

Connery, J. E.: Pernicious anemia, New York State Jour. Med., March 15, 1931; Jour. Amer. Med. Assoc., 97, 605, 1931.

Connery, J. E., and Goldwater, L. J.: Pernicious anemia, Jour. Amer. Med. Assoc., 98, 1060, 1932.

Connery, J. E., and Jolliffe, N.: Pernicious anemia, Amer. Jour. Med. Sci., 181, 830, 1931.

Conyers, J. H., and Daniels, C. W.: Granuloma inguinale, Brit. Guiana Med. Ann., 8, 13, 1896.

Cooke, J. V.: Syphilis, Nelson Loose-Leaf Med., 2, 330 A. Chickenpox, Ann. Int. Med., 2, 518, 1928.

Cooke, R. A.: Hay-fever, Laryngoscope, 25, 108, 1915.

Cooke, W. E.: Filariasis, Lancet, 1, 390, 1928.

Cooke, W. E., and Willoughby, H.: Blackwater fever, Lancet, 1, 334, 1929.

Cooper, H. A., and Gunn, J. A.: Encephalitis, Lancet, 2, 901, 1931.

Coppolino, J. F.: Syphilis, Amer. Jour. Dis. Child., 39, 288, 1930.

Corbitt, H. B., and Myers, C. N.: Syphilis, Med. Times, 51, 282, 1923.

Corbus, B. C.: Gonorrhea, Jour. Amer. Med. Assoc., 98, 532, 1932.

Corey, E. L., and Britton, S. W.: Agranulocytosis, Amer. Jour. Physiol., 102, 699, 1932.

Cornwall, E. E.: Heart failure, Med. Rec., 92, 451, 1917.

Corson, J. E.: Trypanosomiasis, Ann. Trop. Med. and Parasit., 22, 379, 1928; ibid., 25, 63, 1931.

Cort, E. C.: Blackwater fever, Amer. Jour. Trop. Med., 9, 401, 1929. Flagellate dysentery, Jour. Amer. Med. Assoc., 90, 1430, 1928.

Costa, Boyer, and van Deinse: Bacillary dysentery, Compt. rend. Soc. de Biol., 93, 122, 1925.

Cottrell, J. E., and Wood, F. C.: Angina pectoris, Amer. Jour. Med. Sci., 181, 36, 1931.

Coulter, J. S : Pneumonia, Handbook Physical Ther. Amer. Med. Assoc., Chicago, 1932.

Cowen, H. W.: Psoriasis, Lancet, 2, 267, 1932.

Cowgill, G. R., and Anderson, W. E.: Constipation, Jour. Amer. Med. Assoc., 98, 1866, 1932.

Cowgill, G R., and Sullivan, A. J.: Constipation, Jour. Amer. Med. Assoc., 100, 795, 1933.

Cowie, D. M.: Smallpox, Cecil's Textbook of Medicine, Phila., W. B. Saunders Co., 1933, p. 312.

Cowie, D. M., and Hicks, W. C.: Urinary infection, Jour. Lab. and Clin. Med., 17, 681, 1932.

Coyne, A. E.: Beriberi, Ind. Med. Gaz., 62, 17, 1927.

Craig, C. F.: Amebic dysentery, Jour. Amer. Med. Assoc., 98, 1615, 1932.

Craven, E. B., Jr.: Syphilis, Bull. Johns Hopkins Hosp., 48, 131, 1931.

Crawford, A. S.: Cerebrospinal fever, Jour. Amer. Med. Assoc., 98, 1531, 1932.

Crawford, J. H., and McIntosh, G. F.: Heart failure, Arch. Int. Med., 36, 530, 1925; Jour. Clin. Invest., 1, 333, 1925.

Criep, L. H., and McElroy, W. S.: Hay-fever, Arch. Int. Med., 42, 865, 1928.

Criep, L. H., and Wechsler, S.: Urticaria, Jour. Allergy, 2, 479, 1931.

Crile, G. W.: Thyrotoxicosis, Jour. Amer. Med. Assoc., 97, 1616, 1931

Crohn, B. B.: Achylia, Amer. Jour. Med. Sci., 156, 656, 1918.

Cross, F. B.: Pneumonia, Med. Jour. and Rec., September 7, 1927.

Crossen, H. S.: Gonorrhea, Diseases of Women, St. Louis, C. V. Mosby Co., 1926, pp. 260, 264, 434. Dysmenorrhea, Diseases of Women, St. Louis, C. V. Mosby Co., 1926, p. 856.

Cruchet, R.: Tetanus, Brit. Med. Jour., January 16, 1932
Crutchfield, E. D.: Granuloma inguinale, Jour. Amer. Med. Assoc., 87, 1785, 1926 (discussion).
Csépai and Pinter-Kováts: Diabetes mellitus, Münch. med. Wchnschr., 74, 1011, 1927.
Cudlipp, J. S.: Snake-bite, United Fruit Co., Med. Dept. Bull., 1929, p. 332.
Cumston, G. C.: Undulant fever, Med. Jour. and Rec., 121, 219, 1925.
Curtis, G. M., *et al.:* Thyrotoxicosis, Jour. Amer. Med. Assoc., 101, 901, 1933.
Cutler, M.: Blood flukes, Jour. Amer. Med. Assoc., 86, 816, 1926.
Cutting, *et al.:* Obesity, Jour. Amer. Med. Assoc., 101, 193, 1933.
Dabney, W. C.: Epidemic pleurodynia, Amer. Jour. Med. Sci., 96, 488, 1888.
Dakin, H. D., *et al.:* Pernicious anemia, Proc. Soc. Exper. Biol. and Med., 28, 2, 1930.
Dameshek, W.: Anemia, Jour. Amer. Med. Assoc., 100, 540, 1933.
Danforth, W. C., and Davis, C. H.: Obstetrical anesthesia, Jour. Amer. Med. Assoc., 81, 1090, 1923.
Darling, S. T.: Hookworm, Nelson Loose-Leaf Med., 2, 477.
Darling, S. T., Barber, M. A., and Hacker, H. P.: Hookworm, Jour. Amer. Med. Assoc., 70, 499, 1918.
Darling, S. T., and Smillie, W. G.: Hookworm, Jour. Amer. Med. Assoc., 76, 419, 1921.
Darré, H., and Laffaille, A.: Undulant fever, Bull. de l'Acad. de méd., 100, 999, 1928.
Dattner, B.: Syphilis, Klin. Wchnschr., 7, 921, 1928.
Dautrebande, L.: Thyrotoxicosis, Presse méd., 2, 1361, 1928.
David, N. A., Johnstone, H. G., Reed, A. C., and Leake, C. D.: Amebiasis, Jour. Amer. Med. Assoc., 100, 1658, 1933.
Davidson, E. C.: Burns, Surg., Gyn., and Obst., 41, 202, 1925.
Davidson, L. S. P.: Pernicious anemia, Edinburgh Med. Jour., 39, Nos. 7 and 8, 1932.
Davidson, S.: Pernicious anemia, Lancet, 2, 1395, 1931.
Davies, D. S.: Blood flukes, Trans. Roy. Soc. Trop. Med. and Hyg., 20, 436, 1927.
Davies, G. R.: Whooping cough, Amer. Jour. Dis. Child., 23, 423, 1922.
Davies, H. M.: Tuberculosis, Lancet, 2, 274, 1932.
Davis, C. C.: Stokers' cramps, Jour. Amer. Med. Assoc., 83, 2112, 1924.
Davis, C. H.: Obstetrical anesthesia, Amer. Jour. Obst. and Gyn., 14, 806, 1927.
Davis, E., and Sharpe, J. C.: Urinary infection, Jour. Amer. Med. Assoc., 99, 2097, 1932.
Davis, R. C.: Measles, Med. Clin. N. A., 7, 1259, 1924.
Dawson, W. T., and Garbade, F. A.: Malaria, Jour. Amer. Med. Assoc., 94, 704, 1930.
Deaderick, W. H.: Quinine prophylaxis, Nelson Loose-Leaf Med., 2, 241. Blackwater fever, Nelson Loose-Leaf Med., 2, 257.
De Bellard, E. P.: Bacillary dysentery, Gaceta Medica de Caracas, 32, 196, 1925.
De Boinet: Simple goiter, Bull. de l'Acad. Imp. de Méd., October 26, 1858 (cited by Kimball, O. P., *q. v.*).
Debré, R., and Ravine, J.: Measles, Bull. et mém. Soc. méd. de Hôp. de Paris, 47, 226 1923.
De Buys, L. R.: Malaria, Jour. Amer. Med. Assoc., 75, 1003, 1920.
De Buys, L. R., and Dwyer, H. L.: Worms, Amer. Jour. Dis. Child., 18, 269, 1919.
De Castro, A. B.: Oriental sore, Ind. Med. Gaz., 66, 391, 1931.
De Eds, F.: Poliomyelitis, Arch. Int. Med., 34, 511, 1924.
Deeks, W. E.: Amebic dysentery, Ann. Trop. Med. and Parasit., 8, 321, 1914.
Deeks, W. E., and Connor, R. C.: Malaria, Malaria, Its Cause, Prevention and Cure, United Fruit Co., 1930.
Deeks, W. E., and James, W. M.: Blackwater fever, Med. Press and Circ., London, 92, 393, 1911.
De Finis, G.: Undulant fever, Pediatria, 31, 11, 1923.
Degqwitz, R.: Measles, Deutsch. med. Wchnschr., 48, 26, 1922; Jour. Infect. Dis., 41, 304, 1927.
De Langen, C. D.: Strongyloides, Neded. van d. Dienst d. Volksgczondheid in Med.-Indie, Batavia, 1928.
DeLee, J. B.: Preparation of vulva, Textbook of Obstetrics, Phila., W. B. Saunders Co., 1933, p. 297. Obstetrical anesthesia, Textbook of Obstetrics, Phila., W. B. Saunders Co., 1933, p. 317.
De Mello, L.: Scabies, Arch. Dermat. and Syph., 23, 863, 1931.
Dennett, R. H., and Wetchler, S.: Chorea, Jour. Pediat., 1, 203, 1932.
Dennie, C. C., and McBride, W. L.: Syphilis, Jour. Amer. Med. Assoc., 83, 2082, 1924.
De Rezende, C.: Rheumatic fever, Brazil-med., 41, 1005, 1927.
De Rezende, M. O.: Mucocutaneous leishmaniasis, Ann. Paulist. med. e cirurg., 16, 135, 1925.
De Rudder: Chorea, Klin. Wchnschr., 5, 1522, 1926.
Desnoes, P. H.: Seasickness, Jour. Amer. Med. Assoc., 86, 319, 1926.
De Souza, J. S.: Measles, Arch. de méd. d. enf., 35, 633, 1932.
De Takáts, G.: Varicose veins, Jour. Amer. Med. Assoc., 96, 1111, 1931
Deuskar, V. N.: Amebic dysentery, Ind. Med. Gaz., 61, 165, 1926.
Dévé, F.: Hydatid cyst, Presse méd., 35, 193, 1927.
Devi, A. L.: Oriental sore, Ind. Med. Gaz., 64, 139, 1929.

De Witt, L. M., Suyenaga, S., and Wells, H. G.: Tuberculosis, Jour. Infect. Dis., 27, 115, 1920.

De Wolf, H. F., and Van Cleve, J. V.: Lymphogranuloma inguinale, Jour. Amer. Med. Assoc., 99, 1065, 1932.

D'Hérelle, F.: Plague, Presse méd., 33, 1393, 1925 (this was discussed in the Jour. Amer. Med. Assoc., Paris correspondence, 85, 1653, 1925).

Dick, G. F., and Dick, G. H.: Measles, Jour. Infect. Dis., 15, 85, 1914. Scarlet fever, Jour. Amer. Med. Assoc., 81, 1166, 1923; ibid., 83, 84, 1924; ibid., 84, 802, 1925; ibid., 84, 803, 1925; ibid., 84, 1477, 1925; ibid., 85, 1693, 1925. Diphtheria, Jour. Amer. Med. Assoc., 92, 1901, 1929.

Dickson, E. C.: Coccidioidal granuloma, Arch. Int. Med., 16, 1028, 1915.

Dieckmann, W. J.: Eclampsia, Amer. Jour. Obst. and Gyn., 22, 351, 1931.

Dieckmann, W. J., and Crossen, R. J.: Hyperemesis, Amer. Jour. Obst. and Gyn., 14, 3, 1927.

Diehl, H. S.: Catarrhal fever, Jour. Amer. Med. Assoc., 84, 1629, 1925.

Dilling, W. J., and Gemmell, A. A.: Quinine stillbirths, Amer. Jour. Obst. and Gyn., 36, 352, 1929.

Doan, C. A.: Agranulocytosis, Jour. Amer. Med. Assoc., 99, 194, 1932.

Dobell, E.: Amebic dysentery, The Amebae Living in Man, 1919.

Doble, F. C.: Syphilis, Lancet, 1920, 243.

Dobson, H. V.: Achylia, Jour. Pharm. and Exp. Ther., 30, 447, 1927.

Docherty, J. F.: Hookworm, Jour. Amer. Med. Assoc., 81, 454, 1923.

Dochez, A. R.: Scarlet fever, Proc. Soc. Exp. Biol. and Med., 4, 184, 1924.

Dochez, A. R., and Sherman, L.: Scarlet fever, Jour. Amer. Med. Assoc., 82, 542, 1924.

Dodds, E. C., et al.: Thyrotoxicosis, Lancet, 2, 608, 1932.

Doktorsky, A., and Platt, S. S.: Acne, Jour. Amer. Med. Assoc., 101, 275, 1933.

Dollert, F. F.: Hiccup (personal communication to the author).

Dopter, C.: Meningitis, Ann. de l'Inst. Past., 24, 96, 1910.

Dorne and Stein: Gonorrhea, Illinois Med. Jour., March, 1924.

Doull, J. A., and Fales, W. T.: Diphtheria carrier, Amer. Jour. Hyg., 3, 604, 1923.

Doull, J. A., and Lara, H.: Diphtheria carrier, Amer. Jour. Hyg., 5, 508, 1925.

Dragstedt, L. R., and Peacock, S. C.: Tetany, Amer. Jour. Physiol., 64, 424, 1923.

Dreyer, G., and Vollum, R. L.: BCG, Lancet, 1, 9, 1931.

Driver, J. R., and Weller, J. N.: Lupus erythematosus, Arch. Dermat. and Syph., 23, 87, 1931.

Driver, J. R., Gammel, J. A., and Karmosh, L. J.: Syphilis, Jour. Amer. Med. Assoc., 87, 1821, 1926.

Dry, T. J.: Scurvy, Arch. Int. Med., 51, 679, 1933.

Dublin, L. I.: Tuberculosis, Statistical Bull. Met. Life Ins. Co., December, 1932.

Dudley, D. G.: Anthrax, Jour. Amer. Med. Assoc., 70, 15, 1918.

Dudley, S. F.: Diphtheria, Lancet, December 26, 1931.

Duke, W. W.: Asthma, Allergy, St. Louis, C. V. Mosby Co., 1925, p. 238; Jour. Lab. and Clin. Med., 13, 1012, 1928. Hay-fever, Jour. Amer. Med. Assoc., 94, 767, 1930; Asthma, Hay-fever, Urticaria, etc., St. Louis, Mosby, 1925.

Dulitskiy, S. O.: Measles, Jour. Po Rann. Detskonw Voz., 12, 322, 1932.

Duncan, G. G.: Diabetes mellitus, Amer. Jour. Med. Sci., 175, 196, 1928.

Duncan, G. G., and Rudy, A.: Cirrhosis, Amer. Jour. Med. Sci., 172, 351, 1926.

Duncan, J. W., and Harding, V. J.: Hyperemesis, Canada Med. Assoc. Jour., 7, 1057, 1918.

Dundas-Grant, J.: Tuberculosis, Lancet, 2, 999, 1932.

Dundee, J. C.: Tuberculosis, Amer. Rev. Tuberc., 25, 469, 1932.

Dunham, K., and Asbury, E.: Tuberculosis, Jour. Amer. Med. Assoc., 99, 360, 1932.

Dunhill, T. P.: Adenoma, Brit. Jour. Surg., 17, 424, 1928.

Durand, M., et al.: Lymphogranuloma inguinale, Bull. et mém. Soc. med. d. hôp. de Paris, 35, 274, 1913.

Durham, E. C.: Syphilis, Amer. Jour. Syph., 9, 463, 1925.

Dye, W. H.: Trypanosomiasis, Trans. Roy. Soc. Trop. Med. and Hyg., 20, 74, 1926.

Dyer, R. E., et al.: Typhus, Jour. Amer. Med. Assoc., 99, 795, 1932.

Dyer, R. E., Rumreich, A. S., and Badger, L. F.: Rocky Mountain spotted fever, Jour. Amer. Med. Assoc., 97, 589, 1931.

Dyke, S. C.: Diabetes, Lancet, 1, 978, 1932.

Eason, J.: Peptic ulcer, Lancet, 2, 1272, 1932.

East and Cullinan: Chorea, Lancet, 2, 190, 1930.

Eastman, N. J.: Eclampsia, Amer. Jour. Obst. and Gyn., 22, 756, 1931.

Ebaugh, F. G.: Syphilis, Jour. Amer. Med. Assoc., 94, 455, 1930 (discussion).

Eberson, F.: Poliomyelitis, Jour. Lab. and Clin. Med., 18, 565, 1933.

Ecke, A., and Taubert, R.: Obstetrical anesthesia, Zentralbl. f. Gynäk., 50, 1111, 1926.

Edgar, J. C.: Pituitrin in labor, Jour. Amer. Med. Assoc., 60, 1733, 1913 (abstract).

Edmunds, C. W., and Cooper, R. G.: Diphtheria, Jour. Amer. Med. Assoc., 85, 1798, 1925.

Edwards, P. W.: Tuberculosis, Lancet, 1, 709, 1932.

Eggleston, C.: Heart failure, Arch. Int. Med., 16, 1, 1915; Jour. Amer. Med. Assoc., 74, 733, 1920. Syphilis, Jour. Amer. Med. Assoc., 81, 1752, 1923 (discussion). Myocarditis, Cecil's Textbook of Medicine, Phila., W. B. Saunders Co., 1933, p. 1103.

Eggleston, C., and White, T. J.: Heart failure, Jour. Amer. Med. Assoc., 89, 583, 1927.
Egloff, W. C., *et al.*: Hypertension, Jour. Amer. Med. Assoc., 96, 1941, 1931.
Einer, H.: Eclampsia, Zentralbl. f. Gynäk., 31, 1125, 1907.
Einhorn, M., and Rafsky, H. A.: Constipation, Jour. Amer. Med. Assoc., 86, 1754, 1926.
Eismayer, G.: Diabetes, Klin. Wchnschr., 11, 860, 1932.
Eldridge, W. W.: Erysipelas, Ann. Clin. Med., 4, 333, 1925. Syphilis, Jour. Amer. Med. Assoc., 89, 100, 1927 (discussion).
Eley, R. C.: Erysipelas, Amer. Jour. Dis. Child., 39, 529, 1930.
Eley, R. C., and Clifford, S. H.: Hemophilia, Amer. Jour. Dis. Child., 42, 1331, 1931.
Elgood, C.: Whooping cough, Brit. Med. Jour., 1, 963, 1925.
Eliason, E. L., and Ferguson, L. K.: Purpura, Ann. Surg., November, 1932, p. 801.
Eliot, M. M.: Rickets, Jour. Amer. Med. Assoc., 85, 656, 1925.
Eliot, Ellsworth, and Colp: Cirrhosis, Surg., Gyn., and Obst., 28, 309, 1919.
Elliott, A. R.: Essential hypertension, Amer. Jour. Med. Sci., 174, 244, 1927.
Elliott, A. R., and Jenkinson, E. L.: Leukemia, Med. Clin. N. A., 17, 327, 1933.
Elliott, J. A.: Syphilis, South. Med. Jour., September, 1929, 785.
Elliott, T. R.: Tuberculosis, Lancet, 1926, 1, 126.
Elvehjem, C. A., and Sherman, W. C.: Anemia, Jour. Biol. Chem., 98, 309, 1932.
Emery, Rasis, and Morin: Syphilis, Bull. Soc. franç. de dermat. et syph., 37, 905, 1930.
Emge, L. A., and Cooley, C. L.: Obstetrical analgesia, California and West. Med., 31, September, 1929.
Emmerich and Loew: Hay-fever, Münch. med. Wchnschr., 60, 2676, 1913.
Engering: Gonorrhea, Zeitschr. f. Hyg. u. Inf. Krankh., 100, 314, 1923.
Engman, M. F.: Syphilis, Nelson Loose-Leaf Med., 2, 263.
Engman, M. F., Jurstad, L. H., and Engman, M. P., Jr.: Syphilis, Jour. Amer. Med. Assoc., 97, 1503, 1931.
Eppinger, H.: Nephritis, Zur Pathologie und Therapie des menschlichen Ödems, Berlin, 1917.
Eppinger, H., Mark, R. E., and Wagner, R. I.: Diabetes mellitus, Klin. Wchnschr., 4, 1870, 1925.
Epstein, A. A.: Nephritis, Amer. Jour. Med. Sci., 1917, 154, 638; Med. Clin. N. A., 5 1068, 1921; Jour. Amer. Med. Assoc., 87, 913, 1926.
Epstein, J.: Whooping cough, Arch. Pediat., January, 1933, p. 38.
Étienne, G.: Poliomyelitis, Bull. de l'Acad. de méd., 90, 102, 1923; Médecine, 7, 349 1926.
Evans, G.: Rheumatic fever, Brit. Med. Jour., 2, 93, 1926.
Ewing, R.: Dysmenorrhea, Jour. Indust. Med., September, 1931, 244.
Eyding, A.: Pernicious anemia, Münch. med. Wchnschr., Nr. 33, 1283, 1933.
Faber, H. K., and Dickey, L. B.: Thrush, Jour. Amer. Med. Assoc., 86, 900, 1925.
Faber, H. K., and Clark, E. B.: Thrush, Amer. Jour. Dis. Child., 34, 408, 1927.
Faber, H. K., and Struble, H. P.: Whooping cough, Jour. Amer. Med. Assoc., 85, 815, 1925.
Faber, K.: Tuberculosis, Acta Tuberc. Scandinav., 1, 1, 1925; Lancet, 2, 62, 1925.
Fahr, Th.: Nephritis, Virchow's Arch., 239, 32, 1922.
Fahrni, G. S.: Thyrotoxicosis, Canada Med. Assoc. Jour., 27, 42, 1932.
Fairbrother, R. W., and Morgan, W. T. J.: Poliomyelitis, Lancet, 2, 584, 1931.
Fairhall, L. T., and Shaw, C. P.: Lead poisoning, Jour. Indust. Hyg., 6, 159, 1924.
Fairley, N. H.: Blood flukes, Proc. Roy. Soc. Med., 13, 1, 1919.
Falconer, D. G.: Pernicious anemia, Practitioner, December, 1931, p. 686.
Falta: Diabetes mellitus, Wien. Arch. f. inn. Med., 8, 13, 1924; Klin. Wchnschr., 3, 1315, 1924.
Fantus, B.: Catarrhal fever, Jour. Amer. Med. Assoc., 75, 1694, 1920. Constipation, Useful Cathartics, Amer. Med. Assoc., 1927; Malaria, Scabies, Urticaria, Rheumatic fever, Constipation, General Technic of Medication, Amer. Med. Assoc., Chicago, 1930.
Farquharson, R. F., and Graham, D.: Pernicious anemia, Canad. Med. Assoc. Jour., 23, 237, 1930.
Faust, E. C.: Strongyloides, Jour. Amer. Med. Assoc., 98, 2276, 1932.
Favry, J.: Syphilis, Deutsch. med. Wchnschr., 44, 1217, 1918; ibid., 45, 1358, 1919.
Fay, T.: Brain volume, Jour. Amer. Med. Assoc., 80, 1445, 1923. Epilepsy, Amer. Jour. Psychiat., 8, 783, 1929; Arch. Neurol. and Psychiat., 23, 920, 1930; Jour. Amer. Med Assoc., 100, 1450, 1933.
Feil, H.: Heart block, Jour. Amer. Med. Assoc., 80, 26, 1923.
Feinberg, S. M.: Allergy, Jour. Lab. and Clin. Med., 13, 220, 1927.
Feinberg, S. M., Osborne, S. L., and Afremow, M. L.: Asthma, Jour. Amer. Med. Assoc. 97, 880, 1931.
Feinblatt, H. M., and Eggerth, A. H.: Tuberculosis, Arch. Int. Med., 36, 121, 1925.
Feldmann, V.: Syphilis, Ann. dermat. et de syph., 10, 275, 1929.
Felsen, J.: Colitis, Arch. Int. Med., 48, 786, 1931.
Felton, L. D.: Pneumonia, Boston Med. and Surg. Jour., 190, 819, 1924; Jour. Amer. Med. Assoc., 94, 1893, 1930.
Fenn, G. K., and Gilbert, N. C.: Angina pectoris, Jour. Amer. Med. Assoc., 98, 99, 1932.

Fernan-Nuñez, M.: Malaria, Amer. Jour. Trop. Med., 3, 269, 1923. Worms, Arch. Int. Med., 40, 46, 1927; Jour. Amer. Med. Assoc., 88, 903, 1927. Relapsing fever, Wisconsin Med. Jour., 30, 556, 1931.

Ferrell, J. A.: Hookworm disease, Jour. Amer. Med. Assoc., 62, 1937, 1914.

Ferry, N. S., and Fisher, L. W.: Measles, Jour. Amer. Med. Assoc., 86, 932, 1926.

Fetterman, J. L., and Kumin, H. J.: Epilepsy, Jour. Amer. Med. Assoc., 100, 1005, 1933.

Fetterolf, G., and Sponsler, M. B.: Hay-fever, Arch. Otolaryngol., 2, 132, 1925.

Figley, K. D.: Hay-fever, Jour. Allergy, 2, 39, 1930.

Findlay, G. M.: Kala-azar, Trypanosomiasis, Recent Advances in Chemotherapy, P. Blakiston's Son and Co., Phila., 1930. Lymphogranuloma, Lancet, 2, 11, 1932.

Fineberg, M. H.: Hypertension, Jour. Amer. Med. Assoc., 94, 1822, 1930.

Finger, J.: Obstetrical anesthesia, Monatschr. f. Geburtsh. u. Gynäk., 73, 162, 1926.

Finkelstein, A. S.: Whooping cough, Jour. Med. Soc. New Jersey, 28, 96, 1931.

Finkelstein, G. S.: Measles, Urach. Delo, 14, 753, 1931.

Finkelstein, H.: Anemia of infancy, Säuglingskrankheiten, 3rd Ed., 1924, p. 767 (cited by Bass and Denzer, q. v.).

Finland, M.: Pneumonia, New England Jour. Med., 202, 1244, 1930.

Finland, M., and Sutliff, W. D.: Pneumonia, Jour. Amer. Med. Assoc., 100, 560, 1933.

Finlayson: Bacillary dysentery, Brit. Med. Jour., 1, 46, 1917.

Fischer, M. H.: Eclampsia, Detroit Med. Jour., 16, 1, 1916.

Fishberg, M.: Tuberculosis, Jour. Amer. Med. Assoc., 72, 1882, 1919.

Fisk, E. L.: Essential hypertension, Amer. Med., 18, 446, 1923.

Fist, H. S.: Burns, Jour. Amer. Med. Assoc., 88, 1483, 1927. Obstetrical analgesia, California and West. Med., 32, May, 1930.

Fitzgibbon, G.: Eclampsia, Lancet, 1, 666, 1923.

Fitz-Hugh, T.: Agranulocytosis, Amer. Jour. Roentgenol. and Radium Therapy, 27, May, 1932 (discussion).

Fitz-Hugh, T., Jr., and Krumbhaar, E. B.: Agranulocytosis, Amer. Jour. Med. Sci., 183 104, 1932.

Flack, M.: Meningitis, English Report, p. 45.

Fleischmann, P.: Angina pectoris, Deutsch. med. Wchnschr., Nr. 4, 1932.

Fletcher, W., and Travers, E. A. O.: Malaria, Brit. Med. Jour., 1, 629, 1923.

Flexner, S.: Meningitis, Jour. Exper. Med., 17, 553, 1913. Bacillary dysentery, Jour. Amer. Med. Assoc., 76, 108, 1921. Encephalitis, Jour. Amer. Med. Assoc., 91, 21, 1928.

Fliess: Dysmenorrhea (cited by Mayer, E., Jour. Amer. Med. Amer. Assoc., 62, 6, 1914).

Flothow, P. G.: Buerger's disease, Amer. Jour. Surg., 10, 8, 1930.

Foerster, H. R.: Sporotrichosis, Jour. Amer. Med. Assoc., 87, 1605, 1926.

Fogelson, S. J.: Peptic ulcer, Amer. Jour. Nursing, 32, 921, 1932; Jour. Amer. Med. Assoc. 96, 673, 1931; Wisconsin Med. Jour., 30, 971, 1931.

Folin, D., et al.: Eczema-dermatitis, Jour. Biol. Chem., 75, 263, 1927.

Fong, T. C. C.: Syphilis, Med. Jour. and Rec., July 18, 1928.

Fontana, L.: Trypanosomiasis, Arch. Med. Belges, 77, 271, 1924.

Foote, J. A.: Erysipelas, South. Med. Jour., 23, 29, 1930.

Forbes, R. P., and Green, B.: Measles, Jour. Amer. Med. Assoc., 89, 1601, 1927.

Fordyce, J. A.: Syphilis, Brit. Jour. Dermat., 36, 47, 1924.

Fordyce, J. A., and Rosen, I.: Syphilis, Arch. Dermat. and Syph., 9, 355, 1924.

Forestier, J.: Varicose veins, Jour. Amer. Med. Assoc., 90, 1932, 1928.

Forkner, C. E.: Leukemia, Med. Clin. N. A., 15, 1057, 1932.

Forkner and Scott: Leukemia, Jour. Amer. Med. Assoc., 97, 3, 1931.

Forkner, C. E., Scott, T. F. M., and Wu, S. C.: Erythremia, Arch. Int. Med., 51, 616, 1933.

Foshay, L.: Diabetes mellitus, Amer. Jour. Physiol., 73, 470, 1925; Arch. Int. Med., 40, 661, 1927. Tularemia, Jour. Amer. Med. Assoc., 98, 552, 1932; Jour. Infect. Dis., 51, 286, 1932.

Foster, N. B.: Adenoma, Nelson Loose-Leaf Med., 3, 263 (November, 1928). Thyrotoxicosis, Nelson Loose-Leaf Med., 3, 299 B (November, 1928). Diabetes mellitus, Jour. Amer. Med. Assoc., 84, 719, 1925. Nephritis, Epilepsy and the Convulsive State (many authors), Baltimore, Williams and Wilkins, 1931.

Foti, P., and Javarone, N.: Kala-azar, Pediatria, 29, 145, 1921.

Fourche, J. A., and Haveaux, G.: Trypanosomiasis, Bull. Soc. Path. exot., 24, 557, 1931.

Fourneau, E., Tréfonel, J., and Valée, J.: Trypanosomiasis, Ann. de l'Inst. Pasteur, 1924, 2, 81.

Fournier, L.: Syphilis, quoted by Osler, W., and Churchman, J. W., Osler's Mod. Med., 2nd Ed., 2, 209, 1914.

Fournier, L., and Guenot, L.: Syphilis, Presse méd., 27, 554, 1919.

Fouts, P. J., and Zerfas, L. G.: Pernicious anemia, Jour. Amer. Med. Assoc., 101, 188, 1933.

Fox, H.: Herpes zoster, Jour. Amer. Med. Assoc., 79, 1979, 1922. Acne, Jour. Amer. Mcd. Assoc., 81, 1417, 1923. Granuloma inguinale, Jour. Amer. Med. Assoc., 87, 1785, 1926.

Fox, J. C.: Syphilis, Amer. Jour. Syph., 9, 436, 1925.

Fox, J. T.: Epilepsy, Lancet, 1927, 2, 589.

Fradkin, W. Z., and Gray, T.: Colitis, Jour. Amer. Med. Assoc., 94, 849, 1930.

Francis, E.: Tularemia, U.S.P.H. Rep., 34, 2061, 1919; ibid., 36, 1731, 1921.

Frank, E., Nothmann, M., and Wagner, A.: Diabetes mellitus, Klin. Wchnschr., 5, 2100, 1926.

Frankl, G., Herzog, H., and Nobel, E.: Diphtheria, Wien. med. Wchnschr., 78, 1155, 1928.

Fraser, A. R.: Granuloma inguinale, Jour. Urol., 13, 227, 1925.

Frazier, C. H., and Moser, W. B.: Thyrotoxicosis, Jour. Amer. Med. Assoc., 90, 657, 1928.

Freeman, J.: Allergy, Brit. Med. Jour., April 5, 1930, p. 744; Lancet, 1, 561, 1932.

Freeman, M. J., Taylor, G. G., and White, C.: Syphilis, Amer. Jour. Syph., 15, 207, 1931.

Freeman, R. G.: Urinary infections, Arch. Pediat., 41, 171, 1924.

Freeman, W.: Syphilis, Jour. Amer. Med. Assoc., 88, 1064, 1927; ibid., 101, 301, 1933.

Freeman, W., Fong, T. C., and Rosenberg, S. J.: Syphilis, Jour. Amer. Med. Assoc., 100, 1749, 1933.

Frehse, K.: Erysipelas, Münch. med. Wchnschr., August 14, 1931.

Frei, W.: Lymphogranuloma inguinale, Klin. Wchnschr., 4, 2148, 1925.

Freude, E.: Herpes zoster, Münch. med. Wchnschr., 38, 1617, 1931.

Fricke: Preparation of vulva, cited by Williams, J. W. (*q. v.*).

Friedemann, U., and Deicher, H.: Sclaret fever, Deutsch. med. Wchnschr., 51, 1935, 1925.

Frissell, L. F., and Hajek, J.: Diabetes mellitus, Jour. Amer. Med. Assoc., 86, 1903, 1926.

Fuld, E.: Constipation, Klin. Wchnschr., 4, 2182, 1925.

Fuller, A. T.: Ketogenic diet, Lancet, 1, 276, 1933; ibid., 1, 855, 1933.

Fulton, M. N.: Pleurisy, Jour. Amer. Med. Assoc., 97, 1959, 1931.

Gabritschewsky: Scarlet fever, Zentralbl. f. Bakteriol. I., Orig. 41; Berl. klin. Wchnschr., 44, 556, 1907.

Gage, I. M.: Granuloma inguinale, Arch. Dermat. and Syph., 7, 303, 1923.

Gager, L. T.: Essential hypertension, Jour. Amer. Med. Assoc., 90, 82, 1928. Auricular flutter, Ann. Int. Med., 5, 463, 1931.

Gainsborough, H.: Nephritis, Lancet, 1, 1131, 1932.

Gale, A. M., and Gale, C. H.: Thyrotoxicosis, Lancet, 1, 1287, 1931.

Galewsky, E.: Syphilis, Münch. med. Wchnschr., 67, 124, 1920.

Galli-Valeria: BCG, Rev. méd. Suisse rom., 47, March 16, 1927.

Gamble, C. J.: Leukemia, Jour. Amer. Med. Assoc., 88, 87, 1927.

Gänsslen, M.: Pernicious anemia, Deutsch. med. Wchnschr., No. 46, 1, 1931.

Gargill, S. P., and Rudy, A.: Hypertension, Amer. Jour. Med. Sci., 181, 639, 1931.

Garin, C. N., Rousset, J., and Gonthier, B.: Hookworm, Bull. et mém. Soc. med. hôp. de Paris, 20, 1003, 1931.

Garrison, F.: Malarial mosquitoes, History of Medicine, Phila., W. B. Saunders Co., 4th Ed., 1929, p. 583.

Gauthier, A.: Bacillary dysentery, Bull. de l'Acad. de méd., 91, 69, 1924.

Gay, F. P.: Asiatic cholera, Jour. Amer. Med. Assoc., 81, 284, 1923.

Geiger, J. C.: Cyanide poisoning, Jour. Amer. Med. Assoc., 99, 1944, 1932; ibid., 101, 269, 1933.

Gellhorn, G.: Gonorrhea, Jour. Amer. Med. Assoc., 75, 1647, 1920.

Genevrier: Varicose veins, quoted by Blanchod, F. (*q. v.*).

Gennerich, W.: Syphilis, Deutsch. med. Wchnschr., 44, 1243, 1918; Arch. f. derm. u. syph., 165, 209, 1932.

Genoese, G.: Whooping cough, Policlinica, 29, 1105, 1922.

George, I. D.: Snake-bite, United Fruit Co., Med. Dept. Bul., 1929, p. 326.

Gerlach, F., and Kraus, R.: BCG, Ztschr. f. Immunitäts., 59, 306, 1929; Centralbl. f. Bakt. (Abt. 1), 110, 179, 1929.

Gertsmann, J.: Syphilis, Die Malariabehandlung der progressiven Paralyse, Vienna, J. Springer, 1925.

Geyelin, H. R.: Epilepsy, Med. Rec., 99, 1037, 1921.

Geyelin, H. R., and Mackie, T. T.: Diabetes mellitus, New York State Jour. Med., 29, 677, 1929.

Gibbs, O. S.: Phenol Poisoning, Brit. Med. Jour., April 4, 1931.

Giffin, H. Z., and Allen, E. V.: Erythremia, Amer. Jour. Med. Sci., 185, 1, 1933. Polycythemia, Ann. Int. Med., 1, 655, 1928.

Giffin, H. Z., and Conner, H. M.: Polycythemia, Jour. Amer. Med. Assoc., 92, 1505, 1929.

Giffin, H. Z., and Holloway, J. K.: Purpura, Amer. Jour. Med. Sci., 170, 186, 1925.

Giffin, H. Z., and Watkins, C. H.: Anemia, Jour. Amer. Med. Assoc., 95, 587, 1930.

Gilbert, N. C.: Coronary occlusion, Med. Clin. N. A., 17, 545, 1933.

Gilbert, N. C., and Kerr, J. A.: Angina pectoris, Jour. Amer. Med. Assoc., 92, 201, 1929.

Gill, C. A., and Lal, R. B.: Asiatic cholera, Ind. Jour. Med. Res., 18, 1255, 1931.

Gilroy, E.: Pernicious anemia, Lancet, 2, 1093, 1931.

Girard, A. C.: Seasickness, Jour. Amer. Med. Assoc., 46, 1926, 1906.

Giraud, P., and Massot, M.: Kala-azar, Arch. med. des Enfants, 30, 505, 1927.

Girod, R., and Debarge, C.: BCG, Rev. méd. Suisse rom., 47, 1011, 1927.

Glaessner, K.: Peptic ulcer, Lancet, 1, 77, 1932.

Glaser, J.: Glucose administration, Jour. Amer. Med. Assoc., 91, 722, 1928.

Glaser, M. A.: Trigeminal neuralgia, Jour. Amer. Med. Assoc., 96, 916, 1931.

Glaze, A. L.: Eczema-dermatitis, Arch. Dermat. and Syph., 9, 621, 1924.

Gleason, E. B.: Hay-fever, Manual of Diseases of Nose, Throat, and Ear, Phila., W. B. Saunders Co., 3rd Ed., 1914, p. 108; 5th Ed., 1924, p. 112; 7th Ed., 1933, p. 94. Laryngitis, Diseases of Nose, Throat, and Ear, Phila., W. B. Saunders Co., 6th Ed., 1929, p. 259; 7th Ed., 1933, p. 266.

Glover, D. M.: Burns, Surg., Gyn., and Obst., 54, 798, 1932. Stokers' cramps, Jour Indust. Hyg., December, 1931, 347.

Glukhoff, Volkova, Erusalinichik and Panina: Bacillary dysentery, Profilakticheskaya Meditsina, 5, 64, 1926.

Goddard, F. W.: Intestinal flukes, Jour. Parasit., 5, 141, 1919.

Godfrey, E. S.: Diphtheria carrier, Jour. Amer. Med. Assoc., 83, 632, 1924.

Goeckermann, W. H.: Psoriasis, Arch. Dermat. and Syph., 24, 446, 1931.

Gold, H., and de Graff, A. C.: Heart failure, Jour. Amer. Med. Assoc., 90, 1016, 1928; ibid., 95, 1237, 1930.

Gold, H., and Klumpp, M. M.: Diphtheria, Amer. Jour. Med. Sci., 185, 509, 1933.

Gold, H., Kwit, N., and Travell, J.: Heart failure, Proc. Soc. Exper. Biol. and Med., 29, 66, 1931.

Goldberger, J.: Pellagra, Jour. Amer. Med. Assoc., 80, 1866, 1923; Pub. Health Rep., 42, 2706, 1927.

Goldberger, J., and Tanner, W. F.: Pellagra, Pub. Health Rep., 39, 87, 1924; ibid., 40, 54, 1925.

Goldberger, J., and Lillie, R. D.: Pellagra, Pub. Health Rep., 41, 1025, 1926.

Goldberger, J., and Sebrell, W. H.: Pellagra, Pub. Health Rep., 45, 3064, 1930.

Goldberger, J., and Wheeler, G. A.: Pellagra, Pub. Health Rep., 42, 1299, 1927; ibid., 42, 2383, 1927.

Goldberger, J., Waring, C. H., and Tanner, W. F.: Pellagra, Pub. Health Rep., 38, 2361, 1923.

Goldberger, J., Wheeler, G. A., and Tanner, W. F.: Pellagra, Pub. Health Rep., 40, 927, 1925.

Goldbloom, A.: Whooping cough, Jour. Amer. Med. Assoc., 85, 1791, 1925.

Golden, L. A.: Hiccup, New England Jour. Med. and Surg., 204, 1183, 1931.

Goldman, L., and Kully, H. E.: Vincent's angina, Jour. Amer. Med. Assoc., 101, 358, 1933.

Goldring, W., and Chasis, H.: Hypertension, New York State Jour. Med., 31, 1322, 1931.

Gonzaga and Lima: Pub. do Serv. San. do Est, de São Paulo, N. S., 1, 1, 1918.

Goodall, A.: Pernicious anemia, Lancet, 2, 781, 1932.

Goodman, H.: Syphilis, Jour. Amer. Med. Assoc., 74, 803, 1920. Chancroid, Jour. Urol., 13, 489, 1925. Epidermophytosus, Clin. Med. and Surg., 38, 207, 1931.

Goodpasture, E. W.: Yaws, Phil. Jour. Sci., 22, 263, 1923.

Goodrich, C. H.: Thyrotoxicosis, Amer. Jour. Surg., 13, 9, 1931.

Gordon, B., and Cantarow, A.: Tuberculosis, Amer. Rev. Tuberc., 20, 901, 1929.

Gordon, B., Roark, J. L., and Lewis, A. K.: Tuberculosis (calcium), Jour. Amer. Med. Assoc., 86, 1683, 1926.

Gordon, J. E.: Scarlet fever, Jour. Amer. Med. Assoc., 100, 102, 1933.

Gordon, J. E., and Creswell, S. M.: Diphtheria, Jour. Prevent. Med., 3, 21, 1929.

Gordon, J. E., and Meader, F. M.: Chickenpox, Jour. Amer. Med. Assoc., 93, 2013, 1929.

Gordon, M. H.: Hodgkin's disease, Brit. Med. Jour., 1, 179, 1933.

Gordon, R. L.: Urinary tract infection, Jour. Amer. Med. Assoc., 99, 2097, 1932 (discussion).

Gordon, R. M., and Hicks, E. P.: Bilharziasis, Ann. Trop. Med. and Parasit., 24, 443, 1930.

Götzl: BCG, Wien. klin. Wchnschr., 41, 804, 1928.

Gould, W. L.: Epidermophytosus, Jour. Amer. Med. Assoc., 96, 1300, 1931.

Govaerts, P.: Nephritis, Compt. rend. Soc. de biol., 93, 441, 1925.

Grafe, E.: Diabetes mellitus, Joslin's Treatment of Diabetes Mellitus, Phila., Lea and Febiger, 1928, p. 692.

Graham, A. B.: Constipation, Jour. Amer. Med. Assoc., 93, 1188, 1929.

Graham, A. H., Murphree, L. R., and Gill, D. G.: Diphtheria, Jour. Amer. Med. Assoc., 100, 1096, 1933.

Graham, D.: Bacillary dysentery, Lancet, 1, 51, 1918.

Graham, G.: Gout, Proc. Roy. Soc. Med. (Sect. Therap. and Pharm.), 20, 1, 1927

Graham, G., Clark, A., and Robertson, H. E. W.: Diabetes, Lancet, 2, 990, 1932.

Graham, H.: Dengue, Jour. Trop. Med., 6, 209, 1903.

Graham, J. H. P.: Trench fever, Lancet, 2, 703, 1915.

Graham, M., and Golaz, E. H.: Diphtheria carrier, Jour. Amer. Med. Assoc., 79, 1300, 1922.

Graham, R. H.: Scarlet fever, Jour. Amer. Med. Assoc., 85, 95, 1925.

Grant, L.: Hemophilia, Lancet, 2, 1279, 1904.

Gray: Pneumonia, Amer. Jour. Med. Sci., 159, 885, 1920.

Gray, G. A., and Meyer, B. I.: Diphtheria carrier, Jour. Infect. Dis., 28, 323, 1921.

Gray, P. A., and Sansom, W. D.: Diabetes, Jour. Amer. Med. Assoc., 100, 1580, 1933.

Green, J. L., and Scully, F. I.: Flagellate dysentery, Jour. Amer. Med. Assoc., 81, 291, 1923.

Green, R.: Malaria, Lancet, 1, 826, 1932.

Greenbaum, S. S.: Syphilis, Jour. Amer. Med. Assoc., 83, 38, 1924.

Greenbaum, S. S., and Harkins, M.: Boils, Jour. Amer. Med. Assoc., 95, 815, 1930.
Greengard, J.: Diphtheria, Jour. Amer. Med. Assoc., 97, 228, 1931.
Greenthal, R. M.: Chickenpox, Amer. Jour. Dis. Child., 31, 851, 1926.
Greenwood, A. M.: Scabies, Jour. Amer. Med. Assoc., 82, 466, 1924.
Greenwood, M.: BCG, Brit. Med. Jour., 1, 793, 1928.
Greer, A. E.: Epilepsy, Jour. Amer. Med. Assoc., 95, 863, 1930.
Greiff: Diabetes, Klin. Wchnschr., 10, 1955, 1931.
Grieveson, E. R.: Trench fever, Lancet, 2, 84, 1917.
Griffith, A. S.: BCG, Med. Res. Council, Spec. Rep. No. 152, H. M. Stat. Of., 1931; Lancet, 1, 303 and 361, 1932.
Griffith, G. C.: Agranulocytosis, Med. Clin. N. A., 16, 209, 1932.
Grimes, E.: Eczema-dermatitis, Arch. Dermat. and Syph., 24, 725, 1931.
Grinker, R. R.: Epilepsy, Jour. Amer. Med. Assoc., 93, 1218, 1929.
Groover, T. A., et al.: Thyrotoxicosis, Jour. Amer. Med. Assoc., 92, 1730, 1929.
Grossman, H. D.: Lichen planus, Arch. Dermat. and Syph., 26, 46, 1932.
Grove, E. F., and Coca, A. F.: Allergy, Jour. Immunol., 10, 471, 1925.
Grove, J. S.: Trichinosis, Jour. Amer. Med. Assoc., 85, 349, 1925.
Grulee, C. G., and Sanford, H. N.: Anemia, Amer. Jour. Dis. Child., 41, 53, 1931.
Grüzhit: Syphilis, Arch. Dermat. and Syph., 13, 219, 1926 (discussion).
Guelpa, G., and Marie, A.: Epilepsy, Rev. de Thérap., 788, 1911.
Guerner, N.: Typhoid, Compt. rend. Soc. de biol., 96, 333, 1927.
Guggenheim, M.: Constipation, Schweiz. med. Wchnschr., 55, 16, 1925.
Guiffrè, M.: Poliomyelitis, La Pediatria, 13, 689, 1926. Undulant fever, La Pediatria, 35, 345, 1927.
Gunewardene, H. O.: Hypertension, Brit. Med. Jour., 1, 180, 1932.
Gurevich, E.: Scarlet fever, Urach. Gaz., 22, 1653, 1930.
Gutman, A. B., et al.: Thyrotoxicosis, Jour. Amer. Med. Assoc., 101, 256, 1933.
Guttman, M. R.: Poisoning, Jour. Amer. Med. Assoc., 90, 753, 1928.
Gwathmey, J. T.: Obstetrical analgesia, Surg., Gyn., and Obst., 51, 190, 1930; see also Hunt, C. E., Amer. Jour. Obst. and Gyn., 9, 401, 1925.
Gwathmey, J. T., McKenzie, R. A., and Hudson, F. J.: Obstetrical anesthesia, Amer. Jour. Obst. and Gyn., 8, 154, 1924.
Gwathmey, J. T., Donovan, E. P., O'Reagan, J., and Cowan, L. R.: Obstetrical anesthesia, Amer. Jour. Obst. and Gyn., 6, 456, 1923.
Haas, S. O., and Blum, J.: Measles, Jour. Amer. Med. Assoc., 87, 558, 1926.
Haberfeld, W.: Polychthemia, Münch. med. Wchnschr., Nr. 30, 1258, 1931.
Hadden, S. B., and Wilson, G.: Syphilis, Jour. Amer. Med. Assoc., 88, 473, 1927; Amer. Jour. Syph., 15, 316, 1931.
Haden, R. L.: Meningitis, Jour. Amer. Med. Assoc., 73, 983, 1919. Pneumonia, Jour. Lab. and Clin. Med., 10, 337, 1925; Amer. Jour. Med. Sci., 174, 744, 1927. Anemia, Jour. Amer. Med. Assoc., 99, 1398, 1932.
Hadjidakis, G. E.: Obstetrical anesthesia, Wien. klin. Wchnschr., 51, 1482, 1926.
Haggard, H. W., and Greenberg, L. A.: Strychnine poisoning, Jour. Amer. Med. Assoc., 98, 1133, 1932.
Hahn, J. F.: Syphilis, Deutsch. med. Wchnschr., 46, 92, 1920.
Haidvogl, M., and Wiltschke, F.: Diphtheria carrier, Monatschr. f. Kinderhk., 29, 531, 1925.
Haight, C.: Tuberculosis, Amer. Rev. Tuberc., 25, 349, 1932.
Hajare, S. S.: Rabies, Indian Med. Gaz., 68, 212, 1933.
Haldane, J. S.: Pneumonia, Brit. Med. Jour., 1, 181, 1917.
Haldane, J. S., Meakins, J. C., and Priestly, J. G.: Pneumonia, Jour. Physiol., 52, 420, 1919; ibid., 52, 433, 1919.
Haldane, Wigglesworth, and Woodrow: Diabetes mellitus, Proc. Roy. Soc., London, 96, 15, 1924.
Hall, E. M., and MacKay, E. M.: Cirrhosis, Proc. Soc. Exper. Biol. and Med., 28, 166, 1930.
Hall, M. C.: Hookworm, Jour. Agric. Res., 21, 157, 1921; Jour. Amer. Med. Assoc., 77, 1641, 1921.
Hall, M. C., and Shillinger, J. E.: Hookworm, Jour. Agric. Res., 23, 163, 1923; Amer. Jour. Trop. Med., 4, 1, 1924.
Hall, M. C., and Foster, W. D.: Hookworm and roundworm, Jour. Amer. Med. Assoc., 68, 1961, 1917.
Hallay, L.: Erysipelas, Münch. med. Wchnschr., Nr. 16, 674, 1931.
Halpern, L. J.: Measles, Jour. Amer. Med. Assoc., 90, 1109, 1928.
Halt and Fales: Diabetes mellitus, Amer. Jour. Dis. Child., 21, 1, 1921.
Hamblen, E. C., and Hamblin, D. O.: Eclampsia, Amer. Jour. Obst. and Gyn., 23, 592, 1932. Obstetrics, Amer. Jour. Obst. and Gyn., 21, 715, 1931.
Hamburger, W. W.: Arhythmia, Cecil's Textbook of Medicine, Phila., W. B. Saunders Co., 1933, p. 1081.
Hamburger, W. W., et al.: Heart failure, Jour. Amer. Med. Assoc., 98, 1779, 1932.
Hampton, G. G.: Hookworm, Amer. Jour. Trop. Med., 2, 381, 1922.

Handrik, E.: Chickenpox, Monatschr. f. Kinderh., 13, 242, 1914.
Hanes, G. S.: Constipation, Jour. Amer. Med. Assoc., 89, 1039, 1927 (discussion).
Hanington, J.: Trypanosomiasis, Nigeria Ann. Med. and San. Rep. for 1923, Appendix 4, 42, 1924.
Hanzlik, P. J., and Karsner, H. T.: Allergy, Jour. Pharm. and Exper. Ther., 23, 173, 1924.
Hanzlik, P. J., and Scott, R. W.: Rheumatic fever, Jour. Amer. Med. Assoc., 76, 1728, 1921.
Hanzlik, P. J., and Spaulding, J. B.: Syphilis, Amer. Jour. Syph., 16, 335, 1932.
Hanzlik, P. J., Mehrtens, H. G., *et al.:* Syphilis, Jour. Amer. Med. Assoc., 98, 537, 1932; Arch. Dermat. and Syph., 22, 850, 1930; ibid., 22, 861, 1930; Amer. Jour. Syph., 16, 350, 1932.
Harbinson, J. E.: Undulant fever, Ann. Int. Med., 4, 484, 1930.
Harding, V. J., and Van Wyck, H. B.: Eclampsia, Amer. Jour. Obst. and Gyn., 10, 1, 1926; Brit. Med. Jour., October 11, 1930; Hyperemesis, Amer. Jour. Obst. and Gyn., 11, January, 1926.
Hardt, L. L., and Rivers, A. B.: Peptic ulcer, Arch. Int. Med., 31, 171, 1923.
Hare, H. A.: Warts, Practical Therapeutics, Phila., Lea and Febiger, 1927, p. 122. Tuberculosis, Practical Therapeutics, Phila., Lea and Febiger, 1927, p. 180; ibid., p. 1001.
Harkavy, J.: Asthma, Jour. Amer. Med. Assoc., 82, 100, 1924.
Harkavy, J., Hebald, S., and Silbert, S.: Buerger's disease, Proc. Soc. Exper. Biol. and Med., 30, 104, 1932.
Harrar, J. A.: Obstetrical anesthesia, Amer. Jour. Obst. and Gyn., 13, 486, 1927.
Harris, L. I.: Catarrhal fever, Bull. New York Dept. Health, 14, 217, 1924.
Harris, N. G.: Syphilis, Lancet, 1, 1068, 1930.
Harris, S.: Hyperinsulinism, Jour. Amer. Med. Assoc., 83, 729, 1924; ibid., 100, 321, 1933; Endocrinology, 16, 29, 1932.
Harrison, W. J.: Diphtheria, Pub. Health Rep., U.S.P.H.S., 45, 1883, 1930.
Harrold, E. O.: Catharsis, Jour. Amer. Med. Assoc., 88, 1747, 1927.
Harrop, G. A., Jr.: Nephritis, Diet in disease, Philadelphia, P. Blakiston's Son and Co., 1930.
Hart, E. B., Steenbock, H., *et al.:* Anemia, Jour. Biol. Chem., 77, 797, 1928.
Hartsock, C. L.: Simple goiter, Jour. Amer. Med. Assoc., 86, 1334, 1926; also in discussion before the Amer. Col. of Physicians, Cleveland Clinic, February, 22–25, 1927; also quoted by McClure, R. D. (*q. v.*).
Hartwich, A.: Dysentery, Münch. med. Wchnschr., 31, 1217, 1933.
Hashimoto and Iwakiri, I.: Syphilis, Rev. franç. de dermat. et de vén., 8, 131, 1932.
Haskell, B., and Cantarow, A.: Colitis, Amer. Jour. Med. Sci., 181, 180, 1931.
Haskins, J. L.: Syphilis, Psychiat. Quart., 5, 733, 1931.
Hasselmann, C. M., and Hasselmann-Kahlert, M.: Malaria, Phil. Jour. Sci., 37, 75, 1928; Deutsch. med. Wchnschr., 1929, No. 39.
Hasselmann-Kahlert, M.: Leprosy, Deutsch. med. Wchnschr., 57, 724, 1931.
Hatcher, R. A.: Poisoning, Jour. Pharm. and Exper. Ther., 25, 139, 1925.
Hatcher, R. A., and Weiss, S.: Heart failure, Jour. Amer. Med. Assoc., 89, 429, 1927.
Hattinger, A.: Rickets, Zeitschr. f. Kinderhk., 44, 61, 1927.
Hawes, J. B., and Stone, M. J.: Tuberculosis, Jour. Amer. Med. Assoc., 98, 2048, 1932.
Hay, J.: Arhythmia, Lancet, 2, 543, 1924.
Haynes, R. S., and St. Lawrence, W.: Whooping cough, Nelson Loose-Leaf Med., 2, 35.
Hazen, H. H.: Granuloma inguinale, Jour. Amer. Med. Assoc., 99, 1410, 1932.
Head, H., and Fearnsides, E. G.: Syphilis, Brain, 37, 1, 1914.
Healy, J. C.: Paroxysmal tachycardia, New England Jour. Med., 205, 1010, 1931.
Heard, J. D., Marshall, W. R., and Adams, F. S.: Heart block, Amer. Heart Jour., 2, 562 1927.
Hearne, K. G.: Heat stroke, Med. Jour. Australia, 1, 226, 1932.
Heberden, W.: Angina pectoris, Med. Trans. Col. of Physicians, 2, 58, 1768–70.
Hedge, H. M.: Blastomycosis, Jour. Amer. Med. Assoc., 90, 1367, 1928.
Heeres, P. A.: Pernicious anemia, Nederl. Tijdschr. v. Geneesk., Haarlem, 72, 2372, 1928.
Heffernan, P.: Vincent's angina, Lancet, 2, 734, 1932.
Heffron, R., and Anderson, G. W.: Pneumonia, Jour. Amer. Med. Assoc., 101, 1286, 1933.
Heft, H. L., Kahn, and Gies: Diabetes mellitus, Jour. Pharm. and Exper. Ther., 25, 153, 1925.
Hehir, P.: Leprosy, Lancet, 1923, 1, 110.
Heimann-Trosien: Syphilis, cited by Langer, E.: Klin. Wchnschr., 7, 554, 1928.
Heiser, V. G.: Leprosy, Amer. Jour. Trop. Dis., 2, 295, 1914; New York Med. Jour., 103, 289, 1916.
Hektoen, L., and Rappaport, B.: Diphtheria, Jour. Amer. Med. Assoc., 64, 1985, 1915.
Hellerström, S.: Climatic bubo, Acta derma.-venereol. (supp.) 1929, pp. 5–224; ibid., 12, 254, 1931.
Helmholz, H. F.: Urinary infections, Trans. Sec. Child. Dis. Amer. Med. Assoc., 1922, p. 163; Jour. Amer. Med. Assoc., 99, 1305, 1932. Epilepsy, Jour. Amer. Med. Assoc., 88, 2028, 1927.

Helmholz, H. F., and Clark, A. L.: Ketogenic diet, Proc. Staff Meetings, Mayo Clinic, 6, 605 and 609, 1931.

Helmholz, H. F., and Keith, H. M.: Epilepsy, Jour. Amer. Med. Assoc., 95, 707, 1930; Arch. Neurol. and Psychiat., 29, 808, 1933.

Helwig, F. C.: Undulant fever, Jour. Missouri Med. Assoc., 26, 449, 1929.

Hench, P. S., and Rowntree, L. G.: Rheumatic fever, Jour. Amer. Med. Assoc., 95, 1228, 1930 (discussion).

Henderson, Y.: Pneumonia, New England Jour. Med., 206, 151, 1931; Brit. Med. Jour., October 17, 1931. Carbon monoxide poisoning, Jour. Amer. Med. Assoc., 94, 179, 1930. Whooping cough, Jour. Amer. Med. Assoc., 99, 654, 1932.

Henderson, Y., and Haggard, H. W.: Poisoning, Jour. Amer. Med. Assoc., 79, 1137, 1922.

Hendon, G. A.: Sepsis, Trans. South. Surg. Soc., 1924 and 1929; Texas State Jour. Med., 21, 662, 1926; Kentucky Med. Jour., 27, 202, 1929; Ann. Surg., 91, 753, 1930; Jour. Amer. Med. Assoc., 95, 1175, 1930. Hyperemesis, Ann. Surg., 91, 753, 1930. Cirrhosis, Ann. Surg., 91, 753, 1930.

Hendry, A. W.: Diabetes, Lancet, 2, 897, 1932.

Henning, N., and Brugsch, H.: Pernicious anemia, Deutsch. med. Wchnschr., Nr. 18, 1931.

Henricke, S. G.: Whooping cough, Northwest Med., 29, 269, 1930.

Henry, H., and Lewis, F. C.: Scarlet fever, Lancet, 2, 587, 1925.

Hermann and Nathan: Syphilis, Klin. Wchnschr., 4, 1303, 1925; ibid., 4, 1345, 1925.

Hermannsdorfer, A.: Tuberculosis, Ztschr. f. Tuberk., 55, Nr. 1, 1929.

Hermans, E. H.: Climatic bubo, Arch. f. Schiffs. u. Tropen-Hyg., 33, 214, 1929.

Herrera-Vegas, M., and Cranwell, D. J.: Hydatid cyst, Nelson Loose-Leaf Med., 2, 434.

Herrick, W. W.: Sepsis, Nelson Loose-Leaf Med., 1, 106. Meningitis, Jour. Amer. Med. Assoc., 71, 612, 1918; Cecil's Textbook of Medicine, Phila., W. B. Saunders Co., 1933, p. 130.

Herrman, C.: Measles, Abt's Pediatrics, Phila., W. B. Saunders Co., 6, 399, 1925.

Herrman, C., and Bell, T.: Whooping cough, Arch. Pediat., 41, 13, 1924.

Herrmann, G., et al.: Heart failure, Jour. Lab. and Clin. Med., 18, 902, 1933.

Herrmann, G. R., and Ashman, R.: Heart block, Amer. Heart Jour., 1, 269, 1926.

Herrmann, L. G.: Thyrotoxicosis, Surg., Gyn., and Obst., 60, 221, 1932.

Herrold, R. D.: Syphilis, Jour. Amer. Med. Assoc., 86, 413, 1926. Gonorrhea, Ven. Dis. Inform., 11, 55, 1930.

Herrold, R. D., and Culver, H.: Gonorrhea, Jour. Amer. Med. Assoc., 88, 459, 1927.

Herron, W. F., and McEllroy, W. S.: Pernicious anemia, Jour. Amer. Med. Assoc., 100, 1084, 1933.

Hershfield, A. S., Kibler, O. A. ,Colby, S., Koenig, M. T., Schmid, O. W., and Saunders, A. M.: Syphilis, Jour. Amer. Med. Assoc., 92, 772, 1929.

Hertzer, W.: Peptic ulcer, Thesis on a New Method of Treating Ulcer Ventriculi and Duodeni with Pepsin Injections (according to Glaessner), Charlottenburg, 1931.

Hertzler, A. E.: Adenoma, Arch. Surg., 16, 61, 1928.

Herzfeld, A. A.: Poisoning, Jour. Amer. Med. Assoc., 20, 1594, 1921.

Hess, A. F.: Rickets, Cecil's Textbook of Medicine, Phila., W. B. Saunders Co., 1933, p. 612; Jour. Amer. Med. Assoc., 89, 337, 1927; ibid., 91, 783, 1928; ibid., 98, 316, 1932; Amer. Jour. Dis. Child., 28, 517, 1924.

Hess, A. F., and Lewis, J. M.: Rickets, Jour. Amer. Med. Assoc., 99, 647, 1932; ibid., 101, 181, 1933.

Hess, A. F., and Unger, L. S.: Chickenpox, Amer. Jour. Dis. Child., 16, 34, 1918.

Hess, A. F., et al.: Rickets, Jour. Amer. Med. Assoc., 97, 370, 1931.

Hess and Weinstock: Rickets, Amer. Jour. Dis. Child., 32, 483, 1926.

Hess, J. H., et al.: Rickets, Jour. Amer. Med. Assoc., 95, 316, 1930.

Hessler, R.: Dermatitis venenata, Jour. Amer. Med. Assoc., 74, 1475, 1920.

Hewins, W. W., and Acre, R. R.: Syphilis, Urol. and Cutan. Rev., 26, 561, 1922.

Hewitt, L. F : Nephritis, Biochem. Jour., 21, 1109, 1927.

Hewlett, A. W.: Rheumatic fever, Jour. Amer. Med. Assoc., 61, 319, 1913.

Heyn, L. G.: Rheumatic fever, Jour. Amer. Med. Assoc., 63, 1004, 1914.

Heynius van der Burgh, M. R.: BCG, Wien. klin. Wchnschr., 41, 1400, 1928.

Highman, W. J.: Impetigo, Jour. Amer. Med. Assoc., 69, 176, 1917 (discussion). Eczema-dermatitis, Med. Clin. N. A., 14, 1403, 1931.

Hilarowicz, H., and Mozolowski, W.: Peptic ulcer, Zentralbl. f. Chir., 43, 2410, 1925.

Hill, L. W.: Eczema-dermatitis, Jour. Amer. Med. Assoc., 96, 1277, 1931; Jour. Pediat., 2, 133, 1933.

Hill, L. W., and Stuart, H C.: Eczema-dermatitis, Jour. Amer. Med. Assoc., 93, 985, 1929.

Hill, R. B.: Hookworm, Jour. Prev. Med., 1, 537, 1927.

Hiller, R. J.: Hemorrhoids, Amer. Jour. Surg., 16, 64, 1932.

Hilton, S. L.: Constipation, Jour. Amer. Pharm. Assoc., 3, 577, 1914.

Himsworth, H. P.: Diabetes, Lancet, 2, 1103, 1931; ibid., 2, 165, 1932.

Hinman, F.: Urinary infections, Jour. Amer. Med. Assoc., 61, 1601, 1913; ibid., 65, 1769, 1915.

Hirsch, C.: Sea-sickness, Deutsch. med. Wchnschr., Nr. 12, 1931.

Hirschboeck, F. J.: Cardiac neuroses, Jour. Amer. Med. Assoc., 91, 1852, 1928.

Hirschfelder, A. D.: Dysmenorrhea, Minnesota Med., 3, 380, 1920.
Hirschman, L. J.: Constipation, Jour. Amer. Med. Assoc., 89, 1039, 1927.
Hirst, J. C.: Sepsis, Jour. Amer. Med. Assoc., 62, 1873, 1914.
Hoag, L. A., and Rivkin, H.: Tetany, Jour. Amer. Med. Assoc., 86, 1343, 1926.
Hobbs, A. R.: Sepsis, Brit. Med. Jour., October 24, 1931.
Hochrein, M.: Paroxysmal tachycardia, Münch. med. Wchnschr., Nr. 49, 2070, 1931.
Hodgson, E. C., Sen, R. T., and Das, C.: Kala-azar, Ind. Jour. Med. Res., 16, 31, 1928,
Hodson, V. S.: Amebic dysentery, Lancet, 2, 1975, 1924.
Hoedemaker, E. D., and Burns, M. A.: Encephalitis, Jour. Amer. Med. Assoc., 95, 91, 1930.
Hofbauer, J., Hoerner, J. H., and Oliver, K. S.: Labor induction, Amer. Jour. Obst. and Gyn., 14, 137, 1927.
Hofbauer, L.: Asthma, Wien, J. Springer, 1928.
Hoffman, A. M.: Undulant fever, Jour. Amer. Med. Assoc., 92, 2169, 1929.
Hoffman, W. J., and Craver, L. F.: Leukemia, Jour. Amer. Med. Assoc., 97, 836, 1931.
Hoffmann, W.: Chickenpox, Schweiz. med. Wchnschr., 6, 717, 1925.
Hofman: Syphilis, Dermat. Wchnschr., Nr. 40, 1931.
Hogan, J. J.: Delirium tremens, Jour. Amer. Med. Assoc., 67, 1826, 1916.
Holdon, F. C., and Gurnee, W. S.: Gonorrhea, Amer. Jour. Obst. and Gyn., 22, 87, 1931,
Hollaender, L.: Erythremia, Wein. Arch. f. inn. Med., 10, 283, 1925.
Hollingsworth, M.: Stokes-Adams disease, California and West. Med., 26, 802, 1927.
Holman, H. T., and Dean, A. L.: Leprosy, Jour. Cutan. Dis., 37, 637, 1919.
Holst, J., et al.: Thyrotoxicosis, Klin. Wchnschr., 7, 2287, 1928.
Holt, R. L., and Kintner, J. H.: Dengue, Phil. Jour. Sci., 46, 593, 1931; Amer. Jour. Trop Med., 11, 103, 1931.
Holzknecht, G.: Thyrotoxicosis, Strahlentherapie, 30, 605, 1928.
Home, W. E.: Undulant fever, Lancet, 1, 275, 1933.
Hooker, S. B., and Anderson, L. M.: Asthma, Jour. Immunol., 16, 291, 1929.
Höpfner, E.: Cirrhosis, Engebn. d. chir. u. Orth., 1913, 410.
Hoppe, L. D., Goldsmith, L. H., and Freeman, W. T.: Pneumonia, Arch. Pediat., 43, 694, 1926 (contains a bibliography).
Hörlein, H.: Malaria, Beihefte z. Arch. f. Schiffs- u. Trop. Hyg., 30, 305, 1926.
Houck, L.: Syphilis, Med. Klin., 1919, No. 24.
Howard, J. T.: Gall-bladder disease, Jour. Amer. Med. Assoc., 94, 1055, 1930.
Howard, M. Q.: Addiction, Wisconsin Med. Jour., July, 1933, p. 448.
Howard, N. J., et al.: Varicose veins, Arch. Surg., 22, 353, 1931.
Howitt, B. F.: Poliomyelitis, Jour. Infect. Dis., 50, 26, 1932.
Howland, G., Campbell, W. R., Maltby, E. J., and Robinson, W. L.: Hyperinsulinism, Jour. Amer. Med. Assoc., 93, 674, 1929.
Howland, J., and Marriott, W. McK.: Whooping cough, Quart. Jour. Med., 11, 289, 1918.
Hoyne, A. L., and Gasul, B. M.: Measles, Jour. Amer. Med. Assoc., 87, 1185, 1926.
Hoyne, A. L., and Peacock, S.: Measles, Amer. Jour. Dis. Child., 35, 1021, 1928.
Hubbard, R. S.: Hypochlorhydria, Ann. Int. Med., 4, 1203, 1931.
Hudson, G. E.: Goiter, Jour. Amer. Med. Assoc., 97, 1513, 1931.
Hueper, W. C., and Russell, M.: Leukemia, Science News; through Science Suppl., 73, 12, 1931.
Hughes, E., and Birch, C. A.: Gonorrhea, Lancet, 2, 633, 1933.
Hume, W. E.: Paroxysmal tachycardia, Lancet, 2, 1055, 1930.
Hunner, G. L.: Essential hematuria, Amer. Jour. Surg., 16, 279, 1932.
Hunt, C. E.: Obstetrical anesthesia, Northwest. Med., 24, 546, 1925 (quoting Gwathmey).
Hunt, L. W.: Scarlet fever, Jour. Amer. Med. Assoc., 101, 1444, 1933.
Hunt, R.: Myxedema, Arch. Int. Med., 35, 671, 1925.
Hunt, R., McCann, W. S., Rowntree, L. G., Voegtlin, C., and Eggleston, C.: Sepsis Jour. Amer. Med. Assoc., 90, 764, 1928.
Huntoon, F. M.: Pneumonia, Jour. Immunol., 6, 117, 1921.
Hurst, A. F.: Colitis, Brit. Med. Jour., April 25, 1931.
Hutchison, R. H.: Snake-bite (quoted by Cudlipp, J. S., q. v.).
Hutyra, F. V.: BCG, Ztschr. f. Immunitäts-, 62, 74, 1929.
Hyman, H. T., and Fenichel, N. M.: Heart failure, Amer. Jour. Med. Sci., 183, 748 and 753, 1932.
Hyman, H. T., and Kessel, L.: Thyrotoxicosis, Jour. Amer. Med. Assoc., 96, 2014, 1931.
Ignelzi, L. G.: Migraine, Med. Jour. and Rec., May 4, 1932.
Iliescu, C. C., and Sebastini, A.: Paroxysmal tachycardia, Heart, 10, 223, 1923.
Imerman, S. W.: Diabetes mellitus, Jour. Amer. Med. Assoc., 89, 1778, 1927.
Ingals, E. F., and Meeker, W. R.: Angina pectoris, Jour. Amer. Med. Assoc., 70, 969, 1918.
Inouye, Z.: Typhoid, Compt. rend. Soc. de biol., 110, 438, 1932.
Insfrán, J. V.: Hookworm, Jour. Amer. Med. Assoc., 86, 735, 1926.
Irons, E. E.: Asthma, Jour. Amer. Med. Assoc., 96, 1289, 1931.
Irving, S. W.: Dermatitis venenata, Jour. Amer. Med. Assoc., 74, 1475, 1920.
Irwin, P. S.: Tuberculosis, Canad. Med. Assoc. Jour., 24, 245, 1931.

Isaacs, R.: Leukemia, Amer. Jour. Roentgen., 24, 648, 1930.
Isaacs, R., Sturgis, C. C., *et al.*: Pernicious anemia, Jour. Amer. Med. Assoc., 100, 629, 1933.
Iturbe, J.: Blood flukes, Southern Med. Jour., 18, 34, 1925.
Izar, G., and Mastrojeni, G.: Malta fever, Reforma Medica, 43, 100, 1927.
Jackson, A. S.: Simple goiter, Jour. Amer. Med. Assoc., 83, 1864, 1924; Amer. Jour. Med. Sci., 170, 271, 1925. Thyrotoxicosis, Jour. Amer. Med. Assoc., 85, 1660, 1925..
Jackson, H.: Nephritis, Bull. New York Acad. Med., 2, 361, 1926.
Jackson, H., *et al.*: Agranulocytosis, Amer. Jour. Med. Sci., 184, 297, 1932.
Jacobi, H. G.: Polycythemia, Jour. Amer. Med. Assoc., 96, 1138, 1931.
Jacobson, L., and Epplen, F.: Encephalitis, Ann. Int. Med., 4, 145, 1930.
Jacques, L.: Thyrotoxicosis, Surg., Gyn., and Obst., 51, 823, 1930.
Jadassohn, W., and Streit, G.: Tetanus, Klin. Wchnschr., 4, 1498, 1925.
Jakobs, M. F., and Keith, N. M.: Cirrhosis, Med. Cin. N. A., 10, 605, 1926.
James, S. P.: Malaria, Lancet, 1, 1362, 1932 (meeting of Roy. Soc. Trop. Med. and Hyg., London); Quart. Bull. Health Organ. League of Nations, June, 1933, p. 181. Syphilis, Bull. Office internat. d'hyg. pub., 23, 1423, 1931.
James, S. P., Nicol, W. D., and Shute, P. G.: Malaria, Syphilis, Lancet, 2, 341, 1931, ibid. (Special Article), 1, 1061, 1932.
James, W. M., and Deeks, W. E.: Amebic dysentery, Amer. Jour. Trop. Med., 5, 97, 1925.
Jamot and Vernon: Trypanosomiasis, Bull. Soc. de path. exot., 20, 689, 1927.
Jampolis, M., and Londe, S.: Rickets, Jour. Amer. Med. Assoc., 98, 1637, 1932.
Jarotzky, A.: Peptic ulcer, Jour. Amer. Med. Assoc., 84, 695, 1925; Arch. des Mal. de l'App. Digestif, etc., 18, 721, 1928.
Jaso, E.: BCG, Arch. de méd. d. enfants, 34, 169, 1931.
Jenkinson, E. L.: Thyrotoxicosis, Radiology, 4, 453, 1925.
Jensen, K. A., Morch, J. R., and Orskou, J.: BCG, Jour. Amer. Med. Assoc. (abstract), 93, 1268, 1929.
Jessen, H.: Tuberculosis, Münch. med. Wchnschr., 73, 444, 1926.
Joachimoglu, G.: Trigeminal neuralgia, Klin. Wchnschr., 58, 147, 1921.
Jobling, J. W., and Arnold, L.: Pellagra, Jour. Amer. Med. Assoc., 80, 365, 1923.
John, H. J.: Diabetes mellitus, Jour. Lab. and Clin. Med., 11, 548, 1926.
Johns, F. M.: Plague, Nelson Loose-Leaf Med., 2, 124.
Johns, F. M., and Jamison, S. C.: Amebic dysentery, Jour. Amer. Med. Assoc., 84, 1913, 1925.
Johnson, C. A., *et al.*: Barbiturate poisoning, Jour. Amer. Med. Assoc., 95, 576, 1930.
Johnson, G. S., and Jefferson, R. A.: Syphilis, Jour. Nerv. and Ment. Dis., 73, 405, 1931.
Jones, A. A.: Gastritis, Nelson Loose-Leaf Med., 5, 198.
Jones, A. E.: Chancroid, Jour. Amer. Med. Assoc., 88, 1699, 1927.
Jones, H. W.: Pernicious anemia, Jour. Amer. Med. Assoc., 86, 1673, 1926.
Jones, H. W., and Tocantins, L.: Purpura, Jour. Amer. Med. Assoc., 99, 164, 1932; ibid., 100, 83, 1933.
Jones, S.: Seasickness, Brit. Med. Jour., 1, 139, 1925.
Jonnesco, T.: Angina pectoris, Presse méd., 29, 193, 1921.
Jordan, H. P. B., and Dustin, C. C.: Erysipelas, Jour. Amer. Med. Assoc., 82, 874, 1924.
Jordan, S. M.: Peptic ulcer, Jour. Amer. Med. Assoc., 87, 1906, 1926.
Jordan, S. M., and Kiefer, E. D.: Peptic ulcer, Amer. Jour. Surg., 15, 472, 1932.
Jorge, R.: Measles, Bull. Office internat. d'hyg. pub., 24, 978, 1932. Smallpox, Lancet, 1, 215, 1932.
Josephs, H. W., and Davison, W. C.: Bacillary dysentery, Jour. Amer. Med. Assoc., 77, 1863, 1921.
Joslin, E. P.: Diabetes mellitus, Treatment of Diabetes Mellitus, Phila., Lea and Febiger, 1928; Jour. Amer. Med. Assoc., 99, 252, 1932.
Joslin, E. P., *et al.*: Diabetes, Med. Clin. N. A., 15, 829, 1932.
Jötten: Preparation of vulva, Zentralbl. f. Gynäk., 1529, 1912.
Judd, E. S., Allan, F. N., and Rynearson, E. H.: Hyperinsulinism, Jour. Amer. Med. Assoc., 101, 99, 1933.
Kahler, H., and Knollmayer, F.: Syphilis, Wien. klin. Wchnschr., 42, 1342, 1929.
Kahn, I. S.: Hay-fever, Jour. Lab. and Clin. Med., 13, 77, 1927; Jour. Amer. Med. Assoc., 90, 2101, 1928.
Kahn, M.: Tuberculosis, Med. Rec., May 23, 1914.
Kahn, M. H.: Asthma, Arch. Int. Med., 39, 621, 1927.
Kaiser, A. D.: Erysipelas, Arch. Pediat., 32, 519, 1915. Rheumatic fever, Jour. Amer. Med. Assoc., 89, 2239, 1927.
Kantor, J. L.: Peptic ulcer, Jour. Amer. Med. Assoc., 81, 816, 1923; ibid., 88, 2047, 1927.
Kaplan, B., Williamson, C. S., and Geiger, J. C.: Amebic dysentery, Jour. Amer. Med. Assoc., 88, 977, 1927.
Kappis: Milk leg, Deutsch. Ztschr. f. Chir., 223, 317, 1930.
Karamchandani P. V.: Oriental sore, Ind. Med. Gaz., 62, 558, 1927.
Karelitz, S., and Schick, B.: Glucose, Jour. Amer. Med. Assoc., 99, 366, 1932.
Karr, W. G., *et al.*: Diabetes mellitus, Jour. Pharm. and Exper. Ther., 36, 611, 1929; Jour. Lab. and Clin. Med., 18, 1203, 1933.

Kassowitz: Rickets, Ztschr. f. klin. Med., 7, 36, 1884.
Kast, L., Myers, V. C., and Schmitz, H. W.: Peptic ulcer, Jour. Amer. Med. Assoc., 82, 1858, 1924.
Katz, L. N., *et al.:* Heart failure, Amer. Jour. Med. Sci., 184, 810, 1932.
Katzenelbogen, S., and Güder, R.: Constipation, Schweiz. med. Wchnschr., 55, 18, 1925.
Kaunitz, J.: Buerger's disease, Arch. Int. Med., 47, 548, 1931.
Kay: Whooping cough, Ann. Clin. Med., 5, 288, 1926.
Keevil, A.: Trypanosomiasis, Trans. Roy. Soc. Trop. Med. and Hyg., 20, 111, 1926.
Kegel, A. H., *et al.:* Methyl chloride poisoning, Jour. Amer. Med. Assoc., 93, 353, 1929.
Keidel, A., and Kemp, J. E.: Syphilis, Jour. Amer. Med. Assoc., 82, 299, 1924.
Keith, N. M., Barrier, C. W., and Whelan, M.: Nephritis, Jour. Amer. Med. Assoc., 85, 799, 1925.
Keller, W.: BCG, Deutsch. med. Wchnschr., 53, 786, 1927.
Kellersberger, E. R.: Trypanosomiasis, Trans. Roy. Soc. Trop. Med. and Hyg., 20, 185, 1926.
Kelly, M. M.: Epidemic pleurodynia (see Payne, G. C.).
Kemp, J. E., and Stokes, J. H.: Syphilis, Jour. Amer. Med. Assoc., 92, 1737, 1929.
Kempf, G. F., McCallum, J. T. C., and Zerfas, L. G.: Strychnine poisoning, Jour. Amer. Med. Assoc., 100, 548, 1933.
Kerley, C. G.: Cretinism, Arch. Pediat., 43, 94, 1926; ibid., 668, October, 1931; Long Island Med. Jour., November, 1927.
Kermorgant, Y.: Measles, Ann. de l'Inst. Pasteur, 39, 565, 1925; Ann. de Méd., 19, 301 1926.
Kern, H. M.: Varicose veins, Ann. Surg., 697, March, 1931.
Kernohan, J. W., *et al.:* Nephritis, Arch. Int. Med., 44, 395, 1929.
Kerr, W. J.: Nephritis, Amer. Jour. Physiol., 47, 356, 370, 379, 1918.
Kerridge, P. M. T., and Bayliss, L. E.: Nephritis, Lancet, 2, 785, 1932.
Kessel, L., and Hyman, H. T.: Thyrotoxicosis, Arch. Int. Med., 40, 314, 1927.
Khalil, M.: Blood flukes, Lancet, 2, 1235, 1927.
Khalil, M., and Betache, M. H.: Bilharziasis, Lancet, 1, 234, 1930.
Khalil, M., Nazmi, M., *et al.:* Bilharziasis, Deutsch. med. Wchnschr., 55, 1125, 1929.
Kilbourne, N. J.: Varicose veins, Jour. Amer. Med. Assoc., 95, 787, 1930.
Kilduffe, R. A.: Sepsis, Jour. Lab. and Clin. Med., 12, 572, 1927.
Kilmer, T. W.: Whooping cough, Jour. Amer. Med. Assoc., 49, 1750, 1907.
Kim, M. S., and Toy, A. C.: Peptic ulcer, Jour. Amer. Med. Assoc., 97, 1511, 1931.
Kimball, O. P.: Simple goiter, Jour. Amer. Med. Assoc., 91, 454, 1928; ibid., 97, 1877, 1931.
Kimm, H. T., and Van Allen, C. M.: Hemophilia, Jour. Amer. Med. Assoc., 99, 991, 1932.
King, *et al.:* Eclampsia, Amer. Jour. Obst. and Gyn., 23, 867, 1932.
King, J. C.: Trypanosomiasis, Amer. Jour. Med. Sci., 172, 51, 1926.
King, M. J., and Park, W. H.: BCG, Amer. Jour. Pub. Health, 19, 179, 1929.
Kingsbury, A. N., and Amies, C. R.: Malaria, Trans. Roy. Soc. Trop. Med. and Hyg., 25, 159, 1931.
Kingsbury, J. G.: Erythremia, Guy's Hosp. Rep., 76, 90, 1926.
Kingsbury, J., and Peck, S. M.: Chancroid, Jour. Amer. Med. Assoc., 87, 1900, 1926.
Kingston, J. J., and Faber, H. K.: Whooping cough, California State Jour. Med., 21, 429, 1923.
Kinsella, R. A.: Endocarditis, Cecil's Textbook of Medicine, Phila., W. B. Saunders Co., 1933, p. 1124.
Kirshner, H. E.: Tuberculosis, Amer. Rev. Tuberc., 6, 401, 1922.
Kirstein: Sepsis, Arch. Gyn., 125, 399, 1925.
Klare, P., and Reusse, P.: Bronchiectasis, Ztschr. klin. d. Tuberk., 63, 255, 1926.
Klauder, J. V., and Harkins, M. J.: Erysipeloid, Jour. Amer. Med. Assoc., 96, 1205, 1931.
Klein, L.: Pernicious anemia, Lancet, 1, 719, 1932.
Kleine, F. K.: Trypanosomiasis, Lancet, 1, 384, 1924; Deutsch. med. Wchnschr., Nr. 4 u. 5, 1931.
Klemmer, R. N.: Diabetes, Amer. Jour. Med. Sci., 184, 379, 1932.
Klemperer, F.: Tuberculosis, Deutsch. med. Wchnschr., 52, 186, 1926.
Klesk: Bacillary dysentery, Med. Klin., 11, 1147, 1915.
Kline, B. C., and Berger, S. S.: Bronchial spirochetosis, Jour. Amer. Med. Assoc., 85, 1452, 1925.
Kling, C. A.: Chickenpox, Berl. klin. Wchnschr., 50, 2083, 1913.
Koch, R.: Skin disinfection, Mitt. a. d. k. Gsndhtsamt., 1, 271, 1881. Trypanosomiasis, Deutsch. med. Wchnschr., 33, 1889.
Koehler, A. E.: Myxedema, Ann. Clin. Med., 5, 635, 1927.
Kofoid, C. A., and Donat, F.: Trypanosomiasis, Proc. Soc. Exper. Biol. and Med., 30, 489, 1933.
Kofoid, C. A., Kornhauser, S. I., and Plato, J. T.: Amebic dysentery, Jour. Amer. Med. Assoc., 72, 1721, 1919.
Kohler: Peptic ulcer, Mitt. a. d. Grensgeb., 1923.
Kolb, L., and Du Mez. A. G.: Addiction, Pub. Health Rep., 39, 1179, 1924.
Kolle, W.: Syphilis, Deutsch. med. Wchnschr., 32, 1074, 1924.

Kolle, W., and Ritz, H.: Syphilis, Deutsch. med. Wchnschr., 45, No. 18, 1919.
Kolmer, Davis, and Jager: Tuberculosis, Jour. Infect. Dis., 28, 265, 1921.
Kolmer, J. A.: Plague, Infection, Immunity and Biol. Ther., Phila., W. B. Saunders Co.,
  1925, p. 970; Syphilis, Jour. Chemotherapy, 6, 43, 1929; Arch., Dermat. and Syph.,
  21, 394, 1930; Amer. Jour. Syph., 15, 190, 1931. Cerebrospinal fever, Jour. Amer. Med.
  Assoc., 96, 1358, 1931. Vincent's angina, Arch. Dermat. and Syph., 21, 394, 1930.
Kolmer, J. A., Wanna, D., and Koehler, M.: Anthrax, Jour. Infect. Dis., 26, 148, 1920.
Kopeloff, N.: Constipation, Lactobacillus acidophilus, Baltimore, Williams and Wilkins
  Company, 1926.
Kopeloff, N., and Cohen, P.: Constipation, Jour. Amer. Med. Assoc., 94, 1983, 1930.
Kopeloff, N., et al.: Constipation, Psych. Quarterly, 5, 663, 1931.
Koranyi, A.: Leukemia, Berl. klin. Wchnschr., 49, 1357, 1912.
Korchitz, E. U.: Kala-azar, Pensée med. d'Uzbekistane, 1, 36, 1926.
Kosmak, G. W.: Hyperemesis, The Toxemias of Pregnancy, New York, D. Appleton and
  Co., 1922, p. 90 (cited by Titus, P., q. v.).
Kouwenar, D. W.: Hookworm, Geneesk, Tijdschr. v. Nederlandsch-Indie, 65, 646, 1925.
Kracke, R. R.: Agranulocytosis, U. S. Naval Med. Bull., Vol. 30, No. 1.; Amer. Jour. Clin.
  Path., 1, 385, 1931; ibid., 2, 11, 1932.
Kramer, B., Grayzel, H. G., and Shear, M. J.: Tuberculosis, Proc. Soc. Exper. Biol. and
  Med., 27, 144, 1929.
Kramer, F.: Trigeminal neuralgia, Klin. Wchnschr., 58, 149, 1922.
Krause, A. K.: Tuberculosis, Nelson Loose-Leaf Med., 1, 309; Nelson's Medical Service,
  236 (May), 1926.
Krause, P.: Thyrotoxicosis, Strahlentherapie, 27, 393, 1927.
Krause, R., Penna, J., and Cruenca, J. B.: Anthrax, Preusa Med. Argentina, 4, 91, 1917
  (abstract Jour. Amer. Med. Assoc., 69, 1388, 1917); ibid., 4, 455, 1917 (abstract
  Jour. Amer. Med. Assoc., 69, 2076, 1917).
Kretschmer, H. L., and Helmholz, H.: Urinary infections, Jour. Amer. Med. Assoc., 75,
  1303, 1920.
Krogh, A.: Nephritis, Anatomy and Physiology of the Capillaries, New Haven, 1929.
Kühn, M. J.: BCG, Compt. rend. Soc. de biol., 97, 1520, 1927.
Kunde, M. M., Hall, G. W., and Gerty, F. J.: Syphilis, Jour. Amer. Med. Assoc., 89,
  1304, 1927.
Kushelsvskiy, B. P.: Peptic ulcer, Terapeutischesky arkhiv., 9, 281, 1931.
Küstner, H.: Sepsis, Münch. med. Wchnschr., January 15, 1932.
Kyes, P.: Pneumonia, Jour. Med. Res., 38, 495, 1918.
Kyrle, J.: Syphilis, Wien. klin. Wchnschr., 30, 707, 1917.
Labat, G., and Greene, M. B.: Sciatica, Amer. Jour. Surg., 11, 435, 1931.
Labbé, M.: Thyrotoxicosis, Bull. Soc. méd. Hôp. de Paris, 2, 1255, 1928.
Lacapère and Laurent: Syphilis, Bull. Méd., 33, 539, 1919.
Lahey. F. H.: Thyrotoxicosis, Ann. Surg., 1026, May, 1931.
Laignal-Lavastine and Stearne, J.: Encephalitis, Progrès méd., 21, 932, 1932.
Laigret, J.: Trypanosomiasis, Ann. de l'Inst. Pasteur, 40, 173, 1926.
Lain, E. S.: Impetigo, Jour. Amer. Med. Assoc., 69, 176, 1917 (discussion).
Lambert, A.: Delirium tremens, Nelson Loose-Leaf Med., 2, 555; Cecil's Textbook of
  Medicine, Phila., W. B. Saunders Co., 1933, p. 572. Addiction, Jour. Amer. Med.
  Assoc., 53, 985, 1909; ibid., 56, 503, 1911; ibid., 60, 1933, 1913; ibid., 92, 147, 1929;
  ibid., 96, 825, 1931.
Lambert, A. V. S.: Lung abscess, Laryngoscope, 39, 224, 1929.
Lambert, S. M.: Hookworm, Jour. Amer. Med. Assoc., 79, 2055, 1922; ibid., 80, 526,
  1923; ibid., 100, 247, 1933. Sprue, Jour. Amer. Med. Assoc., 80, 1910, 1923.
Lambert, S. W., and Patterson, H. S.: Poisoning, Arch. Int. Med., 16, 865, 1915.
Lamson, P. D.: Eczema-dermatitis, Jour. Amer. Med. Assoc., 97, 1225, 1931.
Lamson, P. D., et al.: Worms, Amer. Jour. Hyg., 13, 568 and 803, 1931.
Lamson, P. D., Brown, H. W., and Ward, C. B.: Hookworm, Jour. Amer. Med. Assoc.,
  99, 292, 1932.
Lamson, P. D., Minot, A. S., and Robbins, B. H.: Hookworm, Jour. Amer. Med. Assoc.,
  90, 345, 1928.
Lamson, R. W.: Asthma, Jour. Lab. and Clin. Med., 14, 931, 1929.
Landsteiner, K., and Scheer, J.: Allergy, Jour. Exper. Med., 48, 315, 1928; ibid., 54, 295,
  1931.
Lange, L., and Clauberg, K. W.: BCG, Beit. z. Klin. Tuber., 70, 346, 1928.
Langer, E.: Syphilis, Klin. Wchnschr., Nr. 12, 554, 1928.
Langley, G. J.: Pneumonia, Lancet, 1, 11, 1924.
Langmead, F. S.: Thyrotoxicosis, Brit. Med. Jour., April 20, 1929.
Lantin, P. T.: Bacillary dysentery, Amer. Jour. Med. Sci., 180, 635, 1930.
Laplace, L. B., and Reisinger, J. A.: Auricular fibrillation, Amer. Jour. Med. Sci., 183, 48,
  1932.
Laptain, J. H. R.: Syphilis, Lancet, 1, 635, 1931.
Lara, C. B.: Leprosy, Jour. Phil. Is. Med. Assoc., 8, 56, 1928; ibid., 9, 336, 1929.
Lara, C. B., and Nicolas, C.: Leprosy, Jour. Phil. Is. Med. Assoc., 9, 321, 1929.

Larimore, J. W.: Ulcerative colitis, Jour. Amer. Med. Assoc., 90, 841, 1928.
Larrabee, R. C.: Purpura, Jour. Amer. Med. Assoc., 80, 838, 1923.
Larson, R. L.: Syphilis, Amer. Jour. Syph., 15, 50, 1931.
Larson, W. P., and Eder, H.: Toxin-ricinoleate, Jour. Amer. Med. Assoc., 86, 998, 1926.
Lasersohn, M.: Syphilis, Jour. Amer. Med. Assoc., 85, 436, 1925.
Lashmet, F. H.: Nephritis, Jour. Amer. Med. Assoc., 97, 918, 1931.
Lassere: Chancroid, Arch. de Méd. et Pharm Nav., 109, 209, 1920.
Laurens, H., and Sooy, J. W.: Purpura, Proc. Soc. Exper. Biol. and Med., 22, 114, 1924
    (also unpublished work cited by Sooy and Moise, *q. v.*).
Lauterburg, M.: Trypanosomiasis, Arch. f. Schiffs.- u. Trop. Hyg., 33, 251, 1929; Deutsch.
    med. Wchnschr. (abstract), 57, 78, 1931.
Lavergne and Florentin: Mumps, Bull. l'Acad. de méd., 93, 362, 1925.
Läwen: Tetanus, Zentlbl. f. Chir., 2370, 1927; ibid., 194, 1928.
Lawrence: Diabetes mellitus, Brit. Med. Jour., 2, 983, 1926; ibid., 1, 595, 1927.
Lawrence, R. D.: Diabetes, Brit. Med. Jour., April 12, 1930.
Lawson, G. B.: Amebic dysentery, Jour. Amer. Med. Assoc., 71, 1049, 1918.
Lawson, G. B., *et al.*: Hemophilia, Jour. Amer. Med. Assoc., 98, 1443, 1932.
Leach, C. N., and Hampton, G. G.: Hookworm, Jour. Amer. Med. Assoc., 80, 8, 1923.
Leach, O. N.: Hookworm, Jour. Amer. Med. Assoc., 78, 1789, 1922.
Leake, C. D.: Secondary anemia, Jour. Pharm. and Exper. Ther., 22, 401, 1923. Amebic
    dysentery, Jour. Amer. Med. Assoc., 98, 195, 1932.
Leake, C. D., and Evans, J. S.: Secondary anemia, Amer. Jour. Med. Sci., 168, 819, 1924.
Leake, C. D., and Leake, E. W.: Secondary anemia, Jour. Pharm. and Exper. Ther., 22
    75, 1923.
Leake, J. P.: Smallpox, Reprint No. 1137, P. H. Reports, U. S. Govt. Print. Office,
    Washington, 1930.
Leavell, H. R., *et al.*: Undulant fever, Jour. Amer. Med. Assoc., 95, 860, 1930.
Lebensohn, J. E.: Sea-sickness, Arch. Ophthalm., 4, 342, 1930.
Le Blanc, E.: Tuberculosis, Münch. med. Wchnschr., 73, 313, 1926.
Leech, C. B.: Rheumatic fever, Jour. Amer. Med. Assoc., 95, 932, 1930.
Leech, P. A.: Rheumatic fever, Jour. Amer. Med. Assoc., 78, 275, 1922.
Lehman, A. M., and Bartholomew, D. C.: Tuberculosis, Jour. Amer. Med. Assoc., 98, 1344,
    1932.
Leifer, A.: Diabetes mellitus, Jour. Amer. Med. Assoc., 90, 610, 1928.
Leiper, R. T.: Blood flukes, Nelson Loose-Leaf Med., 2, 271.
Leiter, L.: Nephritis, Medicine, 10, 135, 1931.
Leitner, P.: Pneumonia, Jahrb. f. Kinderh., 135, 257, 1932.
Lemann, I. I.: Diabetes mellitus, Amer. Jour. Med. Sci., 180, 266, 1930.
Leonard, V.: Urinary infections, Jour. Amer. Med. Assoc., 83, 2005, 1924; ibid., 89, 517
    1927. Skin disinfection, Jour. Amer. Med. Assoc., 94, 1524, 1930.
Leonard, V., and Wood, A.: Urinary infections, Jour. Amer. Med. Assoc., 85, 1855, 1925
Leopold, S. S., and Jonas, L.: Tetany, Amer. Jour. Med. Sci., 183, 418, 1932.
Leopold, S. S., and Miller, T. G.: Asthma, Jour. Amer. Med. Assoc., 88, 1782, 1927.
Leopold, S. S., and Stewart, S. G.: Asthma, Jour. Allergy, 2, 425, 1931.
Lereboullet, P., Boulanger-Pilet and Gournay: Diphtheria, Bull. et mém. Soc. med. d. hôp.
    de Paris, 50, 683, 1926.
Lerman, J., and Meams, J. H.: Thyrotoxicosis, Amer. Jour. Med. Sci., 181, 745, 1931.
Leschke, E.: Lead poisoning, Münch. med. Wchnschr., Nr. 38, 1600, 1931; ibid., Nr. 39,
    1657, 1931.
Leshure, J.: Poisoning, Jour. Amer. Med. Assoc., 88, 168, 1927.
Leslie, G. L.: Tuberculosis, Jour. Amer. Med. Assoc., 100, 313, 1933.
L'Esperance, E.: Hodgkin's disease, Jour. Immunol., 15, 123, 1928; ibid., 16, 27, 1929.
Lethem, W.: Plague, Lancet, 2, 292, 1923.
Letonturier, de Marqueissac and Jamot: Trypanosomiasis, Ann. de l'Inst. Pasteur, 38,
    1053, 1924; Bull. Soc. de path. exot., 17, 692, 1924.
Levine and Blutner: Paroxysmal tachycardia, Brit. Med. Jour., 1, 7, 1927.
Levine, S. A.: Coronary occlusion, Jour. Amer. Med. Assoc., 99, 1737, 1932.
Levine, S. A., and Blotner, H.: Arhythmia, Amer. Jour. Med. Sci., 172, 660, 1926.
Levy, E.: Meningitis, Klin. Jahrb., 25, 121, 1911.
Levy, G.: Syphilis, Cited by Cole, Moore, O'Leary, Parran, Stokes and Wile (*q. v.*).
Levy, L. H.: Constipation, Jour. Amer. Med. Assoc., 75, 177, 1920.
Levy, M. D.: Dengue, Texas State Jour. Med., 19, 182, 1923.
Levy, P. S.: Essential hematuria, Surg., Gyn., and Obst., 34, 22, 1922.
Levy, R. L.: Hookworm, Jour. Amer. Med. Assoc., 63, 1946, 1914. Heart failure, Arch.
    Int. Med., 33, 742, 1924.
Levy, R. L., and Mackie, T. T.: Heart failure, Jour. Amer. Med. Assoc., 89, 432, 1927
    Arhythmia, Jour. Amer. Med. Assoc., 89, 432, 1927.
Levy, R. L., and Moore, R. L.: Angina pectoris, Arch. Int. Med., 48, 146, 1931.
Lévy-Bing, Lehnhoff-Wyld and Gerbay: Syphilis, Ann. d. mal. vén., 14, 520, 1919.
Lewenstein, H.: Encephalitis, Deutsch. med. Wchnschr., 57, 1014, 1931.
Lewis, D. M.: Diphtheria carrier, Med. Jour. and Rec., 119, 132, 1924.

Lewis, D., and Gatewood, W.: Causalgia, Jour. Amer. Med. Assoc., 74, 1, 1920.
Lewis, K. M.: Varicose veins, Ann. Surg., 95, 727, 1932.
Lewis M. S.: Anemia, Jour. Amer. Med. Assoc., 96, 1135, 1931.
Lewis, T.: Auricular fibrillation, Amer. Jour. Med. Sci., 164, 1, 1922.
Lian: Paroxysmal tachycardia, Presse méd., 32, 297, 1924.
Lichtenstein: Hiccup, Klin. Wchnschr., 7, 552, 1928.
Lichtenstein, A.: Measles, Jour. Amer. Med. Assoc., 96, 2102, 1931.
Lichtenstein, J. V.: Syphilis, Arch. Dermat. and Syph., 24, 182, 1931.
Lichtman, S. S.: Cirrhosis, Jour. Amer. Med. Assoc., 97, 1463, 1931.
Lickint, F.: Flagellate dysentery, Münch. med. Wchnschr., Nr. 25, 993, 1932.
Lieb, C. W.: Essential hypertension, Jour. Amer. Med. Assoc., 87, 25, 1926. Nephritis,
    Jour. Amer. Med. Assoc., 87, 25, 1926.
Lignières, J.: Anthrax, Revista de la Assoc. Med. Argentina, 27, 370, 1917 (abstract Jour.
    Amer. Med. Assoc., 69, 2077, 1917). BCG, Bull. de l'Acad. de méd., May 1, 8, 15,
    July 24, 1928; Jour. Amer. Vet. Med. Assoc., 100, 1027, 1928.
Lilienthal, H.: Asthma, Jour. Amer. Med. Assoc., 90, 1192, 1926.
Lincoln, E. M., and Greenwald, C. K.: Tetanus, Proc. Soc. Exper. Biol. and Med., 30,
    1241, 1933.
Lind, S. C.: Rheumatic fever, Ohio State Med. Jour., 95, 1228, 1932.
Linder, G. C., *et al.*: Nephritis, Jour. Exper. Med., 39, 887, 921, 931, 1924.
Lindsay, J. W., Rice, E. C., and Selinger, M. A.: Scarlet fever, Jour. Amer. Med. Assoc.,
    86, 1191, 1926.
Linser, K.: Varicose veins, Dermat. Wchnschr., 81, 1345, 1925.
Linser, P.: Varicose veins, Münch. med. Wchnschr., 66, 795, 1919.
Lipowski, I.: Constipation, Berl. klin. Wchnschr., 46, 1359, 1909; Münch. med. Wchnschr.
    57, 2635, 1910.
Litchfield, L.: Pneumonia, Jour. Amer. Med. Assoc., 71, 503, 1918.
Littman, S., and Hutton, J. G.: Syphilis, Jour. Amer. Med. Assoc., 82, 868, 1924.
Litzenberg, J. C.: Dysmenorrhea, Jour. Amer. Med. Assoc., 73, 601, 1919.
Liu, S. H.: Tetany, Jour. Clin. Invest., 5, 259 and 277, 1928. Nephritis, Arch. Int. Med.,
    40, 73, 1927.
Lloyd, B. J.: Plague, Jour. Amer. Med. Assoc., 85, 729, 1925.
Lockard, L. B.: Tuberculosis, Nelson Loose-Leaf Med., 3, 429.
Lockwood, B. C., and Chamberlin, H. G.: Peptic ulcer, Arch. Int. Med., 32, 74, 1923.
Loeb, R. F., *et al.*: Nephritis, Jour. Clin. Invest., 11, 621, 1932.
Loevenhart, A. S., and Crandall, L. A.: Peptic ulcer, Jour. Amer. Med. Assoc., 88, 1557,
    1927.
Loewenthal, M.: Measles, Brit. Med. Jour., 2, 51, 1924.
Loewy, A., and Zondek, H.: Thyrotoxicosis, Deutsch. med. Wchnschr., 47, 1387, 1921.
Lomholt, S.: Scabies, Lancet, 2, 1251, 1920. Syphilis, Handb. d. Haut.- u. Geschlechtskr.,
    18, 1, 1928; Biochem. Ztschr., 198, 98, 1928; Arch. Dermat. and Syph., 19, 891, 1929;
    Brit. Med. Jour., 2, 887, 1929.
Lopez-Rizal, L., and Sellards, A. W.: Yaws, Phil. Jour. Sci., 30, 497, 1926.
Lopez-Rizal, L., Arguelles, M. V., and Lara, H.: Typhoid, Jour. Phil. Med. Assoc., 7, 7,
    1927.
Lord, F. T., and Nye, R. N.: Pneumonia, Jour. Exper. Med., 34, 201, 1921.
Lord, R. E., and Holmes, G.: Sepsis, Brit. Med. Jour., 1, 335, 1930.
Lorenz, E. F., Loevenhart, A. S., Bleckween, W. G., and Hodges, F. J.: Syphilis, Jour.
    Amer. Med. Assoc., 80, 1497, 1923.
Loucks, R. E.: Thyrotoxicosis, Radiology, 4, 473, 1925.
Loveman, A. B.: Syphilis, Ann. Int. Med., 5, 1238, 1932.
Low, G. C.: Filariasis, Trans. Roy. Soc. Trop. Med. and Hyg., 20, 514, 1927; Lancet, 1, 72,
    1930.
Low, G. C., and Cooke, W. E.: Sprue, Lancet, 2, 960, 1927.
Low, G. C., Cooke, W. E., and Martin, P. H.: Blackwater fever, Lancet, 2, 645, 1928.
Lowenburg, H., and Ginsburg, T. M.: Tetany, Jour. Amer. Med. Assoc., 99, 1166, 1932.
Löwenstein, E.: Diphtheria, Münch. med. Wchnschr., 77, 21, 1930. BCG, Wien. klin.
    Wchnschr., 39, 293, 1926.
Lucherini, T.: Leukemia, Policlinico, 32, 1745, 1925.
Luckhardt, A. B., and Koppányi, T.: Asthma, Proc. Soc. Biol. and Med., 23, 774, 1926.
Lucus, W. P., and Amoss, H. L.: Bacillary dysentery, Jour. Exper. Med., 13, 486, 1911.
Ludlow, A. I.: Roundworms, China Med. Jour., 41, 134, 1927.
Luikart, R.: Hyperemesis gravidarum, Amer. Jour. Obst. and Gyn., 25, 810, 1933.
Luithlen: Food allergy, Wien. med. Wchnschr., 907, 1926.
Lukens, R. M.: Tuberculosis, Jour. Amer. Med. Assoc., 78, 274, 1922.
Lunde, G., *et al.*: Thyrotoxicosis, Biochem. Zeit., 206, 261, 1929.
Lusk, G.: Pneumonia, Elements of the Science of Nutrition, Phila., W. B. Saunders Co.,
    1917, 3rd Ed.
Luten, D.: Heart failure, Arch. Int. Med., 33, 251, 1924.
Lutsch, W.: Amebic dysentery, Münch. med. Wchnschr., 61, March 3, 1914.
Luttinger, P.: Whooping cough, Jour. Amer. Med. Assoc., 68, 1461, 1917; ibid., 78, 1536, 1922.

Lyon, B. B. V.: Gallbladder disease, Non-surgical Drainage of the Gall Tract, Phila., Lea and Febiger, 1923; Jour. Med. Soc. New Jersey, 1931.

Lyon, B. B. V., and Swahn, W. A.: Gallbladder disease, Jour. Amer. Med. Assoc., 85, 1541, 1925.

Lyon, D. M., *et al.*: Nephritis, Lancet, 2, 1009, 1931.

Lyon, G. M.: Cerebrospinal fever, Amer. Jour. Dis. Child., 43, 572, 1932; W. Va. Med. Jour., May, 1932.

Macciotta, G.: Whooping cough, Pediatria, 32, 159, 1924.

MacConkey and Silva: Tetanus, Brit. Med. Jour., 1, 411, 1916.

MacDonald, H.: Catharsis, Jour. Amer. Med. Assoc., 80, 1375, 1923.

Macht, D. I.: Poisoning, Bull. Johns Hopkins Hosp., 26, 98, 1915. Gallstones, Jour. Pharm. and Exper. Ther., 9, 473, 1917. Dysmenorrhea, Jour. Amer. Med. Assoc., 73, 599, 1919.

Macht, D. I., and Finesilver, E. M.: Catharsis, Bull. Johns Hopkins Hosp., 33, 330, 1922.

Maciel, H.: Bilharziasis, Rev. Med.-Cirurg. do Brasil, 39, 43, 1931.

Mackay, H.: Anemia, Medical Research Council Special Report Series, No. 157, London, H. M. Stationery Office, 1931.

Mackay, R. P.: Syphilis, Arch. Neurol. and Psychiat., 26, 102, 1931.

MacKenna, R. M. B.: Lupus erythematosus, Lancet, 1, 126, 1931.

Mackenzie, G. M.: Serum disease, Cecil's Textbook of Medicine, Phila., W. B. Saunders Co., 1933, p. 516.

Mackenzie, G. M., and Hanger, F. M.: Pneumonia, Jour. Amer. Med. Assoc., 94, 260, 1930.

Mackie, F. P.: Cholera, Lancet, 1, 201, 1933.

Maclean, G.: Trypanosomiasis, Ann. Trop. Med. and Parasit., 20, 329, 1926.

Maclean, G., and Fairbairn, H.: Trypanosomiasis, Ann. Trop. Med. and Parasit., 26, 157, 1932.

Macleod, J. J. R.: Diabetes mellitus, Lancet, 2, 383, 1930.

Macphail, N. P.: Malaria, Med. Dept. United Fruit Co. (19th An. Rep.), 1930.

Macrea, D., Jr.: Peptic ulcer, Lancet, 1, 26, 1923.

Madison, F. W.: Agranulocytosis, unpublished observations.

Madison, F. W., and Squier, T. L.: Agranulocytosis, personal communication to the author.

Madsen, T.: Whooping cough, Jour. Amer. Med. Assoc., 101, 187, 1933.

Magath, T. B.: Worms, Jour. Amer. Med. Assoc., 101, 337, 1933.

Magath, T. B., and Brown, P. W.: Worms, Jour. Amer. Med. Assoc., 88, 1548, 1927.

Magliano, H.: Whooping cough, Jour. Amer. Med. Assoc., 87, 2039, 1929 (abstract).

Mainzer, F. S.: Bronchiectasis, Amer. Jour. Surg., 11, 93, 1931.

Mair, W.: Scarlet fever, Lancet, 2, 1390, 1923.

Maitland, T. G.: Sea-sickness, Practitioner, 129, 251, 1932.

Major, R. H.: Thyrotoxicosis, Jour. Amer. Med. Assoc., 80, 83, 1923. Nephritis, Wisconsin Med. Jour., 29, 419, 1930. Lead poisoning, Ann. Med. Hist., N.S., 3, 218, 1931.

Malaret, P. S.: Typhoid, United Fruit Co. Rep., 20, 165, 1931.

Malkani, Moti: BCG, Tubercle, 11, 433, 1930.

Mallory, F. B.: Cirrhosis, Arch. Int. Med., 37, 336, 1926.

Malvoz and Van Beneden: BCG, Ann. de l'Inst. Pasteur, 41, 271, 1927.

Manalang, C.: Hookworm, Amer. Jour. Trop. Med., 7, 57, 1927.

Manifold, J. A.: Malaria, Jour. R. A. M. C., May-June, 1931.

Manoussakis, E.: Malaria, Bull. et mém. Soc. med. hôp. de Paris, 47, 1426, 1931.

Manson-Bahr, P. H.: Malaria, Proc. Roy. Soc. Med. (Sec. Trop. Dis. and Parasit.), 20, 33, 1927; Lancet, 1, 25, 1928; ibid., 2, 496, 1928; ibid., 2, 425, 1931; ibid., 1, 882, 1932.

Manson-Bahr, P., and Morris, R. M.: Amebic dysentery, Lancet, 2, 69, 1926.

Manson-Bahr, P., and Sayers, E. G.: Blackwater fever, Lancet, 1, 273, 1927.

Marchbanks, H. E., *et al.*: Bichloride poisoning, Jour. Amer. Med. Assoc., 96, 611, 1931.

Marchoux, E.: Amebic dysentery, Bull. Soc. de path. exot., 16, 79, 1923; Paris méd., 14, 421, 1924. Malaria, Ann. de l'Inst. Pasteur, 39, 197, 1925.

Marchoux, E., and Cohen: Malaria, Compt. rend. Soc. de Biol., 92, 132, 1925.

Marcuse, H., and Kallmann, F.: Syphilis, Nervenarzt., 2, 149, 1929.

Marie, A.: Syphilis, Bull. de l'Acad. de méd., 106, 248, 1931; Arch. internat. de neurol., 1, 75, 1931; ibid., 1, 229, 1931; ibid., 1, 313, 1931.

Marine, D.: Simple goiter, Bull. Johns Hopkins Hosp., 18, 359, 1907; Jour. Amer. Med. Assoc., 99, 250, 1932.

Marine, D., and Kimball, O. P.: Simple goiter, Jour. Lab. and Clin. Med., 3, 40, 1917; Arch. Int. Med., 25, 661, 1920; Jour. Amer. Med. Assoc., 77, 1068, 1921.

Marine, D., and Lenhart, C. H.: Simple goiter, Bull. Johns Hopkins Hosp., 20, 131, 1909; Jour. Exper. Med., 13, 455, 1911; Arch. Int. Med., 7, 506, 1911.

Marinesco, G., Sager, O., and Façon, H.: Syphilis, Presse méd., 36, 150, 1928.

Mark, R. E., and Wagner, R. I.: Diabetes mellitus, Klin. Wchnschr., 4, 1692, 1925.

Marrack, J. R.: Sea-sickness, Brit. Med. Jour., 1, 178, 1931.

Martin, E., and Jackle, K.: Obstetrical anesthesia, Monatschr. f. Geburtsh. u. Gynäk., 74, 319, 1926.

Martin, L.: Arthritis, Southern Med. Jour., 26, 699, 1933.

Martinez, G. P.: Kala-azar, La Med. ibera, 21, 1927.

Marvin, H. M.: Heart failure, Jour. Amer. Med. Assoc., 87, 2043, 1926; ibid., 87, 1016, 1926; Jour. Clin. Invest., 3, 521, 1927.
Marx, E.: Encephalitis, Münch. med. Wchnschr., 74, 1916, 1927.
Mason, C. C.: Whooping cough, Jour. Amer. Med. Assoc., 81, 2114, 1923.
Mason, E. L.: Purpura, Wisconsin Med. Jour., 31, 447, 1932.
Mateer, J. G., and Baltz, J. I.: Colitis, Ann. Int. Med., 5, 982, 1932.
Mathieu, A., and Sichel, M. S.: Induction of Labor, Surg., Gyn., and Obst., 53, 676, 1931.
Matson, R. W.: Tuberculosis, Amer. Rev. Tuberc., 25, 419, 1932.
Matsumura, S., et al.: Beriberi, Jour. Amer. Med. Assoc., 92, 1325, 1929.
Matthiasson, S.: Hydatid cyst, Ugeskr. f. Leager, 89, 348, 1927.
Maurer, S., et al.: Anemia, Jour. Amer. Med. Assoc., 98, 1069, 1932.
Maver, M. E., and Wells, H. G.: Tuberculosis, Amer. Rev. Tuberc., 7, 1, 1923.
Maxwell, C. H., Jr., and Glaser, J.: Syphilis, Amer. Jour. Dis. Child, 43, 1460, 1932.
Maxwell, J.: Asthma, Brit. Med. Jour., May 10, 1930.
May, E. W.: Rickets, Jour. Amer. Med. Assoc., 96, 1376, 1931.
Mayer, E.: Dysmenorrhea, Jour. Amer. Med. Assoc., 62, 6, 1914.   Tuberculosis, Jour. Amer. Med. Assoc., 97, 1935, 1931; ibid., 98, 221, 1932.
Mayer, E., and Kugelmass, I. N.: Tuberculosis, Jour. Amer. Med. Assoc., 93, 1856, 1929.
Mayes, H. W.: Gonorrhea, New York State Jour. Med., 26, 384, 1926.   Mercurochrome technique, Surg., Gyn., and Obst., 54, 529, 1932; ibid., 55, 771, 1932; Amer. Jour. Obst. and Gyn., 23, 627, 1932.
Maynard, E. P.: Arhythmia, Amer. Jour. Med. Sci., 175, 55, 1928.
Maytum, C. K.: Asthma, Med. Clin. N. A., 15, 201, 1931.
McBride, R. H.: Syphilis, Jour. Amer. Med. Assoc., 84, 729, 1925.
McCafferty, L. K., and MacGregor, J. A.: Syphilis, Amer. Jour. Med. Sci., 170, 22, 1925.
McCann, W. S.: Nephritis, Ann. Int. Med., 5, 579, 1931.
McCarrison, R.: Thyrotoxicosis, Brit. Med. Jour., 1, 178, 1922.   Tetany, The Thyroid Gland, 1917, William Wood and Co., New York.
McCarthy, J. F., and Ritter, J. S.: Gonorrhea, Jour. Amer. Med. Assoc., 98, 687, 1932.
McCay: Nephritis, Scientific Mem. of India, No. 37, 240, 1910.
McClellan, W. S., and DuBois, E. F.: Nephritis, Jour. Biol. Chem., 87, 651, 1930.
McClure, R. D.: Goiter, Wisconsin Med. Jour., 31, 519, 1932.
McCluskey, K. L., and Eichelberger, L.: Tuberculosis, Amer. Rev. Tuberc., 12, 329, 1925.
McConkey, M.: Tuberculosis, Trans. Twenty-fifth An. Meet. Natl. Tuberc. Assoc., 105, 1929.
McConnell, W. T.: Sepsis, cited by Hendon, G. A., Jour. Amer. Med. Assoc., 95, 1175, 1930.
McCord, J. R.: Syphilis, Amer. Jour. Syph., 16, 78, 1932.
McCormick, C. O.: Obstetrical analgesia, Anesth. and Analg., July–August, 1932.
McCormick, R. R.: Herpes zoster, Jour. Amer. Med. Assoc., 96, 766, 1931.
McCowan, P. K., and Northcote, M. L. M.: Syphilis, Lancet, 2, 237, 1932.
McCoy, G. W., and Chapin, C. W.: Tularemia, Jour. Infect. Dis., 10, 61, 1912.
McCoy, G. W., Hasseltine, H. E., Wadsworth, A., and Kirkbride, M. B.: Pneumonia, Jour. Amer. Med. Assoc., 79, 1128, 1922.
McCrae, T., and Caven, W. R.: Syphilis, Amer. Jour. Med. Sci., 172, 781, 1926.
McCrie, J. G.: Pernicious anemia, Brit. Med. Jour., April 30, 1932.
McCullagh, E. P., and McCullagh, D. R.: Tetany, Jour. Lab. and Clin. Med., 17, 754, 1932.
McCulloch, C. C.: Malaria, Amer. Jour. Med. Sci., 155, 10, 1918.
McCulloch, H., and Rupe, W. A.: Heart failure, Amer. Jour. Med. Sci., 162, 231, 1921.
McCurdy, J. R.: Morphine poisoning, Jour. Amer. Med. Assoc., 92, 1927, 1929.
McDonagh, J. E. R.: Chancroid, Venereal Diseases, St. Louis, C. V. Mosby Co., 1920, pp. 267, 268, 363.
McDonald, E.: Urinary infections, Jour. Amer. Med. Assoc., 64, 505, 1915.
McDonald, J. T.: Leprosy, Jour. Amer. Med. Assoc., 75, 1483, 1920.
McDonald, J. T., and Dean, A. L.: Leprosy, Jour. Amer. Med. Assoc., 76, 1470, 1921.
McFarland, A. R.: Syphilis, Jour. Amer. Med. Assoc., 78, 786, 1922.
McGavran, E. G.: Tetany, Jour. Amer. Med. Assoc., 99, 115, 1932.
McGavran, E. G., and Songkla, M.: Tapeworms, Jour. Amer. Med. Assoc., 90, 1607, 1928.
McGee, W. A.: Whooping cough, Jour. Amer. Med. Assoc., 97, 922, 1931.
McGregor, L.: Nephritis, Amer. Jour. Path., 5, 545, 1929.
McGuigan, H.: Poliomyelitis, Proc. Biol. Chem., 2, 67, 1912.
McGuigan, H., and Atkinson, H. V.: Poisoning, Jour. Pharm. and Exper. Ther., 21, 204, 1923.
McGuire, P. F., and Hitchens, A. P.: Diphtheria carrier, Jour. Amer. Med. Assoc., 80, 664, 1923.
McKenney, D. C.: Constipation, Jour. Amer. Med. Assoc., 89, 1039, 1927 (discussion).
McKhann, C. F., and Chu, F. T.: Measles, Amer. Jour. Dis. Child., 45, 475, 1933.
McLean, N.: Trypanosomiasis, Kenya and East African Med. Jour., 8, 180, 1931.
McLean, S.: Worms, Jour. Amer. Med. Assoc., 74, 1774, 1920.

McLester, J. S.: Erythremia, Jour. Amer. Med. Assoc., 62, 1381, 1914. Syphilis, Cecil's Textbook of Medicine, Phila., W. B. Saunders Co., 1933, p. 440. Nephritis, Jour. Amer. Med. Assoc., 99, 192, 1932.
McNair, J. B.: Dermatitis venenata, Jour. Amer. Med. Assoc., 85, 456, 1925.
McNally, W. D.: Tear gas, Jour. Amer. Med. Assoc., 98, 45, 1932.
McNeile, L. G., and Vruwink, J.: Eclampsia, Jour. Amer. Med. Assoc., 87, 236, 1926. Obstetrical anesthesia, California and West. Med., 26, 640, 1927.
McPheeters, H. O., and Merkert, C. E.: Varicose veins, Surg., Gyn., and Obst., 52, 1164, 1931.
McPheeters, H. O., and Rice, C. O.: Varicose veins, Jour. Amer. Med. Assoc., 91, 1090, 1928.
McQuarrie, I.: Epilepsy, Jour. Nutrition, 2, 31, 1929.
McQuarrie, I., and Keith, H. M.: Epilepsy, Amer. Jour. Dis. Child., 34, 1013, 1927; ibid., 37, 261, 1929.
Meader, F. M.: Diphtheria carrier, Jour. Amer. Med. Assoc., 83, 1132, 1924. Scarlet fever, Jour. Amer. Med. Assoc., 94, 622, 1930.
Meaker, S. R.: Gonorrhea, Jour. Amer. Med. Assoc., 87, 1377, 1926.
Meakins, J.: Tetany, Ann. Int. Med., 4, 462, 1930.
Means, J. H.: Myxedema, Jour. Amer. Med. Assoc., 101, 233, 1933.
Means, J. H., and Holmes, G. W. Thyrotoxicosis, Arch. Int. Med., 31, 303, 1923.
Means, J. H., and Lerman, J.: Catarrhal fever, New England Jour. Med., 206, 124, 1932.
Mehrtens, H. G., and Pouppirt, P. S.: Syphilis, Arch. Neurol. and Psychiat., 22, 700, 1929; ibid., 26, 1220, 1931.
Meirowsky: Syphilis, Münch. med. Wchnschr., No. 17, 477, 1920.
Mellon, R. R., et al.: Glucose, Jour. Amer. Med. Assoc., 78, 1026, 1922.
Melnotte, P., and Farjot, A.: Typhoid, Compt. rend. Soc. de biol., 97, 338, 1927.
Meltzer, S. J.: Gallbladder disease, Amer. Jour. Med. Sci., 153, 469, 1917.
Meltzer, S. J., and Auer, J.: Tetanus, Jour. Exper. Med., 8, 692, 1906.
Melville, K. I., and Bruger, M.: Bichloride poisoning, Jour. Pharm. and Exper. Ther., 37, September, 1929.
Melzner, E.: Sepsis, Münch. med. Wchnschr., Nr. 47, 1983 and Nr. 48, 2039, 1931; ibid., Nr. 24, 964, 1932.
Menagh, F. R.: Angioneurotic edema and urticaria, Jour. Amer. Med. Assoc., 90, 668, 1928.
Menard, O. J., and Hurxthal, L. M.: Encephalitis, New England Jour. Med., 205, 759 , 1931.
Mercado: Leprosy, Ind. Med. Gaz., 55, 125, 1920.
Mercado and Heiser: Leprosy, Pub. Health Rep., 28, 1855, 1913.
Mettel, H. B.: Syphilis, Arch. Pediat., 761, December, 1931.
Mettier, S. R., and Minot, G. R.: Anemia, Amer. Jour. Med. Sci., 181, 25, 1931.
Meulengracht, E.: Scurvy, Acta Med. Scandinav., 67, 43, 1927.
Meyer, A. E., et al.: Pernicious anemia, Arch. Int. Med., 50, 538, 1932.
Meyer, J. R., and Pessoa, S. M.: Hookworm, Amer. Jour. Trop. Med., 3, 177, 1923.
Meyer, S., and Reifenberg, H.: Mumps, Ztschr. f. Kinderhk., 42, 163, 1926.
Meyer-Stromfeldt, G.: Chickenpox, Monatschr. f. Kinderh., 35, 111, 1927.
Michael, J. C.: Granuloma inguinale, Jour. Amer. Med. Assoc., 87, 1785, 1926 (discussion). Acne, Arch. Dermat. and Syph., 17, 604, 1928.
Michael, M.: Chickenpox, Arch. Pediat., 34, 702, 1917.
Michel, L. L., and Goodman, H.: Syphilis, Jour. Amer. Med. Assoc., 75, 1768, 1920.
Middleton, W. S.: Pernicious anemia, Wisconsin Med. Jour., 31, 763, 1932.
Middleton, W. S., and Chen, K. K.: Asthma, Arch. Int. Med., 39, 385, 1927.
Miller, C. H.: Gall-bladder disease, Lancet, 1, 767, 1932.
Miller, J. A.: Lung abscess, Laryngoscope, 39, 211, 1929.
Miller, M. D.: Whooping cough, Amer. Jour. Pub. Health, 11, 913, 1921.
Miller, R. H.: Tetanus, Surg., Gyn., and Obst., 36, 90, 1923.
Miller, S.: Undulant fever, Lancet, 1, 1177, 1933.
Miller, T. G.: Asthma, Ann. Clin. Med., 4, 713, 1926. Stokes-Adams disease, Amer Jour. Med. Sci., 157, 181, 1925.
Miller, W. F.: Dysmenorrhea, Jour. Amer. Med. Assoc., 95, 1796, 1930.
Mills, E. S.: Anemia, Amer. Jour. Med. Sci., 182, 554, 1931.
Mills, H. W.: Hydatid cyst, Surg., Gyn., and Obst., 44, 577, 1927.
Minot, G. R.: Pernicious anemia, Jour. Amer. Med. Assoc., 99, 1906, 1932.
Minot, G. R., and Buckman, T. E.: Purpura, Cecil's Textbook of Medicine, Phila., W. B. Saunders Co., 1933, p. 1043. Hemophilia, Cecil's Textbook of Medicine, Phila., W. B. Saunders Co., 1933, p. 1052.
Minot, G. R., and Murphy, W. P.: Pernicious anemia, Jour. Amer. Med. Assoc., 87, 470, 1926; ibid., 89, 759, 1927.
Minot, G. R., et al.: Leukemia, Jour. Amer. Med. Assoc., 82, 1489, 1924.
Mitchell, A. G.: Diabetes mellitus, Jour. Amer. Med. Assoc., 84, 1620, 1925.
Mitchell, A. G., and Guest, G. M.: Nephritis, Jour. Amer. Med. Assoc., 97, 1045, 1931.
Mitchell, A. G., and Ravenel, S. F.: Chickenpox, Arch. Pediat., 42, 709, 1925.

Moehlig, R. C., and Bates, G. S.: Erythremia, Arch. Int. Med., 51, 207, 1933.
Moensch, G. L.: Dysmenorrhea, Jour. Amer. Med. Assoc., 89, 598, 1927.
Mohler, H. K., and Goldburger, H. L.: Diabetes mellitus, Med. Clin. N. A., 15, 2, 1931.
Moine, M.: BCG, Ann. de l'Inst. Pasteur, 41, 214, 1927.
Molitch, M., and Wilson, G.: Angina pectoris, Jour. Amer. Med. Assoc., 97, 247, 1931
Moll, H. H.: Asthma, Brit. Med. Jour., 1, 976, 1932.
Møllgaard, H.: Tuberculosis, Brit. Med. Jour., 1, 643, 1925.
Møllgaard, H.: (in collaboration with Bie, Chiewitz, Gravesen, Fermin, Secher, Strand-
     gaard and Wurtzen). Chemotherapy of Tuberculosis, Copenhagen, Arnold Busck,
     1924.
Molnár, B., Jr.: Nephritis, Wien. klin. Wchnschr., 33, 1111, 1920.
Monash, S., and Traub, E. F.: Lupus erythematosus, Arch. Dermat. and Syph., 24, 110,
     1931.
Montgomery, J. C., and Cole, W. C. C.: Poliomyelitis, Jour. Amer. Med. Assoc., 85,
     890, 1925.
Moore, C. U.: Glucose, Jour. Amer. Med. Assoc., 99, 366, 1932 (discussion).
Moore, J. E.: Gonorrhea, Jour. Amer. Med. Assoc., 75, 911, 1920. Syphilis, Bull. Johns
     Hopkins Hosp., 33, 231, 1922; Jour. Amer. Med. Assoc., 89, 588, 1927; Ven. Dis.
     Inform., 10, 53, 1929.
Moore, J. E., and Keidel, A.: Syphilis, Bull. Johns Hopkins Hosp., 39, 1, 1926.
Moore, J. E., and Kemp, J. E.: Syphilis, Bull. Johns Hopkins Hosp., 39, 16, 1926; ibid.,
     39, 36, 1926.
Moore, J. E., and Wassermann, H.: Syphilis, Jour. Amer. Med. Assoc., 81, 1840, 1923.
Moore, J. E., Robinson, H. M., and Lyman, R. S.: Syphilis, Jour. Amer. Med. Assoc., 83,
     888, 1924.
Moore, J. E., Woo, S. T., Robinson, H. M., and Gay, L. N.: Syphilis, Arch. Dermat. and
     Syph., 23, 74, 1931.
Moore, N. S., and Van Slyke, D. D.: Nephritis, Jour. Clin. Invest., 8, 337, 1930.
Moorer, M. P.: Pruritus, Jour. Amer. Med. Assoc., 83, 766, 1924.
Moragas y Garcia, R.: Kala-azar, Beihefte z. Arch. f. Schiffs- u. Trop. Hyg., 29, 261, 1925.
Morales, E. G., and Mandry, O. C.: Measles, Amer. Jour. Dis. Child., 39, 1214, 1930.
Morawitz, P.: Diabetes mellitus, Münch. med. Wchnschr., 23, 571, 1927.
Moren, J. J.: Encephalitis, Kentucky Med. Jour., 27, 291, 1929.
Morgan, J.: Roundworms, China Med. Jour., 41, 847, 1927.
Morgenroth, J.: Pneumonia, Deutsch. med. Wchnschr., 44, 961, 1918.
Morison, J.: Asiatic cholera, Lancet, December 12, 1931 (editorial).
Moro, E.: Bacillary dysentery, Klin. Wchnschr., 1929, Nr. 52, 2414. Poliomyelitis, Klin.
     Wchnschr., 9, 2383, 1930.
Morris, R. S.: Erythremia, Jour. Amer. Med. Assoc., 101, 200, 1933.
Morris, R. S., Schiff, L., et al.: Pernicious anemia, Jour. Amer. Med. Assoc., 100, 171, 1933
Morris, R. S., et al.: Pernicious anemia, Amer. Jour. Med. Sci., 184, 778, 1932; Jour. Amer.
     Med. Assoc., 98, 1080, 1932.
Morrow, H.: Impetigo, Jour. Amer. Med. Assoc., 69, 176, 1917.
Morrow, H., Walker, E. L., and Miller, H. E.: Chaulmoogra oil, Jour. Amer. Med. Assoc.,
     79, 434, 1922.
Mosenthal, H. O.: Arteriosclerosis, Nelson Loose-Leaf Med., 4, 516. Essential hyper-
     tension, Amer. Jour. Med. Sci., 160, 808, 1920; Jour. Amer. Med. Assoc., 91, 698,
     1928.
Moser: Scarlet fever, Wien. klin. Wchnschr., 15, 10, 1902.
Moser, E.: Peptic ulcer, Med. Klin., 26, 42, 1929.
Moss, W. L.: Yaws, Amer. Jour. Trop. Med., 20, 365, 1926.
Moynihan, B.: Peptic ulcer, Bristol, J. Wright and Sons, 1923.
Much, H.: BCG, München. med. Wchnschr., 77, 2008, 1930.
Mühlens, P.: Malaria, Beihefte z. Arch. f. Schiffs- u. Trop. Hyg., 30, 25, 1926; Deut.
     med. Wchnschr., 53, 2202, 1927; Münch. med. Wchnschr., Nr. 14, 538, 1932.
Mühlens, P., and Fischer, O.: Malaria, Arch. f. Schiffs- u. Trop. Hyg., 31, 7, 1927.
Mühlens, P., Weygandt, W., and Kirschbaum, W.: Syphilis, Münch. med. Wchnschr.,
     67, 831, 1920.
Muir, E.: Leprosy, Lancet, 1, 277, 1924; Trans. Roy. Soc. Trop. Med. and Hyg., 25, 87,
     1931.
Mulherin, W. A., and Mulherin, F. X.: Malaria, Jour. Amer. Med. Assoc., 78, 1873, 1922.
Müller, H.: Syphilis, Deutsch. med. Wchnschr., 44, 1415, 1918.
Müller and Petersen: Diabetes mellitus, Klin. Wchnschr., 5, 1025, 1926.
Müllern-Aspegren: Syphilis, Acta Derm. Vener., 3, 572, 1922.
Mummery, N. H.: Burns, Lancet, 1, 662, 1933.
Mundell, J. J.: Pituitrin in labor, Jour. Amer. Med. Assoc., 68, 1601, 1917.
Munk, F.: Nephritis, Die Nierenerkrankungen, Berlin, 1925.
Munns, J. F., and Aldrich, C. A.: Asthma, Jour. Amer. Med. Assoc., 88, 1233 1927
Munoverro, J. A. A.: BCG, Jour. Amer. Med. Assoc. (abstract), 92, 2065, 1929.
Murphy, D. P., and Drinker, C. K.: Carbon monoxide poisoning, Jour. Ind. Hyg., 12, 92,
     1930.

Murphy, F. D.: Nephritis, Arch. Int. Med., 45, 23, 1930; Wisconsin Med. Jour., July 1933, p. 465.
Murphy, F. D., Grill, J., *et al.*: Hypertension, Ann. Int. Med., 6, 31, 1932.
Murphy, F. D., and Moxon, G. F.: Diabetes mellitus, Amer. Jour. Med. Sci., 182, 301, 1931.
Murphy, F. D., and Warfield, L. M.: Nephritis, Arch. Int. Med., 38, 449, 1926.
Murphy, W. P.: Pernicious anemia, Jour. Amer. Med. Assoc., 98, 1051, 1932. Anemia, Arch. Int. Med., 51, 656, 1933.
Murphy, W. P., and Blotner, H.: Diabetes mellitus, Jour. Clin. Invest., 4, 440, 1927; Jour. Amer. Med. Assoc., 92, 1332, 1929; ibid., 94, 1811, 1930.
Murray, G.: Myxedema, Brit. Med. Jour., 2, 796, 1891.
Muschallik, E.: Quinine in labor, Monatschr. f. Geburtsh. u. Gynäk., 52, 378, 1920.
Musser, J. H.: Angina pectoris, coronary occlusion, Jour. Amer. Med. Assoc., 91, 1242, 1928. Erysipelas, Jour. Amer. Med. Assoc., 88, 1125, 1927. Scarlet fever, Jour. Amer. Med. Assoc., 88, 1125, 1927. Pernicious anemia, Jour. Amer. Med. Assoc. 99, 614, 1932 (discussion).
Myers, G. N.: Diphtheria, Jour. Pharm. and Exper. Ther., 44, 191, 1932.
Myers, H. B., and Thienes, C. H.: Epidermophytosis, Jour. Amer. Med. Assoc., 84, 1985 1925.
Nabarro, D.: Tetanus, Lancet, 1, 450, 1932.
Nabarro, D. N., and Signy, A. G.: Measles, Brit. Med. Jour., October 3, 1931.
Naidu, B. P. B., and Mackie, F. P.: Plague, Lancet, 2, 893, 1931.
Nakamura, T.: Peptic ulcer, Ann. Surg., 79, 29, 1924.
Napier, L. E.: Kala-azar, Ind. Jour. Med. Res., 14, 263, 1926; ibid., 15, 181, 1927; ibid., 16, 141, 1928; ibid., 16, 901, 1929; ibid., 16, 911, 1929; Ind. Med. Gaz., 61, 559, 1926; 63, 687, 1928; Kala-azar (2nd Ed.), London, 1927.
Napier, L. E., and Halder, K. C.: Kala-azar, Ind. Jour. Med. Res., 15, 187, 1927.
Napier, L. E., and Mulliek, M. N.: Kala-azar, Ind. Med. Gaz., 63, 445, 1928; ibid., 64, 315, 1929.
Nass, J.: Carbon monoxide poisoning, Jour. Amer. Med. Assoc., 100, 1862, 1933.
Nassau, E.: Glucose administration, Ztschr. f. Kinderhlk., 41, 413, 1926.
Neal, J. B.: Encephalitis, Jour. Amer. Med. Assoc., 91, 231, 1928. Cerebrospinal fever, Amer. Jour. Pub. Health, 21, 147, 1931.
Neal, J. B., and Bentley, I. A.: Encephalitis, Jour. Amer. Med. Assoc., 28, 897, 1932.
Neill: Leprosy, Ann. Rep., U.S.P.H.S., 21, 1925.
Neisser, E.: Thyrotoxicosis, Berl. klin. Wchnschr., 57, 461, 1920.
Nelson, H. B.: Obstetrics, Amer. Jour. Obst. and Gyn., 23, 752, 1932.
Nelson, M. O.: Syphilis, Amer. Jour. Syph., 15, 185, 1931.
Nelson, T., and Porter, A. D.: Asthma, Lancet, 2, 1342, 1931.
Nesbit, O. B.: Scarlet fever, Jour. Amer. Med. Assoc., 84, 805, 1925.
Netherton, E. W.: Constipation, Med. Jour. and Rec., 119, 134, 1924.
Netter, A., and Debré, R.: Meningitis, Le Méningite Cérébrospinal, Paris, 1911.
Neustaedter, M., and Banzhaf, E. J.: Poliomyelitis, Jour. Amer. Med. Assoc., 68, 1531, 1917.
Nevin, M., Bittman, F. R., and Hazen, E. L.: Tuberculosis, Amer. Rev. Tuberc., 13, 114, 1926.
Newburgh, L. H.: Obesity, Jour. Amer. Med. Assoc., 97, 1659, 1931.
Newburgh, L. H., and Curtis, A. C.: Nephritis, Arch. Int. Med., 42, 801, 1928 (also statement of N.'s opinion in McCann, W. S., *q. v.*).
Newburgh, L. H., Falcon-Lesses, M., and Johnston, M. W.: Nephritis, Amer. Jour. Med. Sci., 179, 305, 1930.
Newbergh, L. H., and Marsh, P. L.: Diabetes mellitus, Arch. Int. Med., 26, 647, 1920; ibid., 27, 699, 1921; ibid., 31, 455, 1923.
Newbergh, L. H., Means, J. H., and Porter, W. T.: Pneumonia, Boston Med. and Surg. Jour., 173, 742, 1915; ibid., 174, 464, 1916; Jour. Exper. Med., 24, 583, 1916.
Newbergh, L. H., and Porter, W. T.: Pneumonia, Jour. Exper. Med., 22, 123, 1915
Newhof, H., and Hirshfeld, S.: Purpura, Ann. Surg., 76, 1, 1922.
Neymann, C. A.: Syphilis, Jour. Amer. Med. Assoc., 101, 301, 1933.
Neymann, C. A., and Koenig, M. A.: Syphilis, Jour. Amer. Med. Assoc., 96, 1858, 1931.
Neymann, C. A., and Osborne, S. L.: Syphilis, Jour. Amer. Med. Assoc., 96, 7, 1931.
Nicolas, C., and Roxas-Pineda, E.: Leprosy, Jour. Phil. Is. Med. Assoc., 8, 135, 1928.
Nicole, J. E., and Fitzgerald, E. J.: Syphilis, Amer. Jour. Syph., 15, 496, 1931.
Nicoll, M.: Plague, Jour. Amer. Med. Assoc., 85, 733, 1925 (discussion).
Nicolle, C., and Conseil, E.: Measles, Bull. et mém. Soc. d. hôp. de Paris, 42, 336, 1918.
Nicholls, L., and Hampton, G. G.: Hookworm, Brit. Med. Jour., 1922, 1, 8.
Niles, H. D.: Herpes zoster, New York State Jour. Med., 32, 773, 1932.
Niles, W. L., and Wyckoff, J.: Pneumonia, Amer. Jour. Med. Sci., 180, 348, 1930.
Nixon, J. A.: Diabetes mellitus, Brit. Med. Jour., February 22, 1932.
Nixon, J. W.: Chaparro amargosa, Texas Sanitarian, August, 1893.
Nixon, P. I.: Chaparro amargosa, Jour. Amer. Med. Assoc., 62, 1530, 1914.
Nobecourt, P.: BCG, Jour. des Prat., 92, 225, 1928; Pediatria, May 17, 1928; Bull. Soc. de pédiat. de Paris, 26, 145, 1928.

Nobl, G.: Varicose veins, Wien. klin. Wchnschr., 39, 1217, 1926; Wien. med. Wchnschr., 76, 1280, 1926.
Noguchi, H.: Yellow fever, Jour. Exper. Med., 29, 547, 1919; ibid., 30, 1, 1919; ibid., 30, 9, 1919; ibid., 30, 87, 1919; ibid., 30, 401, 1919; ibid., 31, 135, 1920; ibid., 31, 159, 1920; ibid., 32, 381, 1920; Jour. Amer. Med. Assoc., 77, 181, 1921; Cecil's Textbook of Medicine, Phila., W. B. Saunders Co., 1927, p. 392.
Noguchi, H., and Battistini, T. S.: Oroya fever, Science, 63, 212, 1926; Jour. Exper. Med, 43, 851, 1926.
Noguchi, H., and Hercelles, O.: Oroya fever, Science, 64, 121, 1926.
Nohlen, A.: BCG, Beit. z. klin. Tuberk., 73, 525, 1930.
Nolf, P.: Bacillary dysentery, Jour. Amer. Med. Assoc., 73, 1177, 1919.
Noon, L.: Hay-fever, Lancet, 1, 1572, 1911.
Noone, E. L., Waltz, A. D., and Donally, J. D.: Worms, Atlantic Med. Jour., 30, 692, 1927.
Norris and Nickelberg: Gonorrhea, Jour. Amer. Med. Assoc., 76, 164, 1921; Arch. Pediat., 39, 281, 1922.
Novak, J.: Dysmenorrhea, Wien. klin. Wchnschr., 26, 2068, 1913.
Nuttall: Trench fever (delousing), Parasitology, 1917, 10.
O'Brien, H. R.: Hookworm, Amer. Jour. Pub. Health, 15, 696, 1925.
O'Conor, V. J.: Urinary infections, Jour. Amer. Med. Assoc., 77, 1088, 1921.
O'Donnell, W. S., and Levin, S. J.: Nephritis, Jour. Amer. Med. Assoc., 96, 837, 1931.
Ogilvie, H. S.: Syphilis, Jour. Amer. Med. Assoc., 63, 1936, 1914.
O'Keefe, E. S., and Rackemann, F. M.: Eczema-dermatitis, Jour. Amer. Med. Assoc., 92, 883, 1929.
Okell, C. C.: Scarlet fever, Lancet, 1, 761–873, 1932.
Okell, C. C., and Parish, H. J.: BCG, Brit. Jour. Exper. Path., 9, 34, 1928.
Okutani, K.: Whooping cough, Amer. Jour. Dis. Child., 37, 420, 1929 (abstract).
O'Leary, P. A.: Syphilis, Jour. Amer. Med. Assoc., 89, 95, 1927; ibid., 97, 1585, 1931; Arch. Dermat. and Syph., 18, 372, 1928.
O'Leary, P. A., and Brunsting, L. A.: Syphilis, New York State Jour. Med., 30, 1223, 1930; Jour. Amer. Med. Assoc., 94, 452, 1930.
O'Leary, P. A., and Montgomery, H.: Syphilis, Jour. Chemotherapy, 6, 39, 1929.
O'Leary, P. A., and Rogin, J. R.: Syphilis, Proc. Staff Meet. Mayo Clin., 7, 273, 1932.
O'Leary, P. A., and Welsh, A. L.: Syphilis, Jour. Amer. Med. Assoc., 101, 498, 1933.
Olitsky, P. K., Rhoads, C. P., and Long, P. H.: Poliomyelitis, Jour. Amer. Med. Assoc., 92, 1725, 1929.
O'Malley, J. J., and Richey, D. G.: Quinine desensitization, Arch. Int. Med., 240, 378, 1919.
Onodera, Wa and Liu: Typhoid fever, Deutsch. Arch. f. klin. Med., 171, 503, 1931.
Opitz and Kotzulla: Tuberculosis, Deutsch. med. Wchnschr., 52, 531, 1926.
Orachowatz, D.: Malaria, Arch. f. Schiffs- u. Trop. Hyg., 32, 119, 1928.
Orator, V.: Peptic ulcer, Arch. f. klin. Chir., 134, 733, 1925.
Orenstein, A. J.: Pneumonia, Jour. Med. Assoc. S. Africa, 5, 339, 1931. Bilharziasis, Jour. Trop. Med. and Hyg., 34, 32, 1931.
Oriel, G. H.: Seasickness, Lancet, 2, 811, 1927.
Osborne, E. D.: Syphilis, Jour. Amer. Med. Assoc., 79, 615, 1922.
Osborne, E. D., and Hitchcock, B. S.: Epidermophytosis, Jour. Amer. Med. Assoc., 97, 453, 1931.
Osgood, H.: Antitoxin reaction, Jour. Amer. Med. Assoc., 81, 1406, 1923.
Osman, A. A.: Nephritis, Lancet, 2, 945, 1930.
O'Sullivan, J. V., and Craner, W. W.: Obstetrics, Lancet, 1, 119, 1932.
Ott: BCG, Ann. de l'Inst. Pasteur, 41, 219, 1927.
Otto, H. L.: Paroxysmal tachycardia, Proc. Soc. Exper. Med., 866, 1925.
Otto, H. L., and Gold, H.: Premature systole, Arch. Int. Med., 38, 186, 1926.
Owen, T.: Erythremia, Jour. Amer. Med. Assoc., 85, 2027, 1925.
Owensby, N. M.: Pellagra, Med. Jour. and Rec., 120, 377, 1924; Jour. Amer. Med. Assoc. 85. 213, 1925.
Pack, G. T., and Craver, L. F.: Polycythemia, Amer. Jour. Med. Sci., 180, 609, 1930.
Page, L.: War gas, Jour. Amer. Med. Assoc., 79, 259, 1922.
Pagniez and Widal: Asthma, Presse méd., 28, 65, 1920.
Paine, J. R., et al.: Agranulocytosis, Jour. Amer. Med. Assoc., 100, 1910, 1933.
Palmer, R. S.: Essential hypertension, Amer. Jour. Med. Sci., 184, 473, 1932.
Palmer, R. S., et al.: Essential hypertension, New England Med. Jour., 201, 709, 1929.
Palmer, W. W.: Obesity, Nelson Loose-Leaf Med., 3, 116.
Papegaaij, J., and Rinsema, P. G.: Syphilis, Nederl. Tijdschr. v. Geneesk., 65, Pt. 2, 560, 1921.
Parade, G. W., and Voit, K.: Stokes-Adams disease, Deutsch. med. Wchnschr., 55, 179, 1929; ibid., 57, 611, 1931.
Pardee, H. E. B.: Heart failure, Jour. Amer. Med. Assoc., 73, 1822, 1919; ibid., 75, 1258. 1920.
Pardo-Castello, V.: Syphilis, Jour. Amer. Med. Assoc., 76, 397, 1921.

Park, W. H.: Toxin-antitoxin, Jour. Amer. Med. Assoc., 79, 1584, 1922. Antitoxin reactions, Jour. Amer. Med. Assoc., 76, 109, 1921. Scarlet fever, Jour. Amer. Med. Assoc., 85, 1180, 1925. Diphtheria, Child Health Bul., Amer. Child. Health Assoc., 6, 73, 1930; Amer. Jour. Dis. Child., 42, 1439, 1931.
Park, W. H., and Freeman, R. G.: Measles, Jour. Amer. Med. Assoc., 87, 556, 1926.
Park, W. H., and Schroder, M. C.: Diphtheria, Amer. Jour. Pub. Health, 22, 7, 1932.
Park, W. H., Bullowa, J. G. M., and Rosenblüth, M. B.: Pneumonia, Jour. Amer. Med. Assoc., 91, 1503, 1928.
Park, W. K.: BCG, Jour. Amer. Med. Assoc., 96, 290, 1931.
Parker, R. R.: Rocky Mountain spotted fever, Arch. Path., 15, 398, 1933.
Parkhurst, H. J.: Acne, Arch. Dermat. and Syph., 25, 213, 1932.
Parkinson, J., and Bedford, D. E.: Arhythmia, Quart. Jour. Med., 21, 21, 1927.
Parkinson, J., and Campbell, M.: Auricular fibrillation, Quart. Jour. Med., 22, 289, 1928-1929.
Parkinson, J., and Nicholl, J. W.: Paroxysmal tachycardia, Lancet, 2, 1267, 1922.
Parounagian, M. B.: Syphilis, Jour. Amer. Med. Assoc., 77, 1706, 1921.
Parsonnet, A. E., and Hyman, A. S.: Stokes-Adams disease, Amer. Jour. Med. Sci., 180, 356, 1930. Diabetes mellitus, Ann. Int. Med., 4, 1247, 1931.
Parsons, L. G.: Anemia, Jour. Amer. Med. Assoc., 97, 973, 1931.
Patch, F. S., and Blew, C. L.: Granuloma inguinale, Canad. Med. Assoc. Jour., 23, 637, 1930.
Patterson, W. G., and Switzer, S. R. L.: Syphilis, Lancet, 2, 348, 1930.
Pattison, C. L.: Tuberculosis, Brit. Med. Jour., 1930, 2, 178.
Payne, G. C., and Armstrong, C.: Epidemic pleurodynia, Jour. Amer. Med. Assoc., 81, 746, 1926.
Peacock: Trench fever (delousing), Jour. Roy. Army Med. Corps., July, 1916.
Pearce, L.: Trypanosomiasis, Jour. Exper. Med., 34, 1921 (Supplement); Proc. Amer. Soc. Pharm. and Exper. Ther., 1924; Rockefeller Inst. Med. Res., Monograph No. 23, 1930.
Pearcy, J. F., and Hayden, D. B.: Seasickness, Jour. Amer. Med. Assoc., 90, 1193, 1928.
Peckham, C. H.: Diabetes mellitus, Bull. Johns Hopkins Hosp., 49, 184, 1931.
Peers, R. A., and Shipman, S. J.: Tuberculosis, Jour. Amer. Med. Assoc., 79, 461, 1922.
Pellini, E. J.: Heart failure, Jour. Amer. Med. Assoc., 76, 774, 1921.
Pelouze, P. S.: Gonorrhea, Jour. Amer. Med. Assoc., 84, 696, 1925.
Pemberton, J. de J.: Purpura, Ann. Surg., 755, October, 1931.
Pemberton, R.: Nephritis, Handbook Physical Therapy, Amer. Med. Assoc., 1932.
Pepper, O. H. P.: Agranulocytosis, California and West. Med., 35, 83, 173, 1931; Jour. Amer. Med. Assoc., 97, 1100, 1931.
Perkins, C. T.: Syphilis, New England Jour. Med., 205, 374, 1931.
Perkins, R. G.: Scarlet fever, Jour. Amer. Med. Assoc., 89, 1239, 1927. Obesity, Pub. Health Rep., 34, 2335, 1919.
Perla, D.: Thrombo-angiitis obliterans, Jour. Amer. Med. Assoc., 84, 1557, 1925.
Permin, G. E.: Tuberculosis, Acta Tuberc. Scandinav., 1, 89, 1925.
Perry, C. B.: Rheumatic fever, Lancet, 1, 861, 1933.
Perry, J. C.: Rocky Mountain spotted fever, California and West. Med., October, 1928.
Pershing, H. T.: Epilepsy, Jour. Amer. Med. Assoc., 69, 869, 1917.
Peshkin, M. M., and Fineman, A. H.: Asthma, Amer. Jour. Dis. Child., 39, 1240, 1930.
Peterman, M. G.: Epilepsy, Amer. Jour. Dis. Child., 28, 28, 1924; Jour. Amer. Med. Assoc., 84, 1979, 1925; ibid., 88, 1868, 1927; ibid., 90, 1427, 1928; ibid., 97, 703, 1931; Wisconsin Med. Jour., March, 1932. Measles, Amer. Jour. Dis. Child., 36, 123, 1928; ibid., 39, 294, 1930.
Peters, J. P., and Bulger, H. A.: Nephritis, Arch. Int. Med., 37, 153, 1926.
Peters, J. P., and Eiserson, L.: Nephritis, Jour. Biol. Chem., 84, 155, 1929.
Petersen, W. F., and Levinson, S. A.: Pneumonia, Jour. Amer. Med. Assoc., 78, 257, 1922.
Petren: Diabetes mellitus, Verhand. d. 34 Kong. d. Deut. Gesell. f. inn. Med., 1922; Acta Med. Scandinav., Suppl. 3, 101, 112; Verd. v. Stoff.-Krank., 8, 5, 1923; Jour. Metab. Res., 5, 1, 1924; Erg. d. inn. Med. u. Kind., 28, 92 1925; Handbuch de. Gesam. Therap., G. Fischer, Jena, 1, 827, 1926; Verd. v. Stoff.-Krank., 8, 2, 1927.
Petroff, S. A.: BCG, Amer. Rev. Tuberc., 20, 275, 1929; Jour. Amer. Med. Assoc., 96, 58, 1931.
Petroff, S. A., Branch, A., and Steenken, W., Jr.: BCG, Proc. Soc. Exper. Biol. and Med., 25, 14, 1927; Amer. Rev. Tuberc., 19, 79, 1929.
Petrowych, A: Flagellate dysentery, Deutsch. med. Wchnschr., Nr. 23, 975, 1931.
Pettey, G. E.: Addiction, Memphis Med. Month., July, 1909; Texas State Jour. Med., June, 1910; New York Med. Jour., Nov. 5, 1910.
Pettit, A.: Poliomyelitis, Bull. Gén. de Therap., 178, 389, 1925.
Pfahler, G. E.: Thyrotoxicosis, Radiology, 18, 879, 1932.
Pfahler, G. E., and Vastine, J. H.: Thyrotoxicosis, Amer. Jour. Roentgenol., 24, 395, 1930
Pfister, M.: Addiction, Münch. med. Wchnschr., Nr. 29, 1161, 1932.
Phelps, B. M., and Hu, C. H.: Hookworm, Jour. Amer. Med. Assoc., 82, 1254, 1924.
Phemister, D. B.: Rickets, Jour. Amer. Med. Assoc., 70, 1737, 1918.
Phemister, Miller and Bonar: Rickets, Jour. Amer. Med. Assoc., 76, 850, 1921

Pierce, N. H.: War gas, Jour. Amer. Med. Assoc., 79, 259, 1922 (discussion).
Pilcher, J.: Poisoning, Jour. Pharm., 3, 19, 1912.
Pilcher, J. D.: Eczema, Jour. Amer. Med. Assoc., 89, 110, 1927.
Pilcher, J. D., and Gerstenberger, H. J.: Chorea, Amer. Jour. Dis. Child., 40, 1239, 1930.
Pilcher, J. D., and Sollmann, T.: Gonorrhea, Jour. Lab. and Clin. Med., 9, 256, 1924; ibid., 10, 38, 1924; ibid., 10, 103, 1924.
Pillsbury, D. M.: Eczema-dermatitis, Jour. Amer. Med. Assoc., 96, 426, 1931.
Pinard, M.: Syphilis, Bull. Soc. franc. de Dermat. et de Syph., July, 1930, 933 (discussion).
Piness, G.: Hay-fever, Jour. Amer. Med. Assoc., 84, 584, 1925.
Piness, G., and Miller, H.: Asthma, Jour. Amer. Med. Assoc., 89, 515, 1927.
Pirquet, C.: BCG, Deutsch. med. Wchnschr., 54, 2118, 1928.
Pitschugin, P. I.: Malaria, Jahrb. f. Kinderheilk., 108, 347, 1925.
Pittaluga, G.: Yellow fever, Siglo Médico, 81, 221, 1928.
Place, E. H.: Scarlet fever, New England Jour. Med., 205, 225, 1931.
Plant, O. H., and Miller, G. K.: Intestinal fermentation, Jour. Pharm. and Exper. Ther., 27, 149, 1926.
Plass, E. D., and Swanson, C. N.: Obstetrical anesthesia, Jour. Amer. Med. Assoc., 87, 1716, 1926.
Platt, R.: Nephritis, Quart. Jour. Med., 23, 129, 1929.
Plaut, F., and Steiner, G.: Syphilis, Ztschr. Neurol. u. Psychiat., 53, 103, 1920.
Plummer, H. S.: Thyrotoxicosis, Jour. Amer. Med. Assoc., 80, 1955, 1923.
Polera, U., and Ranieri, G.: Peptic ulcer, Riv. di Clin. Med., 32, 607, 1931.
Polychroniades, G.: Malaria, Beihefte z. Arch. f. Schiffs.- u. Trop. Hyg., 31, 117, 1927.
Porter, W. B., and Rucker, J. E.: Gonorrhea, Jour. Amer. Med. Assoc., 92, 1513, 1929.
Pottenger, F. M.: Asthma, Amer. Jour. Med. Sci., 167, 203, 1924.
Potter, W. L.: Chancroid, Med. Jour. Australia, 2, 65, 1918.
Potts: Purpura, cited by Mason, E. L., *q. v.*
Poulsen, V.: Urinary infections, Amer. Jour. Dis. Child., 26, 56, 1923.
Poulton, *et al.*: Diabetes mellitus, Proc. Roy. Soc. Med., 24, 1291, 1930, 1931.
Power and Barrowcliff: Chaulmoogra oil, Jour. Chem. Soc., 87, 884, 1905; ibid., 91, 557, 1907.
Power and Gornall: Chaulmoogra oil, Jour. Chem. Soc., 85, 838, 1904; ibid., 85, 851, 1904.
Power, T. D.: Syphilis, Lancet, 1, 338, 1932.
Powers, G. F.: Whooping cough, Amer. Jour. Dis. Child., 30, 632, 1925.
Poynton, F. J.: Chorea, Nelson Loose-Leaf Med., 6, 399.
Prather, E. O., Jr., *et al.*: Rickets, Amer. Jour. Dis. Child., 42, 52, 1931.
Pratt, J. H.: Gout, Nelson Loose-Leaf Med., 3, 37.
Prausnitz, C.: Undulant fever, Med. Klin., 25, 135, 1929.
Pressman, J. J.: Hyperinsulinism; Glucose administration, Amer. Jour. Med. Sci., 179, 520, 1930.
Pribaum: Bacillary dysentery, Zentralbl. f. Bakteriol., 80, 33, 1918; ibid., 81, 37, 1918.
Price, J. P.: Kerosene poisoning, Jour. Amer. Med. Assoc., 99, 214, 1932.
Prodger, S. H., and Ayman, D.: Angina pectoris, Amer. Jour. Med. Sci., 184, 480, 1932.
Pupo, A.: Blastomycosis, Jour. Amer. Med. Assoc., 91, 1733, 1928 (Rio de Janeiro letter).
Pusey, W. A.: Syphilis, Jour. Amer. Med. Assoc., 64, 1961, 1915. Burns, Jour. Amer. Med. Assoc., 65, 291, 1915 (discussion). Warts, Jour. Amer. Med. Assoc., 74, 97, 1920.
Pusey, W. A., Hagner, F. R., *et al.* (Surgeon General's Comm.): Chancroid, Jour. Amer. Med. Assoc., 69, 1004, 1917.
Queoli, C., Jr., and Nelsen, M. T.: Undulant fever, Northwest Med., 31, 12, 1932.
Rabello, E., and Vernet, I.: Leprosy, Third Internat. Confer. on Leprosy, 305, 1923 (quoted by Lara, *q. v.*).
Rabinoff, S.: Chickenpox, Arch. Pediat., 32, 651, 1915.
Rabinowitch, J. M.: Diabetes, Canad. Med. Assoc. Jour., 23, 489, 1930; ibid., 26, 141, 1932.
Rabinowitz, M. A.: Rheumatic fever, Jour. Amer. Med. Assoc., 95, 1228, 1930.
Rackemann, F. M.: Hay-fever, Boston Med. and Surg. Jour., 182, 295, 1920. Asthma, Jour. Immunol., 8, 295, 1923; Jour. Lab. and Clin. Med., 12, 1185, 1927; Jour. Amer. Med. Assoc., 99, 202, 1932.
Rackemann, F. M., and Graham, L. B.: Asthma, Jour. Immunol., 8, 295, 1923.
Rafsky, H. A.: Colitis, Med. Jour. and Rec., July 1, 1931.
Rafksy, H. A., Schwartz, L., and Kruger, A. W.: Peptic ulcer, Jour. Amer. Med. Assoc., 99, 1582, 1932.
Raiziss, G. W., Severac, M., and Moetsch, J.: Syphilis, Jour. Amer. Med. Assoc., 83, 1734, 1924.
Ralli, E. P.: Diabetes mellitus, Jour. Lab. and Clin. Med., 17, 1204, 1932.
Ralli, E. P., and Brown, M. S.: Malnutrition, Med. Clin. N. A., 17, 305, 1933.
Ramirez, M. A.: Asthma, Arch. Int. Med., 42, 368, 1928.
Ramon, G.: Diphtheria, Ann. de l'Inst. Pasteur, 42, 959, 1928; ibid., 45, September, 1930.
Ramon, G., and Helie, G. I.: Diphtheria, Jour. Amer. Med. Assoc., 91, 1028, 1928.

52

Ramsay, G. C.: Yaws. Jour. Trop. Med. and Hyg., 28, 85, 1925.
Ramsdell, R. L., and Magness, W. H.: Pellagra, Amer. Jour. Med. Sci., 185, 568, 1933.
Ramsden, W., Lipkin, I. J., and Whitley, E.: Sepsis, Amer. Jour. Trop. Med., 12, 223, 1918.
Randall, A.: Granuloma inguinale, Amer. Jour. Med. Sci., 168, 728, 1924.
Ransom, B. H.: Roundworms, Nelson Loose-Leaf Med., 2, 414. Guinea worm, Nelson Loose-Leaf Med., 2, 384.
Rappaport, B.: Diphtheria, Jour. Amer. Med. Assoc., 66, 943, 1916.
Rappaport, B. Z., and Reed, C. I.: Allergy, Jour. Amer. Med. Assoc., 101, 105, 1933.
Rappaport, I.: Hypertension, Jour. Amer. Med. Assoc., 92, 1158 and 1697, 1929.
Ratner, B.: Eczema-dermatitis, Jour. Amer Med. Assoc., 97, 1291, 1931 (discussion).
Rauschkolb, J. E.: Chancroids, Arch. Dermat. and Syph., 21, 251, 1930.
Ravdin, I. S.: Cirrhosis, Jour. Amer. Med. Assoc., 93, 1193, 1929.
Ravenel, S. F.: Glucose administration, Jour. Amer. Med. Assoc., 100, 473, 1933.
Ravogli, A.: Burns, Jour. Amer. Med. Assoc., 65, 291, 1915.
Ray, H. H.: Diphtheria, Amer. Jour. Med. Sci., 182, 251, 1931.
Ray, H. H., and Cunningham, J. S.: Chorea, Amer. Jour. Dis. Child., 39, 1205, 1930.
Raynal, J.: Malaria, Bull. Soc. de path. exot., 20, 408, 1927.
Read, C. F.: Syphilis, Arch. Neurol. and Psychiat., 24, 649, 1930; Illinois Med. Jour., 59, 21, 1931.
Read, J. M.: Thyrotoxicosis, Jour. Amer. Med. Assoc., 83, 1963, 1924; ibid., 89, 493, 1927; Arch. Int. Med., 34, 553, 1924.
Reasoner, M. A.: Syphilis, Jour. Amer. Med. Assoc., 68, 973, 1917.
Reasoner, M. A., and Gill, W. D.: Vincent's angina, Jour. Amer. Med. Assoc., 88, 716, 1927.
Reddish, G. F., and Drake, W. E.: Skin disinfection, Jour. Amer. Med. Assoc., 91, 712, 1928.
Redewill, F. H.: Gonorrhea, Amer. Jour. Physiol. Ther., October, 1927.
Redewill, F H., Potter, J. E., and Garrison, H. A.: Gonorrhea, Jour. Urol., 16, 397, 1926.
Redewill, F. H., et al.: Gonorrhea, Jour. Urology, 22, 705, 1929. Urinary infection, Jour. Amer. Med. Assoc., 94, 688, 1930.
Reed, A. C.: Amebic dysentery, Jour. Amer. Med. Assoc., 98, 195 (reference 3), 1932.
Reed, A. C., Anderson, H. H., David, N. A., and Leake, C. D.: Amebic dysentery, Jour. Amer. Med. Assoc., 98, 189, 1932.
Reeves, T. B.: Peptic ulcer, Surg., Gyn., and Obst., 30, 374, 1920.
Regan, J. C.: Anthrax, Jour. Amer. Med. Assoc., 72, 1724, 1919; ibid., 77, 1944, 1921; Amer. Jour. Med. Sci., 162, 406, 1921. Mumps, Jour. Amer. Med. Assoc., 84, 279, 1925.
Regan, J. R.: Epilepsy, Wisconsin Med. Jour., 554, July, 1931.
Reid, W. D.: Heart failure, Jour. Amer. Med. Assoc., 89, 1353, 1927; ibid., 81, 435, 1923.
Reiss and Jungmann: Scarlet fever, Deutsch. Arch. f. klin. Med., 106, 70, 1912.
Reitschel, H.: Measles, Deutsch. med. Wchnschr., 49, 1386, 1923.
Remlinger, P., and Bailly, J.: BCG, Ann. de l'Inst. Pasteur, 41, 286, 1927; Canad. Jour. Res., 44, 54, 1930. Rabies, Compt. rend. Soc. de Biol., 106, 523, 1931.
Rennie, J. B.: Ketogenic diet, Arch. Dis. Child., February, 1933, p. 47.
Reznikoff, P.: Agranulocytosis, Jour. Clin. Invest., 12, 45, 1933.
Ribeyro, R. E.: Oroya fever, Reforma méd., 18, 252, 1932.
Rice, E. M.: Hookworm, Ind. Med. Gaz., 62, 126, 1927.
Richardson, G. L., and Connor, H.: Measles, Jour. Amer. Med. Assoc., 72, 1046, 1916.
Richet, C., Jr., and Couder: Food allergy, Jour. Amer. Med. Assoc. (Paris letter), 99, 573, 1932.
Richter, O., et al.: Anemia, Jour. Lab. and Clin. Med., 17, 1185, 1932. Pernicious anemia, Jour. Amer. Med. Assoc., 98, 1623, 1932.
Richter, E.: Trench fever, Ther. d. Gegenwart, N. F., 19, 89, 1917.
Riecke: Syphilis, Münch. med. Wchnschr., 66, 969, 1919.
Riehl, G.: Burns, Arch. f. Dermat. u. Syph., 153, 41, 1927.
Rienhoff, W. F., Jr.: Adenoma, Bull. Johns Hopkins Hosp., 37, 285, 1925; Arch. Surg., 13, 391, 1926.
Rienhoff, W. F., Jr., and Lewis, D.: Adenoma, Arch. Surg., 16, 79, 1928.
Rigby, H. C., and Rigby, C.: Malaria, South Carolina Med. Assoc. Jour., 25, 579, 1929.
Riggall, C.: Obstetrics, Lancet, 2, 1183, 1932.
Rilliet: Simple goiter, Bull. de l'Acad. Imperial de Méd., 24, 23, 1858–59 (cited by Kimball, O. P., q. v.).
Ritchie, E. B.: Erysipeloid, Arch. Dermat. and Syph., 23, 1069, 1931.
Ritchie, E. B., and Becker, S. W.: Erysipeloid, Jour. Amer. Med. Assoc., 95, 26, 1930.
Rittinger, F. R., and Dembo, L. H.: Food allergy, Amer. Jour. Dis. Child., 44, 1221, 1932.
Rivers, A. B., et al.: Peptic ulcer, Jour. Amer. Med. Assoc., 98, 1156, 1932.
Rivers, T. M., and Tillet, W. S.: Erysipelas, Jour. Exper. Med., 41, 185, 1925.
Rivett, L. C.: Obstetrics, Lancet, 1, 495, 1933 (annotation).
Robbins, F. W., and Seabury, F. P.: Chancroid, Jour. Amer. Med. Assoc., 69, 1217, 1917.
Roberts, E. H.: Tuberculosis, Amer. Rev. Tuberc., 9, 159, 1924.

Roberts, S. R., and Kracke, R. R.: Agranulocytosis, Jour. Amer. Med. Assoc., 95, 780, 1930; Ann. Int. Med., 5, 40, 1931.
Robertson, W.: Burns, Lancet, 1, 830, 1933.
Robinson, G. C.: Heart failure, Amer. Jour. Med. Sci., 159, 121, 1920.
Robinson, G. C., White, P. D., Eggleston, C., and Hatcher, R. A.: Heart failure, Jour. Amer. Med. Assoc., 83, 504, 1924.
Robinson, L. F.: Epilepsy, Jour. Amer. Med. Assoc., 67, 1522, 1916.
Roch, M.: Poisoning, Merck's Rep., 21, 45, 1907 (cited by Sollmann, T., *q. v.*).
Rodriguez, J.: Leprosy, Phil. Is. Med. Assoc., Jour., 5, 40, 1925.
Roehl, W.: Malaria, Beihefte z. Arch. f. Schiffs.- u. Trop. Hyg., 30, 311, 1926; ibid., 31, 48, 1927.
Rogers, L.: Leprosy, Lancet, 1, 288, 1916; ibid., 2, 682, 1917; Ind. Jour. Med. Res., 5, 277, 1917; Brit. Med. Jour., 1, 147, 1919; Ind. Med. Gaz., 55, 125, 1920; Jour. Amer. Med. Assoc., 86, 637, 1926. Sprue, Bowel Diseases in the Tropics, London, Oxford Medical Publications, 1921.
Rogers, L., and Muir, E.: Leprosy, London, Wm. Wood and Co., 1925.
Ronaldson, G. W., and Collier, J. I.: Measles, Brit. Med. Jour., 2, 994, 1930.
Ronnefeldt, F.: Malaria, Münch. med. Wchnschr., 6, 240, 1931.
Root, H. F., and Graybiel, A.: Diabetes mellitus, Jour. Amer. Med. Assoc., 96, 925, 1931.
Rosen, P. S., and Korobicina, L. A.: Scarlet fever, Jour. Amer. Med. Assoc., 84, 1476, 1925.
Rosenberg, D. H., and Bloch, L.: Peptic ulcer, Jour. Lab. and Clin. Med., 18, 1041, 1933.
Rosenblüth, M. B., and Block, M.: Pneumonia, Jour. Amer. Med. Assoc., 98, 396, 1932.
Rosener, L. A.: Anthrax, Sovets. Klin., 15, 122, 1931.
Rosenfeld: BCG, Wien. klin. Wchnschr., 41, 800, 1928.
Rosenow, E. C.: Peptic ulcer, Surg., Gyn., and Obst., 33, 19, 1921. Poliomyelitis, Jour. Amer. Med. Assoc., 94, 777, 1930.
Rosenthal and Behrendt: Diabetes mellitus, Ztschr. f. d. ges. exp. Med., 53, 562, 1926.
Rosenwald, L.: Chancroid, Urologic and Cutaneous Rev., 27, 553, 1923.
Rost: Syphilis, Arch. f. Dermat. u. Syph., 138, 89, 1922.
Rothwell, J. J., and Maloney, E. R.: Syphilis, Amer. Jour. Syph., 9, 413, 1925.
Rougebief, H.: BCG, Ann. de l'Inst. Pasteur., 41, 282, 1927.
Rowe, A. H.: Food allergy, Jour. Amer. Med. Assoc., 91, 1623, 1928; ibid., 97, 1440, 1931; ibid., 99, 912, 1932. Allergic migraine, Jour. Amer. Med. Assoc., 99, 912, 1932.
Rowntree, L. G.: Diabetes insipidus, Jour. Amer. Med. Assoc., 83, 399, 1924. Cirrhosis, Jour. Amer. Med. Assoc., 89, 1590, 1927.
Rowntree, L. G., and Brown, G. E.: Asthma, Endocrinology, 10, 301, 1926.
Rowntree, L. G., Keith, N. M., and Barrier, C. W.: Cirrhosis, Jour. Amer. Med. Assoc., 85, 1187, 1925.
Royer, E. R.: Hookworm, Jour. Amer. Med. Assoc., 75, 1702, 1920.
Rubin, E. H.: Tuberculosis, Amer. Rev. Tuberc., 25, 490, 1932.
Rucker, M. P., and Haskell, C. C.: Pituitrin in labor, Jour. Amer. Med. Assoc., 76, 1390, 1921.
Ruggles, E. W.: Herpes Zoster, Arch. Dermat. and Syph., 23, 472, 1931.
Ruh, H. O., and Hanzlik, P. J.: Urinary infections, Jour. Amer. Med. Assoc., 79, 1980, 1922.
Ruhräh, J.: Hiccup, Jour. Amer. Med. Assoc., 84, 698, 1925.
Rupel, E.: Gonorrhea, Jour. Amer. Med. Assoc., 80, 530, 1923; Jour. Indiana State Med. Assoc., 18, 89, 1925. Chancroid, Jour. Amer. Med. Assoc., 86, 544, 1926.
Rupprecht: Diabetes mellitus, Arch. f. Kinderhlk., 82, 66, 1927.
Russell, F. F.: Typhoid, Nelson Loose-Leaf Med., 1, 53.
Rutschko, I. E., and Melnik, M. I.: Typhoid, Münch. med. Wchnschr., 34, 1355, 1932.
Sabbatani, L.: Poisoning, Gaz. Osp. Clin., 33, No. 58, 1913 (cited by Sollmann, T., Manual of Pharmacology, 4th Ed., Phila., W. B. Saunders Co., 1932, p. 909.)
Sack, W. T.: Eczema-dermatitis, Dermat. Wchnschr., 84, 16, 1927.
Sadler, *et al.*: Induction of labor, Jour. Obst. and Gyn. Brit. Emp., 37, 529, 1930.
Sáenz, B.: Lupus erythematosus, Vida Nueva, 21, 75, 1928.
Sagal, Z.: Constipation, Jour. Amer. Med. Assoc., 88, 1502, 1927.
Sagel, W.: Syphilis, Ztschr. f. d. ges. Neurol. u. Psychiat., 137, 11, 1931.
Saha, B.: Kala-azar, Calcutta Med. Jour., 25, 335, 1931.
Sakel: Addiction, Deutsch. med. Wchnschr., 56, 1777, 1930.
Salant, W.: Hookworm, Jour. Amer. Med. Assoc., 69, 2016, 1917.
Salvesen, H. A.: Tetany, Acta med. Scandinav., 1923, Supplement 6, pp. 1–159. Nephritis, Acta Med. Scandinav., 65, 152, 1926.
Salzer, B. F.: Trichinosis, Jour. Amer. Med. Assoc., 67, 579, 1916.
Sampson, J. J., and Anderson, E. M.: Arrythmia, Jour. Amer. Med. Assoc., 99, 2257, 1932.
Sanders, J. P.: Malaria, Jour. Amer. Med. Assoc., 97, 850, 1931; ibid., 99, 1773, 1932.
Sanders, J. P., and Dawson, W. T.: Malaria, Jour. Amer. Med. Assoc., 99, 1773, 1932.
Sanderson, W., Capon, N. B., and MacWilliam, H. H.: Sepsis, Lancet, 2, 12, 1927.
Sanford, H. N.: Syphilis, Jour. Amer. Med. Assoc., 85, 242, 1925. Obstetrical anesthesia, Jour. Amer. Med. Assoc., 86, 265, 1926.

Sanford, H. N., and Heitmeyer, P. L.: Glucose administration. Jour. Amer. Med. Assoc., 90, 737, 1928.

Sanger, B. J.: Thyrotoxicosis, Arch. Int. Med., 37, 627, 1926.

Sansum, W. D.: Obesity, California and West. Med., 29, 42, 1928. Diabetes mellitus, Colorado Med., October, 1927; Treatment of Diabetes Mellitus, Phila., Lea and Febiger, 1930.

Sansum, W. D., Blatherwick, N. R., and Bowden, R.: Diabetes mellitus, Jour. Amer. Med. Assoc., 86, 178, 1926.

Sargant, W.: Pernicious anemia, Lancet, 1, 230, 1932.

Sauer, L. W.: Whooping cough, Jour. Pediat., 2, 740, 1933; Jour. Amer. Med. Assoc., 100, 239, 1933. Pylorospasm, Amer. Jour. Dis. Child., 22, 166, 1921.

Saunders, J. C.: Diphtheria, Lancet, 2, 1047, 1932.

Savchenko: Scarlet fever, Russk. Vrach., 1905, No. 25, p. 797.

Sawyer, W. A.: Yellow fever, South. Med. Jour., 25, 291, 1932.

Sawyer, W. A., et al.: Yellow fever, Proc. Soc. Exper. Biol. and Med., 29, 62, 1931.

Saxl, P., and Heilig, R.: Heart failure, Wien. klin. Wchnschr., 33, 943, 1920.

Saxtorph: Tuberculosis, Ugeskr. f. Laeger, 80, 1763, 1918.

Saye, L., Domingo, P., and Miralbell, M.: BCG, Res. de la Tuberc., 8, 668, 1927.

Sazerac, R., and Levaditi, C.: Syphilis, Compt. rend. Acad. d. sc., Paris, 172, 1391, 1921; ibid., 173, 338, 1921.

Scales, H. L.: Pneumonia, Jour. Amer. Med. Assoc., April 16, 1932.

Sceleth, C. E.: Addiction, Jour. Amer. Med. Assoc., 66, 860, 1916.

Sceleth, C. E., and Kuh, S.: Addiction, Jour. Amer. Med. Assoc., 82, 679, 1924.

Schamberg, J. F.: Smallpox, Nelson Loose-Leaf Med., 1, 486. Chickenpox, Nelson's Med. Service, 595, May, 1927. Syphilis, Jour. Amer. Med. Assoc., 97, 1523, 1931 (discussion).

Schamberg, J. F., and Wright, C. S.: Lupus erythematosus, Arch. Dermat. and Syph., 15, 119, 1927.

Schelm, G. W.: Syphilis, U. S. Vet. Bur. Med. Bull., 6, 544, 1930.

Schenk, E.: Encephalitis, Münch. med. Wchnschr., Nr. 28, 1177, 1931.

Schereschewsky, J. W.: Heat stroke, Nelson Loose-Leaf Med., 2, 651.

Scherf, D.: Diabetes insipidus, Wien. Arch. f. inners med., 7, 15, 1932.

Schick, B., and Topper, A.: Diphtheria, Amer. Jour. Dis. Child., 38, 929, 1929; Ann. de Méd., 29, 628, 1931.

Schick, B., et al.: Chorea, Amer. Jour. Dis. Child., 45, 1216, 1933.

Schiff, E.: Nephritis, Jahrb. f. Kinderh., October, 1932, p. 1.

Schiff, N. S.: Asthma, Amer. Jour. Med. Sci., 166, 664, 1923. Hay-fever, Ann. Clin. Med. 5, 374, 1926.

Schilling, G. S., et al.: Undulant fever, Jour. Amer. Med. Assoc., 96, 1945, 1931.

Shilling and Jossmann: Blackwater fever, Klin. Wchnschr., 3, 149, 1924.

Schlesinger, H.: Sciatica, Münch. med. Wchnschr., Nr. 31, 1300, 1931. Syphilis, Münch. med. Wchnschr., 78, 1300, 1931.

Schloss, O.: Worms, Amer. Jour. Med. Sci., 139, 675, 1910. Hay-fever, Amer. Jour. Dis. Child., 19, 433, 1920.

Schlossmann: BCG, Deutsch. med. Wchnschr., 54, 1871, 1928.

Schmal: Chorea, Deutsch. med. Wchnschr., 51, 1439, 1925.

Schmitter, F.: Sprue, Jour. Amer. Med. Assoc., 64, 53, 1915.

Schnell, W.: Lice, Deutsch. med. Wchnschr., 47, 1254, 1921.

Schottmüller, H.: Rheumatic fever, Münch. med. Wchnschr., 74, 861, 1927; 76, 499, 1929.

Schowalter, R. P.: Whooping cough, Amer. Jour. Dis. Child., 39, 544, 1930.

Schreiber: Bacillary dysentery, Med. Klin., 27, 1445, 1931.

Schrijner, J.: Peptic ulcer, Nederl. Tijdschr. v. Geneesk., 2, 1757, 1925; Jour. Amer. Med. Assoc. (abstract), 85, 1848, 1925.

Schüffner, W.: Blackwater fever, Trop. Dis. Bull., 29, 342, 1932 (abstract).

Schulemann, W., and Memmi, G.: Malaria, Beihefte z. Arch. f. Schiffs.- u. Trop. Hyg., 31, 59, 1927; Klin. Wchnschr., 6, 1093, 1927.

Schulemann, W., Schönhöfer, F., and Wingler, A.: Malaria, Abhandl. a. d. Gebiet d. Auslandskunde, Hamburg Univ., 26, 507, 1927.

Schultz, E. W.: Urinary infection, California and West. Med., 36, No. 1, January, 1932; ibid., 36, No. 2, February, 1932.

Schultz, E. W., and Gebhardt, L. P.: Poliomyelitis, Proc. Soc. Exper. Biol. and Med., 28, 412, 1931.

Schultz, E. W., and Marx, A.: Hookworm, Amer. Jour. Trop. Med., 4, 469, 1924.

Schultz, M. P.: Rheumatic fever, Arch. Int. Med., 48, 1138, 1931.

Schultz, W.: Agranulocytosis, Deutsch. med. Wchnschr., 48, 1494, 1922.

Schultz, W., and Charlton, W.: Scarlet fever, Ztschr. f. Kinderhlk., 17, 328, 1918.

Schultzer, P.: Scurvy, Lancet, 2, 589, 1933.

Schulze: Syphilis, Deutsch. med. Wchnschr., 51, 1856, 1925.

Schussler, H., Jr.: Varicose veins, Jour. Amer. Med. Assoc., 88, 1983, 1927; ibid., 90 1358, 1928; also a personal communication, 1933.

Schwab, S. I., and Cady, L. D.: Syphilis, Amer. Jour. Syph., 11, 1, 1927.
Schwartz, A.: Syphilis, Ann. de l'Inst. Pasteur, Paris, 45, 386, 1930.
Schwartz, A. B., and Janney, F. R.: Diphtheria, Amer. Jour. Dis. Child., 39, 504, 1930; Wisconsin Med. Jour., 30, 719, 1931.
Schwartz, B.: Trichinosis, Jour. Amer. Med. Assoc., 69, 884, 1917.
Schwartz, N.: Anthrax, New York Med. Jour., 107, 1171, 1918.
Schwartz, S. P., and Jezer, A.: Stokes-Adams disease, Amer. Heart Jour., 7, 652, 1932.
Schwarzmann, J. S.: Angina pectoris, Münch. med. Wchnschr., 35, 1463, 1931.
Schwentker, F. F.: Glucose, Amer. Jour. Dis. Child., 40, 533, 1930.
Schwentker, F. F., and Noel, W. W.: Diph theria, Bull. Johns Hopkins Hosp., 45, 259, 1929; ibid., 46, 359, 1930.
Sclavo: Anthrax, Commun. au VI Congr de la Soc. Ital. de Méd. intern. à Rome, 1895.
Scott, H. H.: Sprue, Trans. Roy. Soc. Trop. Med. and Hyg., February 15, 1923.
Scott, L. C.: Dengue, Jour. Amer. Med. Assoc., 80, 387, 1923.
Scott, L. C., and Herrmann, G. R.: Beriberi, Jour. Amer. Med. Assoc., 90, 2083, 1928.
Scott, W. W., and Birkhaug, K. E.: Skin disinfection, Ann. Surg., 587, February, 1931.
Scott, W. W., and Hill, J. H.: Skin disinfection, Jour. Urol., 14, 135, 1925; Internat. S. Digest, 3, 195, 1927; Jour. Amer. Med. Assoc., 92, 111, 1929.
Scriver, W. de M.: Pylorospasm, Canad. Med. Assoc. Jour., 24, 99, 1931.
Seeger, S. J.: Burns, Surg., Gyn., and Obst., 55, 455, 1932; Wisconsin Med. Jour., 755, November, 1932.
Seides, S.: Pituitrin in labor, Surg., Gyn., and Obst., 36, 108, 1923.
Selinger, J.: Peptic ulcer, Ann. Surg., 96, 204, 1932.
Sellards, A. W.: Asiatic cholera, Cecil's Textbook of Medicine, Phila., W. B. Saunders Co., 1933, p. 273.
Sellards, A. W., and Goodpasture, E. W.: Yaws, Phil. Jour. Sci., 22, 285, 1923.
Sellheim, A.: Seasickness, Jour. Amer. Med. Assoc., 90, 1381, 1928 (Ed. comment).
Selling, L.: Leukemia, Bull. Johns Hopkins Hosp., 21, 33, 1910.
Senear, F. E., and Cornblett, T.: Granuloma inguinale, Arch Dermat. and Syph., 25, 167, 1932.
Senftner and Coughlin: Typhoid fever, Amer. Jour. Hyg., 17, 711, 1933.
Serbinow, P. I., and Schulmann, E. S.: Pinworms, Arch. f. Schiffs.- u. Trop. Hyg., 31, 482, 1927.
Seward, B. T.: Hypertension, Virginia Med. Month., 59, 391, 1932.
Sgalitzer: Polycythemia, Jour. Amer. Med. Assoc., 99, 237, 1932 (Vienna letter).
Shaffer, P. A : Diabetes mellitus, Jour. Biol. Chem., 46, 6, 1921; ibid., 47, 449, 1921; ibid., 49, 143, 1921; ibid., 54, 399, 1922; Med., 2, 375, 1923; also Harvey Lectures, 1922.
Shallenberger, W. F.: Sepsis, Surg., Gyn., and Obst., 39, 291, 1924.
Shapiro, S.: Encephalitis, Jour. Neurol. and Mental Dis., 68, 488, 1928.
Shattuck, G. C.: Liver flukes, Amer. Jour. Trop. Med., 4, 507, 1924.
Shattuck, H. F., Rohdenburg, E. L., and Booker, L. E.: Peptic ulcer, Jour. Amer. Med. Assoc., 82, 200, 1924.
Shaughnessy, H. J., Harmon, P. H., and Gordon, F. B.: Poliomyelitis, Jour. Exper. Med., 4, 463, 1930.
Shaw, E. B., and Thelander, H. E.: Poliomyelitis, Jour. Amer. Med. Assoc., 90, 1923, 1928.
Shaw, E. B., Thelander, H. E., and Fleishner, E. C.: Poliomyelitis, Jour. Amer. Med. Assoc., 85, 1555, 1925.
Sheer, K.: Tetany, Jahrb. f. Kinderh., 97, 130, 1922.
Shelling, D. H.: Tetany, Amer. Jour. Dis. Child., 44, 1071, 1932.
Shelmire, B.: Acne, Jour. Amer. Med. Assoc., 90, 1869, 1928.
Shepard, C. A., and Fleming, W. D.: Sprue, Amer. Jour. Trop. Med., 6, 443, 1926.
Sherman, H. C.: Nephritis, Chemistry of Food and Nutrition, ed. 3, New York, Macmillan Company, 1930, p. 271.
Sherrill: Diabetes mellitus, Jour. Metab. Res., 3, 59, 1923.
Shirer, J. W.: Thyrotoxicosis, Amer. Jour. Med. Sci., 185, 73, 1933.
Shivers, C. H. de T.: Gonorrhea, Jour. Urol., 8, 35, 1922. Syphilis, Arch. Dermat. and Syph., 22, 462, 1930.
Sicard, J. A.: Varicose veins, Marseille méd., No. 3, 67, 1920; Gaz. d. Hôp., 95, 1573, 1922.
Sicard, J. A., and Gaugier, L.: Varicose veins, Le Traitement des Varices par les Injections Locale Sclerosantes, Paris, Masson et Cie, 1927.
Sicard, J. A., Paraf, J., and Forestier, J.: Varicose veins, Jour. méd. franç., 10, 45, 1921.
Sicé, A.: Trypanosomiasis, Bull. Soc. de path. exot., 24, 5, 1931; Ann. de l'Inst. Pasteur, 45, 221, 1930.
Siddall, R. S.: Preparation of vulva, Surg., Gyn., and Obst., 40, 281, 1925.
Sidlick, D. M.: Herpes zoster, Arch. Dermat. and Syph., 22, 91, 1930.
Siegel, A. E., and Ermann, H.: Measles, Amer. Jour. Med. Sci., 179, 192, 1930.
Sielmann, R.: Thyrotoxicosis, Münch. med. Wchnschr., Nr. 33, August 12, 1932, p. 1314.
Sigwald, J.: Hyperinsulinism, L'Hypoglycémie, Paris, 1932.
Silberstein, S.: Syphilis, Arch. f. Dermat. u. Syph., 143, 334, 1923.
Silbert, S.: Thromboangiitis obliterans, Jour. Amer. Med. Assoc., 86, 1759, 1926; ibid., 89, 964, 1927; ibid., 94, 1730, 1930.

Siler, J. F., Hall, M. W., and Hitchens, A. P.: Dengue, Jour. Amer. Med. Assoc., 84, 1163, 1925.

Silverman, I.: Varicose veins, Jour. Amer. Med. Assoc., 97, 177, 1931.

Simmons, J. S.: Skin disinfection, Jour. Amer. Med. Assoc., 91, 704, 1928.

Simmons, J. S., St. John, J. H., and Reynolds, F. H. K.: Experimental Studies in Dengue, Bureau of Printing, Manila, 1931.

Simonds, J. P.: Nephritis, Jour. Amer. Med. Assoc., 98, 803, 1932.

Simpson, C. W.: Obstetrical anesthesia, Jour. Amer. Med. Assoc., 67, 559, 1916 (discussion).

Simpson, V. E.: Nephritis, Kentucky Med. Jour., July, 1931.

Simpson, W. M.: Undulant fever, Ann. Int. Med., 4, 238, 1930; Ohio State Med. Jour., 27, 21, 1931; U. S. Nav. Med. Bull., 29, 581, 1931.

Sinderson, H. C.: Oriental sore, Trans. Roy. Soc. Trop. Med. and Hyg., 19, 232, 1925.

Singer and Winterberg: Paroxysmal tachycardia, Wien. Arch. f. innere med., 3, 229, 1922.

Sinton, J. A.: Malaria, Ind. Jour. Med. Res., 15, 287, 1927; Ind. Med. Gaz., 65, 603, 1930.

Sinton, J. A., and Bird, W.: Malaria, Ind. Jour. Med. Res., 16, 159, 1928.

Sinton, J. A., Smith, S., and Pottinger, D.: Malaria, Ind. Jour. Med. Res., 17, 793, 1930.

Sioli, F.: Malaria, Arch. f. Schiffs.- u. Trop. Hyg., 30, 319, 1926.

Sippy, B. W.: Peptic ulcer, Jour. Amer. Med. Assoc., 64, 1625, 1915.

Skeel, A. J.: Obstetrical anesthesia, Jour. Amer. Med. Assoc., 66, 797, 1916.

Skrotskiy, A. I.: Mumps, Odessky Med. Jour., 4, 8, 1929.

Sliwensky, M.: Malaria, Beihefte z. Arch. f. Schiffs.- u. Trop. Hyg., 31, 129, 1927.

Small, J. C.: Epidemic pleurodynia, Amer. Jour. Med. Sci., 168, 571, 1924; Cecil's Textbook of Medicine, Phila., W. B. Saunders Co., 1933, p. 415. Rheumatic fever, Amer Jour. Med. Sci., 173, 101, 1927.

Smillie, W. G.: Hookworm, Jour. Amer. Med. Assoc., 74, 1503, 1920. Pin and whip worms, Jour. Amer. Med. Assoc., 88, 1747, 1927.

Smillie, W. G., and Pessoa, S. B.: Hookworm, Amer. Jour. Hyg., 3, 35, 1923.

Smillie, W. G, and Augustine, D. L.: Hookworm, Jour. Amer. Med. Assoc., 85, 1958, 1925; Amer. Jour. Dis. Child., 31, 151, 1926.

Smith, A. G., and Rudolf, R. D.: Hypertension, Canad. Med. Assoc. Jour., 19, 282, 1928.

Smith, A. H.: Gout, Jour. Lab. and Clin. Med., 7, 473, 1922.

Smith, C., and Leighton, W. E.: Tetanus, Amer. Jour. Med. Sci., 168, 852, 1924.

Smith, D. T.: Vincent's angina, Jour. Amer. Med. Assoc., 94, 23, 1930.

Smith, D. T., and McConkey, M.: Peptic ulcer, Arch. Int. Med., 51, 413, 1933.

Smith, F. B.: Breast abscess, Amer. Jour. Obst. and Gyn., 24, 123, 1932.

Smith, F. H.: Leukemia, Jour. Amer. Med. Assoc., 64, 1734, 1915.

Smith, F. L.: Varicose veins, Jour. Amer. Med. Assoc., 99, 2008, 1932.

Smith, J. H.: Pellagra, Arch. Int. Med., 48, 907, 1931.

Smith, K. S.: Angina pectoris, Brit. Med. Jour., April 22, 1933; Lancet, 1, 632, 1933.

Smith, L. W, Bowditch, H. I., Leonard, R. D., Emerson, P. W., Wyman, E. T., Barron, E. W., Green, H., Hubbard, E., and Tennis, M.: Whooping cough, Jour. Amer. Med. Assoc., 85, 171, 1925.

Smith, M. I.: Tuberculosis, Amer. Rev. Tuberc., 7, 33, 1923.

Smith, W. A.: Hay-fever, Mil. Surg., 61, 560, 1927.

Smithies, F.: Flagellate dysentery, Amer. Jour. Med. Sci., 156, 173, 1918. Peptic ulcer, Jour. Amer. Med. Assoc., 85, 674, 1925; ibid., 97, 774, 1931 (discussion).

Smorodintsev: Kala-azar, Kazan Med. Jour., 1926.

Smyly, H. J.: Bacillary dysentery, Cecil's Textbook of Medicine, Phila., W. B. Saunders Co., 1933, p. 169. Kala-azar, Ann. Trop. Med. and Parasitol., 21, 171, 1927.

Smyth, F. S., et al.: Eczema-dermatitis, Jour. Amer. Med. Assoc., 97, 1291, 1931.

Snapper, I., and du Preez, J. D. G.: Pernicious anemia, Arch. Int. Med., 47, 771, 1931.

Snell, A. M.: Cirrhosis, Ann. Int. Med., 5, 338, 1931. Tetany, Med. Clin. N. A., 15, 1593, 1932.

Snell, A. M., and Keyes, H. C.: Cirrhosis, Med. Clin. N. A., 16, 1455, 1933.

Snell, A. M., and Rowntree, L. G.: Diabetes mellitus, Endocrinology, 11, 209, 1927.

Soldin, M.: Chickenpox, Med. Klin., 19, 579, 1923.

Solis-Cohen, S.: Gout, Jour. Amer. Med. Assoc., 63, 945, 1914 (discussion). Pneumonia, Ann. Clin. Med., 2, 90, 1923.

Solis-Cohen and Githens: Tuberculosis, Pharmacotherapeutics, New York, D. Appleton, 1928.

Sollmann, T.: Burns, Jour. Amer. Med. Assoc., 68, 1799, 1917; ibid., 68, 1895, 1917; ibid., 72, 992, 1919. Epilepsy, Syphilis, Aspidium, Morphine poisoning, Manual of Pharmacology, 4th ed., Phila., W. B. Saunders Co., 1932.

Sollmann, T., Barlow, O. W., and Biskind, M. S.: Poisoning, Jour. Amer. Med. Assoc., 88, 623, 1927.

Solomon, H. C., Berk, A., Theiler, M., and Clay, C. L.: Syphilis, Arch. Int. Med., 38, 391, 1926.

Solomons, B.: Eclampsia, Amer. Jour. Obst. and Gyn., 25, 172, 1933.

Sonnenberg: Syphilis, Derm. Wchnschr., 85, 1638, 1925.

Sooy, J. W., and Moise, T. S.: Purpura, Jour. Amer. Med. Assoc., 87, 94, 1926.

Soper, F. L.: Hookworm, Amer. Jour. Hyg., 5, 402, 1925.
Soper, H. W.: Gallbladder disease, Amer. Jour. Med. Sci., 169, 398, 1925. Peptic ulcer, Jour. Amer. Med. Assoc., 97, 771, 1931. Colitis, Jour. Amer. Med. Assoc., 98, 1677, 1932.
Sorge, G.: Flagellate dysentery, Policlinico., 38, 156, 1931.
Soskin, S., *et al.*: Diabetes mellitus, Amer. Jour. Med. Sci., 182, 675, 1931.
Spach, A. B.: Angina pectoris, Illinois Med. Jour., 39, 28, 1921.
Speidel, E.: Eclampsia, Amer. Jour. Obst. and Gyn., 9, 320, 1925.
Speidel, F. G.: Pylorospasm, Kentucky State Med. Jour., 21, 512, 1923; also personal communication to the author. Diabetes, Kentucky State Med. Jour , April, 1930.
Spence, H. D. L.: Syphilis, Lancet, 1927, 2, 379.
Spencer, H. J.: Measles, Jour. Amer. Med. Assoc., 89, 1662, 1927.
Spicer, S.: Diphtheria, Jour. Amer. Med. Assoc., 90, 1778, 1928.
Spiegel, L.: Syphilis, Arch. Dermat. and Syph., 23, 266, 1931.
Spiethof: Syphilis, Med. Klin., 21, 1839, 1925.
Spiro, H., and Newman, W. W.: Arhythmia, Jour. Amer. Med. Assoc., 91, 1268, 1928.
Sprague, H. B., and White, P. D.: Paroxysmal tachycardia, Boston Med. and Surg. Jour. 193, 91, 1925; Med. Clin. N. A., 161, 895, 1933.
Sprunt, D. H.: Nephritis, Arch. Int. Med., 46, 494, 1930.
Stander, H. J.: Eclampsia, Amer. Jour. Obst. and Gyn., 13, 5, 1927.
Stander, H. J., and Eastman, N. J.: Eclampsia, Amer. Jour. Obst. and Gyn., 20, 822, 1930.
Stander, H. J., *et al.*: Eclampsia, Amer. Jour. Obst. and Gyn., 19, 26, 1930.
Starling, E. H.: Nephritis, Jour. Physiol., 19, 312, 1895.
Starr, I.: Tachycardia, Amer. Jour. Med. Sci., 186, 330, 1933.
Starr, P., and Gardner, L.: Sprue, Amer. Jour. Trop. Med., 10, 283, 1930.
Stealy, C. L.: Polycythemia, Jour. Amer. Med. Assoc., 98, 1714, 1932.
Stecher, R. M.: Stokes-Adams disease, Amer. Heart Jour., 3, 567, 1928.
Stein, H. B.: Diabetes, Arch. Int. Med., 48, 313, 1931.
Stein, I. F.: Gonorrhea, Surg., Gyn., and Obst., 36, 43, 1923.
Steinfield, E.: Mycoses, Med. Clin. N. A., 15, 2, 1931.
Stephenson, R.: Sepsis, Jour. Amer. Med. Assoc., 100, 100, 1933.
Stepp, W., and Schliephake, E.: Arhythmia, Münch. med. Wchnschr., 72, 1997, 1925.
Stern, F.: Encephalitis, Epidemic Encephalitis, Berlin, Julius Springer, 1928.
Stevens, J. T.: Thyrotoxicosis, Jour. Amer. Med. Assoc., 97, 1689, 1931.
Stevens, W. E., and Heppner, M.: Gonorrhea, Jour. Amer. Med. Assoc., 75, 1477, 1920.
Stevens, W. J.: Obstetrical analgesia, Canad. Med. Assoc. Jour., 26, 178, 1932.
Stewart, Z. W.: Hay-fever, Women's Med. Jour., October, 1931.
St. George, A. V.: Sepsis, Jour. Amer. Med. Assoc., 85, 2005, 1925.
Stieglitz, E. J.: Hypertension, Jour. Amer. Med. Assoc., 95, 842, 1930; Jour. Pharm. Exper. Ther., 46, 343, 1932.
Stiles, C. W.: Hookworm, Jour. Amer. Med. Assoc., 88, 455, 1927; Science, 77, 237, 1933.
St. John, J. H.: Relapsing fever, Cecil's Textbook of Medicine, Phila., W. B. Saunders Co., 1933, p. 432.
Stockton, A. B., and Hoffmann, P. E.: Constipation, Jour. Lab. and Clin. Med., 18, 12, 1932.
Stoddard, C. H.: Cretinism, Wisconsin Med. Jour., 32, 389, 1933.
Stokes, A., *et al.*: Yellow fever, Amer. Jour. Trop. Med., 8, 103, 1928.
Stokes, J. H.: Syphilis, Jour. Amer. Med. Assoc., 72, 241, 1919; Modern Clinical Syphilology, Phila., W. B. Saunders Co., 1934. Eczema-dermatitis, Jour. Amer. Med. Assoc., 98, 1127, 1932.
Stokes, J. H., and Busman, G. J.: Syphilis, Jour. Amer. Med. Assoc., 74, 1013, 1920.
Stokes, J. H., and Chambers, S. O.: Syphilis, Jour. Amer. Med. Assoc., 89, 1500, 1927.
Stokes, J. H., and Schaffer, L. W.: Syphilis, Jour. Amer. Med. Assoc., 83, 1826, 1924; ibid., 85, 1271, 1925.
Stokes, J. H., Miller, T. H., and Beerman, H.: Syphilis, Arch. Dermat. and Syph., 23, 624, 1931.
Stokes, J. H., Cole, H. N., Moore, J. E., O'Leary, P. A., Wile, U. J., Clark, T., Parran, T., Jr., and Usilton, L. J.: Syphilis, Ven. Dis. Inform., a series of papers which appeared throughout 1932.
Stolkind, E.: Erythremia, Proc. Roy. Soc. Med. (Clin. Sec.), 19, 19, 1926.
Stone, C. T., *et al.*: Erythremia, Jour. Amer. Med. Assoc., 101, 495, 1933.
Stone, H. B.: Pruritus, Surg., Gyn., and Obst., 42, 565, 1926.
Stone, W. L.: Tetanus, Jour. Amer. Med. Assoc., 78, 1939, 1922.
Stookey, P. F., Elliott, B. L., and Teachenor, F. R.: Cerebrospinal fever, Jour. Amer. Med. Assoc., 95, 106, 1930.
Storchheim, F.: Epilepsy, Jour. Amer. Med. Assoc., 101, 1313, 1933.
Strada, L., and Lopes, A. J.: Trypanosomiasis, Ann. Soc. belge de Méd. trop., 7, 1, 1927.
Strang, J. M., McClugage, H. B., and Evans, F. A.: Obesity, Amer. Jour. Med. Sci., 179, 687, 1930; ibid., 181, 336, 1931; Jour. Amer. Med. Assoc., 97, 1063, 1931.
Strause, S., and Kelman, S. R.: Essential hypertension, Arch. Int. Med., 31, 151, 1923.
Strauss: Diabetes mellitus, Klin. Wchnschr., 6, 296, 1927.

Strauss, A., Sidlick, D. M., Mallas, M. L., and Crawford, B. L.: Syphilis, Jour. Amer. Med. Assoc., 78, 632, 1922.

Strauss, I.: Sciatica, Jour. Amer. Med. Assoc., 69, 2032, 1917.

Strauss, M. B., and Castle, W. B.: Pernicious anemia, Lancet, 2, 111, 1932; Jour. Amer. Med. Assoc., 98, 1620, 1932.

Strauss, M. B., and McDonald, W. J.: Beri-beri, Jour. Amer. Med. Assoc., 100, 1320, 1933.

Sträussler, E., and Koskinas, G.: Syphilis, Ztschr. f. d. ges. Neurol. u. Psychiat., 97, 176, 1925.

Strehl, H.: Catarrhal fever, Münch. med. Wchnschr., February 12, 1932.

Streicher, M. H., and Kaplan, B.: Colitis, Jour. Amer. Med. Assoc., 94, 10, 1930.

Strickland, C., and Chowdhury, K. L.: Blackwater fever, Ind. Jour. Med. Res., 18, 377, 1930.

Strong, R. P.: Trypanosomiasis, Nelson Loose-Leaf Med., 2, 333. Onchocerciasis, United Fruit Co., 20th Ann. Rep., 152, 1931.

Strong, W. M.: Hookworm, Trans. Roy. Soc. Trop. Med. and Hyg., 20, Nos. 1 and 2, p. 132, 1926.

Struthers, E. B.: Kala-azar, China Med. Jour., 16, 755, 1927; ibid., 44, 1, 1931.

Stumpf, J.: Cholera, Münch. med. Wchnschr., 61, No. 40, 1914.

Sturgis, C. C., and Isaacs, R.: Pernicious anemia, Amer. Jour. Med. Sci., 180, 597, 1930; Ann. Int. Med., 5, 131, 1931.

Sturgis, C. C., and Whiting, W. B.: Myxedema, Jour. Amer. Med. Assoc., 85, 2013, 1925.

Suarez, J.: Filariasis, Amer. Jour. Trop. Med., 10, 183, 1930.

Sudhoff, K.: Epilepsy, Arch. f. Gesell. d. Med., 4, 353, 1910–11; ibid., 6, 454, 1912–13.

Sühs, J.: Ergot in puerperium, Zentralbl. f. Gynäk., 56, 596, 1932.

Suk, V.: Goiter, Lancet, 2, 596, 1932.

Sulzberger, M. B.: Buerger's disease, Jour. Immunol., 24, 85, 1933; Bul. New York Acad. Med., 9, 294, 1933. Diabetes insipidus, Jour. Amer. Med. Assoc., 100, 1928, 1933.

Sulzberger, M. B., and Feit, E.: Buerger's disease, Jour. Immunol., 24, 425, 1933.

Sulzberger, M. B., and Wise, F.: Climatic bubo, Jour. Amer. Med. Assoc., 99, 1407, 1932.

Sunderman, F. W.: Pneumonia, Jour. Clin. Invest., 7, 313, 1929.

Sutliff, W. D., and Finland, M.: Pneumonia, Jour. Amer. Med. Assoc., 96, 1465, 1931.

Sutton, L. P.: Chorea, Jour. Amer. Med. Assoc., 97, 299, 1931.

Sutton, R. L.: Lichen planus, Jour. Amer. Med. Assoc., 62, 175, 1914. Balanitis, Jour. Amer. Med. Assoc., 70, 675, 1918. Warts, Jour. Amer. Med. Assoc., 87, 1127, 1926. Herpes zoster, Diseases of the Skin, St. Louis, C. V. Mosby Co., 1926, p. 283. Acne, ibid., p. 1065. Dermatitis venenata, ibid., p. 376. Seborrheic dermatitis, ibid., p. 233. Impetigo, ibid., p. 336. Tinea versicolor, ibid., p. 1202.

Sweany, H. C., and Wasick, M. M.: Tuberculosis, Amer. Rev. Tuberc., 12, 316, 1925.

Sweet, J. E., and Wilmer, H. B.: Trench fever, Lancet, 1, 252, 1919.

Swellengrebel, N. H., and de Buck, A.: Malaria, Proc. Roy. Acad. Sc. Amsterdam, 34, 1216, 1931.

Swenson: Typhoid fever, Tidsshr. f. d. norske laegefor, 53, 63, 1933.

Swetlow, G I.: Tuberculosis, Amer. Rev. Tuberc., 13, 21, 1926.

Swetlow, G. I., and Schwartz, S. P.: Angina pectoris, Jour. Amer. Med. Assoc , 86, 1679, 1926.

Swift, G. W.: Epilepsy, Surg., Gyn., and Obst., 54, 566, 1932.

Swift, H. F.: Trench fever, Nelson Loose-Leaf Med., 1, 431. Rheumatic fever, Amer. Jour. Med. Sci., 180, 497, 1930.

Swift, H. F., and Ellis, A. W. M.: Syphilis, Arch. Int. Med., 12, 331, 1913.

Swift, H. F., Hitchcock, C. H., and McEwen, C.: Rheumatic fever, Amer. Jour. Med. Sci., 181, 1, 1931.

Sydenstricker, E.: Bronchitis, Bull. New York Acad. Med., 4, 191, 1928.

Sylvester, P. H.: Syphilis, Jour. Amer. Med. Assoc., 87, 298, 1926.

Symmers, D.: Anthrax, Cecil's Textbook of Medicine, Phila., W. B. Saunders Co., 1933, p. 264. Glanders, Cecil's Textbook of Medicine, Phila., W. B. Saunders Co., 1933, p. 260.

Symmers, D., and Lewis, K. M.: Erysipelas, Jour. Amer. Med. Assoc., 89, 880, 1927.

Taege: Syphilis, Münch. med. Wchnschr., 66, 841, 1919.

Taillens, J.: BCG, Rev. Méd. Suisse Rom., 47, 1033, 1927.

Takaki, K.: Beriberi, Sei-I-Kwai Med. Jour., 1885.

Talbot, F. B., Metcalf, K., and Moriarty, M.: Epilepsy, Trans. Amer. Ped. Soc., 38, 30, 1926; Amer. Jour. Dis. Child., 32, 316, 1926; ibid., 33, 218, 1927.

Talbott, J. H, and Michelsen, J.: Stokers' cramps, Jour. Clin. Invest., 12, 533, 1933.

Tallerman, K. H.: Nephritis, Lancet, 2, 60, 1932.

Taralrud, M.: Syphilis, Med. Klin., 27, 320, 1931.

Tatum, A. L., Atkinson, A. J., and Collins, K. H.: Poisoning, Jour. Amer. Med. Assoc., 84, 1177, 1925.

Taube, N.: Buerger's disease, Jour. Amer. Med. Assoc., 96, 1469, 1931.

Taussig, A. E.: Diabetes mellitus, Jour. Amer. Med. Assoc., 89, 149, 1927. Agranulocytosis, Jour. Amer. Med. Assoc., 96, 2151 1931.

Taylor, J.: Bacillary dysentery, in the combined reports in Bull. Of. Internat. d'Hyg., 22, 1882, 1930 (Asheshov, Taylor, Morison and Malone). Plague, Ind. Med. Res. Mem., No. 27, March, 1933.

Taylor, K. P. A.: Epidermophytosis, United Fruit Co., 18th Ann. Rep., 1929, p. 153.

Taylor, L.: Myocarditis, Arch. Int. Med., 14, 769, 1914.

Teague, O.: Plague, Jour. Amer. Med. Assoc., 76, 243, 1921.

Teichmann, T.: Tetanus, Münch. med. Wchnschr., Nr. 4, 135, 1932.

Teissier, P.: Mumps, Bull. Méd., 39, 349, 1925.

Telford, E. D.: Angina pectoris, Lancet, 2, 771, 1932.

Tennent, T.: Syphilis, Jour. Ment. Sci., 77, 86, 1931.

Terrell, E. H.: Hemorrhoids, Jour. Amer. Med. Assoc., 69, 1509, 1917; ibid., 89, 781, 1927 (discussion).

Thalhimer, W.: Secondary anemia, Jour. Lab. and Clin. Med., 10, 129, 1924. Hyperemesis, Amer. Jour. Obst., 9, 673, 1925; Jour. Amer. Med. Assoc., 85, 488, 1925 (discussion).

Thannhauser, S. J.: Pellagra, Münch. med. Wchnschr., Nr. 8, February 24, 1933, p. 291.

Theiler, M.: Yellow fever, Ann. Trop. Med. and Parasit., 24, 249, 1930.

Thieme, O.: Yaws, Arch. f. Schiffs.- u. Trop. Hyg., 29, 162, 1925.

Thomas, H. M., and Rienhoff, W. F.: Thyrotoxicosis, South. Med. Jour., 19, 87, 1926.

Thomas, W. A.: Nephritis, Jour. Amer. Med. Assoc., 88, 1559, 1927; ibid., 97, 1055, 1931. Essential hypertension, Jour. Amer. Med. Assoc., 88, 1559, 1927.

Thomas, W. A., et al.: Nephritis, Arch. Int. Med., 43, 139, 1929.

Thomas, W. S.: Asthma, Amer. Jour. Med. Sci., 171, 719, 1926. Asthma, New York, Paul B. Hoeber, 1928.

Thommen, A. A.: Hay-fever and Asthma (see Cocoa, Walzer and Thommen).

Thompson, J. G.: Blackwater fever, Proc. Roy. Soc. Med. (Sec. Trop. Dis. and Parasitology), 17, 47, 1924.

Thompson, W. O., et al.: Thyrotoxicosis, Endocrinology, 14, 393, 1930; Ann. Int. Med., 5, 1129, 1932; Amer. Jour. Med. Sci., 179, 733, 1930; Arch. Int. Med., 45, 261–420–430–481, 1930; ibid., 46, 946, 1930; ibid., 48, 351, 1931; ibid., 49, 199, 1932.

Thonnard-Neumann, E.: Tetanus, United Fruit Co. Rep., 20, 242, 1931.

Thonnard-Neumann, E., and Valera, F.: Amebic dysentery, United Fruit Co., 19th Ann. Rep., 1930.

Throne, B., and Myers, C. N.: Sycosis, Long Island Med. Jour., August, 1926. Psoriasis, New York State Jour. Med., August 1, 1928.

Throne, B., et al.: Lupus erythematosis, Arch. Dermat. and Syph., 25, 494, 1932.

Thurber, D. S.: Undulant fever, Canad. Med. Assoc. Jour. 23, 665, 1930.

Thurmon, F. M., and Thompson, W. O.: Hypothyroidism, Arch. Int. Med., 46, 879, 1930.

Tileston, W.: Sepsis, Cecil's Textbook of Medicine, Phila., W. B. Saunders Co., 1933, p. 72.

Tinker, M. B., and Sutton, H. B.: Skin disinfection, Jour. Amer. Med. Assoc., 87, 1348, 1926; ibid., 88, 1560, 1927.

Tisdall, F. F., and Brown, A.: Rickets, Amer. Jour. Dis. Child., 34, 721, 1927; ibid., 34, 737, 1927; ibid., 42, 1144, 1931.

Titus, P.: Hyperemesis, Jour. Amer. Med. Assoc., 85, 488, 1925; ibid., 86, 969, 1926. Eclampsia, 86, 969, 1926.

Titus, P., and Givens, M. H.: Hyperemesis, Jour. Amer. Med. Assoc., 78, 92, 1922.

Titus, P., and Dodds, P.: Glucose administration, Amer. Jour. Obst. and Gyn., 14, 181, 1927.

Titus, P., Dodds, P., and Willetts, E. W.: Eclampsia, Amer. Jour. Obst. and Gyn., 15, 303, 1928.

Titus, P., Hoffmann, G. L., and Givens, M. H.: Hyperemesis, Jour. Amer. Med. Assoc., 74, 777, 1920.

Titus, P., et al.: Eclampsia, Amer. Jour. Obst. and Gyn., 19, 16, 1930.

Tobias, N.: Syphilis, Amer. Jour. Syph., 12, 536, 1928.

Todd, A. T., et al.: Diabetes, Practitioner, 128, 531, 1932.

Tolstoi, E., and Corke, D. R.: Rheumatic fever, Jour. Lab. and Clin. Med., 17, 450, 1932.

Toomey, J. A., Fullerton, R. M., and Kishma, M. E.: Scarlet fever, Amer. Jour. Dis. Child., 33, 420, 1927.

Torroella, M. A.: Rickets, Gaceta Medica de Mexico, 58, 765, 1927.

Tourtelles: Leprosy, Ann. d. Dermat. et Syph., Ser. 3, 10, 721, 1899.

Tow, A.: Whooping cough, Amer. Jour. Dis. Child., 29, 477, 1925.

Towle, H. P., and Talbot, F. B.: Eczema-dermatitis, Amer. Jour. Dis. Child., 4, 219, 1912.

Traub, E. F., and Tolmach, J. A.: Herpes zoster, New York State Jour. Med., September 1, 1931.

Trautmann, E.: Migraine, Münch. med. Wchnschr., Nr. 12, p. 513, 1928.

Trudeau, F. B.: Tuberculosis, Jour. Amer. Med. Assoc., 98, 309, 1932.

Tsuchiya, H., and Andrews, J.: Dysentery, Amer. Jour. Hyg., 12, 297, 1930.

Tuft, E. H.: Peptic ulcer, Amer. Jour. Nursing, 32, 925, 1932.

Tunick, I. S., and Nach, R.: Varicose veins, Ann. Surg., May, 1932, 734.

Tunick, I. S., et al.: Varicose veins, Amer. Jour. Surg., 6, 479, 1929.

Tunnicliff, R.: Measles, Jour. Infect. Dis., 37, 193, 1925.
Tunnicliff, R., and Hoyne, A. L.: Measles, Jour. Amer. Med. Assoc., 87, 2139, 1926.
Tunnicliff, R., and Taylor, R.: Measles, Jour. Amer. Med. Assoc., 87, 846, 1926.
Tyrrel, S.: Hay-fever (quoted by Bishop, S. S., q. v.).
Tzanck, A.: Migraine, Bull. et mém. Soc. méd. de hôp. de Paris, 45, 495, 1929.
Ude, W. H., and Platov, E. S.: Erysipelas, Jour. Amer. Med. Assoc., 95, 1, 1930.
Uhlenhuth, P., and Seiffert, W.: Weil's disease, Med. Klin., 24, 584, 1928; Centralbl. f. Bakt., 114, 241, 1929.
Umansky, J.: Malaria, Lancet, 2, 349, 1931.
Underhill, F. P.: War gases, The Lethal War Gases, New Haven, Yale Univ. Press, 1920. Burns, Jour. Amer. Med. Assoc., 95, 852, 1930.
Underhill, F. P., and Kapsinow, R.: Burns, Jour. Lab. and Clin. Med., 16, 823, 1931.
Underhill, F. P., and Ringer, M.: Pneumonia, Jour. Amer. Med. Assoc., 75, 1531, 1920.
Ungley, C. C.: Pernicious anemia, Lancet, 2, 63, 1931; ibid., 1, 227, 1932; ibid., 2, 867, 1932; Quart. Jour. Med., 2, 381, 1933.
Upshaw, C. B.: Eclampsia, Jour. Amer. Med. Assoc., 99, 2088, 1932.
Urbach, E.: Asthma and food allergy, Klin. Wchnschr., 2, 2046, 1930. Eczema-dermatitis, Arch. f. Dermat. u. Syph., November, 1929, 523.
Urbach, E., and Sicher, G.: Eczema-dermatitis, Wien. klin. Wchnschr., 41, 1481, 1928.
Urbanitzky, E.: Dysentery, Münch. med. Wchnschr., 31, 1219, 1933.
Utz, L., and Keatinge, L.: Hodgkin's disease, Med. Jour. Australia, 1, 521, 1932.
Vallery-Radot, P., and Mauric, G.: Asthma, Bull. et mém. de la Soc. méd. des hôp. de Paris, 47, 1046, 1931.
Van Allen, C. M.: Tuberculosis, Jour. Amer. Med. Assoc., 99, 13, 1932.
Van Del, D. T.: Obstetrics, Amer. Jour. Obst. and Gyn., 25, 564, 1933.
Van den Branden, F.: Trypanosomiasis, Bull. Soc. de path. exot., 18, 645, 1925; ibid., 19, 8, 1926.
Van den Branden, F., and Van Hoof, L.: Trypanosomiasis, Ann. Soc. belge de Méd. trop., 4, 205, 1923; Bull. Soc. de path. exot., 16, 606, 1923.
Vanderhoof, D.: Beriberi, Cecil's Textbook of Medicine, Phila., W. B. Saunders Co., 1933, p. 603.
Vander Veer, A., Jr.: Hay-fever, Amer. Jour. Med. Sci., 164, 97, 1922.
Vander Veer, A., Jr., Cooke, R. A., and Spain, W. C.: Hay-fever, Amer. Jour. Med. Sci., 174, 101, 1928.
Van Dolsen, W. W.: Breast abscess, Amer. Jour. Obst. and Gyn., 13, 236, 1927.
Van Hoof, L.: Trypanosomiasis, Final Rep. League of Nations Internat. Comm. on Human Trypan., Geneva, 382, 1928.
Van Hoosen, B.: Obstetrical analgesia, Anesth. and Analg., 7, 151, 1928; ibid., 7, 353, 1928.
Van Leeuwen, W. S.: Asthma, Internat. Clin., September, 1924; Allergic Diseases, Phila., J. B. Lippincott Co., 1925.
Van Leeuwen, W. S., Bien, Z., and Varekamp, H.: Asthma, Ztschr. f. Immunitäts forsh. u. exper. Therap., 37, 77, 1923.
Vanni, V.: Infectious jaundice, Riforma Medica, 40, 916, 1924.
Van Poole, G. M.: Tuberculosis, Laryngoscope, 40, 132, 1930.
Van Slyke, D. D., et al.: Nephritis, Medicine, 9, 257, 1930.
Van Wyck, H. B.: Hyperemesis, Amer. Jour. Obst. and Gyn., 21, 243, 1931.
Vanzant, F. R., et al.: Hypochlorhydria, Arch. Int. Med., 49, 345, 1932.
Vaucel, M., and Boisseau, R.: Trypanosomiasis, Bull. Soc. de path. exot., 24, 528, 1931; ibid. 24, 374, 1931.
Vaucel, M., and Salaön, G.: Trypanosomiasis, Bull. Soc. de path. exot., 24, 834, 1931.
Vaughan, W. T.: Hay-fever, Jour. Amer. Med. Assoc., 97, 90, 1931; Allergy and Applied Immunology, St. Louis, Mosby, 1931.
Vecki, V. G.: Gonorrhea, Jour. Amer. Med. Assoc., 85, 1609, 1925.
Vedder, E. B.: Amebic dysentery, Jour. Amer. Med. Assoc., 62, 501, 1914. Tear gas, The Med. Aspects Chem. Warfare, Baltimore, Williams and Wilkins Co., 1925.
Vedder, E. B., and Sawyer, H. P.: Catarrhal fever, Jour. Amer. Med. Assoc., 82, 764 1924.
Veeder, B. S., and Jeans, P. C.: Syphilis, Abt's Pediatrics, Phila., W. B. Saunders Co., Vol. 5, p. 611, 1924.
Velasco, F. I., Alonso, J. M., Limkako, G., Fernandez, G., and del Rosario, F. T.: Leprosy Jour. Phil. Is. Med. Assoc., 9, 327, 1929.
Vergeer, T.: Tapeworm, Jour. Amer. Med. Assoc., 90, 673, 1928; ibid., 90, 1687, 1928
Vidgoff, B.: Diabetes insipidus, Endocrinology, 16, 289, 1932.
Viko, L. E., et al.: Auricular fibrillation, Arch. Int. Med., 31, 359, 1926.
Vincent, B.: Hemorrhage of newborn, Nelson Loose-Leaf Med., 4, 146.
Vincent, S., and Thompson, J. H.: Hypertension, Jour. Physiol., 66, 307, 1928.
Voegtlin, C., Johnson, J. M., and Dyer, H.: Syphilis, Pub. Health Rep., 37, 2783, 1922.
Voegtlin, C., Smith, M. J., and Johnson, J. M.: Tuberculosis, Jour. Amer. Med. Assoc., 77, 1017, 1921.
Voegtlin, C., Smith, M. I., Dyer, H., and Thompson, J. W.: Syphilis, Pub. Health Rep., 38, 1003, 1923.

Vogel, K. M.: Leukemia, Nelson Loose-Leaf Med., 4, 66.
Vogelsang, T. M., and Haaland, M.: Typhoid, Norsk. Mag. f. Laegevidenskaben, November, 1931.
Voit, K.: Poliomyelitis, Arch. f. exper. Path. u. Pharm., 95, 124, 1922.
Volhard, F., and Fahr, Th.: Nephritis, Die Brightsche Nierenkrankheit, Berlin, 1914.
Von Behring, E.: Toxin-antitoxin, Deutsch. med. Wchnschr., 39, 873, 1913.
Von Berghaus BCG, Deutsch. med. Wchnschr., 56, 1771, 1930.
Von den Velden, R.: Angina pectoris, Deutsch. med. Wchnschr., 57, 619, 672, 712 and 753, 1931.
Von den Steinen: Syphilis, Münch. med. Wchnschr., 74, 1006, 1927.
Von Noorden, C.: Obesity, Med. Klin., 5, 1238, 1926; Wien. med. Wchnschr., No. 1, 1931.
Von Oettingen, W. F.: Syphilis, Physiol. Rev., 10, 221, 1930.
Von Oettingen, W. F., and Sollmann, T.: Intestinal fermentation, Jour. Amer. Med. Assoc., 87, 1990, 1926.
Von Redwitz, E.: Peptic ulcer, Münch. med. Wchnschr., December, 1927.
Von Sholly, A. I., Blum, J., and Smith, L.: Whooping cough, Jour. Amer. Med. Assoc., 68, 1451, 1917.
Waddell, J. A.: Rheumatic fever, Arch. Int. Med., 8, 748, 1911.
Waddell, W. M., Jr., and Eley, R. C.: Chickenpox, Amer. Jour. Dis. Child., 34, 540, 1927.
Wade, H.: Hiccup, Jour. Urol., 28, 381, 1932.
Wade, H. W.: Leprosy, Phil. Jour. Sci., 26, 21, 1925.
Wade, H. W., Lara, C. B., and Nicolas, C.: Leprosy, Phil. Jour. Sci., 25, 661, 1924.
Wagner-Jauregg, J.: Syphilis, Jahrbuch f. Psychiat. u. Neurol., 7, 94, 1887; Psychiat. Neurol. Wchnschr., 20, 132, 1918; ibid., 20, 251, 1919; Ven. Dis. Inform. (U. S. P. H. S.), 8, 393, 1927.
Wainwright, J. M.: Tetanus, Arch. Surg., 12, 1062, 1926.
Waldbott, G. L.: Asthma, Arch. Int. Med., 41, 683, 1928.
Walker, E. L., and Sweeney, M. A.: Chaulmoogra oil, Jour. Infect. Dis., 26, 238, 1920.
Walker, J H. C.: Roundworms, Jour. Roy. Army Med. Corps, 49, 49, 1927.
Wallace, W.: Syphilis, Lancet, 1835, 2, 5.
Waller: Bacillary dysentery, Lancet, 1919, 2, 778.
Wallgren, A.: BCG, Jour. Amer. Med. Assoc., 91, 1876, 1928.
Walravens, P.: Trypanosomiasis, Bull. Soc. de path. exot., 18, 641, 1925.
Walsh, G.: Spider bite, South. Med. Jour., 23, 1038, 1930.
Walshe, F. M. R.: Beriberi, Nelson Loose-Leaf Med., 3, 182.
Walton, D. C.: Burns, Jour. Amer. Med. Assoc., 84, 1569, 1925.
Warfield, L. M.: Hypothyroidism, Jour. Amer. Med. Assoc., 95, 1076, 1930. Nephritis, Wisconsin Med. Jour., 29, 419, 1930 (discussion). Pneumonia, Wisconsin Med. Jour., 32, 324, 474, and 539, 1933.
Waring, J. I.: Beriberi, Amer. Jour. Dis. Child., 38, 52, 1929. Kerosene poisoning, Amer. Jour. Med. Sci., 185, 325, 1933.
Warma, J. D.: Oriental sore, Ind. Med. Gaz., 66, 383, 1931.
Warren: Trypanosomiasis, Jour. Amer. Med. Assoc. (London letter), 98, 1314, 1932.
Warren, L. E.: Constipation, Jour. Amer. Med. Assoc., 84, 1682, 1925.
Warringsholz: Anthrax, Münch. med. Wchnschr., 79, 1523, 1932.
Warthin, A. S.: Tapeworms, Jour. Amer. Med. Assoc., 90, 2080, 1928.
Warwick, W.: Measles, Canad. Med. Assoc. Jour., 21, 694, 1929.
Washburn, A. H.: Purpura, Jour. Amer. Med. Assoc., 94, 313, 1930.
Washburn, B. E.: Hookworm disease, Jour. Amer. Med. Assoc., 68, 1162, 1917.
Waters, C. A., and Firor, W. B.: Agranulocytosis, Amer. Jour. Roentgenol. and Radium Therapy, 27, 740, 1932.
Watkins, C. H., and Giffin, H. Z.: Agranulcytosis, unpublished observations.
Watson, A. J.: Encephalitis, China Med. Jour.; Brit. Med. Jour.; the subject discussed in Jour. Amer. Med. Assoc., 91, 1299, 1928.
Watson, B. P.: Labor induction, Amer. Jour. Obst. and Gyn., 4, 603, 1922.
Watson, E. A.: BCG, Jour. Amer. Vet. Med. Assoc., 71, 732, 1927; ibid., 73, 799, 1928.
Watson, M.: Malaria, Lancet, 2, 1432, 1931; ibid., 1, 1362, 1932 (discussion).
Watson, S. H.: Tuberculosis (Heliotherapy), Jour. Amer. Med. Assoc., 87, 1026, 1926.
Watt, G. L.: Eclampsia, Canad. Med. Assoc. Jour., 27, 51, 1932.
Wauchope, G. M.: Hyperinsulinism, Quart. Jour. Med., N. S., 2, 117, 1933.
Waugh, T. R.: Anemia, Arch. Int. Med., 47, 71, 1931.
Wayson, N. E.: Asiatic cholera, Jour. Amer. Med. Assoc., 69, 267, 1917.
Weaver, G. H., and Crooks, T. T.: Measles, Wisconsin Med. Jour., 23, 555, 1925.
Webb, G. B., and Sevier, J. A.: Tuberculosis, Trans. Assoc. Amer. Phys., 1923.
Webb, G. B., Forster, A. M., and Gilbert, G. B.: Tuberculosis, Jour. Amer. Med. Assoc., 76, 846, 1921.
Weech, A. A.: Chickenpox, Jour. Amer. Med. Assoc., 82, 1245, 1924. Rickets, Bull. Johns Hopkins Hosp., 40, 244, 1927.
Weed, L. H., and McKibben, P. S.: Brain volume, Amer. Jour. Physiol., 48, 512, 1919.
Weeks, C.: Hiccup, Ann. Surg., 93, 811, 1931.
Weeks, C., and Mueller, R. S.: Varicose veins, Surg., Gyn., and Obst., 54, 98, 1932.

Wegner: Rickets, Arch. f. path. Anat., 61, 44, 1874.
Weill-Halle and Turpin: BCG, Paris Méd., 1, 20, 1925; Ann. de l'Inst. Pasteur, 41, 254, 1927; Bull. Acad. de Méd., 97, 25, 1927; Arch. de méd. d'enf., 31, 517, 1928; Presse méd., 37, 1181, 1929; Rev. de la Tuberc., 10, 9, 1929.
Weinfeld, G. F., and Cooperstock, M.: Diphtheria, Amer. Jour. Dis. Child., 38, 35, 1929.
Weinstein, L., et al.: Constip,ation Arch. Int. Med., 52, 384, 1933.
Weis, C. R.: Rheumatic fever, Jour. Amer. Med. Assoc., 99, 21, 1932.
Weise, E. C.: Boils, Jour. Amer. Med. Assoc., 95, 324, 1930; ibid., 95, 1607, 1930.
Weisman, S. A.: Auricular fibrillation, Arch. Int. Med., 49, 728, 1932.
Weiss, S., and Hatcher, R. A.: Heart failure, Jour. Amer. Med. Assoc., 76, 508, 1921.
Wells, H. G.: Tuberculosis, Arch. Int. Med., 7, 721, 1911.
Wells, H. S.: Hookworm, Proc. Soc. Exper. Biol. and Med., 22, 235, 1925.
Wenckebach, K. F.: Arythmia, Jour. Amer. Med. Assoc., 81, 472, 1923. Beriberi, Geneesk. Tijdschr. v. Nederl.-Indië, 72, 915, 1932.
Wenyon, C. M.: Kala-azar, Lancet, 1, 243, 1932.
Wersen: Tuberculosis, Upsala Läkaref. Förhand., 20, 1, 1914.
Wesselhoeft, C.: Mumps, Boston Med. and Surg. Jour., 183, 425, 458, 491, 520, 1920. Diphtheria, Med. Clin. N. A., 15, 951, 1932.
West, R., and Howe, M.: Pernicious anemia, Jour. Biol. Chem., 88, 427, 1930; ibid., 94, 611, 1931.
Westphali, K.: Essential hypertension Ztschr. f. klin. Med., 101, 545, 1925; Deutsch. Arch. f. kln. Med., 152, 331, 1926.
Wetzel, N. C., and Nourse, J. D.: Rheumatic fever, Arch. Path. and Lab. Med., 1, 182, 1928.
Weyer, E. R., Park, W. H., and Banzhaf, E. J.: Poliomyelitis, Jour. Exper. Med., 53, 553, 1931.
Wheeler, G. A.: Pellagra, Pub. Health Rep., 39, 2197, 1924; ibid., 46, 2663, 1931; Nelson Loose-Leaf Med., 3, 191; Science, 76, 101, 1932.
Wheeler, R. E., Doull, J. A., and Frost, W. H.: Diphtheria, Amer. Jour. Hyg., 14, 555, 1931.
Wheelock, M. C.: Strychnine poisoning, Jour. Amer. Med. Assoc., 99, 1862, 1932.
Whipple, G. H., Hooper, C. W., and Robscheit, F. S.: Anemia, Amer. Jour. Physiol., 53, 151, 1920; ibid., 52, 236, 1920.
Whipple, G. H., and Robscheit-Robbins, F.: Anemia, Amer. Jour. Physiol., 72, 408, 1925; ibid., 72, 419, 1925. Secondary anemia, Amer. Jour. Physiol., 72, 395, 1925; ibid., 79, 260, 1927; Proc. Soc. Exper. Biol. and Med., 24, 860, 1926–1927.
Whipple, G. H., et al.: Anemia, Amer. Jour. Med. Sci., 179, 628, 1930.
White, C. E.: Hemophilia, Jour. Oklahoma State Med. Assoc., 25, 304, 1932.
White, C. J.: Lichen planus, Jour. Cutan. Dis., 37, 671, 1919. Warts, Jour. Cutan. Dis., 33, 731, 1915. Epidermophytosis, Arch. Dermat. and Syph., 15, 387, 1927. Eczema-dermatitis, Arch. Dermat. and Syph., 7, 50, 1923; ibid., 12, 896, 1925; ibid., 13, 242, 1926.
White, E. C.: Gonorrhea, Jour. Amer. Med. Assoc., 80, 1261, 1923.
White, J. C.: Syphilis, Jour. Amer. Med. Assoc., 99, 10, 1932.
Whitmore, E. R.: Bacillary dysentery, Nelson Loose-Leaf Med., 2, 161. Malaria, Med. Dept. United Fruit Co. (18th Ann. Rep.), 1929. Blackwater fever, Ann. Int. Med., 2, 316, 1928; Med. Dept. United Fruit Co. (18th Ann. Rep.), 1929, 59.
Whitmore, E. R., Roberts, C. M., and Jantzen, W.: Malaria, Med. Dept. United Fruit Co, (18th Ann. Rep.), 1929.
Whittingham, H. E.: Flagellate dysentery, Brit. Med. Jour., 1923, 1, 799.
Wien, M. S., and Perlstein, S.: Eczema-dermatitis, Arch. Dermat. and Syph., 27, 963, 1933.
Wiener, J. J., and Fishberg, M.: Tuberculosis, Arch. Int. Med., 52, 341, 1933.
Wigglesworth, V. B.: Diabetes mellitus, Biochem. Jour., 18, 1203, 1924.
Wilbert, J.: BCG, Ann. de l'Inst. Pasteur, 39, 641, 1925.
Wilder, R. M.: Epilepsy, Mayo Clin. Bull., 2, 307, 1921. Nephritis, personal communication, 1930.
Wilder, T. S., and Drake, T. G. H.: Pneumonia, Jour. Clin. Invest., 7, 353, 1929.
Wile, U.: Syphilis, Amer. Jour. Med. Sci., 164, 415, 1922.
Wile, U., and Davenport, K. M.: Syphilis, Jour. Amer. Med. Assoc., 97, 1579, 1931.
Wilgus, S. D., and Lurie, L.: Syphilis, Arch. Neurol. and Psychiat., 26, 662, 1931; Illinois Med. Jour., 60, 341, 1931.
Wilkins, L., and Wells, H. S.: Bacillary dysentery, Jour. Amer. Med. Assoc., 82, 1599, 1924.
Wilkinson, J. F.: Pernicious anemia, Brit. Med. Jour., 1, 85, 1931; ibid., 1, 325, 1932.
Wilkinson, J. F., and Brockbank, W.: Pernicious anemia, Clin. Jour., October 1, 1930.
Williams, A. W.: Hydrophobia, Nelson Loose-Leaf Med., 2, 140.
Williams, H. U.: Trichinosis, Report of the Laboratories of the Univ. of Buffalo, Med. Dept. 2, 64, 1903 (quoted by Blumer, G., q. v.).
Williams, J. R., and Swett, M.: Glucose, Jour. Amer. Med. Assoc., 78, 1024, 1922.
Williams, J. W.: Preparation of vulva, Amer. Jour. Med. Sci., 106, 45, 1893; Amer. Jour. Obst., 38, 807, 1898; Textbook of Obst., D. Appleton and Co., New York, 5th Ed. p. 996.

Williams, O. T., and Forsyth, C. E. P.: Tuberculosis, Brit. Med. Jour., 2, 1120, 1909.
Williams, T. J.: Gonorrhea, Amer. Jour. Obst. and Gyn., 16, 861, 1928; ibid., 23, 575, 1932.
Williamson, A. C.: Quinine in labor, Surg., Gyn., and Obst., 34, 812, 1922.
Williamson, T. U., *et al.*: Granuloma inguinale, Jour. Amer. Med. Assoc., 100, 1671, 1933.
Willmore, J. G., and Martindale, W. H.: Amebic dysentery, Brit. Med. Jour., 1, 525, 1926.
Willoughby, H., and Aslett, E.: Amebic dysentery, Jour. Roy. Nav. Med. Serv., 17, 19, 1931.
Wills, L.: Pernicious anemia, Brit. Med. Jour., June 20, 1931; Lancet, 1, 1283, 1933.
Wilson, C. M.: Ketogenic diet, Lancet, 2, 960, 1932.
Wilson, G., and Limberger, W. A.: Epilepsy, Jour. Amer. Med. Assoc., 101, 110, 1933.
Wilson, H.: Hay-fever, Jour. Amer. Med. Assoc., 66, 715, 1916.
Wilson, J. A.: Burns, The Chemistry of Leather Manufacture, New York, The Chemical Catalog Co., Inc., 1928.
Wilson, L. A.: Granuloma inguinale, Jour. Amer. Med. Assoc., 95, 1093, 1930.
Wilson, M. G., Lingg, C., and Croxford, G.: Rheumatic fever, Amer. Heart Jour., 4, 197, 1928.
Wilson, R. H.: Hypertension, Proc. Soc. Exper. Biol. Med., 29, 961, 1932.
Wilson, R. M.: Leprosy, Jour. Amer. Med. Assoc., 80, 1636, 1923; ibid., 87, 1211, 1926.
Winans, H. M.: Hyperinsulinism, Amer. Jour. Med. Sci., 185, 500, 1933.
Winkelstein, A.: Peptic ulcer, Amer. Jour. Med. Sci., 185, 695, 1933.
Winkler, L.: Syphilis, Wien. klin. Wchnschr., 41, 374, 1928.
Wirz, F.: Syphilis, Münch. med. Wchnschr., Nr. 29, 1147, 1932.
Wisart, Johantgen, and Clark: Typhoid, Therapeutic Manual University of Michigan Hosp., Geo. Wahr, Ann Arbor.
Wise, F.: Smallpox, Jour. Amer. Med. Assoc., 75, 335, 1920. Ringworm, Jour. Amer. Med. Assoc., 86, 1409, 1926.
Wise, F., and Parkhurst, H. J.: Stomatitis, Nelson Loose-Leaf Med., 5, 41.
Wiseman, J. R.: Heart failure, Jour. Amer. Med. Assoc., 99, 114, 1932.
Withers, S., Ranson, J. R., and Humphrys, E. D.: Diphtheria carrier, Jour. Amer. Med. Assoc., 87, 1266, 1926.
Wohl, M. G.: Thyrotoxicosis, Med. Clin. N. A., July, 1932, 121.
Wolbach, S. B.: Rocky Mountain spotted fever, Cecil's Textbook of Medicine, Phila., W. B. Saunders Co., 1933, p. 362.
Wolf, M.: Varicose veins, Dermat. Wchnschr., 93, 1859, 1931.
Wolferth, C. C.: Paroxysmal tachycardia, New York Med. Jour., 117, 552–555, 1923.
Wolff, L., and White, P. D.: Auricular fibrillation, Arch. Int. Med., 43, 653, 1929.
Wolff, S.: Bacillary dysentery, Deutsch. med. Wchnschr, 1930, Nr. 52; ibid., 1931, Nr. 52.
Wolffe, J. B., and Bellett, S.: Paroxysmal tachycardia, Ann. Int. Med., 4, 795, 1931.
Wolff-Eisner: Cholera, Therap. d. Gegenw., 17, 92, 1915.
Wollstein, M.: Mumps, Nelson Loose-Leaf Med., 1, 554; Jour. Exper. Med., 23, 353, 1916; ibid., 28, 377, 1918.
Wood, E. J.: Sprue, Nelson Loose-Leaf Med., 5, 465.
Wood, J. E., Jr.: Stokes-Adam's disease, Jour. Amer. Med. Assoc., 98, 1364, 1932.
Woods, A. C., and Moore, J. E.: Syphilis, Jour. Amer. Med. Assoc., 82, 2105, 1924.
Woodyatt, R. F.: Diabetes mellitus, Arch. Int. Med., 28, 125, 1921.
Worster-Drought, C., and Hill, T. R.: Encephalitis, Lancet, 218, 1225, 1930.
Wright, A. D.: Varicose veins, Proc. Roy. Soc. Med., 23, 30, 1930; Brit. Med. Jour., September 26, 1931; Lancet, 1, 457, 1931.
Wright, C. S.: Syphilis, Jour. Amer. Med. Assoc., 89, 424, 1927.
Würtzen, C. H.: Lupus erythematosus, Research on the Effects of Sanocrysin, Copenhagen, Levin and Munksgaard, 1926.
Wyckoff, J., and Goldring, W.: Heart failure, Arch. Int. Med., 39, 488, 1927.
Wyckoff, J., DuBois, E. F., and Woodruff, I. O.: Pneumonia, Jour. Amer. Med. Assoc., 95, 1243, 1930.
Yater, W. M., and Trewhella, A. P.: Angina pectoris, Amer. Jour. Med. Sci., 182, 35, 1931.
Yates, J. L., and Thalhimer, W.: Pernicious anemia, Jour. Amer. Med. Assoc., 87, 2156, 1926.
Yernaux and Barnard: Syphilis, Scalpel, 24, 593, 1919.
Yesko, S. A.: Gonorrhea, Amer. Jour. Dis. Child., 33, 630, 1927.
Yorke, W.: Blackwater fever, Trop. Dis. Bul., 28, 940, 1931.
Yorke, W., and Murgatroyd, F.: Malaria, Ann. Trop. Med. and Parasit., 25, 551, 1931.
Young, C. W.: Kala-azar, Cecil's Textbook of Medicine, Phila., W. B. Saunders Co., 1927, p. 380.
Young, F. F.: Beriberi, Jour. Amer. Med. Assoc., 40, 111, 1903.
Young, H. H.: Gonorrhea, Practice of Urology, Phila., W. B. Saunders Co., 1926, pp. 229, 247; Jour. Amer. Med. Assoc., 87, 1366, 1926. Chancroid, Practice of Urology, Phila., W. B. Saunders Co., 1926, p. 190. Ulcerative colitis, Jour. Amer. Med. Assoc., 87, 1366, 1926. Boils, Jour. Amer. Med. Assoc., 87, 1366, 1926. Sepsis, Jour. Amer. Med. Assoc., 87, 1366, 1926. Erysipelas, Jour. Amer. Med. Assoc., 87, 1366, 1926. Rheumatic fever, Jour. Amer. Med. Assoc., 87, 1366, 1926. Scarlet fever, Jour. Amer. Med. Assoc., 87, 1366, 1926.

Young, H. H., and Birkhaug, K.: Scarlet fever, Jour. Amer. Med. Assoc., 83, 492, 1924.
Young, H. H., Hill, J. H., and Scott, W. W.: Sepsis, Arch. Surg., 10, 813, 1925.
Young, H. H., Scott, W. W., and Hill, J. H.: Urinary infections, Jour. Urol., 12, 237, 1924.
Young, H. H., White, E. C., and Swartz, E. O.: Gonorrhea, Jour. Amer. Med. Assoc., 73, 1483, 1919.
Young, H. H., White, E. C., Hill, J. H., and Davis, D. M.: Urinary infections, Surg., Gyn., and Obst., 36, 508, 1923.
Young, H. H., *et al.*: Gonorrhea, Jour. Amer. Med. Assoc., 98, 715, 1932.
Young, W. A., and Tudhope, G. R.: Amebic dysentery, Trans. Roy. Soc. Trop. Med. and Hyg., 20, 93, 1926.
Ziegler, O.: Tuberculosis, Deutsch. med. Wchnschr., Nr. 1, 1931.
Zimmermann, L.: Measles, Deutsch. med. Wchnschr., 48, 1701, 1922.
Zingher, A.: Schick test, Amer. Jour. Dis. Child., 25, 392, 1923.   Measles, Jour. Amer. Med. Assoc., 82, 1180, 1924.   Toxin-antitoxin, Cecil's Textbook of Medicine, Phila., W. B. Saunders Co., 1927, p. 90.   Antitoxin, Cecil's Textbook of Medicine, Phila., W. B. Saunders Co., 1927, p. 90.   Toxoid, Proc. Soc. Exper. Biol. and Med., 22, 462, 1925.
Zondek, B., and Krohn, H.: Diabetes insipidus, Klin. Wchnschr., 31, 1293, 1932.
Zur Nedden: Burns, Trans. Heidelberg Congr., 1905, p. 216 (cited by Barkan and Barkan, *q. v.*).
Zwick, K. G.: Syphilis, Jour. Amer. Med. Assoc., 83, 1821, 1924.

INDEX

831

53

54